Universal Blood and Body Fluid Precautions

The Centers for Disease Control recommend universal blood and body fluid precautions (also referred to as *universal precautions*) in the care of *all* clients, especially those in emergency care settings, in which the risk of blood exposure is increased and the infection status of the client is unknown. In other words, the nurse should treat all body substances or fluids of all clients as if they are potentially infectious.

The CDC (1988, p.2) recommends that these precautions apply to blood and to body fluids containing visible blood, as well as to semen and vaginal secretions; to tissues, and to the following fluids: cerebrospinal fluid, synovial fluid, pleural fluid, peritoneal fluid, pericardial fluid, and amniotic fluid. Universal precautions do not apply to nasal secretions, sputum, saliva, sweat, tears, urine, feces, and vomitus unless they contain visible blood. Blood is the single most important source of HIV, HBV, and other bloodborne pathogens in the health care setting.

Protective barriers—gloves, gowns, masks, and protective eyewear—reduce the risk of exposure to potentially infective materials. The following specific precautions are recommended.

Wash your hands thoroughly and immediately after accidental contact with body substances containing blood, between clients, and immediately after gloves are removed.

Wear gloves when touching blood and body fluids containing blood, as well as when handling items or surfaces soiled with blood or body fluids as mentioned above.

Change gloves between client contacts.

Use sterile gloves for procedures involving contact with normally sterile areas of the body.

Use examination gloves for procedures involving contact with mucous membranes, unless otherwise indicated, and for other client care or diagnostic procedures that do not require the use of sterile gloves.

Do not wash or disinfect surgical or examination gloves for reuse. Washing with surfactants may cause *wicking*, i.e., the enhanced penetration of liquids through undetected holes in the glove. Disinfecting agents may cause deterioration.

Use general-purpose utility gloves (e.g., rubber household gloves) for housekeeping chores involving potential blood contact and for instrument cleaning and decontamination procedures. Utility gloves may be decontaminated and reused, but should be discarded if they are peeling, cracked, or discolored, or if they have punctures, tears, or other evidence of deterioration.

Wear gloves when performing phlebotomy (venipuncture):
- if the nurse has cuts, scratches, or other breaks in the skin.
- in situations where hand contamination with blood may occur, e.g., with an uncooperative client.
- when the nurse is learning phlebotomy techniques.

Wear gloves when performing finger and/or heel sticks on infants and children.

Wear masks and protective eyewear (glasses, goggles) or face shields to protect the mucous membranes of your mouth, nose, and eyes during procedures that are likely to generate droplets of blood or other body fluids to which universal precautions apply.

Wear a disposable plastic apron or gown during procedures that are likely to generate splatters of blood or other body fluid (e.g., peritoneal fluid) and soil your clothing.

To prevent injuries, place used disposable needle-syringe units, scalpel blades, and other sharp items in puncture-resistant containers for disposal. Discard used needle-syringe units *uncapped* and *unbroken*. Puncture-resistant containers should be located as close as practicable to use areas.

Place mouthpieces, resuscitation bags, or other ventilation devices in areas where the need for emergency mouth-to-mouth resuscitation is predictable—even though saliva has *not* been implicated in HIV transmission.

If a nurse has exudative lesions or weeping dermatitis, it is necessary to refrain from all direct client care and from handling client-care equipment until the condition is resolved.

Handle soiled linen as little as possible and with minimum agitation to prevent gross microbial contamination of the air and of persons handling the linen. Place and transport linen soiled with blood or body fluids in leakage-resistant bags.

Put all specimens of blood and listed body fluids in well-constructed containers with secure lids to prevent leakage during transport. When collecting specimens, take care to avoid contaminating the outside of the container.

Use a chemical germicide that is approved for use as a hospital disinfectant to decontaminate work surfaces after there is a spill of blood or other body fluids. In the absence of a commercial germicide, a solution of sodium hypochlorite (household bleach) in a 1:10 dilution is effective. Before decontaminating areas, first remove visible material. Wear gloves during cleaning and decontaminating procedures.

Follow agency policies for disposal of infective waste both when disposing of, and when decontaminating, contaminated materials.

Carefully pour bulk blood, suctioned fluids, and excretions containing blood and secretions, down drains that are connected to a sanitary sewer.

U.S. Department of Health and Human Services, Public Health Service. Update: Universal precautions for prevention of transmission of Human Immunodeficiency Virus, Hepatitis B Virus, and other bloodborne pathogens in health care settings, *MMWR*, June 24, 1988; 37:1–7.

Centers for Disease Control. Recommendations for prevention of HIV transmission in health care settings. *MMWR Supplement*. August 21, 1987; 36:25–185.

INTRODUCTION
TO NURSING

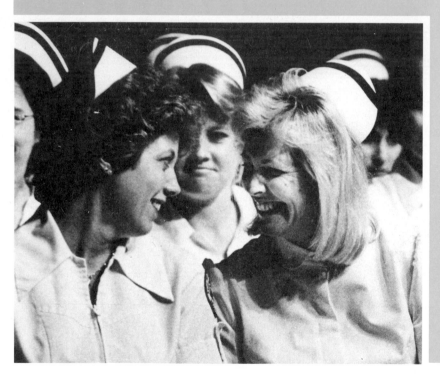

This text is dedicated to the nursing students of today.

You hold the keys to nursing's future.

Introduction to Nursing

Barbara **K**ozier, BA, BSN, RN, MN

Glenora **E**rb, BSN, RN

Patricia McKay **B**ufalino, RN, MN

Addison-Wesley Publishing Company
Health Sciences, Redwood City, California

Menlo Park, California • Reading, Massachusetts • New York
Don Mills, Ontario • Wokingham, U.K. • Amsterdam • Bonn
Sydney • Singapore • Tokyo • Madrid • San Juan

Executive editor: Debra Hunter

Sponsoring editor: Armando Parcés Enríquez

Production supervisor: Judith Johnstone

Interior designer: Paul Quin

Cover designer: Rudy Zehntner

Art coordinators: Brian Jones, Sue Gemmel

Illustrators: Jack P. Tandy, Sue Gemmel

Photographers: William Thompson, Karen Stafford Rantzman, Jeffry Collins, Suzanne Arms, Marianne Gontarz, George Fry, Randy Dean, Bill Murphy, David Barnett, Christopher Scott, Mark Tuschman

Copyeditor: Antonio Padial

Proofreaders: Ann Calandro, Steven Sorensen

Indexer: Steven Sorensen

The photograph on the title page is by Frank Keillor.

The authors and publishers have exerted every effort to ensure that drug selections and dosages set forth in this text are in accord with current recommendations and practice at the time of publication. However, in view of ongoing research, changes in government regulations, and the constant flow of information relating to drug therapy and drug reactions, the reader is urged to check the package insert for each drug for any change in indications or dosage and for added warnings and precautions. This is particularly important where the recommended agent is a new and/or infrequently employed drug.

Library of Congress Cataloging-in-Publication Data

Kozier, Barbara.
    Introduction to nursing / Barbara Kozier, Glenora Erb, Patricia McKay Bufalino.
        p.   cm.
    Includes bibliographies and index.
    ISBN 0-201-12240-5
    1. Nursing.   I. Erb, Glenora Lea, 1937–   . II. Bufalino, Patricia McKay,   III. Title.
    [DNLM: 1. Nursing.   WY 100 K88i]
RT41.K7224 1989
610.73—dc19
DNLM/DLC   88-8194
for Library of Congress   CIP

CDEFGHIJ-MU-943210

ISBN 0-201-12240-5

Addison-Wesley Publishing Company
Health Sciences
390 Bridge Parkway
Redwood City, California 94065

About the Authors

Over one million nursing students have built a solid professional foundation through the brilliant books of Kozier and Erb. **Barbara Kozier** and **Glenora Erb** combine years of teaching experience at the diploma, associate, and baccalaureate degree levels. Barbara Kozier is a member of nursing's honorary society, Sigma Theta Tau. She and Glenora Erb have written nursing texts together for more than twenty years. This author team has created several bestselling texts: *Fundamentals of Nursing: Concepts and Procedures; Techniques in Clinical Nursing: A Nursing Process Approach;* and *Concepts and Issues in Nursing Practice.*

Patricia McKay Bufalino, Associate Professor of Nursing at Riverside Community College, and Mentor for the Statewide Nursing Program through California State University, is the newest addition to this outstanding author team. Also a member of Sigma Theta Tau, she has been involved in nursing associations at regional, state, and national levels. Patricia Bufalino has co-authored the successful *Nursing Care Planning Guides for Adults* and *Critically Ill Adults: Nursing Care Planning Guides.*

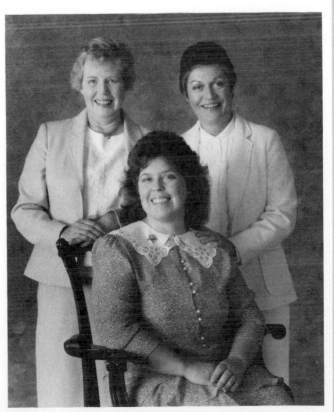

Preface

Nursing practice in 2010 will be intimate, compassionate, empathetic, and truly professional. The knowledge base of practice will be well-delineated and unique; its use will enable the practitioner to offer services for which there is no substitute. Nurses will be well-educated, highly skilled, and capable of managing their own affairs. They will practice in many types of settings and under varying contractual arrangements. Ethics and legal issues will be a major concern. Above all, nursing practice will continue to be directed toward helping others to live lives of the highest possible quality, or enabling them to die with dignity and peace. (Reprinted with permission from M.K. Ayedelotte, "Nursing's Preferred Future," *Nursing Outlook* May/June 1987, 35, 115–120, p. 119. Copyright 1987 American Journal of Nursing Company.)

Since today's nursing students will be the practitioners of 2010, nursing educators presently face a double challenge: preparing students to enter nursing practice in an era of rapid technological growth, and providing a strong foundation for the future. It is not sufficient to prepare students for specific roles in the health care delivery system. Rather, nursing education must prepare practitioners capable of applying learned concepts and skills to new situations and adapting what is known to meet the challenges of the unknown.

A Book for the Beginning Student

Recognizing the challenges of the new millenium, this text provides an introduction to the growing knowledge base of nursing. Taking its cues from today's nurse educators, it focuses on the concepts and skills that *beginning* students must master. The comprehensive Third Edition of *Fundamentals of Nursing* served as a starting point for preparing this shorter text. The authors systematically reviewed and critiqued *Fundamentals* to identify those specific areas essential to a strong foundation in nursing practice. This process established the guidelines for a completely rewritten text that is carefully designed to meet the needs of students in introductory nursing courses.

We have emphasized content essential to practice and commonly presented in introductory nursing courses. Content beyond the scope of the beginning nursing student is mentioned, but not discussed in detail. For example, new students learn that nurses often function as health care providers in client's homes but, since beginning students are not likely to work with home care agencies, home health care is not emphasized here. Similarly, the significance of research in nursing and the roles of nurses in research are presented, but there is no discussion on how to design a research proposal. Likewise, the use of computers in recording and reporting is discussed, while computer systems are not.

Features

To assist the student in applying the concepts and principles discussed in the text, we have incorporated many special features. These include:

Insights. Selected excerpts that provide a sense of what nursing is and what nurses do are strategically placed throughout the book. These Insights, designed in an eye-catching magazine style, complement the concepts presented and promote socialization of the beginning students into nursing. These Insights are excerpted from diverse nursing publications, including the *Journal of Nursing Administration, Nursing Management,* and *Geriatric Nursing.* The authors range from nursing leaders to clients.

Implications for Older Adults. This symbol appears in the margin throughout the text where there are important considerations for older adults. As demographics change, this age group commands special attention because they often represent the largest group of clients in a given health care system. Thus it is very likely that beginning students will be caring for older adults. Whether reading an assigned portion of the text or using the text for reference, the student can quickly locate relevant material about older clients.

Guidelines. This symbol ♠ highlights the instructions that assist student learning. Key concepts and principles discussed in the text are featured in these special boxes. These boxes thus consistently reinforce student learning.

Nursing Diagnosis. DX Common nursing diagnoses, including the newly adopted 1988 NANDA diagnoses, are grouped in special boxes for easy identification. Etiologies, as well as health problems and strengths, are included in the diagnostic statements. Examples of actual and potential diagnoses are given. Where appropriate, collaborative diagnoses have been listed with explanations for the student as to the nursing responsibilities. The 1988 NANDA diagnoses are listed in full on the endsheets at the back of the book.

Outcome Criteria. Desired outcomes that would indicate attainment of client goals are also enclosed in special boxes. These fall in the evaluation section of each chapter, and are cross referenced in the planning section. We emphasize the importance of establishing evaluation criteria during the planning phase of the nursing process.

Procedures. Sixty-three newly revised procedures are provided in this text, since skills are an essential aspect of nursing practice. The procedures are easily located within the text by their yellow backgrounds, and they are listed by number on the endsheets at the front of this book. When teaching skills, instructors may wish to refer students to the "yellow pages" for ready reference. Basic procedures that all beginning students commonly perform (e.g., measuring vital signs, bathing and positioning clients, recording fluid intake and output) are included. Given the increasing acuity of client populations in most clinical agencies, it is likely that even beginning students may be assigned clients with multiple presenting problems. Therefore, this text also includes many of the procedures students will observe or perform less frequently (e.g., administering tube feedings or enemas, changing bowel diversion ostomy appliances, performing oropharyngeal and nasopharyngeal suctioning). A Procedures Supplement containing 75 additional procedures is also available. A list of the Procedures that appear in the Supplement can be found on page *xix* of this book.

Organization

Introduction to Nursing contains nine major content units. As nursing process is the key organizational element of this text, it is introduced early (Unit II). Subsequent units provide applications of the process. Units V, VI, VII, and VIII focus on nursing interventions having to do with health (protecting, promoting, assessing, and supporting behaviors). Unit IX covers the implementing of specific nursing measures, such as medications, wound care, and perioperative care. Appendices, a glossary, and an index further assist the student.

■ **Unit 1, Nursing and Health,** provides an overview of contemporary nursing, as well as health care systems and practices. It also provides information on essential ethical and legal aspects of nursing and introduces the student to selected areas of nursing practice (e.g., education, research, political activism) that impact nursing's future.

■ **Unit 2, The Nursing Process,** provides an indepth discussion of the process as a whole, devoting separate chapters to each of the five components. Thus, the student is given a strong reference point for beginning to integrate newly acquired concepts and skills into developing nursing practice.

■ **Unit 3, Concepts About Humans,** discusses both psychosocial and biophysical concepts. It provides a holistic frame of reference within which the student can come to understand human differences and responses. Specific chapters address self-concept, sexuality, cultural diversity, spiritual practices, and the grieving process.

■ **Unit 4, Communication Processes,** focuses on the skills that beginning students will need—to communicate in a helping relationship, implement a teaching plan, and exchange essential information about the client through recording and reporting. We emphasize the importance of listening and developing objectivity.

■ **Unit 5, Protecting Health,** describes current practices regarding the transfer of microorganisms and provides specific guidelines that nurses should follow to protect themselves as well as their clients from environmental hazards.

■ **Unit 6, Promoting Health,** emphasizes wellness and describes the developmental tasks achieved by healthy individuals at various ages. Examples underscore the consequences when individuals are unable to achieve these tasks. A separate chapter about the family assists the student to recognize the importance of the client's family.

■ **Unit 7, Assessing Health,** builds upon Chapter 8 (Assessing). It features guidelines for performing basic nursing assessment skills and for assisting with selected diagnostic procedures. Content on special procedures is provided to enable students to prepare clients appropriately before procedures, to support clients while the procedure is being performed, and to monitor them afterwards.

■ **Unit 8, Supporting Health,** contains chapters on physiologic needs, and nursing activities to assist clients in meeting these needs. Using the nursing process as a unifying thread, this unit assists the beginning student to recognize the significance of specific assessments, to analyze data and identify relevant nursing diagnoses, to select priorities and strategies when planning care, to perform selected techniques, and to use outcome criteria to evaluate the client's status.

■ **Unit 9, Implementing Special Nursing Measures,** introduces the student to underlying basic principles for commonly performed skills, such as administering medications, providing wound care, and caring for clients before and after surgery. We have integrated current guidelines from the Centers for Disease Control and included rationales for specific interventions.

Teaching/Learning Package

■ **1. Procedures Supplement,** contains 75 additional procedures. This unique supplement is part of our commitment to giving instructors and students maximum flexibility and utility of print resources. Each Procedure is presented in a step-by-step format that systematically reinforces the nursing process. Illustrations further define the techniques.

■ **2. Instructors' Manual,** available to faculty only, covers key concepts and rationales. Teaching objectives are tied to discussion questions, review exercises, and student activities. Special troubleshooting and helpful hint sections offer suggestions for teaching content, which many instructors have told us can be problematic. The manual includes chapter outlines, transparency masters, audiovisual resources, and guidelines for finding primary resource materials.

■ **3. Student Learning Guide,** by Lina K. Sims and Kendra A. Ross, the first care-planning study guide in fundamentals of nursing. It contains learning objectives, chapter overviews, and study questions based on case studies for each chapter. Exercises challenge students to synthesize, apply, and extend text knowledge as they complete care plans from information provided in the case studies.

■ **4. Testbank,** available to faculty only, provides 1000 new items covering a broad range of levels. All questions are presented in NCLEX format. Computerized versions are available for IBM-PC or Apple II users.

■ **5. Transparency Kit,** includes 40 two-color transparencies, featuring some illustrations not found in the main text.

To meet the challenges of nursing today and in the future requires intelligence, flexibility, and resourcefulness. But, just as in the past, these traits are not the essence of nursing. Central to every nursing activity is caring—genuine concern for others. It is our hope that this new text conveys that essence to all who use it.

Acknowledgments

Many persons besides the authors have participated in the development and production of this text. In particular, we would like to express our warmest appreciation and sincere thanks to:

■ Chuck, Charles, Michael, and Jeanne Bufalino, who gave so much of their time when Mom was "working on the book."
■ The contributors to the Third Edition of *Fundamentals of Nursing:* Janice Denehy, Thomas Eoyang, Barbara Germino, Diana Mason, Mary Kelly Memmer, Rita Olivieri, Ross A. Stewart, Susan Talbott, and Holly Skodol Wilson.
■ All the reviewers, whose comments and suggestions were extremely helpful in preparing this manuscript. These colleagues are listed on page *v*.
■ Nancy Evans, our longtime sponsoring editor, whose editorial guidance throughout the development of this manuscript was invaluable. We are very grateful to her, knowing that the strong foundation she helped establish is reflected in the finished product.
■ Armando Parcés Enríquez, our new editor, for his enthusiasm and support in completing this project.
■ Debra Hunter, executive editor, and Glenda Epting, production manager, for their continued support.
■ Brian Jones and Sue Gemmel, whose attention to detail in coordinating the artwork for this text has been invaluable.
■ Laurie Bryant, editorial assistant, for her work in the initial preparation of the art manuscript, and Wendy Earl, for her careful editing of the Procedures.
■ Antonio Padial, for his excellent copyediting, both in this text and over the years we have been associated with him.
■ Ann Calandro, for a great job of reading the galleys.
■ Steven Sorensen, for his usual meticulous reading of the pages and creation of the index.
■ Judith Johnstone, production supervisor and friend, whose ability to "see" how the text is developing is a true gift that she uses so well.

Barbara Kozier
Glenora Erb
Patricia McKay Bufalino

Contents in Brief

Contents in Detail

Appendices   867

Additional Procedures in Supplement

INTRODUCTION TO NURSING

Nursing and Health

CHAPTERS

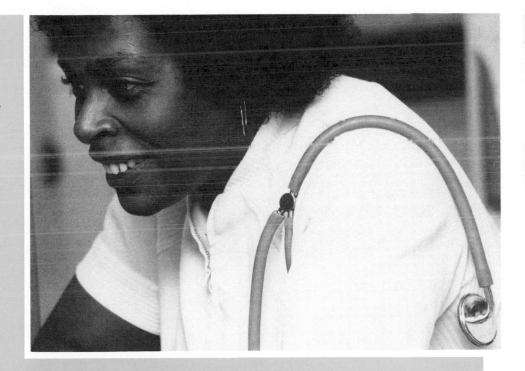

CHAPTER 1

Nursing and Nurses

OBJECTIVES

Identify the essential aspects of nursing and professional growth within nursing.

Explain the significance of conceptual and theoretical frameworks in nursing.

Describe the relationship of the nursing process to conceptual models of nursing.

Describe the relationship of nursing theory to nursing research.

Identify differences in the nurse's role in various practice settings.

Describe the common models for delivery of nursing care.

Explain the significance of nurse practice acts.

Describe the importance of established standards of nursing practice.

Explain career mobility and expanded roles in nursing.

Describe the various educational programs in nursing.

Compare the functions of national and international nurses' associations.

Describe the functions of selected special interest organizations relating to nursing.

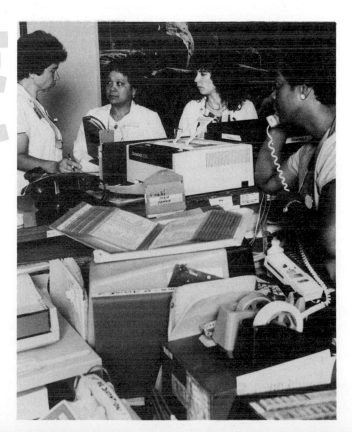

An Emerging Definition of an Evolving Profession

Nursing today is far different from nursing as it was practiced 50 years ago. It takes a vivid imagination to envision how the nursing profession will evolve in the next 50 years in an ever-changing world. To comprehend present-day nursing and at the same time prepare for nursing in tomorrow's world, one must understand not only past events but also contemporary nursing practice and the sociologic factors affecting it.

Florence Nightingale defined nursing over 100 years ago as "the act of utilizing the environment of the patient to assist him in his recovery" (Nightingale 1860). Nightingale considered a clean, well-ventilated, and quiet environment essential for recovery. Often considered the first theorist, Nightingale raised the status of nursing through education. Nurses were no longer untrained housekeepers but people trained in the care of the sick.

Virginia Henderson was one of the first modern nurses to define nursing. One hundred years after Nightingale, Henderson wrote, "The unique function of the nurse is to assist the individual, sick or well, in the performance of those activities contributing to health or its recovery (or to peaceful death) that he would perform unaided if he had the strength, will, or knowledge, and to do this in such a way as to help him gain independence as rapidly as possible" (Henderson 1966, p. 3). Like Nightingale, Henderson described nursing in relation to the patient and his or her environment. Unlike Nightingale, Henderson saw the nurse as concerned with both well and ill individuals, acknowledged that nurses interact with clients even when recovery may not be feasible, and mentioned the teaching and advocacy roles of the nurse.

In the latter half of the twentieth century, a number of nurse theorists developed their own views of nursing. A **nurse theorist** is a person who seeks to define basic principles of nursing practice systematically. Certain themes are common to many of these definitions: that nursing is caring, adaptive, individualized, holistic, family- and community-interrelated; that it involves teaching and direct/indirect services; and that it is a science as well as an art concerned with health promotion, health maintenance, health restoration, and the care of the dying. See Table 1–1 for definitions of nursing by selected nurse theorists.

Professional nursing associations have also examined nursing and developed their definitions of nursing. The American Nurses' Association (ANA) describes nursing practice as "direct, goal oriented, and adaptable to the needs of the individual, the family, and community during health and illness" (ANA 1973, p. 2). In 1980, the ANA published this definition of nursing: "Nursing is the diagnosis and treatment of human responses to actual or potential health problems" (ANA 1980, p. 9). In its 1987 House of Delegates, the ANA adopted a statement on the scope of nursing practice: "There is one scope of clinical nursing practice. The core, or essence, of that practice is the nursing diagnosis and treatment of human responses to health and to illness" (ANA 1987, p. 76). The new statement further describes the differences between professional and technical nurses as to the "depth and breadth to which the individual nurse engages in the total scope of the clinical practice of nursing are defined by the knowledge base of the nurse, the role of the nurse, and the nature of the client population within a practice environment" (ANA 1987, p. 76). The Canadian Nurses' Association (CNA) published a definition in 1984 that serves as the professional standard for nurses in Canada.

The history of nursing is one of constant evolution. The nursing profession owes much to the influence of Florence Nightingale (1820–1910), a woman with a vision. In an era when nursing was regarded with contempt, Nightingale crusaded to change the world's view of the nurse. No longer is nursing held in disrepute as it was in the nineteenth century. Nightingale's belief in education, her development of theories of nursing practice and hygiene techniques, and her campaign to emphasize prevention in health care are important facets of nursing today.

In the early twentieth century, however, people lost view of some of Nightingale's ideas temporarily. Medicine, in its zeal to control disease, frequently emphasized cure rather than prevention. The role of the nurse was that of the physician's handmaiden. Traditionally, nurses were trained in hospital schools, rather than educated in institutions of higher learning. Student nurses frequently worked long hours performing hospital chores rather than spending time and energy with clients or books. Nurses were allowed only to follow orders and not to make independent decisions about client care. Nightingale's intentions for the nursing profession were ignored but fortunately not forgotten. Her vision was shared by nursing pioneers in the years that followed, and this vision is the motivating force behind the campaign today for similar aims. Our changing society, advances in medicine, current goals for human rights, and Nightingale's vision continue to spur change in nursing practice.

Professionalism in Nursing

The growth of professionalism in nursing can be viewed in relation to specialized education, knowledge base, ethics, and autonomy.

Specialized Education

Historically, schools of nursing were run by hospitals. In modern times, however, the trend has been toward nursing education programs in colleges and universities. In the United States today, there are five levels of education in registered nursing: hospital diploma, associate degree, baccalaureate degree, master's degree, and doctoral degree (DeYoung 1985, p. 246).

Programs leading to entry at the master's or doctoral level are designed specifically for non-nurse col-

Table 1—1 Definitions and Descriptions of Nursing

Nursing Theorist and Theory	Definition/Description
Faye Abdellah (1960): Twenty-one nursing problems	Service to individuals and families; therefore, to society. An art and science that mold the attitudes, intellectual competencies, and technical skills of the individual nurse into the desire and ability to help people, sick or well, cope with their health needs. May be carried out under general or specific medical direction.
Virginia Henderson (1966): Fourteen basic needs	The unique function of the nurse: to assist clients, sick or well, in the performance of those activities contributing to health, its recovery, or peaceful death that clients would perform unaided if they had the necessary strength, will, or knowledge. Also, to do so in such a way as to help clients gain independence as rapidly as possible.
Dorothy E. Johnson (1980): Behavioral system theory	An external regulatory force that acts to preserve the organization and integration of the client's behavior at an optimal level under those conditions in which the behavior constitutes a threat to physical or social health, or in which illness is found.
Imogene King (1971, 1981): Goal attainment theory	A helping profession that assists individuals and groups in society to attain, maintain, and restore health. If this is not possible, nurses help individuals die with dignity. Nursing is perceiving, thinking, relating, judging, and acting vis-a-vis the behavior of individuals who come to a nursing situation. A nursing situation is the immediate environment, spatial and temporal reality, in which nurse and client establish a relationship to cope with health states and adjust to changes in activities of daily living if the situation demands adjustment. It is an interpersonal process of action, reaction, interaction, and transaction whereby nurse and client share information about their perceptions in the nursing situation.
Madeleine Leininger (1984): Transcultural care theory	A learned humanistic art and science that focuses on personalized (individual and group) care behaviors, functions, and processes directed toward promoting and maintaining health behaviors or recovery from illness. Behaviors have physical, psychocultural, and social significance or meaning for those being assisted generally by a professional nurse or one with similar role competencies.
Myra Levine (1973): Four conservation principles	A human interaction; a discipline rooted in the organic dependency of the individual on relationships with other human beings. A subculture reflecting ideas and values unique to nurses, even though the values mirror the social template that created them.
Bette Neuman (1982): Systems theory	A unique profession in that it is concerned with all of the variables affecting an individual's response to stressors, which are intra-, inter-, and extrapersonal in nature. The concern of nursing is to prevent stress invasion, or, following stress invasion, to protect the client's basic structure and obtain or maintain a maximum level of wellness. The nurse helps the client, through primary, secondary, and tertiary prevention modes, to adjust to environmental stressors and maintain client system stability.
Dorothea Orem (1985): Self-care theory	A helping or assisting service to persons who are wholly or partly dependent—infants, children, and adults—when they, their parents, guardians, or other adults responsible for their care are no longer able to give or supervise their care. A creative effort of one human being to help another human being. Nursing is deliberate action, a function of the practical intelligence of nurses, and action to bring about humanely desirable conditions in persons and their environments. It is distinguished from other human services and other forms of care by its focus on human beings.
Hildegard Peplau (1952): Psychodynamic nursing	A significant, therapeutic, interpersonal process. It functions cooperatively with other human processes that make health possible for individuals in communities. An educative instrument, a maturing force that aims to promote forward movement of the personality in the direction of creative, constructive, productive, personal, and community living.
Martha Rogers (1970): Unitary human beings, an energy field	A humanistic science dedicated to compassionate concern with maintaining and promoting health, preventing illness, and caring for and rehabilitating the sick and disabled. Nursing seeks to promote symphonic interaction between the environment and the person, to strengthen the coherence and integrity of the human beings, and to direct and redirect patterns of interaction between the person and the environment for the realization of maximum health potential.
Sister Callista Roy (1976, 1984): Adaptation theory	A theoretical system of knowledge that prescribes a process of analysis and action related to the care of the ill or potentially ill person. As a science, nursing is a developing system of knowledge about persons used to observe, classify, and relate the processes by which persons positively affect their health status. As a practice discipline, nursing's scientific body of knowledge is used to provide an essential service to people, that is, to promote ability to affect health positively.

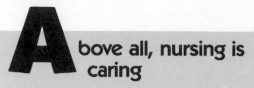

Above all, nursing is caring

Nursing is primary care, secondary care and tertiary care, no matter how those are defined. Nursing is health care and sickness care, prevention, health promotion and rehabilitation. Nursing is community care, home care, institutional care, mental health care, and increasingly, self-care. Nursing is there at the beginning of life and the end. Nursing treats individuals, families, groups, communities, and where it is practiced as administration, institutions. Nurses observe, listen, test, assess, diagnose, monitor, manage, treat and cure. But above all nursing is caring.

As a profession, we have any number of divisions among us, divisions of training, gender, education, philosophy, state, organization, setting and regulation. But the one thing upon which nurses agree is that the essence of the practice, and thus the knowing, is caring. . . . Care [that] is simply technical or merely procedural and not tender and loving is not quality care. Similarly, care which is simply tender and loving but not thoughtful and planned is not good care.

Caring for and about people cannot be dismissed as merely intuitive. But intuition has been defined as "unconscious intelligence." Nursing is not just comfort, care, coordination, collaboration, or just applied psychology, physiology, sociology, anthropology or diluted medical science. Nursing is all of these things and more. It requires an effort of considerable intellectual acuity—which looks to an outsider like intuition—to thread one's way through all the knowledge, technique and tenderness one has and to come out with the right action to serve the patient's particular need.

Source: D. Diers, To profess—To be a professional, *Journal of Nursing Administration,* March 1986, 16(3): 25–30. Reprinted from *The Journal of the New York State Nurses' Association,* December 1984. Excerpt reprinted here by permission.

---

lege graduates. In addition to entry level programs, there are a number of options for advanced education in nursing. These are discussed in the next chapter.

Body of Knowledge

As a profession, nursing is establishing a well-defined body of knowledge and expertise. Conceptual frameworks (discussed later in this chapter) contribute to the knowledge base of nursing and give direction to nursing research and nursing education. Research contributes to the body of nursing knowledge. In the 1940s, nursing research was at a very early stage of development. In the 1950s, federal funding and professional support helped to establish centers for nursing research. Early research focused on the needs and resources of nursing and nursing education. In the 1960s, studies were often related to the nature and veracity of the knowledge base underlying nursing practice (Gortner 1980, p. 205).

During the 1970s, research was largely practice-related. In the 1980s, nursing's involvement in research continues to grow. The ANA Commission on Nursing Research (1981b) identified the following as priorities for nursing research:

1. Promoting health and preventing illness.
2. Decreasing the negative impact of health problems on coping abilities, productivity, and satisfaction.
3. Developing strategies that provide effective nursing care to high-risk vulnerable groups.
4. Developing cost-efficient delivery systems of nursing care.

The establishment of the National Center for Nursing Research in 1986 has meant additional federal support for professional growth.

Ethics

Nurses have traditionally placed a high value on the worth and dignity of others. The nursing profession requires integrity of its members; that is, a member is expected to do what is considered right regardless of the personal cost. Nurses must not only respect the professional judgment of others but also develop nursing standards and establish mechanisms for identifying and dealing with unethical behavior.

Ethical codes change as the needs and values of society change. The nursing profession has developed its own codes of ethics and has set up means to monitor the behavior of its members. See Chapter 5 for additional information on nursing ethics.

Autonomy

A profession is autonomous if it regulates itself and sets standards for its members. Providing autonomy is one of the purposes of a professional association. Nurses, therefore, must work within their professional organizations to attain autonomy for the profession.

To practioners of nursing, autonomy means independence at work, responsibility, and accountability for one's actions. The ANA statement on the scope of practice describes the accountability of professional and technical nurses:

Professional nurses develop nursing policies, procedures, and protocols and set standards for nursing care for all client populations in all practice settings. . . . Technical nurses use policies, procedures, and protocols developed by professional nurses in implementing an individual's plan of care. Technical nurses are accountable for practicing within these guidelines (ANA 1987, p. 77).

Autonomy is more easily achieved and maintained from a position of authority. Therefore, many nurses seek administrative positions rather than expanded clinical competence as a means to ensure their autonomy in the workplace.

Conceptual Frameworks and Theories of Nursing

Conceptual frameworks and models offer ways of looking at a discipline (e.g., nursing) in clear, explicit terms that can be communicated to others. Although most nurses have an idea of what nursing is, its uniqueness needs to be clearly stated to other health care workers and the public. Professionalism and a desire for collegial status with other health professionals have made this need explicit. Nurses must communicate exactly what makes their place in the interdisciplinary team unique and important.

Before one discusses conceptual frameworks, the terms *concept, model, framework, conceptual model* or *framework,* and *theory* must be clarified. A **concept** is an abstract ideal or mental image of phenomena or reality. Many concepts apply to nursing: concepts about human beings, health, helping relationships, and communication. The concepts that influence nursing most significantly and determine its practice include: the *person* receiving nursing care, the *environment* in which the person exists, *health* at the time of interaction with the nurse, and *nursing actions.*

A **model** is a pattern of something to be made, an abstract outline or architectural sketch of a genuine article, or an approximation or simplification of reality. A toy model, such as a toy car, illustrates the definition simply. The model is not actually a car, but its parts represent the features of a real car. A model can also show the features of a discipline. Nursing models include those concepts that the model builder considers relevant and that aid understanding by others.

A **framework** is a basic structure supporting anything. A **conceptual framework** is a set of concepts and statements that integrate the concepts into a meaningful configuration (Fawcett 1984, p. 2). A **conceptual model** gives clear and explicit direction to the three areas of nursing: practice, education, and research. A **theory,** like a conceptual model or framework, is made up of concepts and statements about the concepts; however, a theory accounts for phenomena with much greater specificity. The primary purpose of a theory is to generate knowledge in a field. A conceptual model or framework, by contrast, provides a guide for nursing practice, education, and research.

Some Conceptual Frameworks of Nursing

As there are varying opinions on the nature and structure of nursing, theories continue to be developed. Each theory bears the name of the person or group who developed it and reflects the beliefs of the developer.

Some well-known theories are Virginia Henderson's (1966) complementary-supplementary model, Dorothy E. Johnson's (1966) behavioral systems model, Imogene King's (1981) open systems theory, Madeleine Leininger's (1984) transcultural care theory, Myra Levine's (1973) conservation theory, Betty Neuman's (1982) system model, Dorothea E. Orem's (1985) self-care model, Martha Roger's (1970, 1980) life process theory, and Sister Callista Roy's (1976) adaptation model. Each nursing education program is based on a conceptual framework selected or developed by the program's faculty to guide student learning and to provide a nursing model for graduates.

Relationship to the Nursing Process

Conceptual models for nursing are abstractions that are operationalized or made real by the use of the nursing process. See Chapters 7–12 for detailed information on the nursing process. This systematic process, similar to the scientific or problem-solving process, consists of five steps:

1. *Assessing.* Specific data about a client's health needs are collected during this first step of the nursing process. If the client is seen as having 14 fundamental needs when using a particular model, data are collected about these 14 needs.
2. *Diagnosing.* In this step, the assessment data are analyzed to identify actual, potential, and possible nursing diagnoses. The client's actual or potential health problems are outlined or written as a nursing diagnostic statement in accordance with the nursing model used.
3. *Planning.* Planning also relates directly to the conceptual nursing model. Goals for resolution of client problems, nursing interventions aimed at achieving those goals, and outcome criteria by which the nurse can evaluate whether or not the goals are met are established in accordance with the modes of nursing outlined in the conceptual model.
4. *Implementing.* Implementing the planned interventions draws on scientific knowledge that is not part of the nursing model. The nursing model instructs the nurse what to do and directly influences what nursing interventions are planned, but it does not tell the nurse how to do it.
5. *Evaluating.* Evaluating is a continuous nursing function. How is the client adjusting and reacting? What does the client see as needs? How does the client see these needs changing? Has the client achieved the desired consequences? The answers to these questions help the nurse evaluate the effectiveness of the total nursing process and the nursing model.

Relationship of Nursing Theory to Research

Nursing theory and nursing research are closely related. Scientific knowledge is derived from testing hypotheses generated by theories for nursing. Research determines the utility of those hypotheses, and research findings may be developed into theories for nursing. In the research process, comparisons are made between the observed outcomes of research and the relationship predicted by the hypotheses.

Nursing Practice

Nurses practice in an ever-increasing variety of roles and settings. How individual nurses practice is influenced largely by the setting, the needs of the clients, the nurse practice acts of the area, and the standards of the professional organization.

The Recipient of Nursing Care

The recipients of nursing care are sometimes called *consumers,* sometimes *patients,* and sometimes *clients.* A **consumer** is an individual, a group of people, or a community that uses a service or commodity. A family that uses electricity in its home is a consumer of electricity. People who use health care products or services are consumers of health care.

A **patient** is a person who is waiting for or undergoing medical treatment and care. The word *patient* comes from a Latin word meaning to suffer or to bear. Traditionally, the person receiving health care has been called a patient. Usually, people become patients when they seek assistance because of illness or surgery. Some nurses believe that the word *patient* implies passive acceptance of the decisions and care of health professionals. Additionally, with the emphasis on health promotion and prevention of illness, many recipients of nursing care are not ill. Moreover, nurses interact with family members and significant others in addition to the persons actually receiving nursing care. For these reasons, nurses are increasingly referring to recipients of health care as *clients.*

A **client** is a person who engages the advice or services of another who is qualified to provide this service. The term *client* presents the receiver of health care less as a passive recipient and more as a collaborator in the care, i.e., as a person who is also responsible for his or her health. Thus the health status of a client is the responsibility of the individual in collaboration with health professionals. In this book, *client* is the preferred term, although *consumer* and *patient* are used in some instances.

Focus of Nursing Practice

Nursing involves an interrelationship of many people concerned with a client's responses to potential or actual health problems. Today, there is an emphasis on the whole person; people are seen not merely as physical beings but as biopsychosocial beings. Nursing practice involves a complex of knowledge and skills applied to the whole client. Nurses are also involved with support persons and the community as a whole. For this reason,

nurses must be aware of how the support persons and community affect the client's well-being and consider the well-being of these support persons and the community.

Settings for Nursing Practice

In the past, the acute care hospital was the only practice setting open to most nurses. Today, however, there are employment opportunities not only in acute and long-term chronic or rehabilitation hospitals but also in clients' homes, community agencies, ambulatory clinics or health maintenance organizations (HMOs), and nursing practice centers, for example. Table 1–2 shows areas of registered practice in the United States.

Nurses have different degrees of nursing autonomy and nursing responsibility in the various settings. Today, nurses have a variety of career choices and can pursue any number of interests. They may specialize, for example, in intensive care nursing or respiratory nursing. In addition to providing direct care, they teach clients and support persons, serve as nursing advocates and agents of change, and help determine health policies affecting consumers in the community and in hospitals.

Models for Delivery of Nursing Care

Common configurations for the delivery of nursing care include the case method, the functional method, team nursing, and primary nursing.

Case Method.
The case method, also referred to as total care or total patient care, is one of the earliest models developed. This method is client-centered. One nurse is assigned to and is responsible for the comprehensive care of a group of clients during an 8- or 12-hour shift. For each client, the nurse assesses needs, formulates diagnoses, develops nursing plans, implements care, and evaluates the effectiveness of care. In this method, a client has consistent contact with one nurse during a shift but may have different nurses on other shifts. The case method, considered the precursor of primary nursing, continues to be used in a variety of practice settings, e.g., private duty nursing and intensive care.

With the shortage of nursing personnel during World War II, the case method could no longer be the chief mode of delivering care to clients. To meet staff shortages, managers hired personnel with less educational preparation than the professional nurse and developed on-the-job training programs for auxiliary helpers. The total care method became unfeasible in such situations, and the functional method was developed in response.

Functional Method.
This system of assignment, which evolved from concepts of scientific management used in the field of business administration, focuses on the jobs to be completed. In this task-oriented approach, personnel with less preparation than the professional nurse fulfill less complex care requirements. It is based on a production and efficiency model

Table 1—2   Areas of Registered Nurse Employment

Practice Setting	United States 1984 (percent*)	Canada 1984 (percent*)
Hospitals	68.1	73.0
Nursing homes/homes for the aged	7.7	6.5
Community health	6.8†	9.2
Physicians' and dentists' offices, family practice units	6.6	2.6
Nursing education	2.7	
Educational institutions (Canada)		2.7
Schools	2.9	
Occupational health	1.5	
Other, e.g., self-employed, insurance claims reviewers	3.7	3.1
Not stated	—	2.9

*Rounded to the first decimal
†These figures do not reflect the shift to home health care.
Sources: American Nurses' Association, *Facts about nursing 86–87* (Kansas City Mo.: American Nurses' Association, 1987), p. 101, and Statistics Canada, *Revised registered nurses data series.* Health Manpower Statistics Section (Ottawa: Health Statistics, 1984), Table 6.

that gives authority and responsibility to the person assigning the work, e.g., the head nurse. Clearly defined job descriptions, procedures, policies, and lines of communication are required. The functional approach to nursing is economical and efficient and permits centralized direction and control. Its disadvantages are fragmentation of care (the client receives care from several different categories of nursing personnel) and the possibility that nonquantifiable aspects of care, such as meeting the client's emotional needs, may be overlooked.

■ **Team Nursing.**   In the early 1950s, Eleanor Lambertson (1953) and her colleagues proposed a system of team nursing to overcome the fragmentation of care resulting from the task-oriented functional approach and to meet increasing demands for professional nurses created by advances in technologic aspects of care. **Team nursing** is the delivery of individualized nursing care to clients by a nursing team led by a professional nurse. A nursing team consists of registered nurses, licensed practical nurses, and often nurses' aides. This team is responsible for providing coordinated nursing care to a group of clients during an 8- or 12-hour shift. Compared to the functional system, team nursing emphasizes humanistic values and responds to the needs of both clients and employees. Individualized client care on a personal level rather than task-oriented care on an impersonal level is emphasized. Employees are stimulated to learn and develop new skills by the professional nurse leader, who instructs them, supervises them, and provides assignments that offer the potential for growth.

Basic to team nursing are the team conference, nursing care plan, and leadership skills. The conference, led by the professional nurse team leader, includes all personnel assigned to the team. Discussing the needs of clients, establishing goals, individualizing the plan of care, instructing personnel, and following up are all under the direction of the team leader. In essence, the team leader has a management role that requires a high degree of competence in coordination and leadership.

Although the team nursing approach has worked effectively in many health care agencies, some weaknesses have been observed. The client may still perceive care as fragmented if the team leader does not establish a satisfactory relationship with the client. Teams may not have the appropriate health care personnel, and team members may not have the expertise to meet the needs of a particular client population. Often, there is only one professional nurse, who must assume the role of team leader. When there are no professional nurses assigned to the unit, technical nurses, who are not prepared educationally to fulfill the leadership role required of a team leader, are assigned to this role. To manage effectively, the leader may revert to using a functional mode of delivering care.

■ **Primary Nursing.**   Primary nursing was introduced at the Loeb Center for Nursing and Rehabilitation, Bronx, New York, under the leadership of Lydia Hall (1963). **Primary nursing** is a system in which one nurse is responsible for total care of a number of clients 24 hours a day, 7 days a week. It is a method of providing comprehensive, individualized, and consistent care.

Primary nursing uses the nurse's nursing knowledge and management skills. The primary nurse assesses and prioritizes each client's needs, identifies nursing diagnoses, develops a plan of care with the client, and evaluates the effectiveness of care. Although associates provide some care, the primary nurse coordinates care and communicates information about the client's health to other nurses and other health care professionals. Primary nursing encompasses all aspects of the professional role, including teaching, advocacy, decision making, and continuity of care. The primary nurse is the first-line manager of the client's care with all its inherent accountabilities and responsibilities.

▪ Nurse Practice Acts

Nurse practice acts or nursing licensure laws regulate the practice of nursing in the United States and Canada. Each state in the United States has its own nurse practice act, as does each province in Canada. Although nurse practice acts differ in various jurisdictions, they all have a common purpose: to protect the public.

Nurse practice acts usually define what constitutes nursing practice, describe a "registered nurse" and a "practical or vocational nurse," and establish minimum educational and competency standards that individuals seeking authority to practice must meet. Nurse practice acts are a formalized contract between society and the profession. They serve a public purpose and also meet the needs of the profession. The public is granted a mechanism to ensure minimum standards for entry into the profession and to distinguish the unqualified. The profession achieves partial implementation of its goal of maintaining standards in practice through appropriate entry credentialing (Snyder and Labar 1984, p. 2).

My nurses were able to alleviate the fear

All of the nurses I encountered impressed me with the fact that they were personally interested in my welfare and wished to do everything possible to effect my recovery. There was not a hint of effusiveness in this attitude of personal concern; it was simply that by performing their tasks efficiently, promptly, and cheerfully they seemed to be saying, "We want you to get well. We very much want you to get well." So, human nature being what it is, I said to myself, "Well, if they are all so eager to help me, I'll try that much harder to help myself."

One capacity my nurses possessed that I certainly valued was their ability to alleviate the fear (or should I say terror?) that a patient in my situation sometimes understandably feels. The superb poise of those nurses! They knew my situation was serious, and they were prepared (I fully understood this) to take further action if further action became necessary. But because they remained so calm, I likewise assumed that attitude—and, their words provided the self-confidence that right then was so important to me, an old and very much emaciated man.

Rodney Perkins
Age 77, Indiana

Source: R. Perkins, Older authors of the year, (Second Prize), *Geriatric Nursing,* May/June 1983.

Standards of Nursing Practice

Establishing and implementing standards of practice are major functions of a professional organization. Nursing practice standards provide exact criteria against which clients, nurses, and employers can evaluate care for effectiveness and excellence. In the ANA publication *Standards of Nursing Practice,* the association comments on this responsibility of the nursing profession to society:

Nursing's concern for the quality of its services constitutes the heart of its responsibility to the public. The more expertise required to perform the service, the greater society's dependence upon those who carry it out. Nursing must control its practice in order to guarantee the quality of its service to the public. Behind that guarantee are the standards of the profession, which are directed toward assurance that service of a good quality will be provided. This is essential both for the protection of the public and for the profession itself. A profession which does not maintain the confidence of the public will soon cease to be a social force (ANA 1973, p. 1).

Nursing standards clearly reflect the specific functions and activities that nurses provide, as opposed to the functions of other health workers. The ANA's Standards of Nursing Practice are set forth in Table 1–3, and those of the CNA are summarized in Table 1–4. These standards apply to the practice of all registered nurses.

When standards of professional practice are implemented, they serve as yardsticks for the measurements used in licensure, certification, accreditation, quality assurance, peer review, and public policy (Phaneuf and Lang 1985, p. 7). Licensure, certification, and accreditation are discussed in Chapter 6. Quality assurance and peer review are discussed in Chapter 12.

Career Mobility

The public image of the nurse is that of a hospital staff nurse who has been educated in a hospital school. The general public is often unaware of the variety of roles and educational backgrounds of nurses. Two kinds of mobility are open to the nurse: vertical and horizontal. Vertical mobility means advancing upward within a hierarchy, for example, from staff nurse to head nurse. Horizontal mobility refers to the ability to change practice settings, such as from a nursing home to a community health agency.

Recognizing that nurses require encouragement, motivation, and recognition, some settings provide clinical ladder models for career development. Traditionally, a nurse's clinical competence was rewarded by moving the nurse away from client care into administrative roles. Clinical ladders provide nurses with recognition of their clinical competence while encouraging them to continue clinical nursing practice.

Expanded Nursing Roles

A **role** is a pattern of behavior expected of individuals in specific social situations. An **expanded role** is one that a nurse assumes by virtue of education and experience. The nurse who assumes an expanded role has increased responsibilities and, usually, greater autonomy. Nurses are occupying expanding roles in both hospitals and communities.

Nurse Practitioner. The role of the nurse practitioner is an extension of the nurse's basic caregiving role. Usually, nurse practitioners have advanced educational preparation; often, they have master's degrees in nursing, are graduates of a nurse practitioner program, or have advanced clinical nursing experience beyond the basic level. Nurse practitioners exercise judgment more independently than do other registered nurses in most settings.

Nurse practitioners are employed in hospitals and in communities. They may be generalists, e.g., family nurse practitioners, or specialists, e.g., geriatric nurse practitioners. Nurse practitioners in a community may be employed in health maintenance organizations, health

Table 1—3 **American Nurses' Association Standards of Nursing Practice**

Standard	Rationale	Standard	Rationale
1. The collection of data about the health status of the client/patient is systematic and continuous. The data are accessible, communicated, and recorded.	Comprehensive care requires complete and ongoing collection of data about the client/patient to determine the nursing care and needs of the client/patient. All health status data about the client/patient must be available for all members of the health care team.	5. Nursing actions provide for client/patient participation in health promotion, maintenance, and restoration.	The client/patient and family are continually involved in nursing care.
2. Nursing diagnoses are derived from health status data.	The health status of the client/patient is the basis for determining the nursing care needs. The data are analyzed and compared to norms when possible.	6. The nursing actions assist the client/patient to maximize his health capabilities.	Nursing actions are designed to promote, maintain, and restore health.
3. The plan of nursing care includes goals derived from the nursing diagnoses.	The determination of the results to be achieved is an essential part of planning care.	7. The client/patient's progress or lack of progress toward goal achievement is determined by the client/patient and the nurse.	The quality of nursing care depends upon comprehensive and intelligent determination of nursing's impact upon the health status of the client/patient. The client/patient is an essential part of this determination.
4. The plan of nursing care includes priorities and the prescribed nursing approaches or measures to achieve the goals derived from the nursing diagnoses.	Nursing actions are planned to promote, maintain, and restore the client/patient's well being.	8. The client/patient's progress or lack of progress toward goal achievement directs reassessment, reordering of priorities, new goal setting, and revision of the plan of nursing care.	The nursing process remains the same, but the input of new information may dictate new or revised approaches.

Source. American Nurses' Association, *Standards of nursing practice* (Kansas City, Mo.: American Nurses' Association, 1973). Reprinted with permission.

centers, schools, and physicians' offices. They are usually skilled at making nursing assessments, performing physical examinations, counseling, teaching, and treating (in concert with the physician) minor, self-limiting illnesses or stable, long-term illness.

▪ **Clinical Nursing Specialist.** The clinical nursing specialist has advanced knowledge and skills in a particular area of nursing. An educational prerequisite is usually a master's degree in nursing. These nurses practice in hospitals or communities. In the hospital, such nurses give direct client care, advise other nurses, and coordinate nursing care given by others. The clinical nurse specialist serves as a role model for other nurses and is expected to keep abreast of new developments in the field.

▪ **Nurse Clinician.** The term *nurse clinician* was first used by Frances Reiter in 1966. Such nurses provide bedside or direct care in a specialty area. They may or may not have advanced educational preparation.

▪ **Nurse Anesthetist.** Nurse anesthetists are registered nurses with advanced preparation in an accredited program of anesthesiology. They are licensed to administer anesthetic agents under the supervision of an anesthesiologist (a physician with specialized knowledge of anesthetic agents). Nurse anesthetists often administer anesthetic agents to clients about to undergo minor surgical procedures or examinations in hospitals and community clinics.

Education for Nursing

Nursing functions today are so complex that a nursing student requires knowledge in the biologic, physical, and social sciences in addition to nursing theory and practice. It is not possible for nurses to acquire a safe level of skill through empirical (experience and observation) means alone. They require specific knowledge and skills that can be gained only through an organized nursing curriculum.

The traditional focus of nursing education has been on teaching the skills required in hospitals. However, considerable evidence shows that the need for community and home services is increasing and that using these services overcomes some of the negative aspects of hospitalization, such as separation from family. As a result, nursing curricula now focus more broadly on health as well as illness, on community as well as hospital interests, and on selected principles and applications from the biologic, social, and physical sciences.

Table 1—4 Canadian Nurses Association Standards for Nursing Practice

Criterion Variable	Nursing Standards	Criterion Variable	Nursing Standards
Standards Related to a Conceptual Model for Nursing			of the focus and modes of intervention
	Nursing practice requires the nurse, in any setting at any time, to have:	Implementation of the intervention	4. Perform nursing actions that implement the plan
The goal	1. A clear conception of the distinct goal of nursing	Evaluation	5. Evaluate all steps of the nursing process in accord with her conceptual model for nursing
The client	2. A clear conception of the client toward whom nursing is directed		
The role of the nurse	3. A clear conception of her role as a health professional in response to health needs of society	**Standards Related to the Helping Relationship**	
The source of difficulty	4. A clear conception of the source of client difficulty		Nursing practice requires the nurse to:
The focus and modes of intervention	5. A clear conception of the focus and modes of nursing intervention	Initiation	1. Initiate interaction that helps the client to perceive the experience as understandable, manageable, and meaningful at the outset
The consequences	6. A clear conception of the expected consequences of nursing activities	Maintenance	2. Set mutually agreed upon expectations with the client
Standards Related to the Nursing Process		Termination	3. Ensure a successful termination of the helping relationship
	Nursing practice requires the nurse to:	**Standards Related to Professional Responsibilities**	
Collection of data	1. Collect data in accord with her conception of the client		Nursing practice requires the nurse to:
Analysis of data	2. Analyze data collected in accord with her conception of the goal of nursing, her own role, and the client's source of difficulty	Legal responsibility	1. Conform to statutes, policies, procedures, and directives relevant to the practice setting
Planning of the intervention	3. Plan her nursing action based upon the identified actual and potential client problems and in accord with her conception	Ethical responsibility	2. Conform to the code of ethics of her profession
		Collaboration	3. Function as a member of a health team

Source: Canadian Nurses Association, Ottawa, Ontario, Canada, February 1987.

State laws in the United States and provincial laws in Canada recognize two types of nurses: the licensed practical (vocational) nurse (LPN or LVN) and the registered nurse (RN). Various types of programs exist to prepare technical and professional nurses to enter nursing practice. In addition, advanced educational programs permit nurses to expand their levels of practice.

Licensed Practical Nursing Education

Approved practical or vocational nursing programs are provided by community colleges, vocational schools, hospitals, and a variety of health agencies. These programs usually last one year and provide both classroom and clinical experiences. At the end of the program, the graduate takes examinations to obtain a license as a practical or vocational nurse. In some states and provinces, applicants for licensure are assessed on the basis of their nursing experience rather than their formal education in an approved school.

Licensed practical nurses work in structured care settings, such as hospitals and nursing homes. Their skills are basically those required for bedside nursing under the guidance of a registered nurse. In some areas of the United States, LPN programs are being expanded to the associate degree level.

Registered Nursing Education

Most basic education for registered nurses is provided in three types of programs: diploma, associate degree, and baccalaureate programs. As mentioned earlier in this chapter, there are a few special programs leading to the master's or doctoral degree for persons with nonnursing baccalaureate degrees.

Diploma. Nursing education originated in hospital based programs. First developed by Florence Nightingale (circa 1860), these programs were operated by hospitals to ensure a pool of qualified nurses. Today's diploma nursing programs have changed markedly from the original Nightingale model, becoming hospital-based educational programs that provide a rich clinical experience for nursing students. These programs may last 2 or more years and are often associated with colleges or universities.

▪ Associate Degree. Associate degree programs in nursing were suggested in 1951 by Mildred L. Montag (1980) as a solution to the acute shortage of nurses that grew out of World War II. Associate degree programs are offered in the United States in junior colleges as well as colleges and universities. The graduating student receives an associate degree in nursing (ADN), or an associate of arts (AA), associate of science (AS), or associate in applied science (AAS) degree with a major in nursing. In Canada, associate degrees are not offered, but similar programs confer a diploma upon graduation.

Although ADN programs relieved the post World War II nursing shortage, the utilization of ADN graduates in hospital practice did not fulfill Montag's original intent; ADN and BSN graduates are often used interchangeably. This creates a discrepancy between what competencies are expected of new graduates and their actual competencies. In an effort to resolve this discrepancy, differentiated competency statements (Table 1–5) were developed during two projects sponsored by the Midwest Alliance in Nursing and funded by the W. K. Kellogg Foundation (Primm 1986, pp. 135–37). Because ADN and BSN prepared nurses currently function under the same practice acts, "these differentiated statements provide a basis for discussion of collaborative ADN and BSN nursing practice" (Primm 1986, p. 136) A new organization, the National Organization of ADN Educators, has been formed recently to address issues in modern ADN education.

▪ Baccalaureate Degree. Although baccalaureate nursing education programs were established in universities in the early 1900s, it was not until the 1960s that the number of students enrolled in these programs increased markedly. These programs usually emphasize the theoretical and scientific bases for the nursing process as a framework for clinical instruction.

Most baccalaureate programs also admit registered nurses who have diplomas or associate degrees. Some programs have special curricula to meet the needs of these students. Some universities also offer nursing students the opportunity to pursue a self-paced or independent study program. Many accept transfer credits from other accredited colleges and universities and offer students the opportunity to take challenge examinations when they believe they have the knowledge or skills taught in a course.

Graduate Programs

Education at the graduate level requires independent critical thinking; therefore, nurses who enter graduate study must have sufficient intellectual capacity and scholastic achievement to profit from it. Most graduate programs are conducted by departments within the graduate school of a university, and the applicant must first meet requirements established by the graduate school.

▪ Master's Programs. Master's programs generally take from 1½ to 2 years to complete. Degrees granted are the master of arts in nursing (MA), master of science in nursing (MN), or master of science in nursing (MSN). Master's degree programs focus on medical-surgical nursing, maternal-child nursing, psychiatric–mental health nursing, community health nursing, and subspecialty areas such as cardiovascular nursing, gerontologic nursing, inservice education, and rehabilitation. The functional focus of these programs is primarily on advanced clinical practice, but many also include teaching, supervision, and administration/management in either nursing service or education. Many programs prepare the nurse for expanded roles, such as the clinical nurse specialist and nurse practitioner.

▪ Doctoral Programs. Doctoral programs in nursing, awarding the doctor of philosophy (PhD), doctor of nursing science (DNS or DNSc), or nursing doctorate (ND), began in the 1960s in the United States. These programs further prepare the nurse for advanced clinical practice, administration, education, and research. Before 1960, nurses acquired doctoral degrees in such related fields as psychology, sociology, physiology, and education.

Content and approach vary among doctoral programs. Some focus on usual clinical areas, such as medical-surgical nursing, whereas others emphasize such nontraditional areas as transcultural nursing. Some programs emphasize theory development, but all emphasize research (DeYoung 1985, p. 119). Although master's programs require nurses to specialize in a certain area, doctoral programs narrow the area of specialization even further. A nurse with a doctorate becomes an expert in a given area through research.

Ladder Programs in Nursing

The ladder concept fosters progression of an individual from one educational level to another. The nurse who wishes to progress "up the ladder" can often obtain credit for experience and/or courses at an earlier level. Although associate degree programs were not originally designed to lead to further education, many universities now grant academic credit toward a baccalaureate degree for these years. Often, baccalaureate programs emphasize independent learning and self-pacing, and external degree programs, such as the New York State Regents Program and the California Statewide Nursing Program, provide alternatives to traditional university programs to allow for this independent, self-paced learning.

Continuing Education

The term *continuing education* refers to formalized experiences designed to enlarge the knowledge or skills of practitioners. Compared to advanced education programs, which result in an academic degree, continuing education courses tend to be more specific and shorter. Participants may receive certificates of completion or specialization.

Continuing education is the responsibility of each practicing nurse. Constant updating and growth are

Table 1—5 Differentiated Competency Statements

General Statement

The ADN cares for focal clients who are identified as individuals and members of a family. The level of responsibility of the ADN is for a specified work period and is consistent with the identified goals of care. The ADN is prepared to function in structured health care settings. The structured settings are geographical and/or situational environments where the policies, procedures, and protocols for provision of health care are established and there is recourse to assistance and support from the full scope of nursing expertise.	The BSN cares for focal clients who are identified as individuals, families, aggregates, and community groups. The level of responsibility of the BSN is from admission to post-discharge. The BSN is prepared to function in structured and unstructured health care settings. The unstructured setting is a geographical and/or situational environment which may not have established policies, procedures, and protocols and has the potential for variations requiring independent nursing decisions.

Provision of Direct Care Competencies

The ADN provides direct care for the focal client with common, well-defined nursing diagnoses by:

A. Collecting health pattern data from available resources using established assessment format to identify basic health care needs.
B. Organizing and analyzing health pattern data in order to select nursing diagnoses from an established list.
C. Establishing goals with the focal client for a specified work period that are consistent with the overall comprehensive nursing plan of care.
D. Developing and implementing an individualized nursing plan of care using established nursing diagnoses and protocols to promote, maintain, and restore health.
E. Participating in the medical plan of care to promote an integrated health care plan.
F. Evaluating focal client responses to nursing interventions and altering the plan of care as necessary to meet client goals.

The BSN provides direct care for the focal client with complex interactions of nursing diagnoses by:

A. Expanding the collection of data to identify complex care needs.
B. Organizing and analyzing complex health pattern data to develop nursing diagnoses.
C. Establishing goals with the focal client to develop a comprehensive nursing plan of care from admission to post-discharge.
D. Developing and implementing a comprehensive nursing plan of care based on nursing diagnoses for health promotion.
E. Interpreting the medical plan of care into nursing activities to formulate approaches to nursing care.
F. Evaluating the nursing care delivery system and promoting goal-directed change to meet individualized client needs.

Communication Competencies

The ADN uses basic communication skills with the focal client by:

A. Developing and maintaining goal-directed interactions to encourage expressing of needs and support coping behaviors.
B. Modifying and implementing a standard teaching plan in order to restore, maintain, and promote health.

The ADN coordinates focal client care with other health team members by:

A. Documenting and communicating data for clients with common, well-defined nursing diagnoses to provide continuity of care.
B. Using established channels of communication to implement an effective health care plan.
C. Using interpreted nursing research findings for developing nursing care.

The BSN uses complex communication skills with the focal client by:

A. Developing and maintaining goal-directed interactions to promote effective coping behaviors and facilitate change in behavior.
B. Designing and implementing a comprehensive teaching plan for health promotion.

The BSN collaborates with other health team members by:

A. Documenting and communicating comprehensive data for clients with complex interactions to provide continuity of care.
B. Using established channels of communication to modify health care delivery.
C. Incorporating research findings into practice and by consulting with nurse researchers regarding identified nursing problems in order to enhance nursing practice.

Management Competencies

The ADN organizes those aspects of care for focal clients for whom s/he is accountable by:

A. Prioritizing, planning, and organizing the delivery of standard nursing care in order to use time and resources effectively and efficiently.
B. Delegating aspects of care to peers, LPNs, and ancillary nursing personnel, consistent with their levels of education and expertise, in order to meet client needs.

The BSN manages nursing care of focal clients by:

A. Prioritizing, planning, and organizing the delivery of comprehensive nursing care in order to use time and resources effectively and errficiently.
B. Delegating aspects of care to other nursing personnel, consistent with their levels of education and expertise, in order to meet client needs and to maximize staff performance.

(continued)

Table 1–5 Differentiated Competency Statements *(continued)*

Management Competencies

C. Maintaining accountability for own care and care delegated to others to assure adherence to ethical and legal standards.	C. Maintaining accountability for own care and care delegated to others to assure adherence to ethical and legal standards.
D. Recognizing the need for referral and conferring with appropriate nursing personnel for assistance to promote continuity of care.	D. Initiating referral to appropriate departments and agencies to provide service and promote continuity of care.
E. Working with other health care personnel within the organizational structure to manage client care.	E. Assuming a leadership role in health care management to improve client care.

Source: P.L. Primm, Entry into practice: Competency statements for BSNs and ADNs, *Nursing Outlook,* May/June 1986, 34:135–137. Used by permission. Copyright 1986 American Journal of Nursing Company.

essential to keep abreast of scientific and technologic change and changes within the nursing profession. A variety of educational and health care institutions conduct continuing education programs. They are usually designed to meet one or more of the following needs:

1. To keep nurses abreast of new techniques and knowledge
2. To help nurses attain expertise in a specialized area of practice, such as intensive care nursing
3. To provide nurses with information essential to nursing practice, for example, knowledge about the legal aspects of nursing

Some state laws now require nurses to obtain a certain number of continuing education credits to renew their licenses. In these states, required continuing education (CE) contact hours vary from 15 to 30 hours for every 2-year relicensure period. All, some, or none of these hours may be acquired through home study. Some home study courses are offered through professional journals. A few regions also require a certain number of hours of practice, either independently or in lieu of study hours, before license renewal.

In-Service Education

An in-service education program is administered by an employer; it is designed to upgrade the knowledge or skills of employees. For example, an employer might offer an in-service program to inform nurses about a new piece of equipment, about specific isolation practices, or about a different method of providing nursing, such as primary nursing or implementing a nurse theorist's conceptual framework for nursing.

Nursing Organizations

One way nurses can demonstrate professional commitment is by active involvement in a nursing organization. There are two types of organizations: professional and nonprofessional. "A professional organization is an organization of practitioners who judge one another as professionally competent and who have banded together to perform social functions which they cannot perform in their separate capacities as individuals" (Merton 1958, p. 50). Two examples of professional organizations are the American Nurses' Association (ANA), the professional organization for RNs in the United States, and the Canadian Nurses' Association (CNA) in Canada. The National League for Nursing (NLN) is an example of a nonprofessional nursing organization; many levels of nurses and nonnurses can join. Nursing organizations are established at local, national, and international levels.

National Nursing Students' Association

The National Nursing Students' Association is the official preprofessional organization for nursing students. It was formed in 1953 and incorporated in 1959. Originally, it functioned under the aegis of the ANA and NLN; however, in 1968 it became an autonomous body, although it communicates with the NLN and the ANA. To qualify for membership, a student must be enrolled in a state-approved nursing education program.

International Honor Society: Sigma Theta Tau

Sigma Theta Tau (STT) is the international honor society in nursing. It was founded in 1922 and has its headquarters in Indianapolis, Indiana. The Greek letters stand for the Greek words *storga, tharos,* and *tima* meaning love, courage, and honor. STT is a member of the association of college honor societies. The society's purpose is professional rather than social. STT membership is attained through academic achievement. Students in baccalaureate nursing programs and nurses in master's, doctoral, and postdoctoral programs are eligible to be selected for membership.

The official journal of STT, *Image: Journal of Nursing Scholarship,* is published quarterly. The journal publishes scholarly articles of interest to nurses. The organization also publishes *Reflections,* a quarterly newsletter that provides information about the organization and its various chapters.

American Nurses' Association (ANA)

The American Nurses' Association is the national professional organization for nurses in the United States. It was founded in 1896 as the Nurses Associated Alumnae of the United States and Canada. In 1911, the name was changed to the American Nurses' Association. It was a charter member of the International Council of Nurses along with Great Britain and Germany in 1899. The purposes of the ANA are to foster high standards of nursing practice and to promote the educational and professional advancement of nurses so that all people may have better nursing care. The ANA is composed of the nurses' associations from the 50 states, Guam, the Virgin Islands, Puerto Rico, and the District of Columbia. These state associations are in turn divided into regional and local chapters.

In 1982, the ANA became a federation of state nurses' associations. Individual nurses no longer belong to the ANA but participate by joining their state nursing association. Each state nurses' association, as a member of the federation, is entitled to representation in the ANA House of Delegates, with the number of seats dependent on the number of members in each state organization. The official journal of the ANA is the *American Journal of Nursing.* The official newspaper is the *American Nurse.* The functions of the ANA are shown in Table 1–6.

Table 1–6 Functions of the American Nurses' Association

Establish standards of nursing practice, nursing education, and nursing services.

Establish a code of ethical conduct for nurses.

Ensure a system of credentialing in nursing.

Initiate and influence legislation, governmental programs, national health policy, and international health policy.

Support systematic study, evaluation, and research in nursing.

Serve as the central agency for the collection, analysis, and dissemination of information relevant to nursing.

Promote and protect the economic and general welfare of nurses.

Provide leadership in national and international nursing.

Provide for the professional development of nurses.

Conduct an affirmative action program.

Ensure a collective bargaining program for nurses.

Provide services to constituent state nurses' associations.

Maintain communication with constituent state nurses' associations through official publications.

Assume an active role as consumer advocate.

Represent and speak for the nursing profession with allied health groups, national and international organizations, governmental bodies, and the public.

Source: American Nurses' Association Bylaws, as amended June 8, 1987. Kansas City, Mo.: American Nurses' Association, 1982. Used by permission.

Canadian Nurses' Association (CNA)

The Canadian Nurses' Association is the national nursing association of Canada. Nurses do not join the CNA independently but obtain membership by paying a fee to the provincial chapters. In 1985, 175,000 nurses belonged to provincial chapters and thus to the CNA. In November 1985, the Quebec Nurses' Association withdrew from the CNA. Because of the departure of the Quebec Nurses' Association, the CNA plans to reduce spending severely and is considering a restructuring of the association.

The CNA has developed national standards and a code of ethics, and it offers support to all provincial associations. Through the National Testing Services, the CNA prepares licensure examinations. These examinations are available to all provinces and territories and provide a national standard for licensure of registered nurses. Through the Canadian Nurses' Foundation, research grants, fellowships, and scholarships are offered to Canadian nurses. The official journal of the CNA, *Canadian Nurse,* is published monthly and sent to each nurse member.

National League for Nursing (NLN)

The National League for Nursing, formed in 1952, is an organization of both individuals and agencies. Its objective is to foster the development and improvement of all nursing services and nursing education. People who are not nurses but have an interest in nursing services, for example, hospital administrators, can be members of the league. This feature of the NLN—involving nonnurse members, consumers, and nurses from all levels of practice—is unique.

The NLN is "dedicated to meeting the health needs of the people by improving nursing education and nursing service" (NLN 1975). The NLN has traditionally offered a wide range of services including institutes, workshops, seminars, consultation, accreditation of nursing education programs, testing services, and educational aid. The official journal of the NLN up to 1979 was *Nursing Outlook;* as of 1980, the official magazine became *Nursing and Health Care.*

International Council of Nurses (ICN)

The ICN was established in 1899. Nurses from both the United States and Canada were among the founding members. The council is a federation of national nurses' associations such as the ANA and CNA. In 1985, 97 national associations from different countries were affiliated with the ICN.

The purpose of the ICN is to provide a medium through which national nursing associations can work together and share common interests. Membership in the national association automatically makes a nurse a member of the ICN. The functions of the ICN are:

1. To promote the organization of national nurses' associations and advise them in their continued development.
2. To assist national nurses' associations to play their part in developing and improving health service for the public, the practice of nursing, and the social and economic welfare of nurses.

3. To provide means of communication among nurses throughout the world for mutual understanding and cooperation.
4. To establish and maintain liaison and cooperation with other international organizations and to serve as representatives and spokespeople of nurses at the international level.
5. To receive and manage funds and trusts that contribute to the advancement of nursing or for the benefit of nurses.
6. To do any other things incidental or conclusive to the attainment of the objective of the ICN (ICN 1973).

Special Interest Organizations

A number of nursing organizations in the United States and Canada are involved with special interests of the nurses.

Red Cross. The American Red Cross and the Canadian Red Cross are two of about 120 Red Cross, Red Crescent, Sun Societies, and Red Lion organizations around the world. The original Red Cross organization was founded by Jean-Henri Dunant in 1859. He organized a group of volunteers who worked to help the injured on the battlefield of Solferino in Italy. His work was nonpartisan, and both sides were helped by his group.

Nurses in the American Red Cross pioneered public health nursing in the United States. By 1930, however, most states had their own public health nursing services. At that time, the Red Cross extended its functions in the United States and Canada by establishing home nursing courses, organizing volunteers to assist in hospitals and nursing homes, and organizing disaster nursing and blood programs. Nursing students can volunteer their services to help the Red Cross perform many of these activities.

Alumni Associations. The major purpose of alumni associations is to foster the high ideals of the nursing program from which the nurses graduated. Alumni associations offer an opportunity for nurses to socialize, participate in educational programs, and raise funds for nursing students.

Other Nursing Organizations. During the past 15 years, a number of specialty organizations have formed to meet the needs of groups of nurses. A few of these organizations are the Association of Operating Room Nurses, the National Association of Pediatric Nurse Associates/Practitioners, the American Association of Nurse Anesthetists, the Canadian Orthopaedic Nurses' Association, and American Association of Nephrology Nursing.

World Health Organization (WHO). WHO is one of the special agencies of the United Nations. It is an intergovernmental agency, formed in 1948, whose primary aim is to help all people in the world achieve the highest possible level of health. Its major activities are to provide assistance to countries by improving health standards, education, and training; fighting disease; combating water pollution; and undertaking special projects as needs arise.

Nurses make an essential contribution to the activities of WHO. American and Canadian nurses are frequently asked to go to countries that require assistance in nursing education and public health. About 300 nurses presently work for WHO in countries other than their own.

Chapter Highlights

- Florence Nightingale may be thought of as nursing's first nurse theorist, since she emphasized such independent nursing functions as preventive health care, humanistic care, comfort, and support of the client.
- There are many definitions and descriptions of nursing, but the essence of nursing is caring for and caring about people as holistic beings in matters related to health promotion, health maintenance, health restoration, and dying.
- A desired goal of nursing is professionalism, which necessitates a unique body of knowledge, delineation of specific skills and competencies, autonomous regulation, enforcement of standards of education and practice, attention to the social and general welfare of nurses, formulation of a code of ethics, and an attitude of concern about society as a whole.
- Conceptual models and theories of nursing are essential in clarifying exactly how the nurse's role differs from the roles of other health professionals.
- Nurses use the nursing process to put a conceptual model of nursing into practice.
- Although the majority of nurses today are employed in hospital settings, more nurses are working in other areas, such as home health care and community clinics.
- Nursing practice acts vary among states and provinces, and nurses must be aware of the act governing their practice.
- Standards of nursing practice provide criteria against which the effectiveness of nursing care can be evaluated.
- The career mobility of nurses increases with their education.
- Nurses are fulfilling expanded nursing roles, for instance, those of the nurse practitioner, the clinical nursing specialist, the nurse clinician, and the nurse anesthetist, which allow greater independence and autonomy.
- Educational programs for nurses must reflect the health care demands and needs of a changing society, accommodate changes in the health care delivery system, and adhere to professional standards, yet be responsive to concerns about rising costs of health care.
- Flexibility in nursing curricula and innovation in implementing curricula are needed to upgrade the educational achievement of nursing graduates from programs below the baccalaureate degree level.
- Both professional and nonprofessional nursing organizations and associations fulfill essential functions

for the nursing profession and for individual nurses. Participation in the activities of nursing associations enhances the growth of involved individuals and helps nurses collectively influence policies affecting nursing practice.

Selected References

Aiken, L. H. American Academy of Nursing (ed.). 1982. *Nursing in the 1980s: Crises, opportunities, challenges.* Philadelphia: J. B. Lippincott Co.

American Nurses' Association. December 1965. American Nurses' Association first position on education for nursing. *American Journal of Nursing* 65:106–11.

———. 1973. *Standards of nursing practice.* Kansas City, Mo.: American Nurses' Association.

———. April 1979. Credentialing in nursing: A new approach. Report of the Committee for the Study of Credentials in Nursing. *American Journal of Nursing* 79:674–83.

———. 1980. *Nursing: A social policy statement.* Kansas City, Mo.: American Nurses' Association.

———. 1981a. *Facts about nursing 80–81.* New York: American Journal of Nursing Co.

———. 1981b. *The nursing practice act: Suggested state legislation.* Kansas City, Mo.: American Nurses' Association.

———. 1987. *Facts about nursing 86–87.* Kansas City, Mo.: American Nurses' Association.

———. 1987. *Proceedings of the 1987 house of delegates.* Kansas City, Mo.: American Nurses' Association.

American Nurses' Association Cabinet on Nursing Services. 1984. *Career ladders: An approach to professional productivity.* Kansas City, Mo.: American Nurses' Association.

Austin, J. K., and Champion, V. L. 1983. King's theory for nursing: Explication and evaluation. In Chinn, P. L., editor. *Advances in nursing theory development.* Rockville, Md.: Aspen Systems.

Barritt, E. R. 1973. Florence Nightingale's values and modern nursing education. *Nursing Forum* 12(1):6–47.

Benner, P. 1984. *From novice to expert: Excellence and power in clinical nursing practice.* Menlo Park, Calif.: Addison-Wesley Publishing Co.

Brill, C., and Hill, L. May 1985. Giving the help that goes on giving. *Nursing 85* 15:44–47.

Canadian Nurses' Association. 1980. *A definition of nursing practice: Standards for nursing practice.* Ottawa: Canadian Nurses' Association.

Check, J. F., and Wurzbach, M. E. January/February 1984. How elders view nursing. *Geriatric Nursing* 5:37–39.

Chinn, P. L., and Jacobs, M. K. 1983. *Theory and nursing: A systematic approach.* St. Louis: C. V. Mosby Co.

DeYoung, L. 1985. *Dynamics of nursing.* 5th ed. St. Louis: C. V. Mosby Co.

Diers, D. March 1986. To profess—To be a professional. *Journal of Nursing Administration* 16(3):25–30.

Dugas, B. W. May 1985. Baccalaureate for entry to practice: A challenge that universities must meet. *The Canadian Nurse* 81:17–19.

Europa Year Book. 1985. Vol. 1. International Organizations. London: Europa Publications.

Fawcett, J. 1984. *Analysis and evaluation of conceptual models of nursing.* Philadelphia: F. A. Davis Co.

George, J. B., editor. 1985. *Nursing theories: The base for professional nursing practice.* 2d ed. Englewood Cliffs, N.J.: Prentice-Hall.

Gortner, S. R. July/August 1980. Nursing research: Out of the past and into the future. *Nursing Research* 29:204–7.

King, I. M. 1981. *A theory for nursing: Systems, concepts, process.* New York: John Wiley and Sons.

Hall, L. November 1963. A center for nursing. *Nursing Outlook* 11:805–6.

Henderson, V. 1966. *The nature of nursing: A definition and its implications for practice, research, and education.* New York: Macmillan Co.

Hood, G. May 1985. At issue: Titling and licensure. *American Journal of Nursing* 85:592, 594.

International Council of Nurses 1973. *Constitution and regulations.* Geneva: International Council of Nurses.

Johnson, D. E. 1980. The behavioral system model for nursing. In Riehl, J. P., and Roy, C. Conceptual models for nursing practice. 2d ed. New York: Appleton-Century-Crofts.

Kerr, J. May 1985. Taking the campus to the student. *The Canadian Nurse* 81:30–31.

Kinney, C. D. May/June 1985. A reexamination of nursing role conceptions. *Nursing Research* 34(3): 170–76.

Lambertson, E. 1953. *Nursing team organization and functioning.* New York: Teachers College Press.

LaSor, B., and Elliott, M. R. 1977. *Issues in Canadian nursing.* Scarborough, Ontario: Prentice-Hall of Canada.

Leddy, S., and Pepper, J. M. 1985. *Conceptual bases of professional nursing.* Philadelphia: J. B. Lippincott Co.

Leininger, M. 1984. *Care: The essence of nursing and health.* Thorofare, N.J.: Charles B. Slack.

Levine, M. 1973. *Introduction to clinical nursing.* 2d ed. Philadelphia: F. A. Davis Co.

Lewis, E. P. September/October 1983. News outlook: The issue that won't go away. A report on the 1983 NLN convention. *Nursing Outlook* 31:246–47.

———. September/October 1985. Taking care of business: The ANA House of Delegates. *Nursing Outlook* 33:239–43.

Marram, G.; Barrett, M. W.; and Bevis, E. O. 1979. *Primary nursing: A model for individualized care.* 2d ed. St. Louis: C. V. Mosby Co.

Marriner, A. 1986. *Nursing theorists and their work.* St. Louis: C. V. Mosby Co.

McBride, A. B. September/October 1985. Orchestrating a career. *Nursing Outlook* 33:244–47.

Merton, R. K. January 1958. The function of the professional organization. *American Journal of Nursing* 58:50–54.

Miller, B. K. April 1985. Just what is a profession? *Nursing Success To-day* 2:21–27.

Montag, M. L. April 1980. Looking back: Associate degree education in perspective. *Nursing Outlook* 28:248-50.

National Commission on Nursing: Summary report and recommendations. July 1983. American Hospital Association. Chicago: The Hospital Research and Educational Trust, and American Hospital Supply Corporation.

National League for Nursing. March/April 1975. 1974 Annual Report. *NLN News* 23:3.

———. 1978a. *Characteristics of graduate education in nursing leading to the master's degree.* New York: The League.

———. 1978b. *Competencies of the associate degree nurse on entry into practice.* New York: The League.

———. 1978c. *Roles and competencies of graduates of diploma programs in nursing.* New York: The League.

———. 1979. *Characteristics of baccalaureate education in nursing.* New York: The League.

———. 1985. *Getting the pieces to fit 85/86: A handbook for state associations and school chapters.* New York: National Student Nurses' Association.

Neuman, B. 1982. *The Neuman systems model: Application to nursing education and practice.* New York: Appleton-Century-Crofts.

Nightingale, F. 1860. *Notes on nursing: What it is, and what it is not.* London: Harrison. Reprinted in Bishop, F. L. A., and Goldie, S. 1962. *A bio-bibliography of Florence Nightingale.* London: Dawsons of Pall Mall.

Notter, L. E., and Spalding, E. K. 1976. *Professional nursing: Foundations, perspectives, and relationships.* 9th ed. New York: J. B. Lippincott Co.

Orem, D. E. 1985. *Nursing: Concepts of practice.* 3d ed. New York: McGraw-Hill.

Palmer, I. S. June 1981. Florence Nightingale and international origins of modern nursing. *Image* 8:28–31.

Phaneuf, M. C., and Lang, M. 1985. *Issues in professional nursing practice 7: Standards of nursing practice.* Kansas City, Mo.: American Nurses' Association.

Poulin, M. A. 1985. *Issues in professional nursing practice 5. Configurations of nursing practice.* Kansas City, Mo.: American Nurses' Association.

Primm, P. L. May/June 1986. Entry into practice: Competency statements for BSNs and ADNs. *Nursing Outlook* 34:135–37.

Reiter, F. February 1966. The nurse-clinician. *American Journal of Nursing* 66:274–80.

Riehl, J. P., and Roy, C. 1980. *Conceptual models for nursing practice.* 2d ed. New York: Appleton-Century-Crofts.

Rogers, M. E. 1970. *An introduction to the theoretical basis of nursing.* Philadelphia: F. A. Davis Co.

———. 1980. Nursing: A science of unitary man. In Riehl, J. P., and Roy, C. *Conceptual models for nursing practice.* 2d ed. New York: Appleton-Century-Crofts.

Roy, C. 1976. *Introduction to nursing: An adaptation model.* Englewood Cliffs, N.J.: Prentice-Hall.

———. 1984. *Introduction to nursing: An adaptation model.* 2d ed. Englewood Cliffs, N.J.: Prentice-Hall.

Segal, E. T. June 1985. Is nursing a profession? Yes no. *Nursing 85* 15:40–43.

Snyder, M. E., and LaBar, C. 1984. *Issues in professional nursing practice 1. Nursing: Legal authority to practice.* Kansas City, Mo.: American Nurses' Association.

Storch, J. L. January 1986. In defense of nursing theory. *The Canadian Nurse* 82:16–20.

Stull, M. K. May/June 1986. Entry skills for BSNs. *Nursing Outlook* 34:138, 153.

Styles, M. M. November 1983. The anatomy of a profession. *Heart and Lung* 12:570–75.

Sultz, H. A.; Henry, O. M.; Bullough, B.; Buck, G. M.; and Kinyor, L. J. September/October 1983. Nurse practitioners: A decade of change. Part 3. *Nursing Outlook* 31:266–69.

CHAPTER 2

Changing Nursing Practice

OBJECTIVES

Describe the change process.

Explain the importance of selected historical aspects of nursing.

Identify factors currently influencing nursing practice.

Describe current professional and economic issues in nursing.

Explain the significance of the broadening focus of nursing practice.

Describe the role of research in influencing current and future nursing practice.

List some of the implications for nursing in an increasingly technical society.

Explain why nurses need to be politically active.

Describe the guiding principles of political action.

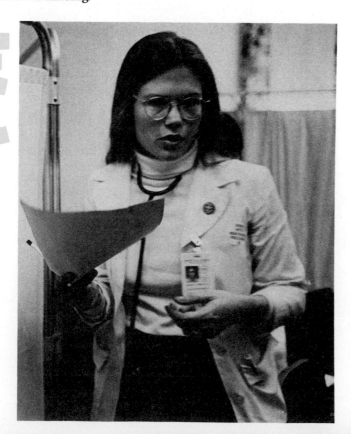

In Chapter 1, we discussed what nursing is and what nurses do. It is not useful, however, to confine ourselves to static definitions. Nurses practice in a changing environment and thus must change with it. This chapter examines the factors and trends that influence nursing practice and require nurses to change in response. It also explores how nurses control nursing practice and influence other facets of our society.

Change

To be effective and influential in today's world, nurses need to understand change theory and apply its precepts in the workplace, in government and professional organizations, and in the community. Planning and implementing change are professional responsibilities as well as largely unrealized power sources that are vital to the practice of nursing. Some synonyms for change are *alter, transform, modify, convert,* and *vary.* All these terms suggest that a fundamental difference or substitution is the outcome of change.

Steps in the Change Process

The following steps are a model of planned change. The model outlines the actions one must take to plan and control change and make it serve a specific purpose (Spradley 1980).

1. Identify symptoms that indicate something needs changing.
2. Diagnose the problem by reviewing the symptoms and gathering additional data.
3. Explore alternative solutions in terms of their risks, benefits, driving and restraining forces, advantages, disadvantages, and probable outcomes. (An effective technique often used by change agents is brainstorming.)
4. Select one course of action from among the identified alternatives.
5. Plan the steps in the change process:
   - Write measurable objectives.
   - Determine a timetable.
   - Plan a budget.
   - Recruit individuals to carry out each aspect of the plan.
   - Ensure ability of the change agents to work with the client system.
   - Evaluate resources (driving forces) and resistance (restraining forces) and plan strategies to manage both.
   - Design a plan to evaluate the outcomes of the change effort.
   - Identify measures to refreeze or establish the change within the client system.
6. Implement the change. (Pilot testing a new idea affords one the opportunity to evaluate it on a small scale and to "sell" it to the larger client system.)
7. Evaluate the outcome(s) on the basis of the measurable objectives and make appropriate adjustments.
8. Refreeze the client system so that the changes are seen as standard operating procedures and the system is once again stable.

Examples of Change

It is exciting to realize how effective nurses can be when they determine the need for change and plan strategies to bring it about. The following examples outline changes initiated by nurses who have identified a need to "do something" in each of four spheres of influence: the workplace, organizations, government, and the community.

The Workplace. At each of three shift meetings Mrs. Hawkins, Head Nurse, listened to nurses complain about problems with getting clients' laboratory work done and reported to the unit in a timely manner. She conferred with other head nurses and with the attending and resident physicians on her unit. It appeared that similar complaints were widespread.

At the next head nurse meeting, Mrs. Hawkins described the problem. The group appointed a task force, with Mrs. Hawkins as Chair, and asked it to present a plan to solve the problem at the next meeting. After gathering more data, the task force invited representatives from the attending and resident staff and the laboratory director to meet with them to review the data, consider alternative solutions, and select a plan to solve the problem.

By the next head nurse meeting, a preliminary plan to alter the system of laboratory reporting had been devised, and all concerned were working cooperatively to implement the plan.

The Professional Organization. Nurses on the Education Committee of a district nurses' association recognized the need to make a public policy statement concerning the care of clients with AIDS. Since the Board of Directors had recently expressed interest in promulgating such policy statements, the committee sensed the timing was right and that the board would welcome its draft despite the controversial subject matter.

Members of the committee researched and drafted a statement. The full committee offered a critique and selected an articulate spokesperson to present the statement to the association president and seek support before asking to have the statement presented to the board. Once the president had approved the statement, it was placed on the agenda for the next board meeting.

After making minor additions, the board approved it for distribution to the lay and nursing press and asked the Education Committee to suggest a nurse to present the statement at a local hearing of the City Council Health Committee.

The Government. While the pressure to contain health care costs escalated through the first half of the 1980s, a coalition representing the shared interests of the ANA, the NLN, and the American Association of

Colleges of Nursing (AACN) mounted a campaign to convince Congress of the cost-effectiveness of a center for nursing research within the National Institutes of Health (NIH). Despite incredible odds, including a presidential veto and opposition from the American Medical Association, the American Association of Medical Colleges, and the NIH administrations, the proposal was passed by Congress in the fall of 1985. The success of this effort demonstrates the effectiveness of carefully planned change including the collaboration of nursing organizations. It also illustrates the clout organized nurses can wield on any level and in any sphere.

▪ The Community.

Every nurse plays several roles besides that of registered nurse. Each resides in a community, and many are parents. Some serve on school boards, belong to the League of Women Voters, or participate in religious, club, or scouting activities. There are numerous opportunities for nurses to contribute to the health and welfare of the communities in which they live. A group of nursing students recognized a health problem within their community and developed a plan to intervene. Many of the students were parents of children in local elementary schools where a high percentage of children were being sent home daily with head lice. Because of previously enacted budget cuts, the district's school nurses were each responsible for between three and five schools. The students volunteered to work with the district nurses to provide screening and health teaching at each of the elementary schools, thereby helping to resolve the community's problem.

All nurses are affected by change; nobody can avoid it. Knowledgeable nurses make rational plans to deal with both opportunities to initiate and guide needed change as well as to respond to change that affects them in the workplace, government, organizations, and the community. To recognize these opportunities for change and respond to the factors that influence nursing from without, it is helpful to consider the history of nursing, current trends in nursing, and present political, social, technological, and economic issues.

Factors Influencing Nursing Practice

To understand nursing as it is practiced today and as it will be practiced tomorrow requires not only a historic perspective of nursing's evolution but also an understanding of some of the social forces presently influencing this profession. These forces usually affect the entire health care system, and nursing, as a major component of that system, cannot avoid the effects.

▪ Historical Development

Nursing as an activity that provides help to those in need has existed since the earliest times. Before the early Christian period (1–500 A.D.), caring for the sick was a function women performed in their homes. Later, religious orders provided nursing functions as part of their activities. The first nursing order, the Augustinian Sisters, was established in the Middle Ages.

Prior to the Protestant Reformation in the sixteenth century, hospital facilities were organized chiefly by the Roman Catholic Church. With the Reformation, beginning in 1517, came a decline in people's interest in and support of the church and religion. This change introduced an era known in nursing history as the "dark period." Hospitals were unsanitary places, dark and foreboding. Nursing was provided by women who were frequently described as drunk, heartless, and immoral. They were expected to carry out the housework of the hospital, launder clothes and bed linens, and do all the cleaning for very little reward. No training was required of nurses, and it was not unusual for a nurse to work from 12 to 40 consecutive hours. This period of decline lasted until the middle of the nineteenth century.

The era of reform in nursing is marked by the work of the British nurse, Florence Nightingale, during the Crimean War (1854–56). Nightingale's efforts made nursing a respectable vocation once again. However, her reform activities did not stop at respectability. Besides crusading for cleanliness and comfort in hospitals, Nightingale also worked toward educating people about health measures to combat the widespread presence of diseases in the cities.

Florence Nightingale believed in prevention of illness and in nursing the whole person, calling upon her fellow nurses to make sure that patients always had fresh air, good water, proper medication, quiet, mobility, and knowledge of how to care for themselves in the future. Many of Nightingale's ideas are now standards of client care. Education of nurses was one of her major goals. Among her many accomplishments was the establishment of the Nightingale School of Nurses at St. Thomas' Hospital, London, in 1860. This school is credited with providing the first planned educational program for nurses. Florence Nightingale also assisted in establishing the first organized home nursing services.

In North America, establishment of nursing and health services was slow prior to the American Revolution (1775–83). One notable organization was the Nurse Society of Philadelphia, which gave women minimal instruction in obstetrics to enable them to provide maternity nursing services in home settings. It was not until the late 1800s that a time of rapid reform of nursing services occurred in the United States and Canada. Schools of nursing with planned educational programs were started. A number of their graduates became the early leaders in the profession.

Two early graduates of the New York Hospital, Lillian D. Wald and Mary Brewster, were the first to offer trained nursing services to the poor in the New York slums. Their home among the poor on the upper floor of a tenement is now famous as a center of public health nursing (the Henry Street Settlement). Soon after, school nursing was established as an adjunct to visiting nursing. Again Wald was involved, along with Lina L. Rogers.

Linda Richards, who graduated in 1873 from the New England Hospital for Women and Children Training School for Nurses in Boston, is cited by many historians

We must nurture a sense of commitment

If nursing is to prosper, and nurses are to become leaders in the emerging health care delivery systems, three developments must be encouraged. All are possible because all exist, although in muted form, today.

First, the profession must recover and nurture a sense of commitment among its members. The knowledge nurses amass and the skills they acquire are more a public *trust* than a private acquisition to be prized and sold on the open market. Opportunities for financial gain and personal advancement in a profession flourish only in the context of the valuable services the profession provides to the public; and the utility and advance of the profession depend upon individual members who have some sense of professional identity, commitment and responsibility. When the professional bond is weak and each practitioner things of himself or herself only as an entrepreneur—uninvested with a public and professional *trust*—the profession is wounded, perhaps mortally.

Second, members of the nursing profession must become far more aware of their responsibilities to one another. Nurses must recognize more fully than they have before their duty to support, nurture, guide and correct one another. Cooperation and mutual growth must be accepted as the norm in professional relationships—not competition, one-upmanship or acquisition of power. Practically speaking, one's own success depends largely upon the knowledge and skill of one's colleagues as well as upon their willingness to share information and insight and to engage in constructive criticism. The collegial relationship is the one, vital, living factor that is completely within the control of nurses.

Third, nurses must address the systems, institutions and structures that shape the environment in which they practice. Advancing technology, shrinking resources and the rapid reorganization of services they engender demand that nurses collaborate with others in the design and development of new systems of care.

L. L. Curtin: A professional and public trust . . . , (Editorial Opinion), *Nursing Management,* November 1986, 17(11): 7–11

---

as America's first trained nurse (Jamieson et al. 1966, p. 224). She is credited with initiating nursing reforms in 12 major hospitals, some of which were specialized mental hospitals. She began training schools for students in mental health nursing. Her programs included a period of training in general hospitals. She also founded the first training school for nurses in Japan.

Some, however, dispute that Richards was the first trained nurse. Evidence in a series of reports of Women's Hospital of Philadelphia suggests that Harriet Newton Phillips was the first trained nurse to receive a certificate from that hospital in 1864 (Large 1976, p. 50). Phillips is also considered the first trained nurse in America to provide community nursing, to do missionary service, and to take postgraduate training. America's first trained black nurse was Mary Mahoney. She also trained at the New England Hospital for Women and Children, graduating in 1879 (Notter and Spalding 1976, p. 15).

Isabel Hampton Robb had been a young schoolteacher in Canada. She decided to change her profession and entered the Bellevue Hospital Training School in New York. After graduation, she nursed in Rome for 2 years, and then she became superintendent of the Illinois Training School at 26 years of age. Three years later she went to Baltimore to organize a new school in connection with Johns Hopkins Hospital. Among her many accomplishments was a nursing textbook, which became the standard text for nursing schools in America.

Mary Adelaide Nutting, also from Canada, was in the first class at Johns Hopkins. After graduation, she established a course of training for students prior to ward experience at Johns Hopkins. Later, she reduced the nursing students' daily work hours from 12 to 8 and lengthened the periord of nurses' training to 3 years.

Mary Agnes Snively graduated from Bellevue and returned to Canada to take charge of the nurses' training at Toronto General Hospital. She is largely credited with directing Canadian nursing education. Among her accomplishments was being the first president of the Canadian Nurses' Association.

During the late 1800s, the need for concerted action by nurses was felt first in England and soon afterward in America. In 1894, the Matrons' Council of Great Britain and Ireland was organized, followed by the American Society of Superintendents of Training Schools for Nurses of the United States and Canada. Alumnae associations joined to form the Nurses' Associated Alumnae of the United States and Canada in 1897. In 1908, the National Association of Colored Graduate Nurses was founded by a group of nurses who felt such an association could further not only the nursing cause but also their own special interests.

Current professional and related groups grew from these early nursing organizations. The Nurses' Associated Alumnae became the American Nurses' Association in 1911. The Society of Superintendents divided nationally and ultimately became the Canadian National Association of Trained Nurses in 1908 (now the Canadian Nurses' Association) and the National League of Nursing Education in 1912 (now the National League for Nursing).

After World War I, the Frontier Nursing Service (FNS) was established by a notable pioneer nurse, Mary Breckinridge. In 1918, she worked with the American Committee for Devastated France, distributing food, clothing, and supplies to rural villages in France and taking care of sick children. In 1921, Breckinridge returned to the United States with plans to provide health care to the people of rural America. She initially prepared herself by taking courses at Teachers College in New York and midwifery training in London, and by developing prominent social contacts for fundraising. Within the FNS, Breckinridge began one of the first midwifery training schools in the United States.

The general trend from the beginning of formal organization (the late 1800s) to the end of World War I was rapid expansion in the establishment of hospitals, with nursing schools dependent upon them for support. Hospitals in turn depended on the schools to carry the chief nursing load. During World War I, greater numbers of young women were accepted for entrance and less consideration was given to selection requirements. Most schools by this time had adopted 3-year programs, but the 8-hour day originally proposed with those programs was less quickly adopted.

By 1920, the hospital system of educating nurses was beginning to be criticized. The effectiveness of the nurse as a teacher of nurses was also being questioned. Therefore, Teachers College of Columbia University in New York City offered a special postbasic course to prepare nurses as teachers. Preparations for a postbasic public health nursing program were also made in response to an influenza epidemic and the development of broader aims by the medical profession. These aims now included teaching the principles of healthful living to individuals, families, and community groups.

During the early 1920s, the Rockefeller Survey (Committee for the Study of Nursing Education) recommended that nursing schools be independent of hospitals and on a college level. As a result, two university schools of nursing were set up, one at Yale University, New Haven, Connecticut, and the other at Western Reserve University, Cleveland, Ohio. The purpose of these experimental schools was to prove the feasibility of planning both classroom instruction and ward practice in accordance with the educational needs of the students. Emphasis was placed on the social welfare and health aspects of nursing.

Another far-reaching result of the Rockefeller Survey was a proposal by the National League of Nursing Education to undertake a comprehensive study of nursing education (1926–34) that would lead to the grading of nursing schools. It was believed that grading would establish standards for education in these schools. This was the beginning of the accreditation function that the National League for Nursing now carries out.

During this period between the two world wars, the concept of the clinical nurse specialist arose. In 1933, the need for "experts in the nursing art and specialists in the clinical branches they represent" was recognized (Stewart 1933, p. 363). This concept, currently seen by many as a new role in nursing, was discussed by nursing leaders in the 1930s and 1940s.

In the early 1940s, it was thought that more emphasis needed to be placed on the clinical specialties in the advanced professional curricula of colleges and universities. The goal of most advanced nursing curricula was to prepare specialists in nursing school administration, teaching, and supervision; in public health; and in hospital administration. Clinical specialties were not emphasized. These specialties gained prominence in the postwar society. Nurses returning from overseas were required to work in clinical areas not familiar to them. One such area was psychiatric nursing, which helped individuals readjust to civilian life. By 1946, many nursing programs in the United States were providing more clinical content in specialty areas.

From its early days to the present, nursing has undergone change in every area. Rapid strides have been made in nursing education programs and in a wide variety of hospital and community nursing services. In spite of these changes, the nursing profession has been characterized by continuity and stability in helping people.

▌Current Influences

It is difficult to escape the influences of society, science, and technology upon nursing. Many factors influence the individual nurse, nursing practice, and, of course, clients. To function effectively in the face of information overload, rapid systems of communication, and advances in research, nurses must develop new practice models. The current major influences can be grouped into nine broad areas: consumer demands, family structure, economics, science and technology, legislation, demography, the women's movement, collective bargaining, and the nursing profession itself.

▌ Consumer Demands.
Consumers of nursing services (the public) have become an increasingly effective force in changing nursing practice. On the whole, people are better educated and have more knowledge about health and illness than in the past. Consumers also have become more aware of others' needs for care. The ethical and moral issues raised by poverty and neglect have made people more vocal about the needs of minority groups and the poor.

The public's concepts of health and nursing have also changed. Most now believe that health is a right of all people, not just a privilege of the rich. The media emphasize the message that individuals must assume responsibility for their own health by obtaining a physical examination regularly, checking for the seven danger signals of cancer, and maintaining their mental well-being by balancing work and recreation. Interest in health and nursing services is therefore greater than ever. Furthermore, many people now want more than freedom from disease—they want energy, vitality, and a feeling of wellness.

Increasingly, the consumer has become an active participant in making decisions about health and nursing care. Planning committees concerned with providing nursing services to a community usually have active consumer membership. Recognizing the legitimacy of public input, many state and provincial nursing associations and regulatory agencies have consumer representatives on their governing boards.

▌ Family Structure.
The need for and provision of nursing services are being influenced by new family structures. An increasing number of people are living

away from the extended family and the nuclear family, and the family breadwinner is no longer necessarily the husband. An extended family consists of parents, children, grandparents, and sometimes aunts and uncles; a nuclear family consists only of parents and their children.

Today, many single men and women rear children, and in many two-parent families both parents work. It is also common for young parents to live at great distances from their own parents. These young families need support services such as day-care centers. Many such families do not have grandparents or other relatives readily available to help in times of illness or to offer advice about childbearing and child health. These parents usually get this advice from physicians and nurses as well as others. Similarly, grandparents who live alone and far from other members of the family require homemaker and visiting nurse services when they are ill since they cannot receive this care from younger members of the family.

Adolescent mothers also need specialized nursing services. These young mothers have the normal needs of teenagers as well as those of new mothers. In 1960, 13.9% of all births were to teenage mothers; this percentage has increased steadily despite the fact that an increasing number of women are choosing to delay motherhood. Many teenage mothers are raising their children alone. This type of single-parent family is especially vulnerable because motherhood compounds the difficulties of adolescence.

■ **Economics.** Another factor that has increased the demand and need for nursing care is the greater financial support provided through public and private health insurance programs. Health services such as emergency room care, mental health counseling, and preventive physical examinations are increasingly being used by people who could not afford them in the past. Federal governments recognized this need and markedly increased their budgets for health care in the 1970s and early 1980s. This increase in expenditure is accompanied by increased employment opportunities for those who provide health services.

Costs of health care have also increased during this period as well. In response to these increasing costs, the Medicare payment system to hospitals was revised in 1982, establishing fees according to diagnostic related groups (DRGs). With the implementation of this legislation, a greater proportion of clients in hospitals are more acutely ill than before, and clients once considered sufficiently ill to be hospitalized are now treated at home.

These changes in acuity present challenges to nurses. Currently, the health care industry is shifting its emphasis from inpatients to outpatients with preadmission testing, posthospitalization rehabilitation, home health care, health maintenance, and physical fitness (Powell 1984, p. 33). Nurses need to identify how their knowledge and skills can fit into these settings. Rogers (1985, p. 10) suggests that before long a large majority of nurses will not work in hospitals. This change in the area of employment has implications for nursing education, nursing research, and nursing practice.

■ **Science and Technology.** Advances in science and technology affect nursing practice. For example, widespread immunization for poliomyelitis decreased the morbidity of that disease and the need for specialized nursing care. As physicians expand their knowledge base and technical skills, nurses acquire complementary knowledge and skills as they adapt to meet the new needs of clients.

In some settings, technologic advances have required that nurses become highly specialized. Nurses frequently have to use sophisticated computerized equipment to monitor or treat clients. As technologies change, nursing education changes, and nurses require increasing education to provide effective, safe nursing practice.

Advances in technology are exemplified by the many machines now used to help clients maintain life. There seems to be no end to the discoveries and the knowledge explosion of the twentieth century. With this knowledge explosion has come the charge that medical services—and some health professionals—have become dehumanized. Yet an increasing understanding of the psychologic, emotional, and spiritual aspects of care has developed to balance the technologic advances. As science and technology create methods of treating disease, it is the responsibility of all health professionals, and nurses in particular, to remember that clients are human beings requiring warmth, care, and acknowledgment of self-worth. Often equipment is frightening to clients and their support persons. Medical vocabulary appears mysterious and is frequently misunderstood. The nurse who deals with clients daily is in an ideal situation to humanize technology as much as possible. To humanize highly technical care, nurses can offer explanations, communicate their support, and recognize the clients' needs to understand and to be supported. This is the "high touch" aspect of a "high tech" environment.

Problems created by technologic change present new challenges to nurses. For example, some industries are hazardous to employees because of dangerous equipment or harmful chemical residues. Trauma (injury) and disease are frequently the direct result of advanced technology; the classic example is automobile accidents, which are among the top five causes of death in North America. In addition, our society frequently creates high levels of stress, which does not promote mental health.

◼ Legislation.

Legislation about nursing practice and health matters affects both the public and nursing. Legislation related to nursing is discussed in Chapter 6. Changes in legislation affecting health also affect nursing. For example, relaxation of laws governing abortions has been associated with reduced maternal morbidity from self-induced abortions.

Legislation regarding the Medicare payment system according to DRGs has had an enormous influence on nursing practice in hospitals and communities. Many clients leave hospitals sooner than they did in the past. As a result, more clients in hospitals are seriously ill, and more clients at home require more complex nursing care than in the past. Although this trend has contributed to a shortage of nurses in acute care settings, it has opened new opportunities for nurses in home health care.

◼ Demography.

Demography is the study of population including statistics about distribution by age and place of residence, **mortality** (death), and **morbidity** (incidence of disease). From demographic data, needs of the population for nursing services can be assessed. For example:

1. The total population in North America has increased since 1900. The proportion of elderly people has also increased, creating an increased need for nursing services for this group.
2. The population is shifting from rural to urban settings. This shift signals increased needs for nursing related to problems caused by pollution and by the effects on the environment of concentrations of people. Thus, most nursing services are now provided in urban settings.
3. Mortality and morbidity studies reveal the presence of "risk factors." Many of these "risk factors," e.g., smoking, are major causes of death and disease that can be prevented through changes in life-style. The nurse's role in assessing risk factors and helping clients to make healthy life-style changes is discussed in Chapter 25.

◼ The Women's Movement.

The women's movement has brought public attention to human rights. Persons are seeking equality in all areas, particularly educational, political, economic, and social equality. Because the majority of nurses are women, this movement has altered the perspectives of nurses about economic and educational needs. As a result, nurses are increasingly asserting themselves as professional people who have a right to equality with men in health professions, and nurses are demanding more autonomy in client care.

The increasing number of women physicians might also affect nursing practice. Women physicians may be less autocratic and more collegial in their professional relationships. As a result, nurses may find support in their quest for autonomy.

◼ Collective Bargaining.

More nurses are using collective bargaining to deal with their concerns. The ANA has participated in collective bargaining for more than 40 years through its economic and general welfare programs on behalf of nurses. Today, some nurses are joining other labor organizations that represent them at the bargaining table. In both the United States and Canada, nurses have gone on strike over certain demands and concerns. Often these concerns go beyond economic reward to issues about safe care for clients. Increasingly, nurses are becoming aware of the strength of organized, large numbers. DeCrosta (1985, p. 20) believes that nurses will increasingly look to unions as they attempt to resist staff cuts and perceived dilution of the quality of nursing care.

◼ The Nursing Profession.

Professional nursing associations have provided leadership that affects many areas of nursing. Voluntary accreditation of nursing education programs by the NLN and by mandatory accreditation licensing boards in each state have also influenced nursing. Many programs have steadily improved to meet the standards for accreditation over the years. As a result, nurse graduates are better prepared to meet the demands of society.

In 1979, the ANA published findings of a committee on credentialing, which recommended the establishment of a center for credentialing in nursing (ANA 1979, p. 682). **Credentialing** is the process of determining and maintaining competence in nursing. The credentialing of expanded nursing roles, such as that of the nurse practitioner, is carried out by the ANA and certain nursing specialty organizations, such as the American Association of Critical-Care Nurses.

To influence health care policy-making, a group of professional nurses organized formally to take political action in the nursing and health care arenas. Nurses for Political Action (NPA) was formed in 1971 and became an arm of the ANA in 1974, when its name changed to Nurses Coalition for Action in Politics (N-CAP). In 1986, the name was changed to ANA-PAC. Through this group, nurses have lobbied actively for legislation affecting health care. A number of nursing leaders hold positions of authority in government. Attaining such positions is essential if nurses hope to exert ongoing political influence.

The drive for increased autonomy comes from the nursing profession itself. During the past 20 years, the increased autonomy of nurses has been evidenced by their function in specialty care units, such as intensive care units, and in their expanded roles, such as that of the nurse practitioner. Many states have rewritten their nurse practice acts to reflect such changes in nursing practice.

Nursing Education

Although current scientific, social, and economic influences may affect the utilization of nursing services, they do not determine nursing practice. Nursing is controlled from within the profession itself. The future of nursing lies not with the leaders of the past or present but rather with today's and tomorrow's nursing students. In recognition of this reality, the nursing profession is particularly interested in the educational preparation of nurses for the future.

Technical and Professional Levels of Practice

In 1985, the ANA House of Delegates proposed that two levels of nurses be delineated: technical and professional. The technical nurse is to be prepared in an associate degree program, and the professional nurse is to be prepared in a baccalaureate degree program. This proposal, if implemented by the state nursing associations, has many implications. One implication concerns "grandfathering" to protect those nurses already licensed to practice. Because at present both technical and professional nurses are licensed as registered nurses, there is substantial agreement about grandfathering those already licensed. But, even with a grandfather clause in place, many nurses fear that they will not be protected from discrimination when they compete with recent graduates for jobs.

Titling and Licensure. The designations *registered nurse* (RN) and *licensed practical* or *vocational nurse* (LPN, LVN) have been used since licensure laws were first enacted. In its 1985 proposal, the ANA endorsed that the professional nurse with a baccalaureate degree be licensed under the legal title *registered nurse* (RN) and that the technical nurse with an associate degree be licensed under the legal title *associate nurse* (AN). As a professional organization, however, the ANA cannot legislate these changes. It is the responsibility of each state to define the legal boundaries of nursing practice and to designate the titles to be used by those practioners who meet the individual state's criteria for licensure. Thus, if this proposal is to be accepted nationally, each state will need to implement its own changes. Such changes have major implications for diploma nurses and LPNs, because their status is not discussed in the proposal. In addition, this proposal means that new standardized examinations must be developed to test the two levels of competencies.

Economic Constraints. Stevens (1985, p. 124) states that "what is best for nursing may not coincide with what is best for society at large," and that "one can no longer assume that the *best* for society—at any price— is a feasible goal." Recognizing that no discipline has ever achieved professional status outside of the traditional academic institutions, Stevens (1985, pp. 125–26) points out that 4-year baccalaureate programs are more costly than 2-year programs, BSN graduates require higher salaries, and the financial resources of the health care industry are shrinking. For these reasons, the nursing profession must substantiate to the general public that the BSN nurse can deliver qualitatively different care from that provided by the ADN nurse. The 2-year associate degree program, however, can potentially effect cost savings that can offset the high cost of educating and hiring the BSN nurse. How the two roles can be redesigned to best complement each other is a question that needs to be answered. The 1987 ANA statement on the scope of practice (see Chapter 1) begins to answer this question and calls for further differentiation between the professional and technical practice of nursing (ANA 1987, pp. 76–79).

Types of Educational Preparation Required

In the future, more nurses will be needed in home and community settings as a result of the prospective payment system in hospitals. What education will best prepare nurses to meet these needs? Because of nurses' greater autonomy in these areas, some nurse educators think that at least a baccalaureate degree is necessary. Others believe that ADN nurses can implement plans of care that are developed by a BSN primary nurse.

Given the expanding knowledge and technologic bases of nursing, it may be expected that curricula will have to be scrutinized to remove extraneous content and to ensure appropriate clinical experiences that relate to the theoretical content presented. Some educators are calling for inclusion of computer courses in nursing programs as society becomes more computer dependent. Before the implementation of the Medicare prospective payment system, many nurses had little knowledge of health care and nursing care economics. Perlich (1986, p. 6) advocates that nursing school curricula be changed to reflect such realities as cost containment and accountability of productivity to educate future nurses as to their role in both influencing and implementing policies in this area.

Post-RN Baccalaureate and Master's Programs. The thrust to make the baccalaureate degree the minimum entry level for professional nursing practice has significantly increased the need for post-RN baccalaureate programs. Providing programs to meet these needs and demands is a challenge for universities, especially since the profile of returning nursing students indicates that most are married women in their 30s and 40s who have dependent children and hold either full-time or part-time jobs (Dugas 1985, p. 18). Universities must be flexible to plan and provide such programs for these adult learners. Some universities now offer courses in off-campus sites for post-RN baccalaureate and MSN students and use distance delivery tech-

niques such as teleconferencing and shipments of basic reference materials to remote areas (Kerr 1985, p. 30).

Specialization

Basic nursing education programs (see Chapter 1) are designed to develop nurses as generalists, not specialists in any aspect of nursing. Traditionally, educators and employers have perpetuated the idea that nurses should be generalists who can rotate among services and shifts with minimal preparation. Yet, with the technological advances affecting nursing practice over the past 10 years, the market demand for nurses with specialized knowledge and skills has grown significantly.

A *specialty* is a defined area of clinical practice that has a narrow in-depth focus. Some clinical specialties are occupational health nursing, emergency and operating room nursing, enterostomal therapy nursing, intravenous therapy nursing, infection control nursing, nephrology nursing, neurology nursing, nurse midwifery, critical care nursing, oncology nursing, and palliative care nursing.

There is a bewildering array of educational programs to prepare specialists. Aims, length, and content of the programs differ. Once prepared, the specialists are employed in a wide number of capacities and have a variety of job titles. There is a need for the national association to establish priorities for specialty development, program standards, credentialing mechanisms, and an accompanying need for employers to provide appropriate economic rewards for the performance of specialty services.

Trends in Nursing

A **trend** is a general direction or a prevailing tendency or inclination. Several trends are apparent in the nursing profession today. Some trends in nursing are subtle and emerge slowly, while others are obvious and seem to surface quickly. Not all trends complement one another; some may seem divergent, if not in conflict. Over time, some aspects of nursing will become prevailing trends, while others may be modified by social forces or disappear altogether. A number of trends are apparent today: the broadening focus of nursing practice, the increasingly scientific basis of nursing practice, the growth of nursing research, the increasing use of technology, and a heightened awareness of the need for "high touch" skills.

Broadening Focus

The focus of nursing has broadened from the care of the ill person (the patient) to the care of people in illness and health, and from care of only the patient to care of the client, the family or support persons, and, in some instances, the community. In the past, nursing, like medicine, was oriented toward disease and illness.

Today, there is increasing recognition of people's need for health care as distinct from illness care and of the nurse's independent functions in this area.

A holistic philosophy is evident in modern nursing care. Today's nurse deals with clients as emotional and social as well as physical beings. Care is directed not toward a particular health problem but toward the response of the total person, the health of the whole person. The broadened focus of care requires an integration of skills and concepts.

Another aspect of the broader nursing focus is the movement of nursing practice into the community. In a sense, this is a return to the beginnings of nursing, e.g., before it became a recognized occupation. Throughout much of this century, however, nurses worked only in institutions; increasingly, nursing services are provided in the community, often in homes and in clinics. These nursing activities not only assist those who are ill but also help those who are healthy to maintain or enhance their health.

Scientific Basis

In the past, nursing was largely either intuitive or relied on experience or observation, rather than on research. Through trial and error, the individual nurses discovered which measures would assist the client, and many nurses became highly skilled in providing care through experience. The past 20 years have brought an increased emphasis on nursing research and on the use of scientific data at the bedside.

Nursing research is more than just scientific investigations conducted by a person educated and credentialed as a nurse. It refers instead to research directed toward building a body of nursing knowledge about "human responses to actual or potential health problems" (ANA 1980, p. 9) and to the effects of nursing action on such human responses. The human responses of people may be reactions of individuals, groups, or families to actual health problems (e.g., the burden a family experiences when they must care for an elderly relative with senile dementia); and concerns of individuals and groups about potential health problems (such as accident prevention or stress management in an industrial setting). The purpose of nursing research is to improve health care while reflecting the traditional nursing perspective. In this perspective, the client is seen as a whole person, with physiologic, psychologic, social, cultural, and economic components.

In addition to reflecting concern for the whole person, a nursing perspective implies 24-hour-a-day responsibility. Thus, this perspective encompasses all of the factors in a client's environment, such as fatigue, noise, sensory deprivation, nutrition, and positioning, that might influence coping patterns. Diers (1979) enumerates three distinguishing properties of nursing research:

1. The final focus of nursing research must be on a difference that matters in improving client care.
2. Nursing research has the potential for contributing to theory development and the body of scientific

nursing knowledge.

3. A research problem is a nursing research problem when nurses have access to and control over phenomena being studied.

The examples in Table 2–1 suggest the diversity of subjects, topics, and settings of actual nursing studies. The sample of contemporary nursing studies in this table only begins to show the diversity of fascinating and ultimately valuable research projects being conducted in the field of nursing. Table 2–2 provides examples of reseach consistent with the priorities for nursing research suggested by the ANA.

Findings from nursing studies are being incorporated into textbooks such as this one, and clinical journals such as the *American Journal of Nursing, Heart and Lung,* and *Gerontological Nursing* are increasingly publishing the results of studies about nursing practice. Nursing journals such as *Advances in Nursing Science, Image,* the *Journal of Research in Nursing and Health, Nursing Research,* and the *Western Journal of Nursing Research* have editorial policies that stress science, research, and nursing scholarship and publish current research studies.

The *Cumulative Index to Nursing and Allied Health Literature,* the *International Nursing Index,* and the *Cumulative Medical Index* are excellent resources for locating research published on a topic or problem of interest. Computerized literature searches, such as Medline and MEDLARS, are available through many school libraries. They, too, help the student or researcher find relevant study reports. Since 1983, research on a variety of topics has been collected in yet another valuable resource, the *Annual Review of Nursing Research.*

It is unrealistic to expect each nurse to conduct a study in the clinical setting. Many constraints in clinical settings must be reckoned with before research can become a legitimate and comfortable activity. However, if nursing is to develop as a research-based practice, it is not unreasonable to expect that nurses:

1. Have some awareness of the process and language of research
2. Be sensitive to issues related to protecting the rights of human subjects
3. Participate in the identification of significant researchable problems
4. Be discriminating consumers of research findings

Bridging the research-practice gap, that is, bringing research into the clinical practice arena, is a key strategy in uniting the scholarly, scientific, and caring aspects of nursing in the future. Table 2–3 summarizes this position in the ANA's "Guidelines for the Investigative Function of Nurses" (1981a), which specify the generally expected research competencies of nurses with associate, bachelor's, master's, and doctoral degrees.

▪ Technology

Technology or mechanization is being applied in the health field extensively. Certain areas of a hospital, e.g., intensive care units and coronary care units, are

Table 2–1 Examples of Nursing Studies

Baker et al. (1983) reported on the use of therapeutic touch by nurses to increase the range of motion of joints and to decrease pain in persons with arthritis.

Baker et al. (1984) studied the effect of types of thermometer and length of time inserted on oral temperature measurements of afebrile subjects.

Baum (1984) studied the physiologic determinants of a clinically successful method of endotracheal suction.

Britten (1985) studied head nurses' perceptions of their role in a decentralized nursing department for her master's thesis at the University of Florida.

Choi-Lao (1981) measured the concentration of halothane anesthetic vapors in the operating environments of two hospitals in Canada by analyzing air samples using a gas chromatographic technique.

Dufault (1983) used observation, interviews, and case studies to conduct a descriptive, longitudinal field study that identified themes and patterns of hope in elderly cancer patients.

Fehring (1983) compared the effects of a particular relaxation technique with the effects of the same technique augmented with biofeedback on the symptoms of psychologic stress among healthy college students. Findings indicate that biofeedback-augmented relaxation was more effective in lowering psychologic stress symptoms.

Hutchinson (1984) reported on the strategies used by neonatal intensive care nurses to contend with the meaninglessness and horror that is often part of their everyday work and that is a critical cause of "burnout."

Itano et al. (1983) conducted a study in which they correlated factors such as locus of control, self-esteem, anxiety, client's understanding of the illness, client's perception of the severity of the symptoms, and client's perception of the nurse's care and concern plus several demographic factors to compliance to therapy among clients with cancer.

Martinson and Anderson (1983) studied the effects of applying different degrees of heat to the abdomens of unrestrained, unanesthetized dogs on skin surface, subcutaneous, intraperitoneal, intestinal, and colonic temperatures. Their findings indicate that a wide range of thermal applications to the abdominal skin of dogs changed skin surface and subcutaneous temperature but did not alter deep abdominal temperature.

Norbeck and Sheiner (1982) used a social support scale to identify sources of social support related to single-parent functioning.

Wilson (1982) used a method of qualitative analysis called "Discovering Grounded Theory" to explain how the presence of people can work effectively to control the behavior of unmedicated schizophrenics in an alternative healing community.

more technological than others. Nurses find themselves in the midst of this rapidly changing, increasingly technologic environment in hospitals and in clients' homes. Many feel they need more education to obtain the knowledge and skills necessary to use the new technology. Indicators of increasing technology are:

1. The proliferation of technologic equipment in hospitals and homes
2. The increasing costs of home and self-care equipment
3. The use of computers in many areas of health care

Table 2—2   ANA Guidelines for Nursing Research

Directions for Research	Examples
Priority should be given to nursing research that generates knowledge to guide practice in:	Examples of research consistent with these priorities include the following:
1. Promoting health, well-being, and competency for personal care among all age groups	1. Identification of determinants (personal and environmental, including social support networks) of wellness and health functioning in individuals and families, e.g., avoiding abusive behavior such as alcoholism and drug use, successfully adapting to chronic illness, and coping with the last days of life
2. Preventing health problems throughout the lifespan that have the potential to reduce productivity and satisfaction.	2. Identification of phenomena that negatively influence the course of recovery and that may be alleviated by nursing practice, for example, anorexia, diarrhea, sleep deprivation, deficiencies in nutrients, electrolyte imbalances, and infections
3. Decreasing the negative impact of health problems on coping abilities, productivity, and life satisfaction of individuals and families	3. Development and testing of care strategies to do the following: • Facilitate individuals' ability to adopt and maintain health-enhancing behaviors (e.g., exercise and alterations in diet) • Enhance clients' ability to manage acute and chronic illness so as to minimize or eliminate the necessity for institutionalization and to maximize well-being • Reduce stressful responses associated with the medical management of patients (e.g., surgical procedures, intrusive examination procedures, or extensive use of monitoring devices)
4. Ensuring that the care needs of particularly vulnerable groups are met through appropriate strategies	4. Enhance the care of clients culturally different from the majority (e.g., black Americans, Mexican Americans, native Americans) and clients with special problems (e.g., teenagers, prisoners, mentally ill), and the underserved (the elderly, poor, and the rural)
5. Designing and developing health care systems that are cost-effective in meeting the nursing needs of the population	5. Design and assess, in terms of effectiveness and cost, the models for delivering nursing care strategies found to be effective in clinical studies
6. Promoting health, well-being, and competency for personal health in all age groups	6. Provide more effective care to high-risk populations (e.g., maternal and child care service to vulnerable mothers and infants, family planning services to young teenagers, services designed to enhance self-care in the chronically ill and the very old)

Source: American Nurses' Association Commission on Nursing Research, *Priorities for the 1980s* (Kansas City, Mo.: American Nurses' Association, 1981). Reprinted with permission.

A good example is the computer, which was relatively new 10 years ago. Today, computers are used on most campuses and in many hospitals and health agencies to keep client records, record and analyze vital signs, regulate medications, diagnose and treat, and analyze laboratory data. Nurses need to be flexible and ready to learn how to operate increasingly complex equipment.

■ Computers in Nursing.   By the turn of the century, most nurses will use computers in many aspects of their professional practice. Already, "user-friendly" machines are of great help to the nurse in assessing, diagnosing, planning, implementing, and evaluating nursing care. The nurse educator and the nurse manager have also discovered the usefulness of computers in managing staffing, budgeting, producing grade reports, writing papers, and improving productivity. In fact, computer skills and knowledge will soon be expected and perhaps required for a great many positions. Those who ignore this technologic revolution may be left behind.

The nurse is clearly the manager of client care. Hospital information flows to and through nursing departments. Nurses who allow computer systems to design their practice may find themselves both frustrated and victimized. Instead, they must take an active role in the design, development, and implementation of any such systems. Those professional nurses who understand the conceptual framework of computer applications will find computers to be an extraordinarily useful tool in their professional practice.

In the past, hospital computer applications have been administrative. Tasks such as patient billing, maintaining financial records, and long-term planning are necessary aspects of the business side of the hospital. As computers get smaller, less costly, more powerful, and easier to use, they will be used increasingly in other areas of the health care system as well. Today, it is common to find a microcomputer system or computer terminal in the nurse's station. It is likely that such machines will become a more integral part of the nurse's activities during the next decade.

■ Using the Computer to Plan Care.   Automated client care systems allow "on line" (i.e., directly connected to the computer) use of standardized nursing care plans (see Figure 2—1). After analyzing the assessment data base and identifying the client's nursing diagnoses, nurses are able to create a care plan easily, customize it for each client, type in additions as needed,

Table 2–3   Investigative Functions of a Nurse at Various Educational Levels

Associate Degree in Nursing

1. Demmonstrates awareness of the value or relevance of research in nursing
2. Assists in identifying problem areas in nursing practice
3. Assists in collecting data within an established, structured format

Baccalaureate in Nursing

1. Reads, interprets, and evaluates research for applicability to nursing practice
2. Identifies nursing problems that need to be investigated and participates in the implementation of scientific studies
3. Uses nursing practice as a means of gathering data to refine and extend practice
4. Applies established findings of nursing and other health-related research to nursing practice
5. Shares research findings with colleagues

Master's Degree in Nursing

1. Analyzes and reformulates nursing practice problems so that scientific knowledge and scientific methods can be used to find solutions
2. Enhances the quality and clinical relevance of nursing research by providing expertise in clinical problems and by providing knowledge about the way in which these clinical services are delivered
3. Facilitates investigations of problems in clinical settings through such activities as contributing to a climate supportive of investigative activities, collaborating with others in investigations, and enhancing nursing's access to clients and data
4. Conducts investigations for the purpose of monitoring the quality of the practice of nursing in a clinical setting
5. Assists others to apply scientific knowledge in nursing practice

Doctoral Degree in Nursing or a Related Discipline

1. Provides leadership for the integration of scientific knowledge with other sources of knowledge for the advancement of practice
2. Conducts investigations to evaluate the contribution of nursing activities to the well-being of clients
3. Develops methods to monitor the quality of the practice of nursing in a clinical setting and to evaluate contributions of nursing activities to the well-being of clients

Graduate of a Research-Oriented Doctoral Program

1. Develops theoretical explanations of phenomena relevant to nursing by empirical research and analytic processes
2. Uses analytic and empirical methods to discover ways to modify or extend existing scientific knowledge so that it is relevant to nursing
3. Develops methods for scientific inquiry of phenomena relevant to nursing

Source: American Nurses' Association Commission on Nursing Research, *Guidelines for the investigative function of nurses* (Kansas City, Mo.: American Nurses' Association, 1981). Reprinted with permission.

---

evaluate and update information at any time, and retrieve data appropriate to each specific nursing diagnosis. Specific ways in which an automated client care plan can facilitate the role of the nurse include the following:

1. Entry of nursing assessments is simplified; e.g., the nurse can touch a computer screen display of possibilities.
2. Laboratory data can be ordered by entering a request at a computer workstation.
3. Laboratory results can be retrieved in a shorter time with less paperwork.
4. The system facilitates complete and legible medication orders.
5. The system promotes consistent doctor's orders (verbal orders are not accepted).
6. The nursing implications of a doctor's order can be sent to the nurse. Client preparation needs for a particular test can be listed automatically in the client's nursing care plan.
7. The use of nursing diagnosis is facilitated; a common format can be used.
8. Current information can be updated easily. Discontinued medication orders can be deleted easily, making all information timely, legible, and complete.

■ **Using the Computer as a Consultant.**   The term *expert system* will no doubt become familiar to those in the health care professions over the next decade. An **expert system** is a computer-based model (using some of the principles of an exciting area of computer science called **artificial intelligence**) that strives to simulate the way human experts in a particular discipline gather data and make decisions. The human expert, for example, a clinical nurse specialist, is an important part of the design of these systems. In effect, the clinical nurse specialist is fulfilling a consulting role through the computer.

COMMES (Creighton On-Line Multiple Modular Expert Systems) is an artificial intelligence system that can simulate a consultation with a professional nurse. To do so, the system must have a current knowledge base and be able to mimic professional decision-making skills while avoiding the risk of providing incorrect or inappropriate data (Ryan 1985). Some expert systems are, in many ways, merely computer data bases that allow retrieval of data in various ways. It is quite likely that, in the near future, expert systems will not only contain the information of a human considered an expert in a particular field but also the logical analysis capability of that human expert and his or her decision-making capability. In this way, the "system" can begin to provide assistance in educational settings, hospital settings, and emergency settings and facilitate client care of consistent quality.

■ **Using the Computer as a Research Tool.** Nursing research is also made easier by the computer's ability to access information in client records. Many

Client name :	Martha Johnson		Rm number	403

Admission date : 05/25/89

Sex : F   Religion : Catholic

Age : 56   Date of birth : 03/13/33

Admitting physician : Dr. Raymond Atkins

Medical diagnosis : Diabetes

Primary nurse : Judy Foster, R.N.

Allergies : Penicillin   Diet : 1500 c ADA

Risk factors : Hearing aid   Vital signs : T.I.D.

Nursing diagnosis : Impairment of skin integrity related to pruritus.

Long-term goals : Client will experience improved skin integrity within 48 hours.

Short-term goals	Nursing interventions	Evaluation
Given the prescribed care, client will experience descreased itching sensation.	1. Infrequent baths. 2. Use cool water. 3. Soap substitute. 4. Blot skin dry. DO NOT RUB! 5. Lubricate skin with lotion after bath.	
Client will understand and implement health teaching.	1. Explain phenomenon of itching. 2. Teach avoidance of excessive warmth. 3. Teach need for increased humidity.	

Figure 2–1 Computer-generated nursing care plan

hospitals maintain extensive computerized records. If access to these data is permitted, the nurse researcher can gather information that may be important in a particular study or project. For example, a researcher interested in determining what interventions were most successful in caring for clients with the nursing diagnosis "impairment of skin integrity" can retrieve the care plans containing this information from the computer-based record. In addition, other key variables, such as the client's age, background, and sex, can be obtained and used to facilitate the analysis of the research problem. Collecting these data manually (if they were available at all) would take a long time.

■ **Using the Computer for Administrative Tasks.** The particular needs of the nursing administrator or manager can often be met by a hospital's computer system. The director of nurses or the division head of client services in a hospital needs data related to staffing, nurse scheduling, budgeting, and the evaluation of client services. If the appropriate information is stored in a computer-based information system, the manager can generate reports on the acuity levels of clients on each unit. These can be used to devise a formula for

determining both the appropriate skill levels and the number of nurses required per shift and per floor. In addition, the scheduling of personnel is often made difficult by changing shifts, different skill levels, vacations, weekends, legal coverage requirements, and so on. Computer-based scheduling models can save much time and provide options that can be difficult to discover if the information is handled manually.

■ **Using the Computer for Education.** In the educational setting, the computer is becoming increasingly important, both as a teaching tool and as a resource for improving faculty and student productivity. It is likely that the use of the computer in these ways will increase dramatically over the next few years as these machines become easier to use. Table 2–4 shows some educational applications that are currently available. Although brief, the list in the table illustrates the variety of computer applications available in health education.

It is quite likely that the microcomputer will become even more pervasive as a resource for educators and students. Additional computer applications programs in nursing and health care will be developed, machines will become easier to use, and professional and academic organizations will begin to require graduates to have some familiarity with them.

■ **The Nurse's Role in Developing Computer Systems.** Nurses can play many roles to integrate the computer into their environment. One method is to become more comfortable with, knowledgeable about, and an advocate of the use of microcomputers. In addition (and perhaps more importantly), nurses need to become involved with the planning, design, and implementation of any computer systems that affect their profession. In most cases, health care applications are designed by persons or groups with computer expertise, who often lack skill in and knowledge of the application area in which they plan to put the computer to use. Sometimes, these developers seek out the active participation of those who will use the implemented system every day. Many times, no such attempt is made. It is essential that nurses demand involvement in the design of any systems that will eventually affect them and/or their clients. Otherwise, they run the risk of having to work with a computer system designed by someone unfamiliar with their needs. The probability of such systems being successful without this involvement is remote.

Nurses as Political Activists

Nurses are increasingly more knowledgeable about and capable of influencing the development of health care policy and the delivery of client care. Unless nurses develop their individual and collective political skills and use them to be advocates for the health of society and to promote the profession, client care and the nursing profession itself will be jeopardized.

Table 2—4 **Selected Computer Applications Available in Health Education**

Computer Program	What It Does	Audience
Calculate with Care	Tutorial for mathematics	Beginning students
NURSESTAR	Review of nursing	RN students
TESTSTAR	Test construction	Nursing facility
Build Medical Vocabulary	Tutorial/drill	Beginning students
Cardiac Arrest Simulation	Tutorial and simulation	Nurses and physicians
Hemodynamic Management	Clinical simulation	Critical care RNs
Clinical Nursing	Computer simulation	Advanced nursing students
Drug Interactions	Database of interactions	Nursing students
Nasogastric Suction	Client care simulations	Nursing students
Chest Suction	Client care simulations	Nursing students
Sugar	Hyperglycemia	Nursing students
Pre-lab Testing	30 pre-lab nursing test	Beginning students
Dosages and Solutions	Medication dosage math	Beginning students
Health History	Taking health historics	Beginning students
Genetic History	Basic human genetics	Nurses
Genetic Training		
Drug Therapy	Tutorial	Nursing students
CPR Certification	CPR exam	Nurses, students
Gross Anatomy	Tutorials	Nursing students
Automated Nurse Staffing	Staffing application	Administrators

Politics Defined

What is politics? For many people the word *politics* evokes images of "crooked deals" hatched by men in "smoke-filled rooms," Watergate, the Iran-Contra dealings, bribes, and powerbrokers. More positive examples of **political action** are legislative initiatives to meet consumer needs and campaigns to elect nurse legislators. Although the words *crafty* and *unscrupulous* are sometimes included in the definition of *political*, a more positive definition is "having practical wisdom." Others describe politics as a means to an end, a process by which one can influence the decisions of others and thus exert control over events (Stevens 1980).

Politics can also be defined as "influencing the allocation of scarce resources" (Talbott and Vance 1981, p. 592). Defined in this way, the word denotes more than action in the governmental arena; it is also applicable to every sphere of life where resources are limited and more than one person or group competes for them (Ehrat 1983). The allocation of scarce resources involves everyone in some way. Consider the following examples:

▪ A student applying for a college loan or competing with other students for his or her fair share of a teacher's time and attention

▪ A patient advocate competing for hospital education funds to do more preoperative teaching

▪ A citizen lobbying against the school board's proposal to divide one RN's time between two large schools

▪ A member of a professional association seeking association action on a practice issue, such as care of clients with acquired immune deficiency syndrome (AIDS)

Nurses' Discomfort with Politics

Despite nurses' experience with the political realities affecting the allocation of scarce resources, many nurses still harbor negative images of anything associated with the word *politics*. For example, it is not unusual to hear a colleague say, "I like her; she does not play politics." Although this remark is meant as a compliment, apolitical nurses in today's world hinder not only themselves and their colleagues but also the profession. For example, the nursing school dean, the head nurse, and the nurse researcher must all be politically skilled if they are to influence who gets how much of such scarce resources as funds for nursing education or nursing salaries, space for classrooms or offices, or release time to conduct research.

Why are nurses reluctant to engage in politics? Why do many view political activity as outside the realm of the professional nurse's role and responsibility? There are a number of reasons why nurses, and many women, have avoided becoming involved in political action. Among these are:

1. There has been minimal recognition of the social activism of many of the profession's early leaders or of the efforts of nurses working together to effect legislative changes on issues relating to nursing and health.
2. Prior to the contemporary wave of activism in women's rights, politics was considered an aggressive, men-only endeavor. Even though more women and nurses are becoming involved in governmental politics, many nurses have difficulty viewing the larger world of politics as an appropriate arena in which to participate. Women are socialized differ-

ently than men; for this reason, few women exert much influence on the male-dominated world of business and the professions.

3. The fact that relatively few nurses know and appreciate their rich heritage also contributes to their discomfort with politics. Nurses who have been leaders and social activists, such as Lavinia Dock, Lillian Wald, Harriet Tubman, and Margaret Sanger, were all skilled politicians. Each was able to make significant contributions to the profession and society because of her political skills. Maybe they had read the wise words of the founder of modern nursing, Florence Nightingale:

> When I entered into service here, I determined that, happened what would, I *never* would intrigue among the Committee. Now I perceive that I do all my business by intrigue. I propose in private to A, B, or C the resolution I think A, B, or C most capable of carrying in Committee, and then leave it to them, and I always win (Huxley 1975, p. 53).

4. Associated with the lack of appreciation of nursing history is the sparse education of nursing students, at the undergraduate and graduate level, on how to be politically astute. There is a critical need for students to have the opportunity to work with faculty and other preceptors who are skilled in the art of influencing governmental, organizational, workplace, and community politics.

Thus, a conscious effort needs to be made to educate nurses and nursing students about effective political action. Clearly, for such education to be effective, nurses must examine who they are as women and men and the values that they have been socialized to hold in relation to team play, power, and competition (Vance et al. 1985). This effort can be facilitated by learning more about how nursing leaders historically have used their political skills to bring about change, not only in the profession and health care but also in the values and actions of society as a whole.

◼ Opportunities for Political Action

◼ **Government.** Most people think of political action in relationship to local, state, or federal government. By voting, responsible citizens convey their opinions to elected and appointed officials on matters of concern. Many women first learn about political action through the educational efforts of the League of Women Voters. Other organizations—including the ANA, CNA, NLN, and NNSA—publish articles on legislative matters and encourage nurses to take action in behalf of health care consumers and the nursing profession. Nursing lobbyists at the state and national level work to influence the development of health policy and legislation, but their success depends on the active support of nurses who back up these paid lobbyists by doing personal lobbying among their own elected officials.

◼ **Workplace.** Since most nurses work in hospitals and too few nurses derive professional satisfaction from working in these bureaucratic institutions, it seems logical that nurses would work together to change the nature of their workplace. Evidence that hospitals can be rewarding places for delivering quality care to clients is documented in the American Academy of Nursing's (1983) study of hospitals with a fine record of attracting and retaining professional nurses.

The politics of client care impinges on the practice of every nurse. For example, as the prospective payment system becomes the norm, hospital stays will be cut more drastically in an effort to reduce health care costs (Shaffer 1984). The need for nurses to be "faster and smarter" in delivering client care and client education will increase. Nurses are already feeling the pressure to prepare clients for discharge days earlier than before. How can nurses ensure that the quality of nursing care is maintained under the new system? One way is for nurses to collaborate with each other and other providers to eliminate nonnursing tasks, such as answering the telephone, emptying the garbage, and transporting nonacute clients. Developing a demonstration project that compares cost and quality of care issues under different hospital unit structures can provide the necessary data and generate support from other providers and administrators for changing the role of staff nurses. This sort of "proactive" planning can empower nurses to take charge of nursing practice in ways that benefit clients and health professionals while conserving scarce resources such as money, time, and supplies.

◼ **Organizations.** Powerful and influential professional associations, such as the ANA and CNA and their affiliated state/province and district associations, provide a collective voice for promoting nursing and quality health care. As such, they exert influence on the individual nurse as well as in the spheres of government, the workplace, the community, and the profession. Associations monitor and influence laws and regulations affecting nursing and health care. Their role in workplace matters ranges from studying practice issues to acting as the collective bargaining agent for nurses. Additionally, the professional nursing organization is often a visible presence in the community because it presents the nursing perspective on health care issues.

◼ **Community.** The community in which the nurse lives and works can include the local neighborhood, the corporate world, the nation, and the international community. The community encompasses the workplace, professional organizations, and government. Many nurses, including Lillian Wald, founder of the Henry Street Settlement and modern public health nursing, view the community as more than a practice setting. Nurses who live in the community where they work can understand and influence the complex interplay among individuals and groups that compete for scarce resources.

Many communities depend on nurses to help with a wide variety of health and social policy decisions, such as environmental pollution and the feminization of poverty (Archer 1985). For example, a nurse who serves as an elected member of her or his community school board can influence decisions that affect the health and health care of students, such as the hiring of nurses for the school system. Nurses' opinions on matters of the public health are frequently sought, and the enterprising nurse looks for opportunities to promote a positive image of nursing while serving the community (Frost 1985). She or he also identifies ways in which fellow citizens can support both consumer health and nursing agendas.

Guiding Principles for Political Action

The following list of "commandments" is designed to help newcomers to political activism consider some ideas to enhance their effectiveness.

1. **Look at the big picture.** Step back and take a look at the larger environment in which you live, work, and study. In the governmental sphere especially, nurses are too often described as concerned only with nursing issues rather than with a broad variety of consumer and health care issues.

   Nurses will not enjoy credibility as health experts unless they become more sensitive to the concerns of others and employ their expertise in all spheres. In the workplace, nurses often focus their attention on their own unit, neglecting to view their position and unit in relationship to the larger organization.

   Astute nurses are aware of the environmental factors that impinge on their work setting. For example, the advent of the prospective payment system has had a major effect on nursing practice and raised many issues regarding the quality of client care. Nurses who make an effort to "take off the blinders" will see and understand the complex forces that affect their practice, the status of the nursing profession, and the nature of health care delivery.

2. **Do your homework.** Homework is not something that ends with graduation. Nurses must take stock of their goals and clarify their personal and professional positions on issues. Taking stock requires setting time aside for reflection. Nurses who use the nursing process as a basis for planning client care can use the same problem-solving approach in their own behalf. For example, developing a strategy to convince the head nurse to support the development of a formal continuing education program for staff nurses requires research and planning and will be most successful if it is based on an understanding of change theory.

3. **Nothing ventured, nothing gained.** Nurses have always been risk takers. Margaret Sanger risked being jailed for promoting birth control. Lavinia Dock and her colleagues chained themselves to the White House fence to call attention to their belief that women should have the vote. Clara Maas lost her life while participating in research on malaria. If you have a dream, an idea, a vision of what might be—make it a reality.

4. **Get a toe in the door.** Incremental changes or actions may have a better chance of success than a major project. Resistance to change is more easily overcome if change is tested by a pilot project. For example, a nursing director is more apt to agree to the introduction of primary nursing on one unit rather than to an overall change in the nursing system of the whole hospital.

5. **"Quid pro quo."** "Something for something." "Scratch my back, and I'll scratch yours." "Everything and everybody has a price." Many nurses are offended by the implications of these aphorisms, believing that they represent a cynical view of human and organizational relationships. Others, however, concede that they represent a realistic view of life. Consider how you relate to your friends and colleagues: Don't you often find yourself making trade-offs?

   When assessing your position within your school of nursing, the clinical area, or among your peers, review your friendships, connections, and pragmatic relationships. Frequently men say, "He owes me one," implying the person has received a favor and will reciprocate. Women and nurses, however, rarely use those words. In fact, they seem uncomfortable with the idea of being "in debt" or owing a favor despite the fact that they participate in give-and-take situations every day. It is important to develop an ease in professional and personal relationships so that one feels connected and supported rather than isolated and resentful.

6. **Walk a mile in another's moccasins.** Nurses learn to evaluate clients, to assess "where they are coming from." But how often do they make similar inquiries of peers, supervisors, or friends? The politically astute nurse who wants to get ahead identifies the goals the head nurse has for the unit and finds ways to support those efforts and get help in meeting personal development goals. Identifying another's agenda can help one plan a win-win situation, one in which the staff nurse or student meets her or his own needs as well as those of the teacher or head nurse.

7. **Strike while the iron is hot.** Any plan for change must include a timetable that identifies the best time for a particular action. Few people would approach the head nurse to discuss the work schedule while a client is in cardiac arrest, but a surprising number of people give little thought to what might be an opportune time to discuss such a topic. Sometimes an eagerness to take action precludes some important questions: "Is this the best time to do this? Will it be received better now or later?"

8. **Read between the lines.** Some people reveal a lot by the information they choose not to share. Just as nurses listen with a "third ear" to their clients, politically astute nurses attend to colleagues, their bosses, and the work environment for cues that help them achieve some measure of control and influence.

9. **Half a loaf is better than none.** It is human nature to want it all, but the reality is that the world is far from perfect. People often need to learn to share the wealth and settle for less than they would like. One way to adjust to this reality is to develop an ability to identify alternative solutions or outcomes. Rather than setting one's heart on a particular goal, it is prudent to outline acceptable alternatives.

10. **Rome was not built in a day.** Because most nurses work in bureaucratic organizations, they need to accept the fact that change does not occur rapidly. Even in a small, flexible organization, change is often slow because the nature of the change process demands that one proceed only after careful deliberation. While political skills are gained only through practice, nurses who ponder and act on the principles that underlie political action gain the ability to view their efforts in perspective.

Chapter Highlights

To be effective and influential in current and future health care delivery systems, nurses need to understand and apply change theory.

Nurses have been effective in promoting change in the workplace, through professional organizations, in the legislative arena, and in the community.

Nursing practice is influenced by: its historical development and current trends and advances in physical and biological science and technology; application of current knowledge from the social and behavioral sciences; demographic, economic, and cultural changes in the population; and the women's movement.

Nursing education focuses on preparing today's nursing students to fulfill current and future expectations and roles.

Apparent trends in nursing today are: the broadening focus of nursing practice, the increasingly scientific basis of nursing practice, the increasing use of technology in nursing, and a heightened awareness of the need for "high touch" skills.

The use of the computer in nursing and health care is expanding and demands that nurses take an active role in developing computer application systems.

Nurses are actively participating in political processes to promote change within the profession and to be influential in policy-making regarding health issues.

Selected References

American Academy of Nursing. 1983. *Magnet hospitals: Attraction and retention of professional nurses.* Kansas City, Mo.: American Nurses' Association.

American Nurses' Association. December 1965. American Nurses' Association first position on education for nursing. *American Journal of Nursing* 65:106–11.

———. April 1979. Credentialing in nursing: A new approach. Report of the Committee for the Study of Credentials in Nursing. *American Journal of Nursing* 79:674–83.

———. 1980. *Nursing: A social policy statement.* Kansas City, Mo.: American Nurses' Association.

———. Commission of Nursing Research. 1981a. *ANA guidelines for investigative functions of nurses.* Kansas City, Mo.: American Nurses' Association.

———. Commission on Nursing Research. 1981b. *Priorities for the 1980s.* Kansas City, Mo.: American Nurses' Association.

———. 1985a. *Facts about nursing 84–85.* Kansas City, Mo.: American Nurses' Association.

———. Center for Research. June 1985b. *DRGs and nursing care.* Kansas City, Mo.: American Nurses' Association.

———. 1987. *Proceedings of the 1987 House of Delegates.* Kansas City, Mo.: American Nurses' Association.

American Nurses' Association Cabinet on Nursing Services. 1984. *Career ladders: An approach to professional productivity.* Kansas City, Mo.: American Nurses Association.

Andreoli, K., and Musser, L. A. January/February 1985. Computers in nursing care: The state of the art. *Nursing Outlook* 33:16–21.

Arbeiter, J. S. November 1984. The big shift to home health nursing, *RN* 47:38–45.

Archer, S. E. 1985. Politics and the community. In Mason, D. J., and Talbott, S. W., editors. *The political action handbook for nurses.* Menlo Park, Calif.: Addison-Wesley Publishing Co.

Aydelotte, M. K. 1983. The future health care delivery system in the United States. In Chaska, N. L. *The nursing profession: A time to speak.* New York: McGraw-Hill.

Ball, M. J., and Hannah, K. 1984. *Using computers in nursing.* Reston, VA: Reston Publishing Co.

Barritt, E. R. 1973. Florence Nightingale's values and modern nursing education. *Nursing Forum* 12(1):6–47.

Baumgart, A. J. June 1985. The time is ripe. *The Canadian Nurse* 81:11.

Benner, P. 1984. *From novice to expert: Excellence and power in clinical nursing practice.* Menlo Park, Calif.: Addison-Wesley Publishing Co.

Brink, P. J., and Wood, M. J. 1983. *Basic steps in planning nursing research.* Belmont, Calif.: Wadsworth, 1983.

Bush, J. March 1985. DRGs challenge nursing curricula. *Journal of Nursing Education* 24:89.

Caterinicchio, R. P., editor. 1984. *DRGs: What they are and how to survive them—A sourcebook for professional nursing.* Thorofare, N.J.: Charles B. Slack.

Crawford, M.; Fisher, M.; and Kilbane, N. Collective bargaining in nursing. In DeYoung, L., editor. 1985. *Dynamics of nursing,* 5th ed. St. Louis: C. V. Mosby Co.

Curtin, L., and Zurlage, C. 1984. *DRGs: The reorganization of health.* Chicago: S-N Publications.

DeCrosta, T. May/June 1985. Megatrends in nursing: Ten new directions that are changing your profession. *Nursing Life* 5:17–21.

Deines, E. October 1985. Coping with PPS and DRGs: The levels of care approach. *Nursing Management* 16:43–43, 46–48, 52.

Diers, D. 1979. *Research in nursing practice.* Philadelphia: J. B. Lippincott Co.

———. June 1985. Nursing intensity and DRGs. Unpublished paper presented at the National League for Nursing Convention.

Dugas, B. W. May 1985. Baccalaureate for entry to practice: A challenge that universities must meet. *The Canadian Nurse* 81:17–19.

Ehrat, K. September 1983. A model for politically astute planning and decision making. *Journal of Nursing Administrative* 13:29–34.

Frost, A. D. 1985. Working together: Local community action. In Mason, D. J., and Talbott, S. W., editors. *The political action handbook for nurses.* Menlo Park, Calif.: Addison-Wesley Publishing Co.

Griffith, H. May 1985. Who will become the preferred provider? *American Journal of Nursing* 85:538–42.

Grobe, S. 1984. *A computer-based resource guide for nurses.* Philadelphia: J. B. Lippincott Co.

Hart, G.; Crawford, T.; and Hicks, B. May 1985. RN to BN: Building on education and experience. *The Canadian Nurse* 81:22–23.

Hood, G. May 1985. At Issue: Titling and licensure. *American Journal of Nursing* 85:592, 594.

Huxley, E. 1975. *Florence Nightingale.* New York: G. P. Putnam's Sons.

Institute of Medicine. 1933. *Nursing and nursing education: Public policies and private actions.* Washington, D.C.: National Academy Press.

Jamieson, E. M.; Sewall, M. F.; and Suhrie, E. B. 1966. *Trends in nursing history.* 6th ed. Philadelphia: W. B. Saunders Co.

Kalisch, B. J., and Kalisch, P. A. 1982. *Politics of nursing.* Philadelphia: J. B. Lippincott Co.

Kerr, J. May 1985. Taking the campus to the student. *The Canadian Nurse* 81:30–31.

Kinney, C. D. May/June 1985. A reexamination of nursing role conceptions. *Nursing Research* 34(3): 170–76.

Lane, B. June 1985. Specialization in nursing. Some Canadian issues. *The Canadian Nurse* 81:24–25.

Large, J. T. October 1976. Harriet Newton Phillips, the first trained nurse in America. *Image* 8:49–51.

Lewin, K. 1951. *Field theory in social science.* New York: Harper and Row.

Maples, L. September/October 1985. Patient-family responses to the DRG system. *Geriatric Nursing* 6:271–72.

Maraldo, P. Fall 1984. Terms of endurance: The future of nursing educaton, *Educational Record* 12–16.

Mason, D. J., and Talbott, S.W., editors. 1985. *The political action handbook for nurses: Changing the workplace, government, organizations, and community.* Menlo Park, Calif.: Addison-Wesley Publishing Co.

McKibbin, R. 1983. Economic and employment issues in nursing education. Kansas City, Mo.: American Nurses' Association.

Mitchell, K. November/December 1984. The next economy: Where will nurses fit? *Heart and Lung* 13:381.

Mussallem, H. K. 1985. *Succeeding Together: Group Action by Nurses.* Geneva: International Council of Nurses.

National Commission on Nursing: Summary report and recommendations July 1983. American Hospital Association. Chicago: The Hospital Research and Educational Trust, and American Hospital Supply Corporation.

———. 1978a. *Characteristics of graduate education in nursing leading to the master's degree.* New York: The League.

———. 1978b. *Competencies of the associate degree nurse on entry into practice.* New York: The League.

———. 1978c. *Roles and competencies of graduates of diploma programs in nursing.* New York: The League.

———. 1979. *Characteristics of baccalaureate education in nursing.* New York: The League.

Nightingale, F. 1860. *Notes on nursing: What it is, and what it is not.* London: Harrison. Reprinted in Bishop, F. L. A., and Goldie, S. 1962. *A bio-bibliography of Florence Nightingale.* London: Dawsons of Pall Mall.

Notter, L. E., and Spalding, E. K. 1976. *Professional nursing: Foundations, perspectives, and relationships.* 9th ed. New York: J. B. Lippincott Co.

O'Neill, P. 1983. *Health crisis 2000.* London: William Heinemann.

Palmer, I. S. June 1981. Florence Nightingale and international origins of modern nursing. *Image* 8:28–31.

Perlich, L. J. M. January 1986. Catalyzing educational change. *Journal of Nursing Administration* 16:6.

Pletsch, P. K. December 1981. Mary Breckinridge: A pioneer who made her mark. *American Journal of Nursing* 81:2188–90.

Powell, D. J. January/February 1984. Nurses—"High touch" entrepreneurs. *Nursing Economics* 2:33–36.

Primm, P. L. May/June 1986. Entry into practice. Competency statements for BSNs and ADNs. *Nursing Outlook* 34:135–37.

Rogers, M. E. 1985. High touch in a high-tech future. Paper presented at the National League for Nursing convention, San Antonio, Texas.

Romano, C.; Ryan, L.; Harris, J.; Boykin, P.; and Power, M. March/April 1985. A decade of decisions: Four perspectives on computerization in nursing practice. *Computers in Nursing* 3(2):64–76.

Rothberg, J. S. 1983. The growth of political action in nursing, *Nursing Outlook* 33:133–35.

Rutkowski, B. L. March/April 1985. DRGs: Now all eyes are on you. *Nursing Life* 5:26–29.

Ryan, S. A. March/April 1985. An expert system for nursing practice: Clinical decision support. *Computers in Nursing* 3(2):77–84.

Sabina, D. J. May 1985. What are the needs of the mature RN students? *The Canadian Nurse* 81:32–33.

Shaffer, F. A. January 1984a. A nursing perspective of the DRG world. Part 1. *Nursing and Health Care* 5:48–51.

Shaffer, F. A., editor. 1984b. *DRGs: Changes and challenges.* New York: National League for Nursing.

Slavinsky, A. T., and Diers, D. May 1982. Nursing education for college graduates. *Nursing Outlook* 30:292–97.

Smith, C. E. January 1985. DRGs: Making them work for you. *Nursing 85* 15:34–41.

Spradley, B. W. 1980. Making change creatively. *Journal of Nursing Administration* 10(5):32–37.

Stevens, B. J. November 1980. Power and politics for the nurse executive. *Nursing and Health Care* 1(4):208–10.

Stevens, K. R. 1983 *Power and influence. A source book for nurses.* New York: John Wiley and Sons.

———. May/June 1985. Does the 1985 education proposal make economic sense? *Nursing Outlook* 33:124–27.

Stewart, I. April 1933. Postgraduate education—new and old. *American Journal of Nursing* 33:363.

Stull, M. K. May/June 1986. Entry skills for BSNs. *Nursing Outlook* 34:138, 153.

Styran, P. May 1985. Winds of change: A university responds to the needs of nurses in the community. *The Canadian Nurse* 81:20–21.

Talbott, S. W., and Vance C. 1981. Involving nursing in a feminist group—NOW. *Nursing Outlook* 29:592–95.

U.S. National Center for Health Statistics. Public Health Service. 1985. *Vital statistics of the United States, 1982.* Vol. 11, Sec. 6. Life tables. DHHS Pub. no. (PHS) 85-1104. Washington, D.C.: U.S. Government Printing Office.

U.S. Department of Commerce. July 1, 1984. *Statistics on elderly population.* Washington, D.C.: Bureau of the Census.

U.S. Department of Health and Human Services. Public Health Service. 1985. *Charting the nation's health trends since 1960.* Hyattsville, Md.: DHHS Pub. no. (PHS) 85-1251.

Vance, C.; Talbott, S. W.; McBride, A. B.; and Mason, D. J. November/December 1985. An uneasy alliance: Nursing and the women's movement. *Nursing Outlook* 33(6):281–85.

Wilson, H. S. 1985. *Research in nursing.* Menlo Park, Calif.: Addison-Wesley Publishing Co.

Wilson, H. S., and Hutchinson, S. A. 1986. *Applying research in nursing.* Menlo Park, Calif.: Addison-Wesley Publishing Co.

CHAPTER 3

Health and Illness

OBJECTIVES

Differentiate between health, illness, and disease.

Identify factors that influence a person's concept of health.

Describe how individual perceptions affect a person's health behavior.

Describe factors affecting compliance.

Identify nursing interventions to enhance compliance.

Describe Suchman's five stages of illness.

Identify common behavior changes in sick persons.

Identify effects of hospitalization on clients.

Describe the effects of illness on family members' roles and functions.

Relate current patterns and trends in health to people's nursing needs.

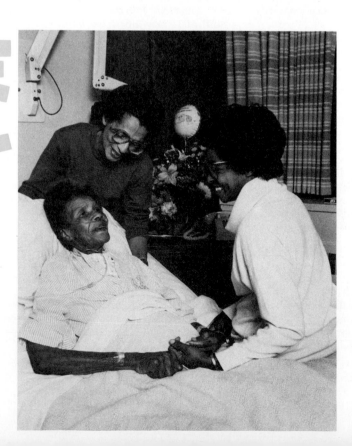

Relationship of Health, Illness, and Disease

The first two chapters of this text describe nurses and nursing in relation to the recipients of nursing care, the clients. The health-illness status of clients significantly influences how nurses relate to those clients. It is therefore appropriate to explore various meanings of health and illness in describing what nursing is and what nurses do. We begin by discussing the relationship of health, illness, and disease.

Health

Health is a highly individual perception. Meanings and descriptions of health vary considerably. An individual's personal definition of health may not agree with that of health professionals. The following factors influence an individual's definition of health.

Developmental Status. The idea of health is frequently related to a person's level of development. The ability to conceptualize a state of health and to respond to changes in health are related directly to age. The nurse's knowledge of an individual's developmental status (see Chapter 26) can facilitate assessment of the appropriateness of the person's behavior and help anticipate future behaviors.

Social and Cultural Influences. Culture and social interactions also influence a person's notion of health. Each culture has ideas about health, and often these are transmitted from parents to children. See Chapter 17 for specific examples.

Previous Experiences. Experiences with health and illness also affect people's perceptions of health. Some people may consider a pain or dysfunction normal because they have experienced it once or often before. Knowledge gained from past experiences helps determine people's definitions of health.

Expectations of Self. Some people expect to be functioning at a high level physically and psychosocially all the time when they are healthy. They perceive any change in that level of functioning, therefore, as illness. Others expect variations in their level of functioning, and their definitions of health accommodate those variations.

Perception of Self. Another factor related to self is how the individual perceives himself or herself generally. These perceptions relate to such aspects of self as esteem, body image, needs, roles, and abilities. When there is any threat or perceived threat to these views of self, the individual usually feels some anxiety and may need to reassess his or her health or to redefine health itself.

Nurses should be aware of their own personal definitions of health and should appreciate that other people have their own individual definitions as well. The person's definition of health influences behavior related to health and illness. By understanding clients' perceptions of health and illness, nurses can provide more meaningful assistance to help clients regain or attain a state of health.

Illness

Illness is a highly personal state in which the person feels unhealthy or ill. Illness may or may not be related to disease. An individual could have a disease, for example, a growth in the stomach, and not feel ill. Parsons defines illness as "a state of disturbance in the normal functioning of the total human individual, including both the state of the organism as a biological system, and of his person and social adjustments" (Parsons 1972, p. 107).

Disease

Disease is a medical term, which can be described as an alteration in body functions resulting in a reduction of capacities or a shortening of the normal life span (Twaddle 1977, p. 97). Intervention by physicians has the goal of eliminating or ameliorating disease processes. Primitive people thought disease was caused by "forces" or spirits. Later, this belief was replaced by the single-causation theory. Increasingly, multiple factors are believed to interact to cause diseases and influence the individual's response to treatment.

Developing a Personal Definition of Health

The following questions can help nurses develop a personal definition of health.

Is a person more than a biophysiologic system?
Is health more than the absence of disease symptoms?
Is health solely the result of the interaction between host, agent, and environment?
Is health the ability of an individual to perform work?
Is health the ability of an individual to adapt to the environment?
Is health a condition of a person's actualization?
Is health a state or a process?
Is health effective functioning of self-care activities?
Is health static or changing?
Are health and wellness the same?
Are disease and illness different?
Are there levels of health?
Are health and illness separate entities or points along a continuum?
Is health socially determined?
How do you rate your health and why?

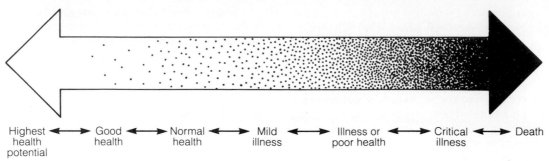

Highest ⟷ Good ⟷ Normal ⟷ Mild ⟷ Illness or ⟷ Critical ⟷ Death
health   health   health   illness   poor health   illness
potential

Figure 3–1 A health-illness continuum representing the holistic health model From J. B. McCann/Flynn and P. B. Heffron. *Nursing: From concept to practice* (Bowie, Md.: Robert J. Brady Company) 1984, p. 34.

Health and Illness

Health and illness can be considered either as points along one continuum (Figure 3–1), as related but separate entities, or as separate entities. (A **continuum** is a grid or graduated scale.) Dunn describes a continuum of well-being (health) in which peak wellness is at one end and death is at the other (Figure 3–2). Jahoda conceptualizes health and illness along separate but coexisting continua (Figure 3–3). The double continuum reflects the fact that people exhibit health and illness in varying degrees at the same time (Jahoda 1958, p. 75). This approach allows one to view a person's strengths (health) and illnesses at the same time. Pender states that health and illness are qualitatively different (separate entities) but related concepts. Illness is represented as discrete life events that are barriers to health. However, poor health can exist without illness (Pender 1982, pp. 38–39).

Illness and Disease

Traditionally, medical practitioners have dealt with diseases as affecting specific parts of the body but not necessarily the whole person. Only recently have medical practitioners started looking at the person as an entity, or whole. Nurses, by contrast, have traditionally viewed the person as an entity, taking a holistic view of people. Nursing practice today is based on the multiple-causation theory of health problems. Unemployment, pollution, life-style, and stressful events, while not diseases, may all contribute to illness. Thus, the concept of illness must include all aspects of the total person as well as the biologic and genetic factors that contribute to disease. Illness, then, is influenced by a person's family, social network, environment, and culture (Kneisl and Ames 1986, p. 18).

Health Beliefs and Behaviors

The **health status** of an individual is the health of that person at a given time. In its general meaning, the term may refer to anxiety, depression, or acute illness and thus describes the individual as a whole; *health status* also can describe such specifics as pulse rate and body temperature.

The health beliefs of an individual are those concepts about health that an individual believes true. Such beliefs may or may not be based on fact. For example, a man may believe that drinking 12 bottles of beer each day will keep his intestines free of infection.

Health behaviors are the actions a person takes to understand his or her health status, maintain an optimal state of health, prevent illness and injury, and reach his or her maximum physical and mental potential. Behaviors such as eating wisely, exercising, paying attention to signs of illness, following treatment advice, and avoiding known health hazards such as smoking are all examples. The ability to relax, emotional maturity, productivity, and self-expression also affect one's health (McCann/Flynn and Heffron 1984, p. 34).

Individual health behaviors may or may not be recommended by health care professionals. For example, the individual who believes that drinking beer will prevent intestinal infections may refuse to accept advice against this practice, even in life-threatening situations.

Health behavior is usually thought of as intended to prevent illness or disease or to provide for early detection of disease. Nurses preparing a plan of care with an individual need to consider the person's health beliefs before they attempt to change health behaviors. Otherwise, the individual may reject the nurses' suggestions

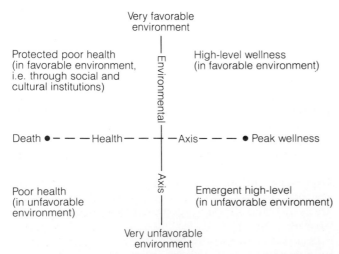

Figure 3–2 Dunn's health grid: its axes and quadrants. From H. L. Dunn, "High-level wellness for man and society," in *American Journal of Public Health,* 1959, 49:788.

and become angry because of intrusion into his or her personal habits.

Variables Affecting Health

Multiple variables influence a person's health status. Some of these are internal factors, such as the person's genetic makeup, and others are external, such as the person's culture and physical environment. *Genetic makeup* influences biologic characteristics, innate temperament, activity level, and intellectual potential. It has been related to susceptibility to specific diseases, such as diabetes and breast cancer. Disease distribution may be associated with *race*. For example, blacks have a higher incidence of sickle-cell anemia and hypertension than the general population, and native American Indians have a higher rate of diabetes.

Certain acquired and genetic diseases are more common in one *sex* than in the other. Disorders more common among females are osteoporosis, rheumatoid arthritis, systemic lupus erythematosus, anorexia nervosa and bulimia, gallbladder disease, and thyroid disease. Those more common among males are stomach ulcers, abdominal hernias, respiratory diseases, arteriosclerotic heart disease, hemorrhoids, and tuberculosis. Obviously, diseases that affect reproductive organs, such as testicular or uterine tumors, are sex dependent.

Distribution of diseases varies with *age*. For example, arteriosclerotic heart disease is common in middle aged males but occurs infrequently in younger persons; such communicable diseases as whooping cough and measles are common in children but are rare in older persons, who have acquired immunity to them. *Developmental level* is also a significant factor. Capabilities for responding to disease are fewer during the first few years of life and again near the end of life. Infants lack physiologic and psychologic maturity. Declining physical and sensory-perceptual abilities in older persons limit their ability to respond to environmental hazards and stressors.

Mind-body relationships—how emotional responses to stress affect body function and what emotional reactions occur in response to body conditions—may also influence health. Emotional distress may increase susceptibility to organic disease or precipitate it. Emotional distress may influence the immune system through central nervous system and endocrine alterations. Alterations in the immune system are related to the incidence of infections, cancer, and autoimmune diseases. Increasing attention is being given to the mind's ability to direct the body's functioning. Relaxation, meditation, and biofeedback techniques are gaining wider recognition by individuals and health care professionals.

A person's *life-style* includes his or her patterns of eating, exercise, methods of coping with stress, and use of tobacco, drugs, and alcohol. Overeating, getting insufficient exercise, and being overweight are closely related to the incidence of heart disease, arteriosclerosis, diabetes, and hypertension. Excessive sugar intake increases the risk of dental caries. Abuse of drugs and alcohol is physically and mentally debilitating. Excessive use of

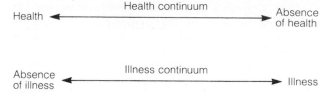

Figure 3–3 Jahoda's coexisting health and illness continua

tobacco is clearly implicated in lung cancer, emphysema, and cardiovascular diseases.

The *physical environment,* including housing and sanitation facilities, also affects health. Air, food, and water pollutants are often directly or indirectly related to various types of cancer. Extreme fluctuations in environmental temperature cause temporary disruptions in a person's internal environment, and the person in such an environment must expend more energy to restore physiologic stability. Persons with minimal physical coping responses are more susceptible to the effects of hypothermia and hyperthermia. Seasonal variations also affect health and the incidence of certain illnesses. For example, drownings and insect bites occur more frequently in the summer, whereas allergic reactions occur more frequently when pollen and related allergens are present.

An individual's *standard of living* (reflecting occupation, income, and education) is related to health, morbidity, and mortality. Hygiene, food habits, and the propensity to seek health care advice and follow health regimens vary among high- and low-income groups. For example, preventing illness may not have as high a priority among the poor as generating and maintaining an income; even when it is a priority, the poor may not be able to afford regular medical examinations, housing, or nutritious foods that promote health. Occupational roles also predispose people to certain illnesses. For instance, some industrial workers may be exposed to carcinogenic agents. More affluent people may fulfill stressful social or occupational roles that predispose them to stress-related diseases. Such roles may also encourage overeating or social use of drugs or alcohol.

How a person perceives, experiences, and copes with health and illness is partly determined by his or her *cultural beliefs.* Some people may perceive home remedies or tribal health customs as superior and more dependable than the health care practices of North American society, whether or not one is more beneficial than the other. Cultural rules, values, and beliefs give people a sense of being stable and able to predict outcomes. The challenging of old beliefs and values by second-generation ethnic groups may give rise to conflict, instability, and insecurity, which may, in turn, contribute to illness.

In addition to transmitting genetic predispositions, the *family* passes on patterns of daily living and lifestyles to offspring. Physical or emotional abuse may cause long-term health problems. Emotional health depends on a social environment that is free of excessive tension and that does not isolate the person from others. A climate of open communication, sharing, and love fosters the fulfillment of the person's optimum potential.

How a person feels about himself or herself (the *self-concept*) affects how that person perceives and handles situations. Such attitudes can affect health practices and the times when treatment is sought. A sense of extreme hopelessness, despair, or fear may cause disease and even death. An example is the anorexic woman who deprives herself of needed nutrients because she believes she is too fat even though she is well below an acceptable weight level.

Having a *support network* (family, friends, or a confidant) and *job satisfaction* helps people avoid illness (Grasser and Craft 1984, p. 210). Support people also help the person confirm that illness exists. Persons with inadequate support networks sometimes allow themselves to become increasingly ill before confirming the illness and seeking therapy. Support people also provide the stimulus for an ill person to become well again. Job satisfaction positively influences both the individual's self-concept and mind-body relationship.

Geography determines climate, and climate affects health. For instance, malaria and malaria-related conditions, e.g., sickle-cell hemoglobin, occur more frequently in tropical than temperate climates (Overfield 1985, p. 84). Multiple sclerosis is more prevalent in northern and central Europe, southern Canada, and the northern United States, for example, than in Asia, Africa, Mexico, and Alaska (Overfield 1985, p. 127).

Factors Influencing Health Behavior

Some factors affecting health status also affect health behavior; cultural and family influences are two examples. However, people can usually control their health behaviors and can choose healthy or unhealthy activities. In contrast, people have little or no choice over their genetic makeup, age, sex, physical environments, culture, or area of residence. This section outlines the factors that affect a person's health beliefs and behavior.

Health Belief Model. In the 1950s, Rosenstock (1974) proposed a **health belief model** intended to predict which individuals would or would not use such preventive measures as screening for early detection of cancer. Becker (1974) modified the health belief model to include these components: *individual perceptions, modifying factors,* and *variables likely to affect initiating action.*

Individual Perceptions. Individual perceptions include:

1. **The importance of health to the person.** Behavior that indicates health is perceived as something of value and includes providing special foods and vitamins to keep children well, having regular dental checkups, and participating in screening tests for cervical cancer, breast cancer, and cardiovascular disorders.
2. **Perceived control.** People who perceive that they have control over their own health are more likely to use preventive services than people who feel powerless. Control over health can relate to such

behaviors as not smoking, maintaining an appropriate weight, using seat belts, or obtaining immunizations for influenza.

3. **Perceived threat of a specific disease.** For example, a man who perceives that many people around him have influenza is more likely to modify his behavior than a man who perceives that most of the people with influenza live in another city.
4. **Perceived susceptibility.** A family history of a certain disorder, such as diabetes or heart disease, may make the individual feel he or she is at high risk.
5. **Perceived seriousness.** In the perception of the individual, does the illness cause death or have serious consequences? Growing concern about the spread of AIDS (acquired immune deficiency syndrome) reflects the general public's perception of the seriousness of this illness.
6. **Perceived benefits of preventive action.** For example, many individuals correctly perceive that not smoking may have beneficial outcomes.
7. **Perceived value of early detection.** This perception can motivate the person to have screening tests and regular physical or dental examinations.

Modifying Factors. Factors that modify a person's perceptions include:

1. **Demographic variables** such as age, sex, and race. An infant, for example, does not perceive the importance of a healthy diet; an adolescent may perceive peer approval as more important than family approval and participate as a consequence in hazardous activities or adopt unhealthy eating and sleeping patterns.
2. **Interpersonal variables.** These include concern of significant others, family patterns of health care (e.g., the members of a family may have dental examinations every 6 months), and interactions with health professionals who are likely to provide information and encourage preventive behavior.
3. **Situational variables.** These include the cultural acceptance of specific health-related behaviors. For example, in some cultures it is considered inappropriate to seek medical advice unless one is seriously ill. Societal norms also influence behavior. For example, a group may convey disapproval when a person drives an automobile after drinking alcohol. Another situational factor that modifies behavior is information from nonpersonal sources, such as newspapers or television broadcasts, which can affect health behavior positively or negatively.

Likelihood of Action. Perceived barriers to action can include cost, inconvenience, unpleasantness, and life-style changes. By contrast, certain cues may trigger action. Such cues may be external or internal, e.g., a birthday may make a person realize that he or she is now at greater risk of developing a particular disease. If the cues are too strong, anxiety can inhibit action rather than encourage it (Pender 1975, p. 388).

The **health belief model** is based on motivational theory. Rosenstock (1974) assumed that good health is an objective common to all people. Becker (1974) added

Individual perceptions   **Modifying factors**   **Likelihood of action**

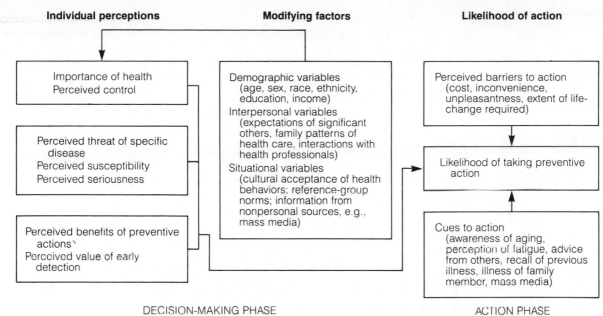

DECISION-MAKING PHASE   ACTION PHASE

Figure 3—4 Pender's modifications to the health belief model. From N. J. Pender, *Health promotion in nursing practice* (Norwalk, Conn.: Appleton-Lange) 1982.

"positive health motivation" as a consideration. Pender (1975) modified the health belief model by adding two further considerations: the importance of health as perceived by the individual and perceived control. See Figure 3–4. Pender believes that preventive well-being (health) behavior occurs in two stages: decision making and action.

Nurses play a major role during the decision-making and action phases. During decision making, nurses help clients monitor health, supply anticipatory guidance, and impart knowledge about health. During the action phase, nurses can reduce barriers to action, e.g., by minimizing inconvenience or discomfort. They can also support preventive actions. For additional information about nursing activities that promote health, see Chapter 25.

▪ Health Care Compliance

Compliance is the extent to which a person's behavior coincides with health practitioners' advice (Yoos 1981, p. 27). Clients' compliance with health care advice is of concern to all health professionals. Yoos reports that 86% of studies of compliance have shown noncompliance in more than 30% of clients (1981, p. 27).

Whether or not a person complies with a therapeutic regimen depends on many variables. Among them are age, education, costs, the complexity of the regimen and its convenience, the individual's value of health, and the inconvenience of the illness itself. In 1974, Becker published a sick role model to explain how people react to illness and to predict whether they will comply with health care advice (Becker 1974). See Figure 3–5. Becker's model indicates that compliance is related to

1. A client's motivation to become well
2. The value a client places on reducing the threat of illness

3. The client's belief that compliance will reduce that threat

Modifying and enabling factors of people's behavior include age, cost, duration, attitudes of health care personnel, interaction with health care personnel, previous health care experiences, and sources of advice. One can use these, Becker believes, to anticipate compliance with health care regimens (Becker 1974).

Researchers have investigated why some people comply with therapeutic regimens and others do not and how to help clients comply with therapeutic regimens. The first step is identifying noncompliance. The nurse can ask the client if he or she is following the regimen. If the client is not complying, the nurse needs to find out why and intervene to assist the client in complying. To enhance compliance, nurses can

1. **Demonstrate caring.** The nurse can do so by showing sincere concern about the client's problems and decisions while accepting the client's right to a course of action. For example, a nurse might tell a client who is not taking his heart medication, "I can appreciate how you feel about this, but I am very concerned about your heart."
2. **Encourage healthy behaviors through positive reinforcement.** If the man who is not taking his heart medication is walking every day, the nurse might say, "You are really doing well with your walking."
3. **Establish why the client is not following the regimen** and, where indicated, provide information, correct misconceptions, attempt to decrease expense, or suggest counseling if psychologic problems are interfering with compliance.
4. **Use aids to reinforce teaching.** For instance, the nurse can leave pamphlets for the client to read later

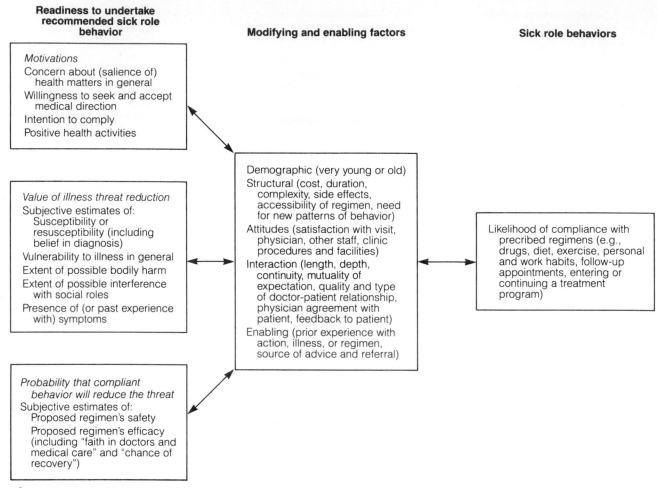

Readiness to undertake recommended sick role behavior

Motivations
Concern about (salience of) health matters in general
Willingness to seek and accept medical direction
Intention to comply
Positive health activities

Value of illness threat reduction
Subjective estimates of:
 Susceptibility or resusceptibility (including belief in diagnosis)
Vulnerability to illness in general
Extent of possible bodily harm
Extent of possible interference with social roles
Presence of (or past experience with) symptoms

Probability that compliant behavior will reduce the threat
Subjective estimates of:
 Proposed regimen's safety
 Proposed regimen's efficacy (including "faith in doctors and medical care" and "chance of recovery")

Modifying and enabling factors

Demographic (very young or old)
Structural (cost, duration, complexity, side effects, accessibility of regimen, need for new patterns of behavior)
Attitudes (satisfaction with visit, physician, other staff, clinic procedures and facilities)
Interaction (length, depth, continuity, mutuality of expectation, quality and type of doctor-patient relationship, physician agreement with patient, feedback to patient)
Enabling (prior experience with action, illness, or regimen, source of advice and referral)

Sick role behaviors

Likelihood of compliance with precribed regimens (e.g., drugs, diet, exercise, personal and work habits, follow-up appointments, entering or continuing a treatment program)

Figure 3–5 Sick role model. From M. H. Becker, *The health belief model and personal health behavior* (Thorofare, N. J.: Slack, Inc., 1974). Copyright Marshall H. Becker. Reprinted by permission of the author.

or make a "pill calendar," a paper with the date and number of pills to be taken.

5. **Establish a therapeutic relationship** of freedom, mutual understanding, and mutual responsibility with the client and support persons. By providing knowledge, skills, and information, the nurse gives clients control over their health and establishes a cooperative relationship, which results in greater compliance (MacElveen-Hoehn 1983, p. 535).

Illness Behaviors

Various scientists have described the stages of illness. By recognizing these stages and the illness behaviors that accompany them, nurses can better understand their clients' behavior and determine ways to assist them. **Illness behavior** is "any activity undertaken by a person who feels ill, to define the state of his health and to discover a suitable remedy" (Igun 1979, p. 445).

How people behave when they are ill is affected by many variables, such as age, sex, occupation, socioeconomic status, religion, ethnicity, psychologic stability,

personality, education, and modes of coping. Suchman (1972, p. 145) describes five stages of illness:

1. **Symptom experience stage.** This is the transition stage during which people come to believe something is wrong. Either a significant person mentions that they look unwell, or people experience some symptoms, which can appear insidiously. The symptom experience stage has three aspects:

 ▪ The physical experience of symptoms (e.g., pain or elevated temperature)
 ▪ The cognitive aspect (the interpretation of the symptoms in terms that have some meaning to the person)
 ▪ The emotional response (e.g., fear or anxiety)

During this stage, unwell persons usually consult others close to them about their symptoms or feelings. People validate with their spouses or support persons that the symptoms are real. At this stage, sick persons sometimes try home remedies, such as laxatives or cough medicines.

2. **Assumption of the sick role.** The second stage signals acceptance of the illness. At this time, individuals decide that their symptoms or concerns are

sufficiently severe to suggest that they are sick. Some people seek professional help quickly; others continue self-treatment, often following the suggestions of family and friends.

In this stage, sick people are usually afraid, but they now accept that they are ill even though they may not be able to accept the possible reasons. In conferring with people close to them, sick persons seek not only advice but also support for the decision to give up some activities and, for example, stay home from work.

At the end of this stage, sick persons experience one of two outcomes. They may find that the symptoms have changed and that they feel better. If family members support the perceptions of such persons, they are no longer considered or consider themselves sick. Then the recovered persons resume normal obligations, such as returning to work or attending a school concert.

If, however, the symptoms persist or increase and if lack of improvement is validated by the family or significant others, then sick people know they should seek some treatment. The choice of a treatment plan is often affected by the known available alternatives and previous experience.

3. **Medical care contact stage.** Sick persons seek the advice of a health professional either on their own initiative or at the urging of significant others. When people go for professional advice, they are really asking for three types of information:

- Validation of real illness
- Explanation of the symptoms in understandable terms
- Reassurance that they will be all right or prediction of what the outcome will be

If the health professional does not validate illness, persons have two recourses: to return to normal activities or to seek other advice. If the symptoms disappear, people often perceive that they are not really ill. If symptoms continue, people usually return to the health professional or go to a second person for care. People who are repeatedly told that they are not ill may seek out quasi-practitioners as a last resort to alleviate the perceived symptoms. Some people will go from health professional to health professional until they find someone who provides a diagnosis that fits their own perceptions.

Most people also want an understandable explanation of their symptoms. When symptoms are not explained, people may assume the health professional does not believe them or perhaps that they are imagining the symptoms. Overly technical explanations, however, often confuse and frighten people.

People often experience anxiety about seeking help with health problems. Even minor symptoms can be construed as serious. Therefore, the client needs reassurance that he or she will be cured. Even when this reassurance cannot be given, most people want to know the likely outcome.

4. **Dependent patient role stage.** When a health professional has validated that the person is ill, the individual becomes a patient, dependent on the professional for help. During this stage, sick persons may or may not be reluctant to accept a professional's recommendations. They may vacillate about what is best for them and alternately accept and reject the professional's suggestions. People vary greatly in the degree of ease with which they can give up their independence, particularly in relation to life and death. Role obligations (such as those of wage earner, father, mother, student, baseball team member, or choir member) complicate the decision to give up independence.

It is also common for the client and the health professional to hold different notions of the nature of the illness. During this stage, a nurse can often provide information that may allay some fears and/ or provide data that support the person. Misconceptions can result from limited information, which clients interpret in the light of their experiences. For example, a woman may be told by a physician that she has a small encapsulated growth in the right groin and that surgical removal is advised. If the individual's mother died after being told she had a growth in her breast, the woman may assume that she also will die.

People have varying dependence needs. For some, illness may meet dependence needs that have never been met and thus provide satisfaction. Other people have minimal dependence needs and do everything possible to return to independent functioning. A few may even try to maintain independence to the detriment of their recovery.

5. **Recovery or rehabilitation stage.** During the fifth stage, the client learns to give up the sick role and return to former roles and functions. For people with acute illnesses, the time as an ill person is

generally short, and recovery is usually rapid. Thus, most find it relatively easy to return to their former life-styles. People who have long-term illnesses and who must make adjustments in life-style may find recovery more difficult. Recovery is particularly difficult for people who have to relearn skills such as walking or talking.

During this stage, readiness for social functioning may not coincide with physical readiness. People may be physically able to go out to dinner but find that functioning socially is still too stressful or they may find that they have the *desire* to perform activities but not the strength. Nurses can help clients function with increasing independence by planning with them those functions they can accomplish by themselves and those with which they need assistance. It is also important for nurses to convey an attitude of hope and to support the client's return to health.

Sick Role Behavior

Sick role behavior is "the activity undertaken by those who consider themselves ill, for the purpose of getting well" (Igun 1979, p. 455). Most North Americans believe that illness, though undesirable, is beyond a person's control and that individuals are not responsible for incurring an illness. Some subcultures view illness as punishment from God, and therefore consider the infirm responsible for their illnesses, because of their sins. This folk belief persists to some degree in American society. A client may say something like, "What have I done to deserve this?" This remark reflects a sense that illness is a punishment. Today, because of the recognition that life-style contributes to illness and disease, some people—for example, the cardiac client who smokes or the overweight person who develops diabetes—are being held increasingly responsible for developing some illnesses.

Nurses can help clients by providing factual information and by not judging the client. It is important to encourage behaviors that promote health and not to reinforce behaviors that may have helped bring about an illness.

The sick person is usually excused from some normal duties. Social pressures on the sick and people's expectations of the sick usually depend on the prognosis and severity of the illness. People who are severely ill and whose prognosis is poor or uncertain are permitted more dependence than people who are less seriously ill. People who are not seriously ill and whose prognosis is good are more likely to be encouraged to fulfill personal and social responsibilities. The person with a cold may still be expected to give a scheduled speech or to take an examination. People who are chronically ill may be permanently exempted from some duties or activities by society.

Some people may express feelings of guilt because they are unable to fulfill their normal responsibilities. Nurses can offer support to clients who cannot fulfill their perceived roles and help them substitute other

appropriate activities, when desirable. For example, a young father who cannot play ball with his son may be able to help his son build a model airplane, thereby fulfilling his perception of the father's role in another way.

Another aspect of the sick role is the obligation of the person to get well as quickly as possible. The sick role is a dependent one, at least in some respects. The person who fears dependence may be threatened by assuming a sick role and having to seek help. This individual might ignore advice despite the most serious consequences. Some people, however, find dependence gratifying. Some clients find dependence so satisfying that they perpetuate the sick role and do not try to get well or continue to complain of symptoms even after they are physically well. Some people in the dependent stage also find it satisfying to control others through excessive demands. With these exceptions, most people usually try to get well as quickly as possible.

Nurses can help clients assume a dependence appropriate to their developmental status and health. Part of the nurse's function is to reinforce both dependence and increasing independence at the appropriate times. For example, a man who is acutely ill may have to be shaved by the nurse; however, once he is stronger the nurse can assist him by providing shaving supplies and later complimenting him on his appearance.

Nurses who are aware of the health facilities available in a community can help people obtain care. Some people require considerable support before seeking assistance. They may fear that the health problem might be serious or they may believe that competent help might not be available. A nurse's function in these instances is to provide accurate information about available health facilities while recognizing clients' beliefs and their right to hold them.

Effects of Hospitalization

Normal patterns of behavior generally change with illness; with hospitalization, the change can be even greater. Hospitalization usually disrupts a person's privacy, autonomy, life-style, roles, and economics.

Privacy. When a client enters a hospital or nursing facility, the loss of privacy is instantly obvious. **Privacy** has been described as a comfortable feeling reflecting a deserved degree of social retreat. Its dimensions and duration are controlled by the individual seeking the privacy. It is a personal, internal state that cannot be imposed from without (Schuster 1976, p. 245).

People need varying degrees of privacy and establish boundaries for privacy; when these boundaries are crossed, they feel invaded. Hospital personnel sometimes show little concern for clients' privacy. Clients are asked to provide information that often they consider private; they may share a room with strangers; and their health is frequently discussed with many health professionals.

The boundaries of privacy are highly individual. The adult who lives alone may be used to privacy while eating, sleeping, and reading. A child from a large family may be accustomed to performing these activities in the presence of others. It is important for nurses to ascertain what privacy means to the individual and to support accustomed practices whenever possible.

▪ Autonomy.

Autonomy is the state of being independent and self-directed without outside control. People vary in their sense of autonomy; some are accustomed to functioning independently in most of their life activities, while others are more accustomed to direction from others. An example of the former is a writer who lives alone and works independently. By contrast, a wife in a patriarchal home may be accustomed to having decisions made by her husband and receiving direction from him.

Hospitalized people frequently give up much of their autonomy. Decisions about meals, hygienic practices, and sleeping are frequently made for them. This loss of individuality is often difficult to accept, and the client may feel dehumanized—"just a piece of machinery." Nurses have been trying to humanize care in recent years by learning about the client as a person and by individualizing nursing care plans.

▪ Life-Style.

Hospitalization marks a change in life-style. Many hospitals determine when people wake up and when they sleep. The woman who normally rises at 8:00 A.M. and the man who usually works until 11:00 P.M. must change their habits. Food in a hospital is usually mass produced, and individual differences in taste are not always accommodated. Occasionally hospitals have relatively large populations from a particular culture and make special food arrangements, for example, a Chinese menu for traditional Chinese clients or Kosher foods for traditional Jewish clients. However, individual preferences are not always met. Nurses can help clients adapt to life in a hospital by:

1. Making arrangements wherever possible to accommodate the client's life-style, such as providing a bath in the evening rather than in the morning
2. Providing explanations about hospital routines
3. Encouraging other health professionals to become aware of the person's life-style and to support healthy aspects of that life-style
4. Reinforcing desirable changes in practices with a view to making them a permanent part of the client's life-style

▪ Economics.

Hospitalization often places a genuine financial burden on clients and their families. Even though many people have health insurance, it may not reimburse all costs; in addition, many lose wages while they are hospitalized. Nurses can be aware of these costs and provide care that is as economical as is safely possible; for instance, they can use only the minimum supplies necessary for safe care. In some agencies, nurses may initiate referrals to the social service department to assist clients in making arrangements to address the financial burdens imposed by hospitalization. When this is not an independent nursing function, the nurse should consult with the client's physician to obtain such a referral.

▪ Effects of Illness on Family Members

A person's illness affects not only the person who is ill but also the family or significant others. The kind of effect and its extent depend chiefly on three factors:

1. Which member of the family is ill
2. How serious and long the illness is
3. What cultural and social customs that family follows

The changes that can occur in the family include:

1. Role changes
2. Task reassignments
3. Increased stress due to anxiety about the outcome of the illness for the client and conflict about unaccustomed responsibilities
4. Financial problems
5. Loneliness as a result of separation and pending loss
6. Change in social customs

Each member of the family is affected differently, depending upon which member of the family is ill, since each plays a different role in the family and supports the family in different ways. Parents of young children, for example, have greater family responsibilities than parents of grown children.

The degree of change that family members experience is often related to their dependence on the sick person. For example, when a child is ill, there are few changes other than added responsibilities directly related to the child's illness. When the mother is ill, however, many changes are often necessary because other family members must assume her functions.

▪ Sick Elderly Persons.

When an elderly person is ill, a son or daughter often assumes the role of parent to the elderly person, providing housing, meals, and assistance with daily needs over a prolonged time. In other words, the parent-child roles are frequently reversed. This role reversal may be only temporary and may end when the illness ends, or it may become permanent.

The whole family, particularly the spouse of the sick person, experiences stress and concern about the outcome of the illness. Usually, the sick person's spouse feels a pending loss or separation most keenly. After a marriage of 50 or 60 years, elderly people may find it difficult to envisage what life will be like without a husband or wife. Younger persons in the family may deal with serious illness in an elderly person by stating, "He has led a good life" or "She had so much pain the past years." In this way, the young prepare themselves for that person's death. This same reasoning is rarely applied to a child or younger adult who is ill.

When an elderly person is ill, adult sons and daughters may face conflicting responsibilities. A daughter who lives some distance away needs to maintain her job and look after her own family, but at the same time her parents need her in another city. How often should she visit? How should she fulfill her responsibilities? These questions pose problems for many families today who live far apart.

The financial problems of the sick elderly can be a major problem for a family as well as a community. Because illness in this age group tends to be chronic, the costs of illness are often considerable. The greatest change in life-style is that the family must now allot time for hospital visits to the elderly relative.

■ **Sick Parents.** When the sick person is a parent, the degree to which the family experiences change is related to the responsibilities the individual has and the number and age of dependents in the person's care. For example, when a father is ill for a long time, his roles are usually taken over by other members of the family, frequently the mother. Such tasks as doing chores in the house or attending a child's basketball games, for example, are either reassigned or not performed at all. Anxiety of family members about the outcome of a parent's illness is usually high, especially if the parent is the wage earner. The implications to the family of prolonged illness or death are great in almost all areas of living because of the needs of the dependents.

Prolonged illness of the mother can have equally serious consequences. Often the children do not understand why their mother is in the hospital, and they may feel lonely and unwanted. Sometimes the mother's functions are taken over by grandparents or by aunts and uncles as well as by the father. When a young mother has a serious illness of unknown outcome, the father and family face worrisome problems of how to manage over a long period of time. Most arrangements have financial implications and involve role changes for the father and children. In this situation, the father must become both father and mother and give up many of his normal social activities. The children may also need to assume more housekeeping functions.

■ **Sick Children.** Because a child is dependent on parents for so many daily needs, both sick children and their families may need to make fewer role adjustments than sick adults and their families. Task reassignments are also generally minimal. Sometimes a younger sibling takes over a paper route for a sick brother or sister, and other members of the family share the sick child's chores.

However, all members of the family experience anxiety if the outcome of the child's illness is in doubt. A permanent disability has implications for schooling, earning a living, and future needs. Financial responsibility for chronic illness or a disability often can be a serious problem for young parents. Other children may feel neglected if an unusual amount of attention is given to the ill child. Husband and wife may also expend most of their energies visiting the hospital and have little time for each other. If extended, this situation can place great stress on a marriage.

When a child is admitted to the hospital, parents and siblings may experience some sense of loss; however, children usually continue with their daily activities, and there frequently is minimal disruption in the home.

Current Health Trends

The health of North Americans is steadily improving. Probable reasons for this improvement are:

1. Earlier preventive efforts based on new knowledge obtained through research
2. Improvements in sanitation, housing, nutrition, and immunization essential to disease prevention
3. Individual measures to promote health and prevent disease, such as the increasing attention that is being paid to exercise, nutrition, environmental health, and occupational health

Risk factors that predispose individuals to illness and disease are being identified, and people are changing their life-styles to avoid becoming ill. Four of the major risk factors responsible for illness and premature deaths cited by the surgeon general (U.S. DHEW 1979, pp. 7–8) are:

1. **Cigarette smoking.** This is clearly identified as a cause of most cases of lung cancer and a major factor increasing the risk of heart attacks.
2. **Alcohol and drug abuse.** Consumption of alcohol and drugs, even among youths, has grown substantially since the 1960s and accounts for significant illness, disability, and death.
3. **Injuries.** The highest death rate from accidents occurs among the elderly, but it is also substantial among those aged 15 to 24. Injuries from accidents may be caused by motor vehicles, firearms, falls, burns, poisons, recreational activities, and adverse drug reactions.
4. **Occupational risks.** Certain occupational hazards, such as exposure to asbestos, rubber, and plastic, are now being identified as potential cancer risks.

All of these risks present challenges to health care workers, especially nurses, in terms of prevention. Measures to enhance health include elimination of cigarette smoking, moderation of alcohol consumption, using seat belts, and periodic screening for such health problems as cancer.

■ Health Behaviors

The number of cigarette smokers in America has declined since 1964 when the Surgeon General's first *Report on Smoking and Health* was released. The sharp rise in smoking among teenage females that occurred in the 1970s has been curbed. However, the ratio of male to female smokers was about equal in 1983, whereas in 1965 male smokers outnumbered female smokers by 150%. In addition, among people who smoke, the percentage who smoke 25 or more cigarettes per day has been increasing (U.S. DHHS 1985, p. 17).

Dietary practices, especially those related to the consumption of saturated fats, have had notable effects on the health of people. Over the past 20 years, the mean serum cholesterol level of adults aged 20 to 74 years has declined for every age group for both men and women. High serum cholesterol levels are associated with heart attacks and strokes. Another indicator of positive health behavior relates to hypertension control. The proportion of people with hypertension who kept their blood pressure below the level of 160/95 mm Hg nearly doubled from 1960–1962 to 1976–1980. This is thought to be due in part to adherence to prescribed medication regimens (U.S. DHHS 1985, p. 18).

Implications for Nursing

As nurses assume an increasingly more visible role in providing health care services, it is helpful to consider the trends and behaviors noted above and to structure nursing services to ensure:

1. Improvement in life-styles to help individuals avoid major risk factors responsible for disease
2. Improvement in the health of adolescents and young adults; their physical, psychologic, and social attitudes; and their health habits to prevent later susceptibility to chronic diseases
3. Education to help youths acquire skills and information to prevent pregnancy, alcohol and drug abuse, and sexually transmitted disease
4. Instruction in accident prevention
5. Instruction to young adults about motor vehicle safety
6. Improved screening programs to assist in the early identification of disease
7. Concerted efforts to reduce respiratory cancer rates by assisting people, especially women between 54 and 64 years of age and teenagers, to stop smoking
8. Increased assistance to help the elderly population with self-care and home management in their homes
9. Guidance to help all people acquire early treatment for illness and comply with therapy
10. Attention to occupational and environmental hazards

Chapter Highlights

- The perspective from which health is viewed has changed; instead of absence of disease, health has come to mean fulfilling one's maximum potential for physical, psychosocial, and spiritual functioning.
- Holistic health practitioners relate the impact of an event to the whole person and encourage the person to take responsibility for and control over his or her health.
- Because notions of health are highly individual, the nurse must determine each client's perception of health in order to provide meaningful assistance.
- Each person's concept of health is molded by social and cultural influences, previous experiences, and expectations of self.
- The health status of a person is affected by many internal and external variables over which the person has varying degrees of control.
- Whether or not people choose to implement health behaviors depends on such factors as the perceived threat of a particular disease, perceived familial susceptibility, perceived seriousness of an illness, and perceived benefits of preventive actions.
- Whether or not people take action to improve their health often depends on the cost, inconvenience, and unpleasantness involved and on the degree of life-style change necessary.
- People realize they are ill when certain symptoms indicate that something is wrong; they accept that they are ill when significant others or a health care professional verifies the illness.
- Increasingly, persons are being held responsible for some illnesses but are excused from certain roles and tasks during the illness; they are obliged, however, to get well as quickly as possible and to seek competent help.
- Nurses need to be aware that the illness of one member of a family affects all other members.
- Nurses need to be aware of a hospitalized client's life-style, roles, economic situation, and need for privacy and autonomy and provide care accordingly.
- Clients may demonstrate certain behavioral changes during illness.
- Health trends indicate that nurses need to assume a major role in helping people make life-style and environmental changes that will prevent accidents, disease, and occupational hazards.

Selected References

Becker, M. H., editor. 1974. *The health belief model and personal health behavior.* Thorofare, N.J.: Charles B. Slack.

Birchfield, M. E. 1985. *Stages of illness: Guidelines for nursing care.* Bowie, Md.: Brady Communications Co.

Brown, N. Spring 1983. The relationship among health beliefs, health values, and health promotion activity. *Western Journal of Nursing Research* 5:155–63.

Carey, R. L. 1984. Compliance and related nursing actions. *Nursing Forum* 21:157–61.

Dixon, J. K., and Dixon, J. P. April 1984. An evolutionary-based model of health and viability. *Advances in Nursing Science* 6:1–18.

Dunn, H. L. June 1959a. High-level wellness in man and society. *American Journal of Public Health* 49:786.

———. November 1959b. What high-level wellness means. *Canadian Journal of Public Health* 50:447.

———. 1961. *High-level wellness.* Arlington, Va.: R. W. Beatty Co.

Grasser, C., and Craft, B. J. G. June 1984. The patient's approach to wellness. *Nursing Clinics of North America* 19:207–18.

Igun, U. A. 1979. Stages in health-seeking: A descriptive model. *Social Science and Medicine* 13A:445–56.

Jahoda, M. 1958. *Current concepts of positive mental health.* New York: Basic Books.

Kneisl, C. R., and Ames, S. W. 1986. *Adult health nursing: A biopsychosocial approach.* Menlo Park, Calif.: Addison-Wesley Publishing Co.

Laken, D. D. January 1983. Protecting patients against themselves. *Nursing 83* 13:26–27.

Leddy, S., and Pepper, J. M. 1985. *Conceptual bases of professional nursing.* Philadelphia: J. B. Lippincott Co.

MacElveen-Hoehn, P. 1983. The cooperation model for care in health and illness, pp. 515-39. In Chaska, N. L., editor. *The nursing profession: A time to speak.* New York: McGraw-Hill.

McCann/Flynn, J. B., and Heffron, P. B. 1984. *Nursing: From concept to practice.* Bowie, Md.: Robert J. Brady Co.

Murray, R. B., and Zentner, J. P. 1985. *Nursing concepts for health promotion.* 3d ed. Englewood Cliffs, N.J.: Prentice-Hall.

Overfield, T. 1985. *Biologic variation in health and illness: Race, age, and sex differences.* Menlo Park, Calif.: Addison-Wesley Publishing Co.

Parsons, T. 1972. Definitions of health and illness in the light of American values and social structure. In Jaco, E. G., editor. *Patients, physicians and illness.* 2d ed. New York: Free Press.

Payne, L. September 1983. Health: A basic concept in nursing theory. *Journal of Advanced Nursing* 8:393–95.

Pender, N. J. June 1975. A conceptual model for preventive health behavior. *Nursing Outlook* 23:385–90.

———. 1982. *Health promotion in nursing practice.* East Norwalk, Conn.: Appleton-Century-Crofts.

Rosenstock, I. M. 1974. Historical origins of the health belief model. In Becker, M. H., editor. *The health belief model and personal health behavior.* Thorofare, N.J.: Charles B. Slack.

Schuster, E. A. October 1976. Privacy: The Patient and Hospitalization. *Social Science Medicine* 10:245.

Shaver, J. F. July/August 1985. A biopsychosocial view of human health. *Nursing Outlook* 33:186–91.

Shillinger, F. L. Spring 1983. Locus of control: Implications for clinical nursing practice. *Image: The Journal of Nursing Scholarship* 25:58–63.

Smith, J. A. April 1981. The idea of health: A philosophical inquiry. *Advanced Nursing Science* 3:43–50.

Suchman, E. A. 1972. Stages of illness and medical care. In Jaco, E. G., editor. *Patients, physicians and illness.* 2d ed. New York: Free Press.

Tatro, S., and Gleit, C. J. March 1983. A wellness model for nursing: Promoting high-level wellness in any setting through independent nursing functions. *Nursing Leadership* 6:5–9.

Trekas, J. September 1984. It takes two to achieve compliance. *Nursing 84* 14:58–59.

Twaddle, A. C. 1977. *A sociology of health.* St. Louis: C. V. Mosby Co.

U.S. Department of Health and Human Services. December 1985. *Health United States 1985.* Pub. no. (PHS) 86-1232. Hyattsville, Md.: Public Health Service.

U.S. Department of Health, Education, and Welfare. 1979. *Healthy people: The Surgeon General's report on health promotion and disease prevention.* Pub. no. 79-55071. Washington, D.C.: U.S. Government Printing Office.

Yoos, L. September/October 1981. Compliance: Philosophical and ethical considerations. *Nurse Practitioner* 6:27, 29–30, 34.

CHAPTER 4

Health Care Delivery Systems

OBJECTIVES

Identify the roles of various health care personnel.

Describe the functions and purposes of various health care delivery systems.

Compare various systems of payment for health care services.

Describe ways in which consumers are influencing changes in health care delivery.

Relate demographic influences to health care delivery.

Describe the effects of specific social changes on health care delivery.

Explain the effects of poverty and unemployment on health care delivery.

Describe effects of the prospective payment system on health care delivery services.

Explain how political decisions affect health care delivery.

Discuss specific health care priorities and the requirements for promoting health and improving health care delivery services in the future.

Describe the implications for nursing of changes in health care delivery systems.

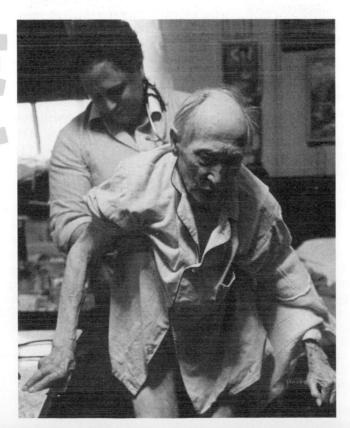

Health Care Team

Health care is the totality of services offered by all health disciplines. The **health care team** consists of health personnel from different disciplines who coordinate their skills to assist a client and/or support persons. The choice of personnel for a particular team depends on the needs of the client. In the present system of health care in North America, health teams commonly include nurses, physicians, pharmacists, dietitians, physiotherapists, respiratory therapists, occupational therapists, paramedical technologists, social workers, and chaplains.

Nurse

The role of the nurse varies with the needs of the situation. The advent of expanded nursing roles has established new dimensions for nursing practice. In the past, nursing was thought to comprise three types of skills: psychomotor, affective, and cognitive. While these skills remain important, with the acceptance of the nursing process as a framework for nursing practice and the recognition of other nursing roles, e.g., manager and counselor, the role of the nurse is seen more broadly today.

Psychomotor skills are the traditional skills of nurses. These skills involve the use of the hands. For example, manipulating equipment or repositioning a client is a psychomotor skill. **Affective skills** include the ability to incorporate cultural, attitudinal, and emotional elements into nursing. The nurse uses affective skills to individualize care. Caring and communicating activities require affective skills. **Cognitive skills** include the ability to think, recall knowledge, apply knowledge, and evaluate. Cognitive skills are required in all aspects of the nursing process.

A number of nursing personnel often participate actively on a health team. Sometimes nurses find it necessary to provide some services normally given by other members of the team, especially in settings where all the health services required by a client are not available 24 hours a day. For example, a nurse might assist a client who has had a cerebrovascular accident (stroke) by giving remedial exercises to restore function of the left arm.

Physician

A **physician** is a person who is licensed to practice medicine in a particular jurisdiction. The physician has successfully completed a course of medical studies. In a hospital setting, the physician is responsible for medical diagnosis and for determining the therapy required by a person who has a disease or injury. The traditional role of the physician is the treatment of disease and trauma (injury). However, many physicians, especially family practice physicians, are now including health promotion and disease prevention in their practice. In a community setting, the physician may be involved in diagnosis and therapy or may play a consulting role. An example of the latter is the physician who specializes in public health and who serves as a consultant to the school nurse. Some physicians extend their roles by employing a **physician's assistant** who is trained to perform certain tasks and authorized to practice under the direction of the physician.

Pharmacist

A **pharmacist** is a person who prepares and dispenses pharmaceuticals in hospital and community settings. The role of the pharmacist in monitoring and evaluating the actions and effects of medications on clients is becoming increasingly prominent. Pharmacists are also actively involved in preparing individual dosages for clients in hospitals that employ the unit dose system. In some settings, pharmacists prepare medications for intravenous therapy. A **clinical pharmacist** is a specialist who guides physicians in prescribing medications. A **pharmacy assistant** is also recognized in some states. This member of the health team administers medications to clients or works in the pharmacy under the direction of the pharmacist.

Dietitian or Nutritionist

When dietary and nutritional services are required, the dietitian or nutritionist may be a member of a health team. A **dietitian** is a person who has special knowledge about the diets required to maintain health and to treat disease. Dietitians in hospitals generally are concerned with therapeutic diets, may design special diets to meet the nutritional needs of individual clients, and supervise the preparation of the meals to ensure that clients receive the proper diet.

A **nutritionist** is a person who has special knowledge about nutrition and food. The nutritionist in a community setting recommends healthy diets and gives broad advisory services about the purchase and preparation of foods. Community nutritionists often function at the preventive level. They promote health and prevent disease, for example, by advising families about balanced diets for growing children and pregnant women.

Physiotherapist (Physical Therapist)

The physiotherapist assists clients with musculoskeletal problems. **Physiotherapists** treat the body by means of heat, water, exercise, massage, and electric current. They provide physical therapy in response to a physician's order. The physiotherapist's functions include assessing clients' mobility and strength, providing therapeutic measures (e.g., exercises and heat applications to improve mobility and strength), and teaching new skills (e.g., how to walk with an artificial leg). Most physiotherapists provide their services in hospitals; however, independent practitioners establish offices in communities and serve clients either at the office or in the home.

Respiratory Therapist

A **respiratory therapist** is skilled in therapeutic measures used in the care of clients with respiratory problems. These therapists are knowledgeable about oxygen therapy devices, intermittent positive pressure breathing respirators, artificial mechanical ventilators, and accessory devices used in inhalation therapy. Programs in respiratory therapy are offered in postsecondary educational institutions. Students complete such programs in 1 to 3 years.

Occupational Therapist

An **occupational therapist** assists clients with some impairment of function to gain the skills to perform activities of daily living. For example, a man with severe arthritis in his arms and hands might be taught how to adjust his kitchen utensils so that he can continue to cook. The therapist also teaches skills that are therapeutic and at the same time provide some satisfaction. For example, weaving is a recreational activity but also exercises the arthritic man's arms and hands. Occupational therapists coordinate their activities closely with those of other members of the health team.

Paramedical Technologists

Laboratory technologists, radiologic technologists, and nuclear medicine technologists are just three kinds of paramedical technologists in an expanding field of medical technology. **Paramedical** means having some connection with medicine. Laboratory technologists examine specimens such as urine, feces, blood, and discharges from wounds to provide the physician with exact information that facilitates the medical diagnosis and the prescription of a therapeutic regimen. The radiologic technologist assists with a wide variety of x-ray film procedures, from simple chest radiography to more complex fluoroscopy and radiography of the client's stomach using a contrast medium. The nuclear medicine technologist, a more recent member of the technology group, uses radioactive substances to provide diagnostic information, for example, about a client's liver, and can administer therapeutic doses of radioactive materials as part of a therapeutic regimen. These technologists have highly specialized skills and knowledge important to client care.

Social Worker

A **social worker** counsels clients and support persons about social problems, such as finances, marital difficulties, and adoption of children. It is not unusual for health problems to produce problems in living. For example, an elderly woman who lives alone and has a stroke resulting in impaired walking may find it impossible to continue to live in her third-floor apartment. Finding a more suitable living arrangement can be the responsibility of the social worker if the client has no support network in place. The current trends toward shorter acute care hospitalizations has lead to an increased need for rehabilitative services in skilled nursing facilities or in the home. For this reason, social workers, who usually make the placement arrangements, are playing an increasingly important role in the health care team.

Chaplains

Hospital chaplains serve as part of the health care team by attending to the spiritual needs of clients. In most facilities, local clergy volunteer their services on a regular or "on-call" basis. Hospitals affiliated with specific religions, as well as many large medical centers, have full-time chaplains on staff. They usually offer regularly scheduled religious services. The nurse is often instrumental in identifying the client's desire to see a chaplain, either by responding promptly to the client's request or by informing the client of the chaplain's services.

Health Care Agencies

Official Agencies

Government (official) agencies are established at the local, state (provincial), and federal levels. Health agencies at the state, county, or city level vary according to the need of the area. Their funds, generally from taxes, are administered by elected or appointed officials. **Local health departments** (county, bicounty, or tricounty) traditionally have responsibility for developing programs to meet the health needs of the people, providing the necessary staff and facilities to carry out these programs, continually evaluating the effectiveness of the programs, and monitoring changing needs. **State health organizations** are responsible for assisting the local health departments. In some remote areas, state departments also provide direct services to people.

The Public Health Service (PHS) of the United States Department of Health and Human Services is an official agency at the **federal** level. Its functions include conducting research and providing training in the health field, providing assistance to communities in planning and developing health facilities, and assisting states and local communities through financing and provision of trained personnel. Also at the national level in the United States are research institutions such as the National Institutes of Health (NIH). The National Institute on Drug Abuse, the National Institute on Alcohol Abuse and Alcoholism, and the National Institute of Mental Health work with federal, regional, and state agencies. The Centers for Disease Control (CDC) in Atlanta, Georgia, administer a broad program related to surveillance of diseases. By means of laboratory and epidemiologic investigations, data are made available to appropriate authorities. The CDC also publishes recommendations about the prevention and control of infections and administers a national health program. The federal government also administers a number of Veterans Administration (VA) hospitals in the United States.

The Canadian Department of Health and Welfare (CDHW) administers such federal programs as native health in the north and health care in the territories. However, provincial governments generally have responsibility for administering health services to the people of each province.

Health and Illness Services

Traditionally, the health care delivery system in North America provides two general types of services: illness care services (restorative) and health care services (preventive). Illness care services help the ill or injured. Health care services promote better health and help prevent disease and accidents. Although most facilities within the system (e.g., hospitals, clinics, and physicians' offices) provide both types of services, illness care services predominate. In recent years, however, there has been increased awareness of the need to promote health and to prevent disease. Considerable emphasis has been placed on the role of the nurse in prevention. Often the community nurse's major function is to promote wellness and prevent illness, for example, through parent and child counseling.

In the past, health care facilities have been influenced largely by the needs of the people providing the service. For example, hospitals have developed in relation to medical and technologic advances and generally reflect the needs of physicians. Also, the public viewed health care facilities as sources of help primarily for the ill or injured. As a result, preventive health care facilities have been slow to develop. This delay can be attributed in great part to three factors:

1. Physicians are largely oriented to illness in their practice.
2. Consumers have been more aware of treatment of illness than of prevention and health promotion.
3. The nurse's role as the chief provider of preventive health care and health promotion has been slow to evolve, and frequently the treatment of illness takes precedence over preventive health care activities.

In the future, increased efforts by nurses, all health professionals, and governments can be instrumental in helping people gain a greater awareness of health as a way of life. Greater emphasis must be given to the ill effects of smoking, excessive consumption of alcohol and narcotics, overuse of prescribed medications, failure to take regular exercise, unbalanced diets, and sexual promiscuity rather than treatment of the consequences of these activities. Measures to prevent disease or reduce risks must also be emphasized. Examples are immunizing children; making childbearing more safe and natural for the mother and infant; reducing the incidence of road accidents, particularly among adolescents; and preventing accidents in the home, especially among children and older people. Prevention of ill health requires the united efforts of all citizens and health care providers.

Agencies Providing Health Care

Health care agencies can be viewed as giving primary, secondary, and tertiary care.

Primary Care.

Primary care agencies are the point of entry into the health care system, i.e., the point at which initial health care is given. Primary care includes health maintenance, health promotion, and disease prevention activities. Settings for primary care are various health centers in the community, homes, schools, physicians' offices, and industry and business. Primary care is frequently inadequate in rural and economically depressed areas, due to lack of physicians. Emergency departments of hospitals are often crowded and overtaxed, in many instances with nonemergency health problems.

Ambulatory care centers are being used more frequently in many communities. They usually have diagnostic and treatment facilities and may or may not be attached to or associated with an acute care hospital. They provide medical, nursing, laboratory, and radiologic services. Some ambulatory care centers provide services to people who require minor surgical procedures that can be performed outside the hospital. After surgery, the client returns home the same day. These centers have two advantages: They permit the client to live at home while obtaining needed health care, and they free costly hospital beds for seriously ill clients. Nurses in ambulatory care centers frequently function as nurse practitioners or clinical nurse specialists, e.g., in gastroenterology or urology.

The term *ambulatory care center* has replaced the term *clinic* in many places. The term *clinic* can refer to a department in a hospital or a group practice of physicians. Traditionally, a hospital clinic was called an outpatient clinic, serving only outpatients, as opposed to those admitted to the hospital (inpatients). The role of the nurse in a clinic may be similar to that of a nurse practitioner or a nurse in a physician's office.

The **physician's office** is a traditional primary care setting in North America. The majority of physicians either have their own offices or work with several other physicians in a group practice. People usually go to a physician because they consider themselves ill, because a relative thinks the client is ill, or because the client needs medical advice.

Nurses employed in physicians' offices have a variety of roles. Some nurses carry out the traditional functions of registering the client, preparing the client for an examination or treatment, and providing information. Other nurses function as nurse practitioners and have the responsibility of providing primary care to clients in stable health.

The **industrial clinic** is gaining importance as a setting for primary care. Employee health has long been recognized as important to productivity. Today, an increasing number of companies are recognizing the value of healthy employees and encouraging healthy lifestyles. Some companies provide exercise facilities, while others provide healthy snacks, such as fruit, instead of coffee. More businesses are prohibiting smoking in the work setting.

Community health nurses in the occupational setting have a variety of roles. Worker safety has been a traditional concern of occupational nurses. Today, nursing functions include health education, screening for such health problems as hypertension and obesity, counseling, and initial care after accidents.

A **health maintenance organization (HMO)** is a group health care agency that provides basic and supplemental health maintenance and treatment services to voluntary enrollees. The enrollees prepay a fixed periodic fee that is set without regard to the amount or kind of services received. The basic idea of the HMO arose in the 1930s, when prepaid health care experiments were sponsored by unions, cooperatives, corporations, municipalities, and other organized groups. HMOs did not become popular, however, until after the passage, in 1973, of the Health Maintenance Organization Act. In 1984, 11 million people were served by HMOs (Curtin and Zurlage 1984, p. 34).

To be federally qualified, an HMO company must meet certain requirements: It must offer physicians' services, hospital and outpatient services, emergency services, short-term mental health services, treatment and referral for drug and alcohol problems, laboratory and radiologic services, preventive dental services for children under 12, and preventive health services. By encouraging preventive health care and by offering ambulatory services, HMOs have reduced the cost of health insurance to the consumer.

A client of an HMO signs a contract to pay a specified amount to the HMO for unlimited care. The plan stresses wellness; the better the health of the person, the less the client needs HMO services and the greater the agency's profit. Because of the emphasis on health promotion and prevention of illness, nurses who work in HMOs focus on these aspects of care, frequently as nurse practioners, client educators, and consultants.

Although not in every community, HMOs have been established across the United States. The largest HMO, the Kaiser-Permanente Medical Care Program, serves clients in California, Oregon, Hawaii, Ohio, and Colorado. A person with private health insurance can obtain services in most hospitals, but the clients of an HMO must use its facilities.

Crisis centers provide emergency services. The clients are often people experiencing life crises. These centers may operate out of a hospital or in the community and usually provide 24-hour telephone service. Some also provide direct counseling to people at the center or in their homes. The primary purpose of a crisis center is to help people cope with an immediate crisis and then provide guidance and support for long-term therapy.

Nurses working in crisis centers need well-developed communication and counseling skills. The nurse must immediately identify the person's problem, offer assistance to help the person cope, and perhaps later provide guidance about resources for long-term support.

■ **Secondary Care.** Secondary care focuses on preventing complications of disease conditions. It has traditionally been the province of hospitals; however, other agencies now increasingly provide this level of service. Secondary care centers of the future will focus on the treatment of temporary dysfunctions that require hospitalization but not highly skilled services and high-risk interventions, the evaluation of long-term illness that requires hospitalization to determine any needed change in treatment, and the provision of counseling and therapy that cannot be provided in a primary care center (Aydelotte 1983, p. 813). Agencies that provide secondary care include hospitals, home health agencies, and ambulatory care centers.

Hospitals traditionally have provided restorative care to the ill and injured. They vary in size from the 12-bed rural hospital to the 1500-bed metropolitan hospital with a 50-bed day surgery center. Hospitals can be classified according to their ownership or control as governmental (public) and nongovernmental (private). Governmental hospitals are either federal, state, city, or county hospitals in the United States and federal or provincial hospitals in Canada. In both countries, governments have traditionally provided hospital facilities for veterans, merchant mariners, and individuals with long-term illness.

Although hospitals are chiefly viewed as institutions that provide care, they have other functions, such as providing resources for health-related research and teaching. Hospital personnel may conduct research and educational programs, or they may provide resources for such personnel as university teachers to carry out research and teaching responsibilities.

Hospitals also are classified by the services they provide. General hospitals admit clients requiring a variety of services, including medical, surgical, obstetric, pediatric, and psychiatric services. Other hospitals offer only specialty services, such as psychiatric or pediatric care.

Hospitals can be further described as acute or chronic. An acute hospital provides assistance to clients who are acutely ill or whose illness and need for hospitalization are relatively short-term, for example, 2 days to perhaps 1 month. From 1968 to 1983, the average short stay in nonfederal United States hospitals decreased from 8.5 days to 6.9 days (U.S. DHHS 1985a, p. 15). Long-term hospitals provide health services for longer periods, sometimes for years or the remainder of the client's life.

Hospitals in the United States are undergoing massive change. In the past, hospitals were virtually the sole providers of secondary care; however, ambulatory care centers and HMOs have forced hospitals to reorganize and adopt different practices. In 1986, many acute care hospital beds remained empty, and some hospitals ran at less than 60% capacity. Some hospitals have merged or sold out to large multihospital for-profit corporations, e.g., Humana, Inc., and Hospital Corporation of America. Other hospitals are providing innovative services, such as fitness classes, day care for elderly people, and nutrition classes. Some hospitals have even established alternative birth centers (ABCs) to attract new families.

In the United States today, all but the most seriously ill are treated outside of a hospital. Because so many of these are elderly, some general hospitals are becoming acute care hospitals solely for the elderly. Because of the increasing acuity of illness among clients, general hospitals are becoming intensive care centers.

▪ Tertiary Care.

Tertiary care is also called rehabilitation or long-term care. It is largely provided through home health care, long-term care facilities, rehabilitation centers, and hospices. **Home health care agencies** are rapidly becoming major tertiary care providers. Home care is one aspect of comprehensive health care. Its purposes include promoting, maintaining, and restoring health, specifically maximizing independent functioning and minimizing the disabling effects of illness, including terminal illness. Services appropriate to the needs of clients and their families are planned, coordinated, and delivered by providers organized for the delivery of home health care through the use of contractual arrangements, employed staff, or a combination of the two (Warhola 1980).

Home care services are appropriate when an individual or family does not need full-time care, observation, or the special facilities of an institution such as a hospital or nursing home, yet does need care that family members or others cannot provide without assistance or teaching. Home care may or may not be associated with a hospitalization. It may precede or follow institutional care in a hospital or long-term care facility, or it may be provided along with ambulatory care (Lundberg 1984). Self-care and care given by health professionals and allied health personnel in the home account for the majority of health care provided in this country today. The time a person spends in a hospital receiving care for acute conditions is generally a very small percentage of his or her life. The need for home care services is increasing as the population of the United States ages and the incidence of chronic illness increases correspondingly (Lundberg 1984). Demand for home care services has increased for three reasons:

1. The costs of health care have inflated markedly, reflecting:
   - ▪ Increased cost of equipment, energy, and labor
   - ▪ Changes in supply and demand
   - ▪ Increased use of highly technical and specialized services
   - ▪ Little out-of-pocket expense to the consumer of health care (Davis 1983)
2. Efforts by the federal government and the health care industry to contain health care costs have resulted in shorter hospital stays and greater awareness and acceptance of home care services by providers and consumers.
3. Broader third-party coverage for care at home has become available.

The nature of home care services has broadened to include both acute, short-term care as well as long-term monitoring of problems associated with chronic illness. Comprehensive home care includes both direct and indirect services.

Direct services involve direct contact between a caregiver and a client for the purposes of administering treatment or nursing care measures, assessment, teaching, counseling, or planning care. Direct services provided may be complex technical procedures, such as intravenous chemotherapy for cancer and respiratory therapy. Such services are becoming more widely available at home. Symptom management, teaching for self-care, monitoring adaptation to long-term illness, family counseling, physical and occupational therapy, and nutritional counseling are direct services provided by a variety of home care agencies. Such basic nursing care measures as bathing, skin care, assistance with ambulation, toileting, feeding, dressing changes, catheter care, and administration of medications have long been and continue to be direct service components of home care. Home care nursing also includes such direct services as providing ongoing assessment, anticipating and planning for problems or crises before they occur, helping clients think through problems and their options for dealing with them, managing symptoms, teaching, counseling, and assisting individuals and families to meet their health care goals.

Indirect services in home care include those measures taken to provide or facilitate direct services in nursing practice (McCorkle and Germino 1984). Consulting with other professionals and allied health personnel about client problems and needs, coordinating care within the home care agency, coordinating community resources and referrals outside the agency, supervising allied health workers providing services, and evaluating the effectiveness of care provided are all examples of indirect services currently provided by home care nurses. In addition, nurses involved in home care may be liaisons with acute care facilities and serve as facilitators and contact persons for clients and families who need access to special health care resources.

▪ Long-Term Care Facilities.

There are a wide variety of **long-term care facilities.** Traditionally, they were all called nursing homes; however, the increase in the elderly and chronically ill population has given rise to a variety of facilities to assist these clients. Long-term care facilities now include skilled nursing facilities for extended care, intermediate care, and personal care for those who are chronically ill or are no longer able to care for themselves without assistance.

Because long-term illness occurs most often in the elderly, many long-term care facilities have programs that are oriented to the needs of this age group. Nursing homes are intended for people who require not only personal services (such as assistance in bathing and dressing, and meal preparation) but also some regular nursing care and occasional medical attention. However, the type of care provided varies considerably. Some admit and retain only residents who can dress themselves and are ambulatory. Other long-term care facilities provide bed care for clients who are more incapacitated. Nursing homes can, in effect, become the clients' home, and consequently the people who live there are frequently referred to as residents rather than patients or clients.

t's not easy outliving your family and friends

As a new graduate, I was certain of one thing: I would never work in a nursing home. Old people depressed me. More than that, they frightened me. The blank expressions of elderly patients who sat alone in hallways and solariums gave me an eerie feeling. I was sure I couldn't help them—even if I wanted to.

Life seemed clearer to these patients, with their serenity and keen insight. Through them, such historical events as World War I, the Great Depression, and the invention of the telephone took on new meanings. They had lived them—I had only read about them.

I began to look past physical diabilities to their extraordinary mental capabilities. Each coped with pain, changes in body image, diminished sensory acuity, loneliness, the death of loved ones, and his own impending death.

Sorrow is intense for these special people as they wrap up their lives. They talk of lost spouses, homes they will never see again, talents they no longer have. In school we are told to concentrate on strengths, not weaknesses, but in the quiet moments it is so necessary to allow the sad feelings to emerge and be acknowledged.

"I'm lonely and blue today," said one 97-year-old when I asked how she was. I encouraged her to go on, and she said, "It's not easy outliving all of your family and friends. I'm alone now and I wish my time would come. I've had a good life and I'm tired now. Please don't tell me not to say this, but I wish I would die." Was I supposed to argue with such insight?

Nursing the older adult poses unique problems, too. One 94-year-old, known all her life for her refined manner and poise, was crippled by advanced osteoarthritis. She could do little for herself, yet, a proud woman, she could not bring herself to ask for help.

By the time she entered the nursing home she was dehydrated, malnourished, and had an impaction and two large pressure sores. It would have been easy to respond with anger or intolerance. ("She knew better. Why didn't she get help sooner?") But after getting to know her, and thinking more about her bitter struggle against dependency, I understood.

I also learned to evaluate each older patient's ability to help with his own care. A blind woman who came to the nursing home for recovery after a cholecystectomy progressed well, but allowed herself to be fed. One day, at a particularly busy dinner hour, I noticed that she was eating without help. She had thought she was supposed to let the nurses feed her. Just because she was elderly and blind, we had assumed the worst.

Source: T. T. Fulmer: Lessons from a nursing home, *American Journal of Nursing*, March 1987, 87(3): 333.

■ Rehabilitation Centers. Rehabilitation centers usually are independent community centers or special units in hospitals. However, rehabilitation ideally starts the moment a client enters the health care system. Thus, nurses are involved in rehabilitation whether they are employed on pediatric, psychiatric, or surgical units of hospitals or in the community. A rehabilitation process usually has four broad objectives:

1. To return affected abilities to the highest possible level of function
2. To prevent further disability
3. To protect the client's present abilities
4. To assist the client to use his or her abilities

The concept of rehabilitation has gained considerable acceptance during the past 40 years. Before that time, it was generally associated with vocational help and social guidance for people who had physical injuries, often as a result of accidents at work. Today, the concept is applied to all illness (physical and mental), to injury, and to chemical addiction. Rehabilitation affects every age group and segment of society. **Rehabilitation** is a process of restoring people to useful function in physical, mental, social, economic, and vocational areas of their lives. Rehabilitation, then, is a process of restoring people to their previous level of health (i.e., to their previous capabilities) or to the level that is possible for them. Rehabilitation, as distinct from maintenance, is an active concept and can be considered largely an educational function. Clients must participate actively in the process if it is to be effective.

■ Hospice Services. A hospice, traditionally, was a place where travelers could rest. Recently, the term has come to mean a health care facility for the dying. The hospice movement subsumes a variety of services given to the terminally ill, their families, and support persons. The movement sprang initially from dissatisfaction with the preoccupation of health personnel with technologic care and insufficient emphasis on caring and psychologic support. In the 1970s, the movement gained momentum. It derived impetus from new attitudes toward death and from the work of such people as Elisabeth Kübler-Ross, whose books challenged prevailing attitudes, and Cicely Saunders, founder of St. Christopher's Hospice in London. Saunders believed that the physical and social environments of dying people are as important as medical interventions on their behalf.

In recent years, hospices have provided a variety of services to terminally ill clients and their families; indeed, hospices have inspired a social movement. Basic to the movement is a humanistic belief in the individuality of people and their needs. Hospice programs are institution and community based. A 1982 survey by the Joint

Commission on Accreditation of Hospitals (JCAH) found that of 1145 hospice services surveyed, 40% were situated in a hospital or institution and 60% were community based (Pryga and Bachofer 1983). Some supply services in the home, either directly or through community resources. Reimbursement for these services is variable, often voluntary.

Hospices are a haven for the dying because they emphasize the needs of the individual and help clients and their families plan for death. The central concept of the hospice movement, as distinct from the acute care model, is not saving life but improving or maintaining the quality of life until death. Important in this care are palliative measures for relief rather than cure. Comfort and relief from pain are frequently the most important needs of the dying. Hospice care addresses the needs of the mind and the spirit as well: It is truly holistic.

Financing Health Care Services

In the United States, medical costs increased 12.5% between 1981 and 1982 (Griffith 1983, p. 262). Funding for personal health care can come from a variety of sources: Governments (social insurance), the client, and health insurance are the major sources.

Social Insurance

Federal funding is largely through the social insurance programs Medicare and Medicaid in the United States, and the National Hospital Insurance program and the National Medical Care Insurance program in Canada. A nationally funded program to cover the health costs of all United States citizens has been discussed for the past 15 years.

United States. In the United States, the 1965 **Medicare** amendments (Title 18) to the Social Security Act provided a national and state health insurance program for the aged. By the mid 1970s, virtually everyone over 65 years was protected by hospital insurance under Part A, which also includes posthospital extended care and home health benefits. Medicaid was established the same year under Title 19 of the Social Security Act. **Medicaid** is a federal public assistance program paid out of general taxes to people who require financial assistance, i.e., low-income groups.

In 1972, Congress directed the Department of Health, Education, and Welfare to create professional standards review organizations (PSROs) to monitor the appropriateness of hospital use under the Medicare and Medicaid programs. In 1974, the National Health Planning and Resources Development Act established health systems agencies (HSAs) throughout the United States for comprehensive health planning. In 1978, the Rural Health Clinics Act provided for the development of health care in medically underserved rural areas. This act opened the door for nurse practitioners to provide primary care.

In addition, disabled or blind persons may be eligible for special payments called **Supplemental Security Income** (SSI) benefits. These benefits are also available to people not eligible for Social Security, and payments are not restricted to health care costs. Clients often use this money to purchase medicines or to cover costs of extended health care.

To control costs of Medicare and Medicaid, the federal government passed legislation in 1983 governing a prospective pricing plan as part of a Social Security amendment. The amount of the reimbursement to hospitals is based on diagnostic related groups (DRGs).

Canada. The Canadian National Hospital Insurance program was started in 1958, and the National Medical Care Insurance program (Medicare) began in 1968. Through these programs, every Canadian can obtain health insurance. Not all hospital and medical services are insured by provincial hospital insurance or Medicare plans; there are slight differences between provinces. Also, not all physicians participate in their provincial or territorial plans, in which case the individual pays the physician directly (Crichton et al. 1984, p. 5). These insurance plans are paid for by federal and provincial governments and by individuals able to pay. In 1984, the Canada Health Act was passed by Parliament to provide federal government reimbursement to provincial governments for health services they provide.

Voluntary Insurance

Health care costs are also covered by private insurance plans. The costs of these insurance plans, such as Blue Shield and Blue Cross, are borne by the individual or shared by the employer and the employee. One type of voluntary health insurance is the prepaid group plan offered by HMOs. Prepaid group plans provide for services required by the participants 24 hours a day. By advance payment, the individual takes out insurance against any health requirements in the future. These plans place heavy emphasis on promotion of health and prevention of disease and injury among participants.

Workmen's Compensation

Workers who are injured on the job may collect workmen's compensation payments during their recovery. In some instances, all health care costs are paid by workmen's compensation. Employer companies contribute to a workmen's compensation fund to make money available when accidents occur.

Charitable Resources

Charitable resources for medical payments are supported by donations from individuals or groups and by bequests. Charitable donations are still made by some philanthropic organizations to assist the poor and to support innovations. On the whole, however, charitable donations as a means of paying for health care are declining in importance.

Current Influences and Changes

Consumer Influences

Rights and Values.
North Americans generally believe that all persons have a right to health care regardless of race, culture, or economic status. In addition, most believe that all persons are entitled to health care that prevents disease, treats disease, and restores ill persons to their previous state of health. In 1966, the World Health Organization stated that health care is a universal human right. This belief has led to the United States Medicare and Medicaid programs, which strive to provide health care to those who cannot afford it. In Canada, the National Hospital Insurance program and the National Medical Care Insurance program (Medicare) provide benefits for all Canadian citizens.

Comprehensive, holistic, and humanistic health care is being emphasized today. People want comprehensive care. They want to have their health care needs met at one time at one agency rather than to seek help for an abdominal pain at one place, for a tooth problem at another place, and for an emotional problem at yet another. Holistic health practitioners emphasize the effects of one problem on the person as biopsychosocial whole. Consumers, therefore, expect health care that reflects this view of the total person and his or her roles and functions. The humanistic values desired include recognition of inherent worth, individual uniqueness, wholeness, freedom of action, equality of status, and shared decision making between the client and health care practitioner.

Mutual Support and Self-Help Groups.
In North America today, there are more than 500 mutual support or *self-help groups* that focus on nearly every major health problem or life crisis people experience. Such groups arose largely because people felt their needs were not being met by the existing health care system. Alcoholics Anonymous, which formed in 1935, served as the model for many of these groups. The National Self-Help Clearinghouse provides information on current support groups and guidelines about how to start a self-help group. Groups vary in effectiveness, but most provide education to encourage self-care as well as social and emotional support. Before referring clients to specific groups, the nurse needs to assess the group's effectiveness and availability to the client.

The consumer self-help movement has generated an abundance of newsletters, hotlines, health and medical self-help books, conferences, and workshops related to health promotion and management of chronic disease. This phenomenon indicates in part that consumers want more information and assistance to gain self-control of their primary health needs.

Health Promotion.
In the past few decades, many North Americans have come to expect more of the health care system than disease prevention or cure.

Consumers today are more aware and knowledgeable about the effects of life-style on health. As a result, they desire more information and services related to health promotion and illness prevention. Although the diagnosis and treatment of illness are still a necessity, the focus of health care has changed. Traditionally, health care was viewed as synonymous with professional and medical care. Now health care professionals are increasingly viewed as a supplementary resource for individuals carrying out their own health maintenance and health promotion activities. As a result, a wide range of health promotion programs have arisen. Some are provided through the traditional health care agencies, but many are developing in community facilities along with physical fitness centers. The media, too, reflect this change. It is not rare for characters in movies, for instance, to exhibit positive health behaviors, such as exercising and not smoking. In Canada, alcohol and tobacco advertisements have been restricted.

Social Influences

Social influences such as the women's movement, changes in family characteristics, increasing population, environmental changes, and cultural diversity all affect the health care delivery system.

Women's Movement.
The women's movement has been instrumental in changing health care practices. Examples are the provision of childbirth services in more relaxed hospital settings or the home, the provision of overnight facilities for parents in children's hospitals, and the attention being paid to premenstrual tension syndrome and unnecessary surgeries (e.g., some radical mastectomies and hysterectomies) performed on women. The literature on the health concerns of women and research into women's unique health experiences are growing. More nursing research is needed in every aspect of women's health. See Chapter 2 for more discussion of the impact of the women's movement.

Family Characteristics.
The characteristics of the North American family have changed considerably in the last few decades. There is a marked increase in single-parent families because of divorce and increased acceptance of children born out of wedlock. Most single-parent families are headed by women. The number of families headed by single females has doubled since 1960 and account for almost 15% of all United States families (U.S. Bureau of the Census 1980). A concern about households headed by females is that many such households have a low standard of living. The incomes of the majority of female heads of households are under the poverty level (Griffith-Kenney 1986, p. 51). Serious illness or hospitalization can create major financial and home management difficulties for single-parent families. See Chapter 30 for additional information on families.

Increasing Population.
Statistics reflect an increase in the total population and indicate the need for increased health services. In both the United States and Canada, there has been tremendous population

growth, particularly since 1945. The impact of the growing elderly population on the health care system is a major social issue. About 30 cents of each health care dollar in the United States are allocated to this group, which now exceeds 28 million and comprises almost 12% of the population (U.S. Department of Commerce 1984).

By the year 2030, it is estimated that the elderly will number 50 million, comprising 17% of the population (U.S. DHEW 1979, p. 71). In Canada, a similar increase in the number of older people is anticipated: from 1.9 million in 1976 (Statistics Canada 1980, p. 10) to 3.2 million by the year 2000. By the year 2031, 21% of the population will be over age 65 (Statistics Canada 1981). Since only 5% of older people are institutionalized because of health problems, substantial home management and nursing support services are required to assist those in their homes and communities.

The frail aged population over age 85 is the second fastest growing population in North America, exceeded only by the "baby boom" generation now between 30 and 45. Numbering more than 2.6 million, this group is expected to increase to 5 million by the year 2000 (U.S. Bureau of the Census 1980). More research into the health and economic conditions of this population is needed.

Because people over 65 are becoming an increasingly large part of the population, their health needs deserve special concern. Long-term illnesses are most prevalent in this group, and these illnesses frequently make special housing, treatment services, and financial support necessary. The elderly need to feel they are still part of a community even though they are approaching the end of their lives. Feelings of being useful, wanted, and productive citizens are essential to their health. Special programs are being designed in communities so that the talents and skills of this group will be used and not lost to society. These programs—e.g., partial employment—are designed especially for the elderly person.

▪ **Environmental Change.** Air and water pollution from industrial waste is a notable change in this century. Many cities publish a daily air quality index so that persons with respiratory disease will know whether the outside air is safe to breathe. Tragic industrial and nuclear leaks are also of concern.

Many work environments also pose health hazards for employees. Coal miners and textile workers are prone to lung disease. Construction workers are prone to asbestosis. Increasingly, the public is demanding smokeless air in work settings. Many corporations and cities have already banned smoking in certain work areas.

▪ **Cultural Diversity.** The health care system of North America reflects largely Western, white values and does not adequately accommodate the values of the many different cultural groups living in this country. Language barriers and inequities in income and education hinder access of minority ethnic groups to health care. The more sophisticated and impersonal health services become, the less accessible they are to ethnic groups, who are often inwardly oriented, have a strong

family tradition, and prefer personalized care from someone who understands them and their families. Many such people look on the modern health care system with distrust. See Chapter 17 for more information about cultural diversity.

▪ Economic Influences

The health care delivery system is very much affected by a country's total economic status. Inflation and the economic recession of the early 1980s have brought increasing concern about escalating health care costs. The United States spends $1 billion a day on health care, and costs are still rising. Medical care costs have increased more than 400% since 1965. Some reasons for this sizable increase are advanced techniques and technology, inflation, increased utilization of health services, and the system of payment for hospitals and physicians.

▪ **Prospective Payment System (PPS).** Efforts to curtail health care costs in the United States were made in 1983, when Congress passed legislation putting the **prospective payment system** into effect. This legislation limits the amount paid to hospitals that are reimbursed by Medicare. Reimbursement is made according to a classification system known as **diagnostic related groups (DRGs).** The system has categories that establish pretreatment diagnosis billing categories.

Under this system, the hospital is paid a predetermined amount for clients with a specific diagnosis. For example, a hospital that admits a client with a diagnosis of uncomplicated asthma is reimbursed a specified amount, such as $1300, regardless of the cost of services, the length of the stay, or the acuity or complexity of the client's illness. In the past, Medicare reimbursed hospitals according to the reasonable cost of services provided to its clients. The hospital billed retrospectively, after the services were rendered. In contrast, prospective payment or billing is formulated before the client is even admitted to the hospital; thus, the record of admission, rather than the record of treatment, now governs payment. DRG rates are set in advance of the prospective year during which they apply and are considered fixed except for major, uncontrollable occurrences. The prospective rates are paid by clients and/or third parties.

This legislation has had a tremendous impact on health care delivery in the United States, since the providers of care, rather than Medicare or other third-party payers, run the risk of monetary losses. If a hospital's cost per case exceeds the defined limit, it incurs a loss; if the cost is less than the defined limit, it receives a surplus. Thus, PPS offers financial incentives for withholding unnecessary tests or procedures and avoiding prolonged hospital stays.

Notable effects of the DRG system to date are earlier discharge of clients, a decline in admissions, and a reduction of services provided and staff, especially nurse's aides and LPN/LVN staff. With the decline in admissions, most clients now admitted are seriously ill and have multiple health problems. Many hospitals are now employing only registered nurses (RNs), believing that RNs can provide the broadest range of nursing care. The earlier discharge of clients has given rise to home care agencies that provide needed home nursing care.

Some disadvantages of the DRG system are (Bentley and Butler 1980):

1. DRGs fail to include all diagnoses and procedures.
2. Assignment to a DRG depends on the documentation of the attending physician and the conventions of the individual coder.
3. DRGs reflect the state of medical practice and technology at the time of their development and do not account for advances in diagnostic procedures or therapies.
4. DRGs provide neither a standard of what should be done nor a measure of the quality of care, since they are based solely on data about length of stay.
5. Since surgical procedures are often associated with high reimbursement rates, there is the possibility that the number of unnecessary surgical procedures will increase.

To protect clients from DRG abuses, Medicare introduced state peer review organizations (PROs). Made up of physicians and other health care professionals, PROs are intended to monitor the hospitals and ensure high-quality care under DRGs. PROs have developed screening guidelines that govern whether admissions or procedures should occur and are used to review records, render payment decisions, and handle difficulties. Some people question the conflict of interest in the dual obligation of PROs, to ensure quality and contain costs (Hamilton 1986, p. 43).

The implication of DRGs for nursing education, practice, and research are many, since the system was developed without explicit attention to nursing costs or the use of nursing resources. The Health Care Financing Administration (HCFA) funds research to study alternative systems for classifying severity of illness through nursing diagnosis (Caterinicchio 1984, p. 130) and to shed light on the relationship between DRGs, nursing resource utilization, and nursing costs (American Nurses' Association 1985).

■ **Unemployment and Poverty.** Unemployment and poverty, whether the result of recessions, new microchip technology, or inadequate education and technical skills, affect which health services are offered and used. Because the unemployed do not receive employment-based health insurance, they do not use health care services to the same extent as the general population. Such people tend to defer needed dental or medical care. Even though some government aid is available, eligibility for government insurance programs and benefits varies considerably from state to state. Chapter 17 includes a discussion of poverty as a subculture. Canada's economic problems are similar to those of the United States; however, the overall effects are not always as apparent because Canada has a smaller population. The National Health Care program in Canada ensures medical care and hospitalization for the poor and unemployed.

The detrimental effects of unemployment and poverty on health have not been properly determined. Some studies reveal a higher incidence of depression, asthma, headache, and backache among the unemployed and higher suicide and homicide rates. When widespread unemployment persists for 2 to 3 years, deaths from heart disease increase (O'Neill 1983, p. 139). When the breadwinner loses a job, the family is forced to change its life-style. Coping methods used to overcome stress may not always be advantageous. For example, mothers may go hungry to see that their children are well fed. Older people may skimp on food to the point of suffering vitamin deficiencies. Poverty not only results in more illness among pregnant mothers, children, and unemployed breadwinners but also exacerbates the effects of alcoholism, such as wife and child abuse (O'Neill 1983). Those who offer health care services to the poor need to consider these factors.

▪ Political Influences

Health care is affected by political decisions. For example, political decisions affect health insurance programs, health care funding, allocation of resources (people, money, and equipment), and laws governing the duties of health care workers and the rights of clients, e.g., of women to have abortions. The attitude of people in government health ministries largely determines whether the focus of health care delivery is primary care, secondary care, or tertiary care. *Political activity by nurses* (see Chapter 2) *is essential.*

Challenges for the Future

Achieving the goal of equal access to appropriate health care for all people in the future requires the efforts of all people and a focus on the following (O'Neill 1983, pp. 117–18):

1. Establishment of community-based health systems in which primary health care is the major function.
2. Redistribution of health and specialty services to overcome regional inequities.
3. Emphasis on self-reliance and participation by the individual and community members in health matters.
4. Increased emphasis on provision of services to specific target groups, such as children and adolescents, the elderly, the disabled, the dying, single mothers, the mentally ill, and working mothers.
5. Increased involvement of existing health organizations and groups.
6. Expanded education of nurse practitioners, nurses, nurse-midwives, and medical practitioners in community and health care as well as traditional hospital and acute care.
7. Expansion of traditional roles and change in the current hierarchical health profession to emphasize cooperation as health care professionals work together to provide leadership in promoting health

I expect the nurse to sit with me when I cry

I expect the nurse to treat me as she would any other human being without regard to age, creed, or color.

I expect the nurse to give me my bath and realize that my circulation is poor although my skin is purplish brown. I also expect the nurse to know that my dry wrinkled skin doesn't need to be bathed every day. Plus, when my skin is bathed, I need an extra amount of lubricating lotion or oil.

I expect the nurse to realize that I don't understand her fancy words and I am embarrassed when I don't know the right words to use when I have to tell her about private parts of my body.

I expect the nurse to look directly at me and talk slowly because I have trouble hearing sometimes. I expect the nurse to answer my light promptly because I can't control my body eliminations well and once I am on the bedpan my back hurts. I expect the nurse to give me a gentle back rub to ease away my pain.

I expect the nurse to understand when I ask her to oil my hair because my scalp is dry, and be aware that it is my subcultural custom to not have my hair dampened when I take a shower.

I expect the nurse to allow me to use my Vicks at night and to recognize my need for liniment to put on my sore aching joints.

I expect the nurse to sit with me when I cry and be there when I need her and to not always send less qualified people to take care of me.

Perlilure Drake
Age 76, Alabama

Source: P. Drake, Older authors of the year, (First Prize), *Geriatric Nursing*, May/June 1983.

care systems that address the needs of clients while meeting society's needs as well.

8. New focus by government on health rather than cure and on the roles that transportation, housing, and industry ministries can play in bringing about a healthy society.

Humanizing Health Care

Although the goal of any health care delivery system (i.e., to protect the healthy and care for the sick) is intrinsically human, the system is perceived as increasingly dehumanizing. Highly specialized techniques and new knowledge emerging during the past 30 years mean that an increasing number of health personnel provide specialized services. They may be highly specialized technicians or technologists who have relatively narrow but exacting jobs, such as respiratory technologists, biomedical electronic technologists, and nuclear medicine technologists. Increased specialization is evident also among physicians. All this specialization means fragmentation of care and sometimes less than desirable total care.

To clients, it may mean receiving care from 5 to 30 people during their hospital experience. This seemingly endless stream of personnel is often confusing and frightening. The client feels like a cog in the wheel and asks, "Who really cares about me?" and "Who is really responsible?" This proliferation of health personnel can impede the smooth flow of information and undermine plans to help the client. The concept of total and humanistic care is more difficult to implement when so many people are involved.

Dehumanization is associated with vulnerability, powerlessness, and loss of identity in large, faceless institutions. The blame usually falls on society in general, technologic change, the rat race, or bureaucratic red tape. Howard and Strauss (1975) discuss ways nurses and other health care professionals can humanize care:

1. Health systems recognize the inherent worth of persons by trying to prolong life, reduce pain, and restore social functioning. Clients themselves emphasize that they should be treated with dignity and respect even if discriminated against in the larger society. The concept of inherent worth needs to apply to professional/client interactions and must be reflected in institutional policy.
2. Humanized care demands an orientation toward clients as individuals. At any given moment, the sum of a person's past and present experience influences the person's feelings, attitudes, and actions.
3. Clients are restricted by such factors as illness, ignorance, and financial constraints. Practitioners are restricted by institutional commitments, colleague pressures, scarce resources for therapy, and cost considerations. Shared decision making and responsibility reflect the ideology that all clients, regardless of education, have a right to participate as much as possible in decisions about their care.
4. Clients expect health care professionals to show sympathy and concern. Otherwise, clients feel depersonalized and dehumanized. In some instances, it may be impossible to put oneself in the client's shoes.

Implications for Nursing

The changes and future trends in the health care system have many implications for nursing practice. Aydelotte (1983, pp. 814–15) described the following:

1. Greater need for nurses to function in primary care
2. Increased demands for nurses to improve their assessment and evaluation skills

3. Increased skills in communication, e.g., a second language or computer skills
4. Increased knowledge and acceptance of cultural diversity
5. Increased acceptance of change
6. Increased use of technology in teaching clients
7. Increased need for leadership skills for functioning in corporate structures

In addition, nurses will need to:

1. Clarify the nurse's unique role in health care delivery. Much of the current work by nurse theorists and nurse researchers has this objective.
2. Expand the nurse's role in primary care in hospitals, homes, and industry and convince the public and government that such services would coordinate care, decrease fragmentation, and be cost efficient.
3. Design nursing strategies to meet the health promotion and health maintenance needs of people, especially the elderly, low-income persons, rural residents, the chronically ill, the unemployed, pregnant women, working women, children, and adolescents.
4. Research the costs of nursing care in relation to DRG categories and conduct research concerning quality assurance to ensure that cost containment measures do not affect the quality of nursing care provided.

Chapter Highlights

- Health care services are provided by a variety of health care personnel in a variety of settings.
- Government health care agencies, established at the local, state (provincial), and federal levels, are supported by revenues obtained through taxes.
- Agencies providing health care can be viewed as giving primary, secondary, and tertiary care.
- Primary care agencies focus on health maintenance, health promotion, and disease prevention.
- Several alternative health care delivery systems, such as health maintenance organizations, preferred provider organizations, and individual practice associations, have arisen in the past decade to encourage preventive health care and to reduce the cost of health care to the consumer.
- Secondary care agencies, such as hospitals and ambulatory care clinics, focus on the treatment of illness and the prevention of complications of disease conditions.
- Tertiary care agencies provide long-term care and rehabilitation services and focus on restoring the client to optimum functioning after physical or mental illness.
- A variety of hospice services meet the special needs of the terminally ill in settings other than acute care agencies; caring and psychologic support are emphasized.
- Health care services are currently financed through social insurance, such as Medicaid and Medicare in the United States and the National Medical and Hospital Insurance programs in Canada; direct client payments; voluntary insurance plans, such as Blue Cross and Blue Shield; and charitable donations.
- The prospective payment system (PPS) was introduced in the United States to curtail the escalating costs of health care.
- Because of fewer hospital admissions, earlier discharges, and staff reductions—the results of PPS—the need for home health care has increased.
- Consumer attitudes—their view of health care as a right and their demand for comprehensive, holistic, and humanistic health care—are noticeably influencing health care delivery.
- Consumers are demanding greater emphasis on health promotion and illness prevention rather than on treatment of disease.
- The idea that health is the responsibility of each individual in society is gaining greater acceptance.
- Social changes, such as the women's movement, the rise in single-parent families and in women working outside the home, cultural diversity, and the growing elderly population, are influencing the type and quantity of health care services needed.
- The unemployed and poverty-stricken have unique health care needs that require increasing attention.
- Future challenges in health care delivery are to promote health as a way of life, to prevent ill health, and to provide community care for all.
- In the future, nurses will need to be prepared to practice in primary care settings and to develop the skills to work in these settings.

Selected References

American Nurses' Association. Center for Research. June 1985. *DRGs and nursing care.* Kansas City, Mo.: American Nurses' Association.

Archer, S. E., and Fleshman, R. P., editors. 1985. *Community health services.* Monterey, Calif.: Wadsworth Health Sciences.

Aydelotte, M. K. 1983. The future health care delivery system in the United States. In Chaska, N. L., editor. *The nursing profession: A time to speak.* New York: McGraw-Hill.

Bentley, J. D., and Butler, P. 1980. Case mix reimbursements: Measures, applications, experiments. *Hospital Financial Management* 3:14.

Caterinicchio, R. P., editor. 1984. *DRGs: What they are and how to survive them—A sourcebook for professional nursing.* Thorofare, N.J.: Charles B. Slack.

Crichton, A.; Lawrence, J.; and Lee, S. 1984. *Doctors and patients negotiate the system of care: Readings. The Canadian Health Care System.* Vol. 1. Ottawa: Canadian Hospital Association.

Curtin, L. L., and Zurlage, C. 1984. *DRGs: The reorganization of health.* Chicago: S-N Publications.

Davis, C. K. 1983. The federal role in changing health care financing. *Nursing Economics* 1:10–17.

Griffith, H. September/October 1983. Competition in health care. *Nursing Outlook* 31:262–65.

———. May 1985. Who will become the preferred provider? *American Journal of Nursing* 85:538–42.

Griffith-Kenney, J. 1986. *Contemporary women's health: A*

nursing advocacy approach. Menlo Park, Calif.: Addison-Wesley Publishing Co.

Hamilton, J. January/February 1986. Consumer alert: DRGs—Are hospitals saving money at your expense? *American Health* 41–45.

Howard, J., and Strauss, A., editors. 1975. *Humanizing health care.* New York: John Wiley and Sons.

Lundberg, C. J. 1984. Home health care: A logical extension of hospital services. *Topics in Health Care Financing* 11:22–33.

McCorkle, R., and Germino, B. 1984. What nurses need to know about home care. *Oncology Nursing Forum* 11(6):63–69.

Morris, E. M., and Fonseca, J. D. 1984. Home care today: An interview. *American Journal of Nursing* 84(3):340–42.

O'Neill, P. 1983. *Health crisis 2000.* London: William Heinemann.

Pryga, E., and Bachofer, H. June 24, 1983. *Hospice care under Medicare.* Working paper. Chicago: Office of Public Policy Analysis, American Hospital Association. Cited in Amenta, M. O. September/October 1984. Hospice U.S.A. 1984: Steady and holding. *Oncology Nursing Forum* 11:68–74.

Rutkowski, B. L. March/April 1985. DRGs: Now all eyes are on you. *Nursing Life* 5:26–29.

Shaffer, F. A., editor. 1984. *DRGs: Changes and challenges.* New York: National League for Nursing.

Smith, C. E. January 1985. DRGs: Making them work for you. *Nursing 85* 15:34–41.

Statistics Canada. 1980. *Perspectives Canada III.* Ottawa: Minister of Supply and Services.

————. 1981. *Canada year book 1980–81.* Ottawa: Statistics Canada.

U.S. Bureau of the Census. 1980. *Statistical abstract of the United States.* 101st ed. Washington, D.C.: U.S. Government Printing Office.

U.S. Department of Commerce. July 1, 1984. *Statistics on elderly population.* Washington, D.C.: Bureau of the Census.

U.S. Department of Health and Human Services. August 1985a. *Charting the nation's health trends since 1960.* Pub. no. (PHS) 85-1251. Hyattsville, Md.: Public Health Service.

U.S. Department of Health, Education, and Welfare. 1979. *Healthy people: The surgeon general's report on health promotion and disease prevention.* Pub. no. 79-55071. Washington, D.C.: U.S. Government Printing Office.

Warhola, C. 1980. *Planning for home health services: A resource book.* Pub. no. (HRA) 80-14017. Washington, D.C.: Public Health Service, Department of Health and Human Services.

Weinstein, S. M. 1984. Specialty teams in home care. *American Journal of Nursing* 84(3):342–45.

CHAPTER 5

Ethical Aspects of Nursing

OBJECTIVES

Define selected terms pertaining to values, rights, and ethics.

Identify various ways in which values, beliefs, and attitudes are learned.

Distinguish between personal and professional values.

Describe reasons for identifying clients' values.

Outline the essentials of the Patient's Bill of Rights established by the American Hospital Association.

Discuss professional and personal rights of nurses.

Identify five rights of students of nursing according to the Student Bill of Rights.

Describe the nurse's role in relation to clients' rights.

Discuss how nurses can protect clients' rights.

Describe the purposes of codes of ethics.

Identify professional values incorporated in nursing codes of ethics.

Explain some ways in which personal values can conflict with professional responsibilities.

Give some examples of ethical issues between nurses and their peers.

Give some examples of ethical issues between nurses and clients, nurses and other health professionals, and nurses and health care agencies.

Describe an approach for resolving ethical dilemmas.

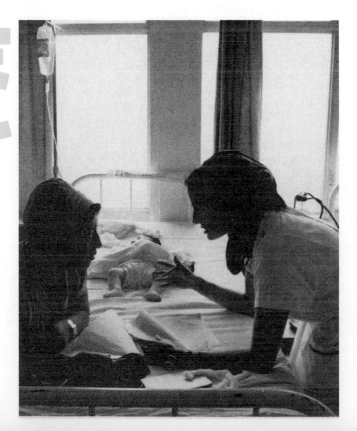

Values, Rights, and Ethics

Nurses are becoming increasingly aware of the values and rights of clients and their support persons and of the ethics involved in nursing practice. A **value** can be defined as something of worth, a belief held dear by a person, or an affective disposition toward a person, object, or idea. Values develop from associations with people, the environment, and self; they are derived from life experiences (Steele and Harmon 1983, p. 1). Values form a basis for behavior; a person's real values are shown by consistent patterns of behavior.

Values exist in some relationship to one another within a person. A **value system** is the organization of a person's values along a continuum of relative importance. There are two types of values: intrinsic and extrinsic. An **intrinsic value** relates to the maintenance of life, e.g., food and water have intrinsic value. An **extrinsic value** originates outside the individual and is not necessary for the maintenance of life, e.g., health, holism, and humanism (Steele and Harmon 1983, p. 2).

A **belief** (opinion) is something accepted as true by a judgment of probability rather than actuality. People hold beliefs that may be true or that can, with reliable evidence, be proved true. Family traditions and folklore are examples of beliefs passed from one generation to another.

Beliefs may or may not involve values. For example, a client may believe that all nurses are honest. The client has accepted that a relationship exists between "nurse" and "honesty"; nurse being the object and honesty the value. The client considers this relationship self-evident. A belief of this type is sometimes called a **value judgment.**

An **attitude** is a feeling tone directed toward a person, object, or idea. Attitudes have behavioral, cognitive, and affective components. The *behavioral* component of an attitude is exemplified by the tendency of the person to take action; it reflects the inclination of the individual to act as a result of his or her attitude. For example, a nurse who dislikes a peer's behavior toward a client is inclined to think, "If she speaks that way to Mr. B again I am going to. . . ." This is the inclination to act, a part of one's attitude toward the peer. The *cognitive* component of an attitude includes the beliefs and factual information associated with the attitude, e.g., nursing is a high-stress occupation. The *affective* component may be the central component of an attitude. It is the feelings that are associated with the belief, knowledge, and the target of the attitude. Feelings vary greatly among people; for example, one client may feel very strongly about the sound from a television in the next room, whereas another client dismisses it as unimportant. The affective component of one's attitudes is usually rooted in a person's values (Muldary 1983, p. 210).

Rights may be defined as "legitimate expectations of persons in a given society at a given time" (Davis and Aroskar 1983, p. 70). Rights can be viewed from legal and personal perspectives. In the legal view, rights provide people with a certain power to control situations; e.g., a person has a legal right to enter a restaurant and purchase a meal. From this viewpoint, rights have certain attendant obligations. The individual with the right to eat in a restaurant is obliged to behave in an appropriate manner and to pay for the meal.

A right may or may not have a *legal* basis. For example, the American Hospital Association's "A Patient's Bill of Rights" (see Table 5–1) states: "The patient has the right to considerate and respectful care." However, lack of consideration during care is not likely to be illegal, although it might be unethical, depending on the situation. By contrast, the right of clients to have their records remain confidential is a legal right in many jurisdictions.

The *personal* concept of rights has much to do with one's values, the way one conducts one's life, the decisions one makes, and one's concepts of right, wrong, good, and evil (Fromer 1981, p. 2). A number of factors influence the development of a personal concept of rights, among them social relationships, parents, culture, and information. Human rights refer to prerogatives of all humans, in particular the right to be respected as a human being. These *human rights,* or the right to be treated as a human, represent a basic respect for humanity, for people as human beings. A nurse who inflicts unnecessary pain or treats a person as a piece of unfeeling machinery fails to recognize the humanity of another person. To be treated as a human is a right of all people.

Ethics is the rules or principles that govern right conduct. The word *ethics* is derived from the Greek *ethos,* meaning custom or character. An ethic is "what ought to be." The term *bioethics* is being used increasingly in the health field. **Bioethics** is the ethics concerning life. Nurses are confronted with bioethical problems in the health care system, e.g., abortion and maintaining life with complex machinery.

Morality is a word often used interchangeably with ethics. **Morality** denotes what is right and wrong in conduct, character, or attitude and what individuals must do to live together in society. The way a person perceives the requirements for living together and responds to them is **moral behavior.** People learn morals during their **socialization,** the process by which individuals learn the knowledge, skills, and dispositions of their social group or society.

Values

Each person, e.g., nurse, client, and physician, has a personal set of values. A **value set** is the group of values a person holds. Individuals incorporate personal values into their lives as a result of observing the behavior and attitudes of parents and teachers and interacting with their cultural, religious, and social environments. Personal values also reflect experiences and a person's intelligence. Similarly, professional values are a reflection and expansion of personal values (Fromer 1981, p. 15). These values are acquired as a nurse is socialized into the nursing profession.

Table 5–1 A Patient's Bill of Rights

1. The patient has the right to considerate and respectful care.
2. The patient has the right to obtain from his physician complete current information concerning his diagnosis, treatment, and prognosis, in terms the patient can be reasonably expected to understand. When it is not medically advisable to give such information to the patient, the information should be made available to an appropriate person in his behalf. He has the right to know by name the physician responsible for coordinating his care.
3. The patient has the right to receive from his physician information necessary to give informed consent prior to the start of any procedure and/or treatment. Except in emergencies, such information for informed consent should include but not necessarily be limited to the specific procedure and/or treatment, the medically significant risks involved, and the probable duration of incapacitation. Where medically significant alternatives for care or treatment exist, or when the patient requests information concerning medical alternatives, the patient has the right to such information. The patient also has the right to know the name of the person responsible for the procedures and/or treatment.
4. The patient has the right to refuse treatment to the extent permitted by law and to be informed of the medical consequences of his action.
5. The patient has the right to every consideration of his privacy concerning his own medical care program. Case discussion, consultation, examination, and treatment are confidential and should be conducted discreetly. Those not directly involved in this care must have the permission of the patient to be present.
6. The patient has the right to expect that all communications and records pertaining to his care should be treated as confidential.
7. The patient has the right to expect that within its capacity a hospital must make reasonable response to the request of a patient for services. The hospital must provide evaluation, service, and/or referral as indicated by the urgency of the case. When medically permissible, a patient may be transferred to another facility only after he has received complete information and explanation concerning the needs for and alternatives to such a transfer. The institution to which the patient is transferred must first have accepted the patient for transfer.
8. The patient has the right to obtain information as to any relationship of his hospital to other health care and educational institutions insofar as his care is concerned. The patient has the right to obtain information as to the existence of any professional relationships among individuals, by name, who are treating him.
9. The patient has the right to be advised if the hospital proposes to engage in or perform human experimentation affecting his care or treatment. The patient has the right to refuse to participate on such research projects.
10. The patient has the right to expect reasonable continuity of care. He has the right to know in advance what appointment times and physicians are available and where. The patient has the right to expect that the hospital will provide a mechanism whereby he is informed by his physician or a delegate of the physician of the patient's continuing health.
11. The patient has the right to examine and receive an explanation of his bill regardless of source of payment.
12. The patient has the right to know what hospital rules and regulations apply to his conduct as a patient.

Source: American Hospital Association. Reprinted with permission of the American Hospital Association, Copyright 1972.

Each person has a relatively small number of values. The origin of these values can be traced to culture, society, institutions, and personality. Values are learned and are greatly influenced by a person's sociocultural environment. For additional information about cultural and ethnic values relative to health and illness, see Chapter 17. Values are learned throughout life; however, many values are learned in early childhood. Acquiring values is usually a gradual process of which the individual is unaware. People do not always realize they have a specific set of values or that they base the decisions they make on values.

Personal and Professional Values

The nurse enters the profession of nursing with values that guide personal actions. Through the process of socialization into the profession, the nurse chooses additional values. Personal and professional values are closely related and often can be the same.

Nurses' personal values influence client-nurse interactions and the practice of nursing. Steele and Harmon (1983, p. 7) believe that nurses can enact their professional roles with minimal discomfort when their personal and professional values are reasonably congruent. Thompson and Thompson (1985, p. 81) agree that nurses who are comfortable with their professional roles probably experience greater satisfaction and possibly provide better care for clients but question the latter point. A nurse who is comfortable with her or his role may not necessarily practice in an ethical manner. For example, the nurse who is comfortable in her or his role may decide not to "make waves" or may fail to take a stand against a decision that goes against her or his sense of ethics.

Personal Values. Most people derive some values from the society or subgroup of society in which they live. Values developed by society ensure its continued functioning and enable people to live harmoniously together. Examples of societal values common to Western civilization are shown in the accompanying box. A person may internalize some or all of these values and perceive them as personal values. In addition to internalizing societal values, people have values that are important to them as individuals. Purtilo (1978, p. 71)

Is health care a right of all people?

The present emphasis on cost and cost-containment produces a . . . concern about its effect on future ethical issues in health care. The conflict between the demands of high-technology medicine and those for positive health promotion introduces politics to ethics. Should nurses be involved? Is health care a right of all people? Who should decide priorities? Who should be involved in the allocation of resources, be they fiscal, human, or material? Are the differences in access to health care a matter of social and moral concerns? If there is a moral obligation to address such concerns, how does nursing deal with it? Should it?

Society's participation in dealing with the many ethical problems regarding health and health care is vital. These problems affect everyone and health professionals can no longer arrogantly assume the roles of both judge and jury. Such participation in decision making should not only be encouraged but extended to include the many health and health promotion issues that arise in the health policies of governments.

Source: R. W. Lubic, Insights from life in the trenches, *Nursing Outlook*, March/April 1988, 36(2): 62. Excerpted from *Making Choices, Taking Chances: Nursing Leaders Tell Their Stories*, 1988, St. Louis: C. V. Mosby Co.

points out that most people find fulfillment only if they can integrate both societal and personal values into a satisfactory life-style. People need societal values to feel like an accepted part of the society and humankind, and they need personal values to individualize themselves.

■ **Professional Values.** Because nursing is a profession based on caring, professional values relate to both competence and compassion. Selected professional values are shown in the accompanying box. Nurses develop these values during socialization into the profession.

Identifying Personal Values

Nurses need to know what values they hold about life, health, illness, and death. To explore personal values, the nurse can begin by answering questions such as (Thompson and Thompson 1985, pp. 77–80): "What ten things do I like to do?' 'What ten things do I like about myself?" "What ten things do I dislike about myself?" An awareness of things the nurse dislikes can lead to thoughts about what she or he may like to change. After initial exercises, the nurse may then list ten values that guide her or his daily interactions or activities. By comparing lists with a trusted friend or in a group that fosters trust and mutual respect, the nurse can see similarities and differences with others. Resulting discussion often reveals reasons for the items listed.

Another strategy for gaining awareness of personal values is to consider individual attitudes to such issues as abortion, unwanted pregnancy, euthanasia, sex-role stereotypes, and sexuality. Examples of some questions and issues adopted from Corey et al. (1984, pp. 57–94) follow. When considering these issues, ask yourself: "Can I accept this or live with this?" "Why does this bother me?" "What would I do or want done in this situation?"

1. *Health.* Consider whether you agree or disagree with the following:
   a. To be most effective in nursing practice, the nurse must be a role model of health.
   b. An obese nurse can effectively instruct an obese client about nutrition and exercise.
   c. A nurse who smokes can effectively help a client to stop smoking.
   d. The nurse who has been pregnant and delivered an infant is most effective in helping a client through this experience.

2. *Differences in life experiences and philosophies.* Indicate with whom you could effectively communicate:
   a. Someone from a strict religious background
   b. Someone of a different race
   c. Someone from a different ethnic group
   d. A physically handicapped person
   e. An elderly person
   f. A child
   g. An obese person
   h. An alcoholic
   i. Someone who has a different sexual orientation
   j. A criminal

3. *Sex-role stereotypes.* Do you agree or disagree with the following statements?
   a. A woman's place is in the home in the role of wife and mother; a man's role is to be the breadwinner.
   b. Husbands and wives should share domestic and child-rearing tasks.
   c. A wife who desires it should be allowed to combine home and a career or school.
   d. A couple should decide which spouse is to be the primary breadwinner and which is to be the primary homemaker.
   e. A woman should do the cooking, not a man.
   f. A husband should make all the financial decisions for the family.

4. *Sexuality.* What are your attitudes toward:
   a. Teenage sex
   b. Casual sex
   c. Sex as an expression of love and commitment
   d. Premarital sex
   e. Extramarital sex for males

f. Extramarital sex for females
g. Group sex
h. Masturbation
i. Homosexuality
5. *Unwanted pregnancy.* In your opinion, what should a female with an unwanted pregnancy do?
   a. Maintain the pregnancy to term
   b. Have an abortion
   c. Marry the father
   d. Put the infant up for adoption if not married
   e. Make own decision regardless of circumstances
6. *Abortion.* Indicate whether you agree or disagree with the following statements.
   a. A woman should have the right to choose abortion.
   b. Abortion at any point during gestation is murder.
   c. Abortion is wrong.
   d. Abortion should be performed if the woman's health is endangered.
   e. A mentally handicapped woman should be encouraged to have an abortion.
   f. Abortion should not be performed after 20 weeks' gestation.
   g. Abortion should be encouraged when parents have genetically transmissible diseases.

7. *Right to die and the choice of suicide.* Do you believe?
   a. Clients have the right to participate in all decisions related to their health.
   b. Clients have the right to refuse extraordinary treatment that is life-sustaining.
   c. Refusing life-sustaining treatment is a form of suicide.
   d. Clients have a right *not* to be interfered with in a rational act of suicide.
   e. Health professionals have a responsibility to assist a client in an act of rational suicide that does not cause injury to others.
   f. Comfort measures should always be provided.
   g. Health professionals should always do their best to sustain a person's life.

Identifying Client Values

People's values change from time to time as their situation in life changes. State of health greatly influences a person's values. For example, a client with failing eyesight will probably place a high value on the ability to see; a client with failing neuromuscular ability will value the ability to stand or walk; and a client with

Selected Societal, Personal, and Professional Values

Societal Values	*Personal Values*	*Professional Values*
Human life	Family unity	Nondiscrimination in providing care
Individual rights	Self-worth	Honesty
Individual autonomy	Worth of others	Respect for persons
Liberty	Independence	Right to privacy
Democracy	Religion	Informed consent
Equal opportunity	Honesty	Self-determination/autonomy of clients
Power	Fairness	Safeguarding the client's welfare
Health	Love	Accountability for actions
Wealth	Sense of humor	Competence
Youth	Safety	Participation in research
Vigor	Peace	Health promotion
Intelligence	Financial security	Health maintence
Imagination	Material things	Health restoration
Education	Money	Alleviation of suffering
Technology	Property of self	
Conformity	Property of others	
Friendship	Leisure time	
Courage	Work	
Compassion	Travel	
Family	Plants	
	Animals	
	Physical activity	
	Intellectual activity	
	Artistic activity	
	Neatness	

chronic pain will value comfort. Normally, people take such things for granted. Nurses, therefore, need to identify the major values, beliefs, and behaviors of clients as they influence and relate to a particular health problem. Reasons for identifying a client's value system include:

1. To help a client discover a new and meaningful value system following injury or illness.
2. To provide information about the client's responses to injury or illness.
3. To help the client explore alternative goals and intervention strategies when valued goals cannot be realized.
4. To plan nursing interventions that support the client's cultural and health care beliefs.

Nurses can use a number of approaches to learn about a client's values (Purtilo 1978, p. 75). Conversing with the client about his or her job, family, pets, hobbies, past achievements, goals, or material possessions can reveal much information, since most clients are eager to talk about what they value. Listening to the client's family and friends often provides clues through casual remarks, such as "I'll tell you something; he used to be a great concert pianist." The nurse thus learns that the client used to value music and may still do so. Reviewing the client's health records can provide information about the client's family background, religion, occupation, age, birthday, and medical history. With this background information, the nurse can initiate conversations that may reveal the client's personal values.

To assist with values clarification, the nurse needs to help clients think about what is and what is not important to them. It may be helpful to ask the following questions:

1. "Are you considering other courses of action?" Make sure that the client is aware of all alternative actions and has thought about the consequences of each.
2. "What do you think you will gain by doing that?" "What benefits do you foresee from doing that?"
3. "Did you have any say in that decision?" "Did you have a choice?"
4. "How do you feel about that decision (or action)?" Because some clients may not feel satisfied with their decision and feel badly about a bad choice, a more sensitive question may be: "Some people feel good after a decision is made; others feel bad. How do you feel?"
5. "What will you say to others (family, friends) about this?"
6. "Will it be difficult to tell your wife (husband, mother, friends) about this?" This helps determine whether the client is prepared to act on the decision.
7. "How many times have you done that before?" or "Would you act that way again?" These questions help the client determine whether he or she consistently behaves in a pattern.

With these questions, the nurse assists the client to think about personal values, never imposing her or his own values on the client. The nurse never offers an opinion, e.g., "It would be better to do it this way," or makes a judgment, e.g., "That's not the right thing to do."

The nurse offers an opinion only when the client asks the nurse for it and then only with care.

Rights

There are three main types of rights: option rights, welfare rights, and legislative rights. **Option rights** are rights of freedom and choice; they express the right of people to live as they choose within prescribed boundaries (Fromer 1981, p. 2). For example, a female nurse working in a hospital can wear any uniform she wishes (her right) provided it is white, clean, and covers her body suitably (boundaries). In this instance the boundaries probably reflect hospital policy and a norm established by many nurses. **Welfare rights** are the legal entitlement to some good, e.g., specific safety standards in a building or a number of years of education (Fromer 1981, p. 3). An example is the right of clients to health care or the right of citizens to safe water. **Legislative rights** are established by law; they are based on the concept of justice. For example, a woman has the legal right not to be raped by her husband.

Clients' Rights

The movement for clients' rights in health care arose in the late 1960s. At that time, the broad goals of the movement were to improve the quality of health care and to make the health care system more responsive to clients' needs. Today, clients are also seeking more self-determination and control over their own bodies when they are ill. Informed consent, confidentiality, and the right of the client to refuse treatment are all aspects of this self-determination. The need for clients' rights is largely the result of two circumstances: the vulnerability of the client because of illness and the complexity of the relationships in the health care setting.

Ill people are frequently unable to assert their rights as they would if they were healthy. Asserting rights requires energy and an underlying awareness of one's rights in the situation. People who are weak or preoccupied about their illness may not be able to assert their rights. In addition, individuals are not always aware of their rights because the health care environment is unfamiliar to them. The need for confidentiality of information about a client's health may not occur to a client.

The complexity and variety of health care relationships also affect the issue of clients' rights. In this day of specialization, the client is one person among many health professionals. The client's needs or priorities can become lost in the communications among health professionals.

In traditional patterns of health care, clients experience losses, e.g., loss of the sense of independence and control. The client may view the care provider as superordinate, an authority, and even a person to be venerated. This traditional pattern encourages client dependence: While the client seeks health or the return to health, the health care providers grant that client only limited rights (Healey 1983, pp. 115–16).

A new pattern of health care relationships is emerging as a result of several forces in society, including more knowledgable consumers and recognition of the role of life-style in preventing and treating diseases. Today, the goals of health care include the return of autonomy and independence to the client and the acceptance of good health as a responsibility of the care provider, the client, and society. These goals cannot be met unless clients accept active responsibility for their health and health care and unless clients and care providers have mutual respect. The clients' rights movement promotes this new health care relationship, and nurses today are combating the undermining of clients' rights by identifying and protecting clients' rights and helping clients assert them (Healey 1983, p. 116).

■ **A Patient's Bill of Rights.** In 1972, the American Hospital Association published "A Patient's Bill of Rights" to promote the rights of hospitalized clients. See Table 5–1. Frequently clients do not know their rights, although many hospitals today give clients upon admission a statement of their rights while in hospital. Some implications for nursing follow.

The right to considerate and respectful care means the client has a right to receive explanations about what will happen, why, and when. The client also has the right to participate in planning his or her care. Considerate and respectful care also includes respect for the dignity of each person. Nurses can convey respect by listening carefully to clients and their support persons and reporting their concerns to the appropriate people.

The responsibility for divulging information about medical diagnoses and treatment belongs to the physician. If a client asks a nurse for this information, the nurse should relay the questions to the physician and document the client's questions and the nurse's actions on the client's record. Nurses should explain independent nursing actions truthfully and completely. Because these activities are solely in the nurse's domain, the nurse has sole responsibility for explaining them.

Dependent nursing functions, i.e., those nursing activities ordered by the physician, should be explained only after the nurse completely understands the physician's and client's positions. Usually, a physician has no objection to a client's understanding the ordered treatments; however, occasionally a physician does not wish a client to be fully informed (e.g., about a medication for a malignancy) before the client has been informed of the diagnosis.

The client's right to give or withhold informed consent includes medical and nursing care. Obtaining informed consent for invasive diagnostic, medical, or surgical procedures is the physician's responsibility. Before a nurse commences any nursing interventions, clients must consent to that care. **Informed consent** has five aspects:

1. Explanation of the proposed treatment
2. Explanation of inherent risks and benefits
3. Alternatives to the proposed treatment

4. Adequate time for client questions
5. Option to withdraw at any time

A client can also withdraw consent after signing a consent form. If a nurse is about to give an injection, for example, and the client says, "I have changed my mind—I don't want that drug," the nurse should not give the injection, report the situation to the charge nurse and/or physician, and record the client's words and the nurse's actions on the client's record. Clients have the right to self-determination. Just as they have the right to informed consent, they also have the right to refuse a treatment. An adult client who is conscious and medically competent has the right to refuse any medical or surgical procedure (Annas 1975, p. 79). When the client refuses treatment, no person has the right to impose the treatment. The client still has the right to the best possible care within the limitations he or she imposes.

People vary in what they consider an invasion of privacy and a threat to dignity. Therefore only the client can decide whether to permit any invasion of privacy. While signing a consent form for an examination or treatment may be giving up certain aspects of privacy, the invasion of the client's privacy must be kept to the minimum. For example, a client who consents to a physical examination is expected to disrobe; however, the nurse can provide some degree of privacy by supplying an appropriate gown, drapes, and a room or enclosed area. When consenting to an examination, the client does not also agree to the presence of people other than those directly involved in the examination. This is important for students to remember; when observing an examination or procedure, always obtain the client's permission to do so.

Confidentiality is closely related to privacy. Only clients have the power to let people not directly involved in their care view their medical records. **Confidentiality** means that information disclosed to a person, e.g., a nurse, will not be disclosed to anyone not directly involved in the client's care. Disclosure of such information is a breach of confidentiality and could lead to legal action against the nurse or the health agency.

The growing use of computers in health care facilities has raised concerns about maintaining the confidentiality of client records. Although computers have facilitated health care in a number of ways, any person who knows an access code can view confidential client information. Therefore, nurses and all health professionals must guard the confidentiality of client records and not give computer codes to unauthorized people.

Clients have a right to know what health care they will need after they are discharged from a hospital. It is often the nurse's responsibility to teach follow-up care and to make appropriate referrals to other health agencies. Discharge planning is discussed in Chapter 10.

Another right not mentioned specifically in the AHA Patient's Bill of Rights is the right of access to medical records. Although in some jurisdictions clients have the right of access to their health records, agency practices vary widely in this regard. Some hospitals, e.g., military hospitals, permit clients to keep records at the bedside. At the other extreme, some agencies release records to clients only if they have a subpoena. A number of state legislatures have passed laws requiring health agencies to establish reasonable policies by which clients are permitted access to their records. Laws about access to records have changed in recent years, and it is generally recognized that only clients can grant others access to their records or permit the release or transfer of their records.

■ **Nursing Implications.** Because nursing research usually focuses on humans, a major nursing responsibility is to be aware of and advocate clients' rights. All clients must be informed about the consequences of consenting to serve as research subjects. All nurses who practice in settings where research is being conducted with human subjects or who participate in such research as data collectors or collaborators play an important role in safeguarding the following rights:

Right not to be harmed. The Department of Health and Human Services defines **risk of harm** to a research subject as exposure to the possibility of injury going beyond everyday situations. The risk can be physical, emotional, legal, financial, or social.

Right to full disclosure. Even though it may be possible to collect data about a client as part of everyday care without the client's particular knowledge or consent, to do so is considered unethical. **Full disclosure** means that deception, either by withholding information about a client's participation in a study, or by giving the client false or misleading information about what participating in the study will involve, will not occur.

Right of self-determination. Many clients in dependent positions, such as people in nursing homes, feel pressured to participate in studies. They feel that they must please those doctors and nurses who are responsible for their treatment and care. The right of **self-determination** means that subjects should feel free from constraints, coercion, or any undue influence to participate in a study.

Right of privacy and confidentiality. Privacy enables a client to participate without worrying about later embarrassment. The **anonymity** of a study is ensured if even the investigator cannot link a specific subject to the information reported. **Confidentiality** means that any information a subject relates will not be made public or available to others. Investigators must inform research subjects about the measures that provide for these rights. Such measures may include using pseudonyms or code numbers or reporting only aggregate or group data in published research.

Nurses who participate in scientific investigations that involve human subjects are in a key position to serve as advocates for research subjects. Certain subjects, including children, fetuses, the mentally disabled, the elderly, captives, the dying, and the sedated or unconscious, are considered particularly **vulnerable subjects.** The guiding principle in these cases is that the less a subject is able to give informed consent, the greater the nurse's responsibility to protect the client's rights.

■ Nurses' Rights

When a nurse's rights (ethical or legal) are violated, the nurse has an obligation to discuss the matter with the appropriate person at the employing agency. If a conflict cannot be resolved, the nurse can report her or his concerns to a professional body, such as the ANA. Most state and provincial associations have mechanisms to deal with legal and ethical issues.

Nurses have rights as citizens and as health professionals. As a citizen, a nurse has all the rights provided under federal and state or provincial law. Upon becoming a nurse, a person does not give up any rights as a citizen. The traditional focus of the profession has been on the nurse's responsibilities and service to others, rather than on the nurse's rights and autonomy. The assertion of nurses' rights should be viewed as a means of improving nursing practice. For example, in a suitable environment, nurses can provide a professional standard of nursing care to clients, whereas in an unsuitable environment, e.g., one lacking staff or equipment, the nurse's right to provide quality care is denied.

Fenner (1980, p. 90) lists four rights of nurses:

1. *To expect own rights to be respected.* This area includes human rights—such as respect for the individual, freedom of choice, and equality, and professional rights—such as the right to set standards of excellence in nurse practice acts and to participate in policy affecting nursing and professional autonomy.
2. *To safe and functional equipment and services.* Implicit in this right is sufficient equipment and sufficient staffing to permit a high standard of professional practice. Also included in this area is the right to work in an environment that minimizes physical and emotional stress. Physical stressors, such as potentially infectious microorganisms, must be identified, and suitable precautions must be taken to protect the health of nurses and other health practitioners.
3. *To compensation for services.* The issue of compensation for services is discussed under contractual agreements in Chapter 6.
4. *To competent assistance.* This right includes not only assistance with the implementation of nursing practice but also support people such as pharmacists, dietitians, and inhalation therapists.

Davis and Aroskar (1983, p. 86) write that the assertion of nurses' rights should not be seen as an end to itself but as a means of improving nursing practice. Therefore, the recognition and implementation of nurses' rights can also result in improved care for clients and their support persons.

■ **Nursing Students' Rights.** In 1970, the Student Bill of Rights was first presented to the ANA House of Delegates. The bill indicates the minimum standards of academic and personal freedom and the rights of students in all educational communities. The National Nursing Students Association (NNSA) also believes that students have the right to qualified instructors, the right to evaluate the performance of their teachers, the right to a curriculum that is relevant to the work situation, and the right to a voice and a vote in determining the content of nursing curricula. In addition, the NNSA supports the right of nursing students to participate in community health projects as a way to meet curriculum objectives and obtain course credits.

In 1974, the United States Congress passed the Family Educational Rights and Privacy Act (Buckley Amendment). Its two major provisions are that the records of a student be available to that student and that the records be private. The records available to the student are educational records, not health records or the private files of teachers. Permission to see the student's file is limited to those involved in the educational process, for example, a nursing instructor who is teaching the student, or the registrar.

In addition, letters of recommendation can be kept from the student only if the student signs a waiver giving up the right to see the letter. Students do not have the right to see confidential materials obtained from parents, such as financial statements. When someone wishes to write a student reference, students have the right to give or withhold permission to examine the information in their files. When the teacher, for example, needs access to the central file to provide reference information about graduates, the student has the right to withhold consent. However, that teacher does not need the student's permission to write a reference without examining the central file. According to the Buckley Amendment, students have the right to challenge factual information, and a conciliation or hearing can subsequently take place.

Students also have other general rights directly involved in their nursing education. They have the right to expect that the curriculum described in the school brochure or calendar will be followed. They have a right to competent instruction. Because students are accountable to clients for care, they must receive sufficient assistance and instruction to give safe care.

Ethics

Because ethics governs right conduct, it deals with what is good and bad and with moral duty and obligation. Ethics is not unlike the law in that each deals with rules of conduct that reflect underlying principles of right and wrong and codes of morality. Ethics evolved to protect the rights of human beings. Nursing ethics provides professional standards for nursing activities; these standards protect both the nurse and the client.

Nursing Codes of Ethics

A **code of ethics** provides a means by which professional standards of practice are established, maintained, and improved. It is essential to a profession. Codes of ethics are formal guidelines for professional action. They are shared by the persons within the profession and should be generally compatible with a professional member's personal values.

A code of ethics gives the members of the profession a frame of reference for judgments in complex nursing situations. No two situations are identical, and nurses are frequently in situations that require judgment about which course of action to take. In these situations, a code of ethics identifies the values and beliefs behind ethical standards (Thompson and Thompson 1985, p. 12).

International, national, state, and provincial nursing associations have established codes of ethics. If a nurse violates the code, the association may expel the nurse from membership. Purposes of ethical nursing codes are:

1. Providing a basis for regulating the relationship between the nurse, the client, coworkers, society, and the profession
2. Providing a standard basis for excluding the unscrupulous nursing practitioner and for defending a practitioner who is unjustly accused
3. Serving as a basis for professional curricula and for orienting the new graduate to professional nursing practice
4. Helping the public understand professional nursing conduct

In 1953, the International Council of Nurses (ICN) developed and adopted its first code of ethics. This code was revised in 1965 and again in 1973. See Table 5–2. The code should be considered together with the relevant data in each situation; thus it provides assistance in setting priorities and in taking action. For the nurse practitioner, the code specifically provides assistance in making judgments and in developing attitudes appropriate to nursing.

The ANA first adopted a code of ethics in 1950, which was revised in 1968, 1976, and 1985. See Table 5–3. This code is designed to provide guidance for nurses by stating principles of ethical concern. In 1980, the Canadian Nurses' Association adopted a code of ethics. It was revised in 1985. See Table 5–4. Nurses have a responsibility to be familiar with the code that governs their nursing practice. In addition, nursing practice is also defined by the particular setting. In a rural, isolated setting, a nurse may be expected to assume responsibilities not normally assumed by urban nurses. For example, the nurse may assess the progress of labor and deliver the infant if the labor is normal. Only if there is a problem is the client flown to a center for a physician's care.

Bioethical Issues in Nursing

Bioethics is the ethics concerned with life, including all life in the environment. Bioethics has come to refer more precisely to the ethics concerned with health care. When referring to ethics in nursing, therefore, one is actually referring to bioethics, although the two terms are often used interchangeably (Thompson and Thompson 1985, p. 219).

Bioethical issues involving nurses surface in nursing practice and in the relationships nurses have with others. Ethical issues arise in almost all areas of nursing prac-

Table 5—2 International Council of Nurses Code for Nurses

The fundamental responsibility of the nurse is fourfold: to promote health, to prevent illness, to restore health, and to alleviate suffering.

The need for nursing is universal. Inherent in nursing is respect for life, dignity, and rights of man. It is unrestricted by considerations of nationality, race, creed, color, age, sex, politics or social status.

Nurses render health services to the individual, the family and the community and coordinate their services with those of related groups.

Nurses and People

The nurse's primary responsibility is to those people who require nursing care.

The nurse, in providing care, promotes an environment in which the values, customs and spiritual beliefs of the individual are respected.

The nurse holds in confidence personal information and uses judgment in sharing this information.

Nurses and Practice

The nurse carries personal responsibility for nursing practice and for maintaining competence by continual learning. The nurse maintains the highest standards of nursing care possible within the reality of a specific situation.

The nurse uses judgment in relation to individual competence when accepting and delegating responsibilities.

The nurse when acting in a professional capacity should at all times maintain standards of personal conduct which reflect credit upon the profession.

Nurses and Society

The nurses shares with other citizens the reponsibility for initiating and supporting action to meet the health and social needs of the public.

Nurses and Co-workers

The nurse sustains a cooperative relationship with co-workers in nursing and other fields. The nurse takes appropriate action to safeguard the individual when his care is endangered by a co-worker or any other person.

Nurses and the Profession

The nurse plays the major role in determining and implementing desirable standards of nursing practice and nursing education.

The nurse is active in developing a core of professional knowledge.

The nurse, acting through the professional organization, participates in establishing and maintaining equitable social and economic working conditions in nursing.

Source: International Council of Nurses, *ICN Code for nurses: Ethical concepts applied to nursing* (Geneva, Switzerland: Imprimeries Populaires, 1973).

tice. Many ethical issues can be viewed in the context of general nursing practice and the people with whom the nurse has contact during practice.

▪ Personal Values and Professional Practice.

With the changing scope of nursing practice and the innovations in medical technology, there is an increasing incidence of conflict between nurses' personal values and practice requirements. On the one hand, employers

have needs and expectations for service from nurses; on the other hand, nurses have the right to be guided by their own personal values. An example of an area of conflict in the contemporary nursing scene is assisting with therapeutic abortions. Nurses have the right to refuse to participate in abortions or any procedure that goes against their personal values, and nurses' employment should not be jeopardized as a result. It is essential, however, that clients' welfare not suffer as a consequence.

Table 5—3 American Nurses' Association Code for Nurses

1. The nurse provides services with respect for human dignity and the uniqueness of the client unrestricted by considerations of social or economic status, personal attributes, or the nature of health problems.
2. The nurse safeguards the client's right to privacy by judiciously protecting information of a confidential nature.
3. The nurse acts to safeguard the client and the public when health care and safety are affected by the incompetent, unethical, or illegal practice of any person.
4. The nurse assumes responsibility and accountability for individual nursing judgments and actions.
5. The nurse maintains competence in nursing.
6. The nurse exercises informed judgment and uses individual competence and qualifications as criteria in seeking consultation, accepting responsibilities, and delegating nursing activities to others.

7. The nurse participates in activities that contribute to the ongoing development of the profession's body of knowledge.
8. The nurse participates in the profession's efforts to implement and improve standards of nursing.
9. The nurse participates in the profession's efforts to establish and maintain conditions of employment conducive to high quality nursing care.
10. The nurse participates in the profession's effort to protect the public from misinformation and misrepresentation and to maintain the integrity of nursing.
11. The nurse collaborates with members of the health professions and other citizens in promoting community and national efforts to meet the health needs of the public.

Source: American Nurses' Association, *Code for nurses* (Kansas City, Mo.: American Nurses' Association, 1985). Reprinted with permission.

Table 5—4   Canadian Nurses Association Code of Ethics for Nursing*

Clients

I. A nurse is obliged to treat clients with respect for their individual needs and values.

II. Based upon respect for clients and regard for their right to control their own care, nursing care should reflect respect for the right of choice held by clients.

III. The nurse is obliged to hold confidential all information regarding a client learned in the health care setting.

IV. The nurse has an obligation to be guided by consideration for the dignity of clients.

V. The nurse is obligated to provide competent care to clients.

VI. The nurse is obliged to represent the ethics of nursing before colleagues and others.

VII. The nurse is obligated to advocate the client's interest.

VIII. In all professional settings, including education, research and administration, the nurse retains a commitment to the welfare of clients. The nurse bears an obligation to act in such a fashion as will maintain trust in nurses and nursing.

Health Team

IX. Client care should represent a cooperative effort, drawing upon the expertise of nursing and other health professions. Acknowledging personal or professional limitations, the nurse recognizes the perspective and expertise of colleagues from other disciplines.

X. The nurse, as a member of the health care team, is obliged to take steps to ensure that the client receives competent and ethical care.

The Social Context of Nursing

XI. Conditions of employment should contribute to client care and to the professional satisfaction of nurses. Nurses are obliged to work towards securing and maintaining conditions of employment that satisfy these connected goals.

Responsibilities of the Profession

XII. Professional nurses' organizations recognize a responsibility to clarify, secure and sustain ethical nursing conduct. The fulfillment of these tasks requires that professional organizations remain responsive to the rights, needs and legitimate interests of clients and nurses.

*This represents only one element of the code—*values. Standards,* which provide more specific directions for conduct than values, and *limitations,* which describe exceptional circumstances in which a value or standard cannot receive its usual application, are provided with each value in the publication cited.

Source: Canadian Nurses Association, Ottawa, Ontario, Canada, February 1985.

Other areas of controversy are euthanasia, prolonging the life of nonresponsive clients by machines, and withholding blood transfusions because of an individual's religious convictions. In the future, conflicts between personal values and professional duty may increase.

For example, a nurse whose personal value system does not support abortion has begun to develop a trusting relationship with a 13-year-old girl admitted to the hospital for a legal abortion. The girl is ambivalent about the abortion; because of her ambivalent feelings and her fear of the procedure, she wants to have the nurse's support. The nurse, as a professional, needs to support the client; however, as a person, the nurse is against abortion and finds it difficult to give the girl complete support. Should the nurse play a strictly professional role and support the abortion, or should the nurse reveal personal feelings about abortion?

A second example is a nurse who is asked to teach birth control and who opposes birth control because of personal values. What are the alternatives? Should the nurse teach the client, thereby compromising personal values? Should the nurse refuse to provide the requested information? Perhaps the nurse should tell the client that she or he doesn't agree with contraception, and then answer the client's questions. Is there a fourth alternative? There are no easy answers in such situations.

Nurses can often avoid ethical conflicts by clarifying, during initial employment interviews, areas in which personal values may conflict with professional respon-

sibility. The nurse can request to be assigned to nursing duties during which conflict is not likely to arise. Nursing students should also make their personal values clear to teachers so as to avoid ethical conflicts. Students who have not anticipated a problem but find themselves facing an ethical conflict involving personal values should write down the alternative actions open to them and then discuss the alternatives with an instructor.

■ **Nurse and Peers.** A nurse who faces a problem with peers may or may not know what course of action to take. One nurse may see another nurse steal medications from the nursing unit drug cupboard. The nurse who is discovered cries and explains that she needs the sleeping pills to sleep during the day while her three children are home from school. She states she uses them only on days before she is to go on night shift. She is the sole support of her children and needs the job. Does the first nurse report the theft or ignore the matter?

A second situation involves a nurse newly employed at a hospital who requests Christmas leave because his father is dying and he wants to spend Christmas with him. Under the special circumstances, the nurse is granted the time. Another nurse finds out that the first nurse's father is not dying and that the nurse plans to spend Christmas vacation skiing with a friend. Does the nurse report the skiing vacation to the responsible nurse or forget the information?

A third example is a white nurse who is afraid to correct a black nurse's error for fear the black nurse will report the white nurse to the Human Rights Commission. Does the white nurse correct the black nurse and risk labor problems and possible firing?

A fourth situation involves a nurse who is employed on a community mental health team. Another nurse discovers that the first nurse spends most of the time at home looking after an ill mother and fabricates reports about visiting clients in their homes. Does the nurse present this information to the members of the community team, discuss the situation with the first nurse, or consider another alternative?

In each of these situations, the nurse's own values or fears lead to ethical conflicts.

█ Nurse and Client.   In some situations, nurses have ethical problems that involve a client, a family, or both. For example, a client requests an abortion. Her husband agrees, but he tells the nurse that he will always be tormented with the thought that he agreed to destroy a human being he helped to create. The wife tells the nurse that her husband was not the father of the unborn baby. Should the nurse tell the father, the physician, or the charge nurse any of this information?

█ Nurse and Other Health Professionals.
Ethical conflicts can arise between nurses and physicians. For example, a surgeon, the chief of staff of surgery, visits a hospital nursing unit one evening to discuss a client's surgery the next day. The nurse smells alcohol on the surgeon's breath, the surgeon's speech is slurred, and his gait is unsteady. Does the nurse report this or ignore it?

█ Nurse and Agency Practice.   Health care agencies exist for a variety of reasons (see Chapter 4), and their policies often reflect the values of the members of a governing board. As an employee of an agency, a nurse may have values that conflict with institutional goals and practices. Sometimes, because of budget restrictions, there may be inadequate equipment or inadequate staff, which can create ethical dilemmas for nurses. Such nurses may work to change agency policy, or they may find it necessary to organize formally and bargain with the employer for safer working conditions.

█ Resolving Ethical Dilemmas

An ethical or moral **dilemma** is a choice between equally undesirable alternatives (Curtin and Flaherty 1982, p. 39). It can also be viewed as "a situation involving a choice between equally satisfactory or unsatisfactory alternatives or a difficult problem that seems to have no satisfactory solution" (Thompson and Thompson 1985, p. 94). In a moral dilemma there is no right or wrong. For example, a nurse is alone at night on a hospital unit and two clients experience cardiac arrest at almost the same time. What does the nurse do? It may be possible to save one client, but not both.

According to Thompson and Thompson (1985, p. 94), for a situation to be a moral dilemma, it must fulfill three criteria:

1. *Awareness of different options.* The individual must be aware of the different options that are open. The awareness may be cognitive (knowing that something is wrong), or it may be affective (feeling that something is wrong).
2. *Moral nature of the dilemma.* Is the dilemma the nurse faces a moral issue? Not all situations that appear confusing to nurses are moral dilemmas, e.g., a conflict between two nurses about how to proceed with specific client care may not be a moral dilemma but simply differing interpretation of facts or even differing assessments. For example, one nurse may believe that a client's respirations indicate the need for oxygen, while another nurse may believe that the administration of morphine sulfate, as ordered by the physician, is indicated. Both nurses may in fact be right.
3. *Two or more options with true choice.* For a situation to be a moral dilemma, one must have a choice between two or more actions. For example, a physician tells a client that when he performed the surgery he did all he could. The nurse present at the conversation knows that a resident physician performed the surgery because the client's physician could not be reached. The nurse's choices are: to tell the client his physician did not perform the surgery, say nothing, report the discussion to the charge nurse, or discuss the conversation with the physician. The nurse in this example has free choice.

To make ethical judgments, one must rely on rational thought, not emotions. Such judgments require conscious, cognitive skills necessary to perceive the client's needs and provide client care (Sigman 1986, p. 21). Every day, nurses make decisions that affect their clients, and these decisions are frequently based on ethics (Sigman 1986, p. 22).

A number of ethical theories and ethical decision-making models can guide nurses in making ethical decisions. Before a nurse can resolve ethical dilemmas, she or he should decide which ethical system is best suited to her or his views. Two prevalent theories that guide decision making are utilitarianism and deontology (Fromer 1986, p. 82).

Utilitarianism can be summarized as "the greatest good for the greatest number." In this approach, moral decisions are based solely on the consequences of an action, not on the inherent rightness of an action. One drawback of this approach is that minority views can be ignored. For example, if three nurses agree on a course of action and the client disagrees, by the utilitarian view the client can be ignored because he or she is not in "the greatest number."

In the **deontologic approach** to ethical problems, certain characteristics make an act right or wrong, regardless of its consequences. These characteristics are values such as truth, justice, and love. One type of deontologic theory is pluralistic; i.e., several principles can

Clinical safety may not be the reason for medical opposition

During the five-year struggle to establish and keep alive the Childbearing Center, I learned a very important lesson that can save countless hours when one is engaged in a battle for change: medical opposition is without exception voiced in terms of desire for clinical quality and safety. Because we nurses are often unsophisticated in overt professional conflict, our tendency is to rise to the bait and search diligently for proof of clinical safety, which early in innovation usually is not yet extant. If such proof is found and presented, one quickly learns that clinical safety is not the real—or at least not the main—reason for opposition.

When your position is challenged or refuted in public forums or before groups, carefully gauge the intensity of emotion displayed. The more strident the attack or argument, the greater the likelihood that self-interest, not concern for quality, is motivating the outburst. I lived through and still experience such attacks, although they have become less frequent. My years in the trenches have taught me that a nurse confronting medical opposition does best to remain calm, polite, and firm in presentation and affect. It does not help to respond in kind even when sorely tempted to do so.

Remember that fear of change and confusion about receiving criticism from consumers may well be motivating the behavior that is being directed at you.

Source: R. W. Lubic, Insights from life in the trenches, *Nursing Outlook,* March/April 1988, 36(2):65. Excerpted from *Making Choices, Taking Chances: Nursing Leaders Tell Their Stories,* 1988, St. Louis: C. V. Mosby Co.

apply in a conflict. Principles such as autonomy and justice can be assigned different priorities, depending on the person solving the dilemma. For example, one nurse may consider the autonomy of the client more important than justice, whereas another nurse may believe the opposite. For this reason, each would approach a problem with different priorities for resolution.

The four most important principles in a deontological approach are autonomy, nonmaleficence, beneficence, and justice. **Autonomy** is personal liberty of action; it implies independence, self-reliance, freedom of choice, and the ability to make decisions (Fromer 1986, pp. 82–83). To be autonomous, a client must be able to act independently, be self-reliant, have freedom to choose a course of action, and be able to make decisions. For a client to be truly autonomous, nurses and all health professionals must respect the autonomy of the client.

Nonmaleficence means the duty to do no harm. This principle is the basis of most codes of nursing ethics. Although this would seem to be a simple principle to follow in nursing practice, in reality it is complex. Harm can mean deliberate harm, risk of harm, and harm that occurs during beneficial actions (Fromer 1986, p. 83). In nursing, intentional harm is always unacceptable. However, the risk of harm is not so clear. A client may be at risk of harm during a nursing intervention that is intended to be helpful. For example, a client may react adversely to a medication. Sometimes, the degree to which a risk is morally permissible can be a conflict.

Beneficence means "doing good." Nurses are obligated to "do good," that is, to implement actions that benefit clients and their support persons. However, in an increasingly technologic health care system, "doing good" can also pose a risk of doing harm. For example, a nurse may advise a client about an exercise program to improve general health but should not do so if the client is at risk of a heart attack.

Justice, the fourth principle, is often referred to as fairness. Nurses frequently face decisions in which a sense of justice should prevail. For example, a nurse is alone on a hospital unit, and one client arrives to be admitted at the same time another client requires a medication for pain. Instead of running from one client to the other, the nurse should weigh the facts in the situation and then act based on the principle of justice.

In resolving ethical problems, nurses need to be aware of the ethical theory with which they are is most comfortable and their own hierarchy of principles or values in that theory. Although codes of ethics offer general guidelines for decision making, more specific guidelines are necessary in many cases to resolve the everyday ethical dilemmas encountered by nurses in practice settings. Suggested guidelines for the nurse to resolve these dilemmas are:

1. **Establish a sound data base.** To do this, the nurse needs to gather as much information as possible about the situation. Aroskar (1980, p. 660) suggests that nurses get answers to the following questions:
   - What persons are involved and what is their involvement in the situation?
   - What is the proposed action?
   - What is the intent of the proposed action?
   - What are the possible consequences of the proposed action?

The following example illustrates the usefulness of a sound data base.

Mrs. Green, a 67-year-old woman, is hospitalized with multiple fractures and lacerations caused by an automobile accident. Her husband, also in the accident, is admitted to the same hospital and dies. Mrs. Green, who was the driver of the automobile, constantly questions the primary nurse about her husband. The surgeon, however, has told the nurse not to tell the client about the death of her husband.

The nurse is not provided with any reason for such a direction and expresses concern to the charge nurse, who says the surgeon's orders must be followed.

In this example, the data base includes:

- *Persons involved.* Client (concerned about husband's welfare), husband (deceased), surgeon, head nurse, and primary nurse.
- *Proposed action.* Withhold information about the husband's death.
- *Intention of proposed action.* Unknown; possibly to protect Mrs. Green from psychologic trauma, overwhelming guilt feelings, and consequent deterioration of her physical condition.
- *Consequences of proposed action.* If information is withheld, the client may become increasingly anxious and angry and may refuse to cooperate with necessary care, delaying recovery.

2. **Identify the conflicts presented by the situation.** A conflict is a clash between opposing elements or ideas. The conflicts for the primary nurse in the example are:
   - Need to be honest with Mrs. Green without being disloyal to the surgeon and the charge nurse
   - Need to be loyal to the surgeon and head nurse without being dishonest to Mrs. Green
   - Conflict about the effects on Mrs. Green's health if she is informed or if she is not informed

3. **Outline alternative actions to the proposed course of action and consider the outcomes or consequences of the alternative actions.** Alternative courses of action to the proposed action for Mrs. Green and their outcomes might include:
   - Follow the surgeon's and charge nurse's advice and do as the surgeon suggests. The outcomes for the nurse would be
     - Approval from the charge nurse and surgeon
     - Risk of being seen as nonassertive
     - Violation of own value to be truthful to Mrs. Green
     - Possible benefit to Mrs. Green's health
     - Possible detriment to Mrs. Green's health
   - Discuss the situation further with the charge nurse and surgeon, pointing out Mrs. Green's rights to autonomy and information. The outcomes might be:
     - The surgeon may acknowledge the client's right to be informed and may then inform the client.
     - The surgeon may state that the client's rights have no legal basis and may adhere to the action originally proposed, based on a judgment about the effects of information on Mrs. Green.

4. **Determine ownership of the problem and the appropriate decision maker.** In some ethical dilemmas, the nurse does not make decisions about her or his own actions but assists the client to make a decision. A series of questions that evolve from decision-making theories can help nurses determine who owns a certain problem (Davis and Aroskar 1983):
   - Who should be involved in making the decision and why?

- For whom is the decision being made?
- What criteria (social, economic, psychologic, physiologic, or legal) should be used in deciding who makes the decision?
- What degree of consent is needed by the subject (client and other)?
- What, if any, moral principles (rights, values) are enhanced or negated by the proposed action?

In the example of Mrs. Green, the surgeon obviously believes the decision is his or hers to make for Mrs. Green, and the charge nurse agrees. However, the criteria used to decide who the decision maker should be are not clear. If the criteria were spelled out, perhaps the conflict about the effects on Mrs. Green's health of knowing or not knowing about her husband's death could be resolved. Is it psychologically advantageous for Mrs. Green to know or not to know? Is it physically advantageous? What will the social and economic effects be?

5. **Define the nurse's obligations.** The nurse has the professional knowledge and expertise to ensure that the client makes an informed decision. Thus the client needs information from the professional's frame of reference about the consequences of decisions. When nurses are determining an ethical course of action, Moser and Cox (1980, p. 43) advise them to list their nursing obligations, to assess the conflicts that will arise if all obligations are met, and to determine the alternatives from which the nurse can choose. Examples of obligations are:
   - To maximize the client's well-being
   - To balance the client's need for autonomy and family members' responsibilities for the client's well-being
   - To support each family member and enhance the family support system
   - To carry out hospital policies
   - To protect other clients' well-being
   - To protect the nurse's own standards of care

The example of Mrs. Green shows that there are no clearly defined right or wrong answers to ethical dilemmas. If there were, they would not be ethical dilemmas. To resolve the ethical dilemma about Mrs. Green, the involved health professionals may need to confer and clearly establish approaches that will be in Mrs. Green's best interests. Once an approach is agreed on, the nurses and physician can devise consistent continuing methods of support for Mrs. Green. That approach may dictate actions by the nurse that conflict with her or his own value system. However, the action chosen for Mrs. Green's best interest takes precedence.

Chapter Highlights

A value is something of worth, a belief held dear by a person, or an affective disposition toward a person, object, or idea.

Values give direction and meaning to life and guide a person's behavior.

A person enters nursing with a personal set of values and acquires professional values that influence nursing actions through socialization in school and in practice settings.

It is important for nurses to clarify personal values to understand how these values guide one's actions and influence decision making.

Nurses may assist clients in clarifying values relative to specific health problems to facilitate decision making.

Rights are personal and legal expectations of persons in a given society at a given time.

Clients' rights include consideration and respect, information about health-illness problems and their treatment, informed consent, privacy, confidentiality, continuity of care, and access to their medical records.

As client advocates, nurses assume responsibilities for protecting clients' rights.

Nurses have both personal and professional rights.

Nursing students have rights relative to their nursing education.

Nursing codes of ethics are formal guidelines for professional actions, designed to protect the rights of clients and nurses.

Bioethical issues in nursing may arise because conflicts between personal values and professional responsibilities or between people involved in client care.

To assist with resolution of an ethical dilemma, nurses should establish a sound data base, identify value conflicts, outline alternative courses of action and projected outcomes, determine who has ownership of the problem, and clarify the nurse's obligations regarding the resolution of the dilemma.

Selected References

American Hospital Association. January 1976. A patient's bill of rights. *Nursing Outlook* 24:29.

American Nurses' Association. 1985. *Code for nurses with interpretive statements.* Kansas City, Mo.: American Nurses' Association.

Annas, G. J. 1975. *The rights of hospital patients: The basic ACLU guide to a hospital patient's rights.* New York: Avon Books.

Aroskar, M. A. April 1980. Anatomy of an ethical dilemma. *American Journal of Nursing* 80:658–63.

Bandman, E. L. and Bandman, B. 1985. *Nursing Ethics in the Lifespan.* Norwalk, Conn.: Appleton-Century Crofts.

Baer, O. J. May/June 1985. Protecting your patients' privacy. *Nursing Life* 5:50–53.

Cory, G.; Corey, M. S.; and Callahan, P. 1984. *Issues and ethics in the helping professions.* 2d ed. Pacific Grove, Calif.: Brooks/Cole Publishing Co.

Curtin, L. L. October 1982. Informed consent: Rights, responsibilities, and roles. *Nursing Management* 13:7–8.

Curtin, L. L., and Flaherty, M. J. 1982. *Nursing ethics: Theories and pragmatics.* Bowie, Md.: Robert J. Brady Co.

Cushing, M. April 1984. Informed consent: An MD responsibility? *American Journal of Nursing* 84:437, 439–40.

Davis, A. April 1984. Patient's right to decide is new value in health care. Part 5. *American Nurse* 16:5–6, 24.

Davis, A. J. and Aroskar, M. A. 1983. *Ethical dilemmas and nursing practice.* 2d ed. Norwalk, Conn.: Appleton-Century-Crofts.

Fenner, K. M. 1980. Ethics and law in nursing professional perspectives. New York: D. Van Nostrand Co.

Fromer, M. J. 1981. *Ethical issues in health care.* St. Louis: C. V. Mosby Co.

———. 1986. Solving ethical dilemmas in nursing practice. In Chinn, P. L., editor. *Ethical issues in nursing.* Rockville, Md.: Aspen Systems Corporation.

Healey, J. M. 1983. Patients' rights and nursing. In Murphy, C. P., and Hunter, H., editors. *Ethical problems in the nurse-patient relationship.* Boston: Allyn and Bacon.

International Council of Nurses. 1973. *ICN code for nurses: Ethical concepts applied to nursing.* Geneva: Imprimeries Populaires.

Johnson, D. W. 1972. *Reaching out: Interpersonal effectiveness and self-actualization.* Englewood Cliffs, N.J.: Prentice-Hall.

Moser, D., and Cox, J. M., editors. May 1980. Perspectives: Resolving an ethical dilemma. *Nursing 80* 10:39–43.

Muldary, T. W. 1983. *Interpersonal relations for health professionals: A social skills approach.* New York: Macmillan Publishing Co.

Murphy, C. P., and Hunter, H. 1983. *Ethical problems in the nurse-patient relationship.* Boston: Allyn and Bacon.

President's Commission for the Study of Ethical Problems in Medicine and Biomedical and Behavioral Research: Making Health Care Decisions. 1982. Washington, D.C.: U.S. Government Printing Office.

Purtilo, R. B. 1978. *Health professional/patient interaction.* 2d ed. Philadelphia: W. B. Saunders Co.

Purtilo, R. B., and Cassel, C. K. 1981. *Ethical dimensions in the health professions.* Philadelphia: W. B. Saunders Co.

Rawnsley, M. M. 1986. The concept of privacy. In Chinn, P. L., editor. *Ethical issues in nursing.* Rockville, Md.: Aspen Systems Corporation.

Sigman, P. 1986. Ethical choice in nursing. In Chinn, P. L., editor. *Ethical issues in nursing.* Rockville, Md: Aspen Systems Corporation.

Silva, M. C. 1985. Comprehension of information for informed consent by spouses of surgical patients. *Research in Nursing and Health* 8:117–24.

Simon, S. B.; Howe, L. W.; and Kirschenbaum, H. 1978. *Values clarification: A handbook of practical strategies for teachers and students.* Rev. ed. New York: Hart Publishing Co.

Steele, S. M., and Harmon, V. M. 1983. *Values clarification in nursing.* 2d ed. Norwalk, Conn.: Appleton-Century-Crofts.

Thompson, J. B., and Thompson, H. O. 1985. *Bioethical decision making for nurses.* Norwalk, Conn.: Appleton-Century-Crofts.

Legal Aspects of Nursing

OBJECTIVES

Describe general legal concepts as they apply to nursing.

Identify essential aspects of privileged communications.

Explain how nurse practice acts legally protect the nurse practitioner.

Differentiate mandatory licensure from permissive licensure.

Describe ways that standards of care, agency policies, and job descriptions affect the scope of nursing practice.

Identify essential types and elements of contracts.

Identify rights and obligations associated with the nurse's legal roles.

Describe collective bargaining with reference to nursing.

Identify specific areas of potential liability in nursing.

Differentiate crimes from torts and give examples of each in nursing.

Differentiate malpractice from negligence.

Explain the nurse's responsibility to report crimes, torts, and unsafe practices of others.

Describe the purpose and essential elements of informed consent.

Explain the nurse's responsibilities in obtaining informed consent from competent adults, minors, mentally ill clients, and unconscious persons.

List information that needs to be included in an incident report.

Describe actions the nurse should take when a client is injured.

Explain the responsibilities of the nurse in witnessing a will.

(continued)

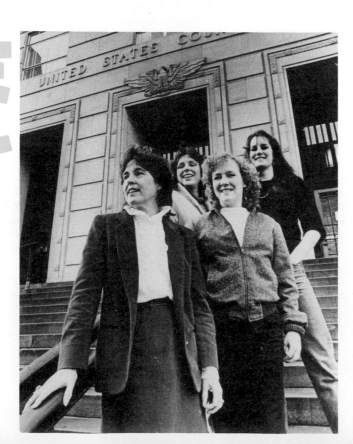

Identify positive and negative aspects of living wills.
Describe the legal implications of euthanasia, no-code, and slow-code orders for nurses.

Compare abortion laws in the United States and Canada.
Describe five legal issues surrounding death.
Explain the intent of Good Samaritan acts.

Describe the purpose of professional liability insurance.
Identify how nursing students can minimize chances for liability.

General Legal Concepts

Nursing practice is governed by many legal concepts. It is important for nurses to know the basics of legal concepts because nurses are accountable for their professional judgments and actions. *Accountability* is an essential concept of professional nursing practice and the law. Knowledge of laws that regulate and affect nursing practice is needed for two reasons:

1. To ensure that the nurse's decisions and actions are consistent with current legal principles
2. To protect the nurse from liability

Nearly every society has rules and regulations that are developed and promulgated by the society itself. These rules and regulations are the laws of the country, and they provide one aspect of social control for people. **Law** can be defined as "a system of principles and processes by which people, who live in a society, attempt to control human conduct in an effort to minimize the use of force as a means of resolving conflicting interests" (Rhodes and Miller 1984, p. 1). The functions of the law with reference to nursing are outlined in the accompanying box.

Sources of Law

The legal systems in both the United States and Canada have their origins in the English common law system. Three primary sources of law are constitutions, statutes, and decisions of courts (common law).

▪ Constitutions.
The Constitution of the United States and the Constitution of Canada are the supreme

---

Functions of the Law in Nursing

The law serves a number of functions in nursing. It:

Provides a framework for establishing what nursing actions in the care of clients are legal.
Differentiates the nurse's responsibilities from those of other health professionals.
Helps to establish the boundaries of independent nursing action.
Assists in maintaining a standard of nursing practice by making nurses accountable under the law.

---

laws of each country. They establish the general organization of the federal governments, grant certain powers to them, and place limits on what federal and state or provincial governments may do. Constitutions create legal rights and responsibilities and are the foundation for a system of justice. The rights created, however, do not relate directly to the nurse-client relationship.

Constitutions have due process and equal protection clauses. The due process clause applies to state or provincial and local agencies, including public hospitals, and to actions that deprive a person of life, liberty, or property. **Due process** has two primary elements:

1. The rules being applied must be reasonable and not vague.
2. Fair procedures must be followed when enforcing the rules.

Equal protection means that like persons must be dealt with in like fashion.

▪ Legislation (Statutes).
Laws enacted by any legislative body are called **statutory laws.** When there is a conflict between federal and state or provincial laws, federal law supersedes. Likewise, state or provincial laws supersede local laws.

The regulation of nursing is a function of state or provincial law. State or provincial legislatures pass statutes that define and regulate nursing, i.e., nurse practice acts. These acts, however, must be consistent with constitutional and federal provisions. Nurses practice acts, Good Samaritan laws, and adult or child abuse laws are examples of statutes that affect nurses.

Legislatures delegate responsibility and power to implement various laws to many administrative agencies who have the time and the expertise to address complex issues. State or provincial administrative agencies oversee the practice of the professions and regulate various aspects of commerce and public welfare. Examples pertinent to nurses are the state boards of nursing and provincial nursing associations, which implement and enforce nurse practice acts.

▪ Common Law.
The body of principles that evolves from court decisions is referred to as **common law,** or decisional laws. Although courts are called upon to interpret and apply constitutional or statutory law, they also are asked to resolve disputes between two parties. In such disputes, statutory and constitutional laws cannot support the case. Common law is continually being adapted and expanded. In deciding specific

controversies, courts generally adhere to the doctrine of *stare decisis*—"to stand by things decided"—usually referred to as "following precedent." In other words, in a current case, the court applies the same rules and principles as applied in similar cases decided previously and arrives at the same ruling. Courts may depart from precedent when slight differences are noted between cases or when it is thought that a particular common-law rule no longer applies to the needs of society. Decisions made by lower courts, for example local courts, must follow the decisions of higher courts, such as state or federal courts.

Principles of Law

The system of law rests on four simple principles that are often cloaked in complex terminology (Fenner 1980, p. 84). These are:

1. *Law is based on a concern for justice and fairness.* The law seeks to protect the rights of one party from the transgressions of another by setting guidelines for conduct and mechanisms to enforce those guidelines.
2. *Law is characterized by change.* Social and technologic changes occur rapidly, and often it is impossible to predict the problems that will follow. Often the legal system reacts rather than acts. For example, after technologic devices such as respirators were developed to prolong life, it became necessary for the law to change its guidelines about indications of death—from cessation of heart function to absence of electric currents from the brain for at least 24 hours.
3. *Actions are judged on the basis of a universal standard of what a similarly educated, reasonable, and prudent person would have done under similar circumstances.* All nurses are expected to function much as another nurse with similar education and experience would function. This rule of reasonable and prudent conduct is the basis for evaluating a person's actions, e.g., for judging whether or not actions were negligent.
4. *Each individual has rights and responsibilities.* Failure to meet one's responsibilities can endanger one's rights. For example, a registered nurse has the right to practice nursing within the constraints of the law (nurse practice acts). If she or he fails to observe these constraints (e.g., prescribes medications or conducts a surgical procedure), the behavior is considered irresponsible, and the right to practice can be revoked.

Privileged Communications

A **privileged communication** is information given to a professional person who is forbidden by law from disclosing the information in a court without the consent of the person who provided it. Legislation regarding privileged communications is highly complicated. A nurse would be unwise to encourage disclosures or advise a

client about the subject. The privileged communication law is for the benefit of the client; a nurse who is given confidential information should be prepared to answer questions fully and honestly if required to testify in a court of law. Many states which have statutes granting privileged communications between clients and health care providers do *not* extend the privilege to nurse-client communication.

The matter of privileged communications is referred to in the ANA's *Code for Nurses,* advising nurses to seek legal counsel in regard to a privileged communication and to become familiar with the rights and privileges of the client and the nurse. In Canada, confidentiality of information is incorporated as an ethic in the legislation on nursing practice. Failure to maintain confidentiality can result in disciplinary action against the nurse.

Legal Dimensions of Nursing

Nurse Practice Acts

Each state in the United States and each province of Canada has nurse practice acts, which protect the nurse's professional capacity and legally control nursing practice through licensing. Nurse practice acts legally define and describe the scope of nursing practice, which the law seeks to regulate, thereby protecting the public as well. Because of the number of acts, there are many definitions and descriptions of nursing.

Many states have an additional acts clause pertaining to acts that may be performed only by certain nurses with education beyond the minimum required for licensure under the act. For example, many of the clauses address the practice of nurse midwives or nurse anesthetists. Some address the nurse practitioner role. These clauses conflict with the ANA policy, which prohibits legal regulation of advanced or specialty nursing practice. The ANA believes it is the function of the professional association, not the law, to establish the scope and desirable qualifications required for each specialized area of practice (Snyder and LaBar 1984, p. 7).

Credentialing

Credentialing is the process of determining and maintaining competence in nursing practice. The credentialing process is one way in which the nursing profession maintains standards of practice and is accountable for the educational preparation of members. Credentialing includes licensure, registration, certification, and accreditation. Principles of credentialing reflect the belief that credentialing exists primarily to protect and benefit the public. See Table 6–1.

■ **Licensure and Registration.** Licenses are legal permits granted by a government agency to individuals to engage in the practice of a profession and to use a particular title. A particular jurisdiction or area is covered by the license. For a profession or occupation to obtain the right to license its members, it generally must meet three criteria:

1. There is a need to protect the public's safety or welfare.
2. The occupation is clearly delineated as a separate, distinct area of work.
3. There is an organization suitable in ability to assume the obligations of the licensing process.

In the United States, nurses are issued a license by individual state boards of nursing or by designated state agencies. **Licensure** is the process by which registered nurses who have successfully completed a course of studies in a school of nursing accredited by the state board of nursing, passed the national qualifying examinations with a score that is acceptable to the individual board and paid the required fee are permitted to practice nursing in that state. A state board may also grant a license to a nurse who holds an active practicing license in another state, through a process of endorsement, without the candidate having to rewrite examinations. The candidate, however, must have attained a passing score on the national examinations that is equal to, or above, that considered acceptable in the state in which she or he wishes to practice.

In Canada, nurses are not licensed except in the province of Quebec. They are, however, **registered** by their provincial nursing association and by the College of Nurses of Ontario. Nurses in the United States are also registered but must in addition be granted a license to practice. **Registration** is the listing of an individual's name and other information on the official roster of a governmental or nongovernmental agency.

There are two types of licensure/registration: mandatory and permissive. Under **mandatory licensure/registration,** anyone who practices nursing must be licensed or, in Canada, registered. The only exceptions are: practice in an emergency, practice by nursing students as part of their education, and practice by nurses employed by the federal government (e.g., nurses who practice in Veterans Administration hospitals and in federal public health agencies must be currently licensed in some jurisdiction but not necessarily where the facility is located).

Under **permissive licensure/registration,** the title RN is reserved for licensed or registered practitioners, but the practice of nursing is not prohibited to others who are not licensed or registered. Registration is permissive in most provinces of Canada. There is a strong movement underway in Canada to make registration mandatory in all provinces.

In each state and province there is a mechanism by which licenses (or registration in Canada) can be revoked for just cause, e.g., incompetent nursing practice; professional misconduct; conviction of a crime such as using illegal drugs or selling drugs illegally; obtaining a license through deception, falsifying school records, or hiding a criminal history; and, in some areas, aiding in a criminal abortion. In each situation, all the facts are generally reviewed by a committee at a hearing. Nurses are entitled to be represented by legal counsel at such a hearing. If the nurse's license is revoked as a result of the hearing,

Table 6-1 Principles of Credentialing

1. In addition to benefiting and protecting the public, credentialing also benefits those who are credentialed.

2. The legitimate interests of the involved occupation or institution and of the general public should be reflected in each credentialing mechanism.

3. Accountability should be an essential component of any credentialing process.

4. A system of checks and balances within the credentialing system should assure equitable treatment for all parties involved.

5. Periodic assessments with the potential for sanction are essential components of an effective credentialing mechanism.

6. Objective standards and criteria and persons competent in their use are essential to the credentialing process.

7. Representation in credentialing systems of the community of interests directly affected by credentialing mechanisms should assure consideration of the legitimate concerns of each group.

8. Professional identity and responsibility should evolve from the credentialing process.

9. An effective system of role delineation is fundamental to any credentialing mechanism for individuals.

10. An effective system of program identification is fundamental to any credentialing mechanism for institutions.

11. Coordination of credentialing mechanisms should lead to efficiency and cost effectiveness and avoid duplication.

12. Geographic, including interstate, mobility should be improved by the credentialing of the individual.

13. Widely accepted definitions and terminology are basic to an effective credentialing system.

14. Communications and understanding between health care providers and society should be facilitated through the credentialing process.

Source: Committee for the Study of Credentialing in Nursing. "The Study of Credentialing in Nursing: A New Approach," Vol. 1. *The Report of the Committee.* Kansas City, Missouri: American Nurses Association, 1979, 43–50.

an appeal can be made to a court, or, in some states, an agency is designated to review the decision before any court action is initiated.

▪ **Certification.** **Certification** is the voluntary practice of validating that an individual nurse has met minimum standards of nursing competence in specialty areas, such as maternal-child health, pediatrics, gerontology, mental health, and school nursing. Certification programs are conducted by the ANA and by specialty nursing organizations. A certification program has not yet been established in Canada, but the CNA is currently considering the establishment of a certification program for nurses in specialized fields of nursing.

▪ Accreditation/Approval of Basic Nursing Education Programs.

Accreditation is a process by which a voluntary organization (e.g., the NLN) or governmental agency (e.g., the state board of nursing) appraises and grants accredited status to institutions and/ or programs or services that meet predetermined structure, process, and outcome criteria (ANA 1979). Minimum standards for basic nursing education programs are established in each state of the United States and in each province in Canada. State accreditation or provincial approval is granted to schools of nursing meeting the minimum criteria. NLN accreditation is concerned with optimum, rather than minimum, standards. In other words, accreditation by the NLN certifies that an educational program not only meets minimum standards but also is considered "good" by national standards.

▪ Standards of Practice

Another way the nursing profession attempts to ensure that its practitioners are competent and safe to practice is through the establishment of standards of practice (see Chapter 1). These standards are often used to evaluate the quality of care provided by nurses. In addition to this basic set of standards, which are applicable in any practice setting, the ANA has developed standards of nursing practice for specific areas such as maternal-child, medical-surgical, geriatric, psychiatric, and community health nursing.

Contractual Arrangements in Nursing

A contract is the basis of the relationship between a nurse and an employer—for example, a nurse and a hospital or a nurse and a physician. A **contract** is an agreement between two or more competent persons, upon sufficient consideration (remuneration), to do or not to do some lawful act. A contract may be written or oral; however, a written contract cannot be changed legally by an oral agreement. If two people wish to change some aspect of a written contract, the change must be written into the contract, because one party cannot hold the other to an oral agreement that differs from the written one.

A contract is considered to be *expressed* when the two parties discuss and agree orally or in writing to its terms, e.g., that a nurse will work at a hospital for a stated length of time and under stated conditions. An *implied* contract is one in which there has been no discussion between the parties, but the law considers that a contract exists. In the contractual relationship between nurse and client, clients have the right to expect that nurses caring for them have the competence to meet their needs.

This *implies* that the nurse has a responsibility to remain competent. The nurse has the associated right to expect the client to provide accurate information as required.

Contract law requires that four elements be met to make a contract valid (Fenner 1980, p. 94):

1. The act contracted for must be legal. The nurse's employment must be legal, and the duties to be performed and services provided must be within the law.
2. The parties to the contract must be of legal age and competent (i.e., free of mental impairment) to enter into a binding agreement.
3. There must be mutual agreement about the service to be contracted for.
4. There must be compensation (or promise of it) for the service to be provided.

These four elements are also required for contracts made by clients (with nurses, other health professionals, or health care institutions) to be valid. For example, the activity contracted for between a client and a hospital is health care, which is legal. Clients who are minors are not usually admitted for care without the consent of their parents or legal guardians. The parties agree to the terms of the contract when the client gives informed consent for care and the hospital offers care. The client promises to reimburse the hospital for its services through insurance coverage or other means.

▪ Legal Roles of Nurses

Nurses have three separate, interdependent legal roles, each with rights and associated responsibilities:

1. **Provider of service.** The nurse is expected to provide safe and competent care so that harm (physical, psychologic, or material) to the recipient of the service is prevented. Implicit in this role are several legal concepts: liability, standard of care, and contractual obligations.

    Liability is the quality or state of being legally responsible to account for one's obligations and actions and to make financial restitution for wrongful acts. A primary nurse or team leader, for example, has an obligation to practice and direct the practice of others under supervision so that harm or injury to the client is prevented and standards of care are maintained. Even when a nurse is directed by a physician, the responsibility for nursing activity is the nurse's. When a nurse is requested to carry out an activity that the nurse believes will be injurious to the client, the nurse's responsibility is to refuse to carry out the order.

    The **standards of care** by which a nurse acts or fails to act are legally defined by nurse practice acts and by the rule of reasonable and prudent action—what a reasonable and prudent professional with similar preparation and experience would do in similar circumstances. A nurse, for example, would be acting illegally in diagnosing or treating a client for a tumor, since these functions are within the scope of the physician's practice, and nurses are constrained from engaging in them. **Contractual**

obligations refer to the nurse's duty of care, that is, duty to render care, established by the presence of an expressed or implied contract discussed earlier.

2. **Employee or contractor for service.** A nurse who is employed by a hospital works as an agent of the hospital, and the nurse's contract with clients is an implied one. However, a nurse who is employed directly by a client, for example, a private nurse, may have a written contract with that client in which the nurse agrees to provide professional services for a certain fee. If the client is dying, the nurse can be protected by a written contract that allows collection of the fee from the client's estate. A nurse might be prevented from carrying out the terms of the contract because of illness or death. However, personal inconvenience and personal problems, such as the nurse's car failure, are not legitimate reasons for failing to fulfill a contract.

Contractual relationships vary among practice settings. An independent nurse practitioner is a contractor for service, whose contractual relationship with the client is an independent one. The nurse employed by a hospital functions within an employer-employee relationship, in which the nurse represents and acts for the hospital and therefore must function within the policies of the employing agency. This type of legal relationship creates the ancient legal doctrine known as **respondeat superior** ("let the master answer"). In other words, the master (employer) assumes responsibility for the conduct of the servant (employee) and can also be held responsible for malpractice by the employee. By virtue of the employee role, therefore, the nurse's conduct is the hospital's responsibility.

This doctrine does not imply that the nurse cannot be held liable as an individual. Nor does it imply that the doctrine will prevail if the employee's actions are extraordinarily inappropriate, i.e., beyond those expected or foreseen by the employer. For example, if the nurse hits a client in the face, the employer could disclaim responsibility, since this behavior is beyond the bounds of expected behavior. Criminal acts, such as assisting with criminal abortions or taking tranquilizers from a client's supply for personal use, would also be considered extraordinarily inappropriate behavior. Nurses can be held liable for failure to act as well. For example, if a nurse sees another nurse hitting a client and fails to do anything to protect the client, the observer may also be considered negligent.

The nurse in the role of employee or contractor for service has obligations to the employer, the client, and other personnel. The nursing care provided must be within the limitations and terms specified. The nurse has an obligation to contract to meet only those responsibilities that she or he is competent to discharge. As an employee, the nurse is expected to uphold the good name of the employer and therefore should not criticize the employer unjustifiably. The employer, in turn, is obligated to provide adequate working conditions, e.g., a safe, functional employment setting.

The nurse is expected to respect the rights and responsibilities of other health care participants. For example, although the nurse has responsibility to explain nursing activities to a client, she or he does not have the right to comment on medical practice in a way that disturbs the client or causes problems for the physician. At the same time, the nurse has the right to expect reasonable and prudent conduct from other health care providers.

3. **Citizen.** The rights and responsibilities of the nurse in the role of citizen are the same as those of any individual under the legal system. Rights of citizenship protect clients from harm and ensure consideration for their personal property rights, rights to privacy, confidentiality, and other rights discussed later in this chapter and in Chapter 5. These same rights apply to nurses. For example, nurses have the right to physical safety and need not perform functions that are considered to pose an unreasonable risk.

Nurses move in and out of these roles when carrying out professional and personal responsibilities. An understanding of these roles and the rights and responsibilities associated with them promotes legally responsible conduct and practice by nurses. See Table 6–2 for examples of the responsibilities and rights associated with each role.

▪ **C**ollective Bargaining

Collective bargaining is a formalized decision-making process between management and labor representatives concerning salaries, work environment, and conditions of employment (Crawford et al. 1985, p. 155). Through a written agreement, both employer and employees legally commit themselves to observe the terms and conditions of employment. Collective bargaining is a controversial issue among nurses. Some nurses argue against collective bargaining on the grounds that it is contrary to the nature of professionalism, it is not necessary, it fosters discord, and it undermines the nurse administrator's role (McClelland 1983, p. 36). Others argue that collective bargaining it is necessary to obtain control of nursing practice and economic security.

The collective bargaining process involves the recognition of a certified bargaining agent for the employees. This agent can be a union, a trade association, or a professional organization. The agent represents the employees in negotiating a contract with management.

When collective bargaining breaks down because an agreement cannot be reached, the employees usually call a strike. A **strike** is an organized work stoppage by a group of employees to express a grievance, enforce a demand for changes in conditions of employment (see the selected working conditions that hinder delivery of nursing services on page 87), or solve a dispute with management (Crawford et al. 1985, p. 162).

Because nursing practice is a service to people (often ill people), striking presents a moral dilemma to many nurses. Actions taken by nurses can affect the safety of people. When faced with a strike, each nurse must make

Table 6–2 Nurses' Legal Roles, Rights, and Responsibilities

Role	Responsibilities	Rights
Provider of service	To provide safe and competent care commensurate with the nurse's preparation, experience, and circumstances To inform clients of the consequences of various alternatives and outcomes of care To provide adequate supervision and evaluation of subordinates for whom the nurse is responsible To remain competent	Right to adequate and qualified assistance as necessary Right to reasonable and prudent conduct from clients, e.g., provision of accurate information as required
Employee or contractor for service	To fulfill the obligations of contracted service with the employer	Right to adequate working conditions, e.g., safe equipment and facilities Right to compensation for services rendered
Citizen	To respect the rights and responsibilities of other health care participants To protect the rights of the recipients of care	Right to reasonable and prudent conduct by other health care givers Right to respect by others of the nurse's own rights and responsibilities

an individual decision as to whether or not to cross a picket line. Nursing students may also be faced with decisions about crossing picket lines in the event of a strike at a clinical agency used for learning experiences. The ANA supports striking as a means of achieving economic and general welfare.

Collective bargaining is more than the negotiation of salary terms and hours of work; it is a continuous process in which day-to-day working problems and relationships can be handled in an orderly and democratic manner. Day-to-day difficulties or grievances are handled through the grievance procedure: a formal plan established in the contract that outlines the channels for handling and settling grievances through progressively higher levels of administration. A **grievance** is any dispute, difference, controversy, or disagreement arising out of the terms and conditions of employment. Grievances fall into four main categories outlined in Table 6–3.

Areas of Potential Liability in Nursing

Crimes and Torts

A **crime** is an act committed in violation of public (criminal) law and punishable by a fine and/or imprisonment. A crime does *not* have to be intended in order to be a crime. For example, a nurse may accidentally give a client an additional and lethal dose of a narcotic to relieve discomfort.

Crimes are classified as either felonies (or in Canada, indictable offenses) or misdemeanors (or in Canada, summary conviction offenses). A **felony** is a crime of a serious nature, such as murder, punishable by a term in prison. In some areas, second-degree murder is called **manslaughter.** A nurse who accidentally gives an additional and lethal dose of a narcotic can be accused of manslaughter. Other examples of felonies are arson, armed

robbery, and, in Canada, criminal abortion and attempted suicide.

Crimes are punished through criminal action by the state or province against an individual. A **misdemeanor** is an offense of a less serious nature and is usually punishable by a fine or short-term jail sentence, or both. A nurse who takes a bottle of wine from a client's locker could be charged with a misdemeanor.

A **tort** is a civil wrong committed against a person or a person's property. Torts are usually litigated in court by civil action between individuals. In other words, the person or persons claimed to be responsible for the tort are sued for damages. Tort liability almost always is based on fault, i.e., something was done incorrectly (an unrea-

Table 6–3 Categories and Examples of Grievances

Category	Examples
Contract violations	Shift or weekend work is assigned inequitably. A nurse is dismissed without cause.
Violations of federal and state law	A female nurse is paid less than a male nurse for the same work. Appropriate payment is not given for overtime work. Minority group nurses are not promoted.
Management responsibilities	Appropriate locker room facilities are not provided. Safe client care is jeopardized by inadequate staffing.
Violation of agency rules	Performance evaluations are conducted only at termination of employment, but the contract requires annual evaluations. A vacation period is assigned without the nurse's agreement, as required in personnel policies.

Source: American Nurses' Association, *The grievance procedure* (Kansas City, Mo.: ANA, 1985), pp. 2–4. Used by permission.

sonable act of commission) or something that should have been done was not done (act of omission).

Torts may be classified as intentional or unintentional. **Intentional torts** include fraud, invasion of privacy, libel and slander, assault and battery, and false imprisonment. **Fraud** is the false presentation of some fact with the intention that it will be acted upon by another person. For example, it is fraud for a nurse applying to a hospital for employment fail to list two past employers for deceptive reasons when she or he is asked to list the previous five employers.

The right to privacy is the right of individuals to withhold themselves and their lives from public scrutiny. **Invasion of privacy** is a direct wrong of a personal nature. It injures the feelings of the person and does not take into account the effect of revealed information on the standing of the person in the community. The right to privacy can also be described as the right to be left alone. Liability can result if the nurse breaches confidentiality by passing along confidential client information to others.

Both libel and slander are wrongful actions that come under the heading of defamation. **Defamation** is communication that is false, or made with a careless disregard for the truth, and results in injury to the reputation of a person. **Libel** is defamation by means of print, writing, or pictures. **Slander** is defamation by the spoken word, stating unprivileged (not legally protected) or false words by which a reputation is damaged. A nurse has a qualified privilege to make statements that could be considered invasions of a client's privacy, both orally and in writing, but only as a part of nursing practice and only to a physician or another health team member caring directly for the client.

In the United States, the terms *assault* and *battery* are often heard together, but each has its own meaning. **Assault** can be described as an attempt or threat to touch another person unjustifiably. Assault precedes battery; it is the act that causes the person to believe a battery is about to occur. For example, the person who threatens someone by making a menacing gesture with a club or a closed fist is guilty of assault. In nursing, a client may perceive that a nurse is *about to* administer an injection without his or her consent.

Battery is the willful touching of a person (or the person's clothes or even something the person is carrying), which may or may not cause harm. To be actionable at law, however, the touching must be wrong in some way, e.g., done without permission, embarrassing, or causing injury. For example, the nurse who administers a hypodermic injection to a client or ambulates a client without his or her consent could be held liable for battery. Liability applies even though the physician ordered the medication or the activity and even if the client benefits from the nurse's action.

In Canada, the term *battery* is not used. Instead assault is classified into three categories: assault with intention to injure (for example, threatening someone by making a menacing gesture with a knife), assault causing bodily injury, and sexual assault. **False imprisonment** is unjustifiable detention that deprives a person of personal liberty for any length of time. For example, a nurse

---

Selected Working Conditions That Hinder Delivery of Nursing Services

Improper use of nurses and other staff

Improper ratio of qualified nurses and unlicensed staff to clients

Lack of involvement of nurses in decision making about delivery of nursing services

Inadequate orientation, in-service, and staff development programs

Inadequate supplies and equipment

Restrictive or rigid policies and procedures

Unsafe and hazardous conditions

Assignment of nonnursing duties

Limited opportunities for nurses to work together as a group to initiate needed changes

(Flanagan 1983)

---

who locks a client in a room unjustifiably is guilty of false imprisonment. False imprisonment accompanied by forceful restraint or threat of restraint is assault and battery (Creighton 1981, p. 207).

Although nurses may suggest to a client under certain circumstances that he or she remain in the room or in bed, the client must not be detained against his or her will. The client has a right to insist upon leaving even though it may be detrimental to health. Detention is legal only when imposed to protect the public or to protect the individual from unintended harm, for example, when a client is drugged and unable to control his or her behavior.

Negligence and malpractice are examples of **unintentional torts** that may occur in health care settings. **Negligence** is "the omission to do something that a reasonable person, guided by those ordinary considerations which ordinarily regulate human affairs, would do, or doing something which a reasonable and prudent person would not do" (Creighton 1981, p. 154). **Malpractice** is that part of the law of negligence applied to the professional person: It is, in effect, any professional misconduct or unreasonable lack of professional skill. A nurse could be liable for malpractice if she or he injured a client while performing a procedure differently from the way other nurses would have done it.

Nurses are responsible for their own actions whether they are independent practitioners or employees of a health agency. The descriptions of negligence and malpractice do not mention good intentions; it is not pertinent that the nurse did not intend to be negligent. If a nurse administers an incorrect medication, even in good faith, the fact that the nurse failed to read the label correctly indicates malpractice if all of the elements of negligence are met.

Another significant aspect of negligence and malpractice is that both omissions and commissions are included. That is, a person can be negligent by forgetting to give a medication as well as by giving the wrong medication. See Table 6−4 for a summary of the differences between intentional and unintentional torts.

Table 6—4 Comparison of Intentional and Unintentional Torts

Intentional	Unintentional (Negligence)
1. They involve the commission of a prohibited act.	1. They can result from either an act of commission or an act of omission.
2. The act in question is willful and deliberate (intentional).	2. The wrong results from failure to use due care.
3. They involve certain specific types of conduct listed as "wrong."	3. They are not spelled out in an all-inclusive list.

▪ Potential Malpractice Situations in Nursing

If a nurse wishes to avoid charges of malpractice, it is helpful to recognize those nursing situations in which negligent actions are most likely to occur and to take measures to prevent them. The most common situation is the **medication error.** Because of the large number of medications on the market today and the variety of methods of administration, these errors may be on the increase. Nursing errors include not reading the medication label, misreading or incorrectly calculating the dosage, not identifying the client correctly, preparing the wrong concentration, or administering a medication by the wrong route (e.g., intravenously instead of orally). Some medication errors are very serious and can result in death. For example, administering dicumarol to a client recently returned from surgery could cause the client to have a hemorrhage. Nurses always need to check medications very carefully. Even after checking, the nurse is wise to recheck the medication order and the medication before administering it if the client states, for example, that he or she "did not have a green pill before."

Sponges or other small items can be left inside a client during an operation because the nurse either failed to count them before the surgeon closed the incision or counted them incorrectly. In either case, the nurse responsible for the **sponge count** can be held liable for malpractice.

A relatively frequent malpractice action attributed to nurses is **burning a client.** Burns may be caused by hot water bottles, heating pads, and solutions that are too hot for application. Elderly, comatose, or diabetic people are particularly vulnerable to burns due to their decreased sensitivity. Hot objects can burn these people before they notice it. A nurse may also be held negligent for leaving a client without taking precautions (giving warnings or providing protections), for example, when using a steam vaporizer.

Clients often fall accidentally, sometimes with resultant injury. Some falls can be prevented by elevating the side rails on the cribs, beds, and stretchers of babies and small children, and of adults when necessary. If a nurse leaves the rails down or leaves a baby unattended on a bath table, that nurse is guilty of malpractice if the **client falls** and is injured as a direct result of not placing the siderails up or leaving the child unattended. Most hospitals and nursing homes have policies regarding the use of safety devices such as side rails and restraints. The nurse needs to be familiar with these policies and to take indicated precautions to prevent accidents.

In some instances, nurses are found guilty of malpractice by ignoring a client's complaints. This type of malpractice is termed **failure to observe and take appropriate action.** The nurse who does not report a client's complaint of acute abdominal pain is negligent, and may be found guilty of malpractice for ensuing appendix rupture and death. By failing to take the blood pressure and pulse and to check the dressing of a client who has just had a kidney removed, a nurse omits important assessments. If the client hemorrhages and dies, the nurse may be held responsible for the death as a result of this malpractice.

Incorrectly identifying clients is a problem, particularly in busy hospital units. Nurses have prepared the wrong client for an operation with unfortunate results such as a healthy gallbladder being removed from the wrong person. Cases of **mistaken indentity** are costly to the client and render the nurse liable for malpractice.

Client property, such as jewelry, money, and dentures, is a constant concern to hospital personnel. Today, agencies are taking less responsibility for property and are generally requesting clients to sign a waiver on admission relieving the hospital and its employees of any responsibility for property. There are, however, situations in which the client cannot sign a waiver, and the nursing staff must follow prescribed policies for safeguarding the client's property. In hospital units, dentures are often a major problem; they can be lost in bedding or left on a meal tray. Nurses are expected to take reasonable precautions to safeguard a client's property, and they can be held liable for its **loss or damage** if they do not exercise reasonable care.

▪ Reporting Crimes, Torts, and Unsafe Practices

Nurses may need to report nursing colleagues or other health professionals for practices that endanger the health and safety of clients. For instance, alcohol and drug use, thcft from a client or agency, and unsafe nursing practice should be reported. Reporting a colleague is not easy. The person reporting may feel disloyal, incur the disapproval of others, or endanger her or his chances for promotion. When reporting an incident or series of incidents, the nurse must be careful to describe observed behavior only and not make inferences as to what might be happening. In cases of substance abuse, states such as California have established voluntary programs that allow nurses to receive help in resolving their problems without losing their licenses to practice.

Selected Legal Facets of Nursing Practice

Informed Consent

Informed consent is an agreement by a client to accept a course of treatment or a procedure after complete information, including the risks of treatment and facts relating to it, has been provided by the physician. Informed consent, then, is an exchange between a client and a physician. Usually the client signs a form provided by the agency. The form is a record of the informed consent, not the informed consent itself.

Obtaining informed consent is the responsibility of a physician. Although this responsibility is delegated to nurses in some agencies, this practice is undesirable. The nurse's responsibility is often to witness the giving of informed consent. This involves witnessing the exchange between the physician and the client, witnessing the client's signature, and establishing that the client really did understand, i.e., was really informed.

If a nurse witnesses only the client's signature and not the exchange between the client and the physician, the nurse should write "witnessing signature only" on the form (Northrop 1984, p. 223). If the nurse finds that the client really does not understand the physician's explanation, then it is important to notify the physician. Northrop (1984, p. 223) describes three major elements of informed consent:

1. The consent must be given voluntarily.
2. The consent must be given by an individual with the capacity and competence to understand.
3. The client must be given enough information to be the ultimate decision maker.

To give informed consent voluntarily, the client must not feel coerced. Sometimes fear of disapproval by a health professional can be the motivation for giving consent; such consent is not voluntarily given.

To give informed consent, the client must receive sufficient information to make a decision; otherwise, the client's right to decide has been usurped. Information needs to include benefits, risks, and alternative procedures. It is also important that the client understand. Technical words and language barriers can inhibit understanding. If a client cannot read, the consent form must be read to him or her before it is signed. If the client does not speak the same language as the health professional who is providing the information, an interpreter must be acquired.

If a client is given sufficient information, he or she can make decisions regarding health. To do so, the client must be competent and an adult. A competent adult is a person over 18 years of age who is conscious and oriented. A person under 18 years who is considered "an emancipated minor," i.e., self-supporting or married, can also give consent. A client who is confused, dis-oriented, or sedated is not considered functionally competent at that time.

There are three groups of people who cannot provide consent. The *first* is minors. In most areas, consent must be given by a parent or guardian before minors can obtain treatment. The same is true of an adult who has the mental capacity of a child if a guardian has been appointed. In some states, however, minors are allowed to give consent for such procedures as blood donations, treatment for drug dependency and sexually transmitted disease, and procedures for obstetrical care. The *second* group is persons who are unconscious or injured in such a way that they are unable to give consent. In these situations, consent is usually obtained from the closest adult relative if existing statutes permit. In an emergency, if consent cannot be obtained from the client or a relative, then the law generally agrees that consent is assumed. The *third* group is mentally ill persons who have been judged to be incompetent. States and province mental health acts or similar statutes generally provide definitions of mental illness and specify the rights of the mentally ill under the law as well as the rights of the staff caring for such clients.

Recordkeeping

The client's medical record is a legal document and can be produced in court as evidence. Often the record is used to remind a witness of events surrounding a lawsuit, since it usually takes several months or years for the suit to go to trial. The effectiveness of a witness's testimony can depend on the accuracy of such records. Nurses, therefore, need to keep accurate and complete records of nursing care provided to clients. Failure to keep proper records can constitute negligence and be the basis for tort liability. Insufficient or inaccurate assessments and documentation can hinder proper diagnosis and treatment and result in injury to the client. Types of records and essential facts about recording are discussed in Chapter 22.

Controlled Substances

United States and Canadian laws regulate the distribution and use of controlled substances such as narcotics, depressants, stimulants, and hallucinogens. Misuse of controlled substances leads to criminal penalties. Controlled substances are kept in securely locked drawers or cupboards, and only authorized personnel have access to them. See Chapter 44 for the legal aspects of drug administration.

The Incident Report

An **incident report** is an agency record of an accident or incident. This report is used to make all the facts about an accident available to agency personnel, to contribute to statistical data about accidents or incidents, and to help health personnel prevent future accidents.

Information to Include in an Incident Report

Identify the client by name, initials, and hospital or identification number.

Give the date, time, and place of the incident.

Describe the facts of the incident. Avoid any conclusions or blame. Describe the incident as you saw it even if your impressions differ from those of others.

Identify all witnesses to the incident.

Identify any equipment by number and any medication by name and number.

Document any circumstance surrounding the incident; e.g., another client (Mrs. Losas) was experiencing cardiac arrest.

All accidents are usually reported on incident forms. Some agencies also report other incidents, e.g., the occurrence of client infection or the loss of personal affects. The accompanying box lists the information to be included in an incident report. The report should be completed as soon as possible, always within 24 hours of the incident.

Incident reports are often reviewed by an agency committee, which decides whether to investigate the incident further. The nurse may be required upon further investigation to answer such questions as: Why do you believe the accident occurred? How could it have been prevented? Should any equipment be adjusted? The nurse who believes she or he may be dismissed or that suit may be brought should obtain legal advice. Even if the agency clears the nurse of responsibility, the client or the client's family may file suit. The plaintiff, however, bears the burden of proof that the accident occurred because reasonable care was not taken. Even if the accepted standard of care was not given, the plaintiff must prove that the accident was the direct result of unacceptable standards of care and that the accident caused physical, emotional, or financial injury.

When an accident occurs, the nurse should first assess the client and intervene to prevent injury. If a client is injured, nurses must take steps to protect the client, themselves, and their employer. Most agencies have policies regarding accidents. It is important to follow these policies and not to assume one is negligent. Although this may be the case, accidents do happen even when every precaution has been taken to prevent them.

Wills

A **will** is a declaration by a person about how the person's property is to be disposed of after his or her death. In order for a will to be valid, the following conditions must be met:

1. The person making the will must be of sound mind, that is, able to understand and retain mentally the general nature and extent of his or her property, the relationship of the beneficiaries and of relatives to whom none of the estate will be left, and the disposition he or she is making of the property. A person, therefore, who is seriously ill and unable to carry out usual roles may be still able to direct preparation of a will.

2. The person must not be unduly influenced by anyone else. Sometimes a client may be persuaded by someone who is close at that particular time to make that person a beneficiary. Clients sometimes are persuaded to leave their estates to persons looking after them rather than to their relatives. Frequently, the relatives contest the will in such situations and take the matter to court, claiming undue influence.

Nurses may be requested from time to time to witness a will, although most agencies have policies that nurses not do so. In most states and provinces, a will must be signed in the presence of two witnesses. In some situations, a mark can suffice if the person making the will cannot write a signature. If a nurse is a witness to a will, the nurse should note on the client's chart the fact that a will was made and the nurse's perception of the physical and mental condition of the client. This record provides the nurse with accurate information if the nurse is called as a witness later. The record may also be helpful if the will is contested. If a nurse does not wish to act as a witness, for example, if in the nurse's opinion undue influence has been brought on the client, then it is the nurse's right to refuse to act in this capacity.

Euthanasia and the Right to Die (Living Wills)

Euthanasia is the act of painlessly putting to death persons suffering from incurable or distressing disease. It is commonly referred to as mercy killing. Regardless of compassion and good intentions or moral convictions, euthanasia is *legally wrong* in both Canada and the United States and can lead to criminal charges of homicide or to a civil lawsuit for withholding treatment or providing an unacceptable standard of care. Because advanced technology has enabled the medical profession to sustain life almost indefinitely, people are increasingly considering the meaning of quality of life. For some people, the withholding of artificial life-support measures or even the withdrawal of life support is a desired and acceptable practice for clients who are terminally ill or who are incurably disabled and believed unable to live their lives without some happiness and meaning.

Voluntary euthanasia refers to situations in which the dying individual desires some control over the time and manner of death. All forms of euthanasia are illegal except in states where right-to-die statutes and living wills exist. Right-to-die statutes legally recognize the client's right to refuse treatment.

Living wills (an individual's signed request to be allowed to die when life can be supported only mechanically or by heroic measures) and right-to-die statutes have received increasing attention in recent years. Most nurses agree that people have a right not to participate in medical treatment or to refuse treatment once it has started. When a person is being maintained on life-sustaining machines, however, a conflict may arise between

Adults are legally competent unless courts rule otherwise

Patients' degree of mental or physical competency or ability to make health care decisions has a significant relationship to the nursing care that they receive. The extent of some patients' ability to participate is questionable. These patients include the mentally ill, mentally retarded, comatose or unconscious patients and the incapacitated elderly. Many nurses automatically assume that these patients are incompetent, and thus make no effort to involve them in their care and treatment decisions. But talking to the elderly patient's son or daughter about the nursing care plan and interventions without consulting the patient not only demonstrates a lack of respect for the patient, but [also] gives the patient no opportunity to be involved and make informed choices. These are legal rights of patients.

The legal definition of competence is determined by the state legislature. All states define a legally competent individual as one who has reached the age of majority, which is usually set at 18 years of age. Therefore, anyone over the age of majority is presumed competent; all who are under it are presumed incompetent. On reaching the age of majority, one gains legal rights and responsibilities, including the right to vote, to enter into a contract, to choose and enter a profession, to own and manage property, and to consent to and/or refuse health care, even life sustaining care.

State legislatures have created some exceptions to the presumed incompetent status of minors. Minors are considered to be competent, if, for example, they marry, become parents, live independently, or seek certain health care treatments, such as mental health counseling or contraception.

In American jurisprudence, adults are presumed legally competent unless declared incompetent through a formal judicial process. A presumption is a given. It can be challenged by evidence or circumstances showing that the presumption is not valid. But until that point, validity is presumed. To determine if a patient is incompetent, courts rely on opinions of the patient's physicians, other health care providers, consulting psychiatrists, family, and the patient. Nurses are frequently being called on to testify at such hearing. . . .

Even patients judicially declared incompetent may still have the capability to be involved in health care treatment decisions. The right of involuntarily committed [incompetent] mentally ill patients to refuse antipsychotic medications has been upheld in recent cases. Yet, unless declared incompetent by a formal hearing, adult patients are legally presumed competent even if they are clearly without decision-making capability in the opinion of their caregivers. . . .

Legal scholars have identified three approaches to determining a patient's decision-making capability: outcome, status, and functional ability. This last approach, which focuses on the individual's actual functioning in decision-making situations, is the approach of choice and includes four tests: evincing a choice; evincing an understanding of relevant information and issues; rationally manipulating the relevant information; and appreciating the nature of the situation, including the nature and consequences of refusing treatment.

Legal competency is not the same as mental or physical competency. It is a legal concept, representing a legal status. It is the presumed status of every adult patient for which nurses care.

Source: C. E. Northrop, Nursing practice and the legal presumption of competency, (Legal Outlook), *Nursing Outlook*, March/April 1988, 36(2): 112.

a physician's ability to prolong life physiologically and the individual's right to die with dignity. Living wills grew out of this conflict. California was the first state to enact legislation, the California Natural Death Act of 1976, that gives legal recognition to a person's desire to control his or her right to die. Since then, 14 other states and the District of Columbia have enacted similar laws. Some oppose these laws, contending there is no need for such laws, the laws exclude family from the decision, and the law hastens death. For a sample living will, see Figure 6–1.

Nurses need to familiarize themselves with statutes that authorize living wills in the state where they are employed. Where statutes do exist, policy and procedures are usually detailed specifically. They may include the need to obtain a court order, a medical opinion, the agreement of an ethics or medical committee, family confirmation, or some combination of these. The statutes usually grant civil and criminal immunity to those who carry out living-will requests.

No-Code and Slow-Code Orders

Physicians may order "no code" or "slow code" for clients who are in a stage of terminal, irreversible illness or expected death. **No code** means no effort is to be made to resuscitate the client. No-code orders may also be written as *"no heroics"* or *DNR* (do not resuscitate or do not make resuscitative efforts). **Slow code** means "half-hearted" resuscitation measures are to be initiated and implemented. "Slow-code" orders are frequently not written orders, but are conveyed in an informal manner (i.e., the physician issuing the order does *not* want it to be written as a verbal or telephone order) and are *not* legally acceptable.

The American Heart Association (AHA) has issued "Standards and Guidelines for Cardiopulmonary Resuscitation and Emergency Cardiac Care" outlining the medicolegal considerations and offering recommendations about DNR orders for physicians (AHA 1986, p. 2880). Although these standards, like those of any pro-

- ▪ TO MY FAMILY, MY PHYSICIAN, MY LAWYER, MY CLERGYMAN
- ▪ TO ANY MEDICAL FACILITY IN WHOSE CARE I HAPPEN TO BE
- ▪ TO ANY INDIVIDUAL WHO MAY BECOME RESPONSIBLE FOR MY HEALTH, WELFARE OR AFFAIRS

Death is as much a reality as birth, growth, maturity and old age—it is the one certainty of life. If the time comes when I, _____, can no longer take part in decisions for my own future, let this statement stand as an expression of my wishes, while I am still of sound mind.

If the situation should arise in which there is no reasonable expectation of my recovery from physical or mental disability, I request that I be allowed to die and not be kept alive by artificial means or "heroic measures." I do not fear death itself as much as the indignities of deterioration, dependence and hopeless pain. I, therefore, ask that medication be mercifully administered to me to alleviate suffering even though this may hasten the moment of death.

This request is made after careful consideration. I hope you who care for me will feel morally bound to follow its mandate. I recognize that this appears to place a heavy responsibility upon you, but it is with the intention of relieving you of such responsibility and of placing it upon myself in accordance with my strong convictions that this statement is made.

Signed _____

Date _____

Witness _____

Witness _____

Copies of this request have been given to:

_____

_____

_____

_____

Figure 6–1 A sample living will. *Source:* Concern for Dying, 250 W. 57th St., New York, N.Y. 10107. Reprinted with permission.

fessional organization, are not legally binding, they are persuasive to a judge and jury. They indicate that CPR is intended to prevent *unexpected* death and that its intent is not to continue life when death is *expected*. The implications of the AHA no-code standards for nurses include:

1. Ensure that the DNR order is written on the client's order sheet and progress notes. Verbal orders can be easily misunderstood and disclaimed.
2. If the physician refuses to write such an order, follow agency policies and procedures. Some agencies have established formal protocols for nurses to follow. Because such procedures are usually carefully reviewed by legal counsel, they can minimize the risk of legal liability substantially.
3. If the agency does not have a well-established procedure, seek a legal opinion through the agency attorney or state or provincial nursing association.
4. If none of the above steps provides the nurse with sufficient guidelines, the nurse must make a personal decision based on moral values and sense of humanity. Even when there are appropriate guidelines, the guidelines may conflict with the nurse's personal ethics. Thus, DNR orders may create an

ethical dilemma as well as a legal dilemma for the nurse.

Abortions

Abortion laws provide specific guidelines for nurses about what is legally permissible. In 1973, when the *Roe vs. Wade* and *Doe vs. Bolton* cases were decided, the Supreme Court of the United States held that the constitutional rights of privacy give a woman the right to control her own body to the extent that she can abort her fetus in the early stages of pregnancy. The state, however, has a legitimate interest in controlling abortion during later stages of pregnancy. The results of the Supreme Court rulings are:

1. It is not legally permissible for the state to restrict or regulate abortions during the first trimester (first 3 months) of pregnancy except to require that the abortion be performed by a licensed physician.
2. During the second trimester of pregnancy (4 to 6 months), the mother's privacy rights must yield to *reasonable* restrictions designed to protect the health and safety of the mother. Restrictions include that the facility in which the abortion is performed be licensed.
3. During the third trimester of pregnancy, the state has the right to prohibit abortion. The rationale for this ruling is that by this stage of pregnancy the state's interest in protecting the viable but unborn child outweighs the woman's right to privacy.

Since these rulings, many states have enacted statutes. In addition, the Supreme Court no longer requires that the parents of a pregnant minor consent to abortion, nor that the father of the woman's child (whether he is her husband or not) consent; however, there are opportunities to appeal these waivers.

Many statutes also include **conscience clauses,** upheld by the Supreme Court, designed to protect nurses and hospitals. These clauses give hospitals the right to deny admission to abortion clients and give health care personnel, including nurses, the right to refuse to participate in abortions. When these rights are exercised, the statutes also protect the agency and employee from discrimination or retaliation. In Canada, abortion is a criminal offense that can result in up to 2 years in prison *unless* the abortion is approved by a medical abortion committee in an approved hospital.

Death and Related Issues

Legal issues surrounding death include the death certificate, labeling of the deceased, autopsy, organ donation, and inquest. By law, a **death certificate** must be made out when a person dies. It is usually signed by the attending physician and filed with a local health or other government office. The family is usually given a copy to use for legal matters, such as insurance claims.

Nurses have a duty to handle the deceased with

dignity and label the corpse appropriately. Mishandling can cause emotional distress to survivors. Mislabeling can create legal problems if the body is inappropriately identified and prepared incorrectly for burial or a funeral. Usually, the deceased's wrist identification tag is left on, and another tag is tied to the client's ankles, in case one of the tags becomes detached. Tags tied to the ankles are preferred, since any tissue damage they cause will be concealed by bed linen or clothing. A third tag is attached to the shroud. All identification tags should include the client's name, hospital number, and physician's name.

An **autopsy** or **postmortem examination** is an examination of the body after death. It is performed only in certain cases. The law describes under what circumstances an autopsy must be performed, e.g., when death is sudden or when it occurs within 48 hours of admission to a hospital. The organs and tissues of the body are examined to establish the exact cause of death, to learn more about a disease, and to assist in the accumulation of statistical data.

It is the responsibility of the physician or, in some instances, of a designated person in the hospital to obtain consent for autopsy. Consent must be given by the decedent (before death) or by the next of kin. Laws in many states and provinces prioritize the family members who can provide consent as follows: surviving spouse, adult children, parents, siblings. After autopsy, hospitals cannot retain any tissues or organs without the permission of the person who consented to the autopsy.

■ **Organ Donation.** Under the Uniform Anatomical Gift Act in the United States or the Human Tissue Act in Canada, any person 18 years or older and of sound mind may make a gift of all or any part of his or her body for the following purposes: for medical or dental education, research, advancement of medical or dental science, therapy, or transplantation (Annas et al. 1981, p. 227). The donation can be made by a provision in a will or by signing a cardlike form in the presence of two witnesses. This card is usually carried at all times by the person who signed it. In most states and provinces, the gift can be revoked either by destroying the card or by an oral revocation in the presence of two witnesses. Nurses may serve as witnesses for persons consenting to donate organs. In some states (e.g., California) health care workers are required to ask survivors for consent to donate the deceased's organs.

■ **Inquest.** An **inquest** is a legal inquiry into the cause or manner of a death. When a death is the result of an accident, for example, an inquest is held into the circumstances of the accident to determine any blame. The inquest is conducted under the jurisdiction of a coroner or medical examiner. A **coroner** is a public official, not necessarily a physician, appointed or elected to inquire into the causes of death, when appropriate. A **medical examiner** is a physician who usually has advanced education in pathology or forensic medicine. Agency policy dictates who is responsible for reporting deaths to the coroner or medical examiner.

Legal Protections for Nurses

Good Samaritan Acts

Good Samaritan acts are laws designed to protect health care providers who provide assistance at the scene of an emergency against claims of malpractice unless it can be shown that there was a gross departure from the normal standard of care or willful wrongdoing on their part. **Gross negligence** usually involves further injury or harm to the person. For example, an injured child left on the side of the road may be struck by an automobile when the nurse leaves to obtain help.

In the United States, most state statutes do not require citizens to render aid to people in distress. Such assistance is considered more of an *ethical* than a *legal* duty. A few states, however, have enacted legislation that requires people trained in health care to stop and aid the injured. To encourage citizens to be good Samaritans, most states have now enacted legislation releasing the good Samaritan from legal liability for injuries caused under such circumstances, even if the injuries resulted from negligence of the person offering emergency aid.

In Canada, some provinces specify in traffic acts that it is the responsibility of people to give aid at the scene of an accident. Alberta is the only province that exempts physicians and nurses from liability unless gross negligence is proved. However, lawsuits against good Samaritans are rarely successful.

It is generally believed that a person who renders help in an emergency, at the level of helping that would be provided by any reasonably prudent person under similar circumstances, cannot be held liable. The same reasoning applies to nurses, who may be the people best prepared to help at the scene of an accident. If the level of care a nurse provides is of the caliber that would have been provided by any other nurse, then the nurse will not be held liable.

Professional Liability Insurance

Because of the increase in the number of malpractice lawsuits against health professionals, nurses are advised in many areas to carry their own liability insurance. Most hospitals have liability insurance that covers all employees, including all nurses. However, some smaller facilities, such as "walk-in" clinics, may not. Thus the nurse should always check with the employer at the time of hiring to see what coverage the facility provides. A physician or a hospital can be sued because of the negligent conduct of a nurse, and the nurse can also be sued and held liable for negligence or malpractice. Because hospitals have been known to countersue the nurse when she or he has been found negligent and the hospital was required to pay, nurses are advised to provide their own insurance coverage and not rely on hospital-provided insurance.

Liability insurance coverage usually defrays all costs of defending a nurse, including the costs of retaining an attorney. The insurance also covers all costs incurred by the nurse up to the face value of the policy, including a settlement made out of court. In return, the insurance company may have the right to make the decisions about the claim and the settlement.

Instructors of nursing and nursing students are also vulnerable to lawsuits. In hospital nursing education programs, instructors and students are often specifically covered for liability by the hospital. An instructor, however, can still be sued by a hospital in cases of negligence and malpractice.

Students and teachers of nursing employed by community colleges and universities are less likely to be covered by the insurance carried by hospitals and health agencies. It is advisable for these people to check with their school about the coverage that applies to them. Increasingly, instructors are carrying their own malpractice insurance in both the United States and Canada. In the United States, insurance can be obtained through the ANA or private insurance companies; in Canada, it can usually be obtained through provincial nurses' associations. Nursing students in the United States can also obtain insurance through the NNSA. In some states, hospitals do not allow nursing students to provide nursing care without liability insurance.

Legal Responsibilities of Nursing

Carrying Out Physician's Orders

Nurses are expected to know basic information about procedures and medications ordered by the physician. It is the nurse's responsibility to seek clarification of ambiguous or seemingly erroneous orders from the prescribing physician. Clarification from any other source is unacceptable and regarded as a departure from competent nursing practice.

If the order is neither ambiguous nor apparently erroneous, the nurse is responsible for carrying it out. For example, if the physician orders oxygen to be administered at 4 liters per minute, the nurse must administer oxygen at that rate, and not at 2 or 6 liters per minute. If the orders state that the client is not to have solid food after a bowel resection, the nurse must ensure that no solid food is given to the client. Nurses also have a responsibility to check for changes in orders from previous shifts of duty.

Becker (1983, pp. 21–23) outlines four orders that nurses must question to protect themselves legally:

1. Question any order a client questions. For example, if a client who has been receiving an intramuscular injection tells the nurse that the doctor changed the order from an injectable to an oral medication, the nurse should recheck the order before giving an injection.

2. Question any order if the client's condition has changed. The nurse is considered responsible for notifying the physician of any significant changes

Nurses and physicians have a mutual ethical concern

The Judicial Council of the AMA has an "opinion" that addresses physicians' interprofessional relations with nurses. The opinion recognizes a mutual ethical concern for patients that bonds medicine and nursing: "Where orders appear to the nurse to be in error or contrary to customary medical and nursing practice, the physician has an ethical obligation to explain those orders to the nurse involved. When a nurse recognizes or suspects error or discrepancy in a physician's orders, the nurse has an obligation to call this to the attention of the physician. The ethical physician should neither expect nor insist that nurses follow orders contrary to standards of good medical and nursing practice." . . .

Such a position serves to demonstrate the cooperation that must exist among physicians and nurses to maintain the necessary high standards essential to patient care. In addition, it embraces the notion that when nurses observe unsafe medical activities, whether these activities directly involve them or not, they have both a legal and an ethical duty to make reasonable attempts to resolve the dilemmas by first attempting to discuss them with the primary physicians. If the physicians fail to respond to these requests, the nurses should follow through by using the appropriate internal hospital channels.

Source: M. Cushing, When hospitals don't listen to nurses' complaints, (The Legal Side), *American Journal of Nursing,* December 1987, 1547–49.

in the client's condition, whether the physician requests notification or not. For example, if a client who is receiving an intravenous infusion suddenly develops a rapid pulse, chest pain, and a cough, the nurse must notify the physician immediately and question continuance of the ordered rate of infusion. If a client who is receiving morphine for pain develops severely depressed respirations, the nurse must withhold the medication and notify the physician.

3. Question and record verbal orders to avoid miscommunications. In addition to recording the time, the date, the physician's name, and the orders, the nurse documents the circumstances that occasioned the call to the physician, reads the orders back to the physician, and documents that the physician confirmed the orders as the nurse read them back.

4. Question standing orders, especially if the nurse is inexperienced. *Standing orders* give the nurse added responsibility to exercise appropriate judgment when implementing them. The nurse is delegated the authority to, for example, adjust the amount of a medication or other substances and make decisions about when a medication is needed. Nurses need to take the same precautions when implementing these orders as when implementing any other orders. In

addition, the nurse who does not feel confident about exercising discretionary judgment should request specific guidelines from the physician or assistance from a more experienced nurse. In some states, standing orders are not allowed except in intensive care or coronary care units.

Implementing Delegated and Independent Nursing Interventions

Nurses implementing care need to take the following precautions (Grane 1983, pp. 17–20; Rhodes and Miller 1984, pp. 153–60):

1. Know their job description. This enables nurses to function within the scope of the description and know what is and what is not expected. Job descriptions vary from agency to agency.

2. Follow the policies and procedures of the agency in which they are working.

3. Always identify clients, particularly before initiating major interventions, e.g., surgical or other invasive procedures, or when administering blood transfusions.

4. Make sure the correct medications are given in the correct dose, by the right route, at the scheduled time, and to the right client. See Chapter 44 for more detailed information about the administration of medications.

5. Perform procedures appropriately. Negligent incidents during procedures generally relate to equipment failure, improper technique, and improper performance of the procedure. For instance, the nurse must know how to safeguard the client in the event that a respirator or other equipment fails.

6. Promptly and accurately document all assessments and care given. Records must show that the nurse provided and supervised the client's care daily.

7. Report all incidents involving clients. Prompt reports enable those responsible to attend to the client's well-being, to analyze why the incident occurred, and to prevent recurrences.

8. Build and maintain good rapport with clients. Keeping clients informed about diagnostic and treatment plans, giving feedback on their progress, and showing concern for the outcome of their care prevent a sense of powerlessness and a build-up of hostility in the client.

9. Maintain clinical competence in their area of practice. For students, this demands study and practice before caring for clients. For graduate nurses, it means continued study, including maintaining and updating clinical knowledge and skills.

10. Know their own strengths and weaknesses. For example, a nurse who recognizes that she or he has difficulty calculating medication dosages should always ask someone to check the calculations before proceeding.

11. When delegating nursing responsibilities, make sure that the person who is delegated a task understands what to do and that the person has the required knowledge and skill. The delegating nurse can be held liable for harm caused by the person to whom the care was delegated.

12. Be alert when implementing nursing interventions and give each task their full attention and skill.

Ways nurses can protect themselves legally are summarized in the listed "Legal Precautions for Nurses."

Legal Precautions for Nurses

Function within the scope of their education and job description. Follow the procedures and policies of the employing agency.

Take appropriate steps to obtain complete nursing histories. Observe and monitor the client adequately.

Communicate and record significant changes in the client's condition to the physician. Carry out physicians' orders promptly and correctly, provided the orders are not ambiguous or considered dangerous for the client.

Check any orders that a client questions. Identify clients before initiating major interventions.

Give medications as ordered to the right client. Perform procedures appropriately.

Protect clients from falls and preventable injuries. Document all nursing assessments and interventions accurately and promptly.

Ask for assistance and supervision in situations for which they feel inadequately prepared. Delegate tasks to persons with the knowledge and skill to carry them out.

Build and maintain good rapport with their clients.

Legal Responsibilities of Students

Nursing students are responsible for their own actions and liable for their own acts of negligence committed during the course of clinical experiences. When they perform duties that are within the scope of professional nursing, such as administering an injection, they are legally held to the same standard of skill and competence as a registered professional nurse (Rhodes and Miller 1984, p. 163). Lower standards are *not* applied to the actions of nursing students.

In cases arising from negligent acts by nursing students, the student has traditionally been treated as an employee of the hospital, which was held liable under the doctrine of *respondeat superior*. Today, associate degree and baccalaureate nursing students are not usually considered employees of the agencies in which they receive clinical experience, since these nursing programs contract with agencies to provide clinical experiences for students. In future cases of negligence involving such students, the hospital or agency (e.g., public health agency) and the educational institution will be held potentially liable for negligent actions by students (Rhodes and Miller 1984, p. 164).

Students in clinical situations must be assigned activity within their capabilities and be given reasonable guidance and supervision. Nursing instructors are responsible for assigning students to the care of clients and for providing reasonable supervision. Failure to provide reasonable supervision and/or the assignment of a client to a student who is not prepared and competent can be a basis for liability.

To fulfill responsibilities to clients and to minimize chances for liability, nursing students need to:

1. Make sure they are prepared to carry out the necessary care for assigned clients.
2. Ask for additional help or supervision in situations for which they feel inadequately prepared.
3. Comply with the policies of the agency in which they obtain their clinical experience.
4. Comply with the policies and definitions of responsibility supplied by the school of nursing.

Students who work as part-time or temporary nursing assistants or aides must also remember that *legally* they can perform only those tasks that appear in the job description of a nurse's aide or assistant. Even though a student may have received instruction and acquired competence in administering injections or suctioning a tracheostomy tube, she or he cannot legally perform these tasks while employed as an aide or assistant.

Chapter Highlights

Accountability is an essential concept of professional nursing practice under the law.

Nurses need to understand laws that regulate and affect nursing practice to ensure that the nurses' actions are consistent with current legal principles and to protect the nurse from liability.

Nurse practice acts legally define and describe the scope of nursing practice that the law seeks to regulate.

Competence in nursing practice is determined and maintained by various credentialing methods, such as licensure, registration, certification, and accreditation, which protect the public's welfare and safety.

Standards of care published by national and state or provincial nursing associations and agency policies, procedures, and job descriptions further delineate the scope of a nurse's practice.

The nurse has specific legal obligations and responsibilities to clients and employers and as a citizen.

Collective bargaining is one way nurses can improve their working conditions and economic welfare.

Nurses can be held liable for the death of clients; for intentional torts, such as fraud, invasion of privacy, defamation, assault and battery, and false imprisonment; and for unintentional torts or negligence.

Negligence or malpractice of nurses is established when the nurse (defendant) owed a duty to the client, the nurse failed to carry out that duty, the client (plaintiff) was injured, and the client's injury was caused by the nurse's failure to carry out her or his duty.

One standard used to determine a nurse's liability for negligence is what would have been done in similar circumstances by a reasonable and prudent professional with similar preparation and experience.

The nurse is responsible for ensuring that the physician obtains informed consents from clients (or from the closest relative in emergencies or from parents or guardians when the client is a minor) before treatment regimens and procedures begin.

Informed consent implies that the consent was given voluntarily; the client was of age and had the capacity and competence to understand; consent was given after an explanation of the benefits, risks, and other facts relating to the procedure; and the client understood the explanations.

The client's medical record is a legal document and can be produced in court as evidence; nurses, therefore, must keep accurate and complete records of nursing care provided to clients.

An incident report needs to include assessment data, witnesses to the situation, descriptive facts of the incident, and surrounding circumstances.

The nurse who witnesses a client's will must ensure that the client is of sound mind and not unduly influenced by others; the nurse must also document the client's physical and mental status on the nursing records.

Living wills are receiving increasing attention; because statutes that authorize living wills vary, nurses need to familiarize themselves with their specifications.

The legality of no-code and slow-code orders is not well established; nurses are advised to follow the American Heart Association standards for no-code orders.

Abortion laws are clearly established in the United States; in Canada, abortion must be approved by a medical abortion committee in an approved hospital.

Nurses must be knowledgable about their responsibilities in regard to legal issues surrounding death: death certificate, labeling of the deceased, autopsy, organ donation, and inquest.

Good Samaritan acts protect health professionals from claims of malpractice when they provide assistance at the scene of an emergency, provided there is not willful wrongdoing or gross departure from normal standards of care.

Practicing nurses who are not covered by liability insurance in their employing agency can obtain liability insurance through professional nursing associations.

Registered nursing students are accountable for all their actions; they are legally held to the same standard of skill and competence as registered nurses.

Nursing students need to make sure they are prepared to provide the necessary care for assigned clients and ask for help or supervision in situations for which they feel inadequately prepared.

Selected References

American Heart Association. June 6, 1986. Standards and guidelines for cardiopulmonary resuscitation and emergency cardiac care. *Journal of the American Medical Association.* 255:2841–3044.

American Nurses' Association. 1975. *Human rights guidelines for nurses in clinical and other research.* Publication no. D-46 5M 7/75. Kansas City, Mo.: American Nurses' Association.

———. 1985. *The code for nurses.* Kansas City, Mo.: American Nurses' Association.

———. April 1979. Credentialing in nursing. A new approach. Report of the Committee for the study of Credentialing in Nursing. *American Journal of Nursing* 79:674–83.

———. 1985. *The grievance procedure.* Kansas City, Mo.: American Nurses' Association.

American Nurses' Association Cabinet on Economic and General Welfare. 1985. *The nature and scope of ANA's economic and general welfare program.* Kansas City, Mo.: American Nurses' Association.

Annas, G. J.; Glantz, L. H.; and Katz, B. F. 1981. *The right of doctors, nurses and allied health professionals.* New York: Avon Books.

Baer, O. J. May/June 1985. Protecting your patient's privacy. *Nursing Life* 5:50–53.

Becker, M. January/February 1983. Five orders you must question to protect yourself legally. *Nursing Life* 3:21–23.

Cournoyer, C. P. March/April 1985. Protecting yourself legally after a patient's injured. *Nursing Life* 5:18–22.

Crawford, M.; Fisher, M.; and Kilbane, N. 1985. Collective bargaining in nursing. In DeYoung, L., editor. *Dynamics of nursing.* 5th ed. St. Louis: C. V. Mosby Co.

Creighton, H. 1981. *Law every nurse should know.* 4th ed. Philadelphia: W. B. Saunders Co.

Cushing, M. August 1985. Incident reports: For your eyes only? *American Journal of Nursing* 85:873–74.

———. February 1986. How courts look at nurse practice acts. *American Journal of Nursing* 86:131.

Davis, A. January/February 1985. Informed consent: How much information is enough? *Nursing Outlook* 33:40–42.

Fenner, K. 1980. *Ethics and the law in nursing.* New York: D. Van Nostrand Co.

Flanagen, L. 1983. *Collective bargaining and the nursing profession.* Kansas City, Mo.: American Nurses' Association.

Kravitz, M. November 1985. Informed consent: Must ethical responsibility conflict with professional conduct? *Nursing Management* 16:34A–B, 34D–H.

Lewis, E. P. September/October 1985. Taking care of business: The ANA house of delegates. *Nursing Outlook* 33:239–43.

McClelland, J. Q. November 1983. Professionalism and collective bargaining: A new reality for nurses and management. *Journal of Nursing Administration* 13:36–38.

Northrop, C. 1984. Legal aspects of nursing. In McCann Flynn, J. B., and Heffron, P. B., editors. *Nursing: From concept to practice.* Bowie, Md.: Robert J. Brady Co.

———. January 1985. The ins and outs of informed consent. *Nursing 85* 15:21.

A *Nursing Life* poll report on ethics. March/April 1983. Do you make your patient live ... or let him die? *Nursing Life* 3:54–55.

Oberst, M. November/December 1985. Another look at informed consent. *Nursing Outlook* 33:294–95.

Rhodes, A. M., and Miller, R. D. 1984. *Nursing and the Law.* 4th ed. Rockville, Md.: Aspen Systems Corporation.

Snyder, M. E., and LaBar, C. 1984. *Issues in professional nursing practice 1. Nursing: Legal authority for practice.* Kansas City, Mo.: American Nurses' Association.

The Nursing Process

CHAPTERS

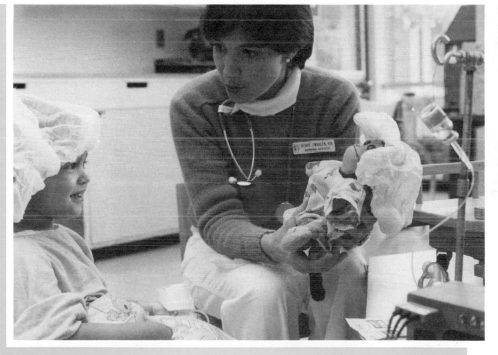

CHAPTER 7

The Nursing Process

OBJECTIVES

Describe the characteristics of the nursing process.

Identify nursing activities involved in each component of the nursing process.

List advantages of the nursing process to the client.

List advantages of the nursing process to the nurse.

Give a historical account of how the nursing process developed.

Describe how nursing and other theories relate to the nursing process.

Compare the scientific method, problem-solving method, decision-making process, and the nursing process.

Describe how the nursing process comprises a framework for accountability.

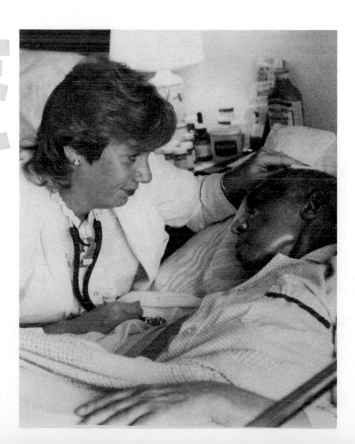

Historical Perspective

Before the nursing process was developed, nurses tended to provide care that was based on medical orders written by physicians and focused on specific disease conditions rather than on the person being cared for. Nursing practice that was provided independently of the physician was often guided by intuition rather than based on a scientific method.

The term **nursing process** and the framework it implies are relatively new. In 1955, Hall originated the term *nursing process.* Since then, various nurses have described the process of nursing in different ways. In 1967, the nursing faculty of the Catholic University of America proposed four components of the nursing process: assessment, planning, intervention, and evaluation (Yura and Walsh 1983).

As nurses used this process, an additional component was added. In 1982, the National Council of State Boards of Nursing defined and described the five-step nursing process in terms of nursing behaviors: assessing, analyzing, planning, implementing, and evaluating (National Council of State Boards of Nursing 1982). In this context, **analyzing** is used to describe an activity required to develop a nursing diagnosis. Nursing theorists may use different terms to describe these steps. In spite of these differences, the activities of the nurse using the process are similar. To avoid misunderstanding, nurses should be familiar with alternate terms that describe steps in the process. For example, *diagnosing* (nursing diagnosis) may be called *analyzing* (analysis) and *implementing* (implementation) may be called *intervening* (intervention).

Components

A **process** is a series of planned actions or operations directed toward a particular result. The **nursing process** is a systematic, rational method of planning and providing nursing care. Its goal is to identify a client's actual or potential health care needs, to establish plans to meet the identified needs, and to deliver specific nursing interventions to meet those needs.

To carry out the nursing process, at least two people must participate: the client and the nurse. The client may be an individual, a family, or even a community. The client participates as actively as possible in all phases of the nursing process. The nurse requires interpersonal, technical, and intellectual skills to use the nursing process.

Interpersonal skills include communicating; listening; conveying interest, compassion, knowledge, and information; developing trust; and obtaining data in a manner that enhances the individuality of the client, promotes the integrity of the family, and contributes to the viability of the community. **Technical skills** are necessary to use equipment and perform procedures. **Intellectual skills** required by a nurse include problem solving, critical thinking, and making nursing judgments.

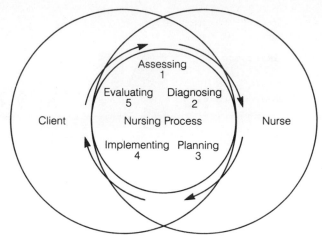

Figure 7—1   The interrelationship of the client, the nurse, and the nursing process

Interaction between the client and the nurse is essential when using the nursing process, as illustrated in Figure 7—1. An overview of the nursing process follows. See also Tables 7—1 and 7—2 for examples of nursing activities and concepts associated with each component of the process. Each component is discussed in depth in subsequent chapters of this unit.

1. **Assessing** is collecting, verifying, and organizing data about a client's health status. Data about the physical, emotional, developmental, social, intellectual, and spiritual aspects of the client are obtained from a variety of sources and are the basis for actions and decisions taken in subsequent phases. Skills of observation, communication, and interviewing are essential to perform this phase of the nursing process.

2. **Diagnosing** is an analytical process that results in a diagnostic statement or nursing diagnosis. A **nursing diagnosis** is a statement of a client's potential or actual alteration of health status that nurses are licensed and able to treat. In this phase, the nurse sorts and clusters the assessment data to identify health problems and their etiologies.

3. **Planning** involves a series of steps in which the nurse sets priorities, writes goals or expected outcomes, and establishes a written guide for nursing interventions designed to solve or minimize the identified problems of the client and to coordinate the care provided by all health team members. In collaboration with the client, the nurse develops specific interventions for each nursing diagnosis.

4. **Implementing** is putting the nursing care plan into action. During the implementation phase, the nurse continues to collect data and validates the nursing care plan. Continued data collection is essential not only to keep track of changes in the client's condition but also to obtain evidence for the evaluation of goal achievement in the next phase.

5. **Evaluating** is reassessing the client after nursing intervention and comparing the response to predetermined standards. These standards are often referred to as **outcome or evaluative criteria.** The nurse determines the extent to which the goals or

Table 7–1 Overview of the Purposes and Activities of the Nursing Process

Component and Purpose(s)	Activities
Assessing	
To establish a data base	Collect data
	Verify conflicting data
	Obtain nursing history
	Perform physical health examination
	Review records, e.g., laboratory records
	Consult other health team members
	Consult support persons
	Review literature
Diagnosing	
To identify the client's health care needs and to prepare diagnostic statements	Validate data
	Sort and group data
	Interpret data
	Label groups of data with a diagnostic statement
Planning	
To identify the client's goals and appropriate nursing interventions	Set priorities
	Write evaluation goals and outcome criteria
	Select nursing strategies
	Consult other health personnel
	Write nursing care plan
	Delegate nursing actions
Implementing	
To carry out planned nursing interventions to help the client attain goals	Reassess client
	Update data base
	Review and revise care plan
	Perform planned nursing interventions
Evaluating	
To determine the extent to which goals of nursing care have been achieved	Collect data about the client's response
	Compare the client's response to evaluation (outcome) criteria
	Analyze the reasons for the outcomes
	Modify the care plan

predetermined outcomes of care have been achieved, partially achieved, or not met.

The nursing process is an adaptation of problem-solving techniques and systems theory. It can be viewed as parallel to but separate from the medical process. Table 7–3 lists the two processes for comparison. Both processes begin with data gathering and analysis and base an action (intervention or treatment) on a problem statement (nursing or medical diagnosis). Both processes include an evaluative component. Whereas, however, the focus of the medical process is on the disease process, the nursing process is directed toward a client's *response* to illness.

Each step or phase of the nursing process affects the others; they are closely interrelated. For example, if an inadequate data base is used during assessment, the nursing diagnoses will be incomplete; this incompleteness will be reflected in the planning, implementation, and evaluation phases. Incomplete assessment necessarily means equivocal evaluation because the nurse will have insufficient criteria against which to evaluate changes in the client and the effectiveness of interventions.

Importance

The nursing process is important to both the client and the nurse. The following advantages have been described (Atkinson and Murray 1983).

Advantages for the Client

1. **Quality client care.** The nursing care is planned to meet the unique needs of the individual, family, or community. Continuous evaluation and reassessment of the client's changing needs ensure an appropriate level of care.
2. **Continuity of care.** The written care plan is accessible to all persons involved in the client's care and prevents each client from having to repeat information and preferences to each caregiver.
3. **Participation by the clients in their health care.** The process can help clients to develop skills related to their health care and to become more committed to the goals of care.

Advantages for the Nurse

1. **Consistent and systematic nursing education.** The NLN, which administers a voluntary accreditation of nursing education programs, requires graduates to be competent in the use of the nursing process (NLN 1978). In addition, licensure examinations for nurses in the United States are organized around nursing process activities.
2. **Job satisfaction.** Well-written care plans give nurses confidence that nursing interventions are based on correct identification of the client's problems, thus preventing uncoordinated, trial-and-error nursing. Plans also can instill a sense of pride when the goals of care are accomplished.
3. **Professional growth.** By evaluating the effectiveness of the nursing interventions, the nurse learns which interventions are effective and which ones can be adapted to meet the needs of other clients. This process enhances the skill and expertise of the nurse. In addition, the shared knowledge and experience gained in collaborating with colleagues when formulating a care plan enhance the nurse's knowledge.
4. **Avoidance of legal action.** When every step of the nursing process is used in delivering nursing care, the nurse is carrying out her or his legal obligations to the client. Failure to conduct a complete nursing assessment or failure to document data appropriately can have adverse legal consequences (Philpott 1985, p. 79).

Table 7—2   Selected Knowledge and Abilities Needed for the Nursing Process

Component	Knowledge	Abilities
Assessing	Biopsychosocial and spiritual systems of humans Developmental needs of humans Health Illness Pathophysiology Family system Culture and values of self and client	Observe systematically Communicate verbally and nonverbally Listen attentively Establish a helping relationship Develop trust Conduct a health interview Perform a nursing physical health assessment
Diagnosing	Common health problems that nurses can identify and treat Etiologic factors of health problems Signs or characteristics of common health problems Risk factors associated with potential health problems Normal measurement standards Individual coping mechanisms	Understand and evaluate cues Differentiate between cues* and inferences† Think critically Identify patterns and relationships Organize and group data Make inferences Reason inductively and deductively Make decisions or judgments
Planning	Client's strengths and weaknesses Values and beliefs of the client Scope of nursing practice Resources available to implement nursing strategies Roles of other health care personnel	Problem solve Make decisions Write client goals that relate to the nursing diagnosis Write measurable outcome criteria that relate to the goals Select and create nursing strategies that are safe and appropriate to meet client goals Write nursing orders Elicit the cooperation and participation of the client and other health care personnel
Implementing	Physical hazards and safety Asepsis Procedures Use of equipment Organization Management Learning Change theory Advocacy Client rights Client's developmental level	Observe systematically Communicate effectively Maintain a helping relationship Perform psychomotor techniques Teach self-care Convey caring Act as a client advocate Counsel clients Delegate Supervise and evaluate the work of others Implement medical orders
Evaluating	Client goals and outcome criteria Client responses to nursing intervention	Obtain relevant data to compare with outcome criteria Draw conclusions about goal attainment Relate nursing actions to outcome criteria Reassess the nursing care plan

*Cue: A fact that one acquires through the use of the five senses.
†Inference: The nurse's judgment or interpretation of a cue.

5. **Accountability and responsibility.** The nursing process holds the nurse accountable and responsible for assessing, analyzing, planning, implementing, and evaluating client care.

Theories That Guide the Process

A **theory** is a scientifically acceptable general principle that governs practice or is proposed to explain observed facts. Various theories guide how the nursing process is implemented. Some of these are nursing theory, problem-solving and decision-making theory, perception theory, communication theory, and human needs theory. Communication theory is discussed in Chapter 20, and human needs theory in Chapter 13.

Nursing Theory

As noted in Chapter 1, conceptual frameworks for nursing are abstractions that are operationalized by using the nursing process. For example, if the client is viewed as having 14 fundamental needs, data are collected about these 14 needs. If a self-care model is used, data are

Table 7—3   Comparison of the Nursing Process and the Medical Process

Nursing Process	Medical Process	Nursing Process	Medical Process
1. Assessing Collection of data from: a. Nursing history b. Health examination c. Review of records d. Consultation with other team members e. Review of literature	1. Assessing Collection of data from: a. Medical history b. Physical examination c. Diagnostic tests d. Review of literature	4. Implementing a. Preimplementation strategies b. Implementation c. Postimplementation strategies: update data base, review and revise care plan	4. Therapy a. Physician's orders b. Medical therapy c. Referrals
2. Analyzing (nursing diagnosis) a. Analysis and synthesis b. Identification of health problems c. Formulation of nursing diagnosis	2. Medical diagnosis* a. Organization of data b. Analysis and interpretation of the data c. Formulation of a diagnosis	5. Evaluating a. Collection of data about the client's response b. Comparison of the data to the established objectives and goals c. Determination of the effectiveness of the nursing plan d. Analysis of variables affecting the outcomes e. Modification of the care plan	5. Evaluating a. Establishment of the effectiveness of the medical therapy in terms of the goals b. Analysis of variables c. Revision of the plan of therapy as necessary
3. Planning a. Establishment of priorities b. Establishment of goals c. Development of objectives d. Written nursing care plan e. Delegation of nursing activities	3. Medical planning a. Establishment of priorities b. Establishment of goals for therapy c. Written plan of therapy		

*Medical diagnosis has four or five phases:
1. Suspected diagnosis following the patient's initial complaint
2. Tentative diagnosis following the medical history
3. Provisional diagnosis following the physical examination
4. Definitive diagnosis following diagnostic tests
5. Anatomic diagnosis following a postmortem

collected about the client's abilities to perform self-care, and the nurse's intervention is focused on the individual's self-care deficits. Nursing theory instructs the nurse *what* to do and directly influences which interventions are planned; however, it does not tell the nurse *how* to intervene. For example, a planned intervention may be to teach a client and his wife how to give insulin injections. What to do is evident, but how to do it is not. To implement this plan effectively, the nurse needs further knowledge about communication, helping relationships, learning, teaching strategies, techniques for giving injections, and so on. This knowledge is drawn from sources other than the nursing model.

Problem-Solving and Decision-Making Theory

Problem solving and decision making are used in applying the nursing process. Although these two terms are often used interchangeably, they are separate processes that are related in some situations. Solving a problem may require making a number of decisions, and making a decision may involve solving a number of problems. In addition, not all decisions involve problem solv-

ing; for example, making the decision that a client can safely remain in a chair for another 15 minutes. Also, not all problems involve deliberate decision making, e.g., stopping a client from pulling out a urinary catheter. This action is usually automatic or habitual and does not involve a conscious decision by the nurse.

Problem-Solving Process. There are various approaches to problem solving. Four of the most commonly used are trial and error, intuition, experimentation, and the scientific method.

Trial-and-Error Problem Solving. One way to solve problems is to try a number of approaches until a solution is found. However, the reason one solution works is not known when alternatives in care are not considered systematically. Trial-and-error methods in nursing care can be dangerous because the client might suffer harm if an approach is inappropriate.

Intuitive Problem Solving. Experienced nurses develop a sense of what nursing measures might help in certain situations. This sense is in part intuitive. A nurse who bases decisions on intuition alone rather than data has difficulty in maintaining credibility, since her or his actions are not based on knowledge from research, and, as a result, they cannot be defended using any nursing care standard. Some nurse researchers, however, are investigating the role of intution in nursing.

Experimentation. Experimentation is more controlled than trial and error. It is based on knowledge and research, and it is therefore more ethical than trial-and-error or intuitive problem solving. Examples of experimentation are pilot projects or limited trials in an effort to solve a problem. For example, a nurse caring for a client with intractable pain may try one specific nursing intervention for 3 days to reduce the pain. If the pain is not reduced, the nurse may then implement a second plan for another 3 days.

Scientific Method. The **scientific method** is a logical, systematic approach to solving problems. The classic scientific method is most useful in a laboratory where the scientist is working in a controlled situation. The classic scientific method has the following steps:

1. Identifying the general problem, including defining the problem and developing hunches about it
2. Collecting all relevant data from appropriate sources
3. Formulating a **hypothesis:** an assumption made to test the logic of a proposition
4. Preparing a plan of action to test the hypothesis
5. Testing the hypothesis
6. Interpreting the test results and then evaluating the hypothesis
7. Concluding the study or revising the plan of action in the light of new data

Modified Scientific Method (Problem-Solving Process). Health professionals require a modified approach of the scientific method for solving problems. This modified scientific problem-solving method is used in the nursing process but can also be used for problems relating to personnel, equipment, or other situations. Like the scientific process, it has seven steps. See Table 7–4 for a comparison of the problem-solving process, the nursing process, and the scientific method.

▪ **Decision-Making Process.** Decision making is a process of choosing a particular and best action to meet a desired goal. Three conditions must prevail:

freedom, rationality, and voluntary (Schaefer 1974, p. 1852). Freedom means that the individual makes the decision without pressure from others and has the authority to make the decision. Rationality, in the context of decision making, means that the best or optimal decision is made and that it is consistent with the decision maker's values and preferences. Rationality involves both deliberation and judgment. Voluntary is making a choice voluntarily.

Decision making involves two types of reasoning: inductive and deductive. In **inductive reasoning,** generalizations are formed from a set of facts or observations. When viewed together, certain bits of information suggest a particular interpretation. For example, the nurse who observes that a client has dry skin, poor turgor, sunken eyes, and dark amber urine may make the generalization that the client is dehydrated.

Deductive reasoning, by contrast, is reasoning from the general to the specific. The nurse starts with a conceptual framework, e.g., Maslow's hierarchy of needs or a self-care action framework, and makes descriptive interpretations of the client's condition in relation to that framework. The nurse who uses the needs framework might categorize data and define the client's problems in terms of elimination, nutrition, or protection needs.

▪ Perception Theory

Perception is a major means by which people gain information about themselves, their needs, and the environment. **Perception** is the process of selecting, organizing, and interpreting sensory stimuli into a meaningful and coherent picture of the world. When looking around, a person sees a whole range of different objects, forms, and colors. People also see depth; all objects appear three-dimensional. Why does the world look the way it does to a person? A superficial answer is that things look the way they do because that is the way they are; they mirror reality.

Perception, however, is more complex than a response to sensory stimuli. It is also the interpretation of the sensation in the light of previous learning. Perception is a person's conscious awareness of reality and

---

Table 7–4 Comparison of Steps in the Problem-Solving Process, the Nursing Process, and the Scientific Method

Problem-Solving Process	Nursing Process	Scientific Method
1. Encounter the problem	1. Assessing	1. Recognize and define the problem
2. Collect data		2. Collect data from observation and experimentation
3. Analyze information and identify exact nature of the problem	2. Diagnosing	3. Formulate hypothesis
4. Determine a plan of action	3. Planning	4. Select plan to test the hypothesis
5. Carry out the plan	4. Implementing	5. Test the hypothesis
6. Evaluate the plan and its outcomes	5. Evaluating	6. Interpret test results (evaluate whether the hypothesis is correct)
7. Terminate or modify the plan		7. Conclude or modify hypothesis

is based on an individual's knowledge and past experiences.

To enhance the ability to collect data and the accuracy of inferences made about the client, the nurse must continually strive to increase her or his observational or perceptual field. This can be achieved by:

1. Using all senses when collecting data.
2. Avoiding focusing attention on only particular events or aspects of a stimulus.
3. Not expecting certain types of stimulation or responses to occur.
4. Asking for feedback about the client's perceptions, sharing and comparing perceptions, and reaching a common understanding. When eliciting feedback, the nurse can say, "I don't understand" or nonverbally indicate a question with a raised eyebrow or other gesture.
5. Increasing her or his knowledge about human behavior.
6. Being aware of her or his own values, beliefs, and biases, which may affect how the nurse interprets what she or he sees and hears. Nurses need to overcome the tendency to attend only to a person's positive attributes (that is, those that are similar to the nurse's own values) or to attend overly to negative attributes (that is, those in conflict with the nurse's values).

A Framework for Accountability

Accountability is the condition of being answerable and responsible to someone for specific behaviors that are part of the nurse's professional role. The nursing process provides the framework for nurses to help clients with their health needs and to produce a record of the actions and their effectiveness. An implicit part of applying the nursing process is having the knowledge and skills to make the required decisions and to implement the required nursing actions. Therefore, nurses are also accountable to themselves for having the knowledge and skills to use the nursing process in a specific situation.

Nurses are also accountable to the client, to their professional statutory nursing body, to colleagues, and to the employing agency. The nursing process provides a framework for accountability in all areas. The professional nurse is accountable for activities in all five phases of the nursing process. When **assessing,** the nurse is accountable for collecting information, encouraging client participation, and judging the validity of the collected data. Moreover, the nurse is accountable for gaps in data or conflicting data, inaccurate data, and biased data.

During the second phase, **diagnosing,** nurses are accountable for the judgments made about the client's health problems, i.e., the diagnostic statements. When making judgments, nurses are accountable for considering a broad spectrum of client sociocultural backgrounds. Accountability at the **planning** stage involves determining priorities, establishing client goals, predicting outcomes, and planning nursing activities. These are all incorporated into a written nursing care plan available to all involved nurses.

Nurses are accountable for all their actions in **implementing** nursing care. Even when a nurse delegates an activity to another person, the nurse is still accountable for the delegated action as well as for the act of delegating. When establishing the degree to which the objectives have been attained in the **evaluating** phase of the process, the nurse is accountable for the success or failure of the nursing actions. The nurse must be able to explain why a client goal was not met and what phase or phases of the nursing process require changing.

Chapter Highlights

▪ The nursing process is a systematic, rational method of planning and providing nursing care.

▪ The goal of the nursing process is to identify a client's actual or potential health care needs, to establish plans to meet the identified needs, and to deliver specific nursing interventions to meet those needs.

▪ The basic components of the nursing process are assessing, diagnosing, planning, implementing, and evaluating.

▪ Specific nursing activities are associated with each component of the nursing process.

▪ The nursing process can be applied to individuals, families, and communities.

▪ Assessing is collecting, verifying, and organizing data about a client's status.

▪ Diagnosing is the process of developing a statement (nursing diagnosis) about a client's potential or actual health problem that nurses are licensed and able to treat.

▪ Planning involves setting priorities, writing goals, and establishing a written guide for nursing intervention designed to solve or minimize identified problems.

▪ Implementing is putting the nursing care plan into action.

▪ Evaluating is assessing the client's response to nursing interventions and comparing the response to predetermined criteria.

▪ The nursing process is similar to the problem-solving process and the scientific method.

▪ The nursing process provides a framework for nurses' accountability.

Selected References

American Nurses' Association. 1980. *Nursing: A social policy statement.* Publication no. NP-63. Kansas City, Mo.: American Nurses' Association.

Atkinson, L. D., and Murray, M. E. 1983. *Understanding the nursing process.* 2d ed. New York: Macmillan Co.

deChesnay, M. Winter 1983. Problem solving in nursing. *Image: The Journal of Nursing Scholarship* 25:8–11.

George, J. B., editor. 1985. *Nursing theories: The base for professional nursing.* 2d ed. Englewood Cliffs, N.J.: Prentice-Hall.

Hall, L. June 1955. Quality of nursing care. *Public health news.* Newark, N.J.: State Department of Health.

Iyer, P. W.; Taptich, B. J.; and Bernocchi-Losey, D. 1986. *Nursing Process and Nursing Diagnosis.* Philadelphia: W. B. Saunders.

Law, G. M. October 5-11, 1983. Accountability in nursing: Providing a framework . . . the nursing process and accountability are inextricably linked. Part 2. *Nursing Times* 79:34–36.

Leddy, S., and Pepper, J. M. 1985. The nursing process. Chapter 12 in *Conceptual bases of professional nursing,* pp. 211–26. New York: J. B. Lippincott Co.

McCann-Flynn, J. B., and Heffron, P. B. 1984. *Nursing: From concept to practice.* Bowie, Md.: Robert J. Brady Co.

Masson, V. March/April 1985. Nurses and doctors as healers. *Nursing Outlook* 33:70–73.

National Council of State Boards of Nursing. 1982. *Test plan for the National Council licensure examination for registered nurses.* Chicago: National Council of State Boards of Nursing.

National League for Nursing. 1978. *Competencies of the associate degree nurse on entry into practice.* Publication no. 23-1731C. New York: National League for Nursing.

Philpott, M. 1985. *Legal liability and the nursing process.* Toronto: W. B. Saunders Co., Canada.

Schaefer, J. October 1974. The interrelatedness of decision making and the nursing process. *American Journal of Nursing* 74:1852–55.

Yura, H., and Walsh, M. B. 1983. *The nursing process: Assessing, planning, implementing, evaluating.* 4th ed. Norwalk, Conn.: Appleton-Century-Crofts.

CHAPTER 8

Assessing

OBJECTIVES

Explain the purpose of the assessment phase of the nursing process as it relates to the other phases.

Identify common health areas the nurse assesses.

Give examples of objective and subjective data and variable and constant data.

Identify primary and secondary sources of data.

Describe essential skills required for data collection.

Identify five methods of data collection and give examples of how each is useful.

Compare the nursing assessment (history) and the medical history.

Compare directive and indirective approaches to interviewing.

Compare closed and open-ended questions, providing examples and listing advantages and disadvantages of each.

Describe important aspects of the interview setting.

Give reasons for consulting as a part of data collection.

Describe the techniques used to perform a physical assessment.

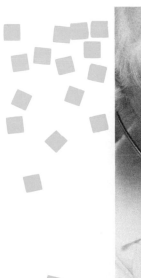

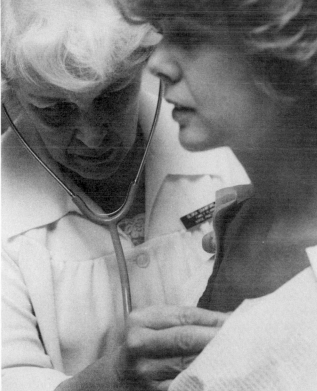

Purpose of Assessing

Assessing is the first phase of the nursing process, involving data collection and verification. Assessing is necessary before analyzing the data to identify the client's nursing diagnoses. Assessing is also carried out during other phases of the nursing process, i.e., implementing and evaluating, although some nurses refer to this as reassessing.

The purpose of assessing is to establish a data base about a client's health, including potential and actual health problems. Nurses are primarily accountable for the diagnosis and management of a client's health care in the areas of daily living and health. Nurses also make assessments in the biomedical realm and consider the implications of those data on daily living and the achievement of developmental tasks (Carnevali 1983, p. 110–11).

The term **data** includes all relevant information about a client. It consists of information, facts, and findings, including an individual's strengths and needs. A **data base** (or the **baseline data**) consists of available information about a client; it includes the physician's history and physical examination, the nursing assessment, physical health examination, and material contributed by other health personnel.

Data collection is the process of gathering information about a client's health status. Data collection must be both systematic and continuous. Systematic data collection can largely prevent the omission of significant data, and continuous data collection maintains the currency of the data, reflecting a client's changing health.

Assessing involves active participation by the client and the nurse. The client may be one or more individuals, a family, or even a community. Both the nurse and the client enter the relationship with specific knowledge and previous experiences that influence their perceptions and interpretations. It is important for nurses to be aware that their interpretations may not be fact; for example, a nurse seeing a man holding his arm to his chest might believe that the client is experiencing chest pain when in fact he has a painful hand. Or a nurse might interpret a client's wish not to talk as depression when the client is in fact very tired. To avoid misinterpretation, verification or validation of the data (with the client or another nurse) is helpful.

Types of Data

Data can be objective or subjective. **Objective data** are detectable by an observer or can be tested by using an accepted standard. They can be seen, heard, felt, or smelled. For example, a discoloration of the skin, a blood pressure reading, or the act of crying are objective data. **Subjective data,** however, are apparent only to the person affected and can be described or verified only by that person. Itching, pain, and feeling worried are exam-

ples of subjective data. Objective data are sometimes called *signs* or *overt data,* and subjective data are sometimes called *symptoms* or *covert data.*

Data can also be described as **variable** or **constant.** Blood pressure, for example, varies from day to day or even by the hour and needs updating. Constant data are unchanging, for example, a date of birth.

A common error in assessing is to offer opinions, generalizations, and interpretations as data. For example, a nurse may describe a client as "uncooperative" rather than record the specific behavior (e.g., refusing to take a deep breath and to cough after surgery). A specific description of the behavior is more useful than an interpretation because the causes of specific behavior can be explored. Perhaps the client refuses to cough because she is afraid of rupturing a suture line, or perhaps she experiences severe pain upon coughing. "I do not want to cough; it hurts too much" is a noninterpretive reporting of the problem. Another common error is obtaining incomplete information, i.e., leaving out information about pain because the client does not mention it and the nurse did not ask.

Clients may generalize or be nonspecific, describing the reason for their hospitalization as a "spell" or as "chest pain." It is important for the nurse to elicit specifics from the client. For example, the chest pain needs to be documented by how the client described it, where it was felt, how it was relieved, when it occurred, and whether it was a new experience. Data should also be concise. The nurse should briefly summarize the information collected using correct medical terms.

Sources of Data

Sources of data are *primary* or *secondary.* See Table 8–1. The client is the primary source of data. Secondary or indirect sources are significant others, other health personnel, records and reports, and relevant literature.

Client

The chief source of data is usually the client unless the client is too ill, young, or confused to communicate clearly. The client can usually provide subjective data

Table 8–1   Sources of Data

Primary Source	Secondary Source
Client	Significant others
	Health personnel
	Health records
	Reports of diagnostic tests

Adapted from R. F. McCain, Nursing by assessment—not intuition, *American Journal of Nursing,* April 1965, 65:82–84. Reprinted in M. F. Meyers, *Nursing fundamentals* (Dubuque, Iowa: Wm. C. Brown Publishers, 1967). Used by permission. Copyright 1965 American Journal of Nursing Company.

that no one else can offer. However, a stoic client may understate symptoms, while another person may exaggerate.

Significant Others

Significant others or support persons know the client well and often can provide data. They may supplement information or verify information provided by the client. They might convey information about the stresses the client was coping with before the illness, family attitudes to illness and health, and the client's home environment.

Health Personnel

Health personnel are often sources of information about a client's health. Nurses, social workers, physicians, and physiotherapists, for example, may have information from either previous or current contact with the client. A physician who knows the client's home setting may provide valuable data about the family and environmental stressors.

Medical Records

Medical records are often a source of a client's present and past health and illness patterns. These records can provide nurses with information about a client's coping behaviors (see Chapter 16), health practices, and previous illnesses. The appropriateness of the information in medical records to the present situation must always be considered. For example, if the most recent medical record is 10 years old, it is likely that the client's health practices and perhaps even coping behaviors have changed.

Other Records and Reports

Other records and reports can also provide pertinent health information. Laboratory data can confirm or conflict with a nurse's findings during the nursing assessment. When laboratory data conflict, the nurse must collect more data to verify findings. Any laboratory data about a client must be compared to established norms for that particular test and for the client's age and sex. Laboratory tests vary among agencies, and norms can therefore be different.

In most settings, laboratory tests are ordered by physicians and independent nurse practitioners, although this practice varies greatly. In some agencies, nurses are expected to order and/or carry out specific tests, e.g., urinalysis and routine blood tests. Other records and reports, e.g., a social agency's report on a client's living conditions or a home health care agency's report on a client's coping at home, can also be helpful to the nurse conducting an assessment.

Literature

The review of nursing and related literature, such as professional journals and reference texts, can provide additional information for the data base. A literature review includes but is not limited to the following information:

1. Standards or norms against which to compare findings, e.g., height and weight tables, normal developmental tasks for an age group
2. Cultural and social health practices
3. Spiritual beliefs
4. Additional required assessment data
5. Nursing interventions and evaluation criteria relative to a client's health problems
6. Information about medical diagnoses, treatment, and prognoses

Methods of Data Collection

The major methods of collecting data are observing, interviewing, consulting, and examining. While these nursing activities are often carried out during the implementing and evaluating phases of the nursing process as well, they are the main nursing activities during the assessing phase. During assessment, observation occurs whenever the nurse is in contact with the client and/or support persons. The primary interviewing process during the assessment phase is obtaining the nursing history. Examining during the assessment phase is the major method used in the physical health examination.

Observing

To **observe** is to gather data by using the five senses. Although nurses observe mainly through sight, all of the senses are engaged during careful observations. A nurse who observes that a client's face is flushed must relate that observation to body temperature, activity, environmental temperature, and blood pressure. Because observation involves selecting, organizing, and interpreting data, there is a possibility of error. For example, a nurse might not notice certain signs simply because they are unexpected in a certain client or situation or because they do not conform to preconceptions about a client's illness.

Observation is a conscious, deliberate skill that is developed only through effort and with an organized approach. Nurses often need to focus on specific stimuli in a clinical situation; otherwise they are overwhelmed by a multitude of stimuli. Observing, therefore, involves discriminating among stimuli, that is, separating stimuli in a meaningful manner. For example, nurses caring for newborns learn to ignore the usual sounds of machines in the nursery but respond quickly to an infant's cry or movement.

Nursing observations should be organized so that no significant data are missed. Most nurses develop an individual sequence for observing events, for example:

1. Clinical signs of client distress, e.g., pallor or flushing, labored breathing, and behavior indicating pain or emotional distress
2. The status of the client, e.g., pulse, blood pressure, and respirations
3. The functioning of associated equipment, e.g., intravenous equipment and oxygen
4. Threats to the client's safety, real or anticipated, e.g., a lowered side rail
5. The immediate environment, including people in it
6. The larger environment, i.e., the community

▮ Interviewing

An **interview** is a planned communication or a conversation with a purpose. Some possible purposes are to gather data, to give information, to identify problems of mutual concern, to evaluate change, to teach, to provide support, and to provide counseling or therapy. Although nurses should not lose sight of these purposes during an interview, they are sometimes obliged to alter plans momentarily. If, for example, a client expresses worry about surgery, the nurse pauses to explore the client's worry and to provide support. Simply to note the worry without dealing with it can leave the impression that the nurse does not care about the client's concerns or dismisses them as unimportant. This impression could lessen the client's willingness to accept assistance from the nurse at a later date.

Interviewing can be viewed as a process that is applied in most phases of the nursing process. One example of the interview is the nursing history, which is the primary tool for data collection during the assessment phase of the nursing process. There are two approaches to interviewing: directive and nondirective. The **direct interview** is highly structured and elicits specific information. The interviewer establishes the purpose of the interview and controls the interview, at least at the outset, by asking closed questions that call for specific responses. Directive interviews are frequently used to gather or provide information. During a **nondirective interview,** the nurse allows the client to control the purpose, subject matter, and pacing. The nurse clarifies and encourages communication by using open-ended questions (see the next section). Nondirective interviewing is used for problem solving, counseling, and performance appraisal (Stewart and Cash 1985, p. 17).

▮ Kinds of Interview Questions. Although there are many ways to categorize questions, in this book they are classified as open-ended or closed and neutral or leading. The type a nurse chooses depends on the needs of the client at the time. For example, the nurse asks direct questions in an emergency because information must be obtained quickly. **Closed questions** are restrictive and generally require only short answers giving specific information. The highly stressed

person and the person who has difficulty communicating finds closed questions easier to answer than open-ended questions. The amount of information gained is generally limited. Examples of closed questions are: "What medication did you take?," "Are you having pain now?," or "How long has it been since you had your last physical examination?"

An **open-ended question** is broad, specifies only the topic to be discussed, and invites answers longer than one or two words. It often elicits expressions of feeling and descriptive or comparative responses. Such questions give the client the freedom to divulge only information he or she is ready to disclose. The response may also convey attitudes and beliefs the client holds. The chief disadvantage of the open-ended question is that the client may spend time conveying irrelevant information. Examples of open-ended questions are: "How have you been feeling lately?" and "How do you feel about coming to the hospital?"

The nurse often finds it more effective to use a combination of directive and indirective approaches throughout an interview. The interview situation usually determines the predominant approach used. For example, the nurse uses a directive approach to assess a client's health status after surgery: "Are you having any pain? Show me where it is." The directive approach is also used in emergencies, when the nurse must assess the client's health status quickly, or learn what events preceded the emergency. For example, when a client is found lying on the floor of a hospital room, the nurse might interview others present: "When did he fall? Did he say anything? What had he been doing?" The indirective approach is used when there is no emergency and to determine the client's feelings and needs. For example, a nurse might ask: "How are you feeling today? Is there anything I can do for you?" See Table 8–2 for

---

Table 8–2 Examples of Direct and Indirect Questions

Direct	Indirect
Nurse: Where is your pain? Client: It's in the calf of my right leg. Nurse: How long have you had this pain? Client: It started about 2 weeks ago. Nurse: When does the pain occur? Client: After I've walked up a flight of stairs or about one block.	Nurse: Tell me about your pain. Client: It's in the calf of my right leg. It starts after I've walked about a block or up a flight of stairs. Nurse: Uh hmm. Client: It started about 2 weeks ago. I was hoping it would go away, but it's getting worse. I don't know what to do. My wife's an invalid and she relies on me to do the shopping and everything. I hope it's not serious.

Table 8–3   Selected Advantages and Disadvantages of Open and Closed Questions

Open Questions		Closed Questions	
Advantages	**Disadvantages**	**Advantages**	**Disadvantages**
1. They let the interviewee do the talking.	1. They take more time.	1. Questions and answers can be controlled more effectively.	1. They may provide too little information and require follow-up questions.
2. The interviewer is able to listen and observe.	2. Only brief answers may be given.	2. They require less effort from the interviewee.	2. They may not reveal how the interviewee feels.
3. They are easy to answer and nonthreatening.	3. Valuable information may be withheld.	3. They may be less threatening, since they do not require explanations or justifications.	3. They do not allow the interviewee to volunteer possibly valuable information.
4. They reveal what the interviewee thinks is important.	4. They often elicit more information than necessary.	4. They take less time.	4. They may inhibit communication and convey lack of interest by the interviewee.
5. They may reveal the interviewee's lack of information, misunderstanding of words, frame of reference, prejudices, or stereotypes.	5. Responses are difficult to document and require skill in recording.	5. Information can be asked for before the information is volunteered.	5. The interviewer may dominate the interview with questions.
6. They can provide information the interviewer may not ask for.	6. The interviewer requires skill in controlling an open-ended interview.	6. Responses are easily documented.	
7. They can reveal the interviewee's degree of feeling about an issue.	7. Responses require psychologic insight and sensitivity from the interviewer.	7. They are easy to use and can be handled by unskilled interviewers.	
8. They can convey interest and trust because of the freedom they provide.			

Table constructed, with permission, from material on pp. 80–85 of Stewart, Charles J., and William B. Cash, Jr., *Interviewing: Principles and practices*, 4th ed. © 1985 Wm. C. Brown Publishers, Dubuque, Iowa. All rights reserved.

examples of directive and indirective interviewing interactions and Table 8–3 for advantages and disadvantages of closed and open-ended questions.

A client can answer a **neutral question** without direction or pressure from the nurse. Examples are: "How do you feel about that?," "Why do you think you had the operation?," and "What happened then?" A **leading question** directs the client's answer. Examples are: "Wouldn't you rather have had the operation then?" and "You will take your medicine, won't you?"

▪ **Planning the Interview and Setting.**   It is important to plan an interview before beginning it. The nurse reviews what information is already available, e.g., a postoperative record, information about the current illness, or literature about the client's health problem. The nurse also reviews the data collection form to make sure that the data to be collected are really needed and will serve some purpose related to the client's care. If a form is not available, most nurses prepare an interview guide to remember areas of information and determine what questions to ask. The guide includes a list of topics and subtopics rather than a series of questions.

Each interview and its setting is influenced by time, place, and seating arrangement. In all instances, the client should be made to feel comfortable and unhurried. Interviews with hospitalized clients should ideally be scheduled for times when the client is physically com-

fortable and free from pain and when interruptions by friends, family, and other health professionals are absent or minimal.

The place of the interview must have adequate privacy to promote communication. A well-lighted, well-ventilated, moderate-sized room that is relatively free of noise, movements, and interruptions encourages communication. Constant interruptions, such as telephone calls, the noise of traffic outside a window, or people moving about in or near the location can disrupt thought patterns, concentration, and moods and may convey the impression that the nurse is uninterested or too busy. In addition, a place where others cannot overhear or, if possible, see the client is desirable. Most people are inhibited when answering personal questions in the hearing of others and expressing strong feelings in the sight of others.

When interviewing a client the nurse can sit at a 45 degree angle to the bed. This position is less formal than sitting behind a table in the room or standing at the foot of the bed. During an initial admission interview, a client may feel less confronted if there is an overbed table between the client and the nurse (Davis 1984, p. 66). Sitting on a client's bed hems the client in and makes staring difficult to avoid. It also violates principles of medical asepsis (see Chapter 23).

The distance between the interviewer and interviewee is also important. This distance should be neither too small nor too great. Most people feel comfortable 1 to 1.2 meters (3 to 4 feet) apart during an interview. A distance of 1.5 to 1.8 meters (5 to 6 feet) encourages the client to talk longer (Davis 1984, p. 66). Height also affects communication. By standing and looking down at a client, the nurse may intimidate the client. Status is associated with greater space and the freedom to move about (Davis 1984, p. 68). Therefore, the client may perceive the nurse who stands during an interview as having greater status.

▪ **Nursing Assessment.** The data collected during an interview between the nurse and client constitute a **nursing assessment,** formerly called a nursing health history. The nurse obtains information about the client, the client's health, responses to illness, sociocultural factors, health beliefs and practices, coping patterns, and day-to-day activities. A nursing assessment differs from a medical history in that it focuses on the meaning of illness and hospitalization to the client and the family as a basis for planning (McPhetridge 1968, p. 68).

The objectives of a nursing assessment are to identify the client's patterns of health and illness, the presence of risk factors for physical and behavioral health problems, any deviations from normal, and the client's available resources for adaptation (Perry 1982, p. 43). There are many nursing models and frameworks that guide data collection through structured assessment tools. One example is Gordon's framework of eleven functional health patterns:

1. *Health-perception-health-management   pattern.* Describes client's perceived pattern of health and well-being and how health is managed
2. *Nutritional-metabolic pattern.* Describes pattern of food and fluid consumption relative to metabolic need and pattern indicators of local nutrient supply
3. *Elimination pattern.* Describes patterns of excretory function (bowel, bladder, and skin)
4. *Activity-exercise pattern.* Describes pattern of exercise, activity, leisure, and recreation
5. *Cognitive-perceptual pattern.* Describes sensory-perceptual and cognitive pattern
6. *Sleep-rest pattern.* Describes patterns of sleep, rest, and relaxation
7. *Self-perception-self-concept pattern.* Describes self-concept pattern and perceptions of self (e.g., body comfort, body image, feeling state)
8. *Role-relationship pattern.* Describes pattern of role-engagements and relationships
9. *Sexuality-reproductive pattern.* Describes client's patterns of satisfaction and dissatisfaction with sexuality; describes reproductive patterns
10. *Coping-stress-tolerance pattern.* Describes general coping pattern and effectiveness of the pattern in terms of stress tolerance
11. *Value-belief pattern.* Describes patterns of values, beliefs (including spiritual), or goals that guide choices or decisions (Gordon 1982, p. 81)

Nursing assessment forms assist the nurse in collecting data about dysfunctional as well as functional behavior. Then, using a framework to analyze data, nurses are able to discern emerging patterns. Figure 8–1 is an example of an eclectic nursing admission assessment form that reflects Gordon's and other frameworks.

Consulting

A **consultation** is a deliberation by two or more people. Consulting differs from referring in that when *consulting,* the responsibility for the client's care remains with the nurse who seeks the consultation. *Referring* is the transfer of a client's care to another person, e.g., a nurse practitioner may refer a client to a physician, and a hospital nurse may refer a client to a home health care agency or nurse. Nurses consult a variety of health personnel, including other nurses, throughout the nursing process. Nurse consultants have specialized knowledge and skills. Some nurse consultants are employed by agencies; others are in independent practice.

Nurses do not consult only other nurses; they frequently consult physicians, social workers, and other health personnel. Some agencies have a protocol to be followed when consulting a health professional not presently involved in a client's care. For example, if a nurse wants to discuss a client's depression with an agency psychiatrist, she or he may need to send an agency form to the psychiatrist requesting a consultation. However, many consultations are arranged less formally. For example, a nurse may discuss a client's problem with the physician when he or she comes to see the client.

The client is not always an active participant in the consulting process. In many instances, a nurse consults on behalf of the client, e.g., when a client's desire to be discharged from the hospital is discussed with a physician. In other instances, the client is an active participant, e.g., the client, physiotherapist, and the nurse discuss the best way for the client to move from a bed to a chair.

Nurses generally consult for the following reasons: to verify findings, to implement change, and to obtain additional knowledge. Nurses frequently ask other nurses to verify assessment data, e.g., an extremely low blood pressure or an exceptionally fast pulse rate, when their findings are unexpected or when they are uncertain about them. Sometimes nurses discuss a client's nursing care plan with another nurse, often to make sure the best possible plan has been arranged or to implement a change in the plan. A second person's ideas can generate new approaches to the client's care.

Examining

Increasingly, nurses are carrying out physical health examinations of clients during the nursing assessment phase of the nursing process to verify data obtained in the nursing assessment. The examination includes the assessment of all body parts and the taking of vital signs, height, and weight. The nurse may focus on a specific problem area noted from the nursing assessment, such as the inability to urinate, or may perform a screening

Dear Patient:

Your nurses will be planning your hospital care to meet your individual needs. We would appreciate your help in answering the following questions. This information will help us learn about your general health and your condition. As nurses, we are concerned about your response to the diagnosis and treatment of your actual and/or potential problems.

This information is confidential. You do not have to answer any questions, or complete the form unless you want to. Thank you.

Instructions for completing the form.

1. If you have been hospitalized at UCSF within the past month, you do not need to fill out the entire form, only update the sections that have changed.
2. Complete the white sections on both sides of this page. The grey sections will be completed by your nurse.
3. A relative or friend may ask you the questions and/or write your answers for you.
4. If the question requires a yes/no answer, please circle the correct answer.
5. When you answer the questions which ask about changes or difficulties, please answer in relation to the last year.
6. After you complete the form, or if you choose not to complete it, please return it to the person who gave it to you.
7. After you are in your room your nurse will review your answers and will develop a plan of care with you.

HEALTH PERCEPTION / HEALTH MANAGEMENT

What language do you find it easiest to read & write? ✓ English; Other _____

If you have any problem completing this form, please return it to the person who gave it to you.

Who should we call in case of emergency? *Joe Smith* ... phone; days *345-5495* nights _____

What has caused this hospitalization? *no energy and shortness of breath*

What do you expect to happen during this hospitalization? *get well, maybe get a new heart valve*

Have you ever been in the hospital before? no yes ✓ *1984 - left hip replacement*

How is your general health? good ✓ fair poor   Do you have any chronic medical problems? (no) yes

What are the most important things you do to keep healthy? *eat a good diet*   Do you feel these things make a difference? no (yes)

Do you smoke? (no) yes... _____ packs/day _____ ...use alcohol? (no) yes _____ drinks/day *no drinking*

...use drugs which are not prescribed for you? (no) yes...type _____

NUTRITIONAL-METABOLIC

Do you follow a special diet? (no) yes...describe *no sugar - I have diabetes*

In the past year did you lose weight? no (yes)...amount? *5 lbs* gain weight? (no) yes...amount? _____

Any changes in your appetite or thirst? (no) yes...describe _____

Any difficulties with food, eating, or swallowing? (no) yes...describe _____

ELIMINATION

Any changes or difficulties with your bowel habits? (no) yes...describe _____

Do you often have diarrhea or constipation? (no) yes...describe _____

Do you use laxatives or other aids for regularity? (no) yes...describe _____

Have you experienced any changes or difficulties with urinary elimination? no (yes)...describe *go too often*

ACTIVITY / EXERCISE

What is your occupation *cattle rancher and farmer*

Do you have enough energy for the day-to-day activities you want to do, i.e. work, recreation, fixing meals, dressing. yes (no)...describe *can't do my daily chores anymore*

Do you feel you get enough exercise? yes no   What exercise do you usually do? _____ How often? _____

For each of the following activities, please check whether you consider yourself independent, needing assistance, or unable to do. If you are not independent, please explain.

	Indep	Need Assist	Unable
Bath/shower	✓		
Dressing yourself	✓		
Eating	✓		
Using the bathroom	✓		
Moving to/from bed or chair	✓		

move slow since my operation

Have you fallen recently? no yes

EQUIPMENT NEEDED IN

	Hospital	Home
Crutches	___	___
Walker	___	___
Wheelchair	___	___
Highrise toilet seat	___	___
Other _____		

Figure 8–1 Nursing Admission Assessment. Courtesy of Department of Nursing, The Medical Center at the University of California, San Francisco.

REST/SLEEP

Do you have any difficulty sleeping? (no) yes . . . describe *I do not sleep much, never have*

Is there anything you do or use to help you sleep? no yes . . . describe _____

COGNITIVE-PERCEPTUAL

Any difficulty hearing? no (yes) . . . describe *a little hard of hearing*

Do you use an aid? (no) yes . . . type_____ Do you have any difficulty seeing? no yes

When were your eyes last checked? *don't know* Do you wear (glasses) contacts? no (yes) . . . type _____

Have you experienced any changes in your memory lately? (no) yes . . . describe _____

Do you sometimes have difficulty learning new things? (no) yes . . . describe _____

What is the easiest way for you to learn them? *have people tell me — don't read much*

Do you regularly experience pain or discomfort? (no) yes . . . describe/manage _____

ROLES-RELATIONSHIPS

With whom do you live? *wife and 6 of my 13 children*

Whom do you define as your family or support system? /X same as above; others . . . *children are ages 16-35*

How does your family or significant other(s) feel about your illness/condition? *scared*

Are you experiencing any family difficulties as a result of your illness/condition? (no) yes . . . describe_____

Do others depend on you for things? no (yes) . . . how are they managing? ✓ no problems; ___ experiencing some difficulty . . . describe _____

Does anyone come into your home to help you (e.g. visiting nurse, housekeeper, etc.)? (no) yes . . . who and how often?

Other questions you'd like answered or specific things you'd like to learn while you're in the hospital? (no) yes . . . (if yes) list _____

Name of person who filled out form (if different than patient): _____

Relationship to patient _____ Date _____

The following personal questions are optional. Please fill in those which you feel will assist your nurse in planning your care.

SELF-PERCEPTION/SELF CONCEPT

Has this illness/condition caused changes in your body or the things you can do? no (yes) . . . describe _____ *too weak to do day to day work on the farm*

Has it effected you emotionally? (no) yes . . . describe _____

Has it caused changes in the way you feel about yourself or your body? (no) yes . . . describe _____

Have any of these changes been a problem for you? (no) yes . . . describe _____

SEXUALITY-Reproduction

Some people have concern that their surgery/condition may affect their sexual relationship(s). Is this a concern for you? (no) yes . . . describe _____

(Women only) Is there a chance you might be pregnant? no yes _____

COPING-STRESS

Who is most helpful in talking things over? *my son Tom* Is s/he available to you now? no (yes)

Other than your illness/condition, have there been any big changes in your life in the last year or so? no (yes) . . . describe *can't do my work*

When you have problems or stress in your life, how do you generally handle them/it? *no problems*

Most of the time does this help? yes no . . . describe *too busy to worry about things*

Being in the hospital is stressful for many people. Is there anything we can do to make it easier for you? _____ *let my family visit*

VALUE-BELIEF

Do you consider religion/spirituality important in your life? (yes) somewhat no

Would you like to see a hospital chaplin? no (yes)

Admitted to: __525 W__ from: __home__ Time: __1500__ Ht: __171__ Wt: __95.3 kg__
T: __36.5__ P: __80 R__ R: __16__ B/P: L: __124/80__ R: _____ Oriented to: __✓__ phone; __✓__ TV; __✓__ bed; __✓__
visiting hours; __✓__ call light; __✓__ meal times/menu; __✓__ care of valuables; __✓__ smoking; __✓__ dentures; __✓__

Completed by: __Mary Jones__ Date/Time: __7/23/89 1400 hrs__
Allergies: __none__

NURSING ADMISSION ASSESSMENT

MEDICATION HISTORY

NAME	DOSE	FREQUENCY	LAST TAKEN	PURPOSE/PROBLEM TAKING
Tolinase	250 mg	qd	7/22	diabetes
Lasix	20 mg	qd	7/22	for bad heart valve
Slow K	20 mEq	qd	7/22	to replace K+
NTG 1/150	ī	prn	2 months ago	angina

GENERAL APPEARANCE: (size; posture; mobility; expression; mental status; orientation) Large, slightly obese elderly 81 year old male. Alert and oriented × 3. Moves well but stiff in joints. Pleasant but not talkative.

HEENT: (trach; eyes; cranial facial abnormalities) Wears corrective glasses for reading.

NEUROLOGICAL: (gait/balance; LOC; speech disorders) Slight limp. Independent.

MUSCULO-SKELETAL: (atrophy; swelling/edema, ROM; prosthetic devices) (L) hip replacement 18 months ago s̄ complications. No pedal edema.

SCREENING EXAM

CARDIOVASCULAR: (pulses: 4+=bounding, 3+=v.strong, 2+=normal, 1+=weak/thready, 0=unable to palpate; rhythm/regularity of heart; color)

Pulse	R	L	Equal	Pulse	R	L	Equal	Rythm: (Regular) Irregular
Temp.	2+	2+		Fem.	3+	4+		loud murmur in aortic area
Carotid	2+	2+		Pop.	2+	0		
Brachial	2+	2+		D.P.	2+	0	(L) limbs	
Radial	2+	2+		Post tib.	2+	0	cooler than (R)	

PULMONARY: (breath sounds; cough or sputum; chest symmetry; respiratory effort) ō cough. Equal expansion. Rales in bases bilaterally which do clear with coughing.

GASTRO-INTESTINAL/GU/GYN: (size; tenderness; distention; ascites; bowel sounds; ostomy; tubes) Abdomen soft, non tender. Last BM 7/22 a.m.

GU/GYN: (date of last period, urgency, frequency, burning, vag. discharge) ↑ frequency c̄ Lasix noted by patient.

INTEGUMENTARY: (Norton Scale; on figure in box note location of any items with the appropriate letter and check in box by the letter) _____ Pink, intact, good turgor.

═══	Numbness	B	Bruise
ooo	Pins and needles	D	Decubitus
xxx	Burning	L	Laceration
+++	Aching	R	Rash
///	Stabbing	S	Scar

602-02 9/85

PRESSURE SORE RISK ASSESSMENT SCORING SCALE: Total score: _____ (circle #'s then total)

Phy. Cond.	Ment. Cond.	Activity	Mobility	Incontin.	If $\leq$ 14, initiate a diagnosis.
(4 good)	(4 alert)	(4 ambulatory)	4 (full)	(4 not)	
3 (fair)	3 (apathetic/withdrawn)	3 (wk/help)	(3)(sl. limited)	3 (occassionally)	
2 (poor)	2 (confused)	2 (chair/bound)	2 (v. limited)	2 (usual/urine)	
1 (very bad)	1 (stuporous/unresponsive)	1 (bedfast)	1 (immobile)	1 (urine & stool/doubly)	

Signatures _____ Mary Jones RN _____ Date _7/23/89_

_____   _____

UNIT SPECIFIC INFORMATION

Pt. admitted for cardiac catheterization and probable aortic valve replacement. Pt has hx (6 mos.) of angina. Over past year patient has noted marked decrease in energy and episodes of SOB on exertion.

Signature _____ Mary Jones RN _____ Date _7/23/89_

_____   _____

examination that includes essential functioning of various body parts or systems.

The nursing admission assessment form shown in Figure 8–1 is an example of a screening examination. Data obtained during the examination are recorded on this form and can be analyzed by comparing the client's status to norms or standards, such as ideal height and weight standards or norms for temperature or blood pressure levels. The data are used to determine the person's general health status and to identify relevant nursing diagnoses. To conduct the examination, the nurse uses techniques of inspection, auscultation, palpation, and percussion.

◼ **Inspection.** **Inspection** is visual examination, that is, assessing using the sense of sight. It includes looking with the naked eye and using a lighted instrument such as an otoscope, which assists with visual examination of the ear. Inspection is an active, not a passive, process. The nurse must know what to look for and where. Nurses use inspection frequently to assess color, rashes, scars, body shape, facial expressions that may reflect emotions, and body structures, e.g., the inner eye. Inspection should be systematic, so that no area is missed.

◼ **Auscultation.** **Auscultation** is the process of listening to sounds produced within the body. Auscultation may be direct or indirect. Direct auscultation is the use of the unaided ear, e.g., to listen to a respiration wheeze or the grating of a moving joint. Indirect auscultation is the use of a stethoscope, which amplifies the sounds and conveys them to the nurse's ears. A stethoscope is used primarily to listen to sounds from within the body, e.g., bowel sounds or valve sounds of the heart.

The stethoscope should be 30 to 25 cm (12 to 14 in) long, with an internal diameter of about 0.3 cm (1/8 in). It should have both a flat-disc and a bell-shaped diaphragm. See Figure 8–2. The flat-disc diaphragm best transmits high-pitched sounds, e.g., bronchial sounds, and the bell-shaped diaphragm best transmits low-pitched sounds, such as some heart sounds. The earpieces of the stethoscope should fit comfortably into the nurse's ears. The diaphragm of the stethoscope is placed firmly but lightly against the client's skin. If a client is very hairy, it may be necessary to dampen the hairs with a cloth so that they will lie flat against the skin and not cause scratching sounds.

Auscultated sounds are described according to their pitch, intensity, duration, and quality. The **pitch** is the frequency of the vibrations (the number of vibrations per second). Low-pitched sounds, e.g., some heart sounds, have fewer vibrations per second than high-pitched sounds, such as bronchial sounds. The **intensity** (amplitude) refers to the loudness or softness of a sound. Some body sounds are loud, e.g., bronchial sounds heard over the trachea, while others are soft, e.g., normal breath sounds heard in the lungs. The **duration** of a sound is its length (long or short). The **quality** of sound is a subjective description of a sound, e.g., whistling, gurgling, or snapping.

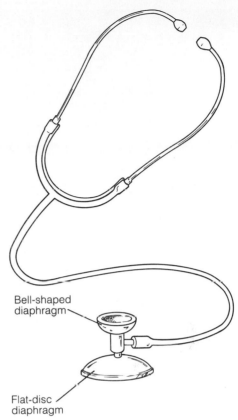

Bell-shaped diaphragm

Flat-disc diaphragm

Figure 8–2 A stethoscope with a flat-disc and bell-shaped diaphragm

◼ **Percussion.** **Percussion** is an assessment method in which the body surface is struck to elicit sounds that can be heard or vibrations that can be felt. A commonly used percussion technique is to place the middle finger of the nondominant hand, referred to as the **pleximeter,** on the client's skin. Only the distal phalanx of this finger should be in contact with the skin. Using the tip of the flexed middle finger of the other hand, called the **plexor,** the nurse strikes the pleximeter between the nail and the distal interphalangeal joint. See Figure 8–3. The striking motion should come from the wrist; the forearm remains stationary. The angle between the plexor and the pleximeter should be 90 degrees, and the blows must be firm, rapid, and short to obtain a clear sound.

Percussion is used to determine the size and shape of internal organs by establishing their borders. It indicates whether tissue is fluid-filled, air-filled, or solid. Percussion elicits five types of sound: flatness, dullness, resonance, hyperresonance, and tympany. **Flatness** is an extremely dull sound produced by very dense tissue such as muscle or bone. **Dullness** is a thudlike sound produced by dense tissue such as the liver, spleen, or heart. **Resonance** is a hollow sound such as that produced by lungs filled with air. **Hyperresonance** is not produced in the normal body. It is described as booming and can be heard over an emphysematous lung. **Tympany** is a musical or drumlike sound produced from an

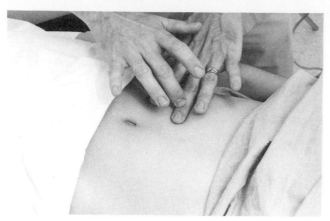

Figure 8—3 The position of the fingers for percussion. Only the middle finger of the nondominant hand is in contact with the skin.

air-filled stomach. On a continuum, flatness reflects the most dense tissue (least amount of air) and tympany the least dense tissue (the most amount of air). A percussion sound is described according to its intensity, pitch, duration, and quality.

■ **Palpation.** **Palpation** is the examination of the body using the sense of touch. The pads of the fingers are used because their concentration of nerve endings makes them highly sensitive to tactile discrimination. Palpation is used to determine:

1. Texture, e.g., of the hair
2. Temperature, e.g., of a skin area
3. Vibration, e.g., of a joint
4. Position, size, consistency, and mobility of organs or masses
5. Distention, e.g., of the urinary bladder
6. Presence and rate of peripheral pulses
7. Tenderness or pain

There are two types of palpation: light and deep. *Light* (superficial) palpation should always precede *deep* palpation, because heavy pressure on the fingertips can dull the sense of touch. For light palpation, the nurse extends the fingers of the dominant hand parallel to the skin surface and presses gently downward while moving the hand in a circular fashion. If it is necessary to determine the details of a mass, the nurse presses lightly several times rather than holding the pressure.

Deep palpation is done with two hands (bimanually) or one hand. In deep bimanual palpation, the nurse extends the dominant hand as for light palpation, then places the fingerpads of the nondominant hand on the dorsal surfaces of the distal interphalangeal joint of the middle three fingers of the dominant hand. See Figure 8–4. Pressure is applied by the top hand while the lower hand remains relaxed to perceive the tactile sensations. For deep palpation using one hand, the fingerpads of the dominant hand press over the area to be palpated. Often the other hand is used to support a mass or organ from below. See Figure 8–5. Deep palpation is a technique used more commonly by nurse practitioners and clinical specialists than by nurses in general practice.

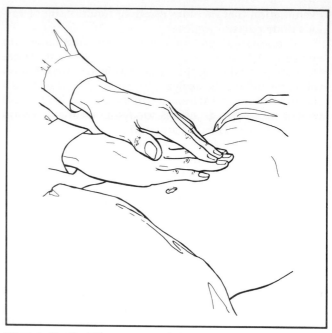

Figure 8—4 The position of the hands for deep bimanual palpation

The effectiveness of palpation depends largely on the client's relaxation. Nurses can assist a client to relax by:

1. Gowning and/or draping the client appropriately
2. Positioning the client comfortably
3. Ensuring that their own hands are warm before beginning, e.g., running them under warm water if they are cold
4. Commencing palpation with areas that are not painful

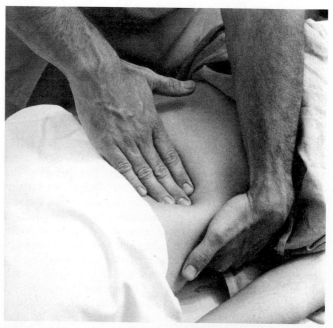

Figure 8—5 Deep palpation using one hand below to support while the hand above palpates the organ

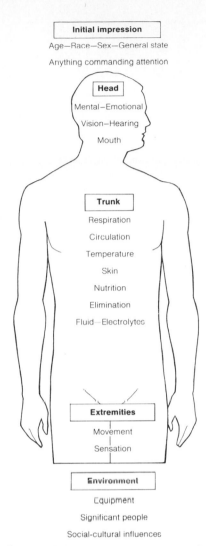

Figure 8—6 entries surrounding image:

Initial impression

Age—Race—Sex—General state

Anything commanding attention

Head

Mental—Emotional

Vision—Hearing

Mouth

Trunk

Respiration

Circulation

Temperature

Skin

Nutrition

Elimination

Fluid—Electrolytes

Extremities

Movement

Sensation

Environment

Equipment

Significant people

Social-cultural influences

Figure 8—6 A tool for assessment. *Source:* Adapted from H. Wolff and R. Erickson, The assessment man, *Nursing Outlook,* February 1977, 25:103. Copyright 1977 American Journal of Nursing Company. Reprinted with permission.

During palpation, the nurse should be sensitive to the client's verbal and facial expressions indicating discomfort.

Physical examination is carried out systematically. Generally, the examiner records a general impression about the client's overall appearance and health status, e.g., age, body size, mental and nutritional status, speech, and behavior. Then the examiner takes measurements such as vital signs, height, and weight. Next, the examiner conducts a physical examination beginning at the head and ending at the toes (head-to-toe or **cephalo-**

caudal examination). See Figure 8—6 for a sample head-to-toe assessment.

Chapter Highlights

Assessment is the collection, verification, and documentation of data about a client's health status.

Assessing involves active participation by the client and the nurse.

Methods used for data collection are informal conversation, formal interview, nursing assessment (history), physical health examination, and consultation.

The data base should be accurate, complete, and brief. The nurse needs to use appropriate medical terminology when compiling the data base.

The data base should include objective and subjective data.

Skills required for data collection are communicating, interviewing, observing, and examining.

Selected References

Benjamin, A. 1981. *The helping interview.* 3d ed. Boston: Houghton Mifflin Co.

Carnevali, D. L. 1983. *Nursing care planning: Diagnosis and management.* 3d ed. Philadelphia: J. B. Lippincott Co.

Davis, A. J. 1984. *Listening and responding.* St. Louis: C. V. Mosby Co.

Gordon, M. 1982. *Nursing diagnosis process and application.* New York: McGraw-Hill Book Co.

La Monica, E. L. 1985. *The humanistic nursing process.* Monterey, Calif.: Wadsworth Health Sciences.

McPhetridge, L. M. January 1968. Nursing history: One means to personalize care. *American Journal of Nursing* 68:68–75.

Orem, D. E. 1985. *Nursing: Concepts of practice.* 3rd ed. New York: McGraw-Hill.

Perry, A. G. 1982. Analysis of the components of the nursing process. In Carlson, J. H., Craft, C. A., and McGuire, A. D., editors. *Nursing diagnosis.* Philadelphia: W. B. Saunders Co.

Philpott, M. 1985. *Legal liability and the nursing process.* Toronto: W. B. Saunders Co., Canada.

Roy, Sr. C. 1984. *Introduction to nursing: An adaptation model.* 2d ed. Englewood Cliffs, N.J.: Prentice-Hall.

Stewart, C. J., and Cash, W. B. 1985. *Interviewing principles and practices.* 4th ed. Dubuque, Iowa: Wm. C. Brown Publishers.

Yura, H., and Walsh, M. B. 1983. *The nursing process: Assessing, planning, implementing, evaluating.* 4th ed. Norwalk, Conn.: Appleton-Century-Crofts.

CHAPTER 9

Diagnosing

OBJECTIVES

Describe characteristics of definitions of nursing diagnoses.

Identify basic steps in the diagnostic process.

Describe how the nurse identifies the client's health problems and strengths.

State the two essential parts of a nursing diagnostic statement.

Identify guidelines for writing diagnostic statements.

Discuss the advantages of using nursing diagnoses.

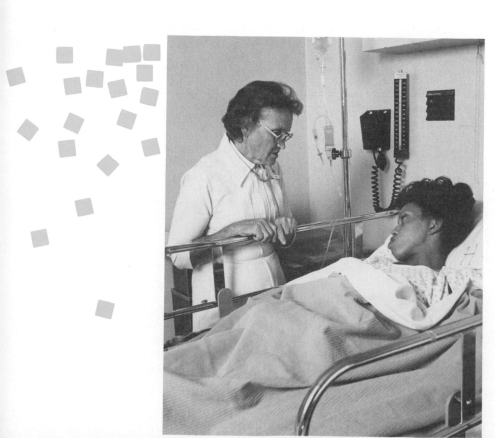

Nursing Diagnosis

Definitions

The term **diagnosis** is derived from the Greek word *diagignoskein,* which means "to distinguish." The process of diagnosing is used in several professions to identify aspects of the client's condition that are of concern to that professional. In fact, anyone who makes a statement or conclusion about the nature of a condition, situation, or problem is diagnosing. Automobile mechanics diagnose the nature or cause of automobile conditions; social workers diagnose economic and social situations; and nurses diagnose the health status of clients requiring nursing care. The term *diagnosis,* therefore, is not restricted to one particular profession and must be qualified by a professional designation, such as medical diagnosis or nursing diagnosis.

Many definitions of *nursing diagnosis* have been developed. Each has different emphases, but all have many similarities. In 1973, the First National Conference on the Classification of Nursing Diagnosis accepted this definition: A **nursing diagnosis** "is the judgment or conclusion [that] occurs as a result of nursing assessment" (Gebbie and Lavin 1975). To Gordon (1976, p. 1299), **nursing diagnoses,** or clinical diagnoses made by professional nurses, describe a combination of signs and symptoms that indicate actual or potential health problems that nurses by virtue of their education and experience are able, licensed, and accountable to treat.

In 1980, the ANA declared that "nursing is the diagnosis and treatment of human responses to actual or potential health problems" (ANA 1980). Clearly, the ANA sees diagnosis as a nursing function even though it is still not unusual for people to believe that diagnosis is the prerogative of the physician. In 1982, the National Conference Group on the Classification of Nursing Diagnoses accepted the name North American Nursing Diagnosis Association (NANDA), thus recognizing the participation and contributions of Canadian as well as United States nurses. Through the efforts of this group, much progress has been made in defining, classifying, and describing nursing diagnoses. NANDA serves as a clearinghouse to disseminate information about nursing diagnoses and publishes a quarterly newsletter, supports research to stimulate study of nursing diagnoses, and sponsors biennial conferences to update the list of accepted nursing diagnoses. See the inside of the cover for the current NANDA list of accepted nursing diagnoses.

The Diagnostic Process

Diagnosis is a process of analysis and synthesis. **Analysis** is the separation into components; i.e., breaking down the whole into its parts. **Synthesis** is the opposite; i.e., putting together the parts into the whole. The cognitive skills required for analysis and synthesis are objectivity, critical thinking, decision making, and inductive and deductive reasoning (Andrews 1982,

p. 90). Nurses use these skills when making nursing diagnoses.

Registered nurses are the persons responsible for making nursing diagnoses. Even though other nursing personnel may contribute data to the process of diagnosing and may implement specified nursing care, the responsibility for formulating a diagnostic statement rests with the registered nurse. This restriction is supported by licensing laws and national standards of practice.

Nursing diagnoses differ from medical diagnoses in several ways. For a summary, see Table 9–1. A nursing diagnosis may be related to a medical diagnosis but is separate and distinct from it. A client who has one or more medical diagnoses and medical orders will likely also have one or more nursing diagnoses and nursing orders. These diagnoses and orders are complementary rather than contradictory. Nursing diagnoses relate to the nurse's **independent functions,** i.e., the areas of health care that are unique to nursing and are separate and distinct from the care included in medical management. Even though the nurse is obligated to carry out medical orders, i.e., **dependent functions,** the nurse is also obligated to diagnose and prescribe within the limits of nurse practice acts.

Determining the Client's Health Problems and Strengths

A **health problem** is any condition or situation in which a client requires help to maintain or regain a state of health or to achieve a peaceful death. It does not always refer to an undesirable state but does refer to a situation for which the client needs nursing assistance. Nursing diagnoses describe **actual health problems**

Table 9–1 Comparison of Nursing and Medical Diagnoses

Nursing Diagnosis	Medical Diagnosis
Describes an individual's response to a disease process, condition, or situation	Describes a specific disease process
Is oriented to the individual	Is oriented to pathology
Changes as the client's responses change	Remains constant throughout the duration of illness
Guides independent nursing activities: planning, intervening, and evaluating	Guides medical management, some of which may be carried out by the nurse
Is complementary to the medical diagnosis	Is complementary to the nursing diagnosis
Has no universally accepted classification system; such systems are in the process of development	Has a well-developed classification system accepted by the medical profession

(deviations from health), **potential health problems** (risk factors that predispose persons and families to health problems), and areas of enriched personal growth.

The domain of nursing diagnosis includes only those health states that nurses are able and licensed to treat. For example, nurses are not educated to diagnose or treat diseases such as diabetes mellitus; this task is defined legally as within the practice of medicine. Yet nurses can diagnose ineffective coping by the client, alterations in nutrition, and potential for injury, all of which may accompany diabetes mellitus. Addressing these problems is within the nurse's capabilities and the scope of the nurse's licensing laws. Nursing diagnosis is a judgment made only after a thorough, systematic analysis of all data collected.

Comparing Data against Standards

The nurse compares the client's data to a wide range of standards, such as normal vital signs, laboratory values, basic food groups, growth, and development. The nurse also uses knowledge—e.g., of physiology, psychology, and sociology—as well as past experience when comparing the data.

When comparing data against standards, the nurse must consider the client's view of "normal," which may differ from that of the nurse. For example, a client may think it is perfectly normal to bathe once a month, whereas the nurse may believe once a day is normal. What is considered normal varies according to the client's expectations, culture, values, economics, and knowledge. The nurse must also consider the client's previous condition.

▪ Clustering Data.

Clustering or grouping data is a thought process of determining the relatedness of facts and finding patterns in the facts. **Cues** (facts that the nurse acquires by using the five senses) are examined to determine whether any patterns are present, whether the cues are isolated incidents, and whether the cues are significant. To relate and group data, the nurse must consider nursing diagnostic categories or areas of nursing responsibility. Gordon (1982, p. 13) states that clustering information involves a search in the nurse's memory stores for previously learned meaningful groups of clinical cues that are associated with a diagnostic category.

Data clustering involves making inferences. An **inference** is the nurse's judgment or interpretation of cues. Data clustering or grouping for Mr. Joe Smith is illustrated in Table 9–2. The data are clustered according to nursing diagnostic categories.

▪ Identifying Gaps and Inconsistencies in the Data.

Gaps are missing information needed to determine a data pattern. For example, during the assessing phase, data about a client's definition of health are essential if the nurse is to understand his statement "I am sick all the time." Sometimes, essential data may be com-

pletely missing (e.g., information about a 15-month-old child's mobility may not specify whether she crawls or walks). Such information is necessary to assess the child's developmental stage.

Inconsistencies are conflicting data. For example, a nurse may learn from the nursing history that the client reports not seeing a doctor in 15 years, yet during the physical health examination he states, "My doctor takes my blood pressure every week." This inconsistency must be clarified before a valid pattern can be established.

▪ Health Problems.

During data processing, the nurse groups data according to categories, most likely with certain problems in mind. However, for health problems (existing or potential) to have a successful outcome, the client must accept the existence of the problem. The nurse, by contrast, determines whether the client needs help dealing with the problem. See Table 9–2 for examples of Mr. Joe Smith's problems.

▪ Strengths.

At this stage, the nurse and client also establish the client's strengths, resources, and abilities to cope. Generally, people have a clearer perception of their problems or weaknesses than of their strengths and assets, which are often taken for granted. By taking an inventory of strengths, the client can develop a more well-rounded self-concept and self-image. Strengths can be an aid to mobilizing health and regenerative processes.

A client's strengths might be that his weight is within the normal range for his age and height, thus enabling him to cope better with surgery. In another instance, a client's strengths might be that she is allergy-free and a nonsmoker. The same client's resources could be a supportive family and an ability to cope.

A client's strengths can be found in the nursing assessment record (health, home life, education, recreation, exercise, work, family and friends, religious beliefs, and sense of humor, for example), the health examination, and the client's records. See Table 9–2 for examples of Mr. Joe Smith's strengths.

Formulating Nursing Diagnoses

After clustering and analyzing the assessment data, the nurse formulates causal (etiologic) relationships between the health problem and the factors related to it. These etiologic factors may be environmental, sociologic, psychologic, physiologic, or spiritual. More than one factor may be related to one health problem. It is important to determine whether or not the problem can be resolved by independent nursing interventions. If it cannot, the nurse should refer the client to the appropriate health team member or collaborate with that person in planning care.

By including the etiologic factors in diagnostic statements, the nurse can structure an individualized plan of care for the client. For example, the diagnosistic category "impaired physical mobility" tells the nurse the problem but does not suggest the direction the nurs-

Table 9–2 Formulating Nursing Diagnoses for Mr. Joe Smith

Diagnostic Category	Grouping Data	Determining Strengths and Health Problems	Formulating Nursing Diagnostic Statements
Activity intolerance	Shortness of breath Lacks energy to do daily chores Does not smoke	Does not smoke (strength) Activity intolerance (problem)	Activity intolerance related to shortness of breath and lack of energy secondary to decreased strength of cardiac contraction
Ineffective air-way clearance	Rales in bases of both lungs relieved by coughing	Able to expel secretions by coughing (strength) Secretions in lung bases (problem)	Potential ineffective airway clearance postoperatively related to chest incision
Potential for injury	Left hip replacement Movement slightly limited Joint stiffness Slight limp	Carries out daily activities independently (strength) Movement slightly limited (problem)	Potential for injury (trauma) related to joint stiffness and limp from hip replacement surgery
Alteration in nutrition	Is diabetic Takes tolazamide (Tolinase) daily "No sugar" in diet "Eats a good diet" Overweight for height Weight loss of 5 pounds in past year	Controls diabetes with Tolinase and "no sugar" (strength) Weight loss of 5 pounds in past year (strength) Overweight (problem)	Alteration in nutrition: more than body requirements related to imbalance of intake versus activity expenditure
Knowledge deficit	Takes furosemide (Lasix) daily Takes Slow K daily Urinates frequently	Complies with medical regime (strength) Does not relate urinary frequency to diuretic (problem)	Knowledge deficit: side-effects of diuretic therapy
Alteration in peripheral tissue perfusion	Vital signs normal Heart rhythm regular Loud heart murmur (aortic area) Femoral pulses stronger than normal Absent pulses (popliteal, dorsalis pedis, posterior tibial) in left leg Left leg cooler than right leg Integument pink and intact	Vital signs within normal range (strength) Skin intact and of good color (strength) Impaired circulation in left leg (problem)	Alteration in peripheral tissue perfusion (left leg) related to impaired arterial circulation
Fear	Hospitalized for cardiac catheterization and possible aortic valve replacement States family "scared" about illness Wants to see chaplain Wants family to visit Perceives son Tom as helpful Says is usually too busy to worry about things	Perceives family as supportive (strength) Says family anxious about illness. Did not indicate own feelings (problem)	Fear related to cardiac catheterization, possible surgery, and its outcome
Comfort	History of angina (6 months) Takes nitroglycerin for angina	Has not needed nitroglycerin for 2 months (strength)	Potential alteration in comfort (angina) related to excessive activity or stress

ing intervention should take, whereas "impaired physical mobility related to neuromuscular impairment" (the more complete diagnostic statement) suggests a direction for plans and interventions to deal with the problem. Obviously, the specific etiologic factor identified, *neuromuscular impairment,* suggests a different direction than the another etiologic factor (e.g., *fear of falling*) would. See Table 9–2 for Mr. Joe Smith's nursing diagnostic statements.

Writing a Diagnostic Statement

Characteristics of a Diagnostic Statement

The nursing diagnostic statement has some very concrete characteristics. It is clear and concise, specific and client-centered, related to one client problem, and based on reliable and relevant assessment data. The diagnostic statement provides information about a client's actual or potential health problem that is within the scope of independent nursing intervention. It is the written outcome of the second phase of the nursing process. The nursing diagnostic statement has two parts:

1. Statement of the client's response (the health problem or strength)
2. Etiology (factors contributing to or probable causes) of the response

The two parts are joined by the words *related to* rather than *due to,* which implies a direct cause-and-effect relationship. In contrast, the phrase *related to* implies a relationship. If one part of the diagnostic statement changes, so may the other part. Examples of nursing diagnoses demonstrating these two parts are:

1. Ineffective breathing pattern (response) related to pain (etiologic factor)
2. Disturbance in self-concept (response) related to loss of arm (etiologic factor)
3. Grieving (response) related to anticipated loss (etiologic factor) secondary to husband's illness

The etiology of the problem (contributing or causative factors) identifies one or more probable causes of the health problem and gives direction to the required nursing therapy. **Etiology** may include behaviors of the client, environmental factors, or interactions of the two. For example, the probable causes of alteration in health maintenance include perceptual or cognitive impairment, lack of gross or fine motor skills, lack of material resources, and ineffective individual coping. See Table 9–3. Differentiating among possible causes in the nursing diagnosis is essential because each may require different nursing therapies.

The **defining characteristics** (cluster of signs and symptoms) are the supporting data that lead the nurse to choose a diagnostic category label. Each nursing diagnostic category is associated with signs and symptoms that occur as a clinical entity. Nursing diagnostic categories are similar to the medical diagnostic categories. For example, the medical diagnostic category *myocardial infarction* (heart attack) has a standardized set of signs and symptoms that are universally understood and accepted. Likewise, the nursing diagnostic category *alteration in health maintenance* has a standardized cluster of signs and symptoms. See Table 9–3. Although these signs and symptoms are frequently not included in the client's care plan, their presence should be documented in the nursing assessment to validate the nurse's selection of the diagnosis.

Potential nursing diagnoses are used when a client's responses can be predicted or when health promotion can contribute to well-being. Predictable responses are based on a client's health history, known complications of a disease process, or the nurse's experience. For example, a client who has smoked two packages of cigarettes per day for 40 years may have a postoperative nursing diagnosis of "potential impaired gas exchange related to smoking."

Possible nursing diagnoses are used when evidence about a response is unclear or when the related factors are unknown. The nurse writes the diagnosis on the client's care plan and collects more data either to support or refute the possible response. For example, an elderly widow who lives alone is admitted to hospital. The nurse notices that she has no visitors and is pleased with attention and conversation from the nursing staff. Until more data are collected, the nurse may write a nursing diagnosis of "Possible social isolation related to

Table 9–3   Components of a Nursing Diagnostic Category

Diagnosis	Definition	Etiology	Defining Characteristics
Health maintenance, alteration in	Inability to identify, manage, and/or seek out help to maintain health	Lack of or significant alteration in communication skills (written, verbal, and/or gestural) Lack of ability to make deliberate and thoughtful judgments Perceptual or cognitive impairment Complete or partial lack of gross and/or fine motor skills Ineffective individual coping; dysfunctional grieving Lack of material resources Unachieved developmental tasks Ineffective family coping: disabling spiritual distress	Demonstrated lack of knowledge regarding basic health practices Demonstrated lack of adaptive behaviors to internal or external environmental changes Reported or observed inability to take the responsibility for meeting basic health practices in any or all functional pattern areas History of lack of health-seeking behavior Expressed interest in improving health behaviors Reported or observed lack of equipment, financial, and/or other resources Reported or observed impairment of personal support system

Source: M. J. Kim, G. K. McFarland, and A. M. McLane, editors, *Pocket guide to nursing diagnoses,* 2d edition (St. Louis: C. V. Mosby Co., 1987). Used by permission.

unknown factors." Identifying a possible nursing diagnosis alerts other nurses to structure their nursing assessments to gather more data in this area to confirm or rule out the possible diagnosis.

▮ Guidelines for Writing a Diagnostic Statement

Clear, concise, client-centered nursing diagnoses can be written by following the guidelines presented in Table 9–4. Some common errors in writing diagnostic statements are:

1. Writing the client's response as a need instead of a problem
2. Using judgmental statements
3. Placing the etiologic factor before the client's response

4. Using statements that provide no specific direction for planning independent nursing interventions
5. Using medical rather than nursing terminology
6. Starting the diagnosis with a nursing intervention
7. Using a single symptom as the client's response

Data interpretation errors occur when the meaning of cues is misinterpreted. The nurse can avoid inaccurate interpretation of cues by determining how the client perceives the health problem, its probable cause, and actions taken to remedy it. For example, the nurse observes that a client repeatedly gets out of bed after the physician has ordered complete bed rest. The nurse may interpret this behavior as noncompliance. However, the client may be experiencing diarrhea and may be embarrassed to use the bedpan or may be refusing to accept a dependent sick role. Another source of diagnostic errors in data interpretation is overgeneralization from one isolated observation of client behavior. For

Table 9–4 Guidelines for Writing a Nursing Diagnostic Statement

Guideline	Correct Statement	Incorrect and/or Ambiguous Statement
1. State in terms of a problem, not a need	Actual fluid volume deficit (problem) related to fever	Fluid replacement (need) related to fever
2. State so that it is legally advisable.	Impaired skin integrity related to immobility (legally acceptable)	Impaired skin integrity related to improper positioning (implies legal liability)
3. Use nonjudgmental statements.	Spiritual distress related to inability to attend church services secondary to immobility (nonjudgmental)	Spiritual distress related to strict rules necessitating church attendance (judgmental)
4. Make sure that both elements of the statement do *not* say the same thing.	Potential impairment of skin integrity related to immobility	Potential impairment of skin integrity related to ulceration of sacral area (response and probable cause are the same)
5. Make sure that the client's response precedes the contributing or causal factor.	Noncompliance with diet (response) related to lack of knowledge (contributing factor)	Lack of knowledge (contributing factor) related to noncompliance with diet (response)
6. Use statements that provide guidance for planning independent nursing interventions.	Social isolation related to loss of speech (loss of speech provides direction for planning alternative communication methods)	Social isolation related to laryngectomy (the nurse can do nothing about the laryngectomy)
7. Word diagnosis specifically and precisely to provide direction for planning nursing intervention.	Alteration in respiratory function related to chronic allergy secondary to pollen from roses (specific)	Alteration in respiratory function related to the environment (vague)
8. Use nursing terminology rather than medical terminology to describe the client's response.	Potential ineffective airway clearance (nursing terminology)	Potential pneumonia (medical terminology)
9. Use nursing terminology rather then medical terminology to describe the probable cause of the client's response.	Potential ineffective airway clearance related to accumulation of secretions in lungs (nursing terminology)	Potential ineffective airway clearance related to emphysema (medical terminology)
10. Do not start the nursing diagnosis with a nursing intervention.	Potential alteration in nutrition: less than body requirements related to inadequate intake of protein (directs but does not state nursing intervention)	Provide high-protein diet because of potential alteration in nutrition (starts with nursing intervention)
11. Avoid using a symptom such as nausea as the client's response. A symptom does not reflect a pattern and requires additional data collection	Insufficient data for a diagnosis	Nausea related to medication

example, one episode of angry behavior does not mean that the client is hostile.

Advantages of Using Nursing Diagnoses

Among the advantages of using nursing diagnoses are:

1. Nursing diagnoses facilitate communication among nurses and with other health team members. A diagnosis identifies a client's health status, strengths, and health problems.
2. They strengthen the nursing process and provide direction for planning independent nursing interventions.
3. They help the nurse focus on independent nursing actions.
4. They help identify the focus of a nursing activity and thus facilitate peer review and quality assurance programs. **Peer review** is the appraisal of a nurse's practice, education, or research by coworkers of equal status. **Quality assurance** is the evaluation of nursing services provided and the results achieved against an established standard.
5. They facilitate nursing intervention when a client moves from one hospital unit to another or from hospital to home. The nursing diagnoses guide the planning of the nursing interventions that the client requires after discharge.
6. They facilitate comprehensive health care by identifying, validating, and responding to specific health problems (Griffith and Christensen 1982).

Chapter Highlights

- A nursing diagnosis is a statement of an actual or potential health problem amenable to independent nursing intervention.
- The diagnostic process is one of analysis and synthesis.
- The cognitive skills for analysis/synthesis are objectivity, critical thinking, decision making, and deductive and inductive reasoning.
- A nursing diagnostic statement has two parts: statement of the client's response and the etiologic factors contributing to or probably causing the response.
- A nursing diagnostic statement should be clear, concise, patient-centered, related to one problem, and based on reliable and relevant assessment data.
- Nursing diagnoses provide direction for planning independent nursing interventions.

Selected References

American Nurses' Association. 1980. *Nursing: A Social policy statement.* Kansas City, Mo.: American Nurses Association.

Andrews, P. B. Analysis and Synthesis. 1982. In Griffith, J. W., and Christensen, P. J., editors. *Nursing process: Application of theories, frameworks, and models.* St. Louis: C. V. Mosby Co.

Caine, R. M., and Bufalino, P. M. 1987. *Nursing Care Planning Guides for Adults.* Baltimore: Williams & Wilkins.

Carnevali, D. L.; Mitchell, P. H.; Woods, N. F.; and Tanner, C. A. 1984. *Diagnostic reasoning in nursing.* Philadelphia: J. B. Lippincott Co.

Doenges, M. E.; Jeffries, M. F.; and Moorehouse, M. F. 1984. *Nursing care plans: Nursing diagnoses in planning patient care.* Philadelphia: F. A. Davis Co.

Fadden, T. C., and Seiser, G. K. April 1984. Nursing diagnosis: A matter of form. *American Journal of Nursing* 84:470–72.

Gebbie, K., and Lavin, M. A., editors. 1975. *Classification of nursing diagnoses.* Proceedings of the First National Conference. St. Louis: C. V. Mosby Co.

Gordon, M. August 1976. Nursing diagnosis and the diagnostic process. *American Journal of Nursing* 76:1298–300.

——— . 1982. *Nursing diagnosis: Process and application.* New York: McGraw-Hill.

Griffith, J. W., and Christensen, P. J., editors. 1982. *Nursing process: Application of theories, frameworks, and models.* St. Louis: C. V. Mosby Co.

Hurley, M. E., editor. 1986. *Classification of nursing diagnoses. Proceedings of the sixth conference. North American Nursing Diagnosis Association.* St. Louis: C. V. Mosby Co.

Kim, M. J.; McFarland, G. K.; and McLane, A. M., editors. 1984. *Pocket guide to nursing diagnoses.* St. Louis: C. V. Mosby Co.

Kritek, P. B. 1985. Nursing diagnosis in perspective: Response to a critique. *Image: The Journal of Nursing Scholarship* 17:3–8.

La Monica, E. L. 1985. *The humanistic nursing process.* Belmont, Calif.: Wadsworth Health Sciences.

Mundinger, M. O., and Jauron, G. D. February 1975. Developing a nursing diagnosis. *Nursing Outlook* 23:94–98.

Shamansky, S. L., and Yanni, C. R. Spring 1983. In opposition to nursing diagnosis: A minority opinion. *Image: The Journal of Nursing Scholarship* 15:47–50.

Shoemaker, J. 1984. *Essential features of nursing diagnoses.* In Kim, M. J.; McFarland, G. K.; and McLane, A. M., editors. *Classification of nursing diagnoses: Proceedings of the Fifth National Conference.* St. Louis: C. V. Mosby Co.

Swearingen, P. L. 1986. *Manual of nursing therapeutics: Applying nursing diagnoses to medical disorders.* Menlo Park, Calif.: Addison-Wesley Publishing Co.

Tartaglia, M. J. March 1985. Nursing diagnosis: Keystone of your care plan. *Nursing 85* 5:34–37.

Yura, H., and Walsh, M. B. 1983. *The nursing process: Assessing, planning, implementing, evaluating.* 4th ed. Norwalk, Conn.: Appleton-Century-Crofts.

CHAPTER 10

Planning

O B J E C T I V E S

Describe the planning phase of the nursing process.

Identify four components of planning.

Identify criteria that assist the nurse and client to set priorities.

State the purposes of establishing client goals.

Describe the relationship of goals to the nursing diagnoses.

Differentiate between goals and outcome criteria.

Give guidelines for writing goals and outcome criteria.

Describe three aspects of planning nursing strategies.

Identify major purposes of a written care plan.

Identify various formats used for nursing care plans.

State guidelines for writing nursing care plans.

Describe effective approaches to discharge planning.

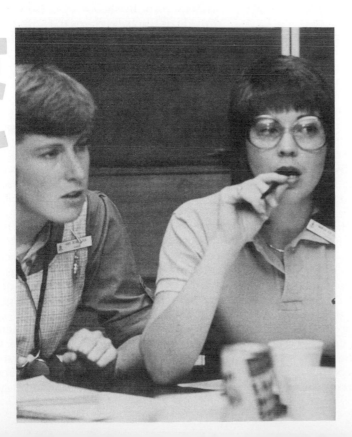

Definition and Process

Planning, the third step of the nursing process, involves identifying client goals and outcome criteria and designing the nursing strategies or interventions required to prevent, reduce, or eliminate client health problems (nursing diagnoses). The following people can be involved in planning nursing strategies: one or more nurses; the client, support persons, and/or caregivers; and sometimes members of other health professions. Although the planning process is basically the responsibility of the nurse, input from the client and/or support persons is essential if a plan is to be effective. It is no longer sufficient that nurses plan *for* the client; whenever possible, the client should participate actively.

Components of Planning

The four components of planning in the nursing process are setting priorities, establishing client goals and outcome criteria, planning nursing strategies, and writing a nursing care plan.

Setting Priorities

Priority setting is the process of establishing a preferential order for nursing strategies. To set priorities, the nurse and the client must first decide which nursing diagnosis deserves attention first, which second, and so on. Diagnoses can be grouped as having high, medium, or low priority. The priorities assigned to problems should not remain fixed. Nursing priorities change as a client's health problems and therapy change.

Setting priorities does not mean that all the high-priority diagnoses should be resolved before any others are considered. A high-priority diagnosis may be dealt with partially and then a diagnosis of lesser priority may become the focus of attention. In addition, the nurse may address more than one diagnosis at a time. Because client problems are usually multiple, this is often the case. See Table 10–1 for the assignment of priorities to the diagnostic statements for Mr. Joe Smith.

Setting priorities is made easier by using a framework, nursing model, or theory. One frequently used framework is Maslow's hierarchy of needs. See Figure 13–1. Maslow's physiologic needs, such as air, food, water, etc., are basic to life and receive higher priority than the need for security or activity. Life-threatening problems have the highest priority.

The client may set priorities differently from the nurse. For example, one nursing diagnosis may relate to smoking and another to nutrition. The nurse may give the smoking problem a higher priority than the problem of obesity, but the client may see the problem of obesity as more important. Sometimes, the client's perception of what is important conflicts with the nurse's knowledge of potential future problems or complications. For example, an elderly female may not regard ambulation

or turning and repositioning every 2 hours as important, preferring to be undisturbed. The nurse, knowing the potential complications of prolonged bed rest (e.g., muscle weakness and decubitus ulcers), should inform the client of these complications and implement necessary interventions to prevent such debilitating effects. Where there is a difference of opinion, the client and nurse should discuss it openly or resolve the conflict. However, in a life-threatening situation, the nurse needs to take the initiative.

Life-threatening situations require that the nurse establish priorities quickly. This also applies to situations that affect the integrity of the client, i.e., that could have a negative or destructive effect on the client. If money, equipment, or personnel are scarce, then a health problem may, of necessity, be given a lower priority. Client resources, such as finances or coping abilities, may also influence the setting of priorities. For example, a client who is unemployed may defer dental treatment; a client whose husband is terminally ill and dependent on her may consider nutritional guidance directed toward weight loss as too much to handle under her stressful circumstances.

Each client feels comfortable with a certain pace of action. Some clients may want to discuss the problem with family members or think about it overnight. Others may want "to get on with it." The nurse must adjust the plan to permit sufficient time for the necessary nursing strategies to modify the nursing diagnosis.

The priorities for treating nursing diagnoses must be congruent with treatment by other health professionals. For example, a high priority for the client might be to become ambulatory; however, if the physician's therapeutic regimen calls for extended bed rest, then ambulation must assume a lower priority in the nursing strategy plan. In such a case, however, the nurse can provide or teach exercises to facilitate ambulation later, provided the client's health permits. The diagnostic statement related to ambulation is not ignored; it is merely deferred.

Establishing Client Goals and Outcome Criteria

A goal is a hoped-for outcome; in terms of the nursing process, a **goal** is the desired outcome of nursing interventions. In the past, nursing goals were often written to direct the nursing care provided to clients. For example, a nursing goal might have been stated as follows: "Increase the client's exercise" or "Increase fiber in diet." From these nursing goals, specific nursing activities were derived, such as ambulating the client at specified intervals, offering instruction about needed dietary adjustments, and ensuring that high-fiber foods were provided.

Reflecting the emphasis on client-centered care, nurses have begun to state goals in terms of desired **client behavior,** not in terms of nursing activities. The term *outcome* means the result of an activity rather than the activity itself. Goals are broadly stated and cannot

Table 10–1 Assigning Priorities to Diagnostic Statements for Mr. Joe Smith (before cardiac catheterization)

Diagnostic Statement List	Priority Rating	Rationale
Activity intolerance related to shortness of breath and lack of energy secondary to decreased strength of cardiac contractions	Medium priority	Lack of energy is the client's stated major concern. Too much activity can create excessive cardiac demands, resulting in further decreased cardiac output with lowered blood pressure and inadequate circulation. However, because Mr. Smith is able to handle basic activities of daily living, strategies to deal with this diagnostic statement can be deferred until after cardiac catheterization and/or cardiac surgery.
Potential ineffective airway clearance postoperatively related to chest incision	Low priority	Until surgery is performed, ineffective airway clearance is not likely, since he is currently able to clear his airways by coughing.
Potential for injury (trauma) related to joint stiffness and limp from hip replacement surgery	High priority	The client is independent and moves slowly to accommodate his limitations. However, new surroundings and a sedative given before cardiac catheterization increase his risk of injury.
Knowledge deficit: side-effects of diuretic therapy	Medium priority	Although the client complies with his medical regimen, he does not seem to understand the side-effects of the prescribed diuretic, e.g., its relation to increased urination.
Alteration in peripheral tissue perfusion (left leg) related to impaired arterial circulation	High priority	Decreased circulation and tissue perfusion to the client's left leg can result in damage to the tissues of the limb.
Fear related to cardiac catheterization, possible heart surgery, and its outcome	High priority	Extreme fear could impair his coping capacity.
Potential alteration in comfort (angina) related to excessive activity or stress	Medium priority	Angina has not been a problem for 2 months, but it could recur with the stress of hospitalization and planned treatments.

be evaluated as to whether they have been met or not unless specific **outcome (or evaluation) criteria** accompany the goals.

Goals may be short-term or long-term. A short-term goal might be, "Client will raise right arm to shoulder height by Friday." In the same context, a long-term goal might be, "Client will regain full use of right arm." Because a great deal of the nurse's time is focused on the immediate needs of the client, most goals are short-term. In addition, the nurse is better able to evaluate the client's progress or lack of it with short-term goals.

A **client goal,** then, is a broad statement about the expected or desired change in the status of the client after he or she receives nursing interventions. Since goals are broad indicators of performance, the use of such verbs as *increase, decrease, maintain, improve, develop,* and *restore* is appropriate. (See some examples of client goals in the accompanying box.) Client goals are structured to:

1. Provide direction for planning nursing interventions that will achieve the anticipated changes in the client.
2. Provide direction for establishing evaluation criteria to measure the effectiveness of the interventions.

Client goals should address the client behavior identified in the first clause of the nursing diagnosis, i.e., the client's response to a health problem. For example, if the first clause of the nursing diagnosis is "Self-care deficit: feeding," the goal might be stated as follows: "Client will demonstrate increased ability to feed self."

If this goal is to be measurable, specific client outcomes (evaluation criteria) must be identified so that the nurse can decide whether or not the goal has been met and, thus, whether the health problem identified in the nursing diagnosis has been resolved. Some nurses make the outcome criteria part of the goal statement (e.g., "The client will demonstrate increased ability to feed self *as evidenced by* his ability to use utensils with sponge-wrapped handles and drink fluids through a straw."). The phrase "as evidenced by" specifies the observable outcomes by which the goal can be evaluated. Other nurses list these criteria separately under

Examples of Client Goals

The client will:

Increase activity tolerance
Maintain urinary elimination pattern
Restore fluid volume
Decrease potential for injury
Develop coping abilities
Improve nutritional pattern

the goal (e.g., "Will use a straw to drink from a glass" and "Will feed self using utensils with sponge-wrapped handles.").

In addition to being important during the planning phase of the nursing process, **outcome criteria** are also essential during the evaluation phase of the nursing process. Outcome criteria serve four purposes:

1. They provide direction for nursing interventions.
2. They provide a time span for planned activities.
3. They serve as criteria for evaluation of goal achievement.
4. They give the client and nurse a sense of achievement.

When establishing outcome criteria during the planning phase of the nursing process, the nurse asks two questions:

1. How will the client look or behave if the desired goal is achieved?
2. What must the client do and how well must he or she do it before the goal is attained?

Well-stated outcome criteria relate to the established goal, are possible to achieve, and are specific, concrete, and measurable, i.e., the outcome can be seen, heard, felt, or measured by another person.

Examples of client goals and outcome criteria associated with the diagnostic statements for Mr. Joe Smith are shown in Table 10–2. Note that the diagnostic statements have been reordered according to established priorities. Refer to the guidelines below when writing client goals and specifying outcome criteria.

▇ Planning Nursing Strategies

Nursing strategies are nursing actions designed to achieve established client goals. Selecting nursing strategies is a decision-making process. Planning nursing strategies involves generating a number of alternative nursing actions likely to solve the client's problem, considering the consequences of each alternative action, and choosing one or more nursing strategies.

Sometimes a nurse, particularly a nurse with limited experience, may wish to generate nursing strategies with other nurses or consult care planning texts to obtain the best alternatives. The client and/or support persons should be included in this discussion whenever possible. Often, the nurse and the client can establish a number of nursing strategies for each problem statement. However, too many alternatives can be confusing. Usually, it is sufficient to develop three to five alternative nursing strategies for each health problem. See Table 10–3.

The next step is to consider the consequences of each action, including the risks as well as the expected benefits. Often, each action will have more than one consequence. For example, the strategy "Provide accurate information" could result in the following client behaviors:

1. Increased anxiety
2. Decreased anxiety
3. Wish to talk with the physician
4. Desire to leave hospital
5. Relaxation

Establishing the consequences of each strategy requires nursing knowledge and experience. The nurse's experience may suggest that providing information before the client's bedtime may increase the client's worry and tension and that maintaining the usual rituals before sleep is more effective. Perhaps some alternative nursing actions should be implemented during the day to facilitate sleep at night, e.g., providing accurate information during the day and increasing daytime activity.

After considering the consequences of the alternative nursing strategies, the nurse chooses one or more that she or he considers likely to be most effective. Although the nurse bases this decision on knowledge and experience, the client's input is very important. For example, a client may say: "I always have a sandwich and glass of milk before going to bed when I am home. I know I'll sleep if I can have that." Maintaining this routine may indeed help the client sleep, and this action might be the first choice as a nursing strategy.

When choosing the best nursing strategy to help the client attain the desired goal, the nurse should evaluate each alternative as to its safety, achievability with the resources available, validity with regard to nursing knowledge and experience or knowledge from relevant sciences, appropriateness for the client's age and health, and congruence with the client's values and beliefs, other therapies, and the stated policy of the agency.

▇ Writing the Nursing Care Plan

The **nursing care plan** is a written guide that organizes information about a client's health; it outlines the actions nurses should take to address the client's identified nursing diagnoses and meet the stated goals. It is

GUIDELINES

Writing Goals and Outcome Criteria

Write goal statements and outcome criteria in terms of client behavior. Avoid statements that direct the nurse what to do for or to the client.

Make sure that the goal statement clearly relates to the nursing diagnosis and that the outcome criteria relate to the goal.

Make sure that the outcome criteria realistically reflect the client's capabilities/limitations and the designated time span.

Ensure that the goals and outcome criteria are compatible with the work and therapies of other professionals.

Keep the goal statement related to only one diagnosis to ensure that outcome criteria selected and planned nursing interventions are clearly related to the diagnosis.

When writing *outcome criteria,* use observable, measurable terms; avoid words that are vague and require interpretation or judgment by the observer.

Table 10–2 Goals and Outcome Criteria for Mr. Joe Smith (before cardiac catheterization)

Diagnostic Statement*	Client Goals	Outcome Criteria
1. Fear related to cardiac catheterization, possible heart surgery, and its outcome	Experience increased emotional comfort and feelings of control	Verbalizes specific concerns Communicates thoughts clearly and logically Facial expressions, voice tone, and body posture correspond to verbal expressions of increased emotional comfort or feelings of control After instruction, describes the cardiac catheterization procedure and what is expected of him before and after the procedure
2. Alteration in peripheral tissue perfusion (left leg) related to impaired arterial circulation	Improve circulation to left leg and foot	Skin intact, pink, and moist Skin temperature warm (as other foot) Left dorsalis pedis, posterior tibial, and popliteal pulses palpable and of same strength as corresponding right pulses Verbalizes factors that improve and inhibit peripheral circulation Capillary refill of left toenails within 1 to 3 seconds
3. Potential for injury (trauma) related to joint stiffness and limp from hip replacement surgery	Prevent injury	Moves in and out of bed and ambulates without falling or injuring self
4. Activity intolerance related to shortness of breath and lack of energy secondary to decreased strength of cardiac contraction	Avoid performance of activities causing shortness of breath and excessive cardiac workload	Rests after meals No shortness of breath during activities Pulse and blood pressure remain stable at 80 beats per minute and 124/80 mm Hg

*Note new order of diagnostic statements to reflect highest priorities.

also referred to as the *client care plan*, since its focus is the client.

The responsible nurse (head nurse, primary nurse, or team leader) starts the care plan as soon as a client is admitted to the health care agency. It is constantly updated and revised throughout the client's stay, in response to changes in the client's condition and evaluations of goal achievement. The purposes of a written care plan are:

1. To provide direction for *individualized care* of the client.
2. To provide for *continuity of care.*
3. To provide *direction about what needs to be documented* on the client's progress notes.
4. To serve as a *guide for assigning staff* to care for the client.

The nursing care plan is organized according to each client's unique nursing care needs. Although many agencies have devised standardized care plans as guides for providing essential nursing care to specified groups of clients, such plans should be used in conjunction with a plan developed for each client. Standardized plans, developed and accepted by the nursing staff of the agency, ensure that the minimally acceptable standards of care are provided. These plans, however, do not ensure individualized care.

The written plan is a means of communicating and organizing the actions of a constantly changing nursing staff. The initial plan, updated to show nursing interventions and new assessment data, is often conveyed to all nursing staff at change-of-shift reports, nursing rounds, and client care conferences. It specifically outlines which observations to make and what nursing actions to carry out. Thus, the plan serves as a guideline for what should be charted (see Chapter 22). Certain aspects of the client's care may need to be delegated to someone who can make necessary judgments about the client's responses. The care plan should also include instructions to be given to the client and/or family members.

Although formats differ from agency to agency, the nursing care plan is generally organized into four categories: nursing diagnoses or problem list, planned goals,

Table 10–3 Developing Alternative Nursing Strategies

Diagnostic Statement	Client Goal	Alternative Nursing Strategies
Sleep pattern disturbance related to anxiety	Obtain 6 to 9 hours of sleep	Provide warm milk and a snack in the evening. Provide more activity during daytime. Provide accurate information. Provide soft music. Provide a hypnotic. Encourage verbalization of worries.

nursing strategies/interventions/nursing orders, and outcome or evaluation criteria. Some agencies have a fifth category, assessment, to highlight the key data nurses need to obtain for baseline and ongoing assessments. Others use only three categories, including the specified outcome criteria to be evaluated with the planning or goal-setting.

To help students learn to write care plans and apply their knowledge, educators often modify this plan by adding another category, the "rationale" for each nursing diagnosis and/or intervention. See Table 10–4 for a sample nursing care plan format, which is structured with five columns to provide a rationale for each nursing order. A **rationale** is the scientific reason for selecting a specific nursing action. Including the rationale helps the student nurse to understand why a specific nursing diagnosis or intervention is relevant for the client. Students may also be required to cite supporting literature for this stated rationale.

Many agencies use a nursing Kardex or Rand system for organizing and storing nursing care plans. A nursing *Kardex* or *Rand* is a file of specially designed 6- x 11-inch index cards containing the care plans for a group of clients. Most of these cards include not only space for the nursing diagnoses, goals, nursing actions, and evaluations but also a concise profile of the client (including name, medical diagnosis, religion, marital status, occupation, allergies, and next of kin). It may also include information about medications the client is receiving, parenteral therapy and other treatments, current operations, and planned laboratory and diagnostic studies. With knowledge of the time and frequency of tests, treatments, and other activities, the nurse can coordinate all care for the client and organize her or his clinical assignments.

Some health care agencies have adopted 8½- x 11-inch nursing care plan records that correspond to the standard chart size and require that the plan be written in ink so that it can be retained as part of the client's permanent legal record. In other agencies, problem-oriented medical records (POMR) are used; in this situation, the nursing care plan is documented in a SOAP format. See Chapter 22. In still other agencies, medical orders are not included on the nursing care plan.

Nursing interventions include those activities that maintain or restore the client's usual patterns, alleviate symptoms, and prevent additional problems. The collection of additional data is often necessary to define a nursing diagnosis better or to learn how to manage a problem. For example, if the nurse notices that a client appears withdrawn, worried, and tense, the nurse needs additional data from the client to clarify the factor contributing to this behavior. The nurse may write a tentative nursing diagnosis of "anxiety related to unknown factors" and then write nursing interventions that guide the nursing staff toward identifying the etiology. For example, a planned intervention may state, "Talk with client to determine cause of anxiety."

If the nurse needs information about how to manage a problem, data may be collected from many sources. One example is "RN to consult physician about method of cleaning ulcer." In other situations, the nurse may consult with other health professionals, such as a pharmacist about the side effects of a medication, a dietitian about the foods allowed on a certain diet, or a physical therapist about appropriate exercise.

Planned nursing interventions may also specify the need to distribute information about continuing management of a problem to the client's support persons or other health team members. For example, a family member may need to learn how to help the client manage a long-term illness, or a visiting nurse association may need information about follow-up nursing care requirements for a client who is being discharged. To ensure clarity and completeness, the nurse can use the following guidelines when writing nursing care plans:

1. Date and sign the plan. The date the plan is used is essential for evaluation, review, and future planning. The signature of the responsible nurse demonstrates accountability to the client and to the nursing profession, since the effectiveness of nursing actions can be evaluated.

2. Use the category headings "Nursing Diagnoses," "Goals," "Nursing Orders/Interventions," and "Evaluation" and include a date for the evaluation of each goal.

3. Indicate that goals are met or revised by your signature or some other method specified by the agency.

4. List the nursing interventions designed to meet each goal in order of priority. For example, the nursing orders for a client with a decubitus ulcer might include "Apply an occlusive dressing for 24 hours" and "Clean the ulcer with Betadine solution daily." The appropriate sequence is to clean the ulcer before applying the dressing, and the orders should be listed in that sequence.

5. Use standardized medical or English symbols and key words rather than complete sentences to communicate your ideas. For example, write, "Turn and reposition q2h" rather than "Turn and reposition the client every two hours."

6. Refer to procedure books or other sources of information rather than including all the steps on the written care plan. For example, write: "See unit procedure book for tracheostomy care," or attach a standard nursing plan about such procedures as radiation-implantation care and preoperative or postoperative care. Using these adjuncts for commonalities of care among clients not only saves the nurse time but also focuses the care plan on the unique differences that individualize the care of clients.

7. Tailor the plan to the unique characteristics of the client by ensuring that the client's choices, such as preferences about the times of care and the methods used, are included. This reinforces the client's individuality and sense of control.

8. Ensure that the care plan incorporates *preventive* and health maintenance aspects as well as restorative. For example, carrying out the order "Provide active-assistance ROM exercises to affected limbs q2h" prevents joint contractures and maintains muscle strength and joint mobility.

Table 10—4 Nursing Interventions with Rationale for Mr. Joe Smith

Diagnostic Statement	Goals	Nursing Interventions	Rationale	Outcome Criteria
1. Fear related to cardiac catheterization, possible heart surgery, and its outcome	Experience increased emotional comfort and feelings of control	Establish a trusting relationship with the client and family	Mistrust in health care providers increases fear	Verbalizes specific concerns
		Encourage client and family to express feelings and concerns	Expression of feelings often relieves tension and enables supportive feedback or correction of misinformation	Communicates thoughts clearly and logically Facial expressions, voice tone, and body posture correspond to verbal expressions of increased emotional comfort or feelings of control
		Discuss the cardiac catheterization procedure and what is expected of him before and after the procedure	Knowledge of the procedure and of what is expected of him will reduce fears of the unknown and feelings of powerlessness	After instruction, describes the cardiac catheterization procedure and what is expected of him before and after the procedure
		Encourage conversation with another client who has recuperated from similar surgery	Another client who has recuperated from heart surgery can provide more hope about the outcome of surgery than the nurse	
2. Alteration in peripheral tissue perfusion (left leg) related to impaired arterial circulation	Improve circulation to left leg and foot	Consult with physician about exercise program, such as walking and range-of-motion exercises to hip, knee, and ankle	Walking and range-of-motion exercises increase peripheral circulation, but because the conditions causing impaired arterial circulation are unknown, the physician must prescribe them	Skin intact, pink, and moist Skin temperature warm (as other foot) Left dorsalis pedis, posterior tibial, and popliteal pulses palpable and of same strength as corresponding right pulses
		Keep the extremity in a *dependent* position (i.e., lower than the heart)	A dependent position facilitates arterial blood flow by gravity	Capillary refill of left toenails within 1 to 3 seconds
		Use Doppler ultrasound stethoscope (DUS) to assess blood flow in left dorsalis pedis, posterior tibial, and popliteal arteries q2h	The DUS detects and indicates movement of blood through arteries by a pulsating sound. When pulses are not palpable, the DUS can determine blood flow	
		Instruct client to keep his legs warm, e.g., wear warm socks but discourage use of external heat sources	Warmth increases circulation; because decreased sensation is often associated with impaired perfusion, external heat may not be perceived and cause burning	
3. Potential for injury (trauma) related to joint stiffness and limp from hip replacement surgery	Prevent injury	Closely assess ambulation and transfers during first few days	Close supervision enables assessment of independence and safety in mobility	Moves in and out of bed and ambulates without falling or injuring self
		Keep bed at lowest level	Low level facilitates safer transfers into and out of bed	
		Encourage to request assistance to ambulate during the night	New surroundings can cause confusion in older people and be the cause of accidents	
		Closely attend or put side rails up when client is sedated	Sedation can alter perception and impair motor abilities	

(continued)

Table 10—4 Nursing Interventions with Rationale for Mr. Joe Smith (*continued*)

Diagnostic Statement	Goals	Nursing Interventions	Rationale	Outcome Criteria
4. Activity intolerance related to shortness of breath and lack of energy secondary to decreased strength of cardiac contraction	Avoid performance of activities causing shortness of breath and excessive cardiac workload	Organize client care and provide undisturbed rest periods Discuss energy conservation methods such as taking periodic rest periods	A balance of activity and rest is necessary to stabilize cardiac effort Implementing energy conservation methods reduces the cardiac workload and deleterious effects of reduced cardiac output	Rests after meals No shortness of breath during activities Pulse and blood pressure remain stable at 80 beats per minute and 124/80 mm Hg
		Tell the client to reduce the intensity, duration, and frequency of activity if he experiences chest pain, shortness of breath, dizziness, or abnormal pulse and blood pressure after activity	These signs indicate inadequate cardiac output	
		Monitor vitals signs q2h and report decreasing blood pressure, increasing heart rate, or increasing respiratory rate	These signs are indicative of additional reduced cardiac output and cardiac failure	

9. Include collaboration and coordination activities in the plan. For example, the nurse may write plans to ask a nutritionist or physical therapist about specific aspects of the client's care.
10. Include plans for the client's discharge and home care needs. It is often necessary to consult and make arrangements with the community health nurse, social worker, and agencies that supply client information and needed equipment.

Discharge Planning

Because the average client stay in acute care hospitals has become shorter due to cost-containment efforts, people are sometimes discharged still needing care. Such care is increasingly being delivered in the home. **Discharge planning,** the process of anticipating and planning for needs after discharge from a hospital or other facility, is becoming a crucial part of comprehensive health care and should be addressed in each client's care plan. Effective discharge planning begins with the admission of the person and continues with ongoing assessment of both client and family needs, until discharge. It involves a comprehensive assessment not only of physical care needs but also of the availability of family and friend caregivers, the home environment as described by the client and family, client and family resources, and community resources.

Some large hospitals have **discharge planners,** nurses whose primary responsibility is to assess anticipated needs after discharge. In most settings, however, staff, head nurses, and clinicians, with the help of social workers, are doing discharge planning. To facilitate collecting the assessment data needed for effective discharge planning, hospital staff may establish liaisons with community-based nurses who can visit the home before the client's discharge, thereby having the opportunity both to anticipate needs and plan with the family in advance of discharge.

Effective two-way communication is obviously essential for the coordination of information and planning. The nurse can be effective in helping family members think through their typical day and week and process the changes they can anticipate when the ill person is at home. Thinking through "what-if" situations (e.g., What if the client falls? What if there is an emergency? What if the caregiver needs to go to the store or do other essential errands?) helps families to confront what is happening to them at their own pace and in their own style and to plan for anticipated problems, thereby experiencing a sense of control and confidence (McCorkle and Germino 1984). It also provides the nurse an opportunity to identify the learning needs of clients and families. These learning needs can be met by individualized teaching prior to discharge or, if necessary, after discharge by the home health nurse. (See Chapter 21.)

When possible, referrals and other actions should be initiated before the day of discharge so that prepa-

Patient Name: *Mr. Donald Phillips*

Medical Record Number: *S447652001*

(addressograph stamp)

INTER-AGENCY REFERRAL FORM
ALLIED HEALTH INFORMATION

Address Reply To:
STANFORD UNIVERSITY HOSPITAL
Patient Care Planning Program
300 Pasteur Drive
Stanford, CA 94305-5232

Medicare No. 0721569702	Medi-Cal No.	From (Ward or Clinic) 4 SOUTH	(415) 725- 4499

Admission Date: 7/15/89	Discharge Date: 8/1/89	Medications Administered Day of Discharge:

Name and Address of Nearest ~~Relative or~~ Friend:
KAY JONES (neighbor)
14 MONTGOMERY ST., MENLO PARK, CA

COUMADIN 5mg @ 0900 hrs.

NURSING EVALUATION

	GOOD	FAIR	POOR
Vision	✓		
Hearing		✓	
Speech			✓
Bladder Control			✓
Bowel Control		✓	
Date of last BM	7/31/89		

MOBILITY			PERSONAL NEEDS	
	Walks		Call Bell	
	Cane	A	Feeds Self	
	Crutches		Eating Device	
	Walker	A	Commode	
A	Wheelchair		Bedpan	
A	Bed/Chair	I	Urinal	
	Bedfast	A	Bathing	
		I	Wash Face	
CODE:		A	Shave/Make-Up	
I = Independent		I	Comb Hair	
A = Assist		A	Brush Teeth/Dentures	
D = Dependent				

PATIENT USES:	YES	NO	COMMENTS
Glasses	✓		
Hearing Aide	✓		
Dentures	✓		
Catheter (condom)	✓		Type: Δ'd:
Tubes		✓	Type: Δ'd:
Prosthesis		✓	Type:
Colostomy		✓	Δ'd:

PATIENT IS:	YES	Describe Atypical Behavior
Alert/Appropriate		
Confused		
Combative		
Noisy		
Withdrawn	✓	DEPRESSED ABOUT DYSPHASIA
Wanderer		

SKIN (describe), DRESSING CHANGES, or TREATMENTS:
SKIN DRY BUT INTACT. SLING APPLIED TO (L) ARM

Myra Brown RN 7/31/89
SIGNATURE — TITLE — DATE

PHYSICAL AND OCCUPATIONAL THERAPY:
ROM exercises to (L) arm and (L) leg daily. Quadriceps exercises to (R) leg. *Larry Agnew, PT 7/31/89*
SIGNATURE — TITLE — DATE

DIET: *NO RESTRICTIONS*

TEACHING:
SIGNATURE — TITLE — DATE

SOCIAL (Current/future living arrangements; family composition, etc.) AND OTHER PERTINENT INFORMATION:
THIS 86 YR. OLD WIDOWER LIVES ALONE. HAS ONE DAUGHTER (IN NEW YORK CITY) WHO IS EXPLORING LONG TERM CARE FACILITIES IN THIS AREA. CLIENT'S ATTEMPTS TO VERBALIZE NEED TO BE ENCOURAGED. HE UNDERSTANDS SLOW, DISTINCT SPEECH. *Myra Brown RN 7/31/89*
SIGNATURE — TITLE — DATE

REPLY TO BE COMPLETED WITHIN 4 WEEKS:

SIGNATURE — TITLE — DATE

Figure 10—1 Patient Referral Form (Courtesy of Stanford University Hospital, Stanford, California)

rations for the client's return home are complete when he or she arrives. In this way, the client's and family's anxiety about the return is kept to a minimum. Referrals of a hospitalized client for home care are often initiated and implemented by the nurses caring for that client, but signed physician's orders for care are required if care is to be reimbursed by third-party payment. The physician may order treatments, medications, adjunctive therapies (e.g., physical, occupational, or speech therapy), and skilled nursing care. See Figure 10–1 for a sample home health referral form.

Chapter Highlights

Planning is the process of designing nursing strategies required to prevent, reduce, or eliminate a client's health problems.

Planning can involve the nurse, the client, support persons, and caregivers.

Nursing strategies are planned around a client's diagnostic statements and goals.

Four components of planning are setting priorities, establishing client goals, planning nursing strategies, and writing a nursing care plan.

Nursing diagnoses are assigned high, medium, and low priorities in consultation with the client, if health permits.

Client goals are used to plan nursing strategies that will achieve anticipated changes in the client.

Client goals are derived from the first clause of the nursing diagnosis.

Outcome criteria describe specific and measurable client responses and help the nurse evaluate the effectiveness of the nursing intervention.

Goal statements and outcome criteria are written in terms of the client's behavior.

Establishing the consequences of each nursing strategy requires nursing knowledge and experience.

The nursing care plan provides direction for individualized care of the client.

Planned nursing interventions are the specific actions to take by the nurse to help the client meet established health care goals.

Shorter acute care hospitalizations necessitate careful discharge planning.

Selected References

Atkinson, L. D., and Murray, M. E. 1983. *Understanding the nursing process.* 2d ed. New York: Macmillan Co.

Caine, R. M. and Bufalino, P. M. 1987. *Nursing Care Planning Guides for Adults.* Baltimore: Williams & Wilkins.

Carnevali, D. L. 1983. *Nursing care planning: Diagnosis and management.* 3d ed. Philadelphia: J. B. Lippincott Co.

Carpenito, L. J. 1987. *Nursing diagnosis: Application to clinical practice.* 2d ed. Philadelphia: J. B. Lippincott Co.

Griffith, J. W., and Christensen, P. J. 1982. *Nursing process: Application of theories, frameworks, and models.* St. Louis: C. V. Mosby Co.

La Monica, E. L. 1985. *The humanistic nursing process.* Monterey, Calif.: Wadsworth Health Sciences.

Lederer, J. et al. 1986. Care planning pocket guide: A nursing diagnosis approach. Menlo Park, Ca.: Addison-Wesley Publishing Co.

McCorkle, R. and Germino, B. 1984. What nurses need to know about home care. *Oncology Nursing Forum* 11(6):63–69.

Moughton, M. September 1982. The patient: A partner in the health care process. *Nursing Clinics of North America* 17:467–79.

Yura, H., and Walsh, M. B. 1983. *The nursing process: Assessing, planning, implementing, evaluating.* 4th ed. Norwalk, Conn.: Appleton-Century-Crofts.

CHAPTER 11

Implementing

OBJECTIVES

Describe two processes that continuously operate throughout the implementation phase of the nursing process.

Describe three categories of skills used to implement nursing strategies.

Identify four cognitive skills nurses use when implementing nursing strategies.

Give reasons why the need for health teaching by nurses has increased.

Describe key aspects of the counseling process.

Identify essential aspects of managing.

List guidelines for implementing nursing strategies.

State the significance of documenting nursing actions accurately.

Describe factors to be considered when delegating nursing activities.

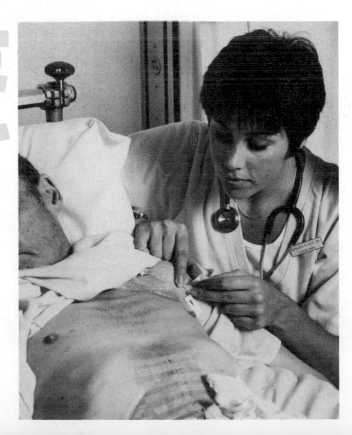

Implementing Defined

Implementing, also called intervening, is putting the nursing strategies listed in the nursing care plan into action. According to Marriner (1983), implementing involves carrying out nursing orders *and* physician's orders. The client's degree of participation often depends on his or her health status. For example, because an unconscious man is unable to participate in his care, he needs to have care given to him. By contrast, an ambulatory client may require very little care from the nurse and carry out health care activities independently. Implementing is the nursing action taken to attain the desired outcome or the client's goals.

Types of Nursing Actions

The terms *independent, dependent,* and *collaborative* or *interdependent* are often used to describe nursing actions. An action, in this context, is an activity appropriate to a person's role. An **independent nursing action** is an activity that the nurse initiates as a result of her or his own knowledge and skills. The nurse determines that the client requires certain nursing interventions, either carries these out or delegates them to other nursing personnel, and is accountable for the decision and the actions. To be *accountable* is to be answerable. An example of an independent action is planning and providing special mouth care.

Dependent nursing actions are those activities carried out on the order of the physician, under the physician's supervision, or according to specified routines. An example of a dependent action is giving an antibiotic by injection to a client as a result of a physician's written order. The dependent activity in nursing practice is usually directly related to the client's disease, and its importance should not be minimized. In addition to the task of carrying out the physician's order, the nurse who performs a dependent nursing action also conducts the appropriate nursing activities associated with the order. In the example above, for instance, the nurse would also monitor the client for signs of improvement, worsening infection, or toxic effects of the antibiotic.

Collaborative nursing actions are those activities performed either jointly with another member of the health care team or as a result of a joint decision by the nurse and another health care team member. Collaborative nursing activities sometimes illustrate the overlapping responsibilities of health personnel and reflect the collegial relationship between health professionals. For example, a nurse and a respiratory therapist together may decide on a schedule of breathing exercises for a woman. The therapist may initially teach the exercises to the client, and the nurse reinforces the learned behavior and assists the client in the therapist's absence.

Protocols

A **protocol** is a written plan specifying the procedure to be followed in a particular situation. For example, agencies often have protocols regarding a client's admission and discharge. Nurse practitioners in a community clinic may have protocols about which clients to refer to the physician and which clients to treat directly. Nurses in a home setting usually have protocols about the procedure to follow when a client dies. Nurses in hospitals frequently have protocols regarding the steps to follow when a postoperative client returns to the unit.

Standing Orders

A **standing order** is a written document about policies, rules, regulations, or orders regarding client care. Standing orders give nurses the authority to carry out specific actions under certain circumstances, often when a physician is not immediately available. In a hospital coronary care unit, a common example is the administration of emergency antiarrhythmic medications when a client's cardiac monitoring pattern changes.

Process of Implementing

The process of implementing normally includes reassessing the client, validating the nursing care plan, determining the need for nursing assistance, implementing the nursing strategies, and communicating the nursing actions. Reassessing the client and validating the nursing care plan are subprocesses that operate continuously throughout the implementing phase.

Reassessing the Client

As was mentioned in Chapter 8, assessing or reassessing is carried out throughout the nursing process whenever the nurse has contact with the client. While providing care nurses continue to collect data about changes (subtle or acute) in the client's level of wellness, i.e., health problems as well as reactions, feelings, and strengths. Following an extensive assessment during the first phase of the nursing process, reassessing in later phases usually focuses on more specific needs or responses of the client, i.e., fluid intake, pain, pulse rate, and urine output. Through this mechanism, nurses are able to determine whether planned nursing strategies are currently appropriate for the client.

Validating the Nursing Care Plan

A nursing care plan must be a flexible tool. When new data are collected, they should be compared with the data base. Sometimes, the new data are incongruent. The nurse must judge the value of the new data and determine whether the nursing care plan is still valid. When a client's health status changes, i.e., when physical or psychosocial responses change, the nursing care plan needs to be adjusted. If the data regarding the client's health status are unchanged, the nurse proceeds with the implementing process. For information on modifying or changing the nursing care plan, see Chapter 12.

Determining the Need for Assistance

When implementing some nursing strategies, the nurse may require assistance for one of the following reasons: The nurse is unable to implement the nursing strategies safely alone (e.g., turning an obese client in bed) and to reduce stress upon a client (e.g., turning a person who has acute pain when moved). In addition, a nurse should obtain assistance if she or he lacks the knowledge or skills to implement a particular nursing activity. For example, a nurse who is not familiar with a particular model of oxygen mask needs assistance the first time she or he applies it. For additional information about the need for assistance, see the section on delegating, later in this chapter.

Implementing Nursing Strategies

Nursing strategies are implemented to help the client meet his or her health goals. Specific activities are discussed later in this chapter. There are four primary areas of nursing practice: health promotion, health maintenance, health restoration, and care of the dying. Nursing actions in each of these areas can be independent, dependent, or collaborative.

Communicating Nursing Actions

Nursing actions are communicated in writing and often verbally *after* they have been carried out. Nursing actions must not be recorded in advance because the nurse may determine upon reassessing the client that the action should not or cannot be implemented. For example, a nurse is authorized to inject 10 mg of morphine sulfate subcutaneously to a client, but the nurse finds that the client's respiratory rate is 4 breaths per minute. This finding contraindicates the administration of morphine (a respiratory depressant). The nurse withholds the morphine and reports the client's respiratory rate to the responsible nurse and/or physician. A nurse might also find that a planned nursing action cannot be implemented, e.g., the client objects, the nurse is unable to perforate the skin with a needle, the nurse encounters an obstruction when inserting a rectal tube. Nursing activities, therefore, are always recorded after they are completed, when the nurse can accurately record exactly what occurred.

In some instances, it is important to record a nursing action immediately after it is implemented. This is particularly true of medications, treatments, etc., because recorded data about a client must be up to date, accurate, and available to other nurses and health care professionals. Immediate recording helps safeguard the client, for example, from receiving a second dose of medication.

The nurse may record certain nursing actions, e.g., giving mouth care every 2 hours or turning a client, at the end of a shift; in the meantime, the nurse maintains a personal record of these interventions so that they can be accurately recorded later. Many agencies have special forms for this type of recording. See Chapter 22 for additional information regarding recording.

Nursing actions are often communicated verbally as well as in writing. When a client's health is changing rapidly, the charge nurse and/or the physician may want to be kept up to date with verbal reports. Verbal reports are given to another nurse or other health professionals. Nurses also make verbal reports regarding clients at a change of shift and upon a client's discharge to another unit or health agency. For additional information about assessing the client's response, see Chapter 8; for information on recording and reporting, see Chapter 22.

Implementing Skills

Three types of skills are needed to implement nursing actions: cognitive, intrapersonal, and technical skills. The necessary **cognitive** (intellectual) skills for implementing are problem solving, decision making, critical thinking, and creativity. They are crucial to safe, intelligent nursing care. Problem solving and decision making are discussed in Chapter 7.

Critical thinking is a pattern of thinking based on knowledge, experience, and the abilities to conceptualize and analyze relationships. To conceptualize means to form a concept. A **concept** is an abstract idea generalized from particular instances. Critical thinking involves organizing information, picking out relevant information, relating, conceptualizing, and making judgments. Critical thinking enables nurses to make decisions quickly without bias.

Creativity, often called **creative thinking,** is establishing new relationships and new concepts, solving problems innovatively. When thinking creatively, the individual cannot always weigh alternatives or establish the logic behind all actions. For nurses, planning nursing strategies and changing nursing actions provide opportunities for creative thinking. Creative thinking helps nurses change a nursing activity efficiently.

Interpersonal skills are all the activities people use when communicating directly with one another. They may be verbal and nonverbal. The effectiveness of a nursing action often depends largely on the nurse's ability to communicate with others. Even when giving a medication to a client, the nurse needs to understand the client and in turn to be understood. A nurse who is delegating a nursing action also needs to be understood.

Interpersonal skills are necessary for all nursing activities: caring, comforting, referring, counseling, and supporting are just a few. They include conveying knowledge, attitudes, feelings, interest, and appreciation of the client's cultural values and life-style. Before nurses can be highly skilled in interpersonal relations, they must have self-awareness and sensitivity to others. See Chapter 20 for more detailed explanations of interpersonal skills.

Technical skills are "hands-on" skills such as manipulating equipment, giving injections, and bandaging, moving, lifting, and repositioning clients. These tasks are also called procedures or psychomotor skills. The term *psychomotor* includes the intrapersonal component, e.g., the communication need of the client. Technical skills require considerable knowledge on the part of the nurse, including the principles behind the steps of the procedure, knowledge about equipment and supplies, and in some instances knowledge as to when the procedure is required. Knowledge of the principles underlying the procedure is of particular importance because it enables the nurse to adapt a procedure to the individual client safely. For example, if a female client cannot turn on her left side for an enema, the nurse can adjust the client's position and still administer the enema effectively if the nurse understands the position of the rectum and large intestine in the body and the flow of fluids by gravity.

When the nurse carries out procedures requiring technical skills, it is important for the nurse to make significant assessments of the client *before* and *during* the procedure. Before a nurse initiates any procedure, it is necessary to relate her or his own knowledge and competence to the needs of the client. Sometimes assistance is necessary to prevent undue stress on the client and to ensure that the procedure is both safe and effective. It is equally important to evaluate the effectiveness of the procedure.

Technical skills frequently require manual dexterity. The number of technical skills expected of a nurse has increased greatly in recent years. Acute care hospitals have become highly technologic. Because of the trend toward increased use of technology, humanizing nursing has become a recognized need for clients. See Chapter 2.

Implementing Activities

To implement nursing care, the nurse generally performs the following activities: communicating, caring, teaching, counseling, managing, and using technical skills. Effective communication is an essential element of all helping professions, including nursing. *Communication* shapes relationships between nurses and clients, nurses and support persons, and nurses and colleagues. It plays a role in every action the nurse undertakes. The communication process, listening and responding skills, and ways to establish helping relationships are discussed in detail in Chapter 20.

The nurse communicates the nursing strategies planned and implemented for each client to other health care personnel. Planned nursing strategies are written on the client's care plan (see Chapter 10). Once the strategies are implemented, the nurse documents them on the client's record. Assessment findings, procedures implemented, and the client's responses are all recorded.

The terms *nursing care* and *caring* have been used by nurses for more than a century. Leininger (1984, p. 3) states: "Care is the essence and the central, unifying, and dominant domain to characterize nursing: it is an essential human need for the full development, health maintenance, and survival of human beings in all world cultures ... yet care has not received the same degree of attention by professionals and the public as cure." In an address to the 75th Annual Registered Nurses' Association of Nova Scotia, Benner (1984, p. 3) made this statement: "Caring is often frankly curative because it facilitates healing." Leininger (1984, p. 6) says that there can be no curing without caring, but there may be caring without curing.

Definitions and a clear understanding of the terms *care* and *caring* have been lacking. Systematic research is needed to describe caring behaviors, values, and practices in nursing so that this knowledge can be incorporated into nursing education and practice areas. A number of researchers are conducting investigations in this area. In her transcultural care theory, Leininger (1984, pp. 5–6) points out that human caring, although a universal phenomenon, varies among cultures in its expressions, processes, and patterns; it is largely culturally derived.

Differences in caring values and behaviors lead to differences in the expectations of those seeking care. For example, cultures that perceive illness primarily as a personal and internal body experience tend to use more medications and physical techniques than cultures that view illness as an extrapersonal experience. Leininger identifies many caring and nursing care constructs. Examples are comfort, compassion, concern, coping behaviors, empathy, enabling, health acts (consultative, instructive, maintenance), involvement, love, nurturance, presence, sharing, tenderness, touching, and trust. Each of these constructs has many subdescriptions. Leininger believes the goal of health care personnel should be to work toward an understanding of care and the health of different cultures so that each culture's care, values, beliefs, and life-styles will be the basis for providing culture-specific care.

Teaching is an interactive process between a teacher and one or more learners in which specific learning objectives or desired behavior changes are achieved (Redman 1984, p. 15). The focus of the behavior change is usually the acquiring of new knowledge or technical skills. See Chapter 21 for detailed information about the teaching/learning process. Shorter hospital stays and the increased longevity of clients with chronic illnesses mean that clients and families must be prepared to manage convalescence and living with disabilities at home. Nurses, therefore, must ensure that discharge teaching is a priority when implementing care.

Counseling is the process of helping a client to recognize and cope with stressful psychologic or social problems, to develop improved interpersonal relationships, and to promote personal growth. It involves providing emotional, intellectual, and psychologic support.

In contrast to the psychotherapist, who counsels individuals with identified problems, the nurse counsels primarily healthy individuals with normal adjustment difficulties. The focus is on helping the person develop new attitudes, feelings, and behaviors rather than on promoting intellectual growth. The client is encouraged to look at alternative behaviors, recognize the choices, and develop a sense of control.

Managing is an important nursing function. The nurse manages the nursing care of individuals, families, and communities. The nurse-manager also delegates nursing activities to ancillary workers and other nurses, and supervises and evaluates their performance. Managing requires knowledge about organizational structure and dynamics, authority and accountability, leadership, change theory, advocacy, delegation, and supervision and evaluation.

Nurses function in various types of organizations. Some are *autocratic* with one person having primary knowledge and power while other persons are subordinate. Some are *bureaucratic* with control through policy, structured jobs, and compartmentalized actions. Others *decentralize* control and emphasize self-direction and self-discipline of members. Still others can be viewed as components of *systems* that interact interdependently and adapt dynamically to change. This organization is particularly useful for the nurse who manages the care of individuals, families, and communities. On a larger scale, the nurse-manager must work in the organizational framework of the employing agency.

Authority is the right to act and command. It is an integral component of managing. Authority is conveyed through leadership actions; it is determined largely by the situation, and it is always associated with responsibility and accountability.

Accountability means being responsible for one's actions and accepting the consequences of one's behavior. Accountability can be viewed within a hierarchical systems framework, starting at the individual level, through the institutional/professional level, and then to the societal level (Sullivan and Decker 1985, p. 18). At the individual or client level, accountability is reflected in the nurse's ethical decision-making processes, competence, commitment, and integrity. At the institutional level, it is reflected in the statement of philosophy and objectives of the nursing department and nursing audits. At the professional level, it is reflected in standards of practice developed by national or provincial nursing associations. At the societal level, it is reflected in legislated nurse practice acts.

As a manager, the nurse acts as a change agent. A **change agent** is any individual or group operating to change the status quo in a system so that the individuals involved must relearn how to perform their role(s) (Zaltman and Duncan 1977, p. 17). By using the nursing process, the nurse promotes change in the health of clients. The nurse as a teacher or counselor facilitates change in the client's knowledge, skill, feelings, and attitudes. On a larger scale, the nurse can be instrumental in promoting change at the institutional, professional, or societal levels.

An **advocate** is one who pleads the cause of another or argues or pleads for a cause or proposal. The nurse acts as a client advocate by informing clients of their rights, by making sure they have the necessary knowledge to make informed decisions, and by supporting clients in the decisions they make. See Chapter 5 for further information.

Because it is often impossible to provide all of the nursing care needed by a group of clients, the nurse as a delegator must assign aspects of the client's care to other nursing personnel. Delegation is a major tool in making the most efficient use of time. **Delegation** is the sharing of responsibility and authority with others and holding them accountable for performance (Sullivan and Decker 1985, p. 168). Delegation is a high-level implementation skill. The nurse as a delegator must have the following information:

1. Needs of the client and family
2. Goals of the client
3. Nursing activity that can help the client meet the goals
4. Skills and knowledge of various nursing personnel

The nurse delegator must also determine how many nursing personnel are needed. This information may be indicated on the client's records. Other sources of this information are the client, the charge nurse, other nursing personnel, and the nurse-delegator's own judgment. Nurses may require assistance to give clients care quickly in certain situations. Assistance may also be necessary to ensure the client's safety; for example, a nurse administering an intramuscular injection to a 3-year-old might need help to prevent injury to the child. If in doubt, nurses should always obtain aid to safeguard the client.

Once a nurse-delegator establishes that assistance is required, it is important to identify what type of help is needed, e.g., lifting or holding; how long help is required; when it is required; and what assistance is available. The nurse must arrange for assistance, usually by asking the appropriate person on the unit, before commencing the nursing activity. Delegation does not mean that a nurse-delegator never gets involved in direct client care. Often the nurse-delegator performs nursing activities appropriate to her or his knowledge and skills. An important aspect of delegation is the development of the potential of nursing personnel. By knowing the backgrounds, experiences, knowledge, skills, and strengths of each person, a nurse can delegate responsibilities that help develop their competencies.

Nursing personnel to whom aspects of care have been delegated need to be supervised and evaluated. The amount of supervision required is highly variable, depending on the knowledge and skills of each person. The nurse-delegator contributes to this evaluation process, since she or he is the person who assigns the activity and observes the performance. Because individual motivation varies, the nurse-delegator needs to realize that not all persons perform equally. Thus, the nurse should evaluate assigned personnel according to standards of performance stated in job descriptions rather than by comparing one person to another. It is essential, too, that the nurse-delegator realize people require ongoing feedback about the care they give. Feedback should be given in an objective manner and include both positive and negative input.

Guidelines for Implementing Nursing Strategies

At times the task of learning what the nurse should or should not do may seem overwhelming to the student. The following guidelines serve as a blueprint for nursing activities.

1. Nursing actions are related to the knowledge and skill of the nurse. If they are to be safe for the client, nursing activities must be purposeful and have a scientific basis.
2. Nursing actions are adapted to the individual. A client's beliefs, values, age, health status, and environment are factors that can affect a nursing action.
3. Nursing actions should always be safe. Nurses and clients need to take precautions to prevent injury. For example, when changing a sterile dressing, the nurse practices sterile technique to prevent infection; when turning a client, the nurse protects the client's skin from abrasions, which could also lead to infection.
4. Nursing actions often require teaching, supportive, and comfort components. These independent nursing activities can often enhance the effectiveness of a specific nursing action.
5. Nursing actions should always be holistic. The nurse must always view the client as a whole and consider his or her responses in that light.
6. Nursing actions should respect the dignity of the client and enhance his or her self-esteem. Providing privacy and encouraging the client to make his or her own decisions are ways of respecting dignity and enhancing self-esteem.
7. The client's active participation in implementing nursing actions should be encouraged as health permits. Active participation enhances the client's sense of independence and control.
8. Nursing actions resulting from a physician's order (dependent actions) must be carried out accurately unless the nurse believes the order is unsafe for the client. Actions considered unsafe for a client must be discussed with the responsible nurse and/or physician.

Chapter Highlights

- Implementing is putting planned nursing strategies into action.
- Reassessing and validating the nursing care plan occur continuously during the implementing phase.
- Cognitive, interpersonal, and technical skills are used to implement nursing strategies.
- Cognitive skills include problem solving, decision making, critical thinking, and creativity.

- Creative thinking helps the nurse and the client to establish innovative nursing actions.
- Implementing activities are communicating, caring, teaching, counseling, managing, and using technical skills.
- Communication is essential for all nursing activities and for establishing relationships.
- The implementing phase of the nursing process is terminated with the documentation of the nursing activities.
- All nursing activities, all assessment data, and all client responses to the nursing activities require documentation.
- Teaching plays an increasing role in most nursing activities.
- Counseling is a helping process designed to promote personal growth and to help the client cope with stress; it requires therapeutic communication skills and leadership skills on the nurse's part.
- Managing nursing interventions requires knowledge of organizational structure, authority, accountability, leadership, change, advocacy, delegation, and supervision and evaluation.
- Nurses are accountable for all their nursing actions.

Selected References

Benner, P. E. June 5, 1984. *The primacy and power of caring in health promotion and healing.* Lecture given at the 75th Annual Registered Nurses' Association of Nova Scotia.

Bradley, J. C. March/April 1983. Nurses' attitudes toward dimensions of nursing practice. *Nursing Research* 32:110–14.

Carpenito, L. J. 1987. *Nursing diagnosis, application to clinical practice.* 2d ed. Philadelphia: J. B. Lippincott Co.

Cushing, M. October 1982. The legal side: Failure to communicate. *American Journal of Nursing* 82:1597.

DeYoung, L. 1985. *Dynamics of nursing,* 5th ed. St. Louis: C. V. Mosby Co.

La Monica, E. L. 1985. *The humanistic nursing process.* Belmont, Calif.: Wadsworth Health Sciences.

Leininger, M. 1984. *Care: The essence of nursing and health.* Thorofare, N.J.: Charles B. Slack.

Marriner, A. 1983. *The nursing process: A scientific approach to nursing care.* 2d ed. St. Louis: C. V. Mosby Co.

———. 1986. *Nursing theorists and their work.* St. Louis: C. V. Mosby Co.

Rabinow, J. September/October 1982. Delegating safely within the law. *Nursing Life* 2:48–49.

Redman, B. K. 1984. *The process of patient education.* 5th ed. St. Louis: C. V. Mosby Co.

Sullivan, E. J., and Decker, P. J. 1985. *Effective management in nursing.* Menlo Park, Calif.: Addison-Wesley Publishing Co.

Watson, J. 1985. *Nursing: Human science and human care—A theory of nursing.* Norwalk, Conn.: Appleton-Century-Crofts.

Yura, H., and Walsh, M. B. 1983. *The nursing process: Assessing, planning, implementing, evaluating.* 4th ed. Norwalk, Conn.: Appleton-Century-Crofts.

Zaltman, G., and Duncan, R. 1977. *Strategies for planned change.* New York: John Wiley and Sons.

CHAPTER 12

Evaluating

OBJECTIVES

Describe five components of the evaluation process.

Describe the steps involved in reexamining the client's care plan both when goals are met and when they are not met.

Differentiate quality assessment from quality assurance.

Describe three approaches to quality evaluation.

Identify essential steps in developing tools to evaluate quality care.

Identify various methods used to evaluate nursing care.

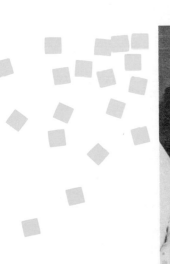

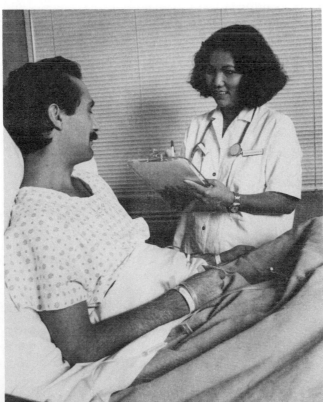

Definition of Evaluation

To evaluate is to judge or to appraise. In the context of the nursing process, evaluation is the fifth and last phase. Here, to **evaluate** means to identify whether or to what degree the client's goals have been met. Evaluating is an exceedingly important aspect of the nursing process because nursing judgments determine whether the nursing interventions can be terminated or must be reviewed or changed.

Evaluating is both a concurrent and a terminal process: It is concurrent in that the nurse normally evaluates during the implementing phase of the process. How is the client reacting to this nursing action? Is the reaction expected or unexpected? At this stage, the nurse may change a nursing action to help the client meet his or her goal. It is a terminal process because after the nurse completes the nursing activity, she or he evaluates whether the client's goals have been met. Often the time frame (if stated) in the outcome criteria is used.

Evaluating is a purposeful and organized activity. Through evaluating, nurses accept responsibility for their actions, indicate interest in the results of the nursing actions, and demonstrate a desire not to perpetuate ineffective actions but to adopt more effective ones.

Process of Evaluating

The evaluation process has six components:

1. Identifying the outcome criteria that will be used to measure achievement of the goals
2. Gathering data related to the identified criteria
3. Comparing the data collected with the identified criteria and judging whether the goals have been attained
4. Relating nursing actions to the outcomes
5. Reexamining the client's care plan
6. Modifying the care plan

The *identification of outcome criteria* used to evaluate the client's response to nursing care is discussed in Chapter 10. See Table 10–2. Criteria serve two purposes: They establish the kind of evaluative data that need to be collected, and they provide a standard against which the data are judged. For example, the goal "Client's urinary elimination pattern will be maintained" does not tell the nurse what data to collect while caring for the client. When these criteria are added, however, any nurse caring for the client knows what data to collect:

Daily fluid intake will be not less than 2500 ml.
Urinary output will be in balance with fluid intake.
Residual urine will be less than 100 ml.

Criteria that are clearly stated, precise, and measurable guide the next step of the evaluation process: *data collection.* Data are collected so that conclusions can be drawn about whether goals have been reached. The nurse collects data in relation to the specified cri-

teria, either by observation, direct communication, and purposeful listening or from reports of other health professionals.

Collection of both objective and subjective data may be necessary. Objective, measurable data are preferred for evaluation purposes; for example, "Respirations increased from 12 to 16 breaths per minute, and pulse rate increased from 70 to 90 beats per minute after client walked around the corridor." However, the nurse often needs to collect subjective data and some objective data that require interpretation. Examples of objective data requiring interpretation are the degree of tissue turgor of a dehydrated client or the degree of restlessness of a client with pain. Examples of subjective data include complaints of nausea or pain by the client.

When objective data require interpretation, the nurse may obtain the views of one or more other nurses to substantiate changes. When subjective data are required, the nurse must rely on either the client's statements (e.g., "My pain is worse now than it was after breakfast") or objective indicators of the subjective data, even though these indicators may require interpretation (e.g., decreased restlessness, decreased pulse and respiratory rates, and relaxed facial muscles as indicators of pain relief). Data collected must be recorded concisely and accurately to facilitate the third part of the evaluating process. Flowsheets and problem-oriented medical records in the SOAP format (discussed in Chapter 22) are recording aids.

If the first two parts of the evaluation process have been carried out effectively, *determining whether a goal has been achieved* is relatively simple. Both the nurse and the client play active roles in this. The data collected are compared with established criteria. Did the client drink 3000 ml of fluid in 24 hours? Did the client walk unassisted the specified distance per day? There are three possible outcomes of evaluation:

1. The goal was met; i.e., the client responded as expected.
2. The goal was partially met; i.e., a short-term goal was achieved, but the long-term goal was not; or, some, but not all, of the outcome criteria were attained.
3. The goal was not met.

See Table 12–1 for evaluation examples of Mr. Joe Smith's outcome criteria.

The fourth aspect of the evaluating process is *determining whether the nursing actions had any relation to the outcome.* It should never be assumed that a nursing action was the cause of or the only factor in meeting, partially meeting, or not meeting a goal. For example, Mrs. Sophi Ringdale was obese and needed to lose 14 kg (30 lb). When the nurse and client drew up a care plan, one outcome criterion was "Loses 1.3 kg (3 lb) by 4/7/88." A nursing strategy in the care plan was "Explain how to plan and prepare a 900-calorie diet." On 4/7/88, the client weighed herself and had lost 1.8 kg (4 lb). The goal had been met, in fact, exceeded. It is easy to assume that the nursing strategy was highly effective. However, it is important to collect more data before drawing that conclusion. Upon questioning the client, the nurse could find any of the following: the client planned a 900-calorie diet and prepared and ate the food; the client planned a 900-calorie diet but did not prepare the correct food; the client did not understand how to plan a 900-calorie diet, so she did not bother with it. If the first possibility is found to be true, the nurse can safely judge that the nursing strategy "Explain how to plan and prepare a 900-calorie diet" was effective in helping the client lose weight. However, if the nurse learns that either the second or third possibility actually happened, then it must be assumed that the nursing strategy did not bring about the outcome. The next step for the nurse is to collect data about what the client actually did to lose weight. The nurse should add these data to the assessment data in the care plan and examine the plan. It is important to establish the relationship (or lack thereof) of the nursing actions to the outcomes.

Evaluating goal achievement provides the feedback necessary to determine if the care plan was effective in resolving, reducing, or preventing the client's problems. It is then necessary for the nurse to *reexamine all aspects of the care plan,* whether or not the goals have been met. Reexamining is a process of reassessing and replanning. See Table 12–1 for an example of evaluating goal achievement for Mr. Joe Smith.

If a goal or goals have been met, one of the following decisions may be made:

1. The nurse may decide that the problem stated in the diagnosis no longer exists. In this instance, the nurse must document that the goal was met and that the care planned to meet this goal is discontinued.
2. The nurse may decide that the problem still exists even though the goal was met. For example, if the criterion is "Client will ingest 3000 ml of fluid daily," and the goal is "Client's state of hydration will be maintained," nursing interventions need to continue even though the goal and criterion have been met.
3. When a long-term goal is met by achieving short-term, progressive goals, the client's problem may remain as an actual problem even though the short-term goals are met.

When goals are not met or only partially met, the nurse needs to reexamine the client's data base, nursing diagnoses statements, goal statements, and nursing strategies. An incomplete or incorrect **data base** influences all subsequent steps of the nursing process and care plan. In some instances, new data may invalidate the data base, necessitating new nursing diagnoses, new goals, and new nursing actions. If the data base is incomplete, new **diagnostic statements** are required. If the data base is complete, the nurse needs to analyze whether the problem was identified correctly and whether the nursing diagnoses are relevant to that data base.

If the nursing diagnostic statement is inaccurate and requires correcting, it is obvious that the **goal statement** needs revision. If the nursing diagnostic statement is appropriate, the nurse then checks that the goal statements are realistic and attainable. Unrealistic, unattainable goals require correction. The nurse should also

Table 12–1   Evaluating Goal Achievement for Joe Smith

Assessment Data	Diagnostic Statement	Goal
Hospitalized for cardiac catheterization and possible aortic valve replacement States family scared about illness Wants to see chaplain Wants family to visit Perceives son Tom as helpful Says is usually too busy to worry about things	Fear related to cardiac catheterization, possible heart surgery, and its outcome	Experience increased emotional comfort and feelings of control
Vital signs normal Heart rhythm regular Loud heart murmur (aortic area) Femoral pulses stronger than normal Absent pulses (popliteal, dorsalis pedis, posterior tibial) in left leg Left leg cooler than right leg Integument pink and intact	Alteration in peripheral tissue perfusion (left leg) related to impaired arterial circulation	Improve circulation to left leg and foot
Left hip replacement Movement slightly limited Joint stiffness Slight limp	Potential for injury (trauma) related to joint stiffness and limp from hip replacement surgery	Prevent injury
Shortness of breath Lacks energy to do daily chores Does not smoke	Activity intolerance related to shortness of breath and lack of energy secondary to decreased strength of cardiac contraction	Avoid performance of activities causing shortness of breath and excessive cardiac workload

(continued)

Table 12—1 Evaluating Goal Achievement for Joe Smith (*continued*)

Nursing Orders	Outcome Criteria	Evaluation
Establish a trusting relationship with the client and family Encourage client and family to express feelings and concerns Discuss the cardiac catheterization procedure and what is expected of him before and after the procedure Encourage conversation with another client who has recuperated from similar surgery	Verbalizes specific concerns Communicates thoughts clearly and logically Exhibits facial expressions, voice tone, and body posture that correspond to verbal expressions of increased emotional comfort or feelings of control After instruction, describes the cardiac catheterization procedure and what is expected of him before and after the procedure	*Goal met* Verbalized concerns: "I'm worried about how my wife will support the family especially if anything bad happens during surgery." Asked questions about cardiac catheterization and surgery Nonverbal and verbal communication were congruent Described what to expect and what is expected of him before and after the cardiac catheterization procedure, e.g., "I know I will be taking a pill to help me relax before the procedure."
Consult with physician about exercise program, such as walking and range of motion exercises to hip, knee, and ankle Keep the extremity in a dependent position (i.e., lower than the heart) Use Doppler ultrasound stethoscope (DUS) to assess blood flow in left dorsalis pedis, posterior tibial, and popliteal arteries q2h Instruct client to keep his legs warm, e.g., by wearing warm socks, but discourage use of external heat	Demonstrates intact, pink, and moist skin Exhibits warm skin temperature (as other foot) Demonstrates palpable left dorsalis pedis, posterior tibial, and popliteal pulses of same strength as corresponding right pulses Verbalizes factors that improve and inhibit peripheral circulation Demonstrates capillary refill of left toenails within 1 to 3 seconds	*Goal partially met* Skin of left foot and ankle intact but pale Skin temperature still cooler in left than right foot Left popliteal pulse palpable but weak Left dorsalis pedis and posterior tibial pulses not palpable Blood flow evident only by DUS Capillary refill in left toenails within 7 seconds
Closely assess ambulation and transfers during first few days Keep bed at lowest level Encourage client to request assistance to ambulate during the night Closely attend client or put side rails up when client is sedated	Moves in and out of bed and ambulates without falling or injuring self	*Goal met* Ambulated and got in and out of bed safely
Organize client care and provide undisturbed rest periods Discuss energy conservation methods, such as taking periodic rests Tell the client to reduce the intensity, duration, and frequency of activity if he experiences chest pain, shortness of breath, dizziness, or abnormal pulse and blood pressure after activity Monitor vitals signs q2h and report decreasing blood pressure, increasing heart rate, or increasing respiratory rate	Rests after meals Experiences no shortness of breath during activities Shows stable pulse rate and blood pressure at 80 bpm and 124/80 mm Hg	*Goal met* Rested after meals and activities Experienced no shortness of breath while performing ADL Pulse rate and blood pressure remained stable at 80 bpm and 124/80 mm Hg

determine whether priorities have changed and whether the client and nurse still agree on the priorities. For example, a priority for the nurse may be to increase the client's fluid intake, but a priority for the client may be to decrease intake because of nausea. (see Table 12–2).

Last, the nurse investigates whether the **nursing strategies** are related to the goals and whether the best nursing strategies were selected. If both the diagnoses

and goals are appropriate, the nursing strategies selected may not have been the best ones to achieve the goal. Before selecting new strategies, the nurse should check whether the planned nursing actions have been carried out. Other personnel may not have carried them out, either because the instructions were unclear or because the interventions were unreasonable in terms of such external constraints as money, staff, and equipment.

Evaluating the Quality of Nursing Care

Over the past 30 years, there has been considerable work on the evaluation of the quality of nursing care to determine what good care is, whether the care nurses give is appropriate and effective, and whether the quality of care provided is good. Evaluating the quality of nursing care is an essential part of professional accountability. Other terms used for this measurement are quality assessment and quality assurance. **Quality assessment** is an examination of services only; **quality assurance** implies that efforts are made to evaluate *and* ensure quality health care.

Historical Perspective

Evaluation of the quality of care is not a new concept. Florence Nightingale's *Notes on Hospitals,* published in 1859, included an evaluation of medical and nursing care. Since that time, evaluation has progressed through a number of stages. Initially, it focused on the environment, e.g., whether equipment was available at the time it was needed. Later, organizational standards in agencies were developed. For example, the ratio of nurses to clients was studied and evaluated in terms of clients' needs. From about 1952 on, the Joint Commission on Accreditation of Hospitals (JCAH) has surveyed hospitals. Objective criteria were applied to evaluate a client's record after discharge from the hospital. This was called a **retrospective audit. Retrospective** means relating to a past event, and **audit** means an examination or review of records. A **nursing audit** is a review of clients' charts to evaluate nursing competence or performance. In 1972 and 1973, the JCAH revised its standards to include the requirement that hospitals be subjected to medical and nursing audits before receiving accreditation.

In 1972, the United States government enacted the Bennett Amendment, which created the Professional Standards Review Organization (PSRO). This program was intended to evaluate the quality of health care partially through peer review. A **peer review** is an encounter between two persons equal in education, abilities, and qualifications, during which one person critically reviews the practices that the other has documented in a client's record. Nursing subsequently developed evaluation programs compatible with the PSRO. These evaluative processes may be **concurrent audits,** in that they review present practices.

Approaches to Quality Evaluation

Three aspects of care can be evaluated. Each has advantages and disadvantages. The **structural approach** focuses on the organization of the client care system, such as administrative and financial procedures that direct the provision of care, staffing patterns, management styles, availability of equipment, and physical facilities. Information about these support structures can be obtained easily. However, proper facilities do not necessarily mean good care. The focus of the **process of care approach** is the nurse's actions, i.e., the performance of the caregiver in relation to the client's needs. This approach may be the most effective in determining the quality of care provided, but it is time-consuming and requires value judgments by appropriate clinical experts.

The focus of the **outcomes of the care received approach** is the client's health status, welfare, and satisfaction, or the results of care in terms of changes in the client. Its advantage is that outcomes may be easily observed, especially in relation to medical care, which focuses on disease entities. In nursing, however, outcomes are more difficult to determine, since nursing takes a more holistic view of the client than medicine

Table 12–2   Modified Care Plan for Joe Smith after Cardiac Surgery (selected examples only)

Assessment Data	Diagnostic Statement	Goal
Rales in bases of both lungs relieved by coughing before surgery Painful chest incision	Potential ineffective airway clearance related to chest incision	Maintain a clear airway
Aortic valve replacement (7/15) Heart rhythm regular at rest Pulse: 80 beats per minute (bpm) BP: 110/80 mm Hg	Potential alteration in cardiac output related to physical exertion and/or shock	Maintain cardiac output and blood volume
Left dorsalis pedis pulse and posterior tibial artery not palpable Skin of left extremity cool and pale	Alteration in tissue perfusion related to impaired arterial circulation	Improve arterial circulation
Aortic valve replacement (7/15)	Potential activity intolerance related to reduced strength of cardiac contraction	Increase activity tolerance *(continued)*

Table 12–2 Modified Care Plan for Joe Smith after Cardiac Surgery (selected examples only) *(continued)*

Nursing Orders	Rationale	Outcome Criteria
Administer analgesics q4h during first 48 hours	Pain relief makes coughing less uncomfortable and more effective	Normal breath sounds auscultated in all areas of both lungs
Splint incision with pillows or hands during coughing	Splinting minimizes pain	
Turn q2h during first 48 hours	Turning prevents the accumulation of secretions in one lung area	
Assist with deep breathing and coughing (DB & C) exercises q2h	DB & C exercises help to move and expel secretions	
Assess vital signs q1h for first 24 hours, q2h if stable for next 48 hours, and q4h thereafter if stable	A lowered blood pressure and rapid pulse indicate lowered blood volume or inadequate cardiac output	Stable vital signs Pulse: 80-100 bpm BP: not less than 110/80 mm Hg Respirations not more than 15 breaths per minute
Assess apical pulse and heart rhythm, not radial pulse		
Report an increase in resting pulse rate above 110 bpm and a BP below 100 mm Hg		
Keep client's legs warm (especially left leg) with blankets or socks	Warmth increases circulation	Left posterior tibial and dorsalis pedis pulses palpable and of same strength as corresponding right pulses
Assess blood flow in left dorsalis pedis artery and posterior tibial artery q2h using DUS	The DUS detects and indicates movement of blood through the arteries	Skin warm, intact, pink Capillary refill of left toenails within 1 to 3 seconds
Keep left leg in dependent position	A dependent position facilitates arterial blood flow by gravity	
Consult physician about a schedule for increasing activity	A gradual increase in activity helps the heart muscle and new valve accommodate increased demands	After activity, heart rate remains below 110 bpm and within 6 bpm of resting pulse after 3 minutes
Monitor and later show the client how to monitor his response to increased activity by: 1. Taking a resting pulse before activity 2. Taking pulse immediately after activity 3. Taking pulse 3 minutes after activity 4. Noting rate decreases, rates about 110, rates not within 6 bpm of resting pulse after 3 minutes	Pulse rate monitoring provides awareness of activities that do not overly exert the heart	
Monitor blood pressure after activity	A drop in blood pressure indicates a reduction in cardiac output	
Starting on 7/19, discuss factors contributing to increased cardiac workload, such as stress, excessive weight, overactivity, large meals	Knowledge of factors contributing to increased cardiac workload may facilitate necessary life-style changes, such as eating smaller meals, losing weight, and altering activity patterns	
Starting on 7/19, discuss the effects of reduced cardiac output such as shortness of breath, pain, fatigue, edema	Knowledge of the effects of reduced cardiac output may motivate him to avoid excessive activity	

takes. Defining emotional, social, and behavioral outcomes is more complex than defining medical outcomes. In addition, client outcomes cannot be wholly attributed to nursing care. The client's own physical and psychologic mechanisms and contributions by family and other health professionals collectively produce outcomes. Timing can be another confounding factor if the outcome is measured at the time of discharge rather than later.

Tools and Methods for Measuring Quality Care

Measuring the quality of care is a complex task. Several established tools are available for measuring the quality of care. Some are process tools, some are outcome tools, and others are process-outcome tools. Each tool consists of standards and criteria. Developing effective quality care evaluation tools is a challenge for the nursing profession. Much work is continuing even on established tools.

Methods of using these tools vary. Some agencies evaluate care by retrospective audits of nursing records using nursing audit committees. Others evaluate using a concurrent audit of process, i.e., direct observation of the nurse or nurses providing the nursing care by educated observers or by peers. Data may also be obtained by questioning and observing clients, questioning the family, and observing the client's environment and the general environment. The time period for measurement also varies. Some tools are designed for use over a 2-hour period; some are designed to evaluate the whole process of care given to the client from admission to discharge.

Chapter Highlights

▪ Evaluation determines whether or to what degree the client goals have been met.

▪ Evaluating is both a concurrent and terminal process.

▪ Evaluating is purposeful and organized.

▪ Identifying outcome criteria is the first aspect of evaluating.

▪ Outcome criteria determine the evaluative data that must be collected to judge whether the goals have been met.

▪ Outcome criteria must be measurable and precise.

▪ Reexamining the client care plan is a process of reassessing and replanning.

▪ Evaluating the quality of nursing care is an essential aspect of professional accountability.

Selected References

American Nurses' Association. 1973. *Standards of nursing practice.* New York: ANA.

———. 1975. A plan for implementation of the standards of nursing practice. New York: ANA.

———. 1976. *Guidelines for review of nursing care at the local level.* New York: ANA.

Curtis, B. J., and Simpson, L. J. October 1985. Auditing a method for evaluating quality of care. *Journal of Nursing Administration* 15:14–21.

Joint Commission on Accreditation of Hospitals. 1975. *Joint commission on accreditation of hospitals.* Chicago: JCAH.

———. 1983. *Manual for hospitals.* Chicago: JCAH.

Maciorowski, L. F.; Larson, E.; and Keane, A. June 1985. Quality assurance: Evaluate thyself. *The Journal of Nursing Administration* 15:38–42.

Phaneuf, M. C. 1972. *The nursing audit: Profile of excellence.* New York: Meredith Corp.

———. 1976. *The nursing audit: Self-regulation in nursing practice.* New York: Appleton-Century-Crofts.

Phaneuf, M. C., and Wandelt, M. 1974. Quality assurance in nursing. *Nursing Forum* 13(4):328–45.

Sundeen, S. J.; Stuart, G. W.; Rankin, E. D.; and Cohen, S. A. 1985. *Nurse-client interaction: Implementing the nursing process,* 3d ed. St. Louis: C. V. Mosby Co.

Wright, D. September 1984. An introduction to the evaluation of nursing care: A review of the literature. *Journal of Advanced Nursing* 9(5):457–67.

Wright, C., and Wheeler, P. March 1984. Auditing community health nursing. *Nursing Management* 15:40–42.

Yura, H., and Walsh, M. B. 1983. *The nursing process: Assessing, planning, implementing, evaluating,* 4th ed. Norwalk, Conn.: Appleton-Century-Crofts.

Concepts About Humans

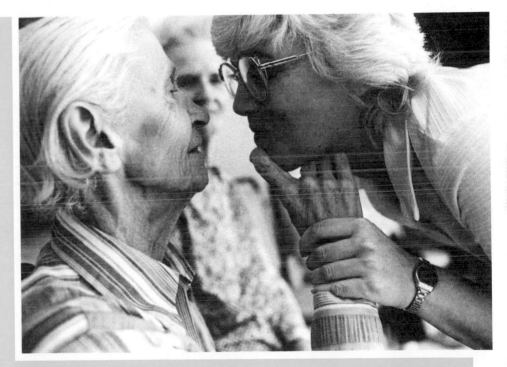

CHAPTER 13

The Holistic Person

OBJECTIVES

Explain the relationship of holism to nursing.

Compare Maslow's hierarchy of needs with Kalish's categories of needs.

Identify selected characteristics of basic human needs.

Identify factors that affect needs satisfaction.

Describe factors influencing priority of needs.

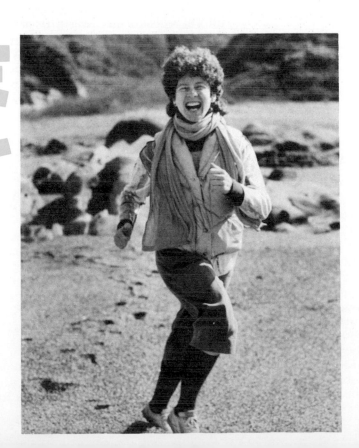

Holism

Nurses are concerned with the individual as a whole, complete, or holistic person, not as an assembly of parts and processes. The terms *holistic* and *holism* are derived from the Greek word meaning "whole." In holistic theory, all living organisms are seen as interacting, unified wholes that are more than the mere sums of their parts. Viewed in this light, any disturbance in one part is a disturbance of the whole system; in other words, the disturbance affects the whole being.

When applied to humans and health, holism emphasizes that "nurses must keep the self-identity of the 'whole' person in mind and must strive to understand simultaneously the relationship of the 'part' of the individual under concern to the totality of that individual's interactions and the relationship of the whole to its parts" (Krieger 1981, p. 4). Therefore, when the nurse studies one part of an individual, she or he must consider how that part relates to all others. The nurse must also consider the interaction and relationship of the individual to the external environment and to others.

Holistic health involves the total person, the whole state of his or her being, and the overall quality of his or her life-style. It includes physical fitness, primary prevention of negative physical and emotional states, stress management, sensitivity to the environment, self-awareness, and spiritual insight (Smith 1984, p. 5). Many holistic health care centers have been established across North America. They help clients to take responsibility for their health, to seek alternative, healthy, self-fulfilling behaviors, and to mobilize inner healing capacities.

Selected Theoretical Views of Human Beings

The nurse's view of human beings influences the nursing interventions she or he provides. Although most nurses agree that humans are biopsychosocial beings, they differ in how they view human beings as recipients of nursing services. Nursing theorists (see Chapter 1) have developed these viewpoints from systems, adaptation, and interactive theories. Table 13–1 summarizes the conceptualizations of selected nursing theorists. This chapter includes selected frameworks that are useful in planning and providing holistic nursing care.

The Person as a System

Humans are open systems with many interrelated subsystems. Because humans are biopsychosocial beings, their biologic, psychologic, social, and spiritual components can be regarded as systems with hierarchic subsystems. The **biologic system** can be subdivided into the neurologic, musculoskeletal, respiratory, circulatory, gastrointestinal, and urinary subsystems, among others. Each subsystem can in turn be subdivided. For example, the urinary system consists of the kidneys, the ureters, and the bladder; the circulatory system consists of the heart and the blood vessels; the neurologic system consists of the brain, the spinal cord, and the nerves.

The **psychologic and social systems** consist of subsystems that include thinking, feeling, and interaction patterns. Names of the psychologic and social subsystems vary considerably according to the individual nursing theorist and model. For example, Johnson (1980, p. 228), who describes the human system in terms of behaviors, lists the following psychologic subsystems: affiliative, dependency, aggressive/protective, and achievement, whereas Orem (1980, p. 316) categorizes the psychologic and social systems as conditions of being alone or with people, situations that threaten the well-being of the individual, and the tendency to conform to the norm.

The Person as an Adaptive System

Adaptation is a process of change allowing the individual to respond to environmental changes yet retain his or her integrity or wholeness (Levine 1969, p. 95). In this sense, **environment** means all the conditions, circumstances, and influences surrounding and affecting the development of an organism or group of organisms. It refers to both the internal and external environments.

Roy states that the person, as an adaptive system, functions as a totality. **Adaptive behavior** is the behavior of the whole person. Roy identifies two major internal processor subsystems of the adaptive system: the regulator and the cognator (Roy and Roberts 1981, p. 43). The individual uses these subsystems to adapt to or cope with internal and external environmental stimuli. The regulator mechanism has neural, endocrine, and perception-psychomotor components. The cognator mechanism encompasses psychosocial pathways and apparatus for perceptual/information processing, learning, judgment, and emotion. These two mechanisms are linked by the process of perception.

The Person as a Personal, Interpersonal, and Social System

According to King (1976, p. 51) the primary concerns of nursing are human behavior, social interaction, and social movements. Therefore, she includes three dynamic interacting systems in her concept of person: individuals (personal systems), groups (interpersonal systems), and society (social systems). Each of these systems has a set of related concepts that King sees as relevant for understanding human beings.

Human Needs

Although each individual has unique characteristics, certain needs are common to all people. Nursing theorists define *need* in various ways. King defines need

Table 13–1 **Selected Nurse Theorists' Concepts and Assumptions About Human Beings**

Theorist	Concepts/Assumptions
Dorothy Johnson (1980, pp. 212–214)	The individual is a behavioral system. The behavioral system is comprised of all patterned, repetitive, and purposeful ways of behaving that characterize each person's life. Subsystems carry out specialized tasks to maintain the integrity of the whole behavioral system and manage its relationship to the environment. Subsystems are: 1. Attachment or affiliative 2. Dependency 3. Ingestive 4. Eliminative 5. Sexual 6. Aggressive/protective 7. Achievement
Imogene King (1981, pp. 143–44)	The individual is a social, sentient, reacting, perceiving, controlling, purposeful, action-oriented, time-oriented being. The individual is conceptualized as a personal system who processes selective inputs from the environment through the senses. The personal system is a unified, complex, whole self who perceives, thinks, desires, imagines, decides, identifies goals, and selects means to achieve them.
Myra E. Levine (1973, pp. 8–10)	The human is a holistic being—a system of systems. The life process of the system is unceasing change that has direction, purpose, and meaning. The change, which is orderly and sequential, occurs through adaptation, which permits the person to protect and maintain his or her integrity as an individual.
Betty Neuman (1974, pp. 101–3; 1980, pp. 119–39)	The total person is a composite of physiologic, psychologic, sociocultural, and developmental variables. Each person has a basic structure or central core of survival factors unique to the individual but in a range common to other humans. The factors include temperature range, genetic response patterns, ego structure, and strengths and weaknesses of body organs. The central core of the person is protected from stressors by concentric rings: 1. A normal line of defense—a normal range of responses or equilibrium state that evolves over time 2. A flexible line of defense—a dynamic, rapidly changing protective buffer that prevents stressors from breaking through the normal line of defense.
Dorothea Orem (1980, pp. 41–51, 120)	The person is a unit that can be viewed as functioning biologically, symbolically, and socially. The individual and the environment form an integrated functional whole or system. People have the ability to perform self-care—activities that individuals initiate and perform on their own behalf to maintain life, health, and well-being. The ability to care for oneself is self-care agency; the ability to care for others is dependent-care agency. *Agency* means action. Self- or dependent-care is undertaken to meet three types of self-care requisites: universal, developmental, and health deviation.
Martha E. Rogers (1970, pp. 47–73)	People are unified entities possessing their own integrity and manifesting characteristics that are more than and different from the sum of their parts. The individual and the environment are continually exchanging matter and energy. The life process of human beings evolves irreversibly and unidirectionally along a space-time continuum. Pattern and organization identify individuals and reflect their innovative wholeness. The human being is characterized by the capacity for abstraction and imagery, language and thought, and sensation and emotion.
Sister Callista Roy, in Riehl and Roy (1980, pp. 179–206)	The person is a biopsychosocial being in a constant interaction with a changing environment. As an adaptive system, the person functions as a totality; adaptive behavior is behavior of the whole person. The person has four modes of adaptation: physiologic needs, self-concept, role function, and interdependence relations. The person has a great potential for self-actualization. The person is an active participant in his or her own destiny.

as "a state of energy exchange within and external to the organism which leads to behavioral responses to situations, events, and persons" (King 1971, p. 80). Roy defines a need as "a requirement within the individual which stimulates a response to maintain integrity" (Roy 1980, p. 184). For the purposes of this book, a **need** is something that is desirable, useful, or necessary.

The humanist Abraham Maslow developed his theory of human needs in the 1940s. To Maslow, needs motivate the behavior of the individual. His model of human needs includes both physiologic and psychologic needs, which he ranks according to how critical to survival they are. Maslow believes that the needs at one level must be met before the needs on the next level can be met. Thus, the physiologic needs must be met before the safety needs are met. Maslow's five categories or levels of needs, in hierarchical order, are (1970, p. 37):

1. Physiologic needs
2. Safety and security needs
3. Love and belonging needs
4. Self-esteem needs
5. Need for self-actualization

Throughout life, people strive to meet their needs at each level; however, the dominant needs *within one level* may vary at different times of life. Maslow sees humans as beings who continue to grow and develop from conception until death. Once a need is completely met, Maslow believes, the individual is no longer aware of it. Needs can be completely met, partially met, or not met at all. An individual usually persists in behavior to meet a need until it is met.

Maslow also states that an individual who apparently meets all of his or her needs still looks further to self-actualization. Maslow discusses two additional needs: the need to know and the need to understand. He believes that these needs are always present and permit people to meet the other needs more efficiently.

Maslow includes air, food, water, shelter, rest and sleep, activity, and temperature maintenance as the basic physiologic needs. A person who is starving or deprived of fluid for an extended time will center all of his or her activities around meeting that need. After the physiologic needs are met, the need to feel safe in one's environment emerges. This need for safety has both physical and psychologic aspects; the person needs to *be* safe and to *feel* safe, both in the physical environment and in relationships.

The third level of needs (for love, affection, and belonging) emerges after the needs for safety are met. According to Maslow, the need for love encompasses both giving and receiving. Belonging needs include attaining a place in a group, e.g., having a family and the feeling of belonging. The need for esteem is at the fourth level. The individual needs both *self-esteem* (i.e., feelings of independence, competence, and self-respect), and *esteem from others,* i.e., recognition, respect, and appreciation.

When the need for esteem is satisfied, the individual strives for **self-actualization.** The self-actualized person has realized his or her full potential. Such a person has the ability to connect the past and the future to the present while living fully in the present, is inner-directed, and is autonomous in contrast to being other-directed. Maslow saw self-actualization as a product of maturity that comes about through relating to people in autonomous and time-competent ways.

Richard Kalish (1977, p. 32) has adapted Maslow's hierarchy and suggests an additional category of needs between the physiologic needs and the safety and security needs. This category includes sex, activity, exploration, manipulation, and novelty. See Figure 13–1. Kalish emphasizes that children need to explore and manipulate their environments to achieve optimal growth and development. He notes that adults, too, often seek novel adventures or stimulating experiences before considering their safety or security needs. Maslow, by contrast, includes the pursuit of knowledge and aesthetic needs in the category of self-actualization needs.

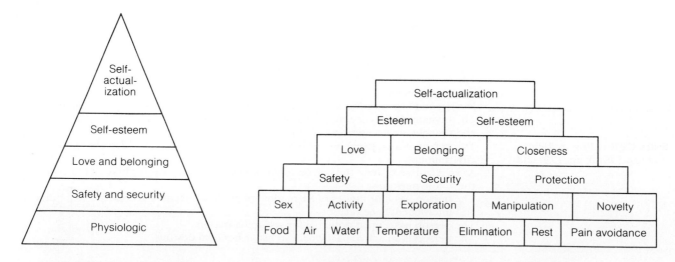

Maslow's hierarchy of needs

Maslow's hierarchy of needs, as adapted by Kalish

Figure 13–1 Maslow's needs (*Source:* As adapted by R. A. Kalish, *The psychology of human behavior*, 5 ed. Pacific Grove, Calif.: Brooks/Cole Publishing Co. Copyright © 1966, 1970, 1973, 1977, 1983 by Wadsworth, Inc.

■ **F**actors Affecting Needs Satisfaction

Gauging whether physiologic needs are met is largely an objective judgment. For example, the nurse can judge whether an individual's need for food has been met by weighing that person, using calipers to measure body fat, or reviewing the results of laboratory tests that analyze the metabolic processes of the body. Gauging whether psychologic needs have been met, however, is largely a subjective judgment. If a person believes a psychologic need (e.g., for love) is not satisfied, then for that person it is not met, regardless of how he or she appears to others. Several factors affect people's abilities to satisfy their needs. Four of these are:

1. Illness
2. Significant relationships
3. Self-concept
4. Development stage

Illness frequently interferes with people's abilities to meet their own needs. Nurses help ill clients to meet their physiologic needs on a number of levels. The man recovering from abdominal surgery probably requires oxygen, intravenous fluids, assistance moving, and reassurance immediately after surgery. Enacting each of these interventions helps to meet a different need. As he recovers, his requirements for nursing help will decrease.

As his physiologic needs are met, the client attends to needs at the next level (e.g., safety needs, according to Maslow) and so on. Ailing people often direct all their energies to meeting physiologic (survival) needs and may not identify needs at higher levels until later.

A second variable affecting needs satisfaction is **significant relationships.** Often these relationships are with family and support persons. Nurses also frequently establish significant relationships with clients because they are present at critical times in people's lives. Through these relationships, nurses can help clients become aware of their needs and establish healthy ways of meeting them.

A person's **self-concept** affects not only his or her ability to meet basic needs but also the awareness of whether or not these needs are satisfied. People who feel good about themselves are more likely to change, to recognize needs, and to establish healthy ways of meeting those needs. Those with a poor self-concept are less likely to meet these needs independently and may require more assistance from the nurse. The self-concept will be discussed with greater depth later in this chapter.

A fourth variable is an individual's **developmental stage.** According to Erikson's model of psychosocial human development (see Table 13–2), if an individual satisfactorily achieves the developmental task of learn-

Table 13–2 Erikson's Eight Stages of Development

Stage	Age	Central Task	Indicators of Positive Resolution	Indicators of Negative Resolution
Infancy	Birth to 18 months	Trust versus mistrust	Learning to trust others Sense of trust in self	Mistrust, withdrawal, estrangement
Early childhood	18 months to 3 years	Autonomy versus shame and doubt	Self control without loss of self esteem Ability to cooperate and to express oneself	Willfulness and defiance
Late childhood	3 to 5 years	Initiative versus guilt	Learning the degree to which assertiveness and purpose influence the environment Beginning ability to evaluate one's own behavior	Lack of self-confidence Pessimism, fear of wrongdoing Overcontrol and overrestriction of own activity
School age	6 to 12 years	Industry versus inferiority	Beginning to create, develop, and manipulate Developing sense of competence and perseverance	Loss of hope, sense of being mediocre Withdrawal from school and peers
Adolescence	12 to 20 years	Identity versus role confusion	Coherent sense of self Plans to actualize one's abilities	Confusion, indecisiveness, and inability to find occupational identity
Young adulthood	18 to 25 years	Intimacy versus isolation	Intimate relationship with another person Commitment to work and relationships	Impersonal relationships Avoidance of relationship, career, or life-style commitments
Adulthood	25 to 65 years	Generativity versus stagnation	Creativity, productivity, concern for others	Self-indulgence, self-concern, lack of interests and commitments
Maturity	65 years to death	Integrity versus despair	Acceptance of worth and uniqueness of one's own life Acceptance of death	Sense of loss, contempt for others

Sources: Adaptation of Erikson's Eight Stages of Development from *Childhood and Society*, 2nd edition, by Erik H. Erikson, by permission of W. W. Norton & Company, Inc. Copyright © 1950, 1963 by W. W. Norton & Company, Inc. Copyright renewed 1978 by Erik H. Erikson. In the British Empire excluding Canada, The Hogarth Press, Ltd., London.

ing to trust, then the basic needs of feeling safe and secure are readily resolved. The person who has already learned to trust others transfers those feelings to the health personnel caring for him or her. As another example, if the developmental tasks of establishing identity and intimacy have been achieved, the individual has an increased sense of belonging and being loved at a time of illness.

Assigning Priorities to Needs

Although Maslow's needs are presented in a hierarchy, sometimes clients and nurses must adjust the priority of the needs. People are continually changing and growing; thus, their needs do not stay constant but also continually change. Depending upon the situation, the nurse may be able to help a client meet several needs at once, partially meet one need and then go on to another, or deal with one need at a time. Needs related to life-threatening situations, e.g., a suffocating client's need for air, always assume first priority.

In many situations one need does not stand out as priority one. In these cases, the client and nurse consider several factors, such as the client's health, the client's and support persons' perceptions about health and areas of need, and the client's sociocultural background. A person may not perceive that he or she has a specific need. If so, the nurse may allocate it a low priority, often deferring action until the person is ready. For example, a man who smokes heavily might not see the need to stop.

Socioeconomic and cultural backgrounds affect how people rank their needs. For example, a man may place his need to return to work ahead of his need to learn exercises. A woman may perceive that getting her husband's breakfast is more important than resting in bed. See Chapter 16 for more information about cultural influences.

Chapter Highlights

- Nursing involves viewing the individual holistically.
- Humans can be viewed as open systems with many interrelated subsystems.
- Maslow defined a hierarchy of human needs, from physiologic (survival) needs to self-actualization.
- People vary in how they rank their needs at any given moment.
- Needs satisfaction can be altered by illness, significant relationships, self-concept, and developmental levels.

Selected Readings

Fawcett, J. 1984. *Analysis and evaluation of conceptual models of nursing*. Philadelphia: F. A. Davis Co.

Holmes, P. April 18–24, 1984. Holistic nursing. *Nursing Times* 80:28–29.

Johnson, D. E. 1980. The behavioral system model for nursing. In Riehl, J. P., and Roy, C., editors. *Conceptual models for nursing practice*. 2d ed. New York: Appleton-Century-Crofts.

Kalish, R. A. 1977. *The psychology of human behavior*. 4th ed. Belmont, Calif.: Wadsworth Publishing Co.

King, I. M. 1971. *Toward a theory for nursing: General concepts of human behavior*. New York: John Wiley and Sons.

———. 1976. The health care system. Nursing intervention subsystem. In Werley, H.; Zuzich, A.; Zajkowski, M.; and Zagornik, A. D., editors. *Health research: The systems approach*. New York: Springer Publishing Co., Inc.

———. 1981. *A theory for nursing: Systems, concepts, process*. New York: John Wiley and Sons.

Krieger, D. 1981. *Foundations for holistic health nursing practices: The Renaissance nurse*. Philadelphia: J. B. Lippincott Co.

Levine, M. E. January 1969. The pursuit of wholeness. *American Journal of Nursing* 69:93–98.

Locheed, T. December 1984. Holistic health: A uniting force for nurses. *The Canadian Nurse* 80:24–25.

Maslow, A. H. 1968. *Toward a psychology of being*. 2d ed. New York: Van Nostrand Reinhold Co.

———. 1970. *Motivation and personality*. 2d ed. New York: Harper and Row.

———. 1971. *The farther reaches of human nature*. New York: Penguin Books.

———. 1980. The Betty Neuman health-care systems model: A total person approach to patient problems. In Riehl, J. P., and Roy, C., editors. *Conceptual models for nursing practice*. 2d ed. New York: Appleton-Century-Crofts.

Orem, D. E. 1980. *Nursing: Concepts of practice*. 2d ed. New York: McGraw-Hill.

Orlando, I. J. 1961. *The dynamic nurse-patient relationship: Function, process and principles*. New York: G. P. Putnam's Sons.

Renshaw, J. April 25–May 1, 1984. Holistic health: The power of the will. Part 2. *Nursing Times* 80:38–39.

Riehl, J. P., and Roy, C. 1980. *Conceptual models for nursing practice*. 2d ed. New York: Appleton-Century-Crofts.

———. 1980. The Roy adaptation model. In Riehl, J. P., and Roy, C., editors. *Conceptual models for nursing practice*. 2d ed. New York: Appleton-Century-Crofts.

Roy, C., and Roberts, S. L. 1981. *Theory construction in nursing: An adaptation model*. Englewood Cliffs, N.J.: Prentice-Hall.

Smith, M. P. August 1984. The new frontier. *RNABC* (Registered Nurses Association of British Columbia) *News* 16:5.

CHAPTER 14

Self-Concept

OBJECTIVES

Differentiate between *self-concept* and *self-esteem*.

Describe the components of self-concept.

Give Erikson's explanation of the effects of psychosocial crises on self-concept and self-esteem.

Describe the effects of communication/coping styles on self-esteem.

Identify four areas involved in the nursing assessment of self-concept.

Describe key data to be included when assessing self-perception.

Describe the essential aspects of assessing roles and relationships.

List important assessment data to be included when identifying clients' stressors and coping strategies.

Identify common stressors affecting self-concept and self-esteem.

List behaviors that could indicate altered self-concept.

Identify nursing diagnoses concerning altered self-concept.

Select appropriate goals for clients with altered self-concept.

Describe nursing actions designed to implement identified goals for clients with altered self-concept.

Describe ways to enhance the self-esteem of older adults.

Identify outcome criteria that permit evaluation of clients with altered self-concept.

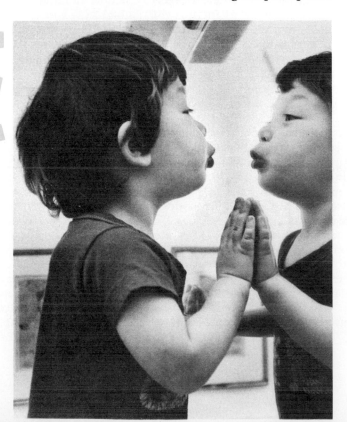

The Self and Related Concepts

Self-concept, self-esteem, and *self-image* are essential to a person's mental and physical health. Individuals with a positive self-concept or high self-esteem are better able to develop and maintain warm interpersonal relationships and resist psychologic and physical illness. Failure to achieve a positive self-image presents major obstacles in the treatment of common disorders such as depression, eating disorders, postvictimization syndrome (abuse or rape), and crisis reactions. Nurses help identify persons with negative self-concept or low self-esteem and assist those clients in developing a more positive view of themselves.

Self-concept is also of personal relevance to the nurse. Nurses who feel positive about themselves are better equipped to meet the needs of others. Such nurses feel good, look good, are effective and productive, and respond to people (including themselves) in healthy and positive ways.

At the various stages of life, people are strongly influenced by general societal expectations regarding role-specific behavior. The larger society and smaller societal groups have expectations that differ in clarity and are communicated with varying degrees of force. Expectations differ by age, sex, socioeconomic status, ethnicity, and career identification. Smaller societal groups such as the family, school, armed forces, work groups, and recreational groups also expect certain behaviors and performance levels of people. Success in meeting such expectations has profound implications for self-esteem.

Because North American society is highly achievement oriented, everything a person does is evaluated, e.g., earning capacity, social skills, performance at school, athletic performance, and sexual performance. A high level of performance is rewarded; poor performance is belittled. As a result, people tend to focus on their failures and shortcomings rather than on their strengths. In many instances a person's actual performance is superior to his or her *perception* of that performance. Compliance with the social expectations for role-specific behavior therefore leads to judgments of personal worth; noncompliance often leads to judgments of personal worthlessness.

Throughout life people face certain *developmental tasks* that, if not successfully achieved, may lead to problems with self, self-concept, and self-esteem. The eight psychosocial stages described by Erikson (1963) (see Chapter 26) provide a convenient and familiar theoretical framework for drawing implications for the development of self-esteem. The success with which a person copes with these developmental crises largely determines the development of self-concept. Inability to cope results in self-concept problems. See Table 14–1 for behaviors indicating successful and unsuccessful resolution of these developmental crises.

Components

The North American Nursing Diagnosis Association (NANDA) suggests four **components of self-concept:** body image, role performance, self-identity, and self-esteem (McLane 1987). Disturbances in one or more of these areas may result in actual or potential health problems. The image of physical self, or **body image,** is the way a person perceives the size, appearance, and functioning of his or her body and its parts. It includes clothing, makeup, hairstyle, jewelry, and other things connected to the person, e.g., artificial limb or wheelchair.

A person's body image develops partly from others' attitudes and responses to his or her body. Cultural and societal values also influence a person's body image. For instance, Western societies value beauty, youth, and wholeness. Generally, a person develops a stable body image over a long time; thus, actual or potential threats to alterations in body image can create considerable anxiety.

A **role** is a set of expectations about how the person occupying one position behaves toward a person occupying another position (Roy 1984, p. 285). Expectations, or standards of behavior, are set by society or the smaller group to which the person belongs. Each person usually has several roles, e.g., husband, parent, brother, son, employee, friend, golf club member. Some roles are assumed for only limited periods, e.g., client/nurse, student/instructor, and the sick role.

Role performance relates what a person does in a particular role to what behaviors are expected of that people in that role. To act appropriately, people need to know who they are in relation to others and what society expects of people holding those positions. When there is role ambiguity, expectations are unclear, and the person does not know what to do or how to do it. The individual is unable to predict the reactions of others to his or her behavior. This ambiguity creates confusion and stress.

A person's **self-identity** is the conscious sense of individuality and uniqueness that evolves continually throughout life. People often view their identity in terms of name, sex, age, race, ethnicity or culture, occupation or roles, talents, and other situational characteristics (e.g., marital status and education). People usually first identify themselves by name and occupation or roles. When interactions progress beyond the superficial, other characteristics may be revealed. Self-identity also includes a person's beliefs and values, personality, and character. In brief, identity is what distinguishes self from others.

Each separate image of and belief about oneself has a bearing on **self-esteem,** or how an individual feels about himself or herself. This appraisal of oneself is not simply a summation of images and beliefs. The various images a person has and the beliefs he or she holds about the self are not given equal weight and prominence (Sanford and Donovan 1984, p. 9). Each individual has

Table 14–1   Examples of Behaviors Associated with Erikson's Stages of Psychosocial Development

Stage: Developmental Crisis	Behaviors Indicating Positive Resolution	Behaviors Indicating Negative Resolution
Infancy: Trust vs mistrust	Requesting assistance and expecting to receive it Expressing belief of another person Sharing time, opinions, and experiences	Restricting conversation to superficialities Refusing to provide a person with information Being unable to accept assistance
Toddlerhood: Autonomy vs shame and doubt	Accepting the rules of a group but also expressing disagreement when it is felt Expressing one's own opinion Easily accepting deferment of a wish fulfillment	Failing to express needs Not expressing one's own opinion when opposed Overconcern about being clean
Early childhood: Initiative vs guilt	Starting projects eagerly Expressing curiosity about many things Demonstrating original thought	Imitating others rather than developing independent ideas Apologizing and being very embarrassed over small mistakes Verbalizing fear about starting a new project
Early school years: Industry vs inferiority	Completing a task once it has been started Working well with others Using time effectively	Not completing tasks started Not assisting with the work of others Not organizing work
Adolescence: Identity vs role confusion	Asserting independence Planning realistically for future roles Establishing close interpersonal relationships	Failing to assume responsibility for directing one's own behavior Accepting the values of others without question Failing to set goals in life
Early adulthood: Intimacy vs isolation	Establishing a close, intense relationship with another person Accepting sexual behavior as desirable Making a commitment to that relationship, even in times of stress and sacrifice	Remaining alone Avoiding close interpersonal relationships
Middle-age adults: Generativity vs stagnation	Being willing to share with another person Guiding others Establishing a priority of needs, recognizing both self and others	Talking about oneself instead of listening to others Showing concern for oneself in spite of the needs of others Being unable to accept interdependence
Elderly adults: Integrity vs despair	Using past experience to assist others Maintaining productivity in some areas Accepting limitations	Crying and being apathetic Not accepting changes Demanding unnecessary assistance and attention from others

specific priorities that influence maintenance of self-esteem.

Assessing Self-Concept

Holistic nursing care includes assessing all clients for strengths and weakness relating to physiologic, psychosocial, and spiritual needs. Specific assessment of disturbances in self-concept is indicated if the client or support persons give cues that a problem might exist or if the client's illness is often associated with self-concept disturbances. Problems with self-concept and self-esteem are frequently manifested by expressions of anxiety, fear, anger, hostility, guilt, and powerlessness. Behaviors reflecting excessive role conflict may also indicate the need for meaningful intervention by nurses.

A trusting client-nurse relationship is essential for an effective assessment of self-concept. Clients tend not to share personal feelings unless the nurse has established an empathetic, nonjudgmental relationship. Disclosure of personal information can be threatening. Some people, particularly those with low self-esteem, may fear that the nurse will not accept or like them if they reveal their true performance capabilities, thoughts, and feelings. Others, especially clients from minority ethnic groups (see Chapter 17), may consider it a breach of family confidence to discuss personal information with health care workers. Nursing assessment involves four areas:

1. Self-perception or self-awareness
2. Role performance and relationships
3. Major stressors and coping strategies
4. Behaviors suggesting altered self-concept

Self-Perception

Assessment of self-perception is twofold. The nurse first ascertains the client's perception of physical self, personal self, and worth and then observes for nonverbal cues that reflect the client's self-perception. To determine the client's perception of **body image,** the nurse either listens to comments made by the client about his or her physical self or to responses the client makes to questions asked by the nurse. Responses such as "I feel ugly," "I'm awkward and clumsy," "I can't do anything now," "No one will like me now," and "I'm afraid my husband won't love me anymore" indicate that the client's self-esteem is threatened or low. The client is focusing on particular disabilities or shortcomings and blocking out accurate perception of the total self.

The nurse should also attend to cues reflecting disturbances in the client's perception of **personal identity** and in **self-esteem.** These aspects of the self-concept may be more difficult to assess. Some people volunteer clearly self-deprecating or overcritical comments about self, indicating low self-esteem, e.g., "People don't like me," or "I'm no good." Others, however, may not provide such information unless asked to do so.

Nonverbal cues—behaviors such as body posture, movements, gestures, tone of voice, speech pattern, and general appearance—tend to be more spontaneous than verbal messages and can provide important clues to the person's self-concept. Nonverbal cues that can indicate low self-esteem include stooped shoulders, lack of attention to hygiene or grooming, avoiding eye contact, hesitant speech, and withdrawing from social interaction. Nonverbal cues can help the nurse confirm the reliability of the client's verbal messages.

Roles and Relationships

The nurse assesses the client's satisfactions and dissatisfactions with role responsibilities and relationships: family roles, work roles, student roles, social roles. Family roles are especially important to clients, since family relationships are particularly close. Relationships can be supportive and growth-producing or, at the opposite extreme, highly stressful if violence and abuse permeate relationships. Assessment of family roles and relationships may begin with structural aspects such as number in the family group, ages, and residence location.

For more information on the family, see Chapter 30. To determine the client's satisfaction or dissatisfaction with work roles and social roles, the nurse might ask some of the following questions:

- How do you get along at work?
- What about your work would you like to change if you could?

- How do you spend your free time?
- Are you involved in any community groups?
- Who is most important to you?
- Whom do you seek out for help?

Major Stressors and Coping Strategies

It is important for the nurse to identify stressors that challenge the client's self-worth. Common stressors that influence a client's self-concept and self-esteem are in the accompanying box. Most people face numerous stress-producing events simultaneously. Illness and hospitalization can compound the effects.

When stressors are identified, the nurse needs to determine how the client perceives the stressor. A positive, growth-oriented perception of stressful events reinforces self-worth; a negative, hopeless, defeatist perception leads to decreased self-esteem. The nurse also should identify the client's coping style and determine whether or not this style is effective by asking the client such questions as:

- When you have a problem or face a stressful situation, how do you usually deal with it?
- Do these methods work?

Stressors Affecting Self-Concept and Self-Esteem

Body-Image Stressors
- Loss of body parts, e.g., amputation, mastectomy, hysterectomy
- Loss of body functions, e.g., from heart disease, renal disease, spinal cord injury, cerebrovascular accident, neuromuscular disease, arthritis, declining mental or sensory abilities
- Disfigurement, e.g., through pregnancy, severe burns, facial blemishes, colostomy, ileostomy, tracheostomy, laryngectomy

Role Stressors
- Loss of parent, spouse, child, or close friend
- Change or loss of job
- Retirement
- Divorce or separation
- Illness
- Hospitalization
- Ambiguous role expectations
- Conflicting role expectations
- Inability to meet role expectations

Identity Stressors
- Change in physical appearance
- Declining physical, mental, or sensory abilities
- Inability to achieve goals
- Relationship concerns
- Sexuality concerns
- Unrealistic ideal self
- Membership in a minority group

Behaviors Associated with Low Self-Esteem

The client:

- Avoids eye contact
- Stoops in posture and moves slowly
- Is poorly groomed and has an unkempt appearance
- Is hesitant or halting in speech
- Is overly critical of self, e.g., "I'm no good," "I'm ugly," or "People don't like me."
- May be overly critical of others
- Is unable to accept positive remarks about self
- Encourages reprimands from others, to punish self
- Apologizes frequently
- Verbalizes feelings of hopelessness, helplessness, and powerlessness, such as "I really don't care what happens," "I'll do whatever anyone wants," "Whatever is destined will happen."
- Verbalizes feelings of worthlessness, such as "Nobody cares about me," "I'm just a burden to everyone," "I'm not worth all that trouble."
- Verbalizes feelings of guilt, such as "It's all my fault," "I am to blame."

- Withdraws from or changes social involvements or relationships
- Fails to complete or follow through with activities
- Avoids initiating conversation or interaction with others
- Exhibits self-destructive behavior, such as excessive use of alcohol, drugs, smoking
- Has negative feelings about own body, e.g., avoids looking at or touching body part, or hides body part; emphasizes previous appearance or function; talks excessively about loss or change
- Is indecisive, e.g., "I can't make up my mind what to do," "I don't understand what's happening."
- Cannot solve problems effectively and does not ask for help
- Displays overdependence, e.g., asks for assistance unnecessarily, seeks attention by speaking loudly, asks irrelevant questions, seeks approval and praise
- Displays lack of energy, e.g., "I feel tired all the time."
- Verbalizes inability to cope
- Expresses or manifests anxiety, fear, anger
- Does not meet role expectations

(NANDA 1986, pp. 534, 537–40; Carpenito 1983, pp. 389–94)

Behaviors Suggesting Altered Self-Concept

Some verbal and nonverbal behaviors associated with low self-esteem are listed in the accompanying box.

Nursing Diagnoses: Disturbances in Self-Concept

Nursing diagnoses for clients with self-concept problems include disturbance in body image, disturbance in self-esteem, disturbance in role performance, and disturbance in personal identity (McLane 1987). Other diagnoses that relate to self-concept include ineffective individual coping, social isolation, powerlessness, sexual dysfunction, anticipatory grieving, and dysfunctional grieving. Sexual dysfunction is discussed in Chapter 15, and grieving in Chapter 19. Examples of specific nursing diagnoses for clients with self-concept problems are shown in the box on page 166.

Planning to Support/Promote Healthy Self-Concepts

The nurse's focus when planning is to assist the client to set goals that reflect a positive resolution of the problem or stressors identified in the nursing diagnosis. Goals should emphasize strengths rather than weaknesses or impairments. Goals may be broadly stated as follows. The client will:

- Have increased awareness of strengths and weaknesses
- Have improved feelings of self-worth
- Perceive and respond to stressors in a constructive manner
- Improve interpersonal relationships

Planning also involves establishing outcome criteria by which to measure goals achievement. For examples of outcome criteria, see the section on evaluation later in this chapter. Once goals for changing self-image are set, the process of modifying self-image begins.

Implementing Nursing Strategies

Assisting people with self-concept disturbances requires skills in communicating and in developing helping relationships (see Chapter 20). Helping clients with self-concept disturbances is akin to promoting health, as discussed in Chapter 25. The client assumes responsibility for implementing the plans. The nurse provides information, education, and ongoing support; suggests strategies to encourage behavioral change; and implements techniques that help the client gain a realistic and acceptable view of self. Selected interventions to help clients with self-concept disturbances follow. Numerous community self-improvement programs are

NURSING DIAGNOSIS

Altered Self-Concept

Disturbance in body image related to: (identify surgical procedure; e.g., mastectomy, colostomy, amputation, facial scarring, etc.) or pregnancy

Disturbance in self-esteem related to:
- loss of job
- unrealistic self-expectations
- unrealistic parental expectations
- divorce

Disturbance in role performance related to:
- change in physical capacity to assume role
- newly assumed work and family roles

Disturbance in personal identity related to loss of job

Ineffective individual coping related to:
- divorce and change in financial status
- death of mother
- inadequate personal resources and social support
- need for mutilating surgery

Social isolation related to alteration in body image

Powerlessness related to:
- inability to perform activities of daily living secondary to arthritis
- inability to perform role responsibilities secondary to progressive debilitating disease

also available, many of them emphasizing the need for individuals to take charge of their lives, to take responsibility for their actions, to think positively rather than negatively, and to become more assertive.

It is important for both the nurse and the client to realize that changes in self-concept require an extended period of time. Although varying from person to person, this may take several months or years. It is essential for the client to learn that self-concept or self-image is not etched in stone; it can change and improve in progressive small steps, particularly if the client desires such change.

Identifying Areas of Strength

Healthy people often perceive their problems and weaknesses more clearly than their assets and strengths. The average well-functioning person with some college education, when asked to write down his or her strengths, may list only five or six; however, the same person might list three to four times as many problems or areas of weakness (Otto 1965, p. 34).

Because people with low self-esteem tend to focus on their limitations, they may list even fewer strengths and many more problems. When a client has difficulty

identifying personality strengths and assets, the nurse provides a framework to follow. Interests, abilities, and past accomplishments and experiences need to be included. An abbreviated framework for identifying personality strengths has been developed at the University of Utah. It is shown in the accompanying box.

Developing Behavior Specificity

Many people overgeneralize and think in unspecific ways. The nurse can assist clients to think more clearly and to become more behavior specific in language and thought. Crouch and Straub (1983, p. 71) offer the following strategies for developing behavior specificity:

1. **Clearly define goals.** For example, in response to the question "How would you like to feel differently about yourself?" the client may give an unspecific, subjective, and unmeasurable answer such as "better" or "not so uptight." To help the client become more behavior specific, the nurse needs to bring unspecific answers into focus. This can be done by inquiring, for example, "How will you know you are better?" or "What do you mean by 'uptight'?"

2. **Help the client think clearly.** Clients with low self-esteem tend to think negatively and irrationally. For example, a client with low self-esteem who has followed through on homework for three out of seven days might say, "There was no excuse; I failed," or "I didn't follow through; I can't do anything right." When responding, the nurse should avoid contradicting the client but need not accept the client's evaluation as accurate. The nurse might ask, "What exactly did you not follow through with?" or "How does not doing the homework perfectly mean you can't do anything right?"

Changing Language Patterns

Helping a client to change language patterns from passive phrases to more active phrases can help the client assume greater responsibility for his or her power. Examples of passive phrases and alternate active phrases are:

It makes me . . . (passive)

I choose to . . . *or* I do. (active)

I have to . . . (passive)

I want to . . . (active)

I can't . . . (passive)

I won't . . . *or* I choose not to . . . (active)

To encourage the use of more active language, the nurse may have the client initially listen for passive language without modifying it and then deliberately notice passive language and modify it. It is also important for the client to gain awareness of his or her overall feeling states when using passive or active language.

■ **E**ncouraging Positive Self-Evaluation

Persons with high self-esteem express positive self-evaluation more frequently than negative self-evaluation. Persons with low self-esteem, however, frequently make negative self-evaluations and rarely give themselves positive feedback. Therefore, clients with low self-esteem need help in developing more positive thoughts and images about themselves.

Several strategies are available for this, including modeling, praise or recognition, positive self-feedback, and visualization. The nurse can **model** positive self-statements for the client by saying such things as "I did a good job painting my recreation room last weekend," or "I am improving my cooking," or "I am proud of the produce I'm getting from my vegetable garden." To help the client make the transition to self-recognition, the nurse may **praise** the client, providing honest, positive feedback, e.g., "I think you did a really fine job," or "It sounds like you worked very hard and have done well."

When clients need guidance in providing **positive self-feedback,** the nurse may choose one or more of the following strategies:

Framework for Identifying Personality Strengths

Spectator sports and similar activities The rationale here is that the client's current interest or participation in spectator sports, as well as past interests which he recalls with pleasure, constitutes a vital spark, is evidence of creative engagement with life, and, in most instances, presages a movement in the direction of health.

Sports and activities Taking part in a program of body-building, conditioning, or rehabilitative exercises or similar physical regimens, including an interest (and anticipated future participation) in sports and outdoor activities.

Hobbies and crafts Participating, or having participated in, some hobby or craft activity, and having the desire to start or resume a hobby, craft, or similar pursuit.

Expressive arts Past or current interest in writing, painting, sketching, or music appreciation with a desire to participate in one of the expressive arts.

Health status Desire to maintain or regain his health, as well as having an interest or ability to carry through with regimens and treatments designed to foster and facilitate health.

Education, training, and related areas Any education is seen as a personality asset—vocational trade or technical training, scholastic honors, self-education or a desire to obtain further education or training.

Work, vocation, job, or position Successful on-the-job performance or enjoyment in his work, a sense of pride in work or duties, earned seniority or recognition for work performed.

Special aptitudes or resources Included here are such diverse factors as sales ability, aptitude for mathematics or some other subject, ability to fix mechanical things, a "green thumb," ability to construct or teach, knowing how to make a good impression on people.

Strengths through family and others Such sources of strengths as a spouse or children, relationships with parents, in-laws, or relatives who give love and understanding.

Intellectual strengths Ability to apply reason to problem solving, do original, creative, and critical thinking; accept new ideas, work on broadening his mind through reading, conversation, and sharing ideas; the capacity to learn and enjoy learning.

Aesthetic strengths Recognizing and enjoying beauty, and being able to use the sense of beauty to enhance the physical environment.

Organizational strengths Capacity for systematic planning, developing sound short- and long range goals, and organizing resources, energy, and time to achieve such goals; the ability to assign and carry out priorities and to coordinate or lead the efforts and labor of others in relation to specific tasks.

Imaginative and creative strengths Such characteristics as creativity, imagination, and inventiveness for the development of new and different ideas in connection with his home, family, work, or social relationships.

Relationship strengths Ability to make people feel comfortable and the capacity to enjoy being with people, being aware of people's needs and feelings, being able to listen, and being patient with children as well as with adults.

Spiritual strengths Religious faith or love of God, membership and participation in church and related activities, and the capacity to express moral and religious values in living, that is, "living what one believes."

Emotional strengths Capacity to give and receive warmth, affection, and love; ability to "take" anger, and to feel and express a wide range of emotions; capacity for empathy.

Other strengths Included here are the ability to use humor, to "laugh" at oneself and take "kidding"; having a liking for adventure or pioneering; having stick-toitiveness, perseverance, and the drive or will needed to get things done.

(Otto 1965, reprinted with permission)

OUTCOME CRITERIA

Disturbance in Self-Concept

The client will:

Discuss limitations in physical mobility

Express feelings and thoughts about body changes

Look at and touch a body deformity

Make decisions regarding a job change and financial arrangements

Participate in self-care

Accept offers of help

Continue preexisting socialization pattern

Begin to assume role-related responsibilities

Discuss own strengths and talents with another person

Share feelings about self with significant others

Discuss options and alternatives when trying to solve problems

1. Ask the client: "Tell me some things you have done recently that you feel good about," or "Tell me some things you like about yourself."
2. Have the client develop a list of accomplishments he or she feels good about and a list of characteristics he or she likes about himself or herself. Encourage frequent reference to this list.
3. Reduce negative self-feedback through thought-stopping techniques. For example, every time the client begins to think negatively about self, ask him or her to say mentally, "Stop," or "No," or "Think about now," and then attend to the details of the present experience.

Because strong positive images or expectations often become self-fulfilling, **visualization** can be used to enhance self-esteem. In visualization, positive images of desired changes are consciously imagined. This can be a powerful tool for achieving goals and gaining a positive self-concept. To strengthen goals with visualization, the client:

1. Sets a positive goal or image, such as "I am talking with someone at a party" or "I am saying to my family that I need some help from them to be able to manage work and home responsibilities."
2. Relaxes and slowly repeats the goal-phrase several times.
3. Closes his or her eyes and visualizes the goal-phrase on a written page.
4. Envisions self as having accomplished the goal.

Because a person's receptivity to positive suggestions is greater when that person is deeply relaxed, deep-breathing exercises, progressive relaxation techniques, meditation, and self-hypnosis are often introduced before imagery techniques are used in individual and group self-involvement programs.

Enhancing Self-Esteem in Older Adults

There is a wide variation in the way older adults perceive themselves; most, however, benefit from having their independence fostered. Low self-esteem is often associated with the dependence that accompanies the declining physical and mental capacities related to aging. The nurse can foster the older adult's independence and a more positive self-concept by doing the following (Hirst and Metcalf 1984, p. 76):

1. Encourage the person to participate in planning his or her care, and involve him or her in decision making, e.g., allowing the person to choose what to wear, which activities to participate in, and what food selections to make.
2. Allow the person to collect numerous objects around him or her. These establish the person's territory or physical space as his or her own.
3. Ask permission before putting the person's clothing (e.g., dressing gown, nightclothes) or other objects into his or her locker or closet. To do so without permission would deny the existence of the person's personal space and can be perceived as disrespectful.
4. Listen to what the person is saying. Elderly people need to know their comments are valued.
5. Allow the person sufficient time to complete an interaction or activity. Older adults are often slow to respond. Attempts to hurry their responses can create anxiety and embarrassment and can lower self-esteem.
6. Receive contributions of thanks or appreciation (e.g., candy or fruit) graciously and sincerely. Having something to contribute helps older adults maintain or enhance their self-esteem.

Evaluation

Examples of desired outcome criteria for clients with self-concept disturbances are shown in the accompanying box. Depending on the specific self-concept disturbance, the meeting of one or more of these criteria supports the nurse's evaluation that the client has achieved the goal of resolving the health problem. When several criteria are designated during the planning phase and only one criterion is met at the time of the nursing evaluation, the nurse may decide that the problem continues. In this case, the nurse may modify or continue the existing nursing care plan.

Chapter Highlights

- A healthy self-concept, or positive self-esteem, is essential to a person's physical and psychologic well-being.
- Components of self-concept include body image, role performance, self-identity, and self-esteem.
- A person's self-perception can differ from the per-

All he would do was nod or stare blankly

Gerald, a 39-year-old construction foreman, was admitted to our hospital to have surgery for a bleeding gastric ulcer. He was married and had two children, aged five and nine, with whom he was very close. His family lived about 200 miles away and could visit only on weekends. The rest of Gerald's family lived in the East.

Gerald was outgoing and charming in a down-home, country sort of way. He was used to being in charge of his life and carried this with him as a patient.

After his second stay in intensive care, Gerald was noticeably withdrawn. He refused to get out of bed, turn, or use his incentive spirometer. His affect was flat and he would not make eye contact with me. I felt frustrated with his uncharacteristically passive behavior because I realized it meant that Gerald was giving up hope of ever getting better.

Various strategies to get him to talk about his feelings didn't work; all he would do was nod his head or stare blankly at the wall. Finally, I said to him: "You just don't care anymore, do you?" He only shook his head no in response.

At that point my emotions got the best of me. I had worked with this man for two months, knew his family, and had developed a relationship with him. Because I felt he was shutting me out, it made me feel sad, frustrated, and angry all at once. At that moment, all the therapeutic interventions I knew deserted me and I responded to Gerald on a gut level. I yelled at him, "Well damn it, Gerald, *we* care!"

A little shaken by my outburst and by his lack of response to it, I left the room, saying that I would return later to take his vital signs. When I did return after about an hour, I noticed that he had been crying. I asked gently, "Gerald, are you OK?" He just reached for my hand, squeezed it, and said, "Thank you."

Not long after that incident, Gerald began to act more like his "old self." He started to take more interest in his care and eventually he recovered and went home.

Source: S. Orlick, The primacy of caring, (A dialogue with excellence), *American Journal of Nursing* (March 1988) 318–19.

---

son's perception of how others see him or her and from how the person would like to be.

- From the hour of birth, interactions with significant others create the conditions that influence self-esteem throughout life.
- The development of self-esteem can be seen as a process of establishing a sense of security, a sense of identity, and a sense of belonging.
- Adults base their self-concept on how they perceive and evaluate their performance in the areas of work, intellect, appearance, sexual attractiveness, particular talents, ability to cope and to resolve problems, independence, and interpersonal interactions.
- Because a healthy self-concept is basic to health, one of the nurse's major responsibilities is to help clients whose self-concept is disturbed develop a more positive and realistic image of themselves.
- A trusting client-nurse relationship is essential for the effective assessment of a client's self-concept, for providing help and support, and for motivating change in client behavior.

Selected References

Carpenito, L. J. 1987. *Nursing diagnosis. Application to clinical practice.* Philadelphia: J. B. Lippincott Co.

Crouch, M. A., and Straub, V. August 1983. Enhancement of self-esteem in adults. *Family and Community Health* 6:65–78.

Erikson, E. H. 1963. *Childhood and society.* 2d ed. New York: W. W. Norton and Co.

Gilbert, R. August 1983. The evaluation of self-esteem. *Family and Community Health* 6:29–49.

Gillies, D. A. September/October 1984. Body image changes following illness and injury. *Journal of Enterostomal Therapy* 11:186–89.

Goldin, J. November/December 1985. The influence of self-image upon the performance of nursing home staff. *Nursing Homes* 34:33–38.

Hirst, S. P., and Metcalf, B. J. February 1984. Promoting self-esteem. *Journal of Gerontological Nursing* 2:72–77.

Kim, M. J.; McFarland, G. K.; and McLane, A. M. 1984. *Pocket guide to nursing diagnoses.* St. Louis: C. V. Mosby Co.

McLane, A. M., ed. 1987. *Classification of nursing diagnoses: Proceedings of the seventh conference.* St. Louis: C. V. Mosby Co.

Muhlenkamp, A. F., and Sayles, J. A. November/December 1986. Self-esteem, social support, and positive health practices. *Nursing Research* 35:334–38.

Norris, J., and Kunes-Connell, M. December 1985. Self-esteem disturbance. *Nursing Clinics of North America* 20:745–61.

North American Nursing Diagnosis Association. 1986. Classification of nursing diagnoses. In Hurley, M. E., editor. Proceedings of the sixth national conference. St. Louis: C. V. Mosby Co.

Oldaker, S. M. December 1985. Identity confusion. Nursing diagnoses for adolescents. *Nursing Clinics of North America* 20:763–73.

Otto, H. A. August 1965. The human potentialities of nurses and patients. *Nursing Outlook* 13:32–35.

Roy, S. C. 1984. *Introduction to nursing. An adaptation model.* 2d ed. Englewood Cliffs, N.J.: Prentice-Hall, Inc.

Sanford, L. T., and Donovan, M. E. 1984. *Women and self-esteem.* New York: Penguin Books.

Stanwyck, D. J. August 1983. Self-esteem through the life span. *Family and Community Health* 6:11–28.

Sexuality

Ross A. Stewart

OBJECTIVES

Describe selected aspects of sexuality.

Identify key aspects of the development of sexuality from the prenatal period to late adulthood.

Compare selected physical and psychologic sexual stimulation patterns.

Identify physiologic changes occurring in males and females during each phase of the sexual response as described by Masters and Johnson.

List factors that affect an individual's sexual attitudes and behaviors.

Give examples of how to obtain data about sexual functioning when conducting a health history.

Identify factors contributing to sexual dysfunction.

List factors that increase and decrease sexual motivation.

Describe common problems of genital sexuality and possible causes.

Identify common illnesses affecting sexuality.

Compare selected intervention models for sexual counseling.

Describe key points about breast and testicular self-examinations to include in health teaching.

Identify essential aspects about selected contraceptive methods to include in health teaching.

Describe guidelines for the prevention of sexually transmitted diseases.

Describe essential outcome criteria that permit evaluation of client progress toward meeting planned goals.

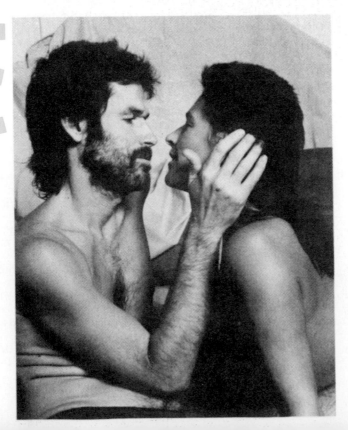

Sexuality is an integral characteristic of every human being. We are all born with the capacity to function as sexual beings. The nurse's clients do not leave their sexuality behind when they enter the health care system. Because nurses give holistic health care, they have a responsibility to promote sexual health care.

As the holistic approach indicates, all aspects of being interact. Thus, sexuality influences and is influenced by the biologic, psychologic, sociologic, and spiritual aspects of being. The need to acknowledge and deal with issues of sexuality in health care practice cannot be overemphasized. Until fairly recently, health care professionals treated sexuality with benign neglect or actively discouraged it as a focus of interest. Nurses have been as slow as other health professionals to identify sexuality as significant to health care.

For nurses practicing in North America today, sexuality is a much more complex issue than it was for nurses in the past. Changes in beliefs, attitudes, and behaviors (and the resulting conflicts) have produced uncertainty and a need to assess nurses' understanding of and attitudes toward the many variations of sexuality. The multicultural nature of North American society has also been a major influence on sexuality, as has the vast increase in mass communication. The impact of such influence groups and movements as the women's movement, gay liberation, handicapped groups, and the "moral majority" has been powerful and is still creating change. To help clients deal with issues of sexual health, nurses must be aware of these multiple factors and must integrate them into effective sexual health care plans.

Sex and Sexuality

The words **sex** and **sexuality** are used interchangeably, and often incorrectly, to define different aspects of sexual being. **Sex** is the term most commonly used to denote biologic male or female status, but it is also used to describe specific sexual behavior, such as sexual intercourse. The more appropriate and descriptive term for sexual issues is **sexuality,** which includes biologic, psychologic, sociologic, spiritual, and cultural variables that influence an individual's personality development and interpersonal relations with others.

Although sexuality is an integral part of the whole human being, it can also be categorized and studied according to three separate aspects: biologic sex, gender identity, and gender role. **Biologic sex** includes all of the human being's genetically determined anatomy and physiology. **Gender identity** is the individual's persisting inner sense of being male or female. Its development is based on biologic sex and sociocultural reinforcement. Congruence between biologic sex and learned sense of sexual self is the most common outcome of this developmental process. Variations of this congruence may occur principally at periods of significant change in the life span (e.g., adolescence, menopause, climacteric, old age). The term *sexual identity* is sometimes equivalent to gender identity but is more commonly used to indicate *sexual orientation* (e.g., heterosexual, bisexual, homosexual). **Gender role** includes all behaviors reflecting the individual's learned sense of masculinity and femininity, sex behavior, sexual relationships, and sexual dimorphism.

The Context of Sexuality

Sexuality and the way people respond to it are influenced by a variety of factors. A review of historical, ethnocultural, religious-ethical, and contemporary perspectives on sexuality helps to place sexuality in the context of the broader human experience.

Historical Perspectives

Sexuality, as a part of the human condition, dates to the beginning of time. Humankind's understanding of sexuality has evolved over time, changing to adapt to changes in knowledge, beliefs, and values. The earliest clear knowledge of sexuality comes from writings, statues, and paintings as old as 10,000 years. Although some early paintings and sculptures indicate an awareness of sexuality, they give no clues as to sexual beliefs or practices. The writings, paintings, and sculptures from 5000 B.C. onward, however, do provide clear information about sexual beliefs, values, laws, and practices; they demonstrate the existence of circumcision, heterosexual genital intercourse, fellatio, anal intercourse, homosexuality, prostitution (male and female), and many other sexual practices. They also indicate variation in attitudes toward and laws about those practices.

Historical records from the period (after the birth of Christ) are even clearer and reveal a great deal about the development of attitudes, beliefs, and laws relating to sexuality. The historical records from Europe (influenced by the Judeo-Christian tradition), the Middle East (predominantly Muslim), India (Hindu), and China (Buddhist and Confucian) show a wide variation in approaches to sexuality. The important message of history is that contemporary approaches to sexuality are part of an ever-evolving process.

Ethnocultural Perspectives

North America is a multicultural, ethnically mixed society. Although the majority of the population traces its roots to Europe, increasingly larger portions of the population in both Canada and the United States have non-European roots. Native Indians, Afro-Americans, Latin Americans, Chinese, East Indians (including Muslim, Hindu, and Sikh), Japanese, and Southeast Asians are some of the ethnic groups that make up significant portions of our society.

All of these groups have their own ethnic and cultural traditions, which influence the ways they view the world and interact with society. Included in these traditions are rules, practices, and values relating to sexuality. Much anthropologic and ethnocultural research indicates that the predominant North American societal

4. Endocrine disorders such as hypothyroidism and Addison's disease

Psychologic factors may include:

1. Doubts about one's ability to perform or about one's masculinity
2. Fatigue, anger, or stress caused by problems at work, in the family, or in interpersonal relationships
3. Traumatic early sexual experiences (e.g., rejection)
4. Pain, fear, or guilt associated with erection
5. Boredom associated with a specific partner

Premature ejaculation occurs when a man is unable to delay ejaculation long enough to satisfy his partner. This usually means that ejaculation occurs after only very limited stimulation of the penis. Often the ejaculation occurs either during penetration (of the vagina, mouth, or anus) or immediately following. The condition may relate to conditioning regarding the need for rapid orgasm or performance demands.

Orgasmic dysfunction, the inability of a woman to achieve orgasm, is of two types: primary and situational. A woman with primary orgasmic dysfunction has never been able to achieve orgasm. A woman with situational dysfunction has experienced at least one orgasm but is at that time nonorgasmic. Orgasmic dysfunction can be caused by drugs, alcohol, aging, and anatomic abnormalities of the genitals. However, most cases have psychologic causes, including hostility between partners, fear or guilt about enjoying the sexual act, and concern about performance.

Vaginismus is the irregular and involuntary contraction of the muscles around the outer third of the vagina when coitus is attempted—that is, the vagina closes before penetration. Its cause can be severe sexual inhibition, often associated with early learning. Other causes can be rape, incest, and painful intercourse. **Dyspareunia** describes the pain experienced by a woman during intercourse as a result of inadequate lubrication, scarring, vaginal infection, or hormonal imbalance.

Nursing Diagnoses

Nursing diagnoses for clients with problems related to sexuality are categorized as *altered sexuality patterns*. This is defined as the state in which an individual expresses concern regarding her or his sexuality. **Sexual dysfunction** is defined by NANDA as a perceived problem in achieving desired sexual satisfaction.

Planning and Implementing for Sexual Health

As in all areas of nursing care, devising strategies to resolve problems related to sexuality requires effective planning and careful implementation (see Chapters 10 and 11). These processes should be based on understanding the nurse's responsibilities, developing self-

awareness, selecting appropriate interventions, and incorporating teaching for sexual health.

Responsibilities of the Nurse

The overall nursing goal for clients with sexual problems is to promote sexual health. Nursing subgoals that define nursing responsibilities include:

1. Developing awareness of one's own sexual attitudes, beliefs, and knowledge
2. Providing accurate sexual information and education to clients
3. Identifying sexual problems and providing intervention as appropriate
4. Enhancing the client's body image and self-esteem

Developing Self-Awareness

To be effective in helping clients with sexual problems, the nurse must first have accurate information about sexuality, identify and accept her or his own sexual values and behaviors and those of others, and be comfortable acquiring and disseminating information about sexuality. Nurses who hold misconceptions may be unable to give clients appropriate advice and assistance. Nurses need to become informed about the anatomy and physiology of sexual organs, psychosocial development of sexuality, psychosocial behaviors, sex-

NURSING DIAGNOSIS

Common Sexual Problems

Examples of nursing diagnoses for clients with sexual problems include:

- Sexual dysfunction related to neurologic deficit secondary to spinal cord injury
- Sexual dysfunction related to neurologic changes secondary to diabetes mellitus
- Sexual dysfunction related to excessive use of alcohol
- Sexual dysfunction related to painful intercourse from inadequate vaginal lubrication
- Disturbance in self-concept: body image or self-esteem related to surgical removal of breast
- Disturbance in self-concept: personal identity related to guilt over enjoyment of sexual activities
- Fear of effects of coitus following heart attack
- Fear of harming fetus by coitus
- Fear of inadequate sexual performance
- Knowledge deficit regarding sexually transmitted diseases
- Knowledge deficit regarding conception
- Knowledge deficit regarding contraception
- Rape trauma syndrome

ual variations among people, and diseases and therapies that can alter sexual behavior.

Awareness of one's own attitudes (feelings, values, and beliefs) about sexuality is also essential. Before the nurse can understand clients' sexuality, she or he must develop an awareness and tolerance of her or his own sexuality. This kind of self-awareness can be acquired via values clarification exercises and discussions (see Chapter 5). Nurses should consider some of their feelings about the following: masturbation, unwanted pregnancy and abortion, contraception, homosexuality and other sexual variations, nudity, sterilization, various modes of sexual stimulation, sexually transmitted diseases, premarital intercourse, unwed parents, and cohabitation. By clarifying her or his own attitudes, the nurse gains a greater understanding and tolerance of sexuality in others.

Selecting Appropriate Strategies for Implementation

Strategies for resolving sexual health problems are many and varied. Major components of any implementation strategy include counseling, education, and referral.

A Model for Implementation

A model to help nurses deliver sexual health care, developed by Mims and Swenson (1978, p. 123), outlines three levels of nursing implementation, all of which require use of the nursing process and communication skills. At the basic level, the nurse helps the client develop awareness of sexuality, which involves his or her knowledge, attitudes, and perceptions. Mims and Swenson believe that all nurses, regardless of educational preparation, should function at this level.

The intermediate level includes giving permission and giving information. Giving permission means that the nurse by attitude or word lets the client know that sexual thoughts, fantasies, and behaviors between informed, consenting adults are sanctioned. Giving permission begins when the nurse acknowledges the client's verbal and nonverbal sexual concerns. For example, an older male with a reduced libido may feel that he cannot discuss sex with the nurse unless the nurse broaches the subject. Other clients may need acknowledgment to feel comfortable about their virginity, homosexual activities, oral-genital sex, or masturbation.

The third level of nursing implementation includes giving suggestions, which involves sexual therapy, educational programs, and research projects. For this level of functioning, the nurse requires advanced and specialized knowledge.

For the client with *sexual dysfunction related to neurologic changes secondary to diabetes mellitus*, implementation might involve teaching about etiology, supportive counseling related to self-image, teaching about continued ability to ejaculate, and providing information about options such as penile prostheses.

Clients with *sexual dysfunction related to neurologic deficits secondary to spinal cord injury* may need special rehabilitation programs, a good example of a third level of implementation.

Teaching About Sexual Health

Providing education for sexual health is an important component of nursing implementation. Many sexual problems exist as a result of sexual ignorance; many others can be prevented with effective sexual health teaching. Examples of important areas of teaching include breast and testicular self-examination, contraception, infertility, and prevention of sexually transmitted diseases.

Contraception is the voluntary prevention of conception or **impregnation** (fertilizing or making pregnant). Contraceptive methods include fertility awareness, mechanical and chemical contraception, and surgical procedures. Increasingly, people are choosing methods that do not employ the use of artificial substances within the body. So-called natural methods have long been preferred by people whose religious beliefs conflict with artificial birth-control methods.

Fertility awareness methods depend upon identification of the days of the month when conception could take place and abstinence during that time. The nurse providing instruction describes the signs of ovulation (see the accompanying box) to the client and explains that, since conception is possible when a woman is ovulating, she should abstain from heterosexual genital intercourse during that time.

Coitus interruptus is another method that does not employ chemical or mechanical barriers. The man withdraws his penis from his partner's vagina prior to ejaculation. While this is one of the oldest methods of birth control, it has certain disadvantages: It requires considerable self-control, the required constraint may decrease sexual gratification, and some semen may escape into the vagina prior to ejaculation.

Mechanical contraceptive methods (using a condom, diaphragm, or sponge) are also current popular choices. The **intrauterine device** (IUD), a preferred mechanical contraceptive method of the 1970s, is now used less frequently because of complications associated with its use and numerous lawsuits against its manufacturers. The **condom** (see Figure 15-1) is a covering

---

Fertility Awareness: Signs of Ovulation

Changes in vaginal mucus: when a woman is not ovulating, her mucus is thick and yellow, and sometimes cloudy; it becomes clearer and thinner near the time of ovulation.

Breast tenderness

Tenderness at either side of the lower abdomen

Midcycle spotting of blood

Changes in basal body temperature: temperature upon arising in the morning drops slightly for 1 to 2 days before ovulation and rises above normal for 1 to 2 days after ovulation.

NURSING DIAGNOSIS

Stress

- Anxiety related to perceived threat to self-concept
- Anxiety related to death of husband
- Ineffective individual coping related to multiple life changes
- Ineffective individual coping related to inadequate support system
- Ineffective family coping related to economic problems
- Ineffective family coping related to prolonged disability

Ineffective individual coping is a "state in which the individual experiences or is at risk of experiencing an inability to manage internal or environmental stressors adequately because of inadequate resources (physical, psychological, or behavioral)" (Carpenito 1987, p. 24). This diagnosis is appropriate when the nurse assesses that the client is not meeting role expectations, is using defense mechanisms inappropriately, or verbalizes an inability to cope. As with most nursing diagnoses, the etiology may be physiologic, psychologic, situational, or maturational. *Ineffective family coping* is defined as the "state in which a family demonstrates destructive behavior in response to an inability to manage internal or external stressors due to inadequate resources (physical, psychological, cognitive, and/or behavioral)" (Carpenito 1987, p. 27.)

Planning

Once nursing diagnoses have been established, goals for changing the existing client responses to the stressor or stressors can be set and strategies for meeting goals planned (see Chapter 10). Plans should be developed in collaboration with the client and significant support persons when possible. The client's state of health (e.g., ability to return to work), level of anxiety, support resources, coping mechanisms, and sociocultural and religious affiliation are considered. The nurse with little experience intervening with clients in stress may wish to consult with a clinical specialist, nurse practitioner, or more experienced nurse to develop effective plans. Examples of possible goal statements appropriate for the sample nursing diagnoses are shown in the accompanying box. See the section on evaluation later in this chapter for outcome criteria which will make these goals measurable.

Implementation

Although stress accompanies every disease and illness, it is also highly individual; a situation that to one person is a major stressor may not affect another. Some methods to help reduce stress will be effective for one person; other methods will be appropriate for a different person. A nurse who is sensitive to clients' needs and reactions can choose those methods of intervention that will be most effective for each individual.

One way to reduce or perhaps eliminate anxiety is for the nurse and client to establish goals that are attainable. Clients must first recognize that they are anxious. This recognition is best brought about in an atmosphere of warmth and trust. Sometimes anxious clients react negatively to nurses because of personal frustration. It is important for nurses to understand this response and react to the behavior in a calm, accepting, and confident manner.

After clients realize that they are anxious, it is important to discuss all the possible reasons for their anxiety. Perley (1984, p. 362) categorizes three underlying states of mind associated with anxiety: *helplessness,* such as that in the person who has recently had a stroke and is unable to perform previous functions; *isolation,* such as that in an adolescent who fears rejection because of a venereal disease; and *insecurity,* such as that in a person who is worried about being unable to earn a living or pay medical bills. When clients can identify the cause of their anxiety, they may find it helpful to explore the cause with the objective of learning better coping strategies. General nursing guidelines to minimize anxiety and stress in clients are:

1. *Support the client and family at a time of illness.* By conveying caring and understanding, the nurse can help clients reduce their stress. Feeling that someone else cares is a source of support to stressed people. Often families require time to talk about their worries and anxieties before they can feel assured and less stressed.
2. *Orient the client to the hospital or agency.* The nurse helps the client adjust to the role change from, for example, independent wage earner to relatively dependent client. The nurse can help family members by giving information, for instance, about visiting hours and specific unit policies.
3. *Give the client in a hospital some way of maintaining identity.* A person's name and clothes are important parts of his or her uniqueness as an indi-

GOAL STATEMENTS

Stress

- The client will experience reduction in level of anxiety.
- The client will resolve anxiety concerning her husband's death.
- The client will be able to cope with multiple life changes.
- The client will receive adequate support for coping.
- The family will be able to cope with existing economic problems.
- The family will be able to cope with the ongoing effects of the father's prolonged disability.

vidual. Nurses can help clients maintain identity by addressing them by the name they prefer and by assisting them to wear their own clothes in a hospital setting, when this is possible.

4. *Provide information when the client has insufficient information.* Fear of the unknown and incorrect information can frequently cause stress. Stressed clients often misunderstand facts related by health personnel. Additional information or clarification can allay stress.

5. *Repeat information when the client has difficulty remembering.* Nurses can assist clients by repeating information when it is requested and assisting people to apply it when they so desire. This problem is particularly prevalent among elderly people who are stressed by a change of setting as well as by their illness.

6. *Encourage the client to participate in the plan of care.* Loss of the right to determine their own destiny can be very stressful to some people, particularly adults who function independently or who assume responsibility for others in their daily lives.

7. *Give the client time to express feelings and thoughts.* Allow time for clients to describe their feelings and worries if they wish. Nurses should be sensitive to clients' needs and neither probe with prying questions nor be too busy to listen.

8. *Ensure that expectations are within the client's capabilities.* Whatever the activity, whether an exercise or recreation, the nurse should make sure that it is possible for the client to accomplish it. If an activity is beyond the client's ability, the client is likely to be more stressed by not achieving the goal.

9. *Be sensitive to specific situations and experiences that increase anxiety and stress for clients.* For example, a man might appear highly stressed each time he receives an intramuscular injection. A careful remark by the nurse about the stress may elicit information that the nurse can use to assist the client.

10. *Assist a client to make a correct appraisal of a situation.* Sometimes, through a lack of knowledge or misinterpretation of a sequence of events, people draw incorrect conclusions. Having valid information might relieve the client's stress.

11. *Provide an environment in which a person can function independently to some degree without assistance.* It may be difficult and stressful for an adult to assume the dependent client role even for a short time. By restoring some degree of independent functioning, such as by adapting eating utensils so that clients can feed themselves, nurses can lower clients' stress levels.

12. *Reinforce positive environmental factors and recognize negative ones to help reduce stress.* Dwelling on problems and difficulties increases stress, but focusing on what can be accomplished positively usually decreases stress.

13. *Arrange for other clients with similar experiences to visit.* Clients with colostomies or similar conditions may be highly stressed and feel that they will never be able to live a normal life again. Meeting

OUTCOME CRITERIA

Stress

The client will:

- Verbally recognize own anxiety
- Verbalize effects of own behavior on significant others
- Verbalize feelings related to event or situation
- Identify past and present coping patterns
- Identify consequences of current coping behavior
- Identify personal strengths
- State an increase in psychologic comfort following exercise program
- Use exercise to reduce anxiety
- Ask for help from others
- Make decisions in anxiety-provoking situations and follow through with appropriate actions

another person who has successfully adjusted to a colostomy can lower the stress greatly.

14. *Bring clients and their families into contact with people in community agencies who can help them make valid plans.* Social workers are familiar with discharge planning and arrangements that a client may need to make. Often people are stressed needlessly because they do not know what help is available to them in the community.

15. *Communicate competence, understanding, and empathy rather than stress and anxiety.* When a nurse conveys stress or anxiety, the client and family may be concerned about the nurse's ability to function where the client's health and life are involved. To reduce a client's stress, nurses need to know themselves well and be able to function in a nondefensive manner that conveys competence and empathy.

In addition to these general guidelines for minimizing anxiety and stress, several health promotion strategies (see Chapter 25) are often appropriate as interventions for clients with stress-related nursing diagnoses. Among these are physical exercise, optimal nutrition, adequate rest and sleep, time management, and relaxation techniques.

Evaluation

Examples of outcome criteria for clients who have stress problems are listed in the accompanying box. These criteria are the measurable or observable signs, symptoms, and behavioral responses that permit the nurse to evaluate the goals established during the planning phase of the nursing process. The criteria listed are not specific to any one goal; they are merely examples of the types of behaviors that a nurse could select as a means of evaluating planned and implemented care. To be valid

Table 16–3 Kinzel's Scale Rating Stress in Nurses

Your Score	Stressful Events	Stress Value
_____	Assuming responsibilities you're not trained to handle	67
_____	Working with unqualified personnel	64
_____	Dealing with nonsupportive supervisors or administrators	61
_____	Working with an inadequate staff	58
_____	Caring for a patient during a cardiac arrest	55
_____	Experiencing conflict with coworkers	52
_____	Dealing with the family of a dying patient	49
_____	Caring for a dying patient	46
_____	Working with broken or faulty equipment	44
_____	Working with inadequate supplies	42
_____	Working an inconvenient shift or schedule	38
_____	Assuming responsibilities without thanks or recognition	36
_____	Dealing with a difficult doctor	34
_____	Trying to communicate within a bureaucracy	31
_____	Discharging a patient inadequately prepared for discharge	28
_____	Caring for a seriously ill patient	25
_____	Spending long periods of time doing paperwork or phone duties	22
_____	Experiencing a problem over salary or promotion	19
_____	Working with a demanding or noncompliant patient	16
_____	Coordinating ancillary personnel	<u>13</u>
_____	YOUR TOTAL TOTAL POSSIBLE	800

Suggested score interpretation

0-133:   The last 24 hours have produced minimal stress, not enough to cause you many problems.

134-266: You're under moderate stress. This is the highest level of stress you should permit on a day-to-day basis.

267-532: You're experiencing high-level stress. You have trouble relaxing and easily become upset. Try relaxation techniques, exercise, and hobbies until you can reduce your stressors.

533-800: You're under extreme stress. Get help fast. You're a prime candidate for burnout.

Source: S. L. Kinzel, What's your stress level? *Nursing Life,* March/April 1982, 2:54-55. Reprinted with permission from the March/April issue of *Nursing Life.* Copyright © 1982 by Springhouse Corporation, 1111 Bethlehem Pike, Springhouse, PA 19477. All rights reserved.

and reliable, outcome criteria need to be individualized for the client.

Stress Management for Nurses

Nurses, like clients, are susceptible to experiencing anxiety and crises. In recent years, more attention has been given to the occupational stress nurses experience. Nursing practice involves many stressors related to both clients and the work environment. Kinzel (1982, p. 55) devised a 20-item, 24-hour scale to help nurses measure their stress levels. See Table 16–3. All 20 items fall into five main categories: inadequate knowledge, inadequate support from peers and supervisors, dealing with death, poor communication, and salary and staffing problems. The purpose of such a scale is to make nurses aware of the source of negative feelings and frustration on the job, to help them make adjustments, and to support colleagues.

Chapter Highlights

Homeostasis is the tendency of the body to maintain a state of relative balance or constancy in response to a changing internal and external environment.

Physiologic homeostasis is maintained by coordinated functioning of the autonomic nervous, endocrine, respiratory, cardiovascular, renal, and gastrointestinal systems.

▪ Homeostatic mechanisms regulate hormone secretion, fluid and electrolyte levels, the functions of body viscera, and metabolic processes that provide energy for the body.

▪ Psychologic homeostasis, or emotional well-being, is acquired or learned through the experience of living and interacting with others.

▪ Stress is a state of physiologic or psychologic tension that affects the whole person—physically, emotionally, intellectually, socially, and spiritually.

▪ A person's response to stressors varies according to the way the stressor is perceived, its intensity and duration, the number of stressors, previous experience, coping mechanisms used, support people available, and age.

▪ A common psychologic response to stress is anxiety, which is manifested in a variety of cognitive, verbal, and motor responses that reduce tension.

▪ Unconscious psychologic defense mechanisms, such as denial, rationalization, compensation, and sublimation, also protect the individual from tension.

▪ Both physiologic and psychologic responses to stressors can be adaptive or maladaptive.

▪ Adaptation is a process of change that occurs in response to stress. It occurs in three interrelated modes: physiologic, psychologic, and sociocultural.

▪ Coping is a more immediate response to stress than adaptation.

▪ Coping strategies can be either effective or ineffective and result in adaptation or maladaptation, respectively.

▪ The nurse can help clients recognize stress and support clients' effective coping mechanisms.

▪ Nursing interventions for stress are aimed at reducing anxiety, at promoting clients' physical and mental well-being so that they handle stress more effectively, and at helping clients learn more effective coping mechanisms.

▪ The nurse, too, is prone to occupational stress and needs to learn effective stress-management techniques.

▪ Selected References

Appelbaum, S. H. 1981. *Stress management for health care professionals.* Rockville, Md.: Aspen Systems Corporation.

Bell, J. M. March/April 1977. Stressful life events and coping methods in mental-illness and wellness behaviors. *Nursing Research* 26:136–40.

Burgess, A. W., and Lazare, A. 1976. *Community mental health: Target populations.* Englewood Cliffs, N.J.: Prentice-Hall.

Byrne, M. L., and Thompson, L. F. 1978. *Key concepts for the study and practice of nursing.* St. Louis: C. V. Mosby Co.

Cannon, W. B. 1939. *The wisdom of the body.* 2d ed. New York: Norton Publishing Co.

Carpenito, L. J. 1987. *Nursing diagnosis: Application to clinical practice.* 2d ed. Philadelphia: J. B. Lippincott Co.

Detherage, K. S., and Johnson, S. S. 1986. Primary prevention in stress and crisis. In Edelman, C., and Mandle, C. L., editors. *Health promotion throughout the life span.* St. Louis: C. V. Mosby Co.

Duldt, B. W. September 1981. Anger: An occupational hazard for nurses. *Nursing Outlook* 29:510–18.

Freud, S. 1946. *The ego and the mechanisms of defense.* New York: International Universities Press.

Graydon, J. E. Summer 1984. Measuring patient coping. *Nursing Papers* 16:3–12.

Guyton, A. C. 1986. *Textbook of medical physiology.* 7th ed. Philadelphia: W. B. Saunders Co.

Hamilton, J. M. July/August 1984. Effective ways to relieve stress. *Nursing Life* 4:24–27.

Holmes, T. H., and Rahe, R. H. August 1967. The social readjustment rating scale. *Journal of Psychosomatic Research* 11:213–18.

Kinzel, S. L. March/April 1982. What's your stress level? *Nursing Life* 2:54–55.

Lazarus, R. S. 1966. *Psychological stress and the coping process.* New York: McGraw-Hill.

Lazarus, R. S., and Folkman, S. 1984. *Stress, appraisal, and coping.* New York: Springer Publishing Co.

Lyon, B. L., and Werner, J. 1987. Stress: Ten years of practice-relevant research. In Werley, H., and Fitzpatrick, J., editors. *Annual Review of Nursing Research.*

Perley, N. Z. 1984. Problems in self-consistency: Anxiety. In Roy, C., editor. *Introduction to nursing: An adaptation model.* Englewood Cliffs, N.J.: Prentice-Hall.

Scully, R. May 1980. Stress in the nurse. *American Journal of Nursing* 80:911–14.

Selye, H. 1956. *The stress of life.* New York: McGraw Hill.

———. 1976. *The stress of life.* Rev. ed. New York: McGraw Hill.

Skinner, K. May 1980. Support group for ICU nurses. *Nursing Outlook* 28:296–99.

Smith, M. J. T., and Selye, H. November 1979. Stress: Reducing the negative effects of stress. *American Journal of Nursing* 79:1953–55.

Taché, J., and Selye, J. 1985. On stress and coping mechanisms. *Issues in Mental Health Nursing* 7:3–24.

Van Os, D.; Clark, C.; Turner, C.; and Herbst, J. August 1985. Life stress and cystic fibrosis. *Western Journal of Nursing Research* 7(3):301–15.

Weisman, A. D., and Worden, J. W. 1976–77. The existential plight in cancer: Significance of the first 100 days. *International Journal of Psychiatry in Medicine* 7:1–15.

Wilson, L. K. May/June 1986. High-gear nursing: How it can run you down and what you can do about it. *Nursing Life* 6:44–47.

CHAPTER 17

Ethnicity and Culture

OBJECTIVES

Describe the concept of culture.

Identify characteristics and universal attributes of culture.

Identify social characteristics common to all ethnic/cultural groups that require consideration by health care providers.

Identify problems unique to ethnic minorities in the provision and use of health care services.

Relate the incidence of specific diseases to certain ethnic or cultural groups.

Identify specific characteristics and values of selected cultural groups that may influence nursing assessment and intervention.

Relate health-related beliefs and practices to economic status.

Contrast the values of the health care culture and selected minority ethnic cultures.

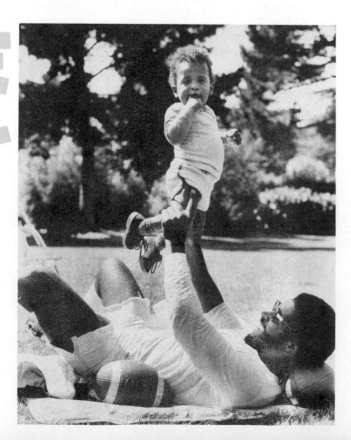

Concepts of Ethnicity and Culture

Definitions

Ethnicity is the condition of belonging to a specific ethnic group. An **ethnic group** is a set of individuals who share a unique cultural and social heritage passed on from one generation to another (Henderson and Primeaux 1981, p. xx). Ethnicity thus differs from race. **Race** denotes a system of classifying humans into subgroups according to specific physical characteristics, including skin pigmentation, stature, facial features, texture of body hair, and head form (Henderson and Primeaux 1981, p. xix). The three racial types that are commonly recognized are Caucasoid, Negroid, and Mongoloid. However, because of the mixture of races, the three groups meld together, and there are many commonalities among groups.

Culture should not be confused with race or ethnic group. **Culture** is the set of beliefs and practices that are shared by people and passed down from generation to generation. Races have different ethnic groups, and the ethnic groups have different cultures. It is therefore important to understand that all white or black people do not have the same culture. North America has people of many different ethnic groups and cultures. Their cultural beliefs and practices can affect health and illness and thus become an important consideration for nurses.

Large cultural groups often have cultural subgroups or subsystems. A subculture is usually composed of people who have a distinct identity and yet are also related to a larger cultural group. A subcultural group generally has ethnicity, occupation, or physical characteristics in common with the larger cultural group. Examples of cultural subgroups are occupational groups (e.g., nurses), societal groups (e.g., feminists), and ethnic groups (e.g., Cajuns, who may be black, French, or German but who share French Acadian heritage and customs). A **bicultural group** is a group of people who embrace two cultures, life-styles, and sets of values (Chen-Louie 1980, p. 4).

Two other terms commonly used with reference to ethnicity and culture are *dominant group* and *minority group.* A **dominant group** is "a collectivity within a society which has a preeminent authority to function as guardians and sustainers of the controlling value system and as prime allocators of rewards in the society" (Schermerhorn 1970, p. 13). A **minority group** or minority is a "group of people who, because of their physical or cultural characteristics, are singled out from the others in the society in which they live for differential and unequal treatment, and who therefore regard themselves as objects of collective discrimination" (Wirth 1945, p. 347). A dominant group is often the largest group in a society, for example, the white middle class of the United States. However, the dominant group is not always the largest; for example, white South Africans are the dominant group and black South Africans are the minority group, yet the blacks far outnumber the whites.

Not uncommonly, people of a minority group often lose the cultural characteristics that distinguish them from the dominant group. This process is referred to as **cultural assimilation** or **acculturation.** Sometimes mutual cultural assimilation occurs, e.g., Chinese people coming to a North American community learn to speak English, and the people in the community learn to cook Chinese dishes.

Ethnocentrism is the belief that one's own culture is superior to all others. This can be seen in the comparison of the values and behavior of other cultures to those of one's own culture, using one's own as the standard. Although all people are subject to ethnocentrism, it is important for nurses to be consciously aware of ethnic and cultural differences and to accept these as appropriate. These differences should not be viewed as good or bad. Many immigrants to the United States and Canada maintain their ethnic and cultural identities in terms of their dress, language, customs, and rituals; accepting these is basic to accepting the client as an individual.

Stereotyping is assuming that all members of a culture or ethnic group are alike. For example, one may assume that all Italians express pain volubly or that all Chinese people like rice. Stereotyping may be based on generalizations founded in research, or it may be unrelated to reality. For example, research indicates that Italians are likely to express pain verbally; however, a particular Italian client may not verbalize pain. Stereotyping that is unrelated to reality may be positive or negative and is frequently an outcome of racism. **Racism** is the assumption of inherent racial superiority or inferiority and the consequent discrimination against certain races. An example of positive stereotyping is "All Jewish people are very clever." An example of negative stereotyping is "All Native Americans are alcoholics." Stereotyping can cause problems in nursing practice, in that the nurse may plan care based on stereotyping rather than on individual assessment of the client.

Ethnoscience is "the systematic study of the way of life of a designated cultural group with the purpose of obtaining an accurate account of the people's behavior and how they perceive and interpret their universe" (Leininger 1970, p. 168). Ethnoscientists attempt to provide an inside view of a culture from the way the people of the culture talk about it. They study and classify data about a cultural or subcultural group so that their report is meaningful to both people within the culture and people outside the culture who try to understand it. Emphasis is placed on the person's point of view, the person's vision, and the person's world.

Nurses can apply much of the knowledge gained by ethnoscientists, specifically about the health-illness behavior systems of people from cultural backgrounds different from their own. In the past decade or more, the client's personal view of illness has received recognition and emphasis. Nurses have, as a result, implemented methods to discover how well clients understand their illnesses, how clients perceive they can be helped by health personnel, and how illness has affected them and their families. In recent years, cultural views affecting health practices and beliefs have been receiving greater recognition. The fact that health beliefs and practices vary among cultures and the implications of this fact for nursing have also received greater attention. To provide effective nursing services to clients, nurses need data about the client's personal and cultural views regarding health and illness. When making nursing care plans, nurses need to consider the client's world and daily experiences. To make valid assessments, nurses need to try to see and hear the world as their clients do. Specific cultural data can provide scientific generalizations about health and illness behavior in different cultures. Clients' needs and behaviors can be better understood when particular health norms are identified.

Characteristics of Culture

A number of universal attributes or characteristics can be used to describe any culture. Among them are:

1. *Culture is learned.* It is not instinctive or innate but learned through life experiences after birth.
2. *Culture is taught.* It is transmitted from parents to children over successive generations. All animals can learn, but only humans can pass culture along. Language is the chief vehicle of culture.
3. *Culture is social.* It originates and develops through the interactions of people.
4. *Culture is adaptive.* Customs, beliefs, and practices change slowly, but they do adapt to the social environment and to the biologic and psychologic needs of people. As life conditions change, some traditional forms in a culture may cease to provide satisfaction and are eliminated.
5. *Culture is integrative.* The elements in a culture tend to form a consistent and integrated system. For example, religious beliefs and practices influence and are influenced by family organization, economic values, and health practices.
6. *Culture is ideational.* Ideational means "forming images or objects in the mind." The group habits that are part of culture are to a considerable extent ideal norms or patterns of behavior. People do not always follow those norms. The norms of their culture may in fact be different from the norms of society as a whole.
7. *Culture is satisfying.* Cultural habits persist only as long as they satisfy people's needs. Gratification strengthens habits and beliefs. Once they no longer bring gratification, they may disappear.

Diversity of North American Society

The populations of the United States and Canada are a mixture of many ethnic groups and cultures. In the United States, white Americans make up 78.13% of the total population; minority groups, 21.87%. The minority population can be further broken down as shown in Figure 17–1. In Canada, British Canadians make up 40.2% of the total population; French Canadians, 26.7%. See Figure 17–1 also. The provision of quality nursing care to all North Americans is a desired goal. Because of the multicultural, multiethnic nature of American society, it is essential that consideration be given to the unique needs of ethnic and cultural groups. The following general considerations can help nurses develop an awareness and sensitivity to some of these specific needs.

Male-Female Roles

Most cultures are patriarchal, i.e., the man is the dominant figure. The degree of dominance of men is variable; when men are highly dominant, women are usually passive. An example of a patriarchal society is the Islamic culture of Iran, where women must be veiled in public and all important decisions are left to the men.

In contrast, the Native American culture is matriarchal, i.e., the woman is the dominant person in the family. Knowing who the decision maker or dominant person in a family is helps nurses understand the meaning of illness to a family and its decision-making process relative to health care. In Mexican American families, the father generally holds the power, whereas in Jewish American families, the mother is generally "the power behind the throne" (Friedman 1981, p. 271).

Language and Communication Patterns

People of an ethnic or cultural group may speak the language of their group fluently and not speak the language of the country. This is particularly true of certain women who, because they stay in the home, have limited interaction with people outside the family. Even the mother of a family who has been in the United States for 30 years may know very little English. The degree to which people learn the language of a new country is highly variable. Some people may become fluent very quickly, while others may learn only enough to get along in their daily activities. When people in the latter group become ill, they are frequently unable to describe their symptoms or answer a health questionnaire. If nurses do not establish that there is a language barrier, a client's needs may not be met. Most health agencies have translators to help nurses and clients, or the nurse may require help from a family member who can translate for the nurse.

Language barriers can be particularly frustrating and anxiety producing when a person is ill and can neither state problems nor understand instructions. It is most difficult for people to convey their emotions about threatening situations in a second language, a crucial factor in cases of emotional and psychiatric illness. Language barriers also arise between people using the same language. The idiomatic English of a regional or cultural group may not be readily understood outside the group. For example, *belly* can mean the abdomen or the entire cavity from the nipple line to the pubic area.

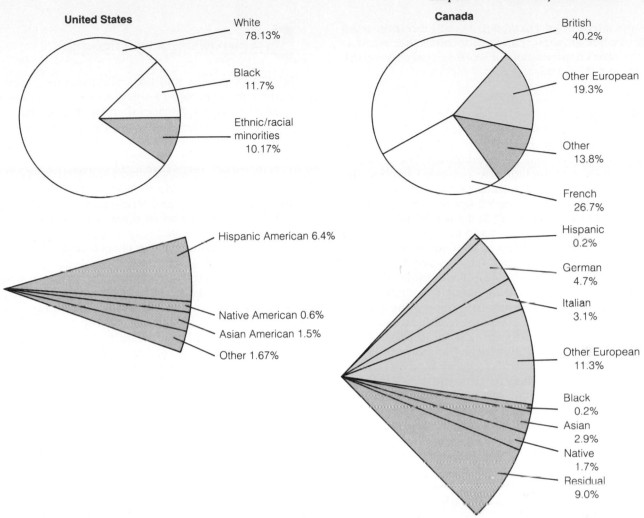

Figure 17–1 Estimates of the distribution of population by ethnic/racial origin based on the United States 1980 census and the Canadian 1981 census. *Sources:* U.S. Department of Commerce, Bureau of the Census, *Census of Population, General Population Characteristics United States Survey* (Washington, D.C.: Government Printing Office, April 1984), Table 40; Statistics Canada, *Census of Canada*, Cat. no. 92-911 (Ottawa: Minister of Supplies and Services, 1984), Table 1. Used by permission.

▪ Territoriality and Personal Space

Both territoriality and personal space are influenced by an individual's culture and ethnicity. **Territoriality** is the pattern of behavior arising from an individual's feeling that certain spaces and objects belong to him or her. **Personal space** is the distance a person prefers to maintain from others when interacting with them. In general, people of Arabic, Southern European, and African origins frequently sit or stand relatively close to each other when talking, whereas people of Asian, North European, and North American countries are comfortable talking farther apart.

▪ Time Orientation

The middle-class group in the United States and in Canada tends to be oriented to the future. People plan for the future, establish long-term goals, and are increasingly concerned about preventing future illness, e.g., by taking calcium to prevent osteoporosis in old age. In daily life, people are oriented to the time of day; meals are taken at a specified time, and clients have appointment times with many health care professionals. The nurse is also highly attuned to time; medications are given at specific times, and work begins and ends at specified times.

However, not all cultures are future oriented. People of other cultures, e.g., Asians, may be oriented to the past. This orientation is illustrated by ancestor worship and the influence that ancient beliefs such as Confucianism have on the present. Other cultures, such as the Native American, are very much oriented to the present. Many Native American homes do not have clocks, and the people live one day at a time with little concern for the future. Hispanic Americans often value relationships with others more than concerns with time.

▪ Work

The attitude of individuals toward work is highly dependent upon their culture. Middle-class Americans generally believe that everyone should be employed and that work should be pleasurable and of value in itself;

this attitude is often referred to as the *Protestant work ethic*. People in some cultures do not value work as much as the compensation for work, i.e., they view work as a means to an end.

Family

The minority client's concept of family can differ from that of white middle-class culture. The minority group family may include the extended family (the nuclear family plus uncles, aunts, grandparents, cousins, and godparents). An associated concept is that family members are most important and must be helped at all costs. When health care is offered to such persons, it is important to consider the needs of the whole family. Sometimes, priorities in such families are detrimental to the health of one of its members. For example, a mother may not think that purchasing elastic stockings for her own ankle edema is as important as purchasing food for an unemployed relative. The home health care nurse in this instance may have to see that the relative's food needs are met before dealing with the mother's health needs.

Cultures that emphasize that the needs of the extended family are as important as personal needs may also hold the belief that personal and family information must stay within the family. Some cultural groups, e.g., the traditional Chinese family, are very reluctant to disclose family information to outsiders, including physicians and nurses. This attitude can present difficulties for psychiatrists and mental health workers who view family interaction patterns as the locus of emotional problems.

Food and Nutritional Practices

The food people eat and the customs associated with food vary widely among subcultures and ethnic groups. For example, the staple food of Asians is rice; of Italians, pasta; and of Europeans, wheat bread. Even families who have been in the United States or Canada for several generations often continue to eat the food of their country (Christian and Greger 1985, p. 213).

Hospitalized clients often have very little choice about the food they are served. The nurse can encourage family members to bring in special meals if the client's condition allows. Instructions about meal planning for clients requiring special diets at home may have to be given to younger family members who are fluent in English or given by a health worker of the same culture, who can act as an interpreter.

When clients are learning about a special diet, nurses must be sensitive to the cultural meanings of food and to the foods a client is accustomed to. For example, it is unwise to recommend a service such as Meals on Wheels if the service is unable to supply the foods to which the client is accustomed, e.g., bean sprouts and vegetables for the Japanese client and fish and rice for the Chinese client.

Susceptibility to Disease

Because of genetic and life-style influences, some ethnic and cultural groups in American society are more susceptible to certain diseases than the general population. Generally, bicultural groups in a lower socioeconomic area have a higher incidence of acquired diseases, such as infections. The following diseases are more prevalent in certain groups than in the general population:

1. *Sickle-cell* disease affects approximately 50,000 Americans of African and Mediterranean descent. It is estimated that between 8 and 10% of the black population in the United States has the sickling trait. The inherited recessive trait is a defect in the hemoglobin molecule. In people with sickle-cell disease, the red blood cells have a 20-day life, in contrast to the normal 120-day life. The symptoms and severity of the disease are variable, depending on the syndrome. Some people are very ill and have a series of crises, while others live fairly long and normal lives (Richardson and Milne 1983, p. 417).

2. *Hypertension* is more prevalent among black and other nonwhite Americans than white Americans, and the incidence is highest in Taiwan and Japan, two highly industrialized nations. It is also more common in recent immigrants to the United States. The pattern of incidence suggests that stress, obesity, and salt intake are implicated in hypertension (Overfield 1985, p. 114).

3. *Diabetes mellitus* is a major health problem of Native Americans. It occurs at an early age, i.e., teens, and the rate of death from diabetes is three to four times higher among Native Americans than the general population. It may be related to a diet high in refined carbohydrates and fats and low in traditional foods as well as a sedentary life-style (Overfield 1985, p. 153).

4. A number of *cancers* vary racially in their incidence; however, diet and some other environmental factors appear to be better predictors of cancer than race (Overfield 1985, p. 91). In the United States, white women have a higher incidence of breast cancer than black women. Skin cancers of all types are less common among blacks than whites; this is thought to be due to the added protection dark pigmentation provides against the sun's rays. Although digestive tract cancers show high and low incidences relative to specific geographic areas and racial groups, diet rather than genetic factors is probably the cause (Overfield 1985, pp. 91–93).

5. Differences among races have been found in *alcohol metabolism*. Many Asians and Native Americans convert alcohol into acetaldehyde more rapidly and convert acetaldehyde to acetic acid more slowly than the general population does. Therefore, Asians and Native Americans experience a rapid onset of and prolonged exposure to high blood acetaldehyde levels, which cause many of the symptoms of alcohol intoxication (Overfield 1985, pp. 83–84).

6. Certain *dermatologic conditions* are more common among blacks than whites. Keloid formation, an exaggerated wound healing process of the skin, is commonly found in blacks. Keloids develop following skin trauma, e.g., surgical incision and burns (Bloch 1976, p. 28). A number of other conditions, e.g., acne vulgaris, can cause postinflammatory pigment changes in the skin among blacks.

7. *Acquired immune deficiency syndrome* (AIDS) is currently more prevalent in the homosexual community than in the heterosexual community in North America, although this is not true in parts of Africa. The majority of people with AIDS are male homosexuals or bisexuals; however, intravenous drug users, the sex partners of people in these groups, and people who received blood transfusions before required screening are also at high risk.

Cultural and Ethnic Groups in North America

This section outlines some selected cultural and ethnic characteristics of significance to nurses. It is important to remember, however, that many people in ethnic and cultural subgroups do not conform to all the practices of their group. This is especially true of second- and third-generation family members who may be assimilated into the dominant cultural group. Table 17-1 presents a summary of the impact of culture on health and illness.

▪ Native Americans

In the United States and Canada, the responsibility for health services for Native Americans rests with the federal government. There are, however, differing health care practices in various geographic locations in the United States. For example, Native Americans living in the eastern states and in most urban areas are not eligible for the services provided by the Indian Health Service, whereas Native Americans living on reservations in the western states are (Spector 1985, pp. 190–91).

Because about 200 different tribes of Native Americans exist in the United States, each with its own language, folkways, religion, mores, and patterns of interpersonal relationships, caution must be used when generalizing about Native American culture. In terms of health care, this variability needs to be considered. For example, the Native American living in isolation on a reservation may retain traditional beliefs (e.g., in cures effected by the tribal medicine man), whereas the urban Native American may have adopted many values of the majority culture in relation to health care. It is not uncommon for Native Americans to accept both kinds of health practices concurrently.

Various tribal groups differ in their traditional values and beliefs. Henderson and Primeaux (1981, pp. 73–74) list the following characteristics, which apply in general to traditional Native Americans: orientation to the present, greater concern with finishing a task than meeting a deadline for completion, valuing the giving rather than the accumulating of goods, respect for age, cooperation rather than competition, harmony with nature, and integration into the extended family. Native Americans are sometimes assumed to be inattentive because some tend not to make direct eye contact when speaking with another person. This practice is based on respect for the other person's privacy and the other person's soul. Some Native Americans believe that direct eye contact may steal the other's soul.

Associated with this belief is the Native American's commitment to autonomy. Each person has the right to speak only for himself or herself, and each person's actions should be self-initiated. Thus, the nurse may have difficulty obtaining a client's history from close family members. Family members may believe they have no right to give personal information about another; they do not mean to be uncooperative but are following an unwritten ethical code.

Native Americans accept that they will die as part of the life cycle and do not worry about how or when or why. They know they will join their ancestors in another world when the Spirit intends. Funerals generally take place in the home and are associated with a large feast and gifts for relatives of the deceased. Burial rituals according to tribal tradition are important to many Native Americans.

Associated with burial is the belief in wholeness. Thus, some Native Americans may want to reclaim amputated limbs and retain them for burial when the person dies. Native Americans also fear the spirits of the dead. It is important to the dying Native American client and family that people be present at the death.

During illness, the Native American client is comforted by visits from relatives and friends. Visits convey caring and enduring bonds of support. Being present is generally more important than talking, and it is not uncommon for large numbers of people to congregate. Most often, one person likes to remain near the client for long periods. The Native American's kinship system can be confusing to nurses of other cultures. A child, for example, may have several sets of brothers or sisters who are not direct relatives but are considered such. These people are all-important to the ill client. The aged, particularly, are looked upon for counsel and wisdom. Friendship ties are strong and can be as meaningful as those of the family or extended family in sustaining the client's recuperative powers.

Various curative and preventive rituals may be conducted to restore balance when illness occurs. These may be carried out by medicine men or family members. Sacred foods, such as cornmeal, may be sprinkled on people's shoulders before they enter a home to prevent disease from entering the home. This sacred food or other substance, such as tobacco or feathers, may be sprinkled around an ill person's bed. It is important for nurses to provide privacy for such ceremonies and to inquire about how long the substance is to be left in place, how to dispose of it, and, if it must be disturbed, exactly how to do so. Items such as herbs are frequently placed near the client on the bedside stand or on the

Table 17–1 Comparison of Health-Related Factors and Subcultures

	Definition of Health	Cause of Illness —Is Prevention Possible; if So, How?	Name of Healer, Healing Practices	Problems of Entry to Health Care System	Communication Patterns	Sexuality and Family Life	Beliefs about Death
Navajo (Native American)	Harmony between individual, earth, and supernatural, as well as the ability to survive difficult circumstances[1,2]	Disease is disharmony and can be caused by violating taboo or attack by witch; illness prevented through elaborate religious rituals; do not believe in germ theory[1,2]	Medicine man, who is more than average human being, is therefore influential figure; medicine man diagnoses and treats problem; treatments include yucca root, massage, herbs, and chanting; his chant states person will get well, and person believes him[1,2]	Language; will first visit medicine man; general beliefs are not compatible with health care system and structure; problems also include money and past experiences of disrespect; fear of spirits of dead may influence decision to leave hospital early[1,2]	Time of silence after each speaker to show respect and reflection on what they said; little eye contact; time orientation not very strict; recording of conversation invasion of privacy[1,2]	Family, extended family, and tribal ties strong; cooperation emphasized; consider children as individuals as soon as they can talk; therefore can make own decisions[1,2]	Fear of spirits of dead; children and family should be with dying person[1]
Hispanic American	Gift from God, also good luck; can tell healthy person by robust appearance and report of feeling well[1,3,4]	Illness is punishment from God for wrongdoing, to be suffered; it can be prevented by eating well, praying, being good, and working; wearing medals may help; physically, illness is an imbalance between "hot" and "cold" properties of body[1,3,4]	Healer called *curandero*; cures hot illness with cold medicine and reverse; classification of hot and cold diseases varies; penicillin is hot medicine; massages and cleanings are common[4]	Language; will first go to woman for advice, then if needed, to "señora," then to curandero, then to physician; many migrant workers are Hispanic, and frequent moves may make access to medical care difficult; belief that hospital is place to go to die causes underuse of system; modesty may result in woman bringing friend to physician with her[1,3,4]	Confidentiality and modesty important; too many questions are insulting; it is more acceptable to make tentative statement to which they can respond; time orientation not strict; politeness essential[1,3–5]	High degree of modesty, may prefer home births for this reason; men are breadwinners, women homemakers; women are healers, men make all decisions[1,3–5]	Afterlife of heaven and hell exists
Traditional black	Harmony with nature, no separation of mind and body[4]	Disease is disharmony caused by spirits and demons; it can be prevented through good diet, rest, cleanliness, and laxatives to clean out system; some use of copper and silver bracelets for prevention	Some belief in voodoo still prevalent; religious healing practiced[4,6]	May seek folk or religious healer first; money and type of service affect decision; emergency room frequent entry point; black women have high "noncompliance" rate[4,6]	Racism toward blacks still prevalent; common names for symptoms should be known by health worker; time orientation not strict	Matriarchy prevalent; almost 30% of black families have woman head of household; therefore women make decisions[4,6]	Death is passage from evils of this world to another state; blacks have shorter life expectancy than national average[6]
Chinese American	Balance of yin and yang (negative and positive energy forces); healthy body is gift from parents and ancestors[4,7,8]	Illness caused by imbalance of yin and yang, which may be due to overexertion or prolonged sitting; disease is prevented through better adaptation to nature[4,7]	Acupuncture and moxibustion (which is a therapeutic application of heat to skin) restore balance of yin and yang; herbal remedies such as ginseng used for many illnesses; healer is called physician[4,7]	Language; traditional Chinese physicians were paid to keep their clients well and cared for sick without fees because illness indicated they had failed in their job; Chinese physicians are available in community and may encourage clients to use Western physician; family spokesman may accompany client to	Open expression of emotions not acceptable; therefore might not complain about pain or symptoms; client may smile when he or she does not understand[4,7]	Women subservient to men; patriarchal family; ancestor worship and respect for obedience for parents observed; divorce considered disgrace[1,4,5]	Reincarnation[7]

Table 17–1 Comparison of Health-Related Factors and Subcultures (continued)

	Definition of Health	Cause of Illness —Is Prevention Possible; if so, How?	Name of Healer, Healing Practices	Problems of Entry to Health Care System	Communication Patterns	Sexuality and Family Life	Beliefs about Death
Low income	Functional definition: if you can work, you are healthy[5,9]	Belief that illness is not preventable; fatalism common; future orientation minimal because present problems are too great[1,5,9]	Will often rely on folk healers and remedies because of belief and problems gaining access to health care system[5]	Western physician[4,7] Use of public funding may limit access and type of care; present time orientation and beliefs about prevention may cause delay in obtaining care; inability to afford health insurance; may lose day's pay to go to physician[5,9]	May use slang and language of subculture; may view providers as authoritarian; time orientation not strict[5]	Many single-parent families with woman head of household[9]	Depends on culture and religion
High income	No data available	General belief in prevention of illness through diet, exercise, and good health habits; motivators such as previous experience or family tradition are influential in actual practice of prevention[5]	Combination of traditional practices of religion and culture, frequent use of health care system and self-help information[5]	Access not too difficult, usually through private physician; most have health insurance through employer[5]	Most like health care culture; cannot be expected to understand jargon	Women more likely to have career by choice than financial necessity	Depends on culture and religion
Health care culture	Optimal level of functioning; more than absence of disease; physical, emotional, social, and mental health included[5]	Scientific approach to cause of illness; prevention involves periodic physical examinations, laboratory studies, inoculations, as well as avoiding smoking and overeating[4]	Healing done by physician, usually takes place in office or hospital; treatments based on scientific knowledge and are frequently embarrassing or uncomfortable; often emotional component of disease is ignored[5]	Physician is main access to system; focus is basically curing illness rather than prevention; encourage management given to population to seek care as soon as symptoms appear; consider health care system as only provider	Widespread use of jargon and specialized language; large percentage of workers from middle class; often expect gratitude for care given; time orientation strict; written records kept[4]	Hierarchy, with physicians making decisions	Death usually means workers have failed to do their job; elaborate means are used to keep people alive; ethical and legal questions are being discussed and tested.

[1] Data from A. T. Brownlee, *Community, culture, and care: A cross-cultural guide for health workers* (St. Louis: C. V. Mosby Co., 1978).

[2] Data from R. Wood, The American Indian and health. In *Ethnicity and health care* (NLN pub. no. 14–1625, 1976), pp. 29–35.

[3] Data from H. Gonzales, Health care needs of the Mexican American family. In *Ethnicity and health care* (NLN pub. no. 14–1625, 1976), pp. 21–28.

[4] Data from R. Spector, *Cultural diversity in health and illness* (New York: Appleton-Century-Crofts, 1985).

[5] Data from R. Murray and J. Zentner, *Nursing assessment and health promotion through the life span* (Englewood Cliffs, N.J.: Prentice-Hall, 1975).

[6] Data from B. Martin, Ethnicity and health care: Afro-Americans. In *Ethnicity and health care* (NLN pub. no. 14–1625, 1976), pp. 47–55.

[7] Data from R. Wang, Chinese Americans and health care. In *Ethnicity and health care* (NLN pub. no. 14–1625, 1976), pp. 9–18.

[8] Data from G. Channing, What Is a Christian Scientist? In Rosten, L., editor: *A guide to religions of America* (New York: Simon & Schuster, 1955).

[9] Data from M. Fromer, Community health care and the nursing process (St. Louis: C. V. Mosby Co. 1979).

Source: Adapted from Joanne Gingrich-Crass, Structural variables: factors affecting adaptation, in S. J. Wold *School nursing: A framework for practice* (St. Louis: C. V. Mosby Co., 1981) pp. 136–41. Copyright © 1981, Susan J. Wold. Reprinted by permission of Susan J. Wold.

Nursing must look beyond material boundaries

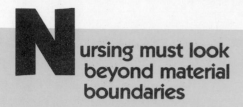

Are national boundaries a major factor in nursing? Although the resources, staffing, and level of function are by no means the same, there are great similarities across boundaries at the practice level. Health needs and health status, however, vary from country to country. We must ask ourselves if the many nurses who come from other countries to study in the United States are receiving the most appropriate educational experience for their future roles. Are our cultural values a source of conflict for these students? And what about all those American nurses who want to travel, lecture, consult abroad? Are cultural awareness and language skills needed? Where is the reciprocity? Is there nothing we can learn from others?

There has been much discussion about the need for better primary health care. As a profession, however, we also have to plan for appropriate care for those in institutions. The right to undergo hip replacement or cataract surgery, for example, cannot continue to belong only to the rich and the powerful who can travel abroad. Nurses must be prepared to better influence the care provided in institutional settings and to work to make it more available and accessible economically as well as geographically.

In July I visited a 100-bed hospital in a semi-rural area of a poor and economically less-developed country. There are usually 125–135 patients for 100 beds. The overflow are on mats on the floor. Many maternity patients, within 6 hours of delivery, are on those mats. They go home as soon after 6 hours as space is needed. The total qualified nursing staff is 9. There are several assistant nurse midwives who do most of the deliveries and routine care. The plumbing does not work, the electricity is erratic, corruption is a problem, and people from the countryside are not prepared to use the sanitary facilities, such as they are. What can be done to help nurses cope with, improve and change the system? Are the learning experiences provided to graduate students from developing countries the most suitable available to help them when they go home? If they do not go home, is that a failure?

Professionally we have to give as well as get and while many think that means going abroad as an expert it also means giving to nurses from other countries who are here. Many nurses remark warmly on the assistance and friendships offered to them during their study time here. Others say they needed someone to listen more, to take a personal interest, to help them to see how their experiences at home could be helpful in their studies.

Some of these people with a good understanding of health needs in their country are not even asked to share that information in their classes. Again, it's the old we-know-best, that-is-not-pertinent attitude that shuts you off from real understanding. It is through those links with students that future links are forged. Look at whom they invite to help them years later. It is people they feel were open and understanding in their student days who will be asked to consult or teach classes in their country later.

Finally, every culture has much to give and much to learn and we need to keep it a two-way street. What goes on in this continent should not always be rapidly spread to others. When attempts are made to move too fast, it can be seen as imperialistic. Challenges for the future within or beyond national boundaries are great in number. There will be no room for boredom and enough to challenge each of us for a long time to come.

Source: C. Holleran, Nursing beyond national boundaries: The 21st century, *Nursing Outlook,* March/April 1988, 36(2):72–75.

---

bed; some may be worn by the client. Nurses need to acquire permission from the client, family, or medicine man if these must be removed.

Healing ceremonies, sometimes referred to as *sings* or *prayers,* may be requested. These vary in length from 30 minutes to 9 days. Space and privacy need to be provided for such ceremonies. In the hospital, the sing usually lasts less than 1 hour. A medicine man may also be requested to perform curative rituals, which vary with the signs and symptoms of the client.

Native Americans believe that a state of health exists when a person is in total harmony with nature. The earth is considered a living organism that has a will and desire to be well, but, just as human beings, may be healthy or not. It is believed that when people harm the earth they harm themselves, and vice versa. Thus, Native Americans believe they should treat the body and the earth with respect.

Many Native Americans view illness not as an altered physiologic state but as an imbalance between the person who is ill and the natural or supernatural forces around the person. Causes of illness relate to this concept. Native Americans believe that if one interferes with this harmony by abusing or offending another person or thing, one may become ill. Even bad thoughts or wishes, such as jealousy or anger, may cause illness. In addition, supernatural or spiritual forces may be involved. In the Papago tribe of southern Arizona, for example, many persons believe that ghosts of the dead, returning as owls or other animals of night, bring sickness. All animals are believed to have supernatural powers, which they can use to send sickness (Winn 1976, p. 281).

Native Americans do not relate disease causation to germ theory. A survey of Native American registered nurses from 23 tribes revealed that none of these tribes had a word for *germ* (Henderson and Primeaux 1981, p. 243). This trait makes it difficult for Native Americans to understand the cause of illnesses such as tuberculosis, for example. Some Navajo Native Americans believed that the signs and symptoms of tuberculosis were the result of lightning. Using the wood of a tree struck by lightning for firewood or other purposes would cause the person to develop abscesses in the lungs (Wauneka 1976, p. 236).

The leading causes of death in the Native American population are accidents, suicide, diabetes, alcoholism, and homicide (Primeaux 1977, pp. 58–59). At least one-third of the Native American population is poverty-stricken. Associated with this income level are poor living conditions, malnutrition, tuberculosis, and high maternal and infant death rates. Native Americans have the highest infant mortality rate in the United States, even though their birth rate is almost twice that of the general population. This mortality rate is attributed to the high incidence of diarrhea in young babies and the harsh environment in which they live (Spector 1985, p. 187).

When caring for Native American clients, nurses need to consider the following:

1. Although most Native Americans recognize the value of Anglo-Western health care, many continue to use traditional medicine and cures either independently or in conjunction with such care.
2. Native American medicine and religion cannot be separated. Native Americans make no distinction between physical and mental illness or between the mind and the body. They live the concept of wholeness.
3. Tribal healing ceremonies and practices are highly ritualistic, religious ways to deal with sickness and death.
4. Tribal rituals that include extended "family" members are one way Native Americans share all aspects of life.
5. Each tribe assigns symbolic meanings to foods or other substances.
6. Such characteristics as not looking others in the eye should not be interpreted as disrespect, inattention, lack of interest, or avoidance.
7. Nurses attempting communication with Native Americans need to be aware of the following factors:
   ▪ It is the custom for the person to speak only for himself or herself.
   ▪ Use of extensive questions during history taking may be construed as an invasion of individual privacy. The history taker may need to rely on observation techniques and make declarative statements, e.g., "You have an obvious cough that keeps you awake at night," to elicit information from the client.
   ▪ Note taking may pose a barrier to communication, since Native Americans tend to value conversation, story telling, and listening.
   ▪ Native Americans often use a very low tone of voice, and the listener is expected to pay attention.

Black Americans

With the arrival of the first African slaves in Jamestown, Virginia, in 1619, a history of deprivation on this continent began for blacks. Even after slavery was abol-

ished, black people endured severe economic and social deprivation. The struggles to overcome these deprivations continue today. However, black American culture now is more similar to white American culture than it was 300 years ago. There is a large black middle class and a large black lower class. There are strong kinship bonds in both low-income and more prosperous black families. These families provide financial support, assist with child care, and serve as buffers against racism and discrimination during children's growing years. A black family may show much cohesion and sharing, particularly in times of trouble.

Often a significant member of a black family must be consulted before important decisions are made. This person may be a father, mother, aunt, son, or grandparent. Nurses need to be sensitive to the fact that a decision may not be made until this person is consulted.

When black Americans who are not familiar with the health care system enter it, they may show defensive behaviors such as hostility and suspicion. These attitudes are often adopted in expectation of being demeaned in some manner. It is important for nurses to recognize the reasons for these responses and learn to relate to all clients as worthy human beings.

Black Americans may believe traditionally that health is maintained by proper diet, which includes a hot breakfast. Some believe that laxatives are important to keep the system running and open (Spector 1985, p. 147). It is important for nurses to understand the values held by a black client and that person's definition of health.

Traditional definitions in black culture stem from the African view of life as a process rather than a state. All things, whether living or dead, were believed to influence each other (Spector 1985, p. 142). Health meant being in harmony with nature; illness was a state of disharmony. Therefore illness could be treated in a number of ways, including reliance on the power of a healer. These beliefs and practices may or may not apply to a particular black client. However, nurses should be aware of any cultural differences and take these into consideration when planning care. See also Table 17–1.

The major health problems of blacks in the United States are hypertension, sickle-cell disease, and cancers of the lungs, oral cavity, larynx, pharynx, esophagus, and urinary bladder. The increase in cancer in these areas is thought to be largely due to the increase in smoking (Orque et al. 1983, p. 106). Poverty among blacks leads to relatively high morbidity and mortality rates among infants and mothers, even though these rates have declined since 1960 (National Center for Health Statistics 1985).

The poor black client may not seek help until a health problem is serious for many reasons, e.g., "finances, child care problems, fear of hospitals, possibility of becoming a 'guinea pig,' and fear of death" (White 1977, p. 30), reasons often cited by poor clients regardless of ethnicity. Many black families in rural areas of the South continue to use folk health practices (Henderson and Primeaux 1981, p. 210) and home remedies. Voodoo and witchcraft are practiced to a minor extent (disease, for instance, may be attributed to a hex). Spiritualists or sorcerers may sometimes be consulted, or clients may vacillate between Western physicians and witch doctors or spiritualists who can remove spells. Historically, churches have been a bulwark of support for blacks, hence religious practices and Bible reading often continue during hospitalization.

Nursing implications relative to the care of the black client include: skin and hair care, assessing skin color, communication, and food preferences. Skin and hair care are discussed in Chapter 34. Many black people are very much aware of any signs of racial discrimination. A sensitive nurse should be alert for situations which may be interpreted as discriminatory and intervene as the client's advocate.

Black clients may favor a traditional rural Southern diet, an urban middle-class diet, or a combination of the two. Soul food is the traditional diet of the Southern black. Pork is the chief meat. Hominy grits, black-eyed peas, and mustard and collard greens are also included. To these are often added cabbage, rice, white potatoes, okra, macaroni, and noodles (Orque et al. 1983, pp. 95–96). Nurses can often assist blacks who are accustomed to eating soul food to adapt special diets to their tastes.

▪ Asian Americans

The term *Asian American* refers to four primary ethnic groups: Chinese, Japanese, Koreans, and Vietnamese. Recently the term *Pacific Asian* has been used to include people originally from the Pacific islands, such as the Philippines, Samoa, and Guam, as well as the other Asian countries. Because of the wide diversity of Asian cultures, full coverage of their views is beyond the scope of this book. This section focuses primarily on Chinese health beliefs and practices, since the traditions of many other Asians derive in part from them. The health beliefs and practices of Japanese Americans, Vietnamese Americans, and Filipino Americans will also be discussed briefly in separate segments.

▪ Chinese Americans.
The Chinese in the United States and Canada are largely concentrated on the west coasts of the countries, on the east coast of the United States, and in large cities such as New York and Chicago. The Chinese population can be considered in three groups: immigrants from rural China who arrived in North America 40 to 50 years ago (who still are largely oriented to Chinese folk medicine), new immigrants from several Asian countries and Hong Kong (who often practice a mixture of Chinese folk and Western medicine), and native North American descendants of nineteenth-century Chinese immigrants (who are oriented to Western medical practices but still may be influenced by their elders in regard to health care).

Prior to the revolution in China, the Chinese family was patriarchal and patrilineal. Respect for ancestors and parents was important, and obedience to the family was practiced. The Chinese frequently had extended families, with several generations living in one household. Family clans were strong social organizations formed of people of the same bloodline with the same surnames. People who came to North America 40 to 50 years ago set up the same traditional families.

Following the revolution, traditional family practices and superstitions became less evident in China and among immigrants. Although family ties continue to be strong, the nuclear family is now more common than the extended family in Chinese-American society. In many Asian families, at least two people are employed full time; they often use their incomes to support the extended family (Wang 1976, pp. 33–41).

Chinese folk medicine originated with Taoist philosophy. It proposes that the universe and health are regulated by two forces, the *yin* and the *yang*. The yin is a negative, female force; some of its characteristics are darkness, cold, and emptiness. The yang represents the positive, maleness, light, warmth, and fullness. When these two energy forces are in balance, health exists.

The Chinese do not consider their bodies to be personal property. The body is viewed as a gift provided by parents and ancestors, and it thus must be cared for. Various parts of the body are controlled by yin and yang. The inside, front part of the body and the five solid organs (*ts'ang*—the liver, heart, spleen, lungs, and kidneys) that collect and store secretions are controlled by yin. The outside, back part of the body, and five hollow organs (*fu*—the gallbladder, stomach, large and small intestines, and bladder) that excrete are controlled by yang. Yin stores the vital strength of life; yang protects the body from outside forces. A person who does not balance yin and yang properly will have a short life. Illness occurs when an imbalance of yin and yang exists. The sole cause of disease is considered to be disrupted harmony.

Chinese staples are polished tofu and rice. In addition vegetables such as bok choy, gai lan, spinach, Chinese cabbage, and mustard greens are favored. Many Chinese do not tolerate milk or cheese well.

Specific health problems more prevalent among the Chinese than the general population are eye problems, tuberculosis, dental caries, malnutrition, and mental illness. Some of these are directly related to the poor environmental conditions of North American Chinatowns rather than to an inherited predisposition. Because of the stress of adjusting to American culture and the lack of family support, mental health problems among aged male Chinese have increased. Another reason for emotional problems is the bicultural conflict between the individual values of freedom, egalitarianism, and individualism and the Chinese values of filial piety, loyalty, and authoritarianism (Orque et al. 1983, p. 196).

Chinese people of the older generations may believe that their blood is not replaceable. Therefore, they are often reluctant to give blood even for a blood test. Like many other people, the elderly Chinese often believe that a hospital is a place to go to die rather than to get well.

Some Chinese American clients follow both Western and Chinese medical advice at the same time. This can produce problems if the therapies are not correlated. For example, a client may receive two forms of the same drug, one from an herbalist and one from the Western physician, thus taking a double dose. Chinese clients should be encouraged to tell a doctor whether they are taking or receiving other therapy.

Pregnant women often observe folk medicine practices (e.g., the use of soy sauce may be restricted so that the baby's skin will not be very dark). In Chinese folk medicine, herbs and acupuncture are used. A folk medicine diagnosis is made chiefly by observing, questioning, listening to the body, and taking the pulse. The prescription is a combination of herbs, which are obtained from a Chinese pharmacy. Acupuncture is used chiefly to treat muscular and skeletal disorders and diseases characterized by excessive yang. Needles are inserted into the body at specific points along certain internal channels, which are called meridians. The internal organs are believed to be connected to the skin points and to the meridians; the acupuncture helps to balance the energy that flows within them. The following are some differences between Western practice and Chinese folk medicine:

1. One dose of an herbal medicine is thought to cure a person or make the person feel better. Thus, the Chinese client may be puzzled by a multiplicity of medicines prescribed in multiple doses.
2. Herbs are generally boiled in water for a prescribed time before being ingested rather than prepared as capsules or pills.
3. Chinese clients may change physicians during an illness in order to find the best cure. When they do so, they may not tell the former doctor because they do not want the doctor to lose face.
4. Some Chinese do not understand or react well to painful diagnostic procedures. They believe that a physician should be able to make a diagnosis solely on the basis of a physical examination. Many may leave the Western health care system to avoid distasteful procedures.
5. Most Chinese believe that it is best to die with the body intact. This belief originates with Confucius, who taught that only those who at the end of their lives return their physical bodies whole and sound shall be truly revered. As a result, Chinese clients may refuse surgery and donation of organs after death.
6. Ginseng is a highly valued herb used as a general strength tonic for the pregnant woman (Chung 1977, p. 71).

■ **Japanese Americans.** Japanese Americans often maintain a number of their cultural values while at the same time acculturating to the larger society. Four values of the Japanese are gaman, haji, enryo, and koko. *Gaman* means self-control. A Japanese person who is stoic when experiencing pain is probably practicing gaman. The client will not verbalize the pain and may try to deal with it. Japanese who carry on in spite of adversity are considered strong (Orque et al. 1983, p. 223).

Haji, or shame, is another important cultural concept. Japanese children are taught not to bring shame on themselves or their families by unacceptable behavior. *Enryo* is a type of behavior that encompasses politeness, respect, deference, reserve, and humility. The opposite of enryo is aggressive, boisterous, loud, rude behavior (Orque et al. 1983, p. 224). For example, a Japanese man might not turn on his signal light because he does not want to bother the nurses. *Koko* is filial piety. The Japanese perceive dependence as natural for the elderly and young children. An elderly person who is dependent still maintains self-esteem. This attitude contrasts to the North American view of dependence as a sign of weakness (Kalish 1967, pp. 65–69). Japanese Americans consider time valuable and like to use it well. They usually follow medication schedules precisely.

■ **Vietnamese Americans.** Thousands of Vietnamese came to the United States following the Vietnam war. Another, smaller group came later. South Vietnamese have a family-centered culture in which the children are taught to value the family's interests over their own (Orque et al. 1983, p. 250). Vietnamese value propriety over time and indirectness over confrontation. In a disagreement, they tend to avoid confrontation to preserve harmony. A Vietnamese client who is embarrassed at a nurse's question may say yes or laugh to lessen his or her embarrassment.

■ **Filipino Americans.** The Filipino culture is diverse. However, its central cultural values are shaped by a fatalistic view that God's will and supernatural forces determine what happens. Filipino culture is family centered, stressing interdependency among members of the family. Filipinos also emphasize achievement and social acceptance. A Filipino client is likely to avoid a disagreement with a nurse and speak evasively. By contrast, the white middle-class American may value an open expression of feelings and thoughts. Because of their fatalistic view, Filipinos often show great patience and endurance when faced with illness.

Hispanic Americans

Hispanic Americans have their origins in a number of Spanish-speaking countries: Mexico, Spain, Cuba, Puerto Rico, and the nations of Central and South America. One of the largest groups for whom Spanish is the dominant tongue is the Mexican American population. Because a full discussion of each Hispanic American culture and its health care implications is beyond the scope of this book, the following pages focus on Mexican American beliefs and practices.

Traditional Mexican American foods are beans and tortillas. For clients requiring a special diet, traditional foods can present problems, requiring special planning in consultation with dietitians. For example, many Hispanics generally prefer rice to potatoes. The manner of preparing the rice is important; it differs from the Asian method. The diet of many low-income Mexican Americans often contains a high proportion of starches: tortillas, beans, corn, and so on. It is usually possible to plan diets to meet clients' preferences and thus increase the chances that the food will be eaten.

Mexican Americans have extended families that play an important part in their lives. The family is usually large, and life revolves around the home. Often the family's needs take precedence over the individual's needs. At a time of illness, the family gives a great deal of support. In the Mexican-American family, the woman is the primary caregiver, and often she decides when medical assistance should be sought.

Many Mexican Americans entered the United States during the early 1900s and brought with them the values, beliefs, and practices of rural Mexico; others are more recent immigrants. Folk concepts of health and illness continue to affect the thinking of some second- and third-generation Mexican Americans today.

Mexican Americans perceive health as the ability to maintain a high level of normal physical activity and illness as a state of discomfort. Some Mexican Americans also believe that certain people can use magical powers to make others ill (Abril 1977, pp. 169–70). Some Mexican Americans believe that illness is due to life-style. They often have precise ideas about the types of rest, activity, recreation, and nutrition that lead to poor and good health (Gonzalez-Swafford and Gutierrez 1983, p. 29). Illness is seen as an imbalance in the individual's body or as a punishment for wrongdoing. The causes of illness can be grouped into four categories (Spector 1985, pp. 161–63):

1. *Imbalance between "hot" and "cold" or "wet" and "dry."* The four humors or body fluids that must be in balance are: blood (hot and wet), phlegm (cold and wet), yellow bile (hot and dry), and black bile (cold and dry). When these fluids are not in balance, illness results. Treatment in hospitals can be based on the principles of hot and cold. For example, illnesses that are classified as hot are treated with food, drugs, and drinks that are classified as cold.

2. *Magic or supernatural forces.* Mal de ojo (evil eye) is disease caused by forces outside the body, such as a person's admiration of part of another person's body, e.g., the hair. The victim can lose the admired part or fall ill. In some places, *mal de ojo* is thought to be prevented by having the admirer touch the admired person while complimenting him or her, and it is believed to be cured with eggs in a ritual. The symptoms of mal de ojo include headaches, fever, fatigue, and prostration.

3. *"Dislocation" of body parts.* One example of a disease of "dislocation" is *empacho,* a disease primarily seen in children. *Empacho* produces swelling of the abdomen as a result of intestinal blockage and is thought to be caused by overeating foods such as soft bread and bananas.

4. *Strong emotional states. Susto,* a disease of emotional origin, is fright caused by natural phenomena such as lightning or loud noises. The symptoms have been described as insomnia, restlessness, and nervousness. It is a common folk disease that is difficult to cure, but it can be treated with herbal tea. *Espanto* is a disease with symptoms similar to those of susto. Its origin is fright caused by seeing supernatural spirits or events. *Coraje* is rage, a response to a particular situation. The victim may continually scream, cry, or yell and display hyperactivity.

Many Mexican Americans, when they are ill, may believe a folk medicine diagnosis rather than a Western diagnosis, even though they may also seek help from a Western physician. Healers within the Mexican American community can be either male (a *curandero*) or female (a *curandera*). They offer a number of treatments; one of the most frequently used is herb tea. Mexican Americans have a personal relationship with the curandero, in contrast to the relationship with health care workers in a hospital.

Puerto Rican beliefs about health and illness are not unlike those of Mexican Americans. Their diseases are also classified as hot and cold; however, food and medications are classified as hot (*caliente*), cold (*frío*), and cool (*fresco*) (Spector 1985, p. 167). Hispanic Americans consider the appearance of blood and the presence of pain as indicators that an illness is severe. If it is "natural" for a condition to occur, it is considered harmless. When it is unnatural and folk methods fail, most Mexican Americans seek medical assistance from Western practitioners.

Mexican Americans are generally proud people. Those who are socially and economically deprived may well have low self-esteem and be reluctant to accept care for which they cannot pay. Therefore, Mexican American clients in the hospital may not ask for help when they have pain; a young Mexican-American male may react with hostility rather than passivity in response to nursing intervention to uphold his self-image.

As do people of diverse ethnic backgrounds, many Mexican Americans look upon the hospital as a place to die. Thus, they may avoid hospitals when they can and enter only with great fear, feeling that death is imminent. Illness is generally regarded not as a personal affair but as a family affair. Therefore, when a person is ill, many relatives generally gather around and visit. Restricting visitors can cause mistrust; nurses need to deal with such a requirement in the context of illness and discuss the matter with the entire family. See Figure 17–2.

As a cultural group, Mexican Americans are very modest. Usually they consider bathing, defecating, and urinating to be very personal matters, yet they may be shy about asking a nurse to leave at such times. The sensitive nurse will provide complete privacy when possible.

Hispanic Americans encounter a number of barriers to health care: language, poverty, and time orientation. To many Hispanic Americans time is relative; the exact time is not a primary consideration. This hinders effective use of a health care system that values promptness

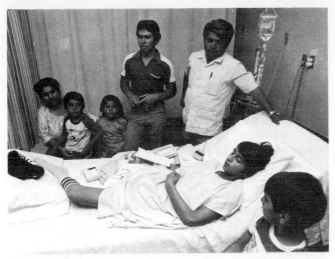

Figure 17—2 Illness is a matter of concern for an entire Hispanic family.

for appointments and mandates specific intervals between doses of medications. Language is another major barrier for many Hispanic Americans seeking help from the health care delivery system. Some do not speak English, and communication is difficult and embarrassing in a system in which the English language predominates. In addition, some Hispanic Americans are below the poverty line. They may not have knowledge of available health resources in the community or the money to use them.

Not all Hispanic Americans identify with their ethnic groups; many identify with white middle-class Americans. The nurse should not stereotype the Hispanic-American or any other client. There are diverse beliefs and practices among various Hispanic-American groups. For example, the majority of Hispanic Americans, though not all, are Roman Catholic (Orque et al. 1983, p. 121). The man in a Hispanic-American family may find it difficult to depend on other family members or even a nurse to do things for him. He expects to decide when and how things should be done, and he should be involved in decisions if health permits.

■ **A**ppalachians

The 24 million Appalachians in the United States, 6 million of whom live in the Southern Appalachian region, are a subculture in American society (Tripp-Reimer and Friedl 1977, p. 41). A family-oriented group, Appalachians include upper, middle, and poor working classes. The upper and middle classes tend to share many values with the rest of the United States, just as the poverty group does with other poverty groups in America. Much of Appalachia is rural, encompassing parts of the states of New York, Pennsylvania, Ohio, Maryland, West Virginia, Virginia, Kentucky, Tennessee, North Carolina, South Carolina, Georgia, and Alabama (Tripp-Reimer and Friedl 1977, p. 43).

The religion of the Appalachians tends to be fundamentalist and fatalistic. Sometimes this fatalism prevents clients from seeking help when they are ill (Lewis

et al. 1985, p. 24). Appalachians value family greatly. The family provides its members with a sense of belonging and a sense of identity. Appalachians value family privacy, a situation that has created some social and cultural isolation. Often many family members accompany a client to a health appointment, and they may wish to stay with the client if he or she is hospitalized. For many Appalachians, socialization begins and ends within the family.

The family is generally large and patriarchal. There are definite divisions between the work of men and women. Family ties are strong, and antagonism against another family may be intense. Time orientation is in the present, and the pressure of finances makes it difficult to plan ahead. Education is usually not a high priority.

Appalachians tend to define an individual as ill only when the person feels ill. They have a general distrust of health organizations and may fear surgery. The health problems of the Appalachians are largely related to their economic circumstances and to their occupations. Nutritional problems are frequently due to the fact that they cannot afford to buy much meat, and the diet may be deficient in protein and iron. Some Appalachians work in coal mines, and prolonged exposure to coal dust can cause sarcoidosis, a disease of the lungs.

When Appalachians feel ill, they tend to try home remedies, e.g., herb teas and tonics. If these cures are not effective, they may seek the advice of a lay practitioner, e.g., a "granny midwife," an herbalist, or a faith healer. In an emergency or during childbirth, an Appalachian may seek "orthodox" medical or nursing help.

The nurse caring for an Appalachian client should be aware of certain customs and values. Appalachians consider direct eye contact to be staring, which is impolite. Nurses should be aware that Appalachians use direct eye contact to express anger or aggression. Nurses should also understand that Appalachians follow the "ethic of neutrality":

■ A person must not be assertive or aggressive.

■ A person should mind his or her own business unless asked to do otherwise.

■ A person should not assume authority over others.

■ Appalachians avoid argument and seek agreement (Hicks 1976).

■ **A**rab Americans

There are approximately 3 million Arabs in the United States, including people who are in America temporarily (Meleis 1981, p. 1181). Most Arabs have a common language and share symbols, mores, and beliefs. Arabs are traditionally future oriented and value the use of time to achieve future goals.

The Arab family is traditionally patriarchal and extended. The male of the household is responsible for earning the living outside the home and for making the decisions; women usually remain at home. Arabs have a need to affiliate with others and use an extensive social network to cope with daily stress (Meleis 1981, p. 1181). Food plays an important part in Arab family life. When family members assemble, it is often around elaborate meals. Love and care are interwoven (Meleis 1981, p. 1182). Christian Arabs consume pork and alcohol, whereas Muslims consume neither. Sometimes Arab Americans find hospital food too bland and prefer to have food brought from home.

Arabs believe that injury or disease affects the whole person. Often Arabs provide a vague description of their illness rather than precise symptoms because they do not have a framework for signs and symptoms. Arabs usually do not refute the germ theory, but they do believe in disease-causing entities such as the evil eye. Arabs also believe that being deprived of food can cause illness.

One health problem that Arabs have in common with other Mediterranean peoples is thalassemia, a genetic condition that results in anemia. It occurs in 7 to 15% of the population in the Middle East (Overfield 1985, p. 85). Arabs do not believe in sharing a problem until help is offered. The person offering help should be able to assess the need without verifying the problem. If a nurse offers an Arab client a choice in care, the client is likely to say "No, thank you." If the nurse accepts this refusal, the client believes the nurse is not interested.

Arabs dislike disclosing information about themselves to strangers and will provide as little information as possible. Nurses must be sensitive to an Arab's dislike of revealing personal information. Sometimes Arabs will defer dealing with a matter until they feel more comfortable sharing information and may rely upon others, i.e., the social network, to give advice at times of stress. Arabs generally respect Western health care. Intrusive procedures are often highly regarded and thought to offer the greatest chance of cure.

Many Arabs regard health care as their right, and some may view health care professionals as their employees. Arab Americans respect expertise, which they regard as knowing about problems, making decisions for others, and being accountable for those decisions (Meleis 1981, p. 1182). Arab Americans may not question caregivers openly because of their respect for authority. Some Arabs wear amulets for protection. Even to say the number "five" is believed to increase protection. Deaths are believed to be the result of the will of God and the inadequacy of equipment and medicine.

Income Groups

The poor and the rich are viewed by some as subcultures of the dominant society. Indeed, many believe economic status to be more influential than culture when predicting responses to health and illness. To describe the lower classes or the upper classes of society as subcultures, one must study both the strengths and the weaknesses of their life situations and behaviors. Unfortunately, many studies dealing with poverty-stricken people tend to focus on only the negative aspects, and little has been written about the health care beliefs, practices, and problems of the rich.

■ High-Income Groups.
Beliefs and behaviors of the rich tend to vary according to whether the persons come from second- or third-generation wealth. Second-generation wealthy persons (new rich) who are close to their parents' value systems tend to value the "work ethic" (Henry and DiGiacomo-Geffers 1980, p. 1426). These persons in their early years had fewer economic advantages and participated in the struggle to get ahead.

In contrast, the third-generation rich (older rich) tend not to value work (Henry and DiGiacomo-Geffers 1980, p. 1426). They have been accustomed to wealth from birth, were raised largely by employed help, and grow up expecting great freedom with little discipline. Having the means to pay for counseling services, a greater percentage of this group tends to seek psychotherapy than does the rest of the population. Grinker (1978, p. 913) summarizes some of the common characteristics of persons within this group who seek psychotherapy: feelings of emptiness and boredom, low self-awareness, lack of introspection, lack of empathy, lack of interest in work, intense pursuit of pleasure and excitement, the belief that they can be happy only with persons like themselves, and the belief that use of their wealth (buying, spending, travel) will solve their emotional problems.

Beliefs about health, illness, and death among the rich depend on their specific religion and culture. Generally the rich tend to believe in the prevention of illness through diet, exercise, and good health habits. They make frequent use of the health care system and self-help information and have ready access to the health care system through private physicians.

Specific problems nurses may encounter with the hospitalized rich are outlined by Henry and DiGiacomo-Geffers (1980, p. 1428). Being accustomed to highly responsive employed help, the rich person tends to have the same expectations of nurses, who then feel they are being treated like servants. This behavior is often an attempt to gain attention and to control the unfamiliar, uncertain environment and sometimes interferes with implementing care because the nurse and client may have different priorities.

Outward appearance is often of critical importance to nationally known people, who are accustomed to being in the limelight. Prior to surgery, some may refuse to remove makeup or dentures, and they must be removed after a general anesthetic agent is administered. In some cases, clients or their families literally redecorate hospital rooms. Drapes and bedcoverings may be changed, paintings hung on the walls, and the room stocked with expensive personal supplies such as liqueurs and floral arrangements. Some clients may request that care be provided only by persons of their own ethnic background. The client may abandon such expectations when he or she understands the need for assigning nurses with appropriate skills for the client's care.

■ Low-Income Groups.
The status of being poor is often referred to as the "culture of poverty," a phrase coined by anthropologist Oscar Lewis in the 1960s. Lewis (1966, p. 19) defined the culture of poverty as a sub-

culture of Western society with its own values and behaviors, which differ from those of the nonpoor and are passed on from generation to generation. This subculture transcends ethnic and regional boundaries. Characteristics of the poor include: lack of participation in the larger society, hostility toward and mistrust of bureaucratic institutions, inadequate use of health services, long periods of unemployment, use of public assistance, abandonment of mothers and children by fathers, lack of privacy, disciplining of children by physical violence, orientation to the present, fatalistic attitudes, and strong feelings of helplessness, dependence, and inferiority (Lewis 1966, pp. 19–25).

Lewis's portrayal of the poor as a subculture is challenged by other researchers, who believe this cultural viewpoint is negative, reflects no attempt to question why these features exist, and fails to recognize the role of the larger society in perpetuating poverty. Some research has shown, for example, that the poor have the same values as the rest of society and that the traits Lewis identified may not be cultural but rather responses to situational circumstances. For example, the negative work behaviors associated with the lower class are not culturally derived but situationally induced. It has been shown that the poor have a strong work ethic, want to work, and do work when given equal opportunity (Mason 1981, p. 83). Lack of societal incentives may prevent the poor from obtaining and holding a job. Situational theorists believe, therefore, that if society were rid of poverty, the former poor would demonstrate middle-class attitudes and behaviors.

Still other researchers suggest that all members of a society share general, abstract values but that specific, concrete values differ among subgroups and social classes. This viewpoint combines the cultural and situational perspectives of poverty into an adaptational perspective. In other words, the poor are considered a special subgroup of society formed in response to social structures that make it impossible for them to actualize the values and behavior forms of the dominant society.

Geographic and social factors influence poverty. Geographic poverty refers to the existence of "pockets of poverty." In the United States, these pockets occur in dense urban areas (e.g., the ghettos) and in rural regions such as Appalachia, the deep South, the lower Southwest, and northern New England. Unless people move out of such regions of poverty, they are likely to remain destitute, since social mobility, education, and employment opportunities are scarce. In spite of reform efforts, local governments have been ineffective in improving conditions in such areas. Massive outside assistance is required to upgrade services in education, sanitation, health, employment, job training, transportation, and welfare.

Social factors of poverty include demographic characteristics that determine what social position a person occupies. Among such characteristics are race, age, family structure and size, education, income, and type of work. Black Americans, Native Americans, and Hispanic Americans are overrepresented in poor populations. People over 65 years of age also account for a substantial number of the impoverished, and the number is increasing in direct relationship to inflation. About one-third of the total poverty population is comprised of youths and children of poor parents. Families in which the mother is the major support are generally poorer than families in which the father is the major support, since employment opportunities and incomes for females are substantially less than for males. Large families with set incomes also are more impoverished. Lower educational attainment and lack of educational opportunities contribute to lower employment opportunities and income. The typical low-income person has less than an eighth grade education and, if employed, works at an unskilled occupation.

Low-income families often define health in terms of work; if people can work, they are healthy. They tend to be fatalistic and to believe that illness is not preventable. Because their present problems are so great and all efforts are exerted toward survival, an orientation to the future may be lacking. Many low-income people do not have regular preventive medical checkups because they cannot afford them. It is more important to them to work than to visit a physician and thus lose a day's pay. Reliance on public assistance and inability to afford health care insurance limit both the low-income person's access to health care and the type of care available.

The environmental conditions of poverty-stricken areas also have a bearing on overall health. Slum neighborhoods are overcrowded and in a state of deterioration. Neglect and disorder are common. Sanitation services tend to be inadequate. Many streets are strewn with garbage, and alleys are overrun by rats. Fires and crime are constant threats. Recreational facilities are almost nonexistent, forcing children to play in streets and alleys. Parents who can work usually work long hours and earn barely enough for subsistence. They are often too tired to spend much time with their children, even though they love them. As a result, preschool children often come and go as they please, and older siblings assume the role of parent for younger children. With all of these problems confronting the poor, it is little wonder that frustration tolerance levels are low, physical abuse is used in discipline, and value is placed on children seeking employment rather than completing their educations.

Recently attention has been focused on a subculture within the poor, the **homeless.** No longer considered derelicts, bums, or drifters, there are an estimated 250,000 to 3 million people who are homeless in the United States, including families, children, military veterans, and persons with serious and persistent alcohol, drug abuse, and mental health disorders (ANA 1987, p. 26). Recognizing that the existing health care system is not accessible to the homeless, the 1987 ANA House of Delegates adopted an emergency resolution on housing and health care for people who are homeless. In this resolution, the delegates pledged to work to ensure that funding is available to provide needed services.

The poor have the same needs and feelings as other people. They are sensitive, concerned, and easily embarrassed. When admitted to health care agencies, they are sometimes treated in humiliating, condescending, and prejudicial ways by misinformed caregivers. Because prejudice is usually based on fear of the unknown, and fear is based on insecurity, it is important for nurses to examine their own values and attitudes. Nurses need to become culturally sensitive and to accept and respect the differences in the life-styles of others.

Middle-Class Anglo-Americans

Middle-class Americans are predominantly descendants of immigrants who came to the United States at least two generations ago. The group is composed largely of white, Anglo-Saxon Protestants (WASPs). Traditionally, the white middle-class American family was patriarchal; the father went to work and the mother was responsible for housekeeping and child-rearing. However, this pattern is changing. The need for extra income, the new assertiveness of women in response to the women's movement, increased awareness of life alternatives, and the rising educational level of women have all contributed to this change. In 1960, only 19% of women with young children were employed outside the home (Hayghe 1976, pp. 12–19); by 1982, 47.8% of women with preschool children were employed (Hayghe 1982, pp. 53–56).

The middle-class American family is generally family oriented. Parents have a strong desire to provide better opportunities for their children than the parents had when they were children. For this reason, they emphasize education. The Protestant work ethic strongly influences the family. A prevailing attitude is that men should work to support their families. Certain work roles are often associated with men and others with women. Middle-class American families are often materialistic. A middle-class person might measure the success of the neighbors by the model of their car or the size of their house. Middle-class Americans are usually future oriented and as such may be very concerned about both the immediate effect of an illness and its implications for the future.

Studies have shown that people differ widely in their personal definitions of health and their health beliefs. Hautman and Harrison (1982, p. 53) found that many people defined good health as the absence of sickness. Some people stated that their health was good because they could function adequately in spite of the presence of such diseases as a prior heart attack or ongoing diarrhea.

Many of the health problems of middle-class Americans are related to life-style. Despite an increasing awareness of the roles of diet and exercise in disease prevention, many middle-class Americans believe serious illness "happens to others but not to me." Studies show that diagnosis of an individual's illness is usually made by the person, explained within his or her personal or cultural folk model, and usually dealt with by self-care (Hautman and Harrison 1982, p. 51). For additional information on health and illness, see Chapter 2.

In the American health care system, many nurses belong to the middle class. A major danger is that nurses may not allow for individual differences and may expect clients' values to conform to their own. Another implication is the cost of health care measures. Many people are conscious of costs, which can affect the degree to which clients follow health care measures. Middle-class clients relate illness to the future and want to deal with future implications early in their illnesses.

The Gay Community

The gay community can be considered a subculture. **Homosexuality** may be defined as repeated and preferential same-sex contacts (Roundtable 1980, p. 69). Gays and lesbians share beliefs, values, and customs of the larger culture; such beliefs are often reflective of their ethnicity, income, or cultural background. However, they may function as members of a gay or lesbian community and as such share values and beliefs common to those communities. One of the most prevalent beliefs of gay and lesbian communities is that sexual and affectional relationships between individuals of the same sex are normal and positive.

Sex roles in the lesbian and gay communities differ from those in the nongay community in that both partners often perform all tasks that are normally assigned by gender in the nongay community. For example, both partners may cook, garden, work, and be supportive. These roles may carry over into the health care setting, where a man may comfort another man or a woman may deal assertively with a situation as well as be supportive of her partner. Health care professionals who are not gay may find these nontraditional sex-role behaviors unsettling.

Areas of concern to both gays and lesbians include health care issues regarding the genitals, sexuality, and sexually transmitted diseases. They may be reluctant to disclose information about sexual behavior to health care professionals, or they may feel anxious about those professionals' attitudes toward sexuality. For instance, the client may not wish to confide in a heterosexual health professional. For these reasons, some areas of the United States have health clinics especially for gay men and lesbians. In addition, many women, including lesbians, prefer women-centered community health centers because they consider traditional health centers sexist. Another concern of some lesbians is alternative modes of fertilization.

A major health problem of gay men is acquired immune deficiency syndrome (AIDS), first noted in 1981. Funding for research, education, and services is vital, since the U.S. Public Health Service has declared AIDS America's number one public health priority. The 1987 ANA House of Delegates adopted a policy statement on AIDS opposing universal mandatory testing and supporting voluntary anonymous HIV (AIDS virus) testing preceded by informed consent and followed by appropriate counseling by qualified health care professionals. The ANA also reaffirmed its commitment to protect the civil and human rights of persons with AIDS and their caregivers (ANA 1987b, pp. 1–2).

It is important for nurses to be informed about homosexuality and to convey a nonjudgmental attitude of acceptance toward homosexual clients and their support persons, helping the latter just as they would the support persons of a heterosexual client. Nurses need to elicit only that information required for the nursing history. The client needs reassurance that the information he or she gives will be kept confidential and conveyed only to health professionals requiring it.

Health Care System as a Subculture

Nurses should remember that the health care system is also a subculture. This system has rules, customs, and a language of its own. When obtaining an education in health care, individuals become acculturated into the system. But clients who enter the system may experience culture shock. For example, the health care culture values cleanliness; thus, nurses wash their hands often and expect their clients to wash daily. This value may not be shared by all clients, and the practice of washing daily may be new for some people.

The health care culture has its own definition of health; often it is defined as "an optimal level of functioning." See Chapter 2 for additional information. Diagnosis and prescription are usually carried out by physicians, often in offices, clinics, or hospitals. Healing practices are based on scientific knowledge. Treatment procedures are frequently embarrassing or uncomfortable. The emotional component of disease is often ignored (Wold 1981, p. 140).

Jargon is widely used in the system and tends to make clients and support persons feel like outsiders. Many health care workers are from the middle class; they often expect gratitude for the care they give. Strict time orientation is adhered to and highly valued. This orientation may conflict with the client's. By keeping written records, caregivers may even be creating conflict with clients' cultural beliefs.

Traditionally, health care workers interpreted the death of a client as failure. This belief is currently being reconsidered. Measures were often taken to preserve the lives of clients but seldom to facilitate death. Currently, clinical nurse specialists called *thanatology nurses* work with families and clients coping with a terminal illness.

By recognizing that they have been acculturated into the health care system, nurses can often identify the values of the system they have adopted. It is then easier to recognize how a client's values differ from those of the system. These differing values may be a source of anxiety or frustration to clients and their support persons.

Where there is a conflict between the client's beliefs and those of the health care system, nurses can try to help the client find a common ground. When the client tries new behavior patterns, nurses can support his or her efforts and provide positive reinforcement. If the client experiences inadequacy or anxiety, nurses can help by openly accepting the client and his or her values, beliefs, and customs.

To provide meaningful nursing care, nurses must be aware of a client's ethnic and cultural values, beliefs, and practices as they relate to his or her health and health care. Additionally, the nurse must develop an awareness of how personal ethnic and cultural values, attitudes, and practices relate to nursing practice. Cultural awareness can be attained by using a values clarification approach (see Chapter 5).

Assessment

A number of assessment guides can help nurses gathering ethnic and cultural data. Basic cultural data that should be collected are summarized in the accompanying box. The purpose of an ethical-cultural assessment is "to identify deviations in cultural parameters with the goal of modifying the client's system or modifying the health care professional's system in order to increase congruence between them" (Tripp-Reimer et al. 1984, p. 81).

A general assessment of the client identifies significant characteristics and suggests areas for in-depth assessment. At this stage, the nurse makes no conclusions but obtains information from the client. The data should be both subjective, preferably in the client's words, and objective. An example of subjective data is this client statement: "I think it is very important to be healthy." An example of objective data is "Attended school to grade 3 in rural Mexico." At this time, it is also important to collect information that affects the nurse-client interaction, e.g., language, etiquette, style of communication.

The general assessment should be followed by an assessment that is specific to the health care area of concern, e.g., preschool immunizations, diabetic teaching, home care. At this time, the nurse obtains information about the client's own reason for seeking out health care, his or her ideas about the current problem and any previous problems, and the treatment he or she anticipates. For example, the client may say, "I came to the center because I feel ill; the world is moving around me. This happened once before. The doctor gave me

Basic Cultural Data

- Ethnic affiliation
- Religious preference
- Family patterns
- Food patterns
- Ethnic health care practices

(Tripp-Reimer et al. 1984, p. 79)

some pills, and it went away." Some questions that may elicit this information are:

1. What do you think caused your problem?
2. What treatment do you think you need now?
3. What are the chief problems your sickness has caused you? (Kleinman et al. 1978, p. 254.)

Nursing Diagnosis

The nursing diagnoses for a client who has special ethnic or cultural needs can relate to any number of factors, such as language and diet. See examples in the accompanying box.

Impaired verbal communication is the "state in which the individual experiences, or could experience, a decreased ability to speak but can understand others" (Carpenito 1987, p. 187). Among the defining characteristics of this nursing diagnosis are the inability to speak the dominant language and difficulty in finding the correct words when speaking, both of which the person of a minority ethnic group or culture might display. In addition to the listed etiologic factor (language barrier), this diagnosis may also be related to fear, shyness, lack of privacy, or lack of support system (all possible etiologic or contributing factors for minority group clients) as well as pathophysiologic and situational conditions.

Ineffective individual and **family coping** were discussed in Chapter 14. **Powerlessness** is the "state in which an individual perceives a lack of personal control over certain events or situations" (Carpenito 1987, p. 474). Its characteristics include expressing dissatisfaction over inability to control what is happening, refusing or being reluctant to participate in decision making, apathy, depression, or resignation to the situation. As discussed earlier in this chapter, people from some cultures are fatalistic about the meaning of illness and the purpose of hospitalization. It would be incorrect for the nurse to make this nursing diagnosis if the client values such a belief.

NURSING DIAGNOSIS

Ethnicity and Culture

- Impaired verbal communication related to language barrier
- Ineffective individual coping related to change in environment
- Ineffective family coping related to absence of extended family
- Powerlessness related to inability to communicate verbally
- Social isolation related to language barrier

Social isolation is the "state in which the individual experiences a need or desire for contact with others but is unable to make that contact" (Carpenito 1987, p. 563). This is a difficult diagnosis to describe. Carpenito comments: "Since social isolation is a subjective state, all inferences made regarding a person's feelings of aloneness must be validated. Because the causes vary and people show their aloneness in different ways, there are no absolute clues to this diagnosis" (1987, p. 563). This diagnosis is most likely for the client whose family or support persons are not nearby during the hospitalization.

Planning

When planning nursing goals, the nurse needs to include appropriate cultural factors relative to the client. According to Tripp-Reimer et al. (1984, p. 81), this stage "is directed at cultural factors that may influence nursing strategies." For example, nurses can ask a client such questions as "What would you normally eat while you have this condition?" or "Is there something I haven't mentioned that you think would be helpful?" These questions demonstrate respect for the client and his or her beliefs or practices.

After obtaining this information, a nurse must organize the data. According to Tripp-Reimer et al., "the nurse is interested in the extent to which the client's beliefs, values, and customs are congruent with a trifold set of standards:

1. Standards of the client's identified culture or ethnic group
2. Standards of the nurse's own culture
3. Standards of the health care facility that serves as the setting for the interaction" (Tripp-Reimer et al. 1984, p. 81)

A nurse may find that the data among the three standards are not congruent. For example, a client always eats rice as a major part of each meal. The nurse learns that this practice is standard for the client's ethnic group, recognizes that this practice differs from her or his own, and realizes that the health care facility cannot provide rice for each meal. Next, the nurse relates this information by determining whether the treatment plan accommodates the client's eating practices. If not, then the nurse can find ways of integrating the client's practice into the nursing care plan, e.g., the client's family might bring cooked rice to the hospital. If, however, rice is contraindicated because of the client's condition, the nurse must establish ways to help the client change if the client is amenable to change or ways to understand the client if the client will not change (Tripp-Reimer et al. 1984, p. 81).

Possible goals for the nursing diagnoses discussed earlier in this chapter are included in the accompanying

GOAL STATEMENTS

Ethnicity and Culture

- The client will be able to communicate basic needs.
- The client will adapt to the change in environment necessitated by hospitalization.
- The family will establish effective coping mechanisms for dealing with the client's hospitalization.
- The client will express feelings of regaining control of situation.
- The client will maintain social contact with visitors and staff.

GUIDELINES

Interacting with Clients of Differing Culture or Ethnicity

1. Convey respect for the individual and respect for his or her values, beliefs, and cultural and ethnic practices.
2. Learn about the major ethnic or cultural groups with whom you are likely to have contact.
3. Be aware of your own communication, e.g., facial expression and body language, and how it may be interpreted. See Chapter 20 for additional information.
4. Be aware of differences in ways clients communicate, and do not assume the meaning of a specific behavior, e.g., lack of eye contact, without considering the client's ethnic and cultural background.
5. Be aware of your own biases, prejudices, and stereotypes.
6. When a client describes a belief that differs from your own, e.g., the cause of his swollen feet, try to relate the client's belief to yours, thus conveying interest and respect for the client's beliefs.
7. Recognize that cultural symbols and practices can often bring a client comfort.
8. Support the client's practices and incorporate them into nursing practice whenever it is possible and they are not contraindicated for health reasons, e.g., provide hot tea to a client who drinks hot tea and never drinks cold water.
9. Do not impose a cultural practice on a client without knowing whether it is acceptable, e.g., Puerto Rican clients prefer not to be touched unnecessarily (Shubin 1980, p. 29).
10. Be aware that the color of a client's skin does not always determine his or her culture.
11. Take time to learn how a client views health, illness, grieving, and the health care system.
12. Be aware of your own attitudes and beliefs about health and objectively examine the logic of those attitudes and beliefs and their origins.
13. Be open to learning about different beliefs and values and learn not to be threatened when they differ from your own.

box. Specific outcome criteria that make these goals measurable are discussed in the section on evaluation, later in the chapter. It is often important to include the client's family in the planning of nursing care, particularly if the client is a member of an extended family and if the family is a major support for the client. When planning care strategies, nurses should consider language barriers and assess the need for an interpreter. Sometimes ethnic clients require information to avoid confusion or embarrassment. For example, an ethnic client who is extremely modest may require considerable preparation and support before having an enema.

Implementation

Successful nursing interventions for ethnic clients require supportive communication by nurses and respect for the client's values, beliefs, and practices. White (1977) stresses the importance of being culturally sensitive. Cultural sensitivity includes: feeling respect for individuals, recognizing that people have their own cultural beliefs and practices, being able to act on behalf of the ethnic client who is being denied safe, quality care, and modifying the care plan by incorporating those client beliefs and practices that are not life threatening (Bello 1976, pp. 36–38, 45). Suggested guidelines for nurses are shown in the accompanying box.

Evaluation

To evaluate the effectiveness of nursing care of clients in special ethnic and cultural groups, the nurse determines the extent to which the goals have been met by comparing the client's current status with predetermined outcome or evaluation criteria (see Chapter 12).

The accompanying box lists outcome criteria that may be used to evaluate the goal statements presented earlier in this chapter.

Nurses must also evaluate their own competence in this area by asking themselves questions such as these: "How well did I communicate?" "How well did I include the client and his or her family in the nursing process?" "How well do I understand the client's values, beliefs, and customs?" "How well did I communicate respect for these?" "Was I able to incorporate any of the client's values, beliefs, and customs into the plan of care?" "How

OUTCOME CRITERIA

Ethnicity and Culture

The client:

- Relates feelings, concerns, requests through interpreter.
- Establishes an effective method of communication with verbal and nonverbal cues.
- Participates in the decision-making process regarding planned care.
- Uses family/friends and unit staff to assist with adaptation to changes in the environment.
- Indicates feelings of greater control over the illness and therapy.
- Interacts with staff through an interpreter or by using nonverbal cues.

The client's family:

- Uses available resources to adapt to the client's hospitalization.
- Employs effective alternative strategies for meeting those needs usually met by the extended family.

well did I communicate my acceptance of values, beliefs, and customs that differ from mine?" "Am I aware of my values, beliefs, and customs?"

Chapter Highlights

North Americans come from a variety of ethnic and cultural backgrounds, and many North Americans retain at least some of their traditional values, beliefs, and practices.

Many minority groups in North America embrace two cultures: the culture of their ethnic origin and the North American culture.

An individual's ethnic and cultural background can influence beliefs, values, and customs.

Through acculturation, most ethnic and cultural minority groups in North America modify some of their traditional cultural characteristics.

Individual factors frequently modify an individual's cultural values, beliefs, and customs.

Stereotyping individuals can lead to incorrect assumptions.

When assessing a client's cultures, the nurse considers values, beliefs, and customs related to health and health care.

Some health problems are more prevalent in certain ethnic groups than in the general population.

Nurses must understand their own cultural values, beliefs, and customs in order to provide meaningful nursing care.

An ethnic and cultural assessment guide can help the nurse gather data about a client.

People can experience culture shock when they enter an unfamiliar environment where previous patterns of behavior are ineffective.

Selected References

Abril, I. F., May/June 1977. Mexican-American folk beliefs: How they affect health care. *The Journal of Maternal Child Nursing* 2:168–73.

American Journal of Nursing. June 1979. Black skin problems. *American Journal of Nursing* 79:1092–94.

American Nurses Association. 1987a. *1987–88 Health Legislation Fact Sheets.* Kansas City, Mo.: ANA.

American Nurses Association. 1987b. *1987 House of Delegates Summary of Proceedings.* Kansas City, Mo.: ANA.

Bello, T. A. February 1976. The third dimension: Cultural sensitivity in nursing practice. *Imprint* 23:36–38, 45.

Bloch, B. 1976. Nursing intervention in black patient care. In Luckraft, D., editor. *Black awareness: Implications for black patient care.* New York: American Journal of Nursing Co.

Carpenito, L. J. 1987. *Nursing Diagnosis.* 2nd ed. Philadelphia: Lippincott.

Chen-Louie, T. T. 1980. Bicultural experiences, social interactions, and health care implications. In Reinhardt, A. M., and Quinn, M. D., editors. *Family-centered community nursing: A sociocultural framework.* St. Louis: C. V. Mosby Co.

Christian, J. L., and Greger, J. L. 1985. *Nutrition for living.* Menlo Park, Calif.: Benjamin/Cummings Publishing Co.

Chung, H. J. March 1977. Understanding the Oriental maternity patient. *Nursing Clinics of North America* 12:67–75.

Friedman, M. M. 1981. *Family nursing theory and assessment.* Norwalk, Conn.: Appleton-Century-Crofts.

Gonzalez-Swafford, M. J., and Gutierrez, M. G. November/December 1983. Ethno-medical beliefs and practices of Mexican-Americans. *Nurse Practitioner* 8:29–30, 32, 34.

Grinker, R. R. August 1978. The poor rich: The children of the super-rich. *American Journal of Psychiatry* 135:913.

Hautman, M. A., and Harrison, J. K. April 1982. Health beliefs and practices in a middle-income Anglo-American neighborhood. *Advances in Nursing Science* 4:49–63.

Hayghe, H. 1976. Families and the rise of working wives: An overview. *Monthly Labor Review* 99:12–19.

———. 1982. Marital and family patterns of worker: An update. *Monthly Labor Review* 105:53–56.

Henderson, G., and Primeaux, M., editors. 1981. *Transcultural health care.* Menlo Park, Calif.: Addison-Wesley Publishing Co.

Henry, B. M., and DiGiacomo-Geffers, E. August 1980. The hospitalized rich and famous. *American Journal of Nursing* 80:1426–29.

Hicks, G. 1976. *Appalachian valley.* New York: Holt, Rinehart and Winston.

Holleran, C. March/April 1988. Nursing beyond national boundaries: The 21st century. *Nursing Outlook* 36, 2:72–75.

Kalish, R. A. 1967. Of children and grandfather: A speculative essay on dependency. *Gerontologist* 7:65–69.

Kleinman, A. et al. February 1978. Culture, illness, and care: Clinical lessons from anthropologic and cross-cultural research. *Annals of Internal Medicine* 88:251–58.

Leininger, M. 1970. *Nursing and anthropology: Two worlds to blend.* New York: John Wiley and Sons.

Lewis, O. October 1966. The culture of poverty. *Scientific American* 215:19–25.

Lewis, S.; Messner, R.; and McDowel, W. August 1985. An unchanging culture: Caring for Appalachian patients and their families. *Journal of Gerontological Nursing* 11:20–24, 26.

Mason, D. J. October 1981. Perspectives on poverty. *Image* 13:82–85.

Meleis, A. I. June 1981. The Arab American in the health care system. *American Journal of Nursing* 81:1180–83.

National Center for Health Statistics. August 1985. *Charting the nation's health trends since 1960.* DHHS publication no. (PHS) 85-1251. U.S. Department of Health and Human Services, Hyattsville, Md.: Public Health Service.

Ohlson, V. M., and Franklin, M. 1985. *An international perspective on nursing practice.* Publication no. NP-68F. Kansas City, Mo.: American Nurses' Association.

Orque, M. S., Bloch, B., and Monrroy, L. S. A. 1983. *Ethnic nursing care: A multicultural approach.* St. Louis: C. V. Mosby Co.

Overfield, T. 1985. *Biologic variation in health and illness.* Menlo Park, Calif.: Addison-Wesley Publishing Co.

Primeaux, M. H. March 1977. American Indian health care practices. *Nursing Clinics of North America* 12:55–65.

Richardson, E. A. W., and Milne, L. S. November/December 1983. Sickle-cell disease and the childbearing family: An update. *American Journal of Maternal/Child Nursing* 8:417–22.

Roundtable. September 15, 1980. Homosexuality 2: When sexual orientation is in doubt. *Patient Care* 58–59 +.

Schermerhorn, R. A. 1970. *Comparative ethnic relations: A framework for theory and research.* New York: Random House.

Shubin, S. June 1980. Nursing patients from different cultures. *Nursing 80* 10:78–81. Canadian edition 10:26–29.

Spector, R. E. 1985. *Cultural diversity in health and illness.* 2d ed. New York: Appleton-Century-Crofts.

Tripp-Reimer, T. Spring 1982. Barriers to health care: Variations in interpretation of Appalachian client behavior by Appalachian and non-Appalachian health professionals. *Western Journal of Nursing Research* 4:179–91.

Tripp-Reimer, T., and Friedl, M. March 1977. Appalachians: A neglected minority. *Nursing Clinics of North America* 12:41–54.

Tripp-Reimer, T.; Brink, P. J.; and Saunders, J. M. March/April 1984. Cultural assessment: Content and process. *Nursing Outlook* 32:78–82.

Wang, R. M. 1976. Chinese Americans and health care. In *Ethnicity and health care.* New York: National League for Nursing.

Wauneka, A. D. 1976. Helping a people to understand. In Brink, P. J., editor. *Transcultural nursing: A book of readings.* Englewood Cliffs, N.J.: Prentice-Hall.

White, E. H. March 1977. Giving health care to minority patients. *Nursing Clinics of North America* 12:27–40.

Winn, M. C. 1976. A proposed tuberculosis program for Papago Indians. In Brink, P. J., editor. *Transcultural nursing: A book of readings.* Englewood Cliffs, N.J.: Prentice-Hall.

Wirth, L. 1945. The problem of minority groups. In Linton, R., editor. *The science of man in the world crisis.* New York: Columbia University Press.

Wold, S. J. 1981. *School nursing: A framework for practice.* St. Louis: C. V. Mosby Co.

CHAPTER 18

Spirituality

OBJECTIVES

Discuss spiritual beliefs and religious practices and doctrines as they relate to health care.

Identify clients who can benefit from spiritual assistance.

Identify essential information to obtain in the nursing history.

Identify clinical signs indicating a spiritual need.

Identify essential aspects of nursing diagnoses related to spiritual distress.

Explain essential aspects to consider when planning for a client's spiritual support.

Explain essential guidelines for nursing implementation related to spiritual needs.

State outcome criteria essential for evaluating the client's progress toward resolving spiritual distress.

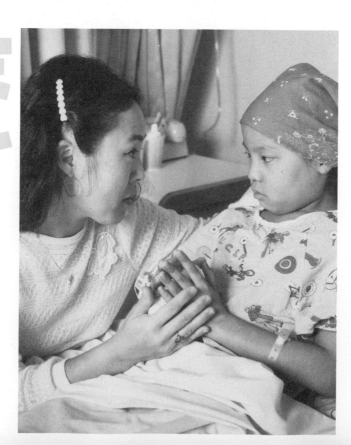

Spirituality and Religion

Spirituality and religion are separate entities, yet some people use the words interchangeably. **Spirituality** is a belief in some higher power, creative force, divine being, or infinite source of energy. For example, a person may believe in "God," in "Allah," or in a "higher power." A **religion** is an organized system of worship. Religions have central beliefs, rituals, and practices usually related to birth, death, marriage, and salvation. To have **faith** is to believe in or be committed to something or someone. In a general sense, religion or spiritual beliefs are an individual's attempt to understand his or her place in the universe, i.e., how that person sees himself or herself in relation to the total environment.

Religion and Illness

Spiritual and religious beliefs are important in many people's lives. They can influence life-style, attitudes, and feelings about illness and death. Some organized religions specify practices about diet, birth control, and appropriate medical therapy. Some religious groups condemn modern science because of "false teachings," such as evolution. Other groups support medical therapy in general but object to specific practices; e.g., the Seventh Day Adventist Church urges its members to avoid all drugs unless they are exceedingly ill.

Spiritual beliefs may assume greater importance at a time of illness than at any other time in a person's life, helping some people accept illness and explaining illness for others. Some clients may look upon illness as a test of faith; i.e., "If I have enough faith I will get well." Viewed from this perspective, illness is usually accepted by the client and his or her support persons and does not shake their religious beliefs.

Other people may look upon illness as punishment and think, "What have I done to deserve this?" These people associate disease with immoral behavior and believe their illness is punishment for past sins. They may believe that through prayer, promises, and perhaps penance, the cause of the disease will disappear. Such people believe that health professionals treat only the symptoms of disease and that they will become well if they are forgiven. If such an individual does not get well, then the support persons either accept the "punishment" or view the "punishment" as unfair.

Usually, spiritual beliefs help people to accept illness and to plan for the future. Religion can help people prepare for death and strengthen them during life. It can provide a meaning to life and to death; a haven of strength, serenity, and faith at a time of crisis; a sense of security; and a tangible network of social support.

Certain spiritual beliefs are in conflict with accepted medical practice. When a person's faith leads him or her to reject certain medical treatment, life may be threatened. For example, many practicing Jehovah's Witnesses will not accept blood transfusions because of religious doctrine.

Spiritual Development

Table 18–1 summarizes human spiritual development from infancy to adulthood.

James Fowler describes the development of faith in people. Fowler believes that faith, or the spiritual dimension, is a force that gives meaning to a person's life. Fowler uses the term *faith* as a form of knowing, a way of being in relation to "an ultimate environment" (Fowler and Keen 1985). To Fowler, **faith** is a relational phenomenon; it is "an active 'mode-of-being-in-relation' to another or others in which we invest commitment, belief, love, risk and hope" (Fowler and Keen 1985). Fowler's stages in the development of faith are given in Table 18–2.

Religious Beliefs Related to Health Care

Meeting the spiritual needs of clients and their support persons is part of the function of nurses as well as designated chaplains and other clergy. The term *clergy* refers to priests, rabbis, ministers, church elders, deacons, and other spiritual advisers. Some religious groups, such as the Church of Latter-Day Saints and the Christian Scientists, do not have ordained clergy, but they do usually have people whose role it is to minister to the ill. Nurses must recognize these people as having legitimate functions.

Although nurses cannot expect to be well versed about the practices of all the religious groups in the United States or Canada, it is important to be familiar with the major religious groups of the community. Representatives of a religion are usually pleased to give nurses information required in the care of clients. Some of the larger religious groups are discussed briefly here. Other reference texts can supply greater detail and information not included in this summary.

The major religions of the United States and Canada are Protestantism, Catholicism, and Judaism. There are many Protestant denominations, e.g., Episcopalians, Methodists, and Baptists. The denominations share some doctrines, but each denomination has its own interpretation of scripture and its own religious practices. Major religions, denominations, and some spiritual groups are listed alphabetically below. Selected facts about each group are included, but no attempt has been made to discuss broad philosophic beliefs or issues.

Agnosticism and Atheism

An **agnostic** is a person who doubts the existence of God or a supreme being or believes the existence of God has not been proven. An **atheist** denies the existence of God. **Theism** is the belief in the existence of a god or gods. The moral and ethical codes of agnostics and atheists are not derived from theistic beliefs.

Table 18—1   Summary of Spiritual Development

Developmental Stage	Characteristics	Developmental Stage	Characteristics
Infants and toddlers	Both infants and toddlers have no sense of right or wrong, spiritual beliefs, or convictions to guide activities. Toddlers may follow rituals (e.g., saying prayers at bedtime) in imitation of their parents. Toddlers may attend a church nursery school, but emphasis is on enhancing their positive self-image.		ments. They realize that their prayers are not always answered on their own terms, and they begin to reason rather than accept a faith blindly. Some children drop or modify certain religious practices (e.g., praying for tangible benefits); others continue to follow religious practices because of dependence on their parents.
Preschoolers	Parental attitudes toward moral codes and religion convey to children what is considered good and bad. Preschoolers copy what they see rather than what they are told. If what they see and what they are told are contradictory, problems arise. They often ask questions about morality and religion (e.g., "Why is [some action or word] wrong?" and "What is heaven?"). They believe that their parents, like God, are omnipotent. Two methods of spiritual education are used with preschool children: indoctrinating them and letting them choose their own way. Preschoolers follow a religion not because they understand it but because it is part of daily life. Three-year-olds like prayers at night and before meals. Five-year-olds often make up prayers themselves. They believe that God or human beings are responsible for such natural events as rain and wind. They may reason, "The rain is God crying; the wind is God blowing air out of His mouth." Many go to church school and participate in religious holidays. They ask many questions about the meaning of the holidays and need explanations about them. However, they are more occupied with such rituals as Santa Claus coming at Christmas than with the reason behind the holiday. When children begin to question such myths as the Easter Bunny, they are ready for a more sophisticated explanation about Easter.		During adolescence, children compare the standards of their parents with others and determine which ones they want to incorporate into their own behavior. Adolescents also compare the scientific viewpoint with the religious viewpoint and try to bring the two together. By 16 years, many adolescents have decided whether to accept the family religion. They may experience personal religious awakenings, such as being saved or converted, either suddenly or gradually. Adolescents with parents of different faiths may choose one faith over the other or no faith. For some, a firm faith provides strength during these turbulent years.
School-age children	Young school-age children expect that their prayers will be answered, good rewarded, and bad punished. During the prepuberty stage, children become aware of spiritual disappoint-	Adults	Young adults who need to answer the religious questions of their own children may find that the teachings of their own early childhood are more acceptable to them now than during adolescence. During the middle years, adults often find that they have more time for religious activities because their children are older. Older adults who have developed religious values often endeavor to broaden them and to understand the newer values of younger people. Elderly adults who do not have mature religious beliefs may experience a feeling of deprivation as they become less active, e.g., because of retirement. During these years, people face death (their own, their spouses', and their friends'). This recognition may make them despondent. The development of a mature religious philosophy can often help older people face reality, participate in life, have feelings of self-worth, and accept death as inevitable.

▪ Baha'i

People following the Baha'i faith use prayer at times of illness. Their beliefs permit use of alcohol and drugs only on a physician's order. It is written in the scriptures that ill persons are to seek competent medical assistance.

▪ Baptist

Baptists believe in the possibility of cure of illness by the "laying on of hands." Although some believe in faith healing to the exclusion of medical therapy, most Baptists seek competent medical help. Some Baptists do

Table 18—2 Fowler's Stages of Spiritual Development

Stage	Age	Description
0. Undifferentiated	0 to 3 years	Infant unable to formulate concepts about self or the environment.
1. Intuitive-projective	4 to 6 years	A combination of images and beliefs given by trusted others, mixed with the child's own experience and imagination.
2 Mythic-literal	7 to 12 years	Private world of fantasy and wonder; symbols refer to something specific; dramatic stories and myths used to communicate spiritual meanings.
3. Synthetic-conventional	Adolescent or adult	World and ultimate environment structured by the expectations and judgments of others; interpersonal focus.
4. Individuating-reflective	After 18 years	Constructing one's own explicit system; high degree of self-consciousness.
5. Paradoxical-consolidative	After 30 years	Awareness of truth from a variety of viewpoints.
6. Universalizing	Maybe never	Becoming an incarnation of the principles of love and justice.

Source: Adapted from J. Fowler and S. Keen, *Life maps: Conversations in the journey of faith* (Waco, Texas: Word Books, 1978).

not drink coffee or tea, and many Baptists do not take alcohol. Birth control, sterilization, and abortion (therapeutic or demand) are left to individual choice. When clients are clearly terminally ill, artificial prolongation of life is discouraged. Full-term stillborn babies are buried; less than full-term fetuses are not. Infant baptism is not practiced.

Black Muslim (Nation of Islam)

The Black Muslim religion is not the same as Islam, although their beliefs are similar. Members emphasize black independence and are encouraged to obtain health care provided by the black community. Black Muslims have a special procedure for washing and shrouding the dead and special funeral rites. Dietary considerations include prohibitions against alcoholic beverages and pork.

Buddhism

Buddhists avoid extremes, and this doctrine applies to the use of drugs, blood, or vaccines. Buddhism does not condone the taking of life in any form. If, however, a client is beyond recovery and can no longer strive toward "enlightenment," euthanasia may be permitted. Likewise, certain circumstances may warrant abortion. Last rite chanting is frequently practiced at the bedside of the deceased. Buddhists generally do not have any dietary restrictions, although members of some sects are strict vegetarians. Many Buddhists do not use tobacco, alcohol, or drugs. Buddhists have special holy days: January 1, February 15, March 21, April 8, May 21, July 15, September 1 and 23, and December 8 and 31. Buddhist clients may need to be asked how they feel about tests and treatments on those days.

Church of Christ, Scientist

Members of the Church of Christ, Scientist, oppose human intervention to cure illness, seeing it as God's will. Sickness and sin are errors of the human mind and can be changed by altering thoughts rather than by medicine. People who strictly follow this religion will not accept a physician's consultation or medical treatment and rarely, if ever, enter a hospital. Christian Scientists do not permit psychotherapy, because in this process the mind is altered by others. A Christian Science "practitioner" can be called to minister to the sick, and spiritual healing is practiced. Physicians and midwives may be used during childbirth, however.

Drugs and blood transfusions are not used, and biopsies and physical examinations are not sought. Tobacco, alcohol, and coffee are considered drugs and not used. Vaccines are accepted only as required by law. Christian Scientists do not have strictly defined policies about birth control, sterilization, or abortion. Autopsy is discouraged but accepted in sudden deaths, and Christian Scientists are unlikely to seek or donate organs for transplant. Whether a person wishes to rely completely upon Christian Science is up to the individual. In some areas, the church operates nursing homes in which there is complete reliance on church doctrine.

Eastern Orthodox

There are a number of Eastern Orthodox denominations, including Greek Orthodox, Russian Orthodox, and Armenian. Most believe in infant baptism by immersion 8 to 40 days after birth. The last rites may be obligatory if death is impending. Dietary restrictions depend on the particular sect. Eastern Orthodox beliefs and practices generally do not restrict medical science; however, the Russian Orthodox church discourages autopsy as well as donation of body parts.

The Greek Orthodox church opposes abortion. The church advocates confession at least yearly. The last rites include administration of Holy Communion (also referred to as the Eucharist or the Lord's Supper), a memorial sacrament in which the worshipper receives consecrated bread (or a thin wafer) representing the body of Jesus Christ, and wine or grape juice representing the blood of Jesus. The church advocates fasting, usually on Wednesdays, Fridays, and during Lent; the church encourages prolonging life, even for terminally ill clients.

Episcopalian (Anglican)

The Episcopal or Anglican religion places no restrictions on the use of medical therapies. It permits birth control and sterilization, autopsy, therapeutic abortion as a life-saving measure, burial or cremation, and genetic counseling. Abortion on demand, however, is regarded as unacceptable. Anglicans celebrate Holy Communion. Some members of this church fast before receiving Communion and abstain from meat on Fridays. The church advocates confession. The rite for anointing of the sick may be performed but is not mandatory.

Hinduism

Hindus follow many dietary practices, and these vary according to sect. Some do not eat veal and beef and their derivatives. Some are strict vegetarians. Alcohol may be consumed at western social functions. Most Hindus accept modern medical practices; artificial insemination is rejected, however, because sterility reflects divine will. When giving a Hindu medications, the nurse avoids touching the client's lips, if possible.

Hindus practice special rites at death. Death is considered rebirth. The priest pours water into the mouth of the corpse and ties a thread around the wrist or neck to indicate blessing. This thread must not be removed. The body is cremated, and the ashes are disposed of in holy rivers. Some injuries, such as loss of a limb, are considered signs of wrongdoing in a previous life, although the afflicted person is not an outcast from society. Hindus believe in a natural division among people, and there is little mixing among castes (hereditary social classes).

Jehovah's Witness

Jehovah's Witnesses are opposed to blood transfusions and organ transplants, although some individuals do agree to them in a crisis. When parents refuse to allow an infant to receive a transfusion, a court order may be sought transferring custody to the courts or to an official of the hospital. Members of the church eat meat that has been drained of blood. Some oppose modern medicine. Infant baptism is not practiced.

Jehovah's Witnesses generally have a neutral attitude toward birth control, believing it is a matter of individual conscience, but sterilization is condemned and prohibited. Both therapeutic and demand abortions are forbidden. Masturbation and homosexuality are condemned. Both burial and cremation are approved. Autopsy is approved only as required by law, and no parts of the body are to be removed. This restriction has implications for donor transplants.

Judaism

There are three main Jewish groups: the Orthodox is the strictest; the Conservative and Reform groups are less so. Jewish law demands that Jews seek competent medical care. Jews allow the use of drugs, blood, and vaccines; biopsies and amputations are also permitted. Some Orthodox Jews believe that the entire God-given body must be returned to the earth, and they require any body tissue to be buried. Donor transplants may therefore not be acceptable to Orthodox Jews. The nurse must ensure that amputated limbs or organs are made available to such Orthodox families for burial. Cremation is discouraged. Autopsy may be permitted in less strict groups as long as parts of the body are not removed. Bodies, even those of fetuses, are washed by the ritual burial society and buried as soon as possible after death.

Therapeutic abortion is permissible if the mother's physical or psychologic health is threatened. Demand abortion is prohibited. Vasectomy is not permitted. Orthodox and Conservative Jews observe kosher dietary laws, which prohibit pork, shellfish, and other foods and the eating of milk products and meat products in the same meal. Reform Jews usually do not observe kosher dietary regulations.

Orthodox and Conservative Jews circumcise male infants on the eighth day of life, although circumcision may be delayed if medically contraindicated. The rabbi and male synagogue members may be present, and a Jewish physician or mohel (ritual circumciser acquainted with Jewish law and hygienic medical technique) performs the rite. Special arrangements generally need to be made for the ceremony, and the physician's approval must be obtained.

Orthodox and some Conservative Jews observe the Sabbath from sundown Friday to sundown Saturday and may resist hospital admission or medical procedures during that period or during major Jewish festivals, unless the treatment is necessary to preserve life. Rosh Hashanah is the first day of the Jewish new year, which usually occurs in September. Ten days later, Yom Kippur marks the end of the time devoted to reflecting upon life.

Lutheran

The Lutheran church imposes no restrictions on medical procedures, including autopsies and therapeutic abortions, and no dietary restrictions. Abortion on demand is not approved, however. Marriage and procreation are discouraged when offspring are likely to inherit severe physical or mental deficits. Birth control and sterilization are left to the individual's conscience. Members are baptized 6 to 8 weeks after birth, and those who wish may be anointed and blessed before death. Burial rites are generally performed on infants who die after 6 to 7 months' gestation.

Mennonite

Members of the Mennonite church are baptized in their middle teens. The church imposes no special dietary restrictions, although some congregations require abstinence from alcohol. No restrictions are placed on medical procedures, although demand abortion is not approved in some sects of the church; in others, it is left to individual conscience. Mennonites oppose the laying on of hands.

Mormon (Church of Jesus Christ of Latter-Day Saints)

Some Mormons believe in cure by the "laying on of hands"; however, there is no prohibition of medical therapy. Alcohol, tobacco, tea, and coffee are prohibited, and meat is eaten sparingly. Mormon clients in the hospital may request the Sacrament of the Lord's Supper by a church priesthood holder. Baptism of the dead is mandatory.

Muslim/Moslem (Islam)

Islam is a major religion of North Africa and the Near East. Rituals and prayers are strictly performed. All pork products are prohibited, and some oppose alcoholic beverages. There is a fasting period in the ninth month of the Mohammedan year (Ramadan), but people who are ill are exempt from it. Circumcision is practiced, and cleanliness is very important.

A fetus aborted 130 days or more after conception is treated as a fully developed human being. Before that time, it is looked upon as discarded tissue. The dying person must confess sins and beg forgiveness. Only relatives and family can touch the body after death. They wash and prepare it and turn it toward Mecca. Islam encourages prolonging life, even for the terminally ill.

Native American

Most Native American tribes have medicine men or shamans, who perform various ceremonies against illness. Believers look to superhuman powers for protection from disease. Many Native Americans today follow modern Christian religions; however, some follow traditional beliefs, and some hold a combination of Christian and traditional beliefs.

Pentecostalist (Assembly of God, Foursquare Church)

The Pentecostal church accepts modern medical practice, including blood transfusions. Members are encouraged to abstain from use of alcohol and tobacco and from eating strangled animals. Some members do not eat pork. Members may pray for divine healing, and in some congregations anointing with oil is practiced.

Roman Catholic

Catholics believe that an infant has a soul from the moment of conception; therefore, a fetus must be baptized unless it is obviously dead, as must all babies whose health or life is endangered. Baptism may be performed by any person (e.g., a physician or nurse in the absence of a priest) who does what the church requires (i.e., pouring water on the baby's head while repeating the prescribed Trinitarian invocation: "I baptize thee in the name of the Father, of the Son, and of the Holy Spirit"). When performed by a nurse or physician, the baptism should be recorded on the infant's chart and the family and priest must be informed.

The Roman Catholic church encourages anointing of the sick both as a source of strength or healing and as a preparation for death. Before changes were instituted by the Second Vatican Council in 1963, this Catholic sacrament was administered to persons only when death was imminent and was referred to as the last rites. Today, the possibility of death may still be a reason for this sacrament, but death need not be the immediate concern. Catholics can now be anointed more than once; many older Catholics, however, may respond to this sacrament with fear or dread, considering it a sign of imminent death. If so, the modern meaning should be explained to minimize apprehension. Anointing of the sick may be preceded by confession and Holy Communion. These sacraments are also performed by a priest or other commissioned person.

The Roman Catholic belief in the "principle of totality" underlies a general acceptance of medical procedures. A donor transplant is accepted as long as loss of the organ does not deprive the donor of life or functional integrity of the body. Biopsies and amputations are accepted in the same light. Autopsy is also accepted; again, all major parts of the body (those retaining human quality) must be given an appropriate burial or cremation.

Strict laws govern birth control, sterilization, and abortion. The only approved method of birth control is abstinence; artificial means are illicit. Sterilization is forbidden unless there is a sound medical indication for it. Some Catholics observe certain dietary and fasting practices, but when ill they are excused from otherwise obligatory fasting or abstaining from meat on Ash Wednesday and Good Friday. Sunday is the day of worship, although church services are held in some churches other days of the week as well.

Salvation Army

The Salvation Army places no restrictions on medical procedures, including transplants and autopsies. Birth control and sterilization are acceptable within marriage. Demand abortions are opposed, but therapeutic ones are approved.

Seventh-Day Adventist (Church of God, Advent Christian Church)

The Adventist church is opposed to infant baptism but conducts baptism of adults by immersion. In dietary matters, it prohibits alcohol, tobacco, narcotics, and stimulants, and some members advocate ovolactovegetarian diets. Some sects practice divine healing and anointing with oil. Saturday is considered the Sabbath by some.

Adventists are encouraged to avoid drugs, but they recognize that blood transfusions, vaccines, and drugs are sometimes necessary. Birth control and sterilization are left to individual conscience. Abortion is approved if the mother's life is endangered or if pregnancy is due to rape or incest. The use of hypnotism is opposed.

Shinto

Some members believe in healing through prayer, and the family is important in providing care and providing emotional support. Shintoists believe in tradition, and they worship ancestors and nature. Physical health may be valued.

Sikh

The Sikhs are a relatively new sect that opposes the caste system in India. Sikhs hold weekly religious services at their temple, from Friday morning through Sunday. During the services, each member reads the holy scripture (the Granth Sahib) in turn for 2-hour periods until the entire scripture is read.

Baptized male Sikhs wear unshorn hair and turbans, which symbolize dedication and group consciousness. A steel bracelet on the right wrist symbolizes restraint, a reminder to do no wrong. No significant dietary restrictions are imposed by the Sikh faith, but many Sikhs are vegetarians. Use of tobacco and alcohol is discouraged.

Taoism

Taoists view illness as part of the health-illness duality. They may accept illness and may view medical treatment as interference. Death is seen as a natural part of life, and the body is kept in-house for 49 days. Taoists believe in an esthetically pleasing environment for meditation.

Unitarian/Universalist

Unitarian/Universalists emphasize reason, knowledge, individual responsibility, and personally established values. There are no dietary restrictions or official sacraments, and no medical practices are prohibited. The Unitarian/Universalist church encourages members to donate parts of their bodies to research and to medical banks.

United Church of Canada

The United Church of Canada is the largest Protestant denomination in Canada. It was formed in 1925 by the amalgamation of the Methodist, Presbyterian, and Congregationalist Churches. It operates some hospitals in underserviced areas of Canada.

Zen

Adherents of Zen practice meditation with the goal of discovering simplicity. When a client is ill, he or she may wish to see a Zen master.

Assessing the Need for Spiritual Assistance

A **spiritual need** is a person's need to maintain, increase, or restore his or her beliefs and faith and to fulfill religious obligations. It is often the nurse who identifies a need for spiritual assistance and obtains the desired help. Sometimes clients ask directly for a visit from the hospital chaplain or their own clergyman. Others may discuss their concerns with the nurse and ask about the nurse's beliefs as a way of seeking an empathic listener. Some people are embarrassed to ask for spiritual counsel but may hint at their concern in such statements as, "I've been wondering what will happen to me when I die," or "Do you go to a church?"

Any client or support person may desire spiritual assistance. The client facing death may have accepted it, but the family and support persons may not. Often relatives are grateful for spiritual support by a nurse or pastor. Assisting them may indirectly assist the client. Among those who may desire spiritual assistance are:

- Clients who appear lonely and have few visitors
- Clients who express fear and anxiety
- Clients about to have surgery
- Clients whose illness is related to the emotions or whose illness has religious or social implications
- Clients who must change their life-style as a result of illness or injury
- Clients preoccupied about the relationship of their religion and health
- Clients whose pastor is unable to visit

The client's religious preference is usually recorded on the hospital admission record and the nursing history. The nurse also can ask if the client follows any religious practices and if he or she would like a pastor, priest, practitioner, or church member to visit. It is important to ask the individual before obtaining assistance. Some people profess no religious beliefs and may be angered if the nurse makes arrangements for a chaplain to visit. The nurse needs to respect the client's wishes and not make a judgment of right or wrong, good or bad.

Nursing Diagnosis

Examples of nursing diagnoses for clients experiencing spiritual distress are given in the accompanying box. As defined by NANDA, **spiritual distress** is the "state in which the individual experiences or is at risk

NURSING DIAGNOSIS

Spiritual Distress

- Spiritual distress related to inability to attend religious services
- Spiritual distress related to conflict between religious doctrine and recommended therapy
- Spiritual distress related to death of husband

of experiencing a disturbance in his belief or value system which provides strength, hope and meaning to his life" (Carpenito 1987, p. 577).

Planning

The goal of plans to decrease spiritual distress should meet one or more of the following needs: providing spiritual resources otherwise unavailable, helping clients fulfill religious obligations, helping clients use inner resources more effectively to meet situations, helping clients maintain or establish dynamic and personal relationships with the deity in the face of unpleasant circumstances, and helping clients find meaning in existence and the present situation. Planning also involves establishing appropriate goals for the nursing diagnoses identified and determining outcome criteria to judge whether the goals are met. For suggestions, see the section on evaluation, later in this chapter.

Implementation

Once spiritual distress has been identified as a relevant nursing diagnosis and specific strategies have been planned, the nurse is ready to implement the plan. To be effective when intervening, nurses should have already examined and clarified their own spiritual beliefs and values (see Chapter 5). A nurse who feels uncomfortable assisting the client spiritually (e.g., reading devotional material or praying with the client on request) should verbalize this discomfort and offer to obtain assistance for the client. It is important to respect the client's beliefs and maintain a supportive relationship. It is equally important for the nurse not to feel guilty about her or his discomfort.

To decrease spiritual distress, nurses should focus attention on the client's perception of his or her spiritual needs rather than on the practices or beliefs of the client's religious affiliation. Individual spiritual beliefs may vary

greatly among members of a given religion. People join religious groups for many reasons (e.g., to have a place of worship, to find an avenue for social action such as helping the poor or homeless, to gain friends for recreational purposes, or to have a place for important life events such as weddings and funerals). Similarly, nurses should not assume that a client has no spiritual needs because the record states no religious affiliation or specifies atheist or agnostic.

To further individualize care, the nurse determines the meaning the client attaches to the situation. Such meanings can influence the client's response to an illness or condition and may either hinder nursing intervention or provide hope, courage, and strength. For example, a person who believes that illness is God's punishment may feel powerless and demonstrate little interest in therapy designed to prevent illness.

When orienting clients to the nursing unit, the nurse can provide information about hospital services to help clients meet spiritual needs and arrange for clients to participate in these as they are able. Many large hospitals have full-time chaplains who assist clients, support persons, and staff with spiritual needs. For smaller hospitals that do not have chaplains, clergy in the community usually provide this service. Many nursing units have a list of clergy who are on call when needed.

Some agencies have a chapel where religious services are regularly held for clients, support persons, and staff. Most hospitals also have quiet rooms that can be used for meditation, counsel, and even worship services. Sometimes a client prefers to meet the chaplain in a quiet, private room, particularly when the client shares his or her hospital room. A hospital may hold nondenominational religious services or several services for different denominations. If a client expresses a desire to attend services, the nurse needs to help organize the client's care so that attendance is possible if health permits.

The nurse sometimes determines that there is a true conflict between spiritual beliefs and medical therapy. In this case, the nurse encourages the client and physician to discuss the conflict and consider alternative methods of therapy. The nurse always supports the client's right to make an informed decision. If the beliefs of the nurse and client conflict, the nurse should discuss this conflict with the nurse in charge and her or his own spiritual leader. It may be preferable for the client to receive care from a nurse with compatible views. The nurse may also wish to discuss her or his feelings with other health professionals, e.g., other nurses on the team.

Evaluation

Examples of outcome criteria for clients who have spiritual distress are listed in the accompanying box.

OUTCOME CRITERIA

Spiritual Distress

The client will:

- Express comfort with spiritual beliefs.
- Continue spiritual practices as appropriate to his or her health status.
- Express decreased feelings of guilt.
- State acceptance of moral decision.
- Display positive affect.
- Express finding positive meaning in the present situation and in his or her own existence.

Chapter Highlights

The spiritual needs of clients and support persons often come into focus at a time of illness.

Nurses must respect the rights of people to hold their own spiritual beliefs and to communicate or not communicate these to others.

Spiritual beliefs and practices are highly personal.

Spiritual and religious beliefs can influence life-style, attitudes, and feelings about illness and death.

Spiritual beliefs often help people accept illness and plan for the future.

Nurses should be aware of their own spiritual beliefs in order to be comfortable assisting others.

Nurses may intervene directly to help clients, support persons, and clergy to meet spiritual needs.

Selected References

Carpenito, L. J. 1987. *Nursing diagnosis: Application to clinical practice.* 2d ed. Philadelphia: J. B. Lippincott Co.

Fehring, R. J., and McLane, A. M. 1986. Value belief—Spiritual distress. *Clinical Nursing* pp. 1843–1857 St. Louis: C. V. Mosby.

Fish, S., and Shelley, J. A. 1978. *Spiritual care: The nurse's role.* Downers Grove, Ill.: InterVarsity Press.

Fowler, J. W., and Keen, S. 1985. *Life maps: Conversations on the journey of faith.* Waco, Texas: Word.

Miller, J. F. 1985. Inspiring hope. *American Journal of Nursing* 85:22–25.

Murray, R. B., and Zentuen, J. P. 1985. *Nursing Concepts for Health Promotion.* 3d ed. Englewood Cliffs, N.J.: Prentice-Hall, Inc.

Pumphrey, J. B. December 1977. Recognizing your patient's spiritual needs. *Nursing 77* 7:64–69.

Ruffing-Rahal, M. A. March/April 1984. The spiritual dimension of well-being: Implications for the elderly. *Home Health-care Nurse* 2:12–13, 16.

Ryan, J. 1984. The neglected crisis. *American Journal of Nursing* 84:1257–1258.

Stoll, R. T. September 1979. Guidelines for spiritual assessment. *American Journal of Nursing* 79:1574–77.

CHAPTER **19**

Loss and Grieving

OBJECTIVES

Recognize selected frameworks for identifying stages of grieving.

List clinical signs of impending and imminent death and of death itself.

Identify clinical symptoms of grief.

Discuss factors affecting a loss reaction.

Recognize common fears associated with dying.

Identify factors contributing to unresolved grief.

Describe guidelines for helping clients to die with dignity.

Identify measures that facilitate the grieving process.

List changes that occur in the body after death.

Describe nursing measures for care of the body after death.

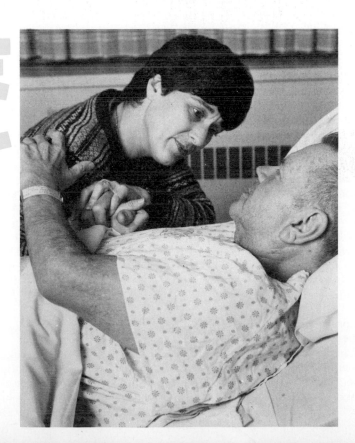

LOSS

Loss is an actual or potential situation in which a valued object, person, or the like is inaccessible or changed so that it is no longer perceived as valuable. People can experience the loss of body image, a significant other, a sense of well-being, a job, personal possessions, beliefs, a sense of self, and so on. Illness and hospitalization often produce losses.

Death is a fundamental loss, both for the dying person and for those who survive. Although death is inevitable for everyone, it is a lonely experience that each person ultimately faces alone. Yet even death, like other losses, can stimulate people to grow in perception of both themselves and others. Death can be viewed not simply as loss of life but as the dying person's final opportunity to experience life in ways that bring meaning and fulfillment.

Types of Loss

There are two general types of loss, actual and perceived. An **actual loss** can be identified by others and can arise either in response to or in anticipation of a situation. For example, a woman whose husband is dying may experience actual loss in anticipation of his death. A **perceived loss** is experienced by one person but cannot be verified by others. Psychologic losses are often perceived losses in that they are not directly verifiable. For example, a woman who leaves her employment to care for her children at home may perceive a loss of independence and freedom. An **anticipatory loss** is experienced before the loss really occurs.

The loss of an **aspect of self** changes a person's body image even though the loss may not be obvious to others. The degree to which these losses affect a person largely depends on the integrity of the person's body image (part of self-concept—see Chapter 14). Sometimes changes in self-image affect a person's social roles, such as employee, father, and husband. Any change that the person perceives as negative in the way he or she relates to the environment can be considered a loss of self.

Losses such as divorce can have considerable impact. A divorce may mean loss of financial security, a home, and daily routines. Therefore, even when the divorce was desired, the sense of loss can last for some time afterward.

During old age, dramatic changes occur in both physical and mental capabilities. Again the self-image is vulnerable, and support and reassurance are important. During this time people usually experience many losses: of employment, of usual activities, of independence, of health, of friends, and of family.

Loss of external objects includes loss of inanimate objects that have importance to the person (e.g., the loss of money for a person without financial means or the burning down of a family's house) and loss of pets that provide love and companionship. **Separation from an accustomed environment** and people who provide security can result in a sense of loss. The 6-year-old sheltered at home is likely to feel loss when first attending school and relating to more people. The university student who moves away from home for the first time may also experiences a sense of loss.

The **loss of a loved one** or valued person through illness, separation, or death can be very disturbing. In illness such as brain damage from viral infection or stroke, a person may undergo personality changes that make friends and family feel they have lost that person. The death of a loved one is a permanent and complete loss. In primitive societies, death was considered a normal, natural event, and life was seldom long. The death of a young man brought greater grief than the deaths of women, children, or elderly people. In contemporary North American society, death is considered unacceptable and usually occurs in private, unless there is an accident. Death often happens in a hospital or in a home in the presence of immediate family.

Loss as Crisis

Loss, especially loss of life or a loved one, can be viewed as a situational or developmental crisis. The loss of a job or the loss of a young child, for example, is usually an unexpected situational crisis. By contrast, losses incurred in the process of normal development—such as the departure of grown children from the home, retirement from a career, and the death of aged parents—are developmental crises that can be anticipated and, to some extent, prepared for.

How individuals deal with loss is closely related to their stage of development, personal resources, and social support systems. In dealing with loss of life, the nurse needs to consider the influence of these factors on the dying person and the surviving loved ones. As with all people in crisis, the experience of a dying person cannot be properly understood apart from the social context (Hoff 1984). In crisis situations, including the crisis of death, it is important for the nurse to consider the entire family as the client of care.

Bereavement and Grief

Bereavement is the subjective response to a loss through the death of a person with whom there has been a significant relationship. **Grief** is the total response to the emotional experience of the loss and is manifested in thoughts, feelings, and behaviors (Martocchio 1985, p. 327). **Mourning** is a behavioral process through which grief is eventually resolved or altered; it is often influenced by culture and custom. Normal bereavement can last as long as a year or more. Dealing with loss through death is complex and intensely emotional and should not be oversimplified.

Age and the Impact of Loss

Age affects a person's understanding of and reaction to loss. With experience, people usually increase their understanding and acceptance of life, loss, and death. As in other aspects of human development, children show more rapid and dramatic variation and changes in their understanding of death. Their understanding is susceptible to influence by outside events, such as life-threatening illness, which usually deepens the child's understanding of death and makes it more like that of an adult (Fetsch 1984). Table 19–1 outlines the development of the concept of death through the life span.

Children differ from adults not only in their understanding of loss and death but also in how they are affected by the loss of others. The child's patterns progress rapidly; adult patterns of growth and development are generally stable. The loss of a parent or other significant person can threaten the child's ability to develop, and regression sometimes results. Assisting the child with the grief experience includes helping the child regain the normal continuity and pace of emotional development.

Adults often assume that children do not have the same need as an adult to grieve the loss of others. In situations of crisis and loss, children are sometimes pushed aside or protected from the pain. They can feel afraid, abandoned, and lonely. Careful work is especially necessary with bereaved children because experiencing a loss in childhood can have serious effects later in life. Research suggests a connection between early loss of a parent through death or divorce and increased risk of depression or suicide in adulthood (Taylor 1983–84).

As people grow, loss comes to be experienced as part of normal development. By middle age, for example, the loss of a parent through death seems a normal occurrence compared to the death of a younger person. Coping with the death of an aged parent has even been viewed as a necessary developmental task of the middle-age adult. Society does not support intense or prolonged mourning for such a normal event (Moss and Moss 1983–84).

For the middle-age adult the loss of a parent can signal the disintegration of the family of origin. It is also a forceful reminder that the adult child is part of the older generation and therefore closer to death. The challenge of this developmental crisis for adult children is to assess the psychologic legacy of the parent, integrating what is valuable into their own identity. If the relationship with the parent was full of conflict, the parent's death can help release the child's energy for more productive use.

For older adults, the loss through death of a long-time mate is profound. Though individuals differ in their ability to deal with such a loss, research suggests an increase in health problems for widows and widowers during the first year following (Richter 1984). Because the majority of deaths occur among the elderly, and because the number of elderly is increasing in North America, nurses need to be especially alert to the potential problems of older grieving adults.

▪ Educating the Nurse About Loss

People in North America are socialized to think of death as the worst occurrence in life. They therefore do their best to avoid thinking or talking about death, especially their own. Death is thought about rarely and almost exclusively in negative terms. Nurses are not immune to such attitudes. They need to take time to analyze their own feelings about death before they can effectively help others with a terminal illness. Nurses who are unconsciously uncomfortable with dying clients tend to impede the clients' attempts to discuss dying and death by:

1. Changing the subject, e.g., "Let's think of something more cheerful," or "You shouldn't say things like that."

Table 19–1 Development of the Concept of Death

Age	Beliefs/Attitudes
Infancy to 5 years	Does not understand concept of death Infant's sense of separation forms basis for later understanding of loss and death Believes death is reversible, a temporary departure, or sleep Emphasizes immobility and inactivity as attributes of death
5 to 9 years	Understands that death is final Believes own death can be avoided Associates death with aggression or violence Believes wishes or unrelated actions can be responsible for death
9 to 12 years	Understands death as the inevitable end of life Begins to understand own mortality, expressed as interest in afterlife or as fear of death Expresses ideas about death gathered from parents and other adults
12 to 18 years	Fears a lingering death May fantasize that death can be defied, acting out defiance through reckless behaviors, e.g., dangerous driving, substance abuse Seldom thinks about death, but views it in religious and philosophic terms May seem to reach "adult" perception of death but be emotionally unable to accept it May still hold concepts from previous developmental stages
18 to 45 years	Has attitude toward death influenced by religious and cultural beliefs
45 to 65 years	Accepts own mortality Encounters death of parents and some peers Experiences peaks of death anxiety Death anxiety diminishes with emotional well-being
65 years +	Fears prolonged illness Encounters death of family members and peers Sees death as having multiple meanings, e.g., freedom from pain, reunion with already deceased family members

2. Offering reassurance, e.g., "You are doing very well."
3. Denying what is happening, e.g., "You don't really mean that," or "You're going to live until you are a hundred."
4. Being fatalistic, e.g., "Everyone dies sooner or later," or "God will take you when He wants you."
5. Blocking discussion, e.g., "I don't think things are really that bad," conveying an attitude that stops further discussion of the subject.
6. Being aloof and distant or avoiding the client.
7. "Managing" the client's care and making the client feel increasingly dependent and powerless.

The curricula of many nursing schools include education about death. Agencies and associations sponsor continuing education programs aimed at reducing death anxiety among nursing staff. Other programs help nurses explore the specific problems of direct contact with terminally ill clients and around-the-clock responsibility for their care. In all such programs nurses learn not only their own attitudes and concerns but also ways to support and comfort each other when they experience anger and frustration in the grief that follows the death of clients whom they cared for and cared about.

Caring for the dying and the bereaved is one of the nurse's most complex and challenging responsibilities, bringing into play all the skills needed for holistic physiologic and psychosocial care. To be effective, nurses must come to grips with their own attitudes toward loss, death, and dying, because these attitudes directly affect their ability to provide care. No single textbook chapter can give nursing students all the information and guidance needed to prepare them to care for dying clients and their families. Each nurse is personally responsible for actively engaging in a career-long process of education through reading, listening, and self-examination.

Grief

Grieving, the normal subjective emotional response to loss, is essential for good mental and physical health. It permits the individual to cope with the loss gradually and to accept it as part of reality. Grief is a social process in that it is best shared and carried out with the assistance of others.

Grief work is important, because bereavement has been shown to have potentially devastating effects on health. Among the symptoms that can accompany grief are anxiety, depression, weight loss, difficulties in swallowing, vomiting, fatigue, headaches, dizziness, fainting, blurred vision, skin rashes, excessive sweating, menstrual disturbances, palpitations, chest pain, dyspnea, and infection (Gonda and Ruark 1984). The bereaved may also experience alterations in libido, concentration, and patterns of eating, sleeping, activity, and communication.

Stages of Grieving

Many authors have described stages or phases of grieving. Perhaps the most famous of them is Kübler-Ross, who has described five stages: denial, anger, bar-

Table 19–2 Kübler-Ross's Stages of Grieving

Stage	Behavioral Responses	Nursing Implications
Denial	Refuses to believe that loss is happening Is unready to deal with practical problems, such as prosthesis after loss of leg May assume artificial cheerfulness to prolong denial	Verbally support client's denial for its protective function Examine your own behavior to ensure that you do not share in client's denial
Anger	Client or family may direct anger at nurse or hospital staff, about matters that normally would not bother them	Help client understand that anger is a normal response to feelings of loss and powerlessness Avoid withdrawal or retaliation with anger; do not take anger personally Deal with needs underlying any angry reaction Provide structure and continuity to promote feelings of security Allow client as much control as possible over his or her life
Bargaining	Seeks to bargain to avoid loss May express feelings of guilt or fear of punishment for past sins, real or imagined	Listen attentively and encourage client to talk to relieve guilt and irrational fears If appropriate, offer spiritual support
Depression	Grieves over what has happened and what cannot be May talk freely (e.g., reviewing past losses such as money or job), or may withdraw	Allow client to express sadness Communicate nonverbally by sitting quietly without expecting conversation Convey caring by touch Help support persons understand importance of being with the client in silence
Acceptance	Comes to terms with loss May have decreased interest in surroundings and support persons May wish to begin making plans, e.g., will, prosthesis, altered living arrangements	Help family and friends understand client's decreased need to socialize and need for short, quiet visits Encourage client to participate as much as possible in the treatment program

gaining, depression, and acceptance. (Kübler-Ross 1969, pp. 38–137). See Table 19–2. Engel (1964, pp. 94–96) has identified six stages of grieving: shock and disbelief, developing awareness, restitution, resolving the loss, idealization, and outcome. See Table 19–3.

Recently, nurses have begun to write about the components of grief. Martocchio (1985) discusses five clusters of grief and maintains that there is no single correct way, nor a correct timetable, by which a person progresses through the grief process. Whether and how a person can succeed in integrating the loss are related to that person's individual development and personal makeup. And individuals responding to the very same loss cannot be expected to follow the same pattern or schedule in resolving their grief, even while they support each other. Martocchio's five clusters of grief include:

1. **Shock and disbelief.** A feeling of numbness is a common response immediately following the death of a loved one. The bereaved may feel depressed, angry, guilty, and sad. Disbelief or denial may persist even though the loss has been accepted intellectually.

2. **Yearning and protest.** The anger that the bereaved feel may be directed at the deceased for having died, at God, at others whose loved ones are still alive, or at the caregivers. The bereaved may begin to fear their own mental deterioration and withdraw from sharing their thoughts and feelings with others.

3. **Anguish, disorganization, and despair.** When the reality of the loss is genuinely admitted, depression can set in. Weeping is common at this time. The bereaved lose interest and motivation in pursuing the future, are unable to make decisions, and lack confidence and purpose. Activities that were once enjoyed with the deceased are now without attraction. Coping strategies such as excessive drinking may compromise health.

4. **Identification in bereavement.** The bereaved may take on the behavior, personal traits, habits, and ambitions of the deceased. Sometimes they may also experience the same symptoms of physical illness.

5. **Reorganization and restitution.** Achieving stability and a sense of reintegration can take a period of time that ranges widely, from less than a year to several years. Although the bereaved are able to experience a sense of well-being and can resume most normal patterns of functioning, the feelings of grief do not simply cease. For many the pain of loss, though diminished, recurs for the rest of their lives.

◼ Assessment

To gather a complete data base that allows accurate analysis and identification of appropriate nursing diagnoses for clients experiencing losses and grieving, the nurse first needs to recognize the state of awareness the client and family manifest, the symptoms of grief, and the factors influencing a loss reaction.

◼ States of Awareness.
In cases of terminal illness, the state of awareness shared by the dying person and the family affects the nurse's ability to communi-

Table 19–3 Engel's Stages of Grieving

Stage	Behavioral Responses
Shock and disbelief	Refusal to accept loss
	Stunned feelings
	Intellectual acceptance but emotional denial
Developing awareness	Reality of loss begins to penetrate consciousness
	Anger may be directed at hospital, nurses, etc.
	Crying and self-blame
Restitution	Rituals of mourning, e.g., funeral
Resolving the loss	Attempts to deal with painful void
	Still unable to accept new love object to replace lost person
	May accept more dependent relationship with support person
	Thinks over and talks about memories of the dead person
Idealization	Produces image of dead person that is almost devoid of undesirable features
	Represses all negative and hostile feelings toward deceased
	May feel guilty and remorseful about past inconsiderate or unkind acts to deceased
	Unconsciously internalizes admired qualities of deceased
	Reminders of deceased evoke fewer feelings of sadness
	Reinvests feelings in others
Outcome	Behavior influenced by several factors, such as: importance of lost object as source of support, degree of dependence on relationship, degree of ambivalence toward deceased, number and nature of other relationships, and number and nature of previous grief experiences (which tend to be cumulative)

Source: From G. L. Engel, Grief and grieving, *American Journal of Nursing,* September 1964, 64:93–98. Copyright 1964 American Journal of Nursing Company. Reprinted with permission.

cate freely with clients and other health care team members and to assist in the grieving process. Three types of awareness that have been described are closed awareness, mutual pretense, and open awareness (Strauss et al. 1970, p. 300).

In **closed awareness,** the client and family are unaware of impending death. They may not completely understand why the client is ill, and they believe he or she will recover. The physician may believe it is best not to communicate a diagnosis or prognosis to the client or family. Nursing personnel are confronted with an ethical problem in this situation, and they have several choices. One course is to answer questions evasively or falsely. But ultimately the client and family will know the truth, and when they do they may recognize that information given them earlier was false. See Chapter 5 for further information on ethical dilemmas.

With **mutual pretense,** the client, family, and health personnel know that the prognosis is terminal but do not talk about it and make an effort not to raise the subject. Sometimes the client refrains from discussing death to protect the family from distress. The client may also sense discomfort on the part of health personnel and therefore not bring up the subject. Mutual pretense permits the client a degree of privacy and dignity, but it places a heavy burden on the dying person, who then has no one in whom to confide fears.

With **open awareness,** the client and people around know about the impending death and feel comfortable about discussing it, even though it is difficult. This awareness provides the client an opportunity to finalize affairs and even participate in planning funeral arrangements.

Not all people can handle open awareness. For example, a 45-year-old man who knows he is dying may be unable to discuss his forthcoming death without becoming angry at people around him. Whether to inform dying clients of their terminality is a difficult issue for physicians. Some authorities believe that terminal clients acquire knowledge of their condition even if they are not directly informed. Others believe that many clients remain unaware of their condition until the end. It is difficult, however, to distinguish what a client knows from what he or she is willing to accept.

■ **Reaction to the Loss.** The nurse assesses the grieving client and/or family members following a loss to determine the phase or stage of grieving. Schulz describes the following clinical symptoms of grief: repeated somatic distress, tightness in the chest, choking or shortness of breath, sighing, empty feeling in the abdomen, loss of muscular power, and intense subjective distress (1978, pp. 142–43). Physiologically, the body responds to a current or anticipated loss with a stress reaction. The nurse can assess the clinical signs of this response. See Chapter 16.

■ **Factors Influencing a Loss Reaction.** The influence of age and developmental level on how a person reacts to loss has already been mentioned. Other factors include the personal significance of the loss, culture, spiritual beliefs, sex role, and socioeconomic status.

The **significance of a loss** depends on the perceptions of the individual experiencing the loss. One person may experience a great sense of loss over a divorce; another may find it only mildly disrupting. A number of factors affect the significance of the loss:

■ The age of the person

■ The value placed on the lost person, body part, etc.

■ The degree of change required because of the loss

■ The person's beliefs and values

Culture influences an individual's reaction to loss. How grief is expressed is often determined by the customs of the culture. It has been suggested that the Protestant ethic (i.e., individualism, self-reliance, independence, and hard work) leads to the practice of handling grief only with significant others, not a larger community (Charmaz 1980, p. 284). In the United States and Canada, unless an extended family structure exists, grief is handled by the nuclear family, which, because of its small size, emphasizes self-reliance and independence.

Many North Americans appear to have internalized the belief that grief is a private matter to be endured internally. Therefore, feelings tend to be repressed and may remain unidentified. People who have been socialized to "be strong" and "make the best of the situation" may not express deep feelings or personal concerns when they experience a serious loss.

Some cultural groups value social support and the expression of loss. In certain black churches, the expression of emotion plays a prominent part. In Hispanic American groups where strong kinship ties are maintained, support and assistance are provided by family members, and the free expression of grief is encouraged.

Spiritual beliefs and practices greatly influence both a person's reaction to loss and subsequent behavior. Most religious groups have practices related to dying, and these are often important to the client and support persons. For additional information, see Chapter 18. For nurses to provide support at a time of death it is important that they understand the client's particular beliefs and practices.

The **sex roles** into which many people are socialized in the United States and Canada affect their reactions at times of loss. Men are frequently expected to "be strong" and show very little emotion during grief, whereas it is acceptable for women to show grief by crying. When a wife dies, the husband, who is the chief mourner, is sometimes expected to repress his own emotions and to comfort sons and daughters in their grieving.

Sex roles also affect the significance of body image changes to clients. A man might consider a facial scar to be "macho," but a woman might consider it ugly. Thus, the woman, but not the man, would see it as a loss.

The **socioeconomic status** of an individual often affects the support system available at the time of a loss. A pension plan or insurance, for example, can offer a widowed or disabled person choices of ways to deal with a loss: A woman who loses a hand and can no longer do her previous work may be able to pursue vocational reeducation; a man whose wife has died can afford to take a cruise or visit relatives in Europe. Conversely, a person who is confronted with both severe loss and economic hardship may not be able to cope with either.

■ **N**ursing Diagnosis

Many of the accepted nursing diagnoses are applicable to grieving clients, depending on the information obtained from individual assessment. Some diagnoses that may be applicable are anticipatory grieving, dysfunctional grieving, impaired adjustment, and social isolation. Anticipatory grieving is often a healthy response. Dysfunctional grieving interferes with performance of usual expected roles.

When changed health status demands modifications in life-style and behavior that the person cannot make, the appropriate nursing diagnosis may be *impaired adjustment.* This diagnosis can be applied to either the person suffering the loss or a significant other. For instance, the husband of a woman hospitalized with a life-threatening illness may feel unable to assume unaccustomed domestic duties such as childcare. And he may be resentful that the disease has removed the person who maintained the stability of family life. Social isolation occurs when the painful nature of grief can cause those experiencing it to withdraw from their normal social support systems.

▪ Planning and Implementation

The goals of grieving are to be able to remember the lost object or person without intense pain and to be able to redirect emotional energy into one's own life and regain the capacity to love. More specifically, the client needs to feel free from emotional bondage to the deceased person, be able to adjust to the changed environment, be capable of developing new relationships and renewing old ones, and feel comfortable with both positive and negative memories of the deceased (Martocchio 1985).

The skills most relevant to situations of loss and grief are attentive listening, silence, open and closed questioning, paraphrasing, clarifying and reflecting feelings, and summarizing. Less helpful to clients are responses that give advice and evaluation, those that interpret and analyze, and those that give unwarranted reassurance (Martocchio 1985). To ensure effective communication, the nurse must make an accurate assessment of what is appropriate for the client.

Communication with grieving clients needs to be relevant to their stage of grief. Whether the client is angry or depressed affects how he or she hears messages and how the nurse interprets the client's statements. Implications for nurse-client communication are related to Kübler-Ross's five stages in Table 19–2.

▪ Evaluation

Evaluating the effectiveness of nursing care of the grieving client is difficult because of the long-term nature of the life transition. Criteria for evaluation must be based on goals set by the client and family, and not on an arbitrary standard of success (Benoliel 1985). A follow-up visit to the surviving family members may be an appropriate nursing measure not only to obtain information for evaluation but also to assist nurses in working through their own grief by expressing their continuing concern for the family. Examples of outcome criteria for grieving clients are:

1. Verbalizes feelings of sorrow (or anger or loss)
2. Verbalizes understanding of feelings experienced
3. Has resumed usual activities
4. Has established new relationships

GUIDELINES

Assisting Clients with Their Grief

The following nursing guidelines may be helpful:

1. Provide opportunity for the persons involved to "tell their story."
2. Recognize and accept the varied emotions that people express in relation to a significant loss.
3. Provide support for the expression of difficult feelings, such as anger and sadness, recognizing that people must do this in their own way and at their own pace.
4. Include children in the grieving process.
5. Encourage the bereaved to maintain established relationships.
6. Acknowledge the usefulness of mutual-help groups.
7. Encourage self-care by family members—in particular, the primary caregiver.
8. Acknowledge the usefulness of counseling for especially difficult problems.

(Benoliel 1985, p. 445)

Care of the Dying Client

Assessment

Nursing care and support for the dying client and his or her family include making an accurate assessment of the physiologic signs of approaching death. In addition to signs related to the client's specific disease, certain other physical signs are indicative of impending death. The four main characteristic changes are: loss of muscle tone, slowing of the circulation, changes in vital signs, and sensory impairment. See the box on page 242 for indications of impending clinical death.

Various consciousness levels occur just before death. Some clients are alert, whereas others are drowsy, stuporous, or comatose. Hearing is thought to be the last sense lost.

▪ Clinical Signs of Death.
The traditional clinical signs of death were cessation of the apical pulse, respirations, and blood pressure. However, since the advent of artificial means to maintain respirations and blood circulation, identifying death is more difficult. In 1968, the World Medical Assembly adopted the following guidelines for physicians as indications of death (Benton 1978, p. 18): total lack of response to external stimuli, absence of breathing and other muscular movement, absence of reflexes, and exhibiting a flat encephalogram. In instances of artificial support, absence of electric currents from the brain (measured by electroencephalography) for at least 24 hours is an indica-

Signs of Impending Clinical Death

1. Loss of muscle tone

- Relaxation of the facial muscles (e.g., the jaw may sag)
- Difficulty speaking
- Difficulty swallowing and gradual loss of the gag reflex
- Decreased activity of the gastrointestinal tract, with subsequent nausea, accumulation of flatus, abdominal distention, and retention of feces, especially if narcotics or tranquilizers are being administered
- Possible urinary and rectal incontinence due to decreased sphincter control
- Diminished body movement

2. Slowing of the circulation

- Diminished sensation
- Mottling and cyanosis of the extremities
- Cold skin, first in the feet and later in the hands, ears, and nose (the client, however, may feel warm due to elevated temperature)

3. Changes in vital signs

- Decelerated and weaker pulse
- Decreased blood pressure
- Rapid, shallow, irregular, or abnormally slow respirations; mouth breathing, which leads to dry oral mucous membranes.

4. Sensory impairment

- Blurred vision
- Impaired senses of taste and smell

tion of death. Only a physician can pronounce death, and only after this pronouncement can life support systems be shut off.

Another definition of death is **cerebral death,** which occurs when the higher brain center, the cerebral cortex, is irreversibly destroyed. The client may still be able to breathe but is irreversibly unconscious. People who support this definition of death believe the cerebral cortex, which holds the capacity for thought, voluntary action, and movement, *is* the individual (Schulz 1978, p. 92).

Nursing Diagnoses

The full range of nursing diagnoses, addressing both physiologic and psychosocial needs, can be applied to the dying client, depending on the assessment data. Three diagnoses that may be particularly appropriate are fear, powerlessness, and hopelessness. Many fears are associated with death, and the nurse needs to determine a client's specific fears. Gonda and Ruark (1984, pp. 31–32) discuss three objects of the dying person's fear: the process of dying, nonexistence, and what comes after death. The nurse is usually better able to assist a client with the complex process of dying than with the spiritual fears of nonexistence and the hereafter.

The dying client or the family may express a lack of control over the situation. Powerlessness is a likely diagnosis when the impending death is sudden and unexpected or when the dying client is a child. However, powerlessness is not limited to such situations. Dying clients who have confronted chronic debilitating diseases may perceive that they can no longer control their conditions.

Feelings of hopelessness often follow an awareness of the reality of the loss and may be expressed in the despair phase of mourning (Gonda and Ruark 1984, p. 38). Real or perceived abandonment can also mean a diagnosis of hopelessness. A loss of belief in religious and spiritual values or powers may be related to the development of hopelessness. The return of realistic hope can be facilitated by the nurse through assisting the client and/or family to focus on the outcomes of specific, short-term goals (Gonda and Ruark 1984, pp. 89–90).

Planning and Implementation

The major nursing responsibility for clients who are dying is to assist the client to a peaceful death. More specific responsibilities are:

1. To provide relief from from loneliness, fear, and depression
2. To maintain the client's sense of security, self-confidence, dignity, and self-worth
3. To maintain hope
4. To help the client accept his or her losses
5. To provide physical comfort

People nearing death need help facing the fact that they will have to depend on others. Some dying clients require only minimal care and can be cared for at home; others need continuous attention and the services of a hospital and its staff. People need help, well in advance of death, in planning for the period of dependence. They need to consider what will happen and how and where they would like to die.

▪ Helping Clients Die with Dignity. *Dignity* may be defined as the ability to function as a significant and integrated person (Sheehy 1981, p. 56). Generally, dependence on others and loss of control over oneself and interactions with the environment are associated with loss of dignity. Dying clients often feel they have lost control over their lives and over life itself. By introducing options available to the client and significant others, nurses can restore and support feelings of control. Some choices that clients can make are: the location of care, e.g., hospital, home, or hospice; times of appointments with health professionals; activity schedule; use of health resources; and times of visits from relatives and friends.

Most clients interviewed about dying indicate that they want to be able to manage the events preceding death so they can die peacefully. Nurses can help clients to find meaning and completeness and to determine their own physical, psychologic, and social priorities. Dying people often strive for self-fulfillment more than self-preservation, and they need to find meaning in continuing to live while suffering. Part of the nurse's challenge, then, is to help maintain, day to day, the client's will and hope.

Salter (1982, p. 21) believes it is important for nurses and clients to focus not on the end, but on three stages of living fully until death:

1. *Developing and growing.* In this stage the client can be assisted to paint, sculpt, go to a library, visit an art gallery, etc. An occupational therapist can help clients do what they still can do and what is pleasurable.
2. *Lying fallow.* In this stage, physiotherapy measures, such as breathing exercises and passive exercises, help the client to relax and enhance self-esteem.
3. *Letting go and becoming dependent.* In this stage, nursing intervention is usually required to meet both physical and psychologic needs.

■ **Hospice and Home Care.** Hospice care, palliative care, and home care focus on support and care of the dying person and his or her family, with the goal of facilitating a peaceful and dignified death. **Hospice caregiving** is based on holistic concepts, in contrast to cure-oriented hospital care (Hadlock 1983, pp. 108–10).

The principles of hospice care can be carried out in a variety of settings, the most common being the autonomous hospice and the hospital-based **palliative-care** unit. Services range from fully comprehensive to a focus on selected areas, such as symptom control and pain management. Home care services for the dying client maintain the client in the natural home environment until that is no longer possible or until death. Hospice care is always provided by a team of both health professionals and nonprofessionals, to ensure a full range of care services. In the United States these services have been delivered primarily through autonomous, community-based hospices, while in Canada most hospice programs are hospital based. This difference may be a function of different methods for funding health care (Corless 1983, pp. 336–39). Both countries have established standards and guidelines for the development and operation of hospice programs (Health and Welfare Canada 1981, National Hospice Organization 1981).

■ **Meeting Physiologic Needs of the Dying Client.** The physiologic needs of the dying are related to a slowing of body processes and to homeostatic imbalances. Interventions include personal hygiene measures, pain control, relief of respiratory difficulties, assistance with movement, nutrition, hydration, and elimination, and measures related to sensory changes. See also Table 19–4.

Many drugs have been used to control the pain associated with terminal illness: morphine, heroin, methadone, alcohol, marijuana, and LSD. In hospitals the most frequently used agents are morphine, methadone, and alcohol. Usually the physician determines the dosage, but the client's opinion should be considered. The client is the one ultimately aware of personal pain tolerance and fluctuations of internal states. Because of decreased blood circulation, analgesics may be administered by intravenous infusion rather than subcutaneously or intramuscularly.

Table 19–4 Physiologic Needs of Dying Persons

Problem	Nursing Interventions
Ineffective airway clearance	Fowler's position: conscious clients
	Throat suctioning: conscious clients
	Low-Fowler's position: unconscious clients
	Oxygen therapy as needed
Impaired physical mobility	Assist client out of bed periodically, if client able
	Regularly change bedridden clients' position
	Support client's position with rolls of blankets or towels as needed
	Lateral position in bed, to decrease aspiration of saliva
	Elevate client's legs when sitting up, to prevent pooling of blood
Alteration in nutrition, less than body requirements	Antiemetics or alcoholic beverages, to stimulate appetite
	High-calorie, high-vitamin diet
Fluid volume deficit, actual or potential	Semisolid, soft, or liquid foods because of decreased gag reflex
	Continuing assessment of gag reflex
Alteration in bowel elimination	Laxatives as needed to prevent constipation
Alteration in urinary elimination	Skin care because of incontinence of urine or feces
	Bedpan, urinal, or commode chair within easy reach
	Call light within reach for assistance onto bedpan or commode
	Absorbent pads placed under incontinent client; linen changed as often as needed
	Catheterization in some cases
	Keep room as clean and odor-free as possible
Sensory-perceptual alteration (visual, tactile)	Clients prefer a light room
	Hearing is *not* diminished; speak clearly and do not whisper
	Touch is diminished, but client will feel pressure of touch

Source: C. R. Kneisl and S. W. Ames, *Adult health nursing. A biopsychosocial approach* (Menlo Park, Calif.: Addison-Wesley Publishing Co., 1986), p. 492. Used by permission.

▪ Spiritual Support. Spiritual support is of great importance in dealing with death. Although not all clients identify with a specific religious faith or belief, the majority have a need for meaning in their lives, particularly as they experience a terminal illness.

The nurse has a responsibility to ensure that the client's spiritual needs are attended to, either through direct intervention or by arranging access to individuals who can provide spiritual care. Nurses need to be aware of their own comfort with spiritual issues and be clear about their own ability to interact supportively with the client. Nurses have a responsibility to not impose their own religious/spiritual beliefs on a client, but to respond to the client in relation to his or her own background and needs. Communication skills are most important in helping the client articulate his or her needs and in developing a sense of caring and trust.

Specific interventions may include facilitating expressions of feeling, prayer, meditation, reading, and discussion with appropriate clergy/spiritual adviser. It is important for nurses to establish an effective interdisciplinary relationship with spiritual support specialists. For a further discussion of spiritual issues, see Chapter 18. Death-related beliefs and practices of selected religious groups are shown in Table 19–5.

Evaluation

Examples of outcome criteria for clients who are dying are listed below. The client:

1. Is free of pain.
2. Participates in self-care activities.
3. Verbalizes feelings of anger, sorrow, or loss.
4. Participates in plans for therapy.
5. Maintains open relationships with support persons and staff.

Care of the Body After Death

Body Changes

Rigor mortis is the stiffening of the body that occurs about 2 to 4 hours after death. It results from a lack of adenosine triphosphate (ATP), which is not synthesized because of a lack of glycogen in the body. ATP is necessary for muscle fiber relaxation. Its lack causes the muscles to contract, which in turn immobilizes the joints. Rigor mortis starts in the involuntary muscles (heart, bladder, etc.), then progresses to the head, neck, and trunk, and finally reaches the extremities.

Because the deceased's family often wants to view the body, and because it is important that the deceased appear natural and comfortable, nurses need to position the body, place dentures in the mouth, and close the eyes and mouth *before* rigor mortis sets in. Rigor mortis usually ceases about 96 hours after death.

Algor mortis is the gradual decrease of the body's temperature after death. When blood circulation terminates and the hypothalamus ceases to function, body temperature falls about 1 C (1.8 F) per hour until it reaches room temperature. Simultaneously, the skin loses its elasticity and can easily be broken when removing dressings and adhesive tape. After blood circulation has ceased, the skin becomes discolored. The red blood cells break down, releasing hemoglobin, which discolors the surrounding tissues. This discoloration, referred to as **livor mortis,** appears in the lowermost or dependent areas of the body.

Tissues after death become soft and eventually liquefied by bacterial fermentation. The hotter the temperature, the more rapid the change. Therefore, bodies are often stored in cool places to delay this process. Embalming reverses the process through injection of chemicals into the body to destroy the bacteria (Pennington 1978, p. 847).

Legal Aspects of Death

Of the many legal ramifications of human death, the most basic for the nurse is that death must be certified by a physician. In circumstances of unusual death, an **autopsy** (postmortem examination) may be required. Nurses have a responsibility to be aware of the legal ramifications of death in the jurisdiction of their practice. Chapter 6 provides legal information about death certificates, labeling the deceased, autopsy, organ donation, and inquest. Wills, euthanasia, and the right to die (living wills) are also discussed in Chapter 6.

Nursing Intervention

Nursing personnel may be responsible for care of a body after death. If the deceased's family or friends wish to view the body, it is important to make the environment as clean and pleasant as possible and to make the body appear natural and comfortable. All equipment and supplies should be removed from the bedside. Some agencies require that all tubes in the body be clamped and remain in place; in other agencies, tubes may be cut to within 2.5 cm (1 in) of the skin and taped in place. Soiled linen is removed so that the room is free from odors.

The body is normally placed in a supine position with the arms either at the sides, palms down, or across the abdomen. The wristband is left on unless it is too tight. One pillow is placed under the head and shoulders to prevent blood from discoloring the face by settling in it. The eyelids are closed and held in place for a few seconds so that they remain closed. If they will not stay closed, a moistened cotton fluff will hold them in place. Dentures are usually inserted to help give the face a natural appearance. The mouth is then closed; a rolled towel under the chin will hold it closed.

Soiled areas of the body are washed; however, a complete bath is not necessary, since the body will be washed by the mortician (also referred to as an undertaker), a person trained in the care of the dead. Absorbent pads are placed under the buttocks to absorb any

Table 19–5 Death-Related Beliefs and Practices of Selected Religious Groups

Group	Afterlife	Rituals/Funerals	Autopsy	Organ Donation	Cremation	Prolonging Life
American Indian	Beliefs vary	Practices vary; most want family present	Prohibited		Practices vary	
Black Muslim		Special procedures for washing and shrouding the dead; special funeral rites				
Buddhist in America	Reincarnation; after reaching state of enlightenment, may attain nirvana	Last rite; chanting at bedside	No restriction		No restriction	Permit euthanasia in hopeless illness
Church of Christ Scientist	Yes	No last rites	Only in sudden death	No	Individual decision	
Church of Jesus Christ of Latter Day Saints (Mormon)	Yes	Baptism essential; preaching gospel to dead also practiced	No restriction	No restriction	Discouraged	
Eastern Orthodox (Greek and Russian Orthodox)	Yes	Last rites (administration of Holy Communion obligatory)	Discouraged		Discouraged	Encouraged
Episcopal (Anglican)	Yes	Last rites not mandatory	No restriction	No restriction	No restriction	
Hindu	Reincarnation; after leading a perfect life, may join Brahma	Priest pours water into mouth of corpse and ties string around wrist or neck as sign of blessing; string must not be removed; family washes body	No restriction	No restriction	Preferred; ashes cast in holy river	
Islam (Moslem, Muslim)	May join Allah by being a good Moslem and observing rituals daily	Dying person must confess sins and ask forgiveness in presence of family; family washes and prepares body (female body cannot be washed by male) and turns body toward Mecca	Prohibited unless required by law	Prohibited	Prohibited	Encouraged
Jehovah's Witness			Prohibited unless required by law. No body parts may be removed	Prohibited	No restriction	
Judaism	Dead will be resurrected with coming of Messiah; man lives on through survival of memory	Body ritually washed by members of Ritual Burial Society; burial as soon as possible after death; dead not left unattended; five stages of mourning extending over a year; no embalming; no flowers at funeral because flowers are a symbol of life	Orthodox prohibit; some liberals permit; no body parts removed	Beliefs vary	Largely prohibited; beliefs vary	
Lutheran	Yes	Last rites optional	No restriction	No restriction	No restriction	
Roman Catholicism	Yes; resurrection with second coming of Christ	Rites for anointing the sick not mandatory; receiving Holy Communion mandatory	Permitted, but all body parts must be given appropriate burial	No restriction	No restriction	Discouraged
Seventh Day Adventist	Dead are asleep until return of Christ, when final rewards and punishments will be given					
Unitarian	Beliefs vary		No restriction	Encouraged	Encouraged	Preferred

Sources: H. M Ross, Societal/cultural views regarding death and dying, *Nursing* 77, December 1977, 7:64–70. Reprinted with permission from the December issue of *Nursing Life*, Copyright © 1977, Springhouse Corporation, 1111 Bethlehem Pike, Springhouse, PA 19477.

feces and urine released because of relaxation of the sphincter muscles. A clean gown is placed on the client and the hair is brushed and combed. All jewelry is removed, except a wedding band in some instances, which is taped to the finger. The top bed linens are adjusted neatly to cover the client to the shoulders. Soft lighting and chairs are provided for the family. All the client's valuables, including clothing, are listed and placed in a safe storage area for the family to take away.

After the body has been viewed by the family, additional identification tags are applied, one to the ankle and one to the wrist if the client's wrist identification band was not left in place. The body is wrapped in a **shroud,** a large rectangular or square piece of plastic or cotton material used to enclose a body after death. Another identification band is then applied to the outside of the shroud. The body is taken to the morgue for cooling, if arrangements have not been made to have a mortician pick it up from the client's room. Agencies vary in their policies about transporting bodies. Some close all room doors before transporting a deceased client through corridors, and service elevators are often used.

Chapter Highlights

- Nurses help clients deal with all kinds of losses, including loss of body image, loss of a loved one, loss of a sense of well-being, and loss of a job.
- Loss, especially loss of a loved one or a valued body part, can be viewed as a crisis, either situational or developmental, and either actual or perceived (both of which can be anticipatory).
- How an individual deals with loss is closely related to the individual's stage of development, personal resources, and social support systems.
- Caring for the dying and the bereaved is one of the nurse's most complex and challenging responsibilities.
- Nurses' attitudes about death and dying directly affect their ability to provide care.
- Nurses must consider the entire family as the client in situations involving loss, especially the crisis of death.
- Grieving is a normal, subjective emotional response to loss; it is essential for mental and physical health.
- Grieving allows the bereaved person to cope with loss gradually and to accept it as part of reality.
- Knowledge of different stages or phases of grieving and factors that influence the loss reaction can help the nurse understand the responses and needs of clients.
- Nurses caring for clients who are suffering loss or dying need effective communication skills.
- Dying clients require physical help and emotional support to ensure a peaceful and dignified death.

Selected References

Alexander, J., and Kiely, J. March/April 1986. Working with the bereaved. *Geriatric Nursing* 7(2):85–86.

Benoliel, J. Q. June 1985. Loss and terminal illness. *Nursing Clinics of North America* 20(2):439–48.

Benton, R. E. 1978. *Death and dying: Principles and practices in patient care.* New York: D. Van Nostrand Co.

Burgess, A. W., and Lazare, A. 1976. *Community mental health: Target populations.* Englewood Cliffs, N.J.: Prentice-Hall.

Charmaz, K. 1980. *The social reality of death.* Reading, Mass.: Addison-Wesley Publishing Co.

Conrad, N. L. June 1985. Spiritual support for the dying. *Nursing Clinics of North America* 20(2):415–26.

Corless, I. B. 1983. The hospice movement in North America. In Corr, C. A., and Corr, D. M., editors. *Hospice care: Principles and practice.* New York: Springer Publishing Co.

Cowan, M. E.; Murphy, S. A.; et al. March/April 1985. Identification of postdisaster bereavement risk predictors. *Nursing Research* 34(2):71–75.

Demi, A. S., and Miles, M. S. 1986. Bereavement. *Annual Review of Nursing Research* 4:105–23.

Engel, G. L. September 1964. Grief and grieving. *American Journal of Nursing* 64:93–98.

Enlow, P. M. July 1986. Coping with anticipatory grief. *Journal of Gerontological Nursing* 12(7):36–37.

Fetsch, S. H. November/December 1984. The 7- to 10-year-old child's conceptualization of death. *Oncology Nurses' Forum* 11(6):52–56.

Field, D. January 1984. "We didn't want him to die on his own"—Nurses' accounts of nursing dying patients. *Journal of Advanced Nursing* 1:59–70.

Gonda, T. A., and Ruark, J.E. 1984. *Dying dignified: The health professional's guide to care.* Menlo Park, Calif.: Addison-Wesley.

Hadlock, D. C. 1983. Physician rules in hospice care. In Corr, C. A., and Corr, D. M., editors. *Hospice care: Principles and practice.* New York: Springer Publishing Co.

Health and Welfare Canada. 1981. Palliative care services in hospitals: Guidelines. Ottawa: Ministry of National Health and Welfare.

Hoff, L. A. 1984. *People in crisis.* Menlo Park, Calif.: Addison-Wesley.

Kennedy, S. R. January/February 1985. Sharing, caring, living, dying. *Geriatric Nursing* 6(1):12–17.

Kübler-Ross, E. 1969. *On death and dying.* New York: Macmillan Publishing Co.

Martocchio, B. C. June 1985. Grief and bereavement: Healing through hurt. *Nursing Clinics of North America* 20(2):327–41.

Moss, M. S., and Moss, S. Z. 1983-84. The impact of parental death on middle-aged children. *Omega* 14(1):65–75.

National Hospice Organization. 1981. Standards of a hospice program of care. Arlington, Va.: National Hospice Organization.

Pennington, E. A. May 1978. Postmortem care: More than ritual. *American Journal of Nursing* 78:846–47.

Richter, J. M. July 1984. Crisis of mate loss in the elderly. *American Nursing Society* 6(4):45–54.

Salter, R. March 1982. The art of dying. *Canadian Nurse* 78:20–21.

Schulz, R. 1978. *The psychology of death, dying and bereavement.* Reading, Mass.: Addison-Wesley Publishing Co.

Sheehy, P. F. 1981. *On dying with dignity.* New York: Pinnacle Books.

Strauss, A. L., et al. 1970. Awareness of dying. In Schoenberg, B., et al., editors. *Loss and grief.* New York: Columbia University Press.

Taylor, D. A. 1983-84. View of death from sufferers of early loss. *Omega* 14(1):77–82.

Communication Processes

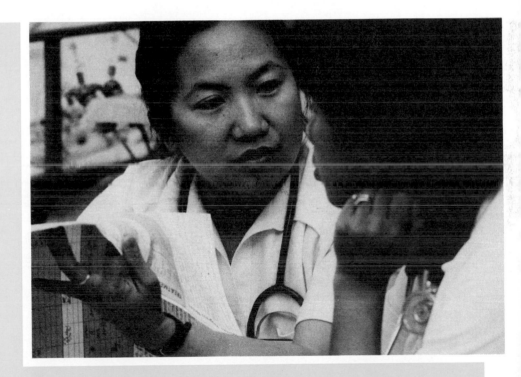

20

Communicating

OBJECTIVES

Describe essential aspects of communication and the communication process.

Differentiate between verbal and nonverbal communication.

Explain the four elements of the communication process outlined in this chapter.

Identify ways in which selected factors influence the communication process.

Give guidelines for assessing problems in communicating.

List examples of nursing diagnoses pertaining to communication.

Describe strategies for planning to resolve communication problems.

Describe effective and ineffective methods used by nurses when communicating with clients

List outcome criteria that can be used to evaluate whether or not communication problems have been resolved.

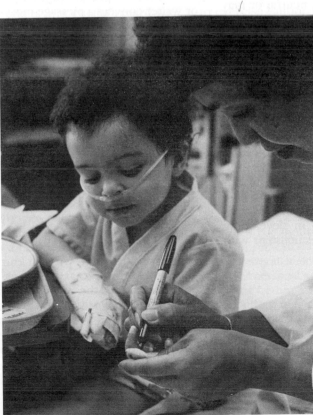

Frequently the receiver is expected to assimilate too much information. The nurse may be talking too quickly or presenting too many ideas at once. This is of particular importance when offering health instruction.

Perceptions

Because each person has unique personality traits, values, and life experiences, each perceives and interprets messages differently. For example, a nurse may draw the curtains around a crying woman and leave her alone. The woman may interpret this in at least three ways: "The nurse thinks I will upset the others around me and that I shouldn't cry." "The nurse doesn't like crying." "The nurse respects my need to be alone." It is important in many situations to validate or correct the perceptions of the receiver.

Personal Space

Personal space is the distance people prefer to stand or sit apart when interacting with others. For middle-class North Americans, various distances, voice tones, and body languages are appropriate in different circumstances. Nurses should assess individual client's comfort levels and attempt to respect that preference as much as is feasible when providing case.

Territoriality

Territoriality is a concept of the space and things that an individual considers as belonging to him or her. Territories marked off by people may be visible to others. For example, a client in a hospital often considers his or her territory as bounded by the curtains around the bed unit or by the walls of a private room. All health care workers must recognize this human tendency to claim territory. Clients often defend their territory when it is invaded by others. For example, a visitor who removes a chair to use at another bed inadvertently violates the territory of the client whose chair was moved.

Roles, Relationships, and Purposes

The roles and the relationship between sender and receiver affect the communication process. Roles such as nursing student and instructor, client and physician, or parent and child affect the content and responses in the communication process. Choice of words, sentence structure, and tone of voice vary considerably from role to role. The specific relationship between the communicators is significant. The nurse who meets with a client for the first time communicates differently from the nurse who has previously developed a relationship with that client. The intended purpose of a communication also alters interactions with others. For example, if the purpose is to acknowledge another's presence, the nurse may say, "Hello, how goes it today?" But if the purpose is to assess the person's pain and the effect of an anal-

gesic, several more specific questions and responses are necessary.

Time and Setting

The time factor in communication includes what precedes and follows the interaction. The hospitalized client who is anticipating surgery or has just received the news that a spouse has lost a job will not be very receptive to information. A client who has had to wait for some time to express needs may respond quite differently from one who has not. The setting also influences communication. The communication process can break down in a room that lacks privacy or is hot, noisy, or crowded.

Nurses' use of time can facilitate or inhibit a client's communication. The nurse who tells a client "I'll be back in a moment" while delivering medications is likely to convey "I haven't time now" or "I've got work to do." This message inhibits client communications. Some clients learn that requests need to be made as soon as the nurse appears. Often their request is accompanied by an apology for taking the nurse's time. However, this nurse can facilitate communication by saying, "Would you tell me now what your concern is about, and then when I've finished delivering medications I'll come back and help you with it."

Attitudes

Attitudes convey beliefs, thoughts, and feelings about people and events. They are communicated convincingly and rapidly to others. Attitudes such as caring, warmth, respect, and acceptance facilitate communication, whereas condescension, lack of interest, and coldness inhibit communication.

Caring and *warmth* convey a feeling of emotional closeness, in contrast to impersonal distance. Caring is more enduring and intense than warmth. It conveys deep and genuine concern for the person. Warmth, by contrast, conveys friendliness and consideration, shown by acts of smiling and attention to physical comfort (Brammer 1985, p. 34). Caring involves giving feelings, thoughts, skill, and knowledge. It requires psychologic energy and poses the risk of gaining little in return, yet, by caring, people usually reap the benefits of greater communication and understanding.

Respect is an attitude that emphasizes the other person's worth and individuality. It conveys that the person's hopes and feelings are special and unique even though similar to those of others in many ways. People have a need to be different from, and at the same time similar to, others. Being too different can be isolating and threatening. Respect is conveyed by listening open-mindedly to what the client is saying, even if the nurse disagrees. Nurses can learn new ways of approaching situations when they conscientiously listen to another person's perspective.

Acceptance conveys neither approval nor disapproval. The nurse willingly receives client's honest feelings and actions without judgment. An accepting attitude allows clients to express personal feelings freely and to be themselves. The nurse may need to restrict acceptance in situations where the client's actions are harmful to self or others.

In contrast, *condescension* is an attitude that conveys superiority over the other person. Clients who feel helpless often perceive nurses to be in a superior position because of their knowledge and skill. In these instances, the nurse may convey condescension by an air of superiority and intellectualism. One common condescending act by nurses is to call clients "honey" or "dear." This casts the nurse in the role of superior mother and the client in the role of inferior child. Another condescending act is patting an elderly client on the head.

Lack of interest also inhibits communication because it conveys the message "I'm not concerned" or "What you say is not important." The nurse conveys lack of interest by forgetting part of the client's conversation or not concentrating on it sufficiently to respond. Being tired near the end of a long day's work or in a hurry to complete tasks may contribute to giving the appearance of not being interested in clients.

Coldness is the opposite of caring and warmth. Nurses convey this attitude by appearing more interested in the technical and procedural aspects of nursing than in the concerns of the person receiving the therapy. For example, the nurse can convey coldness by appearing more concerned about the neatness of the client's bed than about the client's restlessness or more interested in the efficient functioning of a cardiac monitor than in the client's anxiety. A rigid body posture and aloof tone of voice also convey a nurse's lack of genuine concern for the client.

Emotions and Self-esteem

Most people have experienced overwhelming joy or sorrow that is difficult to express in words. Anger may produce loud, profane vocalizations or controlled speechlessness. Fright may produce screams of terror or paralyzed silence. Emotions also affect a person's ability to interpret messages. Large parts of a message may not be heard, or the message may be misinterpreted when the receiver is experiencing strong emotion. This situation occurs frequently in nursing. For example, the client feeling great fear may not remember all the preoperative instructions offered by a nurse.

Self-esteem also influences communication patterns. People whose self-esteem is high communicate honestly, with confidence, and with congruence (agreement or coinciding) between verbal and nonverbal messages. For example, a nurse explaining the importance of preoperative exercises would present a sincere and serious facial expression. Those with low self-esteem or under high stress tend to give double messages; that is, their verbal and nonverbal messages are incongruent (lack consistency). For example, while explaining about a client's colostomy to the client's family, a nurse laughs.

Assessing Communication

When nurses assess the communication of clients, they need to include language development, nonverbal behavior, and communication style.

Language Development

The nurse assesses the following aspects of language development:

- The language skills presented by the client, compared to the language skills normally expected. See Table 20-1 for an overview of language development.
- Adequacy of the language skills in relation to the individual's need.
- The chief method of communicating, e.g., words or gestures.
- Obstacles to language development, such as deafness or absence of environmental stimuli.
- Specific forms of language impairment, e.g., a school-age child's inability to write or lack of abstractions in the language of an adult.

Table 20-1 Language Development

Stage	Normal Behavior
Newborn	At birth—cries as air passes over vocal cords. Within 2 to 3 weeks—cries becomes differentiated.
Infant	At 2 to 3 months—babbling begins. At 7 months—repeats sounds heard from environment. At 10 to 12 months—responds to few familiar words; single words are pronounced. At 15 months—can say about four words.
Toddler	At 2 years—initially has over 50-word vocabulary; this increases progressively to about 800–1000 words by 3 years. Associates symbols with form, e.g., words, pictures. Grammatical errors are common.
Preschooler	At 4 years—vocabulary has grown to about 1600 words. Sentences are complete. By 5 to 6 years—most infantile pronunciations have disappeared.
School-age child	At 6 years—has command of most sentence structures. Speech is less egocentric. Vocabulary continues to increase; comprehension exceeds use. Slang and swear words become part of vocabulary. At 8 to 12 years—boasting commonly occurs.
Adolescent	Uses language of subgroup. Speech reflects consideration of hypotheses.
Adulthood	Has full speech skills. Language often reflects specialized education.

- Cultural influences on language development, e.g., the language used in the home or customs about when and how to speak.

Nonverbal Behavior

In assessing nonverbal communication, the nurse considers:

- Gestures used by the individual.
- Posture and facial expressions employed.
- Use of touch as a means of communication. See the section "Using Touch" later in this chapter.
- The interpersonal distance with which the person feels comfortable, e.g., whether the person assumes an intimate distance for most discussions.
- The grooming and appearance of the individual. These may affect the communication process, e.g., when dress is inconsistent with a setting or presents a stereotype that may evoke biases.

Style of Communication

A person's style of communication is often affected by such factors as his or her health, culture, education, stress level, fatigue, and cognitive ability. In assessing communication style, the nurse considers the following:

- The vocabulary of the individual, particularly any changes from the vocabulary normally used. For example, a person who normally never swears may indicate increased stress or illness by an uncharacteristic use of profanity.
- The use of symbols and gestures to communicate. Some uses of symbols and gestures are culturally determined. For example, a Puerto Rican girl may be taught not to look an adult in the eyes, as a sign of respect and obedience, and the gesture should not be interpreted as a sign of guilt.
- The presence of hostility, aggression, assertiveness, reticence, hesitance, anxiety, or loquaciousness in the communication.
- Difficulties with verbal communication, such as stuttering, inability to pronounce a particular sound, or lack of clarity in enunciation.

Diagnosing Communication Problems

The nursing diagnosis *impaired communication* is the "state in which an individual experiences, or could experience, a decreased ability to send or receive messages, i.e., has difficulty exchanging thoughts, ideas, or desires" (Carpenito 1987, p. 21). This broad diagnostic category includes "impaired verbal communication," which was discussed with reference to language barriers in Chapter 17. A number of conditions may contribute

to the development of communication problems, and the nurse should be especially alert for signs of difficulty in clients with these conditions. Among these are any medical diagnosis (e.g., cerebrovascular accident), pharmacologic intervention (e.g., central nervous system depressants), or surgical procedure (e.g., tracheostomy) that results in cerebral, neurologic, respiratory, auditory, or laryngeal impairments. Similarly, pain, fatigue, memory loss, or psychosocial factors (e.g., fear, shyness, lack of privacy, loneliness, or depression) may be part of the etiology of *impaired communication*.

Planning for Effective Communication

When problems in communication have been identified, the nurse begins planning ways to promote effective communication. Among these ways are developing listening skills and becoming aware of how people respond. With such a knowledge base, the nurse can plan individualized strategies (i.e., specify short-term goals, designate measurable criteria with which to gauge whether the goals have been met, and identify nursing interventions to meet the goals) for effectively communicating with clients.

Attentive Listening

It is essential, in therapeutic communication, that nurses listen and respond to clients purposefully and deliberately. Attentive listening is listening actively, using all the senses, as opposed to listening passively with just the ear. It is probably the most important technique in nursing. Attentive listening is an active process that requires energy and concentration. It involves paying attention to the total message, both verbal messages and nonverbal messages that can modify what is spoken, and noting whether these communications are congruent. Attentive listening means absorbing both the content and the feeling the person is conveying, without selectivity. The listener does not select or listen to solely what he or she wants to hear; the nurse does not focus on her or his own needs but rather on the client's needs. Attentive listening conveys an attitude of caring and interest, thereby encouraging the client to talk. In summary, attentive listening is a highly developed skill, but fortunately it can be learned with practice.

A nurse can convey attentiveness in listening to clients in various ways. Common responses are nodding the head, uttering "uh huh" or "mmm," repeating the words that the client has used, or saying "I see what you mean." Each nurse has characteristic ways of responding, and the nurse must take care not to sound insincere or phony.

Egan (1982, pp. 60–61) has outlined five specific ways to convey physical attending. He defines physical attending as the manner of being present to another or being with another. Listening, in his frame of reference, is what a person does while attending. The five actions of physical attending, which convey a "posture of involvement," arc:

1. *Face the other person squarely.* This position says, "I am available to you." Moving to the side lessens the degree of involvement.
2. *Maintain good eye contact.* Mutual eye contact, preferably at the same level, recognizes the other person and denotes a willingness to maintain communication. Eye contact neither glares at nor stares down another but is natural.
3. *Lean toward the other.* People move naturally toward one another when they want to say or hear something—by moving to the front of a class, by moving a chair nearer a friend, or by leaning across a table with arms propped in front. The nurse conveys involvement when she or he leans forward, closer to the client.
4. *Maintain an open posture.* The nondefensive position is one in which neither arms nor legs are crossed. It conveys that the person wishes to encourage the passage of communication, as the open door of a home or an office does.
5. *Remain relatively relaxed.* Total relaxation is not feasible when the nurse is listening with intensity, but the nurse can show relaxation by taking time in responding, allowing pauses as needed, balancing periods of tension with relaxation, and using gestures that are natural. See Figure 20–3.

These five attending postures need to be adapted to the specific needs of clients in a given situation. For example, leaning forward may not be appropriate at the beginning of an interview. It may be reserved until a closer relationship grows between the nurse and the client. The same applies to eye contact, which is generally uninterrupted when the communicators are very involved in the interaction.

▌Responding

Nurses can learn much by examining and becoming aware of their own reactions (feelings) and responses. Although it is difficult for nurses to see their own nonverbal communication other than by videotape feedback, much can be learned by reflecting on what was heard, what the nurse said, and when and how it was said. Methods such as role playing, process recordings, and audiotapes can be useful.

Nurses need to respond not only to the content of a client's verbal message but also to the feelings expressed. It is important to understand how the client views the situation and feels about it before responding. The content of the client's communication is the words or thoughts, as distinct from the feelings. Sometimes people can convey a thought in words while their emotions contradict the words; i.e., words and feelings are incongruent. For example, a client says, "I am glad he has left me; he was very cruel." However, the nurse observes that the client has tears in her eyes as she says this. To respond to the client's *words,* the nurse might simply rephrase, saying "You are pleased that he has left you."

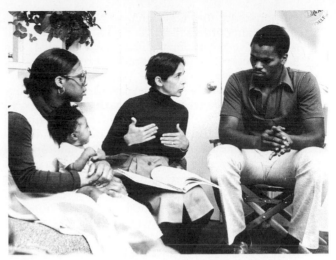

Figure 20–3 The nurse conveys attentive listening through a posture of involvement.

To respond to the client's *feelings,* the nurse would need to acknowledge the tears in the client's eyes, saying, for example, "You seem saddened by all this." Such a response helps the client to focus on her feelings. In some instances, the nurse may need to know more about the client and her resources for coping with these feelings.

Sometimes clients need time to deal with their feelings. Strong emotions are often draining. People usually need to deal with feelings before they can cope with other matters, such as learning new skills or planning for the future. This is most evident in hospitals when clients learn that they have a terminal illness. Some require hours, days, or even weeks before they are ready to start other tasks. Some need only time to themselves, others need someone to listen, others need assistance identifying and verbalizing feelings, and others need assistance making decisions about future courses of action.

▌Developing Helping Relationships

Nurse-client relationships are referred to by some as *interpersonal relationships,* by others as *therapeutic relationships,* and by still others as *helping relationships.* Helping is a growth-facilitating process in which one person assists another to solve problems and to face crises in the direction the assisted person chooses (Brammer 1985, p. 5).

Whatever the practice setting, the nurse establishes some sort of helping relationship in which mutual goals are set with the client, or with support persons if the client is unable to participate. Although special training in counseling techniques and psychiatry is advantageous, there are many ways of helping clients that do not require special training. Shanken and Shanken (1976, pp. 24–27) have outlined 11 of these:

1. *Listen actively.* (See the discussion earlier in this chapter.)
2. *Help to identify what the person is feeling.* Often clients who are troubled are unable to identify or to label their feelings and consequently have difficulty working them out or talking about them.

Responses by the nurse such as "You seem angry about taking orders from your boss" or "You sound as if you've been lonely since your wife died" can help clients recognize what they are feeling and talk about it.

3. *Put yourself in the other person's shoes.* The ability to do this is referred to as **empathy.** According to Egan (1975, p. 76), empathy involves the ability to discriminate what the other's world is like and to communicate to the other this understanding in a way that shows the other that the helper has picked up both the client's *feelings* and the *behavior* and *experience* underlying these feelings.

4. *Be honest.* In effective relationships nurses honestly recognize any lack of knowledge by saying, "I don't know the answer to that right now"; openly discuss their own discomfort by saying, for example, "I feel uncomfortable about this discussion"; and admit tactfully that problems do exist, for instance, when a client says "I'm a mess, aren't I?"

5. *Do not tell a person not to feel.* Feelings expressed by clients often make nurses uncomfortable. Common examples are a client's expressions of anger or worry or a client's crying. When a nurse feels this discomfort, common responses are "Don't worry about it, everything will be fine" or "Please don't cry." Such responses inhibit the client's expression of feelings. Unless feelings are extremely inappropriate, it is best to encourage the client to ventilate (voice) them. Ventilation allows the client to express feelings in words and examine them objectively. Indirectly, such an attitude conveys this message: "Your feelings are not that awful, since I am not bothered by them."

6. *Do not tell a person what he or she should feel.* Statements that indicate to clients how they should feel, rather than how they actually do feel, in essence deny clients' true feelings and suggest that they are inappropriate. Examples are: "You shouldn't complain about pain; many others have gone through this same experience stoically" and "You should be glad that you are alive and not worry about the loss of your arm."

7. *Do not make excuses for the other person.* When a person reacts with an intense feeling such as anger or grief and seems to have lost control of behavior to the astonishment or discomfort of others, a common error is to explain the behavior by offering excuses. Examples are: "Well, Mr. Brown, you're upset about not finishing your lunch, but the dietitian and I gave you too much" and "I guess you've had a tough session in physical therapy." These responses discourage and divert the person from discussing feelings of anger or inadequacy. The helper has made assumptions about the reasons for the client's behavior and therefore inhibits exploration of what the client is really experiencing and feeling.

8. *Be personal.* Personal statements can be helpful in solidifying the rapport between the nurse and the client. The nurse might offer such comments as "I recall when I was in (a similar situation) and I felt angry about being put down." Egan (1982, p. 128) states that the helper "must be spontaneous, open. He can't hide behind the role of counselor. He must be a human being to the human being before him." Egan refers to this quality as *genuineness.* Nurses need to exercise caution when making references about themselves. These statements must be used with discretion. The extreme of matching each of the client's problems with a better story of the nurse's own is of little value to the client.

9. *Use your ingenuity.* There are always many courses of action to consider in handling problems. Whatever course is chosen needs to further achievement of the client's goals, be compatible with the client's value system, and offer the probability of success. The client needs to choose the ways to achieve goals; however, the nurse can assist in identifying options. For example, a client has asked for help because he is depressed and anxious about retirement. The nurse knows he loves animals, young children, and storytelling. In this case, the nurse might direct his thoughts toward acquiring a puppy, writing children's stories, and volunteering at the public library.

10. *Try to summarize to the person at the end of the interview.* Summarizing serves several purposes: it helps to terminate the interview, it reassures the client that the nurse has listened, it checks the accuracy of the nurse's perceptions, it clears the way for new ideas, and it helps the client to note progress and forward direction (Brammer 1985, p. 74). Sometimes clients may spontaneously offer a summary; at other times the nurse must initiate it or ask the client to do so. The nurse may say, "Let's look at what has happened in this interview. What do you think has been accomplished?"

11. *Know your role and your limitations.* Every person has unique strengths and problems. When the nurse feels unable to handle some problems, the client should be informed and referred to the appropriate health professional.

Implementing

Techniques for Therapeutic Communication

Therapeutic communication promotes understanding by both the sender and the receiver. There are a number of techniques that help establish a constructive relationship between the nurse and the client, although use of the techniques is no guarantee of effective communication. So many factors are involved in communication that the nurse is ill-advised to rely on any one technique or even several techniques. Not all people feel comfortable with all techniques, and skill in using them appropriately is essential. The nurse must be comfortable with the technique used and convey sincerity to the client. A phony or false response is usually quickly identified by clients and hinders the development of an effective relationship.

■ **Paraphrasing.** Paraphrasing, also called *restating*, involves listening for the client's basic message and then repeating those thoughts and/or feelings in similar words. Usually fewer words are used. Paraphrasing conveys that the nurse has listened and understood the client's basic message. It may also offer the client a clearer idea of what he or she said. The client's response to the paraphrase may tell the nurse whether the paraphrase was accurate or helpful. (It may be necessary for the nurse to ask for a response.)

Client: I couldn't manage to eat any of my dinner last night—not even the dessert.

Nurse: You had difficulty eating yesterday.

Client: Yes, I was very upset after my family left.

■ **Clarifying.** Clarifying is a method of making the client's message more understandable. It is used when paraphrasing is difficult, when the communication has been rambling or garbled. To clarify the message, the nurse can make a guess and restate the basic message, or confess confusion and ask the client to repeat or restate the message (Davis 1984, p. 9). In the former situation, if the client says, "I didn't sleep at all last night," the nurse might say, "You didn't sleep at all last night." In the latter instance, the nurse might say, "I'm puzzled" or "I'm not sure I understand that" and "Would you please say that again?" or "Would you tell me more?"

Nurses sometimes need to clarify their own messages to clients. The need to do so is generally discovered from the client's nonverbal feedback. Then the nurse might ask a question or say, "It seems to me I didn't make that clear" and repeat or rephrase the message. Sometimes only one word or phrase in a message needs clarifying.

Clarifying also includes *verifying what is implied*. In this instance, the client implies or hints at something without actually saying it. The nurse then tries to clarify the client's statement without interpreting it.

Client: There is no point in asking for a pain pill.

Nurse: Are you saying that no one gives you a pill when you have pain?

or

Nurse: Are you saying that your pills are not helping your pain?

Another clarifying technique is **perception checking,** or *consensual validation*. This verifies the accuracy of the nurse's listening skills by giving and receiving feedback about what was communicated. It involves paraphrasing what the nurse thinks she or he heard and asking the client for confirmation. It is important to allow the client to correct inaccurate perceptions. The advantage of frequent perception checking is that inaccurate perceptions are corrected before communications become confused and misunderstandings arise. Examples of perception checking are: "You sound annoyed with me—is that correct?" or "You seem to have some doubts about the decision you made, and I'd like to see if what I'm hearing is accurate."

■ **Using Open-Ended Questions and Statements.** An open-ended question is one that leads or invites clients to explore (elaborate, clarify, or illustrate) their thoughts or feelings. It allows clients the freedom to talk about what they wish. It also places responsibility on clients to explore and to understand themselves, in contrast to receiving advice from another (Stewart and Cash 1985, p. 79). Examples of open-ended questions are: "How did you feel in that situation?" "What do you think she meant by that remark?" "Would you describe more about how you relate to your child?" "What would you like to talk about today?" Examples of open-ended statements are "I'd like to hear more about that" and "Tell me about . . ."

These questions or statements require more than a "yes" or "no" or other short response, such as "yesterday" or "I don't know." They encourage clients to discover what their thoughts and feelings truly are. Such questions usually begin with "what" or "how." Questions that begin with "when," "where," "who," "do (did, does)" or "is (are, was)" tend to produce short answers that impede self-exploration. Nurses need to use this latter type of question in situations that require information gathering, such as taking a nursing history.

■ **Focusing.** Focusing is used when the client's communication is vague, when the client is rambling, or when the client seems to be talking about numerous things. Focusing can be compared to using a telephoto lens, which focuses sharply on a certain aspect of a view; similarly, the nurse assists or leads the client to focus on one specific aspect of a communication. It is important for the nurse to wait until the client thinks he or she has talked about the main concerns before attempting to focus. The focus may be an idea or a feeling; however, a feeling is often emphasized, to help the client recognize an emotion disguised behind words.

Client: My wife says she will look after me but I don't think she can, what with the children to take care of, and they're always after her about something—clothes, homework, what's for dinner that night.

Nurse: You are worried about how well she can manage.

■ **Being Specific, Tentative, and Informative.** When responding to another person's comments, it is helpful to make statements that are specific rather than general, tentative rather than absolute, and informative rather than authoritarian. Examples are: "You scratched my arm" (specific statement) rather than "You're as clumsy as an ox" (general statement); "You seemed unconcerned about Mary" (tentative statement) rather than "You don't give a damn about Mary and you never will" (absolute statement); and "I haven't finished yet" (informative statement) rather than "Stop interrupting!" (authoritarian statement).

In being informative, the nurse needs to present facts or specific information simply and directly. If the nurse does not know some fact, this is also stated simply, together with a suggestion about where or how the information can be obtained.

Client: I don't know the visiting hours.

Nurse: The visiting hours are 9:00 A.M. to 9:00 P.M. each day.

Client: When will my doctor be in?

Nurse: I don't know. But Ms. Lu, the charge nurse, will be here in a few minutes, and she may know.

Another way to be informative is to make an observation. This indicates that the nurse has noticed a change of behavior but is not placing a value judgment on it. For example: "You have washed your hair" (neutral observation); "Your hair looks better now that you have washed it" (value judgment); "You are holding your arm carefully; is it painful?" (observation; verifying implication).

■ **Using Touch.** Certain forms of touching indicate affection. For example, cheek patting, hand patting, and putting an arm over the person's shoulder are valued forms of affection in North America. The "laying on of hands" is a common expression indicating curative and comforting actions. Tactile contacts vary considerably among individuals, families, and cultures. Some families have a great deal of tactile contact among members. Other families, even within the same culture, have minimal contact. Appropriate forms of touch can be helpful in reinforcing caring feelings by the nurse. See Figure 20–4. The use of touch alone often says much more

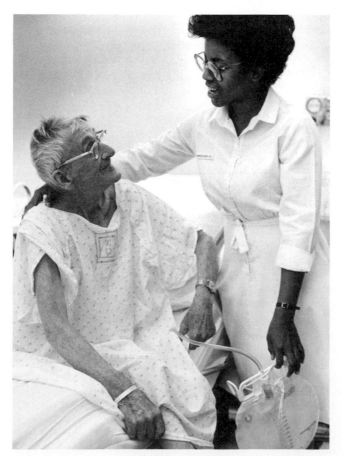

Figure 20—4 Appropriate forms of touch can communicate caring.

than words for clients, such as for those who are terminally ill or who are unable to speak, for whatever reason. It is important, however, for the nurse to be sensitive to the differences in attitudes and practices related to touch among individuals, including the nurse's own attitudes.

■ **Using Silence.** In everyday conversations, natural pauses or silences are often accepted without thought. The listener attentively waits until the talker resumes conversation. These natural pauses are generally used to recall a name or event or to put thoughts or feelings into the most accurate words possible. Pauses or silences that extend for several seconds or minutes, however, make some listeners extremely uncomfortable. The listener who interjects thoughts, questions, or explanations to reduce the discomfort in essence "puts words into the other person's mouth." The unfortunate result is that self-expression is blocked for the initial communicator.

When people are ill, communication about how they feel is often difficult for them. Many prefer to remain stoically silent until they are sure that the nurse is interested or trustworthy. Once communication is initiated, it may be expressed awkwardly, with many pauses. The nurse needs to learn to be silent in these situations and to wait patiently until the person is able to put thoughts and feelings into words.

■ **Providing General Leads.** By providing a general lead, the nurse encourages the client to verbalize and at the same time choose the topic of conversation.

Client: I am sure glad yesterday is over.

Nurse: Perhaps you would like to talk about it.

or

Nurse: Would it help you to discuss your feelings?

■ **Summarizing.** Summarizing the main points of a discussion is a useful technique near the end of an interview, after a significant discussion, or to review a health-teaching session. It clarifies for both the nurse and the client the relevant points discussed and often acts as an introduction to future care planning. For example, the nurse might say, "During the past half hour we have talked about . . . . Tomorrow afternoon we may explore this further" or "In a few days, I'll review what you have learned about the actions and effects of your insulin." A word of caution about summarizing: No new material should be added.

▪ Nontherapeutic Responses

Just as it is important that nurses learn ways of fostering therapeutic exchanges between nurses and clients, it is also helpful for nurses to recognize nontherapeutic techniques that interfere with effective communication. These include failing to listen; giving unwarranted reassurance; using judgmental responses; being defensive; and probing, testing, or challenging.

■ **Failing to Listen.** Because listening is the most effective technique to facilitate communication, the opposite, failing to listen, is the primary inhibitor to communication. It says to the client, "I'm not interested" or "I'm bored" or "You are not important." It suggests that the nurse needs to be entertained, that the nurse's needs require attention, or that the nurse prefers to discuss topics that concern herself or himself.

■ **Unwarranted Reassurance.** Statements such as "You'll feel better soon," "I'm sure everything will turn out all right," "Don't worry," and "You're looking better each day" are futuristic and intended to provide hope for the client. However, they disregard the client's feelings of the moment and in many instances are said when there is no hope of improvement. The client who fears death, for example, needs to express these concerns rather than have them dismissed with false reassurance. The nurse who offers reassurance in this manner needs to examine her or his own feelings and recognize that this type of response is of more help to the nurse than to the client.

■ **Judgmental Responses.** Passing judgment on the client implies that the client *must* think as the nurse thinks—the client's values must be the same as the nurse's—if the client is to be accepted. Approving or disapproving responses, such as "That's good (bad)," "You shouldn't do that," and "That's not good enough," tell clients they must measure up to the nurse's standards rather than to their own goals. Perhaps what the nurse considers "bad" the client considers "good."

Stereotyping responses are judgmental, since they categorize clients and negate the uniqueness of individuals. *Stereotypes* are generalized and oversimplified beliefs we hold about various groups of people, which are based upon experiences too limited to be valid. The less one knows about a person, the more the tendency to stereotype. Examples of stereotyping statements are: "Two-year-olds are brats," "Women are complainers," and "Men don't cry." Communication between nurse and client can be inhibited, depending on how emotionally charged the stereotype is for the nurse. For example, if the nurse is not deeply committed to the "brat" theory, the communication pattern with a 2-year-old who is cooperative may be only temporarily affected. By the same token, the nurse who has marked feelings about men who cry will probably ignore the individualism of a male client who expresses his grief.

Another common error is to offer meaningless stereotyped responses to clients:

Client: I'm sure having a lot of pain.

Nurse: Really? Most people don't have pain after this type of surgery.

Client: I don't have the energy I'd like to have.

Nurse: Rome wasn't built in a day.

Agreeing and disagreeing imply that the client is either right or wrong and that the nurse is in a position to judge this. They can deter the client from thinking through his or her position. Disagreement sometimes causes the client to defend a position.

Client: I don't think Dr. Broad is a very good doctor. He doesn't seem interested in his patients.

Nurse: Dr. Broad is head of the Department of Surgery and is an excellent surgeon.

■ **Defensive Responses.** Many clients offer opinions or comments about their care, directed toward the nurse, the nurse's colleagues, or the institution. Feeling threatened or attacked, the nurse may become defensive and prevent the client from expressing feelings. For example:

Client: The food here is lousy.

Nurse: It's a lot better here than in the county hospital. You should consider yourself lucky.

Client: Those night nurses must just sit around and talk all night. They didn't answer my light for over an hour.

Nurse: I'll have you know we literally run around on nights. You're not the only client, you know.

These responses prevent the client from expressing true concerns. The nurse is saying, "You have no right to complain." Defensive responses protect the nurse from admitting weaknesses in the health care services, including personal weaknesses.

■ **Probing, Testing, and Challenging Responses.** Probing, testing, and challenging are often considered hostile responses. *Probing* is asking for information chiefly out of curiosity rather than with the intent to assist the client. Usually probing is considered prying, and the client feels that his or her privacy is not being respected. Often asking "why" is probing and can place the client in a defensive posture:

Client: I was speeding along the street and didn't see the stop sign.

Nurse: Why were you speeding?

Client: I didn't ask the doctor when he was here.

Nurse: Why didn't you?

Testing is questioning by nurses to make clients admit to something. While testing, the nurse usually asks a question that permits the client only limited answers. Testing often meets the nurse's need rather than the client's. One example of a testing question is: "Who do you think you are?" This question forces the client to admit that his or her status in the health care agency is that of "only a client." Another is "Do you think I am not busy?" which forces the client to admit that the nurse really is busy.

Challenging is giving a response that makes a client prove his or her statement or point of view. Usually the client's feelings are not considered, and he or she feels the necessity to defend a position. Challenging a client's perceptions rarely changes them; often it strengthens them, because the client feels forced to find proof to support the position.

Client: I felt nauseated after that red pill.

Nurse: Surely you don't think I gave you the wrong pill?

Client: I feel as if I am dying.

Nurse: How can you feel that way when your pulse is 60?

Client: I believe my husband doesn't love me.

Nurse: You can't say that; why, he visits you every day.

Evaluating Communication

Techniques that enhance or interfere with therapeutic communication have been discussed as part of implementing nursing care. Nurses often use process recordings to evaluate the effectiveness of their own communications with clients. A **process recording** is a verbatim (word-for-word) account of a conversation. It can be taped or written, and it includes all verbal and nonverbal interactions.

One method of writing a process recording is to make three columns on a page. The first column lists what the client said and did, the second what the nurse said and did, and the third contains interpretive com-

ments about the nurse's responses. See Table 20–2 for a sample format.

Once a process recording has been completed, it should be analyzed in terms of the direction and development of the interaction (process), and the content. The nurse's interaction can be analyzed for process according to a number of questions:

- Was the client's verbal and nonverbal behavior really heard and seen?

- Were any cues missed?

- Were the nurse's verbal responses and behavior congruent?

- Did the client respond to the nurse or independently of the nurse?

- Did the communication process flow smoothly?

- Were the nurse's responses consistent with what the nurse observed and heard? Or were they unrelated, exaggerated, or underresponsive?

- Were the nurses's responses therapeutic or nontherapeutic? See the previous sections on responding therapeutically or nontherapeutically.

Each response can also be analyzed for content in terms of facilitating or inhibiting communication. Table 20–2 also provides a sample analysis.

Table 20–2 Sample Process Recording

Mary Jane Adams, a nursing aide, reports to Irene Olsen, the staff nurse, that Sandra Barrett, the client in room 815, had finished only her orange juice when Ms. Adams collected the breakfast trays. Mrs. Barrett had been admitted two days earlier for diagnostic studies. Concerned about her client, Miss Olsen walks down the corridor to room 815, knocks, and enters. Mrs. Barrett turns away from the window, tears in her eyes, as Miss Olsen enters.

Client	Nurse	Comments
Hello.	Good morning, Mrs. Barrett.	Acknowledging.
I wasn't hungry.	I understand you didn't eat your breakfast.	Making a specific statement, but ignoring the nonverbal.
No. (Eyes fill with tears.)	Is something wrong?	Asking a closed-ended question that fails to facilitate exploration.
(Cries.)	You look sad; as if you're about to cry.	Giving feedback.
(Continues to cry.)	I'll sit here a while with you. (Sits down.)	Offering self.
(Angrily): You can help me by telling me the truth.	(After a 30-second pause): Sometimes it's hard to share the things you're concerned about with someone you don't know well. I'd like to be able to help.	Empathizing. Supporting. Offering self.
Everyone beats around the bush when I ask them what's wrong with me. The head nurse said, "What do *you* think is wrong?" That kind of put-off drives me up the wall!	(Leans forward and maintains eye contact.)	Actively listening and demonstrating interest.

continued

Table 20—2 Sample Process Recording (continued)

Client	Nurse	Comments
	You're angry because you're not getting any answers. It seems as if the staff knows something about your condition and they're keeping it from you.	Paraphrasing.
They all seem to be in cahoots. Nobody tells me anything. (Pause.) (Softly): If the news was good, they wouldn't beat around the bush.		
	I'm wondering if you're worried that because people haven't answered your question it means that you have a serious illness?	Paraphrasing.
Good news is always easy to give.		
	Yes, people do seem to be able to deliver good news easier and faster. I also know that we don't have any news—good or bad—to give you because none of the laboratory or x-ray results are back yet. I know that doesn't help answer your questions, but I hope it relieves you a bit from worrying that there is some bad news that's being withheld.	Giving information. Supporting.
Well, when my father-in-law had surgery for a bleeding ulcer, the x-ray and laboratory results were available immediately.		
	When there's a question of emergency surgery being needed, then tests results are asked for immediately. Usually, though, it's preferable to wait for an accurate reading and a thorough written report.	Giving information.
Are you absolutely sure?		
	You don't sound convinced.	Acknowledging the implied.
Listen, I don't mean to give you a hard time. It's just that . . . it may not seem like an emergency to my doctor or the lab people, but it sure is to me. I can't stand not knowing. I don't know the results of the tests I had yesterday. I don't know how many more tests I have to have. Will I have to have surgery? When can I go home?		
	The problem you need help with now is finding out the answers to four questions: What are the results of yesterday's tests? Is your doctor considering any other tests for you, and if so what are they? Is surgery being planned? And when can you go home? Let's try to figure out how you can get the answers to these questions.	Summarizing. Encouraging problem-solving.
Well, I can't call my doctor on the phone. All his receptionist will do is take the message. And, anyway, I'm afraid that he'll be offended if he thinks I'm complaining about him. You won't tell him, will you?		
	No, not unless you and I decide together that it would be the best solution.	Encouraging collaboration.

continued

Table 20-2 Sample Process Recording (continued)

Client	Nurse	Comments
I suppose I could just try to forget about it and be patient, just like everyone tells me to.		
	You've tried that, but you're still worried, fearful, and angry. Let's think of some other possibilities.	Encouraging further exploration.
Maybe you could call his office for me! Since you're a nurse, they'll probably put your call right through.		
	So far there are three possible solutions—calling his office yourself, waiting until he comes to visit you later this afternoon, or having me call his office. Are there any other possible solutions that we haven't considered?	Focusing on solutions.
I can't think of any others.		
	Okay, then, which do you think would be best?	Demonstrating respect for the client.
I guess I'd feel better if you called his office. I just don't want him to think that I'm criticizing him.		
	You're concerned about what he might think of you because of this phone call. Let's discuss how I should handle the call and what I should say.	Paraphrasing. Encouraging collaboration and problem-solving.

After a few minutes they develop a plan for calling Mrs. Barrett's physician, and Miss Olsen makes the call. The physician has decided to call both the laboratory and the X-ray department for the results of Mrs. Barrett's tests and promises to phone her as soon as he learns the results. They will discuss further possible tests and treatment plans that afternoon when he makes his hospital rounds. Mrs. Barrett asks Miss Olsen to stay with her while she receives the physician's telephone call about the test results.

Courtesy of Carol Ren Kneisl, RN, MS, Nursing Transitions, Williamsville, New York.

▪ Chapter Highlights

▪ Communication incorporates all means of exchanging information between two or more people and is a basic component of human relationships and nurse-client relationships.

▪ Communication is usually categorized as verbal or nonverbal.

▪ Verbal communication is effective when the criteria of simplicity, clarity, timing, relevance, adaptability, and credibility are met.

▪ Nonverbal communication often reveals more about a person's thoughts and feelings than verbal communication; it includes physical appearance, posture and gait, facial expressions, hand movements, and other gestures.

▪ When assessing nonverbal behaviors, the nurse needs to consider cultural influences and be aware that a variety of feelings can be expressed by a single nonverbal expression.

▪ When communication is effective, verbal and nonverbal expressions are congruent.

▪ Communication is a two-way process involving the sender of the message and the receiver of the message.

▪ Because the sender must encode the message and determine the appropriate channels for conveying it, and because the receiver must perceive the message, decode it, and then respond, the communication process includes four elements: sender, message, receiver, and feedback.

▪ Many factors influence the communication process: the ability of the communicator, perceptions, personal space (intimate, personal, social, and public distance), territoriality, roles and relationships, purposes, time and setting, attitudes, emotions, and self-esteem.

▪ There are three broad areas for assessing communication: language development, nonverbal behavior, and style of communication.

▪ Many techniques facilitate therapeutic communication: attentive listening; paraphrasing; clarifying; using open-ended questions and statements; focusing; being specific; using touch and silence; clarifying reality, time, or sequence; providing general leads; and summarizing.

▪ Techniques that inhibit communication include offering unvalidated reassurance, stating approval or disapproval, giving common (not expert) advice, stereotyping, and being defensive.

▪ The effective nurse-client relationship is a growth-facilitating process.

▪ Nurses often use process recordings to analyze both the process and the content of a communication.

◼ **S**elected References

Brammer, L. M. 1985. *The helping relationship: Process and skills,* 3d ed. Englewood Cliffs, N.J.: Prentice-Hall.

Carpenito, L. J. 1987. *Nursing Diagnosis,* 2d ed. Philadelpia: J. B. Lippincott.

Davis, A. J. 1984. *Listening and responding.* St. Louis: C. V. Mosby Co.

Egan, G. 1975. *The skilled helper: A model for systematic helping and interpersonal relating.* Monterey, Calif.: Brooks/Cole Publishing Co.

———. 1982. *The skilled helper. Model, skills, and methods for effective helping,* 2d ed. Monterey, Calif.: Brooks/Cole Publishing Co.

Hall, E. T. 1969. *The hidden dimension.* Garden City, N.Y.: Doubleday and Co.

Lancaster, J. September 1983. Communication: The anatomy of messages. *Nursing Management* 14:42–45.

Leonard, R. November 1985. Speak for yourself. *Nursing 85* 15:30–31.

Muldary, T. W. 1983. *Interpersonal relations for health professionals. A social skills approach.* New York: Macmillan Publishing Co.

Schulman, L. 1984. *The skills of helping individuals and groups,* 2d ed. Itasca, Ill.: F. E. Peacock Publishers.

Shanken, J., and Shanken, P. February 1976. How to be a helping person. *Journal of Psychiatric Nursing and Mental Health Services* 14:24–28.

Stewart, C. J., and Cash, W. B. 1985. *Interviewing principles and practices,* 4th ed. Dubuque, Iowa: Wm. C. Brown Publishers.

Wilkinson, R. April 1986. Communication: Learning from the market. *Nursing Management* 17:42J, 42L.

21

Teaching and Learning

OBJECTIVES

Define terms commonly used in the learning and teaching context.

Describe factors that facilitate or inhibit learning.

Outline five principles of teaching.

Identify the sources of the client's learning needs.

Describe essential aspects of a teaching plan.

Identify four guidelines for ordering the learning experiences.

Identify eight guidelines that help plan teaching intervention.

Identify guidelines for evaluating the effectiveness of the teaching plan.

Describe complete documentation of the teaching process.

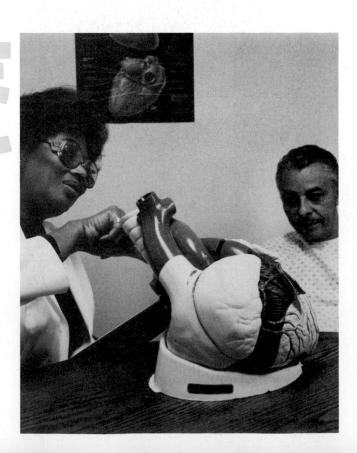

Client Education

In 1972 the American Hospital Association passed the Patients' Bill of Rights mandating client education as a right of all clients. In addition, legislation relating to nursing frequently has included client teaching as a function of nursing, thereby making teaching a legal and professional responsibility (Phillips and Hekelman 1983, pp. 42–46). Client education, a major aspect of nursing practice, is multifaceted, involving promoting, protecting, and maintaining health. It involves teaching about reducing health risk factors, increasing a person's level of wellness, and providing information about specific protective health measures.

Clients have a variety of learning needs. A **learning need** is a need to change behavior. **Learning** is a change in human disposition or capability that persists over a period of time and that cannot be solely accounted for by growth. Learning is represented by a change in behavior (Gagne 1977). An important aspect of learning is the individual's desire to learn and to act on the learning. This is referred to as *compliance.* Compliance is best illustrated when the person recognizes and accepts the need to learn, willingly expends the energy required to learn, and then follows through with the appropriate behaviors that reflect the learning. For example, a man diagnosed as having diabetes willingly learns about the special diet he needs and then plans and follows the learned diet.

Principles of Learning

Learning involves the entire person, and it can affect the person's life-style, methods of handling problems, attitudes, and knowledge. Learning requires energy and the ability to concentrate. To be effective client-teachers, nurses must understand those factors that facilitate learning and those that inhibit it.

Factors Facilitating Learning

Motivation to learn is the desire to learn. Such motivation is generally greatest when a person recognizes a need and believes the need will be met through learning. It is not enough for the need to be identified and verbalized by the nurse; it must be experienced by the client. Often the nurse's task is to help the client personally work through the problem and identify the need. Sometimes clients or families need help identifying relevant situational elements before they can see a need. For instance, clients with heart disease may need to know the effects of smoking and being overweight before they recognize the need to stop smoking or adopt a weight-reduction diet. Or adolescents may need to know the consequences of an untreated sexually trans-

mitted disease before they see the need for treatment.

Readiness to learn involves two facets: emotional and experiential. **Emotional readiness** indicates that the person is willing to put forth the effort needed to learn. **Experiential readiness** involves the person's background of experiences, skills, and attitudes, and his or her ability to learn (Redman 1984, p. 21).

Active involvement in the learning process makes learning more meaningful. For example, if the learner actively participates in planning and discussion, learning is faster and retention is better. See Figure 21–1. Passive learning, such as listening to a lecture or watching a film, does not foster optimal learning.

Once learners have **succeeded** in accomplishing a task or understanding a concept, they gain self-confidence in their ability to learn. This reduces their anxiety about failure and can motivate greater learning. Successful learners have increased confidence with which to accept failure. People learn best when they believe they are **accepted** and will not be judged. The person who expects to be judged as a "poor" or "good" client will not learn as well as the person who feels no such threat.

Feedback is information relating a person's performance to a desired goal. It has to be meaningful to the learner. Feedback that accompanies practice of psychomotor skills helps the person to learn those skills. Support of desired behavior through praise, positively worded corrections, and suggestions of alternative methods are ways of providing positive feedback. Negative feedback such as ridicule, anger, or sarcasm can lead people to withdraw from learning. Such feedback, viewed as a type of punishment, may cause the client to avoid the teacher in order to avoid punishment.

Learning is facilitated by material that is logically organized and proceeds from the **simple to the com-**

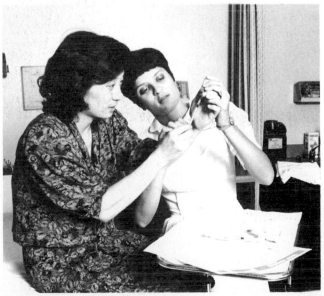

Figure 21–1 Learning is facilitated when the client is interested and actively involved.

plex. Such organization enables the learner to comprehend new information, assimilate it with previous learning, and form new understandings. Of course, simple and complex are relative terms, depending on the level at which the person is learning. What is simple for one person may be complex for another.

Repetition of key concepts and facts facilitates retention of newly learned material. Practice of psychomotor skills improves performance of those skills and facilitates their transfer to another setting. When a person appreciates the **relevance** of specific material, then learning is facilitated. For example, the man who understands the relevance to his health of a special diet is better able to learn about the diet than a person who sees no such connection.

People **retain** information and psychomotor skills **best when the time between learning and use is short;** the longer the time interval, the more that is forgotten. For example, a woman who is taught how to administer her own insulin but is not permitted to do so until discharge from hospital is unlikely to remember much of what she learned. However, if she is allowed to give her own injections while in hospital, her learning will be enhanced.

An **optimal learning environment** has adequate lighting that is free from glare, a comfortable room temperature, and good ventilation. Most students know what it is like to try to learn in a hot, stuffy room; the subsequent drowsiness interferes with concentration. Noise can also distract the student and interfere with listening and thinking. For the best learning in a hospital setting, nurses should choose a time when there are no visitors present and interruptions are unlikely. Privacy is essential for some learning. For example, when a client is learning to irrigate a colostomy, the presence of others can be embarrassing and thus interfere with learning.

Factors Inhibiting Learning

A greatly **elevated anxiety** level can impede learning. Clients or families who are very worried may not hear spoken words or may retain only part of the communication. Extreme anxiety might be reduced by medications or by information that relieves uncertainty. By contrast, clients who appear disinterested and unconcerned may need to be told about potential problems, to increase their anxiety slightly and enhance their motivation to learn.

Learning can be inhibited by **physiologic events** such as a critical illness, pain, or impaired hearing. Because the client cannot concentrate and apply energy to learning, the learning itself is impaired. There are also **cultural barriers** to learning, such as language or values. Obviously the client who does not understand the nurse's language will learn little. Another impediment to learning is differing values held by the client and the health team. For example, a client who does not value being thin may have difficulty learning about a reducing diet.

Teaching

Teaching is a system of activities intended to produce learning. The teaching process is designed to produce specific learning. Teaching is considered one of the functions of nursing. In some states in the United States, teaching is included in the legal definition of nursing, making it a required function under the law.

The teaching/learning process involves dynamic interaction between teacher and learner. Each participant in the process communicates information, emotions, perceptions, and attitudes to the other. The teaching process and the nursing process are very much alike. See Table 21–1. The following **principles of teaching** may be helpful to nursing students:

1. Teaching activities should help the learner meet individual learning objectives. If certain activities do not assist the learner, these need to be reassessed; perhaps other activities can replace them. For example, explanation alone may not be enough to teach a client to handle a syringe. Actually handling the syringe may be more effective.
2. Rapport between teacher and learner is essential. A relationship that is both accepting and constructive best promotes learning.
3. The teacher who can use the client's previous learning in the present situation encourages the client and facilitates the learning of new skills. For example, a person who already knows how to cook can use this knowledge when learning about a special diet.
4. A teacher must be able to communicate clearly and concisely. The words the teacher uses need to have the same meaning to the learner as to the teacher. For example, a client who is taught not to put water on an area of the skin may think it is fine to use a wet cloth to wash the area. The nurse needs to explain

Table 21–1 Comparison of the Teaching Process and the Nursing Process

Step	Teaching Process	Nursing Process
1	Collect data; analyze client's learning strengths and deficits.	Collect data; analyze client's strengths and deficits.
2	Make educational diagnoses.	Make nursing diagnoses.
3	Prepare teaching plan.	Plan nursing intervention.
4	Implement teaching plan.	Implement nursing strategies.
5	Evaluate client learning (effectiveness of teaching plan)	Evaluate effectiveness of nursing interventions.

that no water or moisture should come in contact with the area.

5. The teaching activities should be oriented to the learning objectives. Thus information and skills not related to the learner's objectives need to be eliminated from the teaching process. If they remain, they may confuse the learner or be a distraction from effective learning.

Assessment

Assessing for teaching includes identifying the client's learning needs and collecting relevant data about the client. Smitherman (1981, pp. 125–28) describes three sources for **identifying learning needs:** the client, the client's behavior, and health care professionals. A client aware of a learning need may ask pertinent questions or seek out the needed information in some other way. Learning needs are not always easily detected; frequently, consultation with the client is necessary to confirm or deny the existence of these needs. For example, a client who appears angry may be insecure or worried because he does not understand what is happening, and only after discussion with the client can the nurse be sure that he has a need for information. Anticipatory learning needs related to the client's health problem often are known by health professionals. For example, a client anticipating surgery will probably need to learn about deep breathing and leg exercises. Or a client receiving oxygen who is being discharged from hospital will need to know how to operate the oxygen equipment and the appropriate safety measures to employ while at home.

Particular **client data** that need to be collected and examined include client readiness, client motivation, and personal characteristics such as age and education. Clients who are ready to learn may search out information by asking questions, reading books or articles, talking to others, and generally showing interest. The person unready to learn is more likely to avoid the subject or situation and hope or believe that someone else will take care of the problem (Smitherman 1981, pp. 126–27). In addition, the unready client may change the subject when the nurse introduces it. For example, the nurse might say, "I was wondering about a good time to show you how to change your dressing," and the client responds, "What did you think of the ball game last night?" Clients having surgery may have somatic symptoms (such as headaches, upset stomach, or gas pains) that make it difficult for them to pay attention (Laird 1975, p. 1340).

Nurses can sometimes foster a client's readiness by tactfully calling attention to a learning need (e.g., "Have you thought about learning to change your dressing?"). Two other ways to foster readiness are giving the client information to read and pointing out an opportunity to learn (e.g., "There is a baby bath demonstration at three o'clock today in the next room").

There are two types of motivation: internal and external. **Internal** motivation arises from within the individual. Sometimes clients may even be unaware of their motivation or unwilling to share it. For example, a client may be motivated to learn in order to gain the nurse's approval or in order to return to work. Why a person is motivated is often not clear, and it is unwise to assume a reason. **External** motivation comes from outside the client, such as praise from a support person.

Nurses can often determine whether a client's motivation is internal or external: An internally motivated person often takes the initiative in learning and usually does more than is required. Many externally motivated learners seek frequent feedback and may need to tell others about their learning. Both internal and external motivation are influenced by a person's physical and emotional needs. When clients are tired, worried, or in pain, for example, most of their energy is devoted to those problems, and motivation is usually low.

Nurses can positively influence a client's internal motivation in three ways:

1. By relating the learning to something the client values and helping the client see the relevance of the learning
2. By helping the client to make the learning situation pleasant
3. By encouraging self-direction

To influence the externally motivated learner, a nurse can use **positive reinforcement,** which involves rewarding the learner for achievements, e.g., giving praise or reading a bedtime story to a child. Reinforcement is most effective when given immediately after the desired response. Negative reinforcement, or punishment for undesirable responses, is considered less motivating than positive reinforcement. However, negative reinforcement can be motivating if it is accompanied by encouragement and an explanation of how to correct the response (e.g., "I agree that looks right, but if you place the tube like this the urine should flow more readily").

Nursing Diagnosis

Nursing diagnoses pertinent to a client's learning needs are all grouped under the diagnostic category of *knowledge deficit.* It is extremely important that the nurse specifiy which exact deficits individual clients manifest. Examples are shown in the box on page 270.

Planning

Developing a teaching plan is accomplished in a series of steps. Involving the client at this time promotes the formation of a meaningful plan and stimulates client motivation. The client who participates in the formulation of the teaching plan is more likely to achieve the desired outcomes.

NURSING DIAGNOSIS

Learning

- Knowledge deficit: low-calorie diet related to newly ordered therapy

- Knowledge deficit: diabetic diet related to prescribed treatment

- Knowledge deficit: preoperative care related to impending surgical procedure

- Knowledge deficit: medications related to language differences

- Knowledge deficit: home safety hazards related to denial of declining health

- Knowledge deficit: substance abuse related to lack of motivation to acquire information

Determining Teaching Priorities

The client's learning needs must be ranked according to priority. The client and the nurse should do this together, with the client's priorities always being considered. Once a client's priorities have been addressed, the client is generally more motivated to concentrate on other identified learning needs. For example, a man who wants to know all about diabetes mellitus may not be ready to learn how to give himself injections until his own knowledge needs are met. Nurses can also use theoretical frameworks to establish priorities, such as Maslow's hierarchy of needs. See Chapter 13.

Setting Learning Objectives

The terms *goals* and *objectives* are used interchangeably by some educators and distinguished by others. Used interchangeably, they can be considered as both immediate and long-term aims to be accomplished in a learning situation. However, **goal** is often the more general term, describing a general, long-range intended outcome of learning, whereas **objective** is used to mean a specific, immediate, short-range intended outcome of a learning situation.

The setting of goals and objectives is done by the client (or support persons) and the nurse. **Objectives** relate to immediate client needs, such as perineal care after birth of a baby. **Goals** relate to long-term needs, such as an obese new mother's need to lose weight (in which case the goal may be a specific weight loss through diet and exercise).

The objectives for learning should be both specific and observable in terms of behavior. A specific objective might be "to take 60 mg furosemide (Lasix) upon identifying ankle edema." An objective needs to be stated in terms of client behavior, not nurse behavior. For example, "Will write his own diets as instructed" (client behavior), not "To teach the client about his diet" (nurse behavior).

Objectives should contain three types of information: performance, conditions, and criteria (Mager 1975, p. 21). **Performance,** or behavior, describes what the learner will be able to do after mastering the objective. The objective must reflect an observable activity. The performance may be visible, e.g., walking, or invisible, e.g., adding a column of figures. However, it is necessary to be able to deduce whether an unobservable activity has been mastered from some performance that represents the activity. Therefore, the performance of an objective might be written: "Writes the total for a column of figures in the indicated space" (observable), not "Adds a column of figures" (unobservable).

In some instances it is necessary to state the **conditions** under which a performance is to be carried out so that the objective is clear. For example, "Walks to the end of the hall and back without crutches" describes a performance clearly; "without crutches" is a condition of the objective. Nurses always need to determine the conditions in which an activity will be carried out. Then the objectives for the learning plan can reflect those conditions. For example, if a client lives alone and must irrigate his own colostomy, then "Irrigate his colostomy *independently* as taught" is the correct objective.

Criteria state the standards of performance that are considered acceptable. Each objective should specify a standard against which the performance can be measured. Examples include speed, quality, and accuracy. Learners need to understand the criteria so that they can evaluate their performance validly.

Selecting Teaching Strategies

The method of teaching chosen by the nurse should be suited to the individual, to the material to be learned, and to the teacher. For example, the person who cannot read needs material presented in other ways; a discussion is usually not the best strategy for teaching to give an injection; and a teacher should be a competent group leader in order to use group discussion for teaching. Some people are visually oriented and learn best through seeing; others learn best through hearing and having the skill explained. These attributes should be considered during the planning phase. If this fact is not identified until the teaching plan has been implemented, the plan may need revising.

Ordering the Learning Experiences

Some health agencies have developed teaching guides for lessons that nurses commonly give. These guides save nurses time in constructing their own guides. They also standardize content and assist staff in remembering it (Redman 1984, p. 194). Whether the nurse is implementing a plan devised by another or developing an individualized teaching plan, some guidelines can help the nurse order the learning experiences:

1. Start with something the learner is concerned about, e.g., before learning how to administer insulin to himself, an adolescent wants to know how he can adjust his life-style and still play football.

2. Begin with what the learner knows and proceed to the unknown. This gives the learner confidence. Sometimes a nurse does not know the client's knowledge or skill base and needs to elicit this information either by asking questions or by having the client fill out a form, such as a pretest.

3. Any area of learning that is anxiety provoking should be taught first. A high level of anxiety can impair concentration in other areas. For example, a woman highly anxious about turning her husband in bed might not be able to learn about bathing him until she has successfully learned to turn him.

4. Teach the basics first, then proceed to the variations or adjustments. It is very confusing to learners to have to consider every possible adjustment and variation before the basic concepts are understood. For example, when teaching a female client how to insert a retention catheter, it is best to teach the basic procedure before teaching any adjustments that might be needed if the catheter stops draining after insertion.

Implementation

The nurse needs to be flexible in implementing any teaching plan, since the plan may need revising, e.g., because the client tires sooner than anticipated, the client is faced with too much information too quickly, the client's needs change, or external factors intervene. For instance, the nurse and the client may have planned for the client to learn to administer his own insulin at a particular time, but when the time comes the nurse finds that the client wants additional information before actually giving himself the insulin. In this case, the nurse alters the teaching plan and discusses the desired information, provides written information, and defers teaching the psychomotor skill until the next day.

It is also important for nurses to use teaching techniques that enhance learning and to consider any barriers to learning. See Table 21–2 for barriers to learning. When implementing a teaching plan, the nurse may find the following guidelines helpful.

1. The optimal time for each session depends largely on the learner. Some people, for example, learn best at the beginning of the day, when they are most rested; others prefer late afternoon, when no other activities are scheduled.

2. The pace of each teaching session also affects learning. Nurses should be sensitive to any signs that the pace is too fast or too slow. A client who appears confused or does not comprehend material when questioned may be finding the pace too fast. When the client appears bored and loses interest, the pace may be too slow, the learning period may be too long, or the client may be tired.

3. An environment can detract or assist learning; e.g., noise or interruptions usually interfere with concentration, whereas a comfortable environment promotes learning. Environmental characteristics

Table 21–2 Barriers to Learning

Barrier	Explanation
Acute illness	Requires all resources for survival.
Pain or discomfort	Decreases ability to learn.
Restlessness	Due to stressors such as electrolyte imbalances, can alter orientation, memory, intellectual capacity, judgment, mood, perceptions, motor control, level of consciousness, and concentration.
Age	Vision or hearing can be impaired in the elderly.
Prognosis	Receptivity to learning can be negatively affected when prognosis is poor.
Biorhythms	Mental and physical performances have a circadian rhythm.
Anxiety, denial, hostility, depression, fear, regression, etc.	Such behavioral responses to acute illness can impair learning.
Language, ethnic background, etc.	Can prevent learning.
Iatrogenic barriers	Barriers set up by the nurse, such as talking down to clients, hurried and fragmented teaching, ignoring client cues.

Adapted from Murdaugh, C. L. November / December 1982. Barriers to patient education in the coronary care unit. *Cardiovascular Nursing* 18:33–35.

that should be considered are: lighting, temperature, sound, ventilation, visibility, and a chair or support for the learner.

4. Teaching aids can foster learning. Posters and displays, for example, can help focus a learner's attention. To ensure the transfer of learning, the nurse should use the type of supplies or equipment that the client will eventually use.

5. Learning is more effective when the learners discover the content for themselves. Ways to increase learning include stimulating motivation and stimulating self-direction (Redman 1984, p. 90), e.g., by providing specific objectives, giving feedback, and helping the learner derive satisfaction from learning. Nurses can maximize learner satisfaction by setting realistic goals with the learner (Redman 1984, p. 90).

6. Repetition—e.g., summarizing content, rephrasing (using other words), and approaching the material from another point of view—reinforces learning. For instance, after discussing the kinds of foods that can be included in a diet, the nurse describes the foods again, but in the context of the three meals eaten during one day.

7. It is helpful to employ "advanced organizers" to introduce material to be learned and to present it at a higher level of abstraction, generality, or inclusiveness (Redman 1984, p. 91). Advanced organizers provide a means of relating unknown material

to known material and generating logical relationships. For example: "You understand how urine flows down a catheter from the bladder. Now I will show you how to inject fluid so that it flows up the catheter into the bladder." The details that follow such an introduction are then seen within its framework, and the details have added meaning.

8. Using a layperson's vocabulary enhances communication. So often nurses use terms and abbreviations that have meaning to other health professionals but make little sense to clients. Even words such as *urine* or *feces* may be unfamiliar to clients, and abbreviations such as "RR" (recovery room) or "PAR" (post-anesthesia room) are often misunderstood.

Evaluation

Evaluation is an ongoing and terminal process in which the client, the nurse, and often the support persons determine what has been learned. Both short-term objectives and long-term goals need to be evaluated. Learning is measured against the predetermined objectives. Thus, the objectives not only direct the teaching plan but also provide criteria for evaluation. For example, the objective "Selects foods that are low in carbohydrates" can be evaluated by asking the client to name such foods or to select low-carbohydrate foods from a list.

Following evaluation, the nurse may find it necessary to modify or repeat the teaching plan if the objectives have not been met or met only partially. For the hospitalized client, follow-up teaching in the home may be needed. It is important for the nurse to evaluate her or his own teaching, including the timing, the teaching strategies, the amount of information, and the degree to which the teaching was helpful. The nurse may find, for example, that the client was overwhelmed with too much information, bored, or motivated to learn more. The nurse can use the following guidelines (Smitherman 1981, pp. 141–44) in the evaluation:

1. Forgetting is normal and should be anticipated. Nurses can suggest to clients that they write down information they might forget or provide printed instructions, because such information may be easily forgotten.

2. Both the client and the teacher should evaluate the learning experience. The learner may tell the nurse what was helpful, interesting, and so on. Questionnaires and videotapes of the learning sessions can also be useful.

3. Behavior change does not always take place immediately after learning. Often the person accepts change intellectually first and then may change his or her behavior only periodically (e.g., the person who knows that he or she must lose weight may diet and exercise off and on). If the new behavior is to replace old behavior, it must emerge gradually. Otherwise, the old behavior may prevail. Nurses can assist clients with behavior change by allowing for client vacillation and by providing encouragement.

Documentation

Documentation of the teaching/learning process is essential to provide a legal record of the teaching and to communicate it to other health professionals. The record should detail the client's achievements providing an account of learning. A specific client teaching record or the nurse's notes can be used. The client's reaction to the teaching should also be included, and this reaction should be incorporated into further planning. The responses of support persons should be included as well. Documentation also serves as a reference for client learning and support-person learning. It promotes reevaluation of the teaching plan, suggesting reinforcement of identified areas of learning needs and revision of teaching strategies (Corkadel and McGlashan 1983, pp. 14–15).

Chapter Highlights

Learning is represented by a change in behavior.

A number of factors facilitate learning, including motivation, readiness, active involvement, and success at learning.

Factors such as extreme anxiety, certain physiologic processes, and cultural barriers impede learning.

Teaching is a system of activities intended to produce learning.

Rapport between the teacher and the learner is essential for effective teaching.

Assessment relative to the preparation of a teaching plan must include identification of the client's learning needs and relevant client data.

Readiness is an important aspect of assessment prior to teaching.

Teaching priorities must always be established and must reflect the client's priorities.

Learning objectives guide the content of the teaching plan and are written in terms of client behavior.

Teaching strategies should be suited to the client, the material to be learned, and the teacher.

A teaching plan is a written record that must be revised when the client's needs change or when the teaching strategies prove ineffective.

Evaluation of the teaching/learning process is an ongoing and terminal process.

Selected References

Bille, D. A. March/April 1983. Process-oriented patient education. *Dimensions of Critical Care Nursing* 2:108–15.

Check, J. F., and Wurzbach, M. E. January/February 1984. How elders view learning. *Geriatric Nursing* 5:37–39.

Corkadel, L., and McGlashan, R. January/February 1983. A practical approach to patient teaching. *The Journal of Continuing Education in Nursing* 14:9–15.

Cushing, M. June 1984. Legal lessons on patient teaching. *American Journal of Nursing* 84:721–22.

DeHaes, W. F. M. 1982. Patient education: A component of

health education. *Patient Counseling and Health Education* 4(2):95–102.

Frank-Stromborg, M. January/February 1985. Evaluating patient education material. *Oncology Nursing Forum* 12:65–67.

Frisbie, D. A. November 1984. Looking at teaching through the nursing process. *Journal of Nursing Education* 23:401–403.

Gagne, R. M. 1977. *The conditions of learning.* 3rd ed. New York: Holt, Rinehart and Winston.

Gioiella, E. C., and Bevil, C. W. 1985. *Nursing care of the aging client. Promoting healthy adaptation.* Norwalk, Conn.: Appleton-Century-Crofts.

Laird, M. August 1975. Techniques for teaching pre- and postoperative patients. *American Journal of Nursing* 75:1338–40.

Lewis, S. J. May 1984. Teaching patient groups. *Nursing Management* 15:49-50, 52, 54–56.

Mager, R. F. 1975. *Preparing instructional objectives.* 2d ed. Belmont, California: Fearon Publishers, Inc.

Phillips, J. A., and Hekelman, F. P. September/October 1983. The role of the nurse as a teacher: A position paper. *Nephrology Nurse* 5:42–46.

Redman, B. K. 1984. *The process of patient education.* 5th ed. St. Louis: C. V. Mosby Co.

Smitherman, C. 1981. *Nursing actions for health promotion.* Philadelphia: F. A. Davis Co.

Tiche, S.; Dobson, J.; and Olker, L. April 1984. Pediatric teaching. The small hospital. *American Operating Room Nurses Journal* 39:793–97.

Tyson, J. 1984. Before we educate. *Diabetes Educator* (special issue) 10:23–24.

Woody, A. F., et al. December 1984. Do patients learn what nurses say they teach? *Nursing Management* 15:26–29.

22

Recording and Reporting

OBJECTIVES

Identify seven purposes of client records.

Describe the components of source-oriented medical records and problem-oriented medical records (POMR).

Describe three types of progress records.

Identify abbreviations and symbols commonly used for charting.

Identify measures used to maintain the confidentiality of client records.

Identify measures used to ensure that recording meets legal standards.

List some advantages of flowsheets.

Differentiate between narrative and SOAP recording methods.

Describe the change-of-shift report.

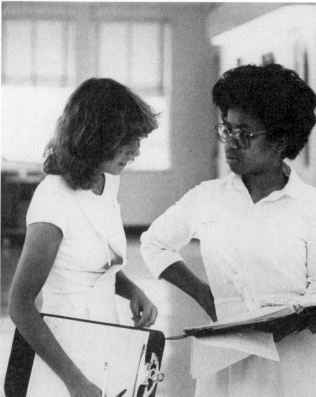

Purposes of Client Records

A client's **medical record,** or **chart,** is an account of the client's health history, current health status, treatment, and progress. It is a highly confidential, legal document used by physicians, nurses, social workers, and other health team members to communicate about that client. When a client goes to a physician's office or enters a hospital, a record is usually started. Records are generally kept in folders, in binders, or on clipboards, and they are updated continually while clients attend the health care facility. When clients are discharged, their records are stored for future reference in the medical records department of the agency.

Although the forms of client records may vary considerably from place to place, nurses are universally required to make entries about clients' health, including, for example, all assessments and interventions. The process of making entries on client records is called **recording** or **charting**.

Client records are kept for a number of purposes: communication, legal documentation, research, statistics, education, audit, and planning client care. The record serves as the vehicle by which different members of the health team **communicate** with each other. Although these members also communicate verbally, the record is an efficient and effective method of sharing information. It also allows health team members on different shifts to convey meaningful data about the client to one another.

The client's record is a **legal document** and is admissible in court as evidence. In some jurisdictions, however, the record is considered inadmissible as evidence when the client objects, because information the client gives to the physician is confidential. A record is usually considered the property of the agency, although there is increasing belief that the client has a right to the information in the record upon request. Legal decisions have recognized this right (Creighton 1981, p. 329).

The information contained in a record can be a valuable source of data for **research.** The treatment plans for a number of clients with the same illness can yield information helpful in treating a particular client. A record made years earlier may also assist members of the health team with a current problem. A client's memory of an illness may provide limited data, but a record of that illness will generally reveal additional and accurate data.

Statistical information from client records can help an agency anticipate and plan for people's future needs. For example, the number of births or kinds of illnesses can be obtained from records. Some statistics, such as records of births and deaths, are required by law. They are filed with a government agency and become a part of the local, national, and international statistics.

Students in health disciplines often use client records as **educational tools.** A record can frequently provide a comprehensive view of the client, the illness, and the kinds of assistance given. In this context, records are used by nursing students, medical students, dietitians, and other health team members.

The client's record is used to monitor the care the client is receiving and the competence of the people giving that care. During nursing **audit,** for example, the nursing interventions are monitored and measured against established standards. Often the audit is a retrospective, in that the care has already been given. A nursing audit carried out by other nurses is sometimes called a **peer review.** Many agencies have audit committees that monitor the practice of individual nurses. Audits are also carried out by outside groups for approval and accreditation purposes.

The entire health team uses data from the client's record to **plan care** for that client. A physician, for example, may order a specific antibiotic after establishing that the client's temperature is steadily rising and that laboratory tests reveal the presence of a certain microorganism. Nurses use data from the history they took on the client's admission to establish an individual nursing care plan. The social worker's data about the client's home environment can assist the nurse in developing an appropriate discharge teaching plan. Data from the physical therapist help the nurse to implement specific physical exercises for the client.

Types of Records

There are two general types of medical records: the traditional or source-oriented medical record and the problem-oriented medical record, also referred to as the **Weed system,** after its originator, L. L. Weed. In the traditional client record, or **source-oriented medical record,** each person or department makes notations in a separate section or sections of the client's chart. For example, the admission department has an admission sheet; the physician has a doctor's order sheet, a doctor's history sheet, and progress notes; nurses use the nurse's notes; and other departments or personnel have their own records.

Source-oriented client records generally have five components: admission sheet, physician's order sheet, history sheet, the nurse's notes, and special records and reports. The **admission sheet** is a part of the record in most agencies. It generally contains demographic data about the client, including an identification number. In hospitals, admission sheets usually set forth the client's full name, address, date of birth, name of attending physician, sex, marital status, nearest relative, occupation and employer, financial status for hospital payments, religious preference, date and hour of admission to the hospital, hospital unit or agency of admission, previous hospital admission, admitting diagnosis or problem, and identification number.

The **physician's order sheet** is a written record of orders. The physician is expected to write the date with the order and sign each order (or sign for several orders written at once). Various agencies have different methods (e.g., using red "flags" on the front or extending out from the chart and/or placing the chart in a designated area of the nursing station) of indicating to the nurse or clerk that there is a new order. When the doctor phones in orders about a client, these are written on the physician's sheet by the recipient of the call and signed by that person, indicating a telephone order. Often the physician is expected to countersign the telephone order within 24 or 48 hours of the call. Before a nurse can accept a verbal order from a physician, however, agency policies and procedures must be checked. Usually, nursing students are not allowed to accept verbal orders.

The **history sheet** is a record of the client's health history, written by the physician. The physician may also use this sheet to record progress notes on the client and future plans, although most agencies have separate records for progress notes. At some facilities, the record of the client's admitting physical examination may also be on the history sheet, which is then usually called the **history and physical** sheet.

The **nurse's notes** are a record of the nursing assessments of the client, identified nursing diagnoses, interventions carried out, and evaluations of the effectiveness of the interventions. In general, nurses' notes record the following kinds of information:

1. Assessments of the client by various nursing personnel, e.g., pale or flushed skin color or dark or cloudy urine
2. Independent nursing interventions, such as special skin care or health teaching, carried out on the nurses' initiative
3. Dependent nursing interventions, such as medications or treatments ordered by a physician
4. Evaluation of the effectiveness of each nursing intervention
5. Measures carried out by the physician (e.g., shortening a postoperative drainage tube) that affect subsequent nursing measures
6. Visits by members of the health team, such as a consulting physician, social worker, or chaplain

Special records and reports also become part of the client's permanent record. These may include consultations from medical specialists, roentgenographic reports, laboratory findings, reports of surgery, anesthesia records, physical therapy records, occupational therapy records, and social service records. In addition, special flowsheets are often used to record certain data about the client. These include graphic records for vital signs, fluid intake and output, and medications.

In a **problem-oriented medical record (POMR or POR),** data about the client are recorded and arranged according to the problems the client has, rather than according to the source of the information. The record integrates all data about a problem, whether gathered by physicians, nurses, or others involved in the client's care. Plans for each active problem are drawn up, and progress notes are recorded for each problem. Unlike the traditional record, which separates the medical data on a problem from the nursing data and other data into different sections of the record, the POR coordinates the care given by all health team members and focuses on the client and his or her health problems.

The POR has four basic components: the defined data base, problem list, initial list of orders or care plans, and progress notes. The **defined data base** consists of all information known about the client when the client first entered the health care agency. It includes the nursing assessment, the physician's history, and the physical health examination. To these are added social and family data from other sources, such as the social worker, and baseline laboratory and roentgenographic data.

The **problem list** is a carefully drawn-up list of problems that is compiled once the data bases have been collected and analyzed. Some problems are obvious on initial contact with the client; others are established as additional data are gathered. Problems are essentially needs that the client is unable to meet without assistance from members of the health care team.

The initial problem list is usually made either by the first health care worker to encounter the client or by the person who assumes primary responsibility for the client's care. Subsequent contributions are made by other members of the health team.

To be complete, the problem list should include socioeconomic, demographic, psychologic, and physiologic problems. The list is usually found at the front of the client's record. Each problem is labeled and numbered so that it can be identified throughout the record. This list has been likened to an index or table of contents. See Figure 22–1. Problems are usually categorized as active or inactive.

Signs, symptoms, and abnormal diagnostic measures, if used, are considered as temporary labels until diagnosis is established. With the development of nursing diagnoses, many nurses are now using the NANDA taxonomy of nursing diagnoses to state nursing problems. Problems statements should refer to one problem only, be written unambiguously (so no interpretation is required) in behavioral terms, and should provide direction for client care.

When several problems have a common etiology or cause, two methods are used to relate the problems: sublisting and cross-referencing. A **sublist** is a group of all manifestations of a major problem that require separate management. Manifestations may be either behavioral or clinical indicators of the same problem. For example, consider the following segment of Figure 22–1:

No.	Client Problem
1	Multiple CVAs resulting in Rt hemiplegia and left-sided weakness
1A	Self-care deficit (hygiene, toileting, grooming, feeding)
1B	Impaired physical mobility
1C	Alteration in urinary elimination: incontinence
1D	Progressive dysphasia

The cross-referencing method lists all problems separately, using consecutive numbers. A "Related to"

No.	Date Entered	Date Inactive	Client Problem	Related to
#1	Mar 9/86		Several CVAs resulting in Rt hemiplegia and left-sided weakness. Redefined Feb 7/87	
#1a	Mar 9/86		Self care deficit (hygiene, toileting, grooming, feeding)	
#1B	Mar 9/86		Impaired physical mobility. Redefined Feb 7/87	
#1C	Mar 9/86		Alteration in urinary elimination: incontinence. Redefined Nov 10/86	
#1D	Mar 9/86		Progressive dysphasia	
#2	Mar 9/86		Alteration in bowel elimination: constipation. Redefined Nov 10/86	
#3	Mar 9/86		History of depression	
#4	Mar 9/86		Essential hypertension	
#5	June 6/86	Nov 86	Altered comfort: pruritis	
#2	Nov 10/86		Potential for constipation	
#1C	Nov 10/86		Nocturnal urinary incontinence	
#1	Feb 7/88		Cerebral vascular disease (multiple CVAs) resulting in bilateral hemiplegia	
#1B	Feb 7/88		Needs major assist. to transfer/unable to walk	

Figure 22–1 A client's problem list using the sublisting method to relate problems. Note that problems 1, 1B, 1C, and 2 were redefined on the dates indicated and listed subsequently. Courtesy of the Nursing Department, University Hospital—UBC site.

column to the right of the "Client Problem" column lists the number of the major problem to which the manifestations are related. For example, Figure 22–1 could also include:

No.	Client Problem	Related to:
1	Multiple CVAs resulting in Rt hemiplegia and left-sided weakness	
2	Self-care deficit (hygiene, toileting, grooming, feeding)	#1
3	Impaired physical mobility	#1
4	Alteration in urinary elimination: incontinence	#1
5	Progressive dysphasia	#1

Major problems can also be cross-referenced to other major problems. An example of this would be:

No.	Client Problem	Related to:
1	Cerebral vascular disease	#4
4	Essential hypertension	#1

"Redefinition" of problems is often necessary to reflect a change in the client's problem or to increase understanding of the problem. Redefining does *not* involve changing the stated nature of the problem; it involves changing the wording of the problem to reflect a change in its frequency or intensity, or increased knowledge. The problem retains the same number (e.g., see Figure 22–1):

No.	Client Problem
1C	Alteration in urinary elimination: incontinence REDEFINED NOV 10/87
1C	Nocturnal urinary incontinence

The **initial list of orders or care plans** is made with reference to the active problems. Care plans or orders are generated by the person who lists the problems. Physicians write physician's orders or medical care plans; nurses write nursing orders or nursing care plans. The written plan in the record is listed under each problem in the progress notes (discussed next) and is not isolated as a separate list of orders or in a separate Kardex.

The plan generated by the physician focuses on three aspects: the *diagnostic workup,* including plans to collect further data to establish a medical diagnosis or to assist in therapeutic management of the client; the *therapy* aspect, which often includes drug therapy and specific treatments; and *patient education,* describing the client's needs for skills and information that will assist in the management of the problem. Nurse-generated plans focus more on how the client's *activities* are to be observed, modified, or assisted. Nurses make many deci-

sions dealing with activity, diet, observation of client behavior (such as vital signs, wound healing, and emotional responses), client education, and other aspects of care.

Progress notes in the POR are made by all members of the health team involved in a client's care: nurse, occupational therapist, dietitian, physician, social worker, and others. All members of the health team add progress notes on the same type of sheet. Progress notes are numbered to correspond to the problems on the problem list.

One systematic format for writing progress notes is referred to as **SOAP** (an acronym for subjective data, objective data, assessment, and planning) charting or recording. The acronyms SOAPIE and SOAPIER refer to formats that add implementation, evaluation, and revision. Many agencies use only the SOAP format. A more recent format is the **APIE** (assessment, plan, implementation, and evaluation), which condenses the client data into fewer statements (Groah and Reed 1983, p. 1184). In APIE, the assessment combines the subjective and objective data with the nursing diagnosis, the plan combines the nursing actions with the expected outcomes, and the implementation and evaluation are the same. See Figure 22–2 for an example of a nurse's progress notes using the SOAP, SOAPIER, and APIE formats.

Subjective data report what the client perceives and the way the client expresses it. **Objective data** include measurements such as vital signs, observations made by health team members using their senses, laboratory and roentgenographic findings, and client responses to diagnostic and therapeutic measures such as medications. Examples of subjective and objective data are provided in Chapter 8.

In the **assessment** stage, the observer makes interpretations and draws conclusions from the subjective and objective data. Again all team members have made assessments, using the knowledge in their possession. At this point the nurse writes a nursing diagnostic statement in accordance with the guidelines discussed in Chapter 9. The **plan** is a plan for action based on the above data. The initial plan is written by the person who enters the problem into the record. All subsequent plans, considered revisions, also are entered into the progress notes. Plans may include: termination of certain activities if the problem is resolved, initiation of new actions if the problem is unchanged, and activities being done to resolve a particular problem.

Implementation, or **intervention,** is documentation of activities in the plan that were actually done for the client. These entries specify which plans were actually carried out. **Evaluation** is documentation of the client's response to the plan, stated in terms of client behavior (e.g., what the client did or said). The question asked at this stage is "Does the client's behavior indicate that the plan was unsuccessful in lessening or alleviating the identified problem?" **Revision,** or **reassessment,** refers to changes that must be made in the initial or original plan. From the evaluation notes and decision, one may determine that the client's condition may have improved or deteriorated. New data may now be available.

SOAP Format

2/13/89 #5 Generalized pruritus

1400   S—"My skin is itchy on my back and arms and it's been like this for a week."

      O—Skin appears clear—no rash or irritations noted. Marks where client has scratched noted on left and right forearms. Allergic to elastoplast but has not been in contact.
No previous history of pruritis.

      A—Alteration in comfort (pruritis): cause unknown

      P—Instructed to not scratch skin
—Applied calamine lotion to back and arms at 1430 hrs.
—Cut fingernails
—Assess further to determine if recurrence associated with specific drugs or foods
—Refer to physician and pharmacist for assessment

                  Tom Ritchie, R.N.

SOAPIER Format

2/13/89 #5 Generalized pruritus

1400   S—"My skin is itchy on back and arms and it's been like this for a week."

      O—Skin appears clear—no rash or irritation noted. Marks where client has scratched noted on left and right forearms. Allergic to elastoplast but has not been in contact.
No previous history of pruritis.

      A—Alteration in comfort (pruritis):

      P—Instruct not to scratch skin
—Apply calamine lotion as necessary
—Cut nails to avoid scratches
—Assess further to determine if recurrence associated with specific drugs or foods
—Refer to physician and pharmacist for assessment

      I —Instructed not to scratch skin
Applied calamine lotion to back and arms at 1430 hrs.
Assisted to cut fingernails
Notified physician and pharmacist of problem

1600   E—States "I'm still itchy. That lotion didn't help."

      R—Remove calamine lotion and apply hydrocortisone ungt. as ordered.

                  Tom Ritchie, R.N.

APIE Format

2/13/89 #5 Generalized pruritus

1400   A—Alteration in comfort; cause unknown. States "My skin is itchy on my back and arms and it's been like this for a week." Skin appears clear
—No rash or irritations noted. Marks where client has scratched noted on left and right forearms. Allergic to elastoplast but has not been in contact. No previous history of pruritis.

      P—Instruct to not scratch skin
—Apply calamine lotion as necessary
—Cut nails to avoid scratches
—Assess further to determine if recurrence associated with specific drugs or foods
—Refer to doctor and pharmacist for assessment

      I —Instructed not to scratch skin
Applied calamine lotion to back and arms at 1430 hrs.
Assisted to cut fingernails
Notified physician and pharmacist of problem

      E—States "I'm still itchy. That lotion didn't help."

                Tom Ritchie, R.N.

Figure 22–2   Examples of nursing progress notes using the SOAP, SOAPIER, and APIE formats.

Types of Progress Records

Three kinds of progress notes are generally recognized: narrative notes, flowsheets, and discharge notes. These are used in both source-oriented and problem-oriented medical records. **Narrative notes** record the client's progress descriptively. They are keyed to client problems and therapy and are filled out by all members of the health team. In POMRs, narrative notes are always written in the SOAP format. In some hospitals, because of DRGs, a note *must* be written every 24 hours.

When specific client variables such as pulse, blood pressure, medications, and progress in learning a new skill need to be recorded accurately, narrative notes are often too long. Instead the **flowsheet,** a graphic record or specially designed page on which data are recorded in appropriate columns, is used to quickly reflect the client's condition. See Figure 22–3 and Figure 22–4.

The time parameters for flowsheets can vary from minutes to months. In a hospital intensive care unit, a client's blood pressure may be monitored by the minute, whereas in an ambulatory clinic, a client's blood glucose level may be recorded once a month. Flowsheets are also often used in POMRs to record the daily nursing care provided. See Figure 22–5.

A **discharge note** may be written by the physician or another member of the health team, depending on the health care agency. In a home visiting service or community clinic, it may be written by the nurse. The discharge note refers to the client problems identified earlier and describes the degree to which each problem has been resolved. If the client has been referred to another agency, this is also noted. Figure 22–6 shows a nursing discharge summary.

Computer Records

Since about 1968, a number of health institutions have introduced computers. Early installations were primarily in hospital business offices. However, increasing numbers of computers are being used in health care planning and delivery as well as in laboratories and physicians' clinics. By the turn of the century, most nurses will use computers in many aspects of their practice. Already, "user friendly" machines, often operated with a light-pen and simple keyboard (see Figure 22–7), are of great help to the nurse in assessing planning, implementing, recording, and evaluating nursing care. Computer skills and knowledge will soon be expected and ▪

THE UNIVERSITY OF BRITISH COLUMBIA
HEALTH SCIENCES CENTRE HOSPITAL
EXTENDED CARE UNIT

FLOW SHEET

Miss Ann Smith

DATE: January, 1989

PARAMETER/PROCEDURE	TIME	17	18	19	20	21	22	23	24	25	26	27	28	29	30	31
B.P. 92 days weekly (Tues/Fri)	1000				180/88			162/90				160/98			160/90	
Weekly diabetic testing for G/A (at lunch)	1200			N/N							+1/N					
Wash perineal area – daily and prn / Heat lamp to area X10–15 mins	1000	JL	JL	JL	CR	CR	CR	CR	YC	YC	YC	PS	PS	PS	SJ	PS
Describe skin condition		excoriated			Red				Less red			Less red			Area	
		open area 2.5 cm			open area 2 cm				open area			open area			clear	
		small amt drainage			no drainage				crusted			healed				

Figure 22–3 A flowsheet on which the parameter of procedures to be measured are written by the nurse. Courtesy of the Nursing Department, University Hospital—UBC site.

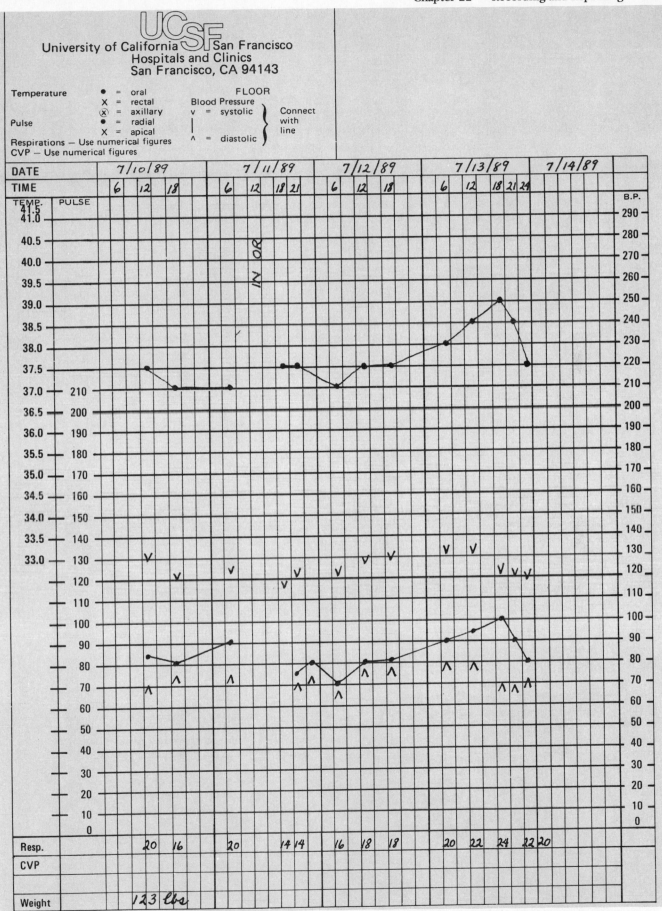

Figure 22—4 A clinical graph record. Courtesy Department of Nursing, The Medical Center at the University of California, San Francisco.

NURSING CARE FLOW SHEET

IMPORTANT CONSIDERATIONS

1. The assigned R.N. is responsible for the documentation of all nursing care. Charting for acute care patients is completed on the Nurses' Notes at least every 24 hrs. Nurses' Notes are completed for long term care patients at least weekly.

2. The initialling of the flow sheet indicates that the required hourly observations of the patient's well-being by nursing staff members have been conducted (including functioning of all equipment, e.g. I.V. infusions).

3. Charting in the Nurses' Notes is necessary when the flow sheet does not adequately reflect the patient's status. NN indicates documentation on Nurses' Notes.

4. Complete all boxes. Use a circle O for areas that are not applicable.

5. Select the abbreviation that most accurately reflects the patient's condition. Place a tick ✔ e.g. eating well ✔ if the statement reflects the patient's condition.

6. Do not chart pedal pulses or dressings on this flow sheet.

IDENTIFYING INFORMATION

Date — Insert new date at 0730. This date is for the time frame 0730-0730.

Time Period — Maximum time period is 12 hours | 0730 / 1930 | Start a new column for shorter time periods that correspond to changes in patient status (e.g. pre-post op).

Initials — Assigned nurse inserts initials and completes the Nurses' Signature Record with a full legible signature.

INSTRUCTION FOR COMPLETION OF SUB-SYSTEMS

Urine — Insert QS if patient voiding adequate amounts.
— Insert HNV if patient has not voided.
— Insert amount if measuring urine (ml.)
— Insert FB if recording amount on Fluid Balance Record.

Stool — Record number with 0 1 SC — Stool Chart.

Diet — Insert T if patient is on a therapeutic diet. Chart in Nurses' Notes when therapeutic diet is initiated or changed.

Turns — Record frequency e.g. q2h etc.

Bedrails — Indicate if one x1 or, if both, x2 are raised.

Mobility — Record highest level of activity achieved. Indicate WC under chair, if using wheelchair.

INSERT ONLY THESE ITEMS INTO BLANK SPACES

Blank spaces are provided for recording other routine nursing care not requiring Nurses' Notes.

1. Heparin Lock Intact.
2. I.V. Intact.
3. TPN Intact.
4. Telemetry Intact.
5. Holter Monitor Intact.
6. Urine Strained.
7. Catheter Care.
8. Calorie Count.

Use a ✔ if no problem observed. Chart in Nurses' Notes NN where a problem exists.

9. Extremity Check: (CWMS) colour/warmth, movement, sensation of area (identify) and side, e.g. CWMS rt. foot.
} Use a ✔ if no problems observed. Document in Nurses' Notes NN if problem observed.

10. Eye Patch Intact.
11. Eye Shield Intact. } (Identify side)
12. Tensor Bandage Intact (Identify side and area).
} Use a ✔ if no problems observed. Document in Nurses' Notes NN if problem observed.

13. Oral Intake.
14. Davol Drain.
15. Penrose Drain.
16. Heyer Drain.
} Insert measured amount. Use the FLUID BALANCE RECORD if patient has an I.V. or a 24 hr. fluid balance is necessary.

17. Cardiac Activity Level.
18. Seizure Level.
} Insert number that indicates assigned level. Indicate measurement in box.

19. Abdominal Girth. (Centimeter, Time)

Figure 22—5 A nursing care flow sheet used in conjunction with the problem-oriented record. Courtesy of the Nursing Department, University Hospital—UBC site.

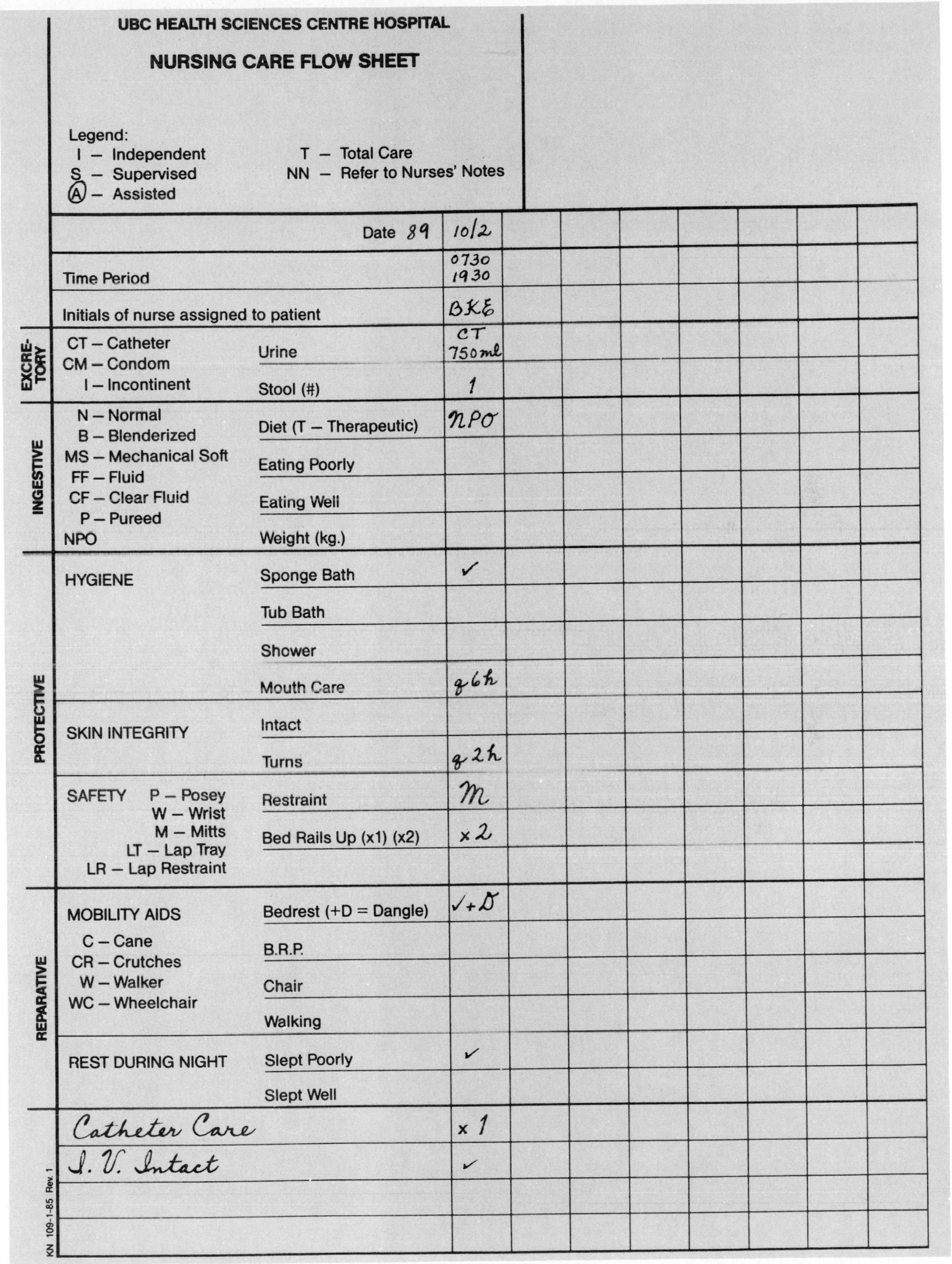

UBC HEALTH SCIENCES CENTRE HOSPITAL

NURSING CARE FLOW SHEET

Legend:
I — Independent   T — Total Care
S — Supervised   NN — Refer to Nurses' Notes
Ⓐ — Assisted

		Date 89	10/2							
	Time Period		0730 1930							
	Initials of nurse assigned to patient		BKE							
EXCRETORY	CT — Catheter CM — Condom I — Incontinent	Urine	CT 750ml							
		Stool (#)	1							
INGESTIVE	N — Normal B — Blenderized MS — Mechanical Soft FF — Fluid CF — Clear Fluid P — Pureed NPO	Diet (T — Therapeutic)	NPO							
		Eating Poorly								
		Eating Well								
		Weight (kg.)								
PROTECTIVE	HYGIENE	Sponge Bath	✓							
		Tub Bath								
		Shower								
		Mouth Care	q6h							
	SKIN INTEGRITY	Intact								
		Turns	q2h							
	SAFETY P — Posey W — Wrist M — Mitts LT — Lap Tray LR — Lap Restraint	Restraint	M							
		Bed Rails Up (x1) (x2)	x2							
REPARATIVE	MOBILITY AIDS C — Cane CR — Crutches W — Walker WC — Wheelchair	Bedrest (+D = Dangle)	✓ +D							
		B.R.P.								
		Chair								
		Walking								
	REST DURING NIGHT	Slept Poorly	✓							
		Slept Well								
	Catheter Care		x 1							
	I. V. Intact		✓							

KN 109-1-85 Rev. 1

Figure 22–5 (continued)

THE UNIVERSITY OF BRITISH COLUMBIA
HEALTH SCIENCES CENTRE
EXTENDED CARE UNIT

NURSING SUMMARY

MISS ANN SMITH
Age 82 years BD: 1 Aug. 06
Admitted: March 5, 1989

DISCHARGE SUMMARY - June 10, 1989

Admitted March 5, 1989 from Victoria General Hospital in Victoria, B.C.

Problems

1. Multiple CVAs with bilateral hemiplegia resulting in need for assistance with ADLs and mobility/transfers--needs 2 person assist to transfer, needs maximum assist with ADLs; dressing, washing and bathing done by staff. She is concerned about her appearance.
2. Continent of urine if routinely toileted during the day--occasionally incontinent of urine at night.
3. Prone to constipation--has soft formed BM q 2-3 days when toileted--needs occasional glycerine suppository and receives Metamucil 15cc daily.
4. Essential hypertension--B.P. ranges from 150/90 to 184/108--monitored 2 days weekly (Tues & Fri.). Receives Nadolol 80 mg daily
5. Has a history of depression--has become lethargic, withdrawn and weepy at times. Minimal response to antidepressant drugs (Amitriptyline 25 mg ghs - was D/C May 19/81). Involved in numerous social groups and 1-1 interaction--responded well to both. Family visited frequently and very supportive.
6. Diet--minced--has occasional difficulty swallowing and tongue mobility due to dysarthria.
7. Progressive dysphasia--speech slurred--difficult to understand; very slow to respond; appreciates help from staff.

Next of Kin

Ray Smith--phone 123-4567 (brother)
Sue Brown--phone 261-0941 (niece)

Medical regime

Metamucil 15 cc daily
Nadolol 80 mg daily
Brandy 30 cc q h.s. prn

Allergies

--elastoplast--suffered period of general pruritis but was unable to relate to specific drugs or food--spontaneously resolved.

Safety Needs

Vision--good/able to read clock on wall and small print
Hearing--able to hear normal conversation
Mechanical aids--side rails and support in chair with pillows and belt restraints
--trunk balance poor
Orientation--well oriented to time, place, person despite deterioration in physical condition

Strengths and Resources

Miss Smith has a very supportive family. She is concerned about her appearance and feels comfortable letting staff know what her needs are.

Resident and family wish Miss Smith to move to LTC facility (X-E.C.U) in South Vancouver as it is much closer for family to visit--family visits 2-3 x weekly.

J. Doe, R.N.

June 10, 1989
Date

J. Doe, R.N.
Signature

Figure 22–6 A nursing discharge summary. Courtesy of the Nursing Department, University Hospital—UBC site.

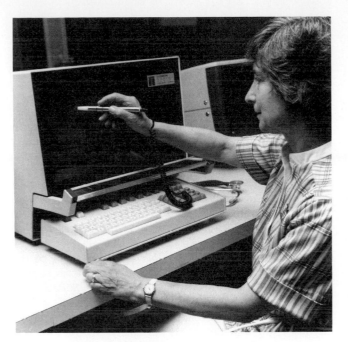

Figure 22—7 An input device

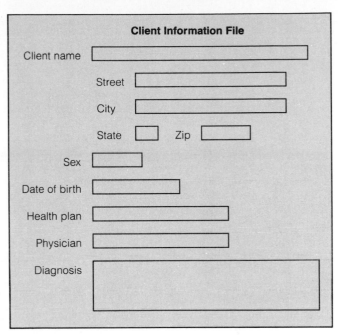

Figure 22—8 Segment of a client's data base

perhaps required for a great many positions in nursing. Those who ignore this technologic revolution may be left behind.

The nurse is clearly the manager of client care. Hospital information flows to and through nursing departments. Nurses who allow computer systems to design their practice may find themselves both frustrated and victimized. Instead, they must take an active role in the design, development, and implementation of any such systems.

In the past, hospital computer applications have been administrative (e.g., tasks such as client billing, maintaining financial records, and long-term planning). As computers get smaller, less costly, more powerful, and easier to use, they are being used increasingly in other areas of the health care system as well. Today, it is common to find a microcomputer system or computer terminal in the nurse's station. It is likely that such machines will become a more integral part of the nurse's activities during the next decade. By using computerized systems, nursing staff are able to create care plans easily, customize them for each client, type in additions as needed, evaluate and update information at any time, and retrieve data appropriate to a specific nursing diagnosis. Such systems can be programmed to provide work lists, as needed, directly from the computer. In this way, lists generated for treatments, procedures, and medications can always be kept up to date. Such an application eliminates the need for multiple flowsheets since all of the same information is available both in the computer and on computer-printed update forms. To record nursing actions, the nurse either enters data directly into the computerized records or completes the computer-generated flowsheet in the client's chart.

A well-designed data base system can make the entry and retrieval of information a relatively easy task for the nurses who use it. Figure 22—8 is an illustration of how a portion of a client's record might appear on the computer screen. The nurse enters the appropriate information into the form by typing it on the computer's keyboard. Changes can be made easily to update this record. Later, as the needs of the nurse dictate, information about a particular client, diagnosis, or physician can be recalled to the screen.

Specific ways in which an **automated client care plan** can facilitate the role of the nurse include the following:

1. Entry of nursing assessments is simplified; e.g., the nurse can touch a computer screen display of possibilities.
2. Laboratory data can be ordered by entering a request at a terminal in the nurses' station, and results can be retrieved over the same terminal in a shorter time with less paperwork.
3. The system facilitates complete and legible medication orders.
4. The nursing implications of a doctor's order can be sent to the nurse. Client preparation needs for a particular test can be listed automatically in the client's nursing care plan.
5. The use of nursing diagnosis is facilitated; a common format can be used.
6. Current information can be updated easily. Discontinued medication orders can be deleted easily, making all information timely, legible, and complete.

With access to a completely automated care plan, the nurse can prepare client discharge summaries that include information from the time of admission. These reports can include all current unresolved nursing diagnoses and the relevant interventions. Computer-generated reports can include relevant information for teaching the client, including instructions about the use of drugs, details of a required diet, activity restrictions, and the date of the next visit to return to the physician's office.

In addition to facilitating individualized client care, computerized records can also be beneficial to nurse-managers who may use stored data to generate reports on the acuity levels of clients on each unit. These can be used to devise a formula for determining both the appropriate skill levels and the number of nurses required per shift and per floor. The scheduling of personnel is often made difficult by changing shifts, different skill levels, vacations, weekends, legal coverage requirements, and so on. **Computer-based scheduling** models can save much time and provide options that can be difficult to discover if the information is handled manually.

Nurses are bound by their professional ethics to maintain a client's privacy. This means that information about a client cannot be disseminated outside of the realm of the caregivers. The use of computer-based informations systems to store client data has increased the risk of an accidental or intentional violation of a client's rights. Just as computers are becoming easier to use, they are becoming easier to abuse. Clients have a right to privacy and confidentiality even where computer-based information systems are used. Nurses should not give their signature codes to anyone or let anyone without an access code use the computer.

In today's information age, health care providers tend to collect more data, share more data bases, and access more client information than in earlier days. Client records are queried for insurance claims, during audits of the nursing (as well as some other) departments, and sometimes on the demand of the courts. There has not been a similar growth in the sophistication of the security systems (both manual and computerized) that are used to limit access to these data. Passwords limiting access to data can often be guessed; disgruntled employees may change, delete, or disseminate data; computer "enthusiasts" may deem it a challenge to "break into" a hospital's computer information system. Nurses must be aware of these problems and risks if they are to fulfill their responsibility to the client. The specific role of the nurse (or student, educator, researcher, manager) does not absolve her or him from the accountability for ensuring a client's right to privacy.

Guidelines About Recording

Because the client's record is a legal document and may be used to provide evidence in court, many factors are considered in recording. Health care personnel not only maintain the confidentiality of the client's record but also meet legal standards in the process of recording. Some of these factors are restricted access, use of ink, signature, errors, blanks, accuracy, appropriateness, completeness, use of standard terminology, and brevity.

The client's record is protected legally as a private record of the client's care. Thus, **access to the record is restricted** to health workers involved in giving care to the client. Insurance companies, for example, have no legal right to demand access to medical records, even though they may be determining compensation to the client. On the other hand, a client who is making a claim for compensation may ask to have the medical history used as evidence. In this instance, the client must sign an authorization for review, copying, or release of information from the record. This form clearly indicates what information is to be released and to whom. In no instance may a nurse allow access to a client's record by family members or any person other than a caregiver.

For purposes of education and research, most agencies allow student and graduate health professionals access to client records. The records are used in client conferences, clinics, rounds, and written papers or client studies. The student or graduate is bound by a strict ethical code to hold all information in confidence. Some agencies code medical records when they are filed, so that the names of clients are removed. This allows records to be used without identifying individuals. When this is not the practice, it is the responsibility of the student or health care professional to protect the client's privacy by not using a name or any statements in the notations that would identify the client. Many agencies also require documentation from the student or health professional wishing to use medical records of discharged clients. A permission note from the student's instructor will confirm the person's status as a student at a particular school.

All entries on the client's record are made in **dark-colored ink** so that the record is permanent and changes can be identified. Dark-colored ink is generally required because it reproduces well on microfilm and in duplication processes. Entries need to be legible. Hand printing or easily understood handwriting is permissible. Each recording on the nursing notes is to be signed by the nurse making it with **name** and **title.** Documentation of the **date** and **time** of each notation is essential not only for legal reasons but also for safe care. For example, the time at which a narcotic was administered to a client needs to be determined before the next one can safely be given. Time can be recorded in the conventional manner (i.e., 9:00 A.M. or 3:20 P.M.) or according to the 24-hour clock (military clock), which avoids confusion about whether a time was A.M. or P.M. See Figure 22–9.

When an **error** is made when charting, a line is drawn through it, and the word "error" is written above it, with the nurse's initials or name (depending on agency policy). Errors should not be erased or blotted out, so there is no doubt about the nursing care given or the charting error made. If the nature of the error is not clear, many attorneys feel it is helpful and legally acceptable to indicate what the error was, in order to protect the client and the nurse. An example might be, "Charted for wrong client." The policy of the agency, however, needs to be checked. If a **blank** appears in a notation, a line is drawn through the blank space, and it is signed.

It is essential that notations on records be **accurate, correct, appropriate, and complete.** Accurate notations consist of facts or exact observations rather than opinions or interpretations of an observation. It is more accurate, for example, to write that the client "refused medication" (fact) than to write that the client "was uncooperative" (opinion); to write that a client "was

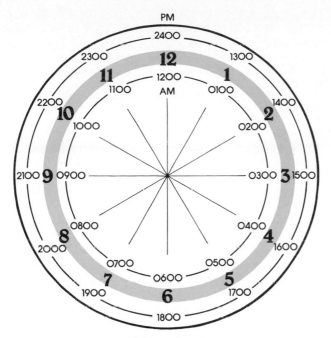

PM

Figure 22–9 The 24-hour clock

crying" (observation) is preferable to noting that the client "was depressed" (interpretation). Opinions or interpretations may or may not be accurate. Similarly, when a client expresses worry about the diagnosis or problem, this should be quoted directly on the record. "Stated: 'I'm worried about my leg.' " Nurses should record what they hear as well as what they observe.

Correct spelling is essential for accuracy in recording. If unsure how to spell a word, the nurse looks it up in a dictionary. Most agency units have one available for this purpose. Two decidedly different medications may have similar spellings (e.g., digitoxin and digoxin). Only information that pertains to the client's health problems and care is recorded. Any other personal information that the client conveys to the nurse is inappropriate for the record. If irrelevant information is recorded, it can be considered an invasion of the client's privacy and/or libelous. A client's disclosure that he or she was a prostitute and has smoked marijuana, for example, *would not* be recorded on the client's medical record unless it had a direct bearing on the client's health problem.

Not all data that a nurse obtains about a client can be recorded. However, the information that is recorded needs to be complete and helpful to the client, physicians, other nurses, and participating health care workers. Incomplete records could be used as evidence in court to show that the client did not receive the quality of care considered to meet generally accepted standards. For example, if a diabetic client's record does not indicate that insulin was given and that the urine was tested, the record could be used as evidence of negligence on the part of the nurse responsible for providing this care. Of course, other examples and evidence would be needed to support a finding of negligence by the nurse. However, the client's record can be used to indicate the kind of care given. A complete notation for a client who has vomited, for example, includes the time,

the amount, the color, the odor, and any other data about the client (e.g., pain).

The following guidelines may assist nurses in selecting essential and complete information to record about clients. Note that the emphasis is on facts that denote a change in the client's health status or behavior or that indicate a deviation from what is usually expected. Essential information includes:

1. Any behavior changes, for example:
   - Indications of strong emotions, such as anxiety or fear
   - Marked changes in mood
   - Change in level of consciousness, such as stupor
   - Regression in relationships with family or friends
2. Any changes in physical function, such as:
   - Loss of balance
   - Loss of strength
   - Difficulty hearing or seeing
3. Any physical sign or symptom that:
   - Is severe, such as severe pain
   - Tends to recur or persist
   - Is not normal, such as elevated body temperature
   - Gets worse, such as gradual weight loss
   - Indicates a complication, such as inability to void following surgery
   - Is not relieved by prescribed measures, such as continued failure to defecate or to sleep
   - Indicates faulty health habits, such as lice on the scalp
   - Is a known danger signal, such as a lump in the breast
4. Any nursing interventions provided, such as:
   - Medications administered
   - Therapies
   - Activities of daily living, if agency policy dictates
   - Teaching clients self-care
5. Visits by a physician or other members of the health team

In a legal battle, incomplete medical records may present difficulties that cannot be overcome. Courts take a dim view of evidence based on recall unsupported by written documentation, especially when a great deal of time has elapsed between the events and the trial. A plaintiff's attorney will never lose an opportunity to point out to the jury that an important event went unrecorded by the providers of care. Some courts have held that lack of exactitude in documentation implies lack of attention. In extreme cases, lack of documentation could be considered evidence of negligence (Cushing 1982).

The nurse needs to use only commonly accepted **abbreviations, symbols,** and **terms** that are specified by the agency. Then, if the record is used in court as evidence, other professionals responsible for interpreting the data can do so correctly. Many abbreviations are standard and used universally; others are confined to certain geographic areas. Some agencies supply a list of the abbreviations they accept. When in doubt about whether to use an abbreviation, the nurse writes the term out in full, until certain about the abbreviation. Table 22–1 lists some commonly used abbreviations (except those used for medications, which are described

Table 22–1 Commonly Used Abbreviations

Abbreviation	Term	Abbreviation	Term
abd	abdomen	nil (ō)	none
ABO	the main blood group system	no. (#)	number
a.c.	before meals (ante cibum)	NPO (NBM)	nothing by mouth (per ora)
ADL	activities of daily living	NS (N/S)	normal saline
ad lib	as desired (ad libitum)	O₂	oxygen
adm	admitted or admission	od	daily (omni die)
A.M.	morning (ante meridiem)	OD	right eye (oculus dexter); overdose
amb	ambulatory	OOB	out of bed
amt	amount	os	mouth
approx	approximately (about)	OS	left eye (oculus sinister)
b.i.d.	twice daily (bis in die)	p.c.	after meals (post cibum)
BM (bm)	bowel movement	PE (PX)	physical examination
BP	blood pressure	per	by or though
BRP	bathroom privileges	P.M.	afternoon (post meridiem)
c̄ (C)	with (cum)	p.o.	by mouth (per os)
C	Celsius (centigrade)	postop	postoperative(ly)
CBC	complete blood count	preop	preoperative(ly)
CBR	complete bed rest	prep	preparation
c/o	complains of	p.r.n.	when necessary (pro re nata)
DAT	diet as tolerated	pr (Pt)	patient
dc (disc)	discontinue	q.	every (quaque)
drsg	dressing	q.d.	every day (quaque die)
Dx	diagnosis	q.h. (q.1h.)	every hour (quaque hora)
ECG (EKG)	electrocardiogram	q.2h., q.3h., etc	every two hours, three hours, etc
F	Fahrenheit	q.h.s.	every night at bedtime (quaque hora somni)
fld	fluid		
GI	gastrointestinal	q.i.d.	four times a day (quater in die)
GP	general practitioner	req	requisition
gtt	drops (guttae)	Rt (rt, R)	right
h. (hr)	hour (hora)	S (s̄)	without (sine)
H₂O	water	SI	seriously ill
h.s.	at bedtime (hora somni)	spec	specimen
I & O	intake and output	stat	at once, immediately (statim)
IV	intravenous	t.i.d.	three times a day (ter in die)
Lab	laboratory	TL	team leader
liq	liquid	TLC	tender loving care
LMP	last menstrual period	TPR	temperature, pulse, respirations
lt (L)	left	Tr.	tincture
meds	medications	VO	verbal order
ml (mL)	milliliter	VS (vs)	vital signs
mod	moderate	WNL	within normal limits
neg	negative	wt	weight

Table 22–2 Commonly Used Symbols

Symbol	Term	Symbol	Number
>	greater than	ō	0
<	less than	ss	½
=	equal to	ī	1
↑	increased	īī	2
↓	decreased	īīī	3
♀	female	īv	4
♂	male	v̄	5
°	degree	v̄ī	6
#	number; fracture	v̄īī	7
ℨ	dram	v̄īīī	8
℥	ounce	īx	9
×	times	x̄	10
@	at		

in Chapter 44). Table 22–2 lists commonly accepted symbols.

Recordings need to be brief as well as complete, to save time in communication. The client's name and the word *client* are omitted. For example, the nurse may write "Perspiring profusely. Respirations shallow, wet, 28/min." Each thought or sentence is terminated with a period.

Records the Nurse Commonly Uses

Client records on which nurses commonly make notations include: the nursing assessment (history) form, flowsheets, nurse's notes (nursing progress notes), the problem list record, the Kardex (Rand) and/or nursing care plan, the discharge note or summary, and consents and releases. **Nursing assessment forms** vary considerably among agencies. Even within an agency, forms may differ among nursing units (e.g, an adult medical-surgical unit, an obstetric unit, a pediatric unit, and a psychiatric unit may want different nursing histories).

Flowsheets commonly used are the clinical record (also called the graphic chart or graphic observation record), the medication record, the fluid intake and output record, and daily nursing care records such as the one shown in Figure 22–5. The **clinical record** indicates: body temperature, pulse rate, respiratory rate, blood pressure readings, and weight. Some agencies also show special medications (such as dicumarol), central venous pressure (CVP), 24-hour fluid intake and output, weight, bowel movement, glucose and acetone in the urine, etc. See Figure 22–4. Before notations are made on a **24-hour fluid balance record,** the nurse records the amount of the client's fluid intake and output on a form kept at the client's bedside. The client and support persons should be taught to use this record. It documents intake and output for the duration of one shift only (8 or 12 hours). The totals for each shift are then recorded on the 24-hour fluid balance record.

In the sample shown in Figure 22–10, the totals for each 8-hour shift (days, evenings, and nights) are recorded, and then the 24-hour totals are calculated. All routes of fluid intake must be measured and recorded: oral, intravenous, and gavage (tube feedings into the stomach). Similarly, all routes of fluid loss or output are measured and recorded: urine, emesis (vomitus), diar-

rhea, and drainage from any tube (such as a T-tube, nasogastric tube, suprapubic drain, wound suction, or bladder or ureteral catheter). When heavy perspiration occurs, this also needs to be estimated. More information about ways to measure and record specific amounts of fluid intake and output is described in Chapter 43.

Nurse's notes and the manner of recording vary, depending on whether a source-oriented medical record or POR is used. In source-oriented medical records, the nursing notes consist of both narrative and chronological charting. **Narrative charting** is a description (narration) of information, and **chronological charting** records data in sequence as time moves forward. The minimum number of words and many abbreviations are used, to keep the information concise. (See "Guidelines about Recording," earlier in this chapter.) Figure 22–11 is an example of narrative nurse's notes. The forms used for the nurse's notes may vary from place to place. Some agencies have separate columns for treatments, nursing observations, and comments. The major disadvantage of narrative charting is that it is difficult for a reader to find all the data about a specific problem without examining all of the recorded information. For this reason, specific flow records are often used for certain information.

In the POR, the nurse's progress notes are written in relation to a specific problem identified on the problem list. Graphic records and flowsheets are used to provide other routine or necessary information. When entering nurse's notes in the POR, the SOAP, SOAPIER, or APIE format is used.

The **Kardex** (see Figure 22–12) is a widely used,

EL CAMINO HOSPITAL

INTAKE AND OUTPUT RECORD

PATIENT LABEL

PATIENT NAME _____

PATIENT # _____

PHYSICIAN _____

	INTAKE				OUTPUT					
TOTAL IV	INTRAVENOUS			TUBE FEED	ORAL	TIME	URINE	NG	EMESIS	BM	MISC.
					DATE:						
						6-2					
						2-10					
						10-6					
						24°					
					DATE:						
						6-2					
						2-10					
						10-6					
						24°					

Figure 22–10 A sample 24-hour fluid intake and output record. Courtesy of El Camino Hospital, Mountain View, California.

DATE		TREATMENTS	DATE		LABORATORY TESTS	DATE TO BE DONE		FAST	DONE
May 23/89	No Code Blue. In case of decease—forms are stamped and on back of chart (see letter from daughter)		June 20	Continuous O₂ @ 4 L/min nasal prongs		Aug 7/89	Swab Lt forearm C&S		✓
			June 22	May get up for walks ē portable O₂		Aug 14/89	Swab Rt eye C&S		✓
						Aug 20/89	Discontinue all blood tests		✓
			Nights	Change O₂ bottle, tubing, and Ventolin tubing and mask Q2d June 2, 4, 6, 8, 10, 12					

DIAGNOSTIC PROCEDURES

						DATE TO BE DONE			
May 25/89	Secretion precaution—sputum		June 21/89	No I.V. infusion unless daughter notified first—family request					
WEIGHT	ASSIST ☐			**ACTIVITY AND HYGIENE** L.B.M. June 22					

SURGICAL PROCEDURES

REFERRALS

DIET			June 22	Reg.—pureed diet Needs to be fed	June 28/89	Toilet program q 2 h		May 22/89	Chest physio & mobilization
								May 23/89	Dietary consult

INTRAVENOUS
None

DIAGNOSIS AND PERTINENT HISTORY

Emphysema & respiratory failure

ALLERGIES	None known.	NEXT OF KIN	Mrs. C. Smith	
		RELATIONSHIP	daughter	
		TELEPHONE	555-5555 (home) 555-1111 (work)	

INTAKE ☐	VITAL SIGNS	daily	AGE	ADMITTING DOCTOR	RESIDENT
OUTPUT ☐			79	Dr. Lonrie	None

BED NO.	NAME				
218 D	Mrs. M. Brown				

KN21-8-80

Figure 22-12 An example of a nursing Kardex. (continued)

are required to listen to the report on all clients, including many not under their care. The tape-recorded report is often briefer and less time-consuming. Some agencies or units combine these methods of giving the change-of-shift report, following the taped report or a brief report to all oncoming staff with a more extensive individual report given by the nurse going off duty to the nurse who will be providing client care during the coming shift. This more detailed report is often given at the bedside, and clients as well as nurses may participate in the exchange of information.

Guidelines that can help nurses prepare and present reports about clients include (Hesse 1983, Smith 1986):

1. Follow a particular order when reporting about a series of clients. For example, follow room numbers in a hospital or times of appointments in a community clinic.
2. Identify the client by name, room number, and bed designation. For example, Ms. Jessie Jones, 702, Bed D. This enables the listeners, especially float nurses or those returning from days off or vacation, to immediately relate subsequent information to this client's case.
3. Depending on the type of unit, provide the reason for admission, that is, the client's medical diagnosis or original complaint. This information may not be necessary in long-term geriatric units or newborn nurseries; in acute-care settings, however, it is often necessary because of multiple tests, consultations, and transfers.
4. Include diagnostic tests and/or results and other therapies performed in the past 24 hours, such as blood transfusions, surgery, initiation of intravenous therapy, narcotics administered, blood gas levels, and group therapy data.
5. Note any significant changes in the client's condition. Oncoming nurses must know about changes for the worse to monitor the client's condition appropriately. Significant improvements toward goal attainment should also be noted so the nurse can provide positive feedback to the client.
6. When reporting about changes, present the pertinent information in this order: assessment, nursing diagnoses (if appropriate), planning, intervention, and evaluation. For example, "Mr. Ronald Oakes said he had an aching pain in his left calf at 1400 hours. Inspection revealed no other signs. Calf pain is related to altered blood circulation. Rest and elevation of his legs on a footstool for 30 minutes provided relief."
7. Provide exact information, such as "Ms. Jessie Jones received Demerol 100 mg. intramuscularly at 2000 hours (8 P.M.)," not "Ms. Jessie Jones received some Demerol during the evening."
8. Do not include unremarkable measurements such as normal temperature, pulse, and blood pressure unless a desired change is involved. For example, a normal body temperature for a client who has had an elevated temperature should be reported.
9. Report the client's emotional responses that need attention before other interventions can be implemented. For example, a client who has just learned

his biopsy results revealed malignancy and who is now scheduled for a laryngectomy needs time to discuss his feelings before the nurse commences preoperative teaching.

Nursing students may want to practice giving report in clinical post-care conferences or by taping themselves giving a simulated report of the current status of their assigned clients.

Chapter Highlights

Written records ensure transmission of information to all health workers caring for the client; are a source of research, educational, and statistical data; and allow the audit of client care standards.

Client records are admissible as evidence in a court of law.

The problem-oriented medical record (POMR or POR) (Weed system) is increasingly recognized as a method that provides a client-centered problem-solving approach to care.

The POR has four basic components: a defined data base, a complete problem list, an initial plan for each identified problem, and progress notes.

Traditional client records are source-oriented records, in that each category of health worker keeps separate records.

Traditional records generally have six parts: admission sheet, face sheet, physician's order sheet, medical history sheet, nurses' notes, and other special records such as the laboratory records.

The Kardex record is widely used for quick access to current data about clients.

Computerized information systems are being used increasingly in health care agencies.

Record entries should be brief, accurate, legible, chronological, made on consecutive lines, and appropriately signed.

Record entries are made after nursing interventions and usually when the client is admitted or transferred.

Because the record is a legal document, nurses sign their names and titles and use standard terms and abbreviations.

Erasures on the client record are not permitted.

Reports about clients need to be concise and pertinent and must include significant changes in the client's condition and therapy.

References

Costello, S., and Summers, B. Y. June 1985. Documenting patient care: Getting it all together. *Nursing Management* 16:31–34.

Creighton, H. 1981. *Law every nurse should know.* 4th ed. Philadelphia: W. B. Saunders Co.

Cushing, M. December 1982. The legal side. Gaps in documentation. *American Journal of Nursing* 82:1899–1900.

Gay, P. March 1983. Get it in writing. *Nursing Management* 14:32–35.

Groah, L., and Reed, E. A. May 1983. Your responsibility in documenting care. *Association of Operating Room Nurses Journal* 37:1174, 1176–77, 1180–85.

Hesse, G. February 1983. A better shift report means better nursing care. *Nursing 83* 13:65. Canadian ed. 13:17.

King, I. M. April 1984. Effectiveness of nursing care: Use of a goal-oriented nursing record in end stage renal disease. *The American Association of Nephrology Nurses and Technicians Journal* 1:11–17, 60.

Rich, P. L. July 1985. With this flow sheet less is more. *Nursing 85* 15:25–29.

Sklar, C. L. May 1984. The patient's record, an invaluable communication tool. *The Canadian Nurse* 80:50, 52.

Smith, C. E. February 1986. Upgrade your shift reports with the three R's. *Nursing 86* 16:63–64.

Weed, L. L. 1971. *Medical records, medical education and patient care: The Problem-oriented record as a basic tool.* Cleveland: Case Western Reserve University Press.

Yarnall, S. R., and Atwood, J. June 1974. Problem-oriented practice for nurses and physicians. General concepts. *Nursing Clinics of North America* 9(2):215–28.

Protecting Health

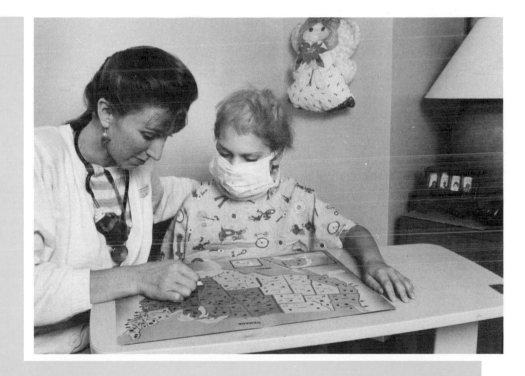

23

Preventing the Transfer of Microorganisms

OBJECTIVES

Describe the importance of biologic safety.

Define selected terms pertaining to protecting health

Identify six links in the chain of infection.

Identify measures that break each link in the chain of infection.

Identify factors influencing a microorganism's capability to produce an infectious process.

Describe four stages of an infectious process.

Identify causal factors of nosocomial infections.

Identify people at risk of acquiring an infection.

Describe the difference between nonspecific and specific defenses of the body.

Identify anatomic and physiologic barriers that defend the body against microorganisms.

Differentiate between natural and acquired types of immunity.

Identify signs of localized and systemic infections.

Explain the concepts of medical and surgical asepsis.

Identify interventions to prevent infections.

Identify interventions to protect body defenses.

Discuss methods for evaluating the effectiveness of protective measures.

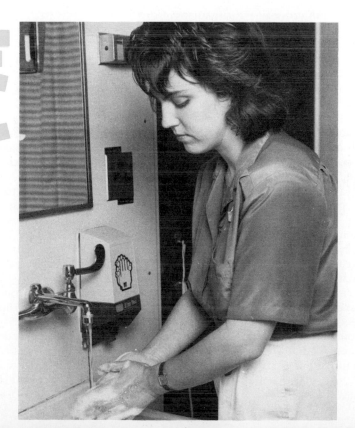

Importance of Biologic Safety

Nurses are directly involved in providing a biologically safe environment and promoting health. Microorganisms exist everywhere in the environment: in water, soil, and within and on the body. The number of microbial colonists on and in the body exceeds the number of body cells by 10 to 1 (Norton 1986, p. 580). Most microorganisms are harmless, and some are even beneficial in that they perform essential functions in the body. Some microorganisms found in the intestines, i.e., enterobacteria, produce substances called bacteriocins, which are lethal to related strains of bacteria. Others produce antibiotic-like substances and toxic metabolites that repress the growth of other microorganisms. Some microorganisms are normal **flora** (the collective vegetation in a given area) in one part of the body and produce infection in another. For example, *Escherichia coli* is a normal inhabitant of the large intestine but a common cause of infection of the urinary tract.

An **infection** is an invasion of body tissue by microorganisms and their proliferation there. Such a microorganism is called an infectious agent. If the microorganism produces no clinical evidence of disease, the infection is called asymptomatic or subclinical. Some subclinical infections can cause significant damage to the host, e.g., cytomegalovirus (CMV) infection in a pregnant woman. A detectable alteration in normal tissue function, however, is called **disease.** Microorganisms vary in their **virulence** (i.e., their ability to produce disease). In general, five groups of microorganisms normally can cause disease: bacteria, viruses, fungi, protozoa, and *Rickettsia.*

Microorganisms also vary in the severity of the diseases they produce and their degree of communicability. For example, the common cold virus is more readily transmitted than the bacillus that causes leprosy (*Mycobacterium leprae*). If the infectious agent can be transmitted to an individual by direct or indirect contact, through a vector or vehicle, or as an airborne infection, the resulting condition is called a **communicable disease.**

Etiology is the study of causes; the etiology of an infectious process is the identification of the invading microorganisms. The control of the spread of microorganisms and the protection of people from communicable diseases and infections are practiced on four levels: international, national, community, and individual. An example of infectious disease control at the international level is the required immunization people must have against certain diseases, such as cholera, before traveling to certain countries. Similarly, international health regulations govern the immunizations required of American and Canadian citizens returning home. National regulations govern, for example, the interstate and interprovincial transportation of food. These regulations protect people from receiving contaminated food. Also, national regulations attempt to control pollution of water, the air, and the environment, subjects currently receiving much publicity.

Communities regulate the disposal of sewage and the purity of drinking water, for example. Such community regulations protect people from infectious disease. Protection from infection is also an individual responsibility. Individuals protect themselves not only by practicing good hygiene (see Chapter 34, "Personal Hygiene") but also by eating a balanced diet and exercising.

Normal Body Defenses

The human normally has microbial flora that reside in and outside the body, e.g., on the skin, on mucous membranes, inside the respiratory passages, and inside the gastrointestinal tract. These microorganisms are called **resident flora** because they are always present, usually in numbers compatible with the individual's health. See Table 23–1. In contrast to resident flora, **transient flora** are microorganisms that are present episodically.

Individuals normally have defenses that protect the body from infection. These defenses can be categorized as nonspecific and specific. Nonspecific defenses protect the person against all microorganisms, regardless of prior exposure. Specific (or immune) defenses, by contrast, are directed against identifiable bacteria, viruses, fungi, or other infectious agents.

Nonspecific Defenses

Nonspecific body defenses include anatomic and physiologic barriers. **Intact skin and mucous membranes** are the body's first line of defense against microorganisms. Unless the skin and mucosa become cracked and broken, they are an effective barrier against bacteria. Fungi can live on the skin, but they cannot penetrate it. The dryness of the skin also is a deterrent to bacteria; they are most plentiful in moist areas, e.g., perineum and axillae. Another deterrent is sebum, which contains an unsaturated fatty acid that kills some bacteria. Resident bacteria of the skin also prevent other bacteria from multiplying. They use up the available nourishment, and the end products of their metabolism inhibit other bacteria. Normal secretions make the skin slightly acidic; acidity also inhibits bacterial growth.

The **nasal passages** have a defensive function. As entering air follows the tortuous route of the passage, it comes in contact with moist mucous membranes and small hairlike projections called cilia. These trap microorganisms, dust, and foreign materials. The **lungs** have alveolar macrophages (large phagocytes) that ingest foreign particles, including microorganisms. Healthy lungs are free of microorganisms. The central nervous system is protected by the skull and spinal column, which prevent microbial entry.

Each body orifice also has protective mechanisms. The **oral cavity** regularly sheds mucosal epithelium to rid the mouth of colonizers. The flow of saliva and its partially buffering action help prevent infections. Saliva

Table 23—1 Common Resident Bacteria of the Body

Body Area	Bacteria	Comment
Skin	*Staphylococcus epidermidis*	Normally nonpathogenic
	Propionibacterium acnes	Uses skin fat and oil for growth
	Staphylococcus aureus	Potential pathogen
	Corynebacterium xerosis	Most numerous in axilla
	Pityrosporum oxale (yeast)	Found on scalp and oily skin
Nasal passages	*Staphylococcus aureus*	Potential pathogen
	Staphylococcus epidermidis	
Oropharynx	*Streptococcus pneumoniae*	Potential pathogen
Bronchi, lungs	None	
Mouth	*Streptococcus*	Adhere to tooth enamel
		Component of plague
	Lactobacillus	Involved in tooth decay
	Neisseria	
	Branhamella	
	Bacteroides	Increased with gum disease
	Actinomycetales	May cause deposition of calcium salts in plaque
Stomach	None	
Esophagus	None	
Small intestine	(See large intestine)	Fewer microorganisms than in large intestine
Large intestine	*Bacteroides*	Ferment food residues
	Fusobacterium	
	Eubacterium	
	Lactobacillus	Produce lactic acid
	Streptococcus	Low pathogenicity
	Enterobacteriaceae	Produce bacteriocins
	Vibrio	
	Escherichia coli	
Urethral orifice	*Staphylococcus epidermidis*	
Urethra	None	
Bladder	None	
Ureters	None	
Kidneys	None	
Vagina	*Lactobacillus*	Balance can be upset by antibiotics
	Bacteroides	
	Clostridium	
Nervous system	None	
Blood, lymph system	None	

contains microbial inhibitors, e.g., lactoferrin, lysozyme, and secretory IgA. Lactoferrin is an iron-binding protein that inhibits the growth of invading microorganisms by making iron unavailable to them. The enzyme lysozyme, present in saliva and tears, functions as an antibacterial agent. Secretory IgA (SIGA) is an immunoglobulin that coats bacteria and thus prevents their attachment to the oral epithelium and to the teeth.

The **eye** is protected from infection by tears, which continually wash microorganisms away and contain inhibiting lysozyme. The **gastrointestinal tract** also has defenses against infection. The high acidity of the stomach normally prevents microbial growth. The role that the normal microorganisms of the small intestine play in the body's defense is unknown. However, the resident flora of the large intestine help prevent the establishment of disease-producing microorganisms. Many enterobacteria produce bacteriocins that are lethal to closely related bacterial strains. (A bacteriocin is a substance released by bacteria that kills other bacteria.) Some enterobacteria release an antibiotic-like substance that kills or inhibits the growth of some bacteria.

The **vagina** also has natural defenses against infection. When a girl reaches puberty, lactobacilli ferment sugars in the vaginal secretions, creating a vaginal pH of 3.5–4.5. This low pH inhibits the growth of many disease-producing microorganisms. A reasonably healthy female normally has a relatively constant number of these lactobacilli in the vagina. However, antibiotic therapy can upset the bacterial balance because the lactobacilli are highly susceptible to antibiotics. Colonization by *Candida albicans* (yeast) often results. The **entrance to the urethra** normally harbors many microorganisms, e.g., "negative staph" (*Staphylococcus epidermidis* coagulase from the skin) and *Escherichia coli* (from feces). It is believed that the urine has a flushing and bacteriostatic action that keeps the bacteria from ascending the urethra.

Inflammation

Inflammation is a local and nonspecific defensive response of the tissues to injury or infection. It is an adaptive mechanism that destroys or dilutes the injurious agent, prevents further spread of the injury, and promotes the repair of damaged tissue. It is characterized by five signs:

1. Pain
2. Swelling
3. Redness
4. Heat
5. Impaired function of the part, if the injury is severe

Commonly, words with the suffix -*itis* describe an inflammatory process. For example, *appendicitis* means inflammation of the appendix; *gastritis* means inflammation of the stomach.

Injurious stressors (inflammatory agents) to body tissues can be categorized as physical agents, chemical agents, and microorganisms. Physical agents include mechanical objects causing trauma to tissues, excessive heat or cold (causing burns or frostbite), and radiation. Chemical agents include external irritants (e.g., strong acids, alkalis, poisons, and irritating gases) and internal irritants (substances manufactured within the body such as excessive hydrochloric acid in the stomach due to altered function). Microorganisms include the broad groups of bacteria, viruses, fungi, protozoa, and *Rickettsia.*

The inflammatory response involves a series of dynamic events commonly referred to as the **three stages of the inflammatory response:**

1. Vascular and cellular responses
2. Exudate
3. Reparative

1. At the start of the **first stage,** constriction of the blood vessels occurs at the site of injury, lasting only a few moments. This initial constriction is rapidly followed by dilation of small blood vessels (occurring as a result of histamine released by the injured tissues). Thus, more blood flows to the injured area. This marked increase in blood supply is referred to as **hyperemia** and is responsible for the characteristic signs of redness and heat.

   Vascular permeability is increased at the injured site with the dilation of the vessels in response to tissue necrosis, the release of chemical mediators (e.g., bradykinin, serotonin, and prostoglandin), and the release of histamine. The result of this altered permeability is an outpouring of fluid, proteins, and leukocytes into the interstitial spaces, clinically manifested by the characteristic inflammatory signs of swelling (edema) and pain. The pain is caused by the pressure of accumulating fluid on local nerve endings and the chemical mediators, which are thought to irritate the nerve endings. Too much fluid pouring into areas such as the pleural or pericardial cavity can seriously affect organ function. In other areas, such as joints, mobility is impaired.

   During the first stage of the inflammatory response, blood flow slows in the dilated vessels. This altered rate of flow facilitates the mobilization of the increased number of leukocytes to the injured tissues. Mobilization of leukocytes includes the two processes of margination and emigration. Normally, blood cells (erythrocytes, leukocytes, and platelets) flow along the center of a blood vessel, while a cell-less stream of plasma flows around them against the walls of the blood vessel. When the blood flow slows, leukocytes (white blood cells) aggregate or line up along this inner surface of the blood vessels. This process is known as **margination.** Leukocytes then move through the blood vessel wall into the affected tissue spaces, a process called **emigration.**

   The actual passage of blood corpuscles through the blood vessel wall is referred to as **diapedesis.** Leukocytes are attracted to injured cells by **chemotaxis.** The action of chemotaxis is not fully understood, but basically leukocytes are drawn toward the source of chemicals released in the injured cells (positive chemotaxis), or they are propelled away from released chemicals (negative chemotaxis).

   In a compensatory response to the exit of leukocytes from the blood vessels, the bone marrow produces large numbers of leukocytes and releases them into the bloodstream (**leukocytosis**). The exact mechanism stimulating this increase is unknown, but it is another sign associated with inflammation. A normal leukocyte count of 4500 to 11,000 per cubic millimeter of blood can rise to 20,000 or more when inflammation occurs.

2. In the **second stage** of inflammation, fluid that escaped from the blood vessels, dead phagocytic cells, as well as dead tissue cells and products that they release, produce the **inflammatory exudate.** A plasma protein called fibrinogen (which is converted to fibrin when it is released into the tissues), thromboplastin (a product released by injured tissue cells), and platelets together form an interlacing network to form a barrier, wall off the area, and prevent its spread. During the second stage, the injurious agent is overcome and the exudate is cleared away by lymphatic drainage.

   The nature and amount of exudate vary in accordance with the tissue involved and the intensity and duration of the inflammation. The major types of exudate are serous, purulent, and hemorrhagic (sanguineous). A **serous exudate** is comprised chiefly of serum (the clear portion of the blood) derived from the blood and serous membranes of the body, such as the peritoneum, pleura, pericardium, and meninges. It is watery in appearance and has few cells. An example is the fluid in a blister from a burn.

   A **purulent exudate** is thicker than serous exudate due to the presence of pus. It consists of leukocytes, liquefied dead tissue debris, and dead and living bacteria. The process of pus formation is referred to as **suppuration**, and the bacteria that produce pus are called **pyogenic bacteria**. Not all microorganisms are pyogenic. Purulent exudates vary in color, some acquiring tinges of blue, green, or yellow. The color may depend on the causative organism.

   A **sanguineous (hemorrhagic) exudate** consists of large amounts of red blood cells, indicating damage to capillaries that is severe enough to allow the escape of red blood cells from plasma.

This type of exudate is frequently seen in open wounds. Nurses often need to distinguish whether the sanguineous exudate is dark or bright. A bright sanguineous exudate indicates fresh bleeding, whereas dark sanguineous exudate denotes older bleeding. Mixed types of exudates are often observed. A sero-sanguineous (consisting of clear and blood-tinged drainage) exudate is commonly seen in surgical incisions.

3. The **third stage** of the inflammatory response, also referred to as the **reparative phase,** involves the repair of injured tissues by regeneration or replacement with fibrous tissue (scar) formation. **Regeneration** is the replacement of destroyed tissue cells by cells that are identical or similar in structure and function. It involves not only replacement of damaged cells one by one but also organization of these cells so that the architectural pattern of the tissue and function are restored.

The **stroma** is the tissue that forms the framework (connective tissue) or ground substance of an organ. The **parenchyma** is the essential functional elements of an organ. Functional cells must have proper relationships between stroma and parenchyma, and among their blood vessels, lymph vessels, nerves, and ducts. All must regenerate concurrently. If one component lags behind the others, a normal product will not be formed.

The ability to reproduce cells varies considerably from one type of tissue to another. For example, epithelial tissues of the skin and of the digestive and respiratory tracts have a good regenerative capacity, provided that their underlying support structures are intact. The same holds true for osseous, lymphoid, and bone marrow tissues. Tissues that have little regenerative capacity include nervous, muscular, and elastic tissues.

When regeneration is not possible, repair occurs by **fibrous tissue formation.** Fibrous (scar) tissue has the capacity to proliferate under the unusual conditions of ischemia and altered pH. The inflammatory exudate with its interlacing network of fibrin provides the framework for this tissue to develop.

Damaged tissues are replaced with the connective tissue elements of collagen, blood capillaries, lymphatics, and other tissue ground substances. In the early stages of this process, the tissue is called **granulation tissue.** It is a fragile, gelatinous tissue, appearing pink or red because of the many newly formed capillaries. Later in the process, the tissue shrinks (the capillaries are constricted, even obliterated) and the collagen fibers contract, so that a firmer fibrous tissue remains. This is called a **cicatrix** or scar.

Although scar tissue has the positive attribute of repairing the injured area, it also can present problems. It can reduce the functional capacity of the tissue or organ. For example, scar tissue in cardiac muscle renders that area weaker. Mechanical obstructions can also arise, for example, in the healing of a duodenal ulcer. Sometimes the pyloric sphincter becomes stenosed as granulation tissue contracts into scar tissue.

▪ Specific Defenses

Specific defenses of the body involve the immune system, which responds to foreign protein in the body (e.g., bacteria or transplanted tissues) or, in some cases, even the body's own proteins. Foreign proteins in the body are called **antigens** and are considered invaders. If the proteins originate in a person's own body, the antigen is called an **autoantigen. Immunity** is the specific resistance of the body to infection (pathogens or their toxins). There are two major types of immunity: active and passive. See Table 23–2. Through **active immunity,** the host produces its own antibodies in response to natural (e.g., infection) or artificial (e.g., vaccines) antigens. With **passive immunity,** the host receives natural (e.g., from a nursing mother) or artificial (e.g., from an injection of immune serum) antibodies produced by another source.

The immune response has two components: antibody-mediated defenses and cell-mediated defenses. These two systems provide distinct but overlapping pro-

Table 23–2 Types of Acquired Immunity

Type	Antigen or Antibody Source	Duration
1. Active	Antibodies are produced by the body in response to infection	Long
a. Natural	Antibodies are formed in the presence of active infection in the body	Lifelong
b. Artificial	Antigens (vaccines or toxoids) are administered to the person to stimulate antibody production	Many years; the immunity must be reinforced by booster inoculations
2. Passive	Antibodies are produced by another source, animal or human	Short
a. Natural	Antibodies are transferred naturally from an immune mother to her baby through the placenta or in colostrum	6 months to 1 year
b. Artificial	Immune serum (antibody) from an animal or another human is injected	2 to 3 weeks

tection. The **antibody-mediated defense** is also referred to as **humoral (circulating) immunity,** since it resides ultimately in the B-lymphocytes and is mediated by antibodies produced by B cells. **Antibodies,** also called **immunoglobulins,** are part of the body's plasma proteins. B cells are one type of lymphocyte; they comprise 30% of blood lymphocytes and are short-lived, having a life span of 15 days. The antibody-mediated response defends primarily against the extracellular phases of bacterial and viral infections.

B cells are activated when they recognize a foreign invader, an antigen. They then differentiate into plasma cells, which secrete antibodies, and serum proteins, which bind specifically to the foreign substance and initiate a variety of elimination responses. The B-cell response to an antigen may produce antibody molecules of five classes of immunoglobulins designated by the letters G, A, M, D, and E and usually written as follows: IgG, IgA, IgM, IgD, and IgE. See Table 23–3. The presence of IgM on laboratory analysis shows current infection. Before an antibody response, the phagocytic cells of the blood bind and ingest foreign substances. The rate of binding and phagocytosis increases if IgG antibodies (which indicate past infection and subsequent immunity) are present.

The first interaction between an antigen and antibody is known as the **primary immune response.** The principal characteristics of this response are a latent period before the appearance of an antibody, the production of only a small amount of antibody (chiefly IgM), and, most importantly, the creation of a large number of memory cells capable of responding to the same antigen in the future. The **secondary immune (or booster) response** takes place on subsequent encounters with the same antigen. The principal characteristics of this response are: rapid proliferation of B cells, rapid differentiation of B cells into plasma cells that promptly produce large quantities of antibody (chiefly class IgG), and release of antibody into the blood and other body tissues, where it can react with the antigen.

The **cell-mediated defense** or **cellular immunity** occurs through the T-cell system. T cells (thymic-lymphoid cells) are present in the thymus gland at birth. These cells leave the thymus to circulate in the blood as long-lived lymphocytes with a life span of up to 5 years. Some settle in lymph nodes and the spleen. T cells comprise 70% of circulating blood lymphocytes. The cell-mediated response defends against viral infection, fungal infection, some bacterial infections, and malignant cells. Malignant cells are thought to arise from changes in normal body cells and therefore are regarded as foreign cells. The response is also responsible for graft rejection.

T cells serve as an immune regulator, primarily by activating the B cells. There are three types of T cells: T helper (Th) cells, which enhance the production of antibodies by the B cells (specifically IgG, IgA, and IgE); T suppressor (Ts) cells, which inhibit antibody production by the B cells; and T cytolytic (Tc) cells, cell-destroying cells, some of which are now called killer T cells. The cytolytic cells travel to the invading antigen, where they produce a variety of powerful chemicals or factors called **lymphokines.** The types and functions of some T-cell lymphokines are shown in Table 23–4. When cell-mediated immunity is lost, as occurs with human immunodeficiency virus (HIV), the individual is "defenseless" against most viral, bacterial, and fungal infection.

Table 23–3 ▪ Antibodies and Their Functions

Antibody	Description	Function
IgM	Principally an antibody of the blood; the first antibody produced in response to an antigen	Provides an early immune response Activates the complement system Stimulates ingestion by macrophages Serves as A, B, and O blood groups' isoantibodies and antibodies to serious infections, such as by Gram-negative microorganisms Responds to artificial immunization
IgG	The most prevalent antibody in the blood and a major antibody in tissue spaces; produced later in the immune response than IgM	Triggers complement fixation Activates macrophage ingestion The only antibody to cross the placental barrier Neutralizes microbial toxins and has antiviral and some antibacterial actions
IgA	Resides under the epithelial mucosal cells, especially of the gastrointestinal tract, but also found in tears, saliva, sweat, colostrum, and breast milk; also produced later in the immune response than IgM	Acts as a protective barrier against microorganisms at several points of entrance Easily crosses cell barriers Protects the mucous membranes of the gastrointestinal and the respiratory tracts Because it is a major antibody of milk and colostrum, may function to protect the gastrointestinal tracts of nursing infants
IgD	Normally present in only minute concentrations in the blood	Unknown
IgE	Normally present in only minute concentrations in the blood	Responds primarily to allergic reactions

Chain of Infection

There are six links in the chain of infection: the etiologic agent, or microorganism; the place where the organism naturally resides (reservoir); a portal of exit from the reservoir; a method (mode) of transmission; a portal of entry into a host; and the susceptibility of the host. See Figure 23–1.

Etiologic Agent

A **parasite** is a microorganism that lives in or on another and obtains its nourishment from it. All viruses are parasites. The extent to which any microorganism or parasite is capable of producing an infectious process depends on the number of organisms present, the virulence and potency of the organisms (pathogenicity), the ability of the organisms to enter the body, the susceptibility of the host, and the ability of the organisms to live in the host's body.

Some microorganisms, such as the smallpox virus, have the ability to infect almost all susceptible people after exposure. By contrast, microorganisms such as the tuberculosis bacillus infect a relatively small number of the population who are susceptible and exposed, usually people who are poorly nourished and living in unsanitary conditions. Some animals and humans are **carriers**, i.e., they carry disease-producing organisms in their bodies although they are not ill themselves. Carriers can pass the microorganisms along to other people. For example, some persons harbor the typhoid bacillus in the gallbladder, excrete it in feces, but manifest no symptoms of the disease.

Reservoir

There are many reservoirs or sources of microorganisms. Common sources are other humans, the

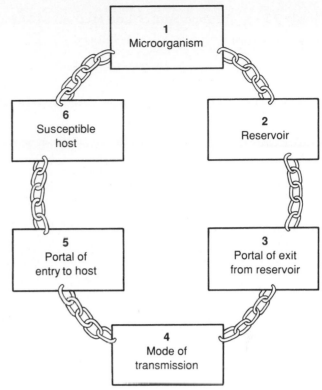

Figure 23–1   The chain of infection

client's own microorganisms, plants, animals, or the general environment. See Table 23–5. People are the most common source of infection for others and for themselves. The person with, for example, an influenza virus frequently spreads it to others. When resistance is lowered by fatigue and other factors, an infection emerges.

Insects, birds, and other animals are common reservoirs of infection. The *Anopheles* mosquito carries the malaria parasite. Food, water, milk, and feces also can be reservoirs. An example is contaminated chicken at a club luncheon. The reservoir must have certain characteristics for the organisms to live and grow. Among these characteristics are: food, water, oxygen (or, for some organisms, absence of oxygen), optimal temperature and pH, and minimal light.

Portal of Exit

Before an infection can establish itself in a host, the microorganisms must leave the reservoir. If the reservoir is within a human, the microorganisms have a number of exits, depending on the site of the reservoir. Common human reservoirs and their associated portals of exit are summarized in Table 23–6.

Method of Transmission

Microorganisms are transmitted by a number of routes, and the same microorganisms can be transmitted by more than one route. There are four main routes

Table 23–4   Types and Functions of Some T-Cell Lymphokines

Lymphokine	Functions
Chemotactic factor (CF)	Attracts macrophages and monocytes to the antigen site
Migration inhibition factor (MIF)	Prevents departure of macrophages from the site
Macrophage activation or aggregation factor (MAF)	Increases phagocytosis of macrophages and agglutinates (clumps) them
Lymphotoxin factor (LT)	Acts as a cytotoxin and directly destroys microorganisms
Transfer factor	Causes nonsensitized lymphocytes at the site to act as a sensitized cell
Interferon (also produced by cells other than lymphocytes)	Blocks viral infection of tissue cells

Table 23–5 Human Source and Method of Transmission of Common Microorganisms

Body Area (Source)	Transport Vehicle	Common Infectious Organisms
Respiratory tract	Droplets expelled while sneezing and coughing	Parainfluenza virus *Klebsiella* species *Staphylococcus aureus*
Gastrointestinal tract	Emesis, feces, drainage (such as from the gallbladder), saliva	Viral hepatitis A *Shigella* species *Salmonella enteritidis*
Urinary tract	Urine	*Escherichia coli* enterococci *Pseudomonas aeruginosa*
Reproductive tract (including genitals)	Urine and semen	*Neisseria gonorrhoeae* *Treponema pallidum* Herpes simplex virus type 2 Viral hepatitis B
Blood	Blood sample, needle used for venipuncture	*Escherichia coli* *Staphylococcus aureus* *Klebsiella* species *Staphylococcus epidermidis*
Tissue	Drainage from a cut or wound	*Staphylococcus aureus* *Escherichia coli* enterococci *Proteus* species

of transmission: contact, vehicle, airborne, and vector-borne. **Contact transmission** is the most important and frequent means of transmission of microorganism (Williams 1983, p. 341). There are three types of contact transmission: direct contact (physical transfer between an infected person and a susceptible host), indirect contact (contact with a contaminated object, e.g., the soiled hands of health care personnel), and droplet contact (close contact with contaminated secretions from an infected person). Most respiratory infections are transmitted by droplet contact.

Vehicle transmission is accomplished through a transporting agent or medium such as food, water, or blood. **Airborne transmission** occurs by dissemination of droplet nuclei or dust particles that contain microorganisms and remain in the air. The microorganisms are then inhaled by a susceptible host. Tuberculosis and varicella are two diseases transported by the airborne route. A **vector** is an animal that transfers microorganisms from a reservoir to a host. Insects and other animals can spread such organisms as certain *Salmonella* species, which are part of the normal flora of some domestic animals but cause gastroenteritis in humans.

Portal of Entry

Before a person can become infected, microorganisms must enter the body. The skin is a barrier to infectious agents; however, any break in the skin can readily serve as a portal of entry. Microorganisms can enter the body through the same routes they use to leave the body. Often, microorganisms enter the body by the same route they used to leave the source.

Susceptible Host

A **susceptible host** is any person who is at risk for infection. **Compromised** hosts are persons "at increased

risk," individuals who for one or more reasons are more likely than others to acquire an infection. Impairment of the body's natural defenses and a number of other factors can affect susceptibility to infection. See "Factors Affecting Risk of Infection," later in this chapter.

Breaking the Chain of Infection

Various practices break the chain of infection or interrupt the infectious disease process. For example, the first link in the chain, the etiologic agent, is interrupted by the use of antiseptics and disinfectants and by sterilization. Nurses carry out practices that break other links in the chain. See Table 23–7. The aim of most hospital precautions is breaking the chain during the mode of transmission phase of the cycle.

Table 23–6 Human Reservoirs and Portals of Exit

Reservoir	Portals of Exit
Respiratory tract	Nose/mouth through sneezing, coughing, breathing, or talking; endotracheal tubes or tracheostomies
Gastrointestinal tract	Mouth: through saliva, vomitus; anus/ostomies: feces; drainage tubes: e.g., nasogastric or T-tubes
Urinary tract	Urethral meatus and urinary diversion ostomies
Reproductive tract	Vagina: vaginal discharge; may be further transported by urine; urinary meatus: semen, urine
Blood	Open wound, needle puncture site, any disruption of intact skin or mucous membrane surfaces

Table 23-7 Nursing Interventions for Infection Control

Link	Interventions	Rationale
Etiologic agent	Ensure articles are properly cleaned and disinfected or sterilized before use.	Proper cleaning, disinfecting, and sterilizing reduce or eliminate microorganisms.
	Educate clients and family members about appropriate methods to clean, disinfect, and sterilize articles.	Knowledge of ways to reduce or eliminate microorganisms reduces the numbers of microorganisms present and the likelihood of disease.
Reservoir	Change dressings and bandages when they are soiled or wet.	Moist dressings are ideal environments for microorganisms to grow and multiply.
	Assist clients to carry out appropriate skin and oral hygiene.	Hygienic measures reduce the numbers of resident and transient microorganisms and the likelihood of infection.
	Dispose of damp, soiled linens appropriately.	Damp, soiled linens harbor more microorganisms than dry linens.
	Dispose of feces and urine appropriately.	Urine and feces, in particular, contain many microorganisms. Feces may also be the source of certain virulent microorganisms, such as the hepatitis A virus in asymptomatic carriers.
	Ensure that all fluid containers, such as bedside water jugs and suction and drainage bottles, are covered or capped. Discard unused portions, IV and irrigation solutions after 24 hrs.	Prolonged exposure increases the risk of contamination and promotes microbial growth.
	Empty suction and drainage bottles at the end of each shift.	Drainage harbors microorganisms that, if left for prolonged periods, proliferate.
Portal of exit	Avoid talking, coughing, or sneezing over open wounds or sterile fields and cover the mouth and nose when coughing and sneezing. Teach clients to cover their mouths when coughing.	These measures limit the number of microorganisms that escape from the respiratory tract.
Mode of transmission	Wash hands between client contacts, after touching body substances, and before performing invasive procedures or touching open wounds. Instruct clients and family members to wash hands before handling food or eating, before and after eliminating, and after touching body substances.	Hand washing is the most effective means of controlling and preventing the spread of microorganisms.
	Place discarded soiled materials in moisture-proof refuse bags.	Moisture-proof bags contain the spread of microorganisms to others.
	Handle bedpans with caution.	Urine and feces in particular contain many microorganisms.
	Initiate and implement isolation precautions when appropriate.	Controlling the mode of transmission of specific microorganisms prevents their spread.
	Wear masks when in close contact with clients who have infections transmitted by droplets from the respiratory tract.	Masks prevent the transmission of airborne microorganisms.
	Wear gloves when handling all body substances. Wear gowns if there is danger of soiling clothing.	Gloves and gowns prevent soiling of the hands and clothing.
Portal of entry	Use sterile technique for invasive procedures such as injections and catheterizations.	Invasive procedures penetrate the body's natural protective barriers to microorganisms.
	Use sterile technique when exposing open wounds or handling dressings.	Open wounds are vulnerable to microbial infection.
	Handle needles and syringes with caution.	Injuries from needles contaminated by blood or body fluids from an infected client or carrier provide a portal of entry into the health care worker.
	Provide each client with his or her own personal care items.	People have less resistance to another person's microorganisms than to their own.
Susceptible host	Maintain the integrity of the client's skin and mucous membranes.	Intact skin and mucous membranes protect against invasion by microorganisms.
	Ensure that the client receives a balanced diet.	A balanced diet supplies essential proteins and vitamins necessary to build or maintain body tissues.
	Educate the public about the importance of immunizations.	Immunizations protect people against virulent infectious diseases.

Factors Affecting Risk of Infection

Whether a microorganism causes an infection depends on a number of factors already mentioned. One of the most important factors is host susceptibility, which is affected by age, heredity, level of stress, nutritional status, immunization status, current medical therapy, and preexisting disease processes.

Age is a factor influencing the risk of infection. Newborns and elderly people have reduced defenses against infection. Infections are a major cause of death of newborns, who have immature immune systems and are protected only for the first 2 or 3 months by immunoglobulins passively received from the mother. Between 1 to 3 months of age, infants begin to synthesize their own immunoglobulins; about 40% of adult levels are reached by 1 year of age (Whaley and Wong 1983, p. 421). Immunizations against diphtheria, tetanus, and pertussis are usually started at 2 months, when the infant's immune system can respond.

With advancing age, the immune responses again become weak. The immune response (cell-mediated immunity) is reduced. Lymphocytes become more diverse with age, and there is a progressive loss of cellular regulation in the body. Although there is still much to learn about aging, it is known that immunity to infection decreases with advancing age. Because of the prevalence of influenza and its potential for causing death, the CDC recommends immunization against influenza for the elderly and for persons with chronic cardiac, respiratory, metabolic, and renal disease. Pneumococcal vaccine is also recommended. Immunization is usually provided in early October or November; annual boosters are required to maintain immunity.

Heredity is a factor influencing the development of infection in that some people have a genetic susceptibility to certain infections. For example, some people may be deficient in serum immunoglobulins, which play a significant role in the internal defense mechanism of the body. The nature, number, and duration of physical and emotional **stressors** can influence susceptibility to infection. Stressors elevate blood cortisone. Prolonged elevation of blood cortisone decreases antiinflammatory responses, depletes energy stores, leads to a state of exhaustion, and decreases resistance to infection. For example, a person recovering from a major operation or injury is more likely to develop an infection than a healthy person.

Resistance to infection depends on adequate **nutritional status.** Because antibodies are proteins, the ability of the body to synthesize antibodies may be impaired by inadequate nutrition, especially when protein reserves are depleted (e.g., as a result of injury, surgery, or debilitating diseases such as cancer). Some **medical therapies** predispose a person to infection. For example, radiation treatments for cancer destroy not only cancerous cells but also some normal cells, thereby rendering them more vulnerable to infection.

Certain **medications** also increase susceptibility to infection. Antineoplastic (anticancer) medications may depress bone marrow function, resulting in inadequate production of white blood cells and lymphocytes necessary to combat infections. Antiinflammatory medications, such as adrenal corticosteroids, inhibit the inflammatory response, an essential defense against infection. Even some antibiotics used to treat infections can have adverse effects. Antibiotics may kill resident flora, allowing the proliferation of strains that would not grow and multiply in the body under normal conditions. Certain antibiotics can also induce resistance in some strain of organisms. Some diagnostic procedures may also predispose the client to an infection, especially when the skin is broken or sterile body cavities are penetrated during the procedure.

Any **disease** that lessens the body's defenses against infection places the client at risk. Examples are chronic pulmonary disease, which impairs ciliary action and weakens the mucous barrier; peripheral vascular disease, which inhibits blood flow; burns, which impair skin integrity; chronic or debilitating diseases, which deplete protein reserves; and such immune system diseases as leukemia and aplastic anemia, which alter the production rate of white blood cells. Diabetes mellitus is a major underlying disease predisposing clients to infection, since compromised peripheral vascular status and increased serum glucose levels increase susceptibility.

Stages of an Infectious Process

The course of an infection has four stages: the incubation period, the prodromal period, the illness period, and the convalescent period.

Incubation Period

The **incubation period** is the time between the entry of the microorganisms into the body and the onset of the symptoms. During this time, the organism adapts to the person and multiplies sufficiently to produce an infection. The length of incubation varies greatly, depending on the microorganism. For example, rubella (measles) develops in 10 to 14 days, whereas tetanus (lockjaw) takes from 4 to 21 days to develop. An average incubation period is 7 to 10 days. In many viral diseases (e.g., chickenpox and measles), persons can transmit infection during the incubation period. A person with hepatitis A is most infectious *before* the onset of any symptoms.

Prodromal Period

The **prodromal period** is the time from the onset of nonspecific symptoms, e.g., fatigue, malaise, elevated temperature, and irritability, until the specific symptoms of the infection appear. Infected persons are most infectious and most likely to spread the infecting organisms during this stage. Because the symptoms are general, precautions to prevent spread are often not taken at this time. A prodromal stage usually lasts a short time, hours or days at the most.

Illness Period

During the **illness period,** specific symptoms develop and become evident. The symptoms of most infectious processes are manifested both in the affected body organ or area (the local inflammatory response or **localized symptoms**) and in the entire body (**systemic symptoms**). During this period, the person often has fever and headache and feels fatigued. Sometimes a skin rash (**exanthema**) or a rash of the mucous membrane (**enanthema**) appears at this stage. The severity of the symptoms and the length of the illness vary with the susceptibility of the person to the etiologic agent.

Convalescent Period

The **convalescent period** extends from the time the symptoms start to abate until the person returns to a normal state of health. Depending on the severity of the illness and the person's general health, convalescence can last from a few days to months. Often it is longer than the person expects.

Nosocomial Infections

Nosocomial infections are infections that were not present or were incubating at the time of admission to a hospital or other medical facility. They include infections clients acquire during their stay in a facility or manifest after discharge. Nosocomial infections may also be acquired by health personnel working in the facility. These infections have received increasing attention in recent years. They are considered more difficult to prevent and treat, more unpredictable, and more resistant to cure than infections contracted in the community (Norton 1986, p. 774). U.S. surveys reveal that nosocomial infections occur in about 5% of all persons admitted to acute care hospitals and in about 8% of persons in long-term care facilities (Norton 1986, p. 774). Clients undergoing surgical procedures have a higher incidence of nosocomial infections than others. One survey indicated that about 70% of all nosocomial infections in a hospital developed in postoperative clients (Simmons 1983, p. 133).

The source of microorganisms that cause nosocomial infections can be the clients themselves (an endogenous source) or the hospital environment and hospital personnel (exogenous sources). Most infections appear to have endogenous sources (Simmons 1983, p. 134). The National Nosocomial Infections study, conducted between 1979 and 1983, found that *Escherichia coli* was the most common infecting organism, followed by *Staphylococcus aureus* and enterococci (Pickering and DuPont 1986, p. 28).

A number of factors contribute to nosocomial infections. **Iatrogenic** (meaning illness due to any aspect of medical therapy) infections are as a direct result of a diagnostic or therapeutic procedure. An example of an iatrogenic infection is bacteremia that results from an intravascular line. Not all nosocomial infections (e.g., the development of a respiratory infection in an immobilized elderly female) are iatrogenic.

Another factor contributing to the development of nosocomial infections is the presence of compromised hosts, i.e., clients whose normal defenses have been lowered by surgery or illness. **Insufficient hand washing** by personnel is perhaps the greatest factor contributing to the spread of nosocomial infections. Personnel can acquire microorganisms from infected clients and pass them on to other clients. The hands of personnel are a common vehicle for the spread of microorganisms. The cost of nosocomial infections to the client, the facility, and funding bodies (e.g., insurance companies and federal, state, or local governments) is very great. Nosocomial infections extend hospitalization time, increase clients' time away from work, cause disability and discomfort, and even result in loss of life.

Assessing Clients at Risk for Infections

The nurse assesses the degree to which a client is at risk of acquiring an infection and the presence of clinical signs of an existing infectious process. To identify clients at risk, the nurse should review the client's chart and structure the nursing interview to collect data regarding the factors influencing the development of infection, especially: existing disease process, history of recurrent infections, current medications and therapeutic measures, current emotional stressors, nutritional status, and history of immunizations.

Physical Health Data

During the physical examination, the nurse inspects the client for local and systemic signs of infection. Signs of a local infection are caused by the inflammatory response and include: swelling, redness, pain or tenderness upon palpation or movement, palpable heat at the infected area, and loss of function of the body part affected, depending on the site and extent of involvement. Signs of a systemic infection include: fever; increased pulse and respiratory rate, if the fever is high; lassitude, malaise, and loss of energy; anorexia and, in some situations, nausea and vomiting; headache; and enlargement and tenderness of lymph nodes that drain the area of infection.

Laboratory Data

Laboratory data that indicate the presence of an infection include:

1. Elevated leukocyte (white blood) cell (WBC) count (4500 to 11,000/cu mm is normal).
2. Increases in specific types of leukocytes as revealed in the differential white blood cell count. Specific types of white blood cells are increased or decreased in certain infections. Normal values are cited for the adult.

   - Neutrophils are increased in acute suppurative infections but may be decreased in acute bacterial infection, especially in older people. Normal range is 54 to 75%.
   - Lymphocytes are increased in chronic bacterial and viral infections. Normal is 25 to 40%.
   - Monocytes are increased in some protozoal and rickettsial infections and in tuberculosis. Normal is 2 to 8%.
   - Eosinophils are generally unaltered in an infectious process. Normal is 1 to 4%.
   - Basophils are generally unaltered in an infectious process. Normal is 0 to 1% (Byrne et al. 1986, p. 78).

3. Elevated **erythrocyte sedimentation rate (ESR)**, commonly referred to as sedimentation rate. The ESR is a measure of the speed with which red blood cells in anticoagulated whole blood settle to the bottom of a calibrated tube. Sedimentation normally takes place slowly, but the rate increases in the presence of an inflammatory process.
4. Urine, blood, sputum, or other drainage cultures that indicate the presence of pathogenic microorganisms.

Nursing Diagnoses for Clients at Risk for Infection

Nursing diagnoses for clients with an infection or at risk for acquiring infection may include potential for infection, potential social isolation, potential diversional activity deficit, and disturbance in self-concept. Any condition in which an individual is at increased risk for being invaded by pathogenic organisms can be identified as the nursing diagnosis "potential for infection." According to NANDA, the presence of one or more of the following risk factors is a defining characteristic of this diagnosis:

1. Inadequate primary defenses, such as broken skin, traumatized tissue, decrease of cilary action, stasis of body fluids, change in pH of secretions, and/or altered peristalsis
2. Inadequate secondary defenses, such as decreased hemoglobin, leukopenia, suppressed inflammatory response, immunosuppression or inadequate acquired immunity, tissue destruction and increased environmental exposure, chronic disease, invasive

procedures, malnutrition, pharmaceutical agents, trauma, rupture of amniotic membranes, and/or insufficient knowledge to avoid exposure to pathogens.

Examples of nursing diagnoses are shown in the accompanying box.

Planning Care for Susceptible Clients

After deriving pertinent causative factors from the data base, nurses plan specific strategies to prevent or treat infection. Overall nursing responsibilities for clients at risk of acquiring an infection or for those with infections include the following:

1. Preventing the spread of an infection
2. Maintaining or restoring the client's body defenses
3. Reducing or alleviating problems associated with the infection

Preventing Infection

Planned nursing strategies to prevent the spread of an infection include use of meticulous medical and surgical asepsis. **Asepsis** is the freedom from infection or infectious material. Hands washed with soap and water or an antiseptic can be considered aseptic; i.e., free from infectious organisms. However, some microorganisms in all probability are still present on washed hands. There are two basic types of asepsis: medical and surgical. **Medical asepsis** includes all practices intended to confine a specific microorganism to a specific area, limiting the number, growth, and spread of microorganisms.

NURSING DIAGNOSIS

Infection

- Potential for infection related to knowledge deficit about required immunization
- Potential for infection related to impaired skin integrity
- Potential for infection related to change in pH of vaginal secretions
- Potential for infection related to decreased ciliary action
- Potential for infection related to suppressed inflammatory response secondary to cortisone therapy
- Potential for infection related to immunosuppression secondary to chemotherapy
- Social isolation related to misinformation by others about transmission of acquired immune deficiency syndrome
- Potential disturbance in self-concept related to acquisition of sexually transmitted disease

In medical asepsis, objects are often referred to as clean or dirty. **Clean** denotes the presence of some microorganisms but the absence of potentially infectious agents. **Dirty** (soiled) denotes the likely presence of disease-producing microorganisms. Aseptic measures are protective as they are designed to reduce the number of potentially infectious agents.

Surgical asepsis, or sterile technique, refers to those practices that keep an area or objects free of all microorganisms; it includes practices that destroy all microorganisms and spores. (A **spore** is a round or oval structure enclosed in a tough capsule. Some microorganisms assume this structure in response to adverse conditions; in this form, they are highly resistant to destruction.) Surgical asepsis is required for invasive procedures, such as injections, intravenous therapy, or urinary catheterization. Initiation of appropriate barrier precautions and client education about immunization, hygiene, sanitation, nutrition, and appropriate food handling practices are other examples of planned nursing strategies to prevent infection.

Supporting Body Defenses

Nursing plans to maintain or restore the client's body defenses include providing adequate fluids and nutrition, promoting rest, and administering and monitoring prescribed antimicrobial therapy. The immunologic system is the body's major defense against infections. The body gradually builds up natural defenses against pathogens with which it comes in contact; **immunizations** give additional protection. A balanced diet enhances the health of all body tissues. Adequate **nutrition** enables tissues to maintain and rebuild themselves and helps keep the reticuloendothelial system functioning well. Adequate **rest and sleep** are essential to health and to one's ability to perform usual activities. See Chapter 37 for additional information. *Stress* predisposes a person to infection. A balance, for example, between work and recreation is important. See the section on psychologic homeostasis in Chapter 16.

Alleviating Associated Problems

Because malaise, fever, pain, and dehydration are often associated with an infection, plans need to incorporate interventions that promote comfort and reduce or prevent these problems. Examples of short-term goals for clients with problems associated with infection are:

▪ The client will maintain healthy skin.

▪ The client's impaired skin areas will heal.

▪ The client will remain free of infection in impaired skin areas.

Specific measures for clients at risk of impaired skin integrity are discussed in Chapter 35. In addition, regular and thorough hygienic practices by or for the client remove transient microorganisms, thereby reducing the likelihood of infection. Hygiene is discussed in Chapter 34.

Implementing Nursing Strategies

Nursing Actions to Prevent Infections

Among the interventions to prevent and/or promptly identify potential infections are:

▪ Wash hands before and after any direct client contact, before any invasive procedure (e.g., urinary catheterization), and after contact with any body substance (e.g., feces, urine, and wound drainage).

▪ Employ practices to reduce the number of organisms in the environment, e.g., change moist dressings frequently. (Drainage on dressings often has a heavy concentration of microorganisms.)

▪ Place soiled materials (e.g., tissues, needles, and dressings) in moisture-resistant containers for appropriate disposal.

▪ Handle needles and syringes carefully to avoid needle-prick injuries. **Do not recap** needles. Many facilities now provide disposal units in all client rooms.

▪ Use surgical asepsis when inserting any intravenous needle or catheter; change intravenous tubing and solution containers according to hospital policy (e.g., every 24–72 hours); and check intravenous solutions for expiration date and clarity.

▪ Inspect skin surfaces every shift or more frequently to check for skin lesions, ulcers, pressure areas, presence of peripheral edema and/or bulging leg veins, and changes in temperature or color of any extremity.

▪ Dry the skin thoroughly after bathing the client and applying lotion to roughened or especially dry areas.

▪ Use pressure-relieving devices and turning clients with impaired physical mobility every two hours to maintain adequate circulation to all pressure points.

▪ Apply prescribed measures to decubitus ulcers (e.g., Maalox, heat lamp, Op Site) according to the physician's order and/or hospital procedure.

▪ Use surgical asepsis when changing dressings.

▪ Monitor for significant changes in vital signs that might indicate the presence of infection (e.g., systemic inflammatory signs: elevated temperature, pulse, and/or respirations; decreased blood pressure).

▪ Place clients at risk for infection in private rooms if possible; at least, move them away from clients with known infection.

▪ Ask the client to move, cough, and breathe deeply at least every 2 hours and use aseptic technique when suctioning clients.

▪ Report the amount and character of secretions expectorated or suctioned and monitor laboratory studies for sputum culture results.

- Provide a fluid intake of 2000–3000 ml/day, unless contraindicated; assist the client to obtain an optimal nutritional intake.

- Prevent urinary infections by using surgical asepsis when inserting the catheter; maintain a closed urinary drainage system with a downhill flow of urine; do not irrigate a catheter unless ordered to do so; provide regular catheter care, cleansing the perineal area with soap and water; and keep the drainage bag and spout off the floor.

- Measure urinary output and observe the characteristics of the urine; obtain specimens by aspiration and monitor lab results; and report to the physician any of the following: client complaints of itching or burning on urination, diminished urinary output or increased specific gravity, urinary frequency, or cloudy, foul-smelling urine.

Nursing Actions for Clients with Infections

Nursing interventions for clients with infections include:

- Assist the physician in aspirating body fluids or tissues, such as spinal or pleural fluid, bone marrow, or liver tissues.

- Obtain blood specimens for differential white blood cell counts or serum immunoglobulins as ordered.

- Perform intradermal skin tests for diagnostic reactions as directed by the physician.

- Initiate and maintain barrier precautions specific to the infecting organism and its mode of transmission.

- Administer prescribed antimicrobial medications and monitor for effectiveness.

- Administer specific immune therapies ordered by the physician, e.g., vaccines, antitoxins or toxoids, and immune antiserums.

- Implement nursing strategies for clients with elevated temperature (see Chapter 31).

- Provide a humidifier to moisten and loosen respiratory secretions and soothe respiratory membranes for clients with coughs and administer expectorants or cough suppressants as prescribed.

- Limit the client's physical activity.

- Immobilize painful body parts, provide relaxation and comfort measures, and administer prescribed analgesics.

- Minimize fluid loss through excessive perspiration, diarrhea, or vomiting by offering fluids; and monitor the client's urinary output in comparison to intake.

- Measure and record the client's vital signs regularly.

- Assess breath sounds if the client has a respiratory infection.

- Obtain specimens for periodic sputum, wound drainage, blood, urine, or fecal cultures to determine the effectiveness of antimicrobial and other therapies.

- Teach the client and family members about the infectious organism, its mode of transmission, and ways to control and prevent its spread. Client education should stress the need for meticulous hand washing after contact with body substances, keeping hands away from drainage areas, and disposing of infectious materials properly. Some clients may need to learn how to take body temperature to monitor a fever; others, how to apply hot or cold compresses to localized infections.

Hand Washing

Hand washing is important in every setting where people are ill, including hospitals. It is considered one of the most effective infection control measures. The goal of hand washing is to remove transient microorganisms that might be transmitted to clients, visitors, or other health care personnel.

Any client may harbor microorganisms that are currently harmless to the client yet potentially harmful to another person or to the same client if they find a portal of entry. It is important that hands be washed at the following times to prevent the spread of these microorganisms: before eating, after using the bedpan or toilet, and after the hands have come in contact with any body substances, such as sputum or drainage from a wound. In addition, health care workers should wash their hands before and after any direct client contact.

For routine client care, the CDC recommends a vigorous hand washing under a stream of water for at least 10 seconds using bar soap, granule soap, soap-filled tissues, or antimicrobial liquid soap (Garner and Favero 1985, p. 7). The CDC recommends antimicrobial hand-washing agents (with any chemical germicides listed with the Environmental Protection Agency):

1. When there are known multiple resistant bacteria
2. Before invasive procedures
3. In special care units such as nurseries and ICUs

This book recommends that the hands be held down (below the elbows) when washing off infectious materials and during routine hand washing so that the microorganisms are washed directly into the sink. For surgical asepsis, the hands should be held above the elbows so that the water runs from the cleanest to least clean area. Procedure 23–1 provides instructions for handwashing.

Isolation Precautions

Isolation practices are indicated when a client has an infection that can be transmitted to others. In 1983, the CDC published recommendations regarding isolation practices in hospitals. Seven categories for isolation were described: strict isolation, contact isolation, respiratory isolation, tuberculosis isolation, enteric precautions, drainage/secretion precautions, and blood/body

PROCEDURE 23-1

Hand Washing

Equipment

- Soap. Liquid soaps are frequently supplied in dispensers at the sink. Antimicrobial soaps are usually provided in high risk areas, eg, newborn nursery.
- Warm running water.
- Towels. Nurses usually dry their hands with paper towels; they discard the towels in the appropriate container immediately after use.

Intervention

1. File the nails short.
   Rationale: Short nails are less likely to harbor microorganisms or scratch a client. Long nails are hard to clean.

2. Remove jewelry, except a plain wedding ring or band, from the hands and arms. Some nurses slide their watches up above their elbows. Others pin the watch to the uniform.
   Rationale: Microorganisms can lodge in the settings of jewelry. Removal facilitates proper cleaning of the hands and arms.

3. Check hands for breaks in the skin, such as hangnails or cuts. Report cuts to the instructor or nurse in charge before beginning work, or check agency policy about cuts. Use lotions to prevent hangnails and cracked, dry skin. A nurse who has open sores may have to change work assignments or wear gloves to avoid contact with infectious material.

4. Turn on the water and adjust the flow so that the water is warm.
   Rationale: Warm water removes less of the protective oil of the skin than hot water.
   There are four common types of faucet controls:
   a. Hand-operated handles.
   b. Knee levers. Move these with the knee to regulate flow and temperature. See Figure 23-2.
   c. Foot pedals. Press these with the foot to regulate flow and temperature. See Figure 23-3.
   d. Elbow controls. Move these with the elbows instead of the hands. This type of handle is most frequently used for surgical asepsis.

5. Wet the hands thoroughly by holding them under the running water. Hold the hands lower than the elbows so that the water flows from the arms to the fingertips.
   Rationale: The water should flow from the least contaminated to the most contaminated area, and the hands are more contaminated than the lower arms.

6. Apply soap to the hands. If the soap is liquid, apply 2-4 mL (1 tsp). If it is bar soap, rub it firmly between

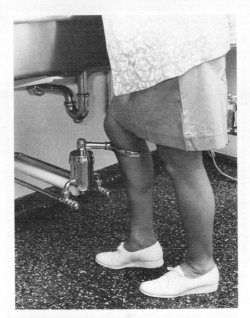

Figure 23-2

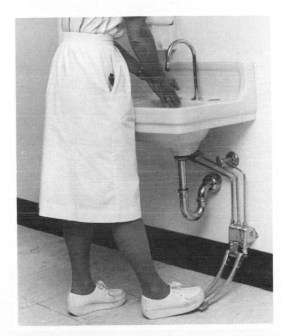

Figure 23-3

the hands, and rinse the bar before returning it to the dish.
Rationale: Rinsing the bar removes microorganisms.

7. Use firm, rubbing, circular movements to wash the palm, back, and wrist of each hand. Interlace the fingers and thumbs, and move the hands back and forth. See Figure 23-4. Continue this motion for 10-15 seconds.

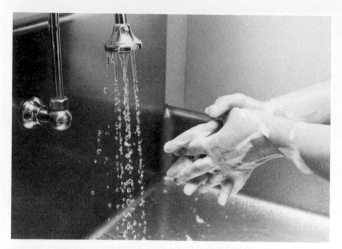

Figure 23–4

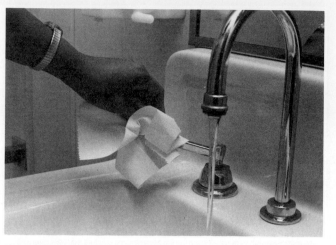

Figure 23–5

Rationale: The circular action helps remove microorganisms. Interlacing the fingers and thumbs cleans the interdigital spaces.

8. Rinse the hands.

9. Most handwashing is for a minimum of 15 seconds. For a more thorough hand washing, extend the time for steps 5 through 8.

10. Dry the hands and arms thoroughly with the paper towel. Discard it in the appropriate container.
   Rationale: Moist skin becomes chapped readily; chapping produces lesions.

11. Turn off the water. Use paper towels to grasp a hand-operated control. See Figure 23–5.
   Rationale: This prevents picking up microorganisms from the faucet handles.

fluid precautions (see Table 23–8). In 1987, the CDC also presented recommendations for universal precautions on all clients to decrease the risk of transmitting unidentified pathogens. The CDC guidelines for universal precautions are shown in the accompanying box.

▪ **Associated Psychologic Problems.** Clients requiring isolation precautions can develop several problems as a result of the separation from others and of the special precautions taken in their care. Two of the most common are sensory deprivation and decreased self-esteem related to feelings of inferiority. **Sensory deprivation** occurs when the environment lacks normal stimuli for the client, e.g., frequent communications with others. The client is usually in a private room and thus has no contact with other clients. Because support persons may need to put on gowns before entering the room, they may not visit as often as usual. Visits by other clients are usually discouraged. Nurses should therefore be alert to common clinical signs of sensory deprivation: boredom, inactivity, slowness of thought, daydreaming, increased sleeping, thought disorganization, anxiety, panic, and hallucinations.

Chapter 14 provides information on the development of self-esteem and self-esteem disturbances. A client's **feeling of inferiority** can be due to the perception of the infection itself or to the required precautions. In North America, many people place a high value on cleanliness, and the idea of being "soiled," "contaminated," or "dirty" can give clients the feeling that they are at fault and substandard. While this is obviously not true, the infected persons may feel "not as good" as others and blame themselves.

Nurses need to provide care that prevents these two

problems and/or deals with them positively. Nursing interventions include:

1. Assess the individual's need for stimulation.
2. Initiate measures to help meet the need, including regular communication with the client and diversionary activities, e.g., toys for a child and books, television, or radio for an adult; provide a variety of foods to stimulate the client's sense of taste; stimulate the client's visual sense by providing a view or an activity to watch.
3. Explain the infection and the associated procedures to help clients and their support persons understand and accept the situation.

GUIDELINES

Universal Precautions (CDC)

▪ Wash hands often.

▪ Wear gloves when hands will be in contact with body substances.

▪ Remove gloves and wash hands after providing care to the client.

▪ Protect clothing with a plastic apron when it is likely that clothing will be soiled with a body substance.

▪ Wear masks and/or plastic goggles when it is likely that mucous membranes and/or eyes will be splashed with body substances (e.g., when suctioning a client with copious secretions).

▪ Discard uncapped needle/syringe units and "sharps" in puncture-resistant containers for this purpose.

PROCEDURE 23–1: VARIATION

Hand Washing Before Sterile Techniques

Hold the hands higher than the elbows during this hand wash. Wet the hands and forearms under the running water, letting it run from the fingertips to the elbows so that the hands become cleaner than the elbows. See Figure 23–6. In this way the water runs from the area with the fewest microorganisms to areas with a relatively greater number. Apply the soap and wash as described earlier in steps 5 through 8, maintaining the hands uppermost. After washing and rinsing, use a towel to dry one hand thoroughly in a rotating motion from the fingers to the elbow. Use a clean towel to dry the other hand and arm. A clean towel prevents the transfer of microorganisms from one elbow (least clean area) to the other hand (cleanest area).

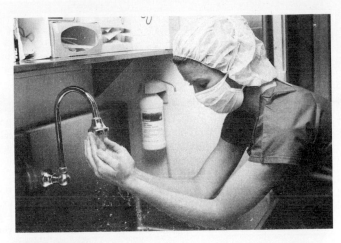

Figure 23–6

4. Demonstrate warm, accepting behavior. Avoid conveying to the client any sense of annoyance about the precautions or any feelings of revulsion about the infection.

■ **Donning and Removing Face Masks.** Masks are worn to prevent the spread of organisms by the droplet contact and airborne routes. The CDC recommends that masks be worn (Garner and Simmons 1983, p. 254):

1. Only by those close to the client if the infection (e.g., acute respiratory diseases in children, measles, or mumps) is transmitted by large-particle aerosols (droplets). Large-particle aerosols are transmitted by close contact and generally travel short distances (about 1 m, or 3 ft).
2. By all persons entering the room if the infection (e.g., diphtheria) is transmitted by small-particle aerosols (droplet nuclei). Small-particle aerosols remain suspended in the air and thus travel greater distances by air.

Masks are worn by all persons entering the rooms of clients who require strict isolation. They are also worn during certain techniques requiring surgical asepsis. During a procedure requiring sterile technique, masks are worn to prevent the airborne or droplet contact transmission of exhaled microorganisms to the sterile field or to a client's open wound. Nurses should wear masks when they are in close contact with clients who require contact isolation, respiratory isolation, and tuberculosis isolation when the client does not cover the mouth when coughing.

Masks must cover the nose and mouth (see Figure 23–7). To don a mask, first hold it by the top strings or loops, position the mask over the bridge of the nose, and tie the upper strings at the top back of the head so that the ties lie above the ears. If glasses are worn, fit the top edge of the mask under the glasses to minimize fogging of the glasses. Then make sure the lower part of the mask is well under the chin, and tie the lower

ties at the nape of the neck. If the mask has a metal strip, adjust it firmly over the bridge of the nose. While wearing the mask, avoid talking as much as possible to keep respiratory airflow at a minimum. Masks become moist and ineffective after a few hours. For this reason, masks should be worn only once and disposed of appropriately. If a mask becomes moist during a lengthy procedure, e.g., an operation, it may be necessary to have another nurse who is not gowned and gloved put a clean, dry mask over the one being worn. Before removing a mask, remove gloves, if used, or wash the hands if they have been in contact with infectious material. After removing the mask, fold it in half with the moist inner surfaces together to contain the microorganisms. Dispose of the mask in the appropriate waste or laundry container.

■ **Gowning for Isolation Precautions.** Clean or disposable gowns or plastic aprons are worn for isolation precautions when the nurse's uniform is likely to become soiled. Gowns are also required when persons enter the room of a client who has an infection, for

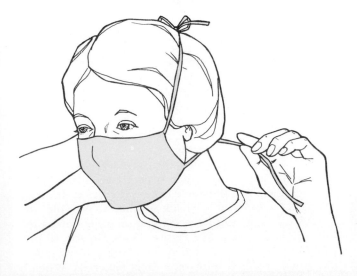

Figure 23–7 A mask covering the nose and mouth

Table 23—8 **Category-Specific Isolation Precautions**

Isolation Category	Purpose	Private Room	Gowns
Strict isolation, e.g., for diphtheria pneumonic plague, smallpox, varicella (chickenpox), zoster	To prevent airborne or contact transmission of highly contagious or virulent microorganisms	Necessary; door must be kept closed	Must be worn by all persons entering room; for smallpox, coverings for cap and shoes are also recommended
Contact isolation, e.g., for acute respiratory infections and influenza in children, pediculosis, wound infections, herpes simplex, impetigo, rubella, scabies	To prevent highly transmissible infections not requiring strict isolation but spread by close or direct contact	Necessary	Must be worn if soiling is likely
Respiratory isolation, e.g., for epiglottitis, measles, meningitis, mumps, pertussis, pneumonia in children	To prevent infections spread by contaminated articles (e.g., tissues) and respiratory droplets that are coughed, sneezed, or exhaled	Necessary	Not necessary
Tuberculosis isolation (AFB isolation) for pulmonary tuberculosis when clients have positive sputum smear or suggestive chest x-ray film	To prevent spread of acid-fast bacilli (AFB)	Necessary, with special ventilation	Necessary only if clothing may become contaminated
Enteric precautions, e.g., for hepatitis A, some gastroenteritis, typhoid fever, cholera, diarrhea with suspected infectious etiology, encephalitis, meningitis	To prevent infections spread through direct or indirect contact with feces	Necessary if client hygiene is poor, e.g., client is incontinent	Same as for tuberculosis isolation
Drainage/secretion precautions, e.g., for any draining lesion, abscess, infected burn, infected skin, decubitis ulcer, conjunctivitis	To prevent infections, spread through direct or indirect contact with material or drainage from body site	Not necessary unless client hygiene is poor	Same as for tuberculosis isolation
Blood/body fluid precautions, e.g., for hepatitis B, syphilis, AIDS, malaria	To prevent infections spread through direct or indirect contact with infected blood or body fluids	Necessary if patient hygiene is poor	Same as for tuberculosis isolation

Source: Adapted from J. S. Garner and B. P. Simmons: CDC guidelines for isolation precautions in hospitals, *Infection Control,* July/August 1983, 4(4):258–60. Used by permission.

example, varicella (chicken pox), that could cause serious illness if spread to others, even though soiling of the clothing is not likely (Garner and Simmons 1983, p. 254). Sterile gowns may be indicated when the nurse is changing the dressings of a client with extensive wounds, e.g., burns. It is recommended that a clean gown be used only once and then discarded in the receptacle designated for the purpose. Gowns may be disposable or reusable after laundering.

Before donning a gown, the nurse washes the hands thoroughly and dons a face mask, if required. When donning the gown the nurse fastens the ties at the neck, overlaps the gown at the back as much as possible, and fastens the waist ties. Overlapping securely covers the uniform at the back. See Figure 23–8. No special precautions are necessary when removing a gown unless the gown is soiled with infectious materials. When a

gown is soiled with infectious material, the nurse removes the gown so that it does not contaminate the uniform.

■ **Donning and Removing Disposable Gloves.** Disposable clean gloves are worn to protect the hands when the nurse is likely to handle any body substances, e.g., blood, urine, feces, sputum, mucous membranes, and nonintact skin. Nurses who have open sores or cuts on the hands should wear gloves for protection. Sterile gloves are used when the hands will come in contact with an open wound or when the hands might introduce microorganisms into a body orifice (see Procedure 23–3, later).

Before donning gloves, don a mask (if required), wash and dry the hands, and don a gown. No special technique is required to don disposable gloves, since they are relatively shapeless and either glove fits either

Masks	Gloves	Hand Washing	Disposal of Contaminated Articles
Must be worn by all persons entering room	Must be worn by all persons entering room	Necessary after touching client or potentially contaminated articles and before caring for another client	Discard in plastic-lined container or bag and label before sending for decontamination and reprocessing
Must be worn if person comes near client	Worn if touching infected material	Same as for strict isolation	Same as for strict isolation
Must be worn by all persons in close contact	Not necessary	Same as for strict isolation	Same as for strict isolation
Necessary if client is coughing and does not always cover mouth	Not necessary	Same as for strict isolation	Clean and disinfect, although these articles rarely transmit disease
Not necessary	Necessary if touching infected material	Same as for strict isolation	Same as for strict isolation
Not necessary	Same as for enteric precautions	Same as for strict isolation	Same as for strict isolation
Not necessary	Necessary if touching infected blood or body fluid	Necessary if hands can become contaminated and before caring for another client	Same as for strict isolation; used needles must be placed in puncture-proof container for disposal

hand. They need to be donned carefully, however, so that they do not tear. If a gown is worn, pull up the gloves to cover the cuffs of the gown. If a gown is not worn, pull up the cuffs to cover the wrists.

No special technique is required to remove gloves, since hands should be washed afterward. However, if there is a reason to prevent soilage of the hands (e.g., the nurse has a cut), grasp the first glove to be removed on its palmar surface just below the cuff, taking care that only glove touches glove and not the skin of the wrist or hand, which is considered clean. See Figure 23–9. Pull the first glove completely off by inverting or rolling the glove inside out. Continue to hold the inverted removed glove with the fingers of the gloved hand. Then place the first two fingers of the bare hand inside the cuff of the second glove and pull the second glove off to the fingers by turning it inside out. This action pulls the first glove inside the second. See Figure 23–10. Using the bare hand, continue to remove the gloves, which are now inside out, and put them in the refuse container. See Figure 23–11. The bare hands, which are considered clean, touch only the insides of the gloves, which are also considered clean. Wash the hands well. Even though gloves were worn, it is considered essential practice to wash the hands following contact with body substances, mucous membranes, or open skin lesions.

■ **Bagging Articles.** Articles contaminated with body substances must be bagged before they are removed from the client's unit. The 1983 CDC guidelines recommend the following methods:

1. A single bag, if it is sturdy and impervious to microorganisms, and if the contaminated articles can be

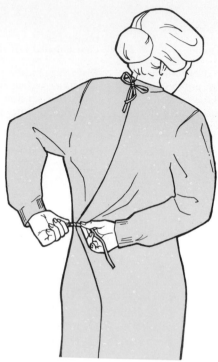

Figure 23-8 Overlapping the gown at the back to cover the nurse's uniform

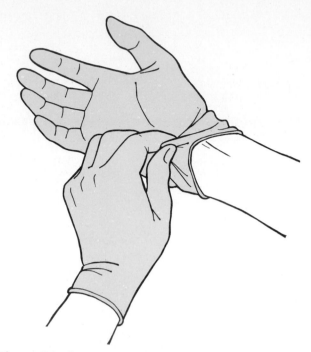

Figure 23-9 Removing the first soiled disposable glove

placed in the bag without soiling or contaminating its outside
2. Double-bagging (placing items into bags inside the client's room and in turn placing those bags inside clean bags held outside the room by another person) if the above conditions are not met

The nurse who cares for the client is responsible for ensuring that all items are placed in the appropriate containers inside the client's room. General guidelines are shown in the accompanying box.

▪ Recommendations for Severely Compromised Clients.
Compromised clients are often infected by their own microorganisms, by microorganisms on the inadequately washed hands of health personnel, and by nonsterile items (food, water, air, and client care equipment). See the accompanying box for the 1983 CDC guidelines for severely compromised clients (Garner and Simmons 1983, p. 254).

▪ Maintaining Surgical Asepsis

An object is sterile only when it is free of all microorganisms. It is well known that surgical asepsis is practiced in operating rooms, labor and delivery rooms, and special diagnostic areas. Less known perhaps is that surgical asepsis is also employed for many procedures in general care areas (i.e., procedures such as administering injections, changing wound dressings, performing urinary catheterizations, and administering intravenous therapy). In these situations, all of the principles of surgical asepsis are applied as in the operating or delivery room; however, not all of the sterile techniques that follow are always required. For example, before an oper-

ating room procedure, the nurse generally puts on a mask and cap, performs a surgical hand scrub, and then dons a sterile gown and gloves. In a general care area, the nurse may only perform a hand wash and don sterile

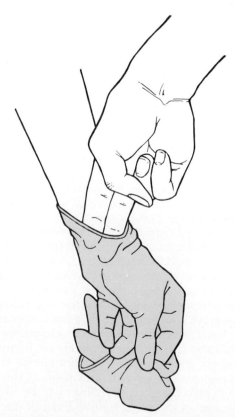

Figure 23-10 Removing the second soiled disposable glove

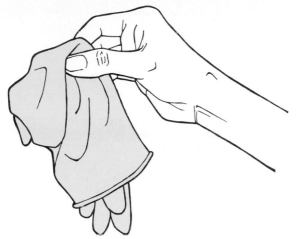

Figure 23–11 Holding soiled disposable gloves with the inside outermost

GUIDELINES

Handling Soiled Items

■ Handle soiled linen as little as possible and with the least agitation possible, to prevent gross microbial contamination of the air and/or persons handling the linen.

■ Place garbage and soiled *disposable* equipment in the plastic bag that lines the waste container. Some agencies separate dry and wet waste material and incinerate dry items, e.g., paper towels and disposable items. They place other waste materials in a central garbage chute or storage area.

■ Place glass bottles or jars in separate plastic or paper containers.

■ Place leftover food in the wet garbage container or flush it down the toilet.

■ Food trays and dishes do not require special precautions unless they are visibly soiled with infectious material. If the client's hygienic practices are unsafe, use disposable dishes (if available) and discard them in the appropriate waste receptacle in the client's unit. Bag and label contaminated nondisposable (reusable) dishes, utensils, and trays before sending them to the food service department.

■ Place dressings in either the wet or the dry waste container, depending on how soiled they are.

■ Place special *nondisposable* equipment in a separate bag to be sent to the central supply area. Place glass and metal equipment in separate bags from rubber and plastic items. Glass and metal can be sterilized in an autoclave, but rubber and plastic are damaged by this process and must be cleaned by other methods, e.g., gas sterilization.

■ Disassemble special procedure trays into component parts. Some components can be discarded; others need to be sent to the laundry or central services for cleaning and decontaminating.

GUIDELINES

Severely Compromised Clients (CDC)

■ Frequent and appropriate hand washing by all personnel before, during, and after client care

■ Private rooms whenever possible

■ Use of sterile gloves, sterile gowns, and masks by people caring for clients with major wounds or burns that cannot be enclosed by dressings.

gloves. The nine basic principles of surgical asepsis, and practices that relate to each principle, appear in Table 23–9 on pages 324–325.

■ **Using Sterile Equipment and Supplies.** Equipment is wrapped in a variety of materials to maintain its sterility. Commercially prepared items are frequently wrapped in plastic, paper, or glass. Commercially prepared sterile liquids for both internal and external use are often supplied in plastic or glass containers. Plastics are often pliable, usually transparent, impervious to dust, and relatively resistant to tearing. Intravenous solutions are commonly packaged in plastic bags. Liquid medications are sterilized in glass containers. Liquids used in hospitals may be prepared commercially or in the hospital. In the past it was not unusual for sterile liquids, e.g., sterile water for irrigations, to be supplied in large glass containers and used many times. This practice is considered undesirable today because once a container has been opened, there can be no assurance that it is sterile. Liquids are preferably packaged in amounts adequate for one use only. Any leftover liquid is discarded. Hospital-packaged liquids are often sterilized in reusable containers; commercially packaged liquids are supplied in disposable containers. These containers normally have a seal over the cap, and often the word *sterile* is clearly marked on the top. If the cap has been tampered with or if the seal is broken, the liquid is considered unsterile. All containers should also be inspected for cracks. Procedure 23–2 provides guidance for using sterile equipment.

■ **Handling Sterile Forceps.** Many styles of forceps are used to handle sterile supplies. Forceps used commonly by nurses are:

1. Hemostat or artery forceps. See Figure 23–25.
2. Tissue forceps. See Figure 23–26.
3. Sponge or transfer (lifting) forceps.

Hemostats and tissue forceps are commonly used for such techniques as changing a sterile dressing and shortening a drain. Transfer forceps are used to move a sterile article from one place to another, e.g., transferring sterile gauze from its package to a sterile dressing tray. Forceps are usually packaged and discarded or re-sterilized after use.

See the box on page 322 for guidelines applying to the use of all types of forceps.

PROCEDURE 23–2

Establishing and Maintaining a Sterile Field

Equipment

- A package containing a sterile drape
- Sterile equipment as needed, eg, wrapped sterile gauze, a wrapped sterile bowl, antiseptic solution, sterile forceps

Intervention

1. Determine that any package containing sterile supplies or equipment is sterile. The package must be clean and dry; if moist, it is considered contaminated and discarded. Check the sterilization expiration dates on the package, and look for any indications that it has been previously opened. Follow agency practice about the disposal of possibly contaminated packages.

Opening a Wrapped Package on a Surface

2. Place the package in the center of the work area so that the top flap of the wrapper opens away from you.
   Rationale: This position prevents subsequent reaching directly over the exposed sterile contents, which could contaminate them.

3. Reaching around the package (not over it), pinch the first flap on the outside of the wrapper between your thumb and index finger. See Figure 23–12. With some folded packages, it may be necessary to grasp the uppermost flap at each corner. Pull the flap open, laying it flat on the far surface.
   Rationale: Touching only the outside of the wrapper maintains the sterility of the inside of the wrapper.

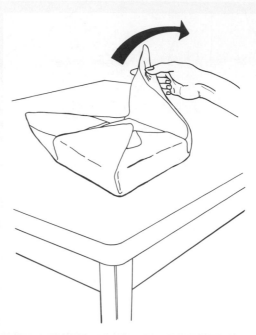

Figure 23–13 Opening the second flap to the side

4. Repeat for the side flaps, opening the top one first. Use the right hand for the right flap, and the left hand for the left flap. See Figure 23–13.
   Rationale: Both hands are used to avoid reaching over the sterile contents.

5. Pull the fourth flap toward you by grasping the corner that is turned down. See Figure 23–14. Make sure that the flap does not touch your uniform.
   Rationale: If the inner surface touches any unsterile article, it is contaminated.

Opening a Wrapped Package While Holding It

6. Hold the package in one hand with the top flap opening away from you.

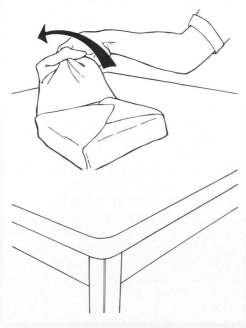

Figure 23–12 Opening the first flap of a sterile wrapped package

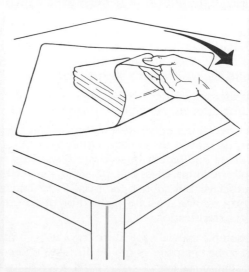

Figure 23–14 Pulling the last flap toward the nurse by grasping the corner

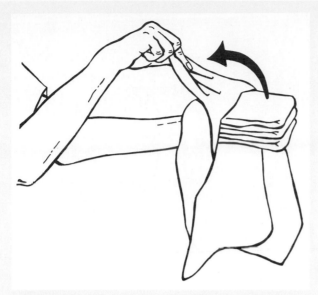

Figure 23—15 Opening a wrapped package while holding it

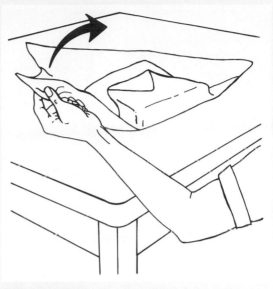

Figure 23—16

7. Using the other hand, open the package as described in steps 3–5, pulling the corners of the flaps well back. See Figure 23–15.
   Rationale: The hands are considered contaminated, and at no time should they touch the contents of the package.

Closing a Wrapped Package

Occasionally, it is necessary to cover up items in sterile wrapper to maintain their sterility for a few minutes, eg, when taking the package to a client's bedside.

8. Pick up the flap closest to you, handling it at the corner (see Figure 23–16), and lay it over the contents. Make sure the corner is folded toward you, as it was before this flap was opened.
   Rationale: This corner is contaminated because it was touched, so it should not touch the package contents.

9. Select the side you opened third. Pinch the side flap from the underside (see Figure 23–17), and lay it over the contents. Use the right hand for the right flap and the left hand for the left flap.
   Rationale: By this method the nurse avoids touching the inner sterile surface of the wrapper and avoids reaching over the sterile contents and thereby contaminating them.

10. Repeat for the other side.

11. Pinch the far flap from the underside by reaching around the package, and bring the flap over the contents. Tuck it in loosely. See Figure 23–18.

12. Use the rewrapped package immediately.
    Rationale: Although the contents are covered, they will not remain sterile for any length of time because the package is loosely wrapped.

13. Reopen the package by using the method described in steps 2–5.
    Rationale: Using the same sequence of steps should keep the contents sterile.

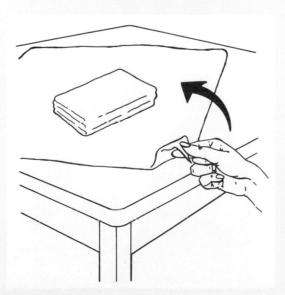

Figure 23—17

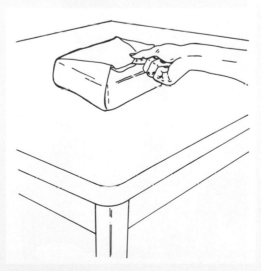

Figure 23—18

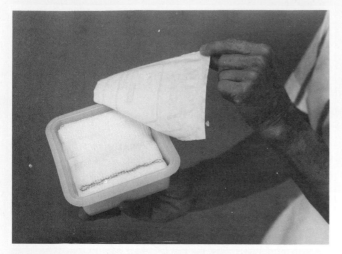

Figure 23—19

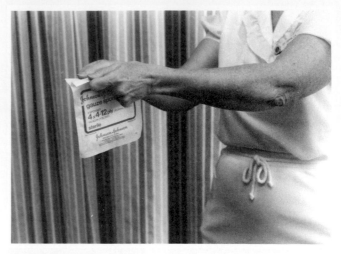

Figure 23—20

Opening Commercially Prepared Packages

Commercially prepared sterile packages and containers usually have manufacturer's directions for opening.

14. If the flap of the package has an unsealed corner, hold the container in one hand, and pull back on the flap with the other hand. See Figure 23—19.

15. If the package has a partially sealed edge, grasp both sides of the edge, one with each hand, and pull apart gently. See Figure 23—20.

Establishing a Sterile Field by Using a Drape

16. Open the package containing the drape as described above.

17. With one hand, pluck the corner of the drape that is folded back on the top.

18. Lift the drape out of the cover, and permit it to open freely without touching any articles. See Figure 23—21.
Rationale: If the drape touches the outside of the package, the nurse's uniform, or any unsterile surface, it is considered contaminated.

19. Discard the cover.

20. With the other hand, carefully pick up another corner of the drape holding it well away from yourself.

21. Lay the drape on a clean, dry surface, placing the bottom (ie, the freely hanging side) farthest from you. See Figure 23—22.
Rationale: By placing the lowermost side farthest away, the nurse avoids leaning over the sterile field and contaminating it.

Adding Wrapped Supplies to a Sterile Field

22. Open each wrapped package as described in the preceding steps.

23. With your free hand, grasp the corners of the wrap-

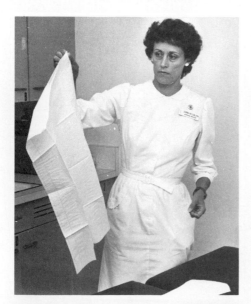

Figure 23—21

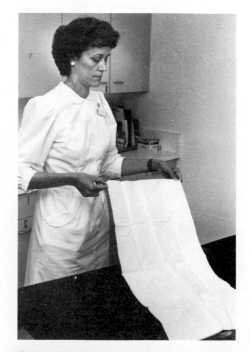

Figure 23—22

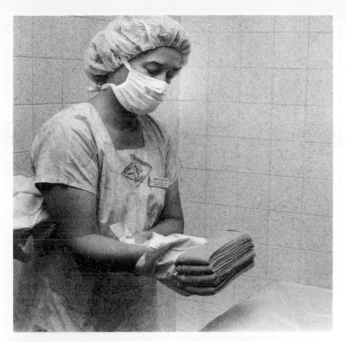

Figure 23—23

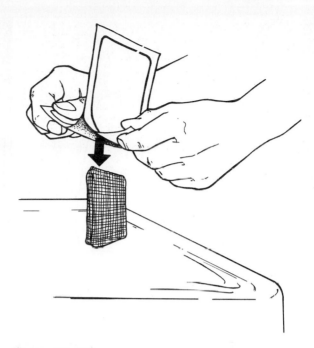

Figure 23—24

per and hold them against the wrist of the hand holding the package. See Figure 23–23.
Rationale: The hand is now covered by the sterile wrapper.

24. Place the sterile bowl, drape, etc, on the sterile field by approaching from an angle rather than holding your arm over the field.

25. Discard the wrapper.

Adding Commercially Packaged Supplies to a Sterile Field

26. Open each package, eg, gauze, as described in step 14 or 15.

27. Hold the package 15 cm (6 in.) above the field, and permit the contents to drop on the field. See Figure 23–24. Keep in mind that 2.5 cm (1 in.) around the edge of the field is considered contaminated.
Rationale: At a height of 15 cm (6 in.), the outside of the package is not likely to touch and contaminate the sterile field.

Adding Sterile Solution to a Sterile Bowl

Sterile liquids (eg, normal saline) frequently need to be poured into metal or nonabsorbent containers within a sterile field. Unwrapped bottles or flasks that contain sterile solution are considered sterile on the inside and contaminated on the outside, since the bottle may have been handled. Bottles used in an operating room may be sterilized on the outside as well as the inside, however, and these are handled with sterile gloves.

Before pouring any liquid, read the label three times to make sure you have the correct solution.

28. Obtain the exact amount of solution, if possible.
Rationale: Once a sterile container has been opened,

its sterility cannot be assured for a future use unless it is used again immediately.

29. From the label, confirm the name of solution and its strength.

30. Remove the lid or cap from the bottle and invert the lid before placing it on a surface that is not sterile.
Rationale: Inverting the lid maintains the sterility of the inside surface because it is not allowed to touch an unsterile surface.

31. Hold the bottle so that the label is uppermost.
Rationale: Any solution that flows down the outside of the bottle during pouring will not damage or obliterate the label.

32. Hold the bottle of fluid at a height of 10–15 cm (4–6 in.) over the bowl and to the side of the sterile field so that as little of the bottle as possible is over the field.
Rationale: At this height there is less likelihood of contaminating the sterile field by touching the field or by reaching an arm over it.

33. Pour the solution gently so as not to splash the liquid.
Rationale: If the sterile drape is on an unsterile surface, any moisture will contaminate the field by facilitating the movement of microorganisms through the sterile drape.

34. Replace the lid securely on the bottle if you plan to use it again. In many agencies a sterile container of solution that is opened is used only once and then discarded.
Rationale: Replacing the lid immediately maintains the sterility of the inner aspect of the lid and the solution.

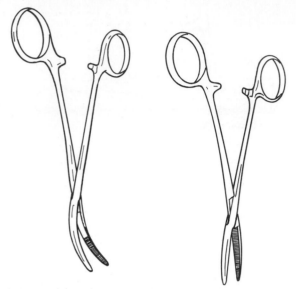

Figure 23—25 Hemostat forceps (curved and straight)

■ **Donning Sterile Gloves (Open Method).**
Sterile gloves may be donned by the open method or
the closed method. The open method is most frequently
used outside the operating room, since the closed method
requires that the nurse wear a sterile gown. Gloves are
worn during many sterile procedures to maintain the
sterility of equipment and protect a client's open wound.

■ **Donning a Sterile Gown and Gloves (Closed
Method).** Sterile gowning and closed gloving are
chiefly carried out in operating or delivery rooms, where
surgical asepsis is necessary. The closed method of gloving can be used only when a sterile gown is worn because
the gloves are handled through the sleeves of the gown.
Prior to these techniques, the nurse dons a hair cover
and a mask and performs a surgical hand wash.

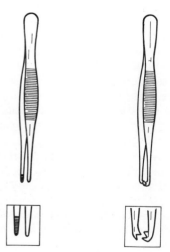

Figure 23—26 Tissue forceps (plain and toothed)

GUIDELINES

Forceps

■ Keep the tips of wet forceps lower than the wrist at
all times, unless wearing sterile gloves. See Figure
23—27. Gravity prevents liquids on the tips from
flowing to the handles and later back to the tips, thus
making the forceps unsterile. The handles are unsterile once they are held by the bare hand.

■ Hold sterile forceps above waist level. There is less
danger of contamination if the forceps are held nearer
to eye level.

■ Hold sterile forceps within sight. While out of sight,
forceps may inadvertently become unsterile. Any such
forceps should be considered unsterile.

■ Remove transfer forceps from their package by lifting
the forceps directly upward. Make sure that the forceps do not touch the edge or inside of the container
or the outside of the wrapper. These areas are not
sterile.

■ When using forceps to lift sterile supplies out of a
commercially prepared package, be sure that the forceps do not touch the edges or outside of the wrapper
which have been handled, and are thus unsterile.

■ When placing forceps whose handles were in contact
with the bare hand on a sterile field, position the
handles outside the sterile area.

■ Deposit a sterile item on a sterile field without permitting moist forceps to touch the sterile field.

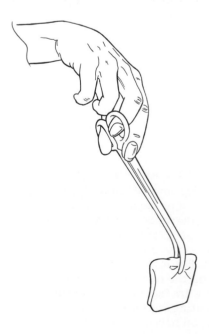

Figure 23—27 Holding forceps with tips lower than the
hand

PROCEDURE 23-3

Donning and Removing Sterile Gloves (Open Method)

Equipment

▪ A package of sterile gloves. Gloves are packaged with a cuff often about 5 cm (2 in.) and with the palms facing upward when the package is opened. The package usually indicates the size of the gloves (eg, size 6 or $7\frac{1}{2}$) so that the nurse can select the appropriate size.

Intervention

Donning Sterile Gloves

1. Place the package of gloves on a clean dry surface. *Rationale:* Any moisture on the surface could contaminate the gloves.

2. Some gloves are packed in an inner as well as an outer package. Open the outer package without contaminating the gloves or the inner package. See "Opening a Wrapped Package" in Procedure 23-2. Remove the inner package from the outer package.

3. Open the inner package as above or according to the manufacturer's directions. Some manufacturers provide a numbered sequence for opening the flaps and folded tabs to grasp for opening the flaps. If no tabs are provided, pluck the flap so that your fingers do not touch the inner surfaces. *Rationale:* The inner surfaces, which are next to the sterile gloves, will remain sterile.

4. If the gloves are packaged so they lie side by side, grasp the glove for your dominant hand by its cuff (on the palmar side) with the thumb and first finger of the nondominant hand. Touch only the inside of the cuff. See Figure 23-28.

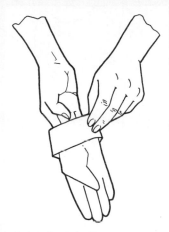

Figure 23-29

or

If the gloves are packaged one on top of the other, grasp the cuff of the top glove as above, using the opposite hand. *Rationale:* The hands are not sterile. By touching only the inside of the glove, the nurse avoids contaminating the outside.

5. Insert the dominant hand into the glove and pull the glove on. Keep the thumb of the inserted hand against the palm of the hand during insertion. See Figure 23-29. Leave the cuff turned down. *Rationale:* If the thumb is kept against the palm, it is less likely to contaminate the outside of the glove.

6. Pick up the other glove with the sterile gloved hand, inserting the gloved fingers under the cuff and holding the gloved thumb close to the gloved palm. See Figure 23-30. *Rationale:* This helps prevent accidental contamination of the glove by the bare hand.

7. Pull on the second glove carefully. Hold the thumb of the gloved first hand as far as possible from the palm. See Figure 23-31.

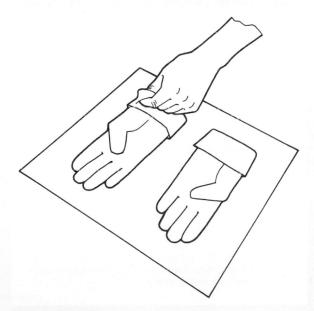

Figure 23-28

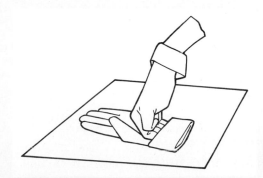

Figure 23-30

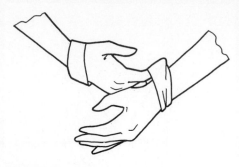

Figure 23–31

Rationale: In this position the thumb is less likely to touch the arm and become contaminated.

8. Adjust each glove so that it fits smoothly, and carefully pull the cuffs up by sliding the fingers under the cuffs.

Removing Used Gloves

9. Pluck either glove near the cuff end and pull the glove over the hand so that the glove inverts itself with the contaminated surface inside.
   Rationale: Sterile gloves are considered contaminated once they have been used.

10. Slide two fingers of the bare hand against the wrist under the cuff of the other glove and slide the second glove off, inverting it over itself and the first glove. Discard the gloves in the designated container.

Table 23–9 Principles and Practices of Surgical Asepsis

Principles	Practices
All objects used in a sterile field must be sterile.	All articles are sterilized appropriately by dry or moist heat, chemicals, or radiation before use.
	Sterile articles can be stored for only a prescribed time; after that, they are considered unsterile.
	Always check a package containing a sterile object for intactness dryness, and expiration date. Any package that appears already open, torn, punctured, or wet is considered unsterile. Never assume an item is sterile.
	Storage areas should be clean, dry, off the floor, and away from sinks.
	Always check the sterilization dates and periods on the labels of wrapped items before using the items.
	Always check chemical indicators of sterilization before using a package. The indicator is often a tape used to fasten the package or contained inside the package. The indicator changes color during sterilization, indicating that the contents have undergone a sterilization procedure. If the color change is not evident, the package is considered unsterile. Commercially prepared sterile packages may not have indicators but are marked with the word *sterile.*
Sterile objects become unsterile when touched by unsterile objects.	Handle sterile objects that will touch open wounds or enter body cavities only with sterile forceps or sterile gloved hands.
	Discard or resterilize objects that come into contact with unsterile objects.
	Whenever the sterility of an object is questionable, assume the article is unsterile.
Sterile items that are out of vision or below the waist level of the nurse are considered unsterile.	Once left unattended, a sterile field is considered unsterile.
	Sterile objects are always kept in view. Nurses do not turn their backs on a sterile field.
	Only the front part of a sterile gown (from the waist to the shoulder) and the front part of the sleeves are considered sterile.
	Always keep sterile gloved hands in sight and above waist level; touch only objects that are sterile.
	Once a sterile field becomes unsterile, it must be set up again before proceeding.
Sterile objects can become unsterile by prolonged exposure to air.	Areas in which sterile procedures are carried out are kept as clean as possible by frequent damp cleaning with detergent germicides.
	The nurse's uniform is kept clean and dry.

continued

Table 23—9 Principles and Practices of Surgical Asepsis (continued)

Principles	Practices
	The nurse's hair is kept clean and short or enclosed in a net to prevent hair from falling on sterile objects. Microorganisms on the hair can make a sterile field unsterile.
	Surgical caps are worn in operating rooms, delivery rooms, and burn units.
	Sneezing or coughing over a sterile field can make it unsterile because droplets containing microorganisms from the respiratory tract can travel 3 feet. Some nurses recommend that masks covering the mouth and the nose should be worn by anyone working over a sterile field or an open wound.
	Nurses with mild upper respiratory tract infections refrain from carrying out sterile procedures or wear masks.
	Anyone working over a sterile field keeps talking to a minimum. The nurse averts the head from the field if talking is necessary.
	The nurse refrains from reaching over a sterile field unless sterile gloves are worn and from moving unsterile objects over a sterile field because microorganisms can fall onto it. Always reach around a sterile field or carefully turn it by reaching under the wrapper or by touching the wrapper edges.
	Sterile objects are moved as little as possible within the sterile field to minimize the danger of contact with unsterile objects.
	Doors are closed and traffic is kept to a minimum in areas where a sterile procedure is being performed because moving air can carry dust and microorganisms.
	Sterile draped tables in the operating room or elsewhere are considered sterile only at surface level.
	Any article that falls outside the edges of a sterile field is considered unsterile.
	Sterile packages are opened by grasping only the outer edges or corners of the coverings.
Fluids flow in the direction of gravity.	Wet forceps are always held with the tips below the handles. When the tips are held higher than the handles, fluid can flow onto the handle and become contaminated by the hands. When the forceps are again pointed downward, the fluid flows back down and contaminates the tips.
	During a surgical hand wash, the hands are held higher than the elbows to prevent contaminants from the forearms from reaching the hands.
Moisture that passes through a sterile object draws microorganisms from unsterile surfaces above or below to the sterile surface by capillary action.	Sterile waterproof barriers are used beneath sterile objects. Liquids (sterile saline or antiseptics) are frequently poured into containers on a sterile field. If they are spilled onto the sterile field, the barrier keeps the liquid from seeping beneath it.
	The sterile covers on sterile equipment are kept dry. Damp surfaces can attract microorganisms in the air.
	When pouring sterile solutions into sterile containers, care is taken to avoid dampening the sterile field.
	One must replace sterile drapes that do not have a sterile barrier underneath when they become moist.
The edges of a sterile field are considered unsterile.	A 2.5 cm (1 in) margin at each edge of an opened drape is considered unsterile, since the edges are in contact with unsterile surfaces.
	All sterile objects are placed more than 2.5 cm (1 in) inside the edges of a sterile field.
The skin cannot be sterilized and is unsterile.	Sterile gloves are worn and/or sterile forceps are used to handle sterile items.
	Prior to a surgical aseptic procedure, the hands are washed to reduce the number of microorganisms on them.
Conscientiousness, alertness, and honesty are essential qualities in maintaining surgical asepsis.	When a sterile object becomes unsterile, it does not necessarily change in appearance.
	The person who sees a sterile object become contaminated must correct or report the situation.
	A sterile field should not be set up ahead of time for future use.

Evaluating the Effectiveness of Protective Measures

Many health facilities have infection control committees whose responsibility is to investigate, control, and prevent infections in the facility. In 1958, the Joint Commission on Accreditation of Hospitals (JCAH) recommended that every hospital set up an infection control committee. The responsibilities of the infection control committee are:

1. To establish a system for reporting infections
2. To keep records of infections
3. To review the hospital's bacteriologic services
4. To review and make recommendations about the hospital's aseptic practices
5. To undertake an educational program for hospital employees

An infection control nurse is a member of the committee. The responsibility of this nurse, often referred to as a nurse epidemiologist, is to:

1. Promote personnel behaviors that help control infection
2. Provide facts and statistical data regarding epidemiologic investigations
3. Supervise the hospital infection control program

How the infection control nurse performs these responsibilities varies from agency to agency. The following are common ways:

▪ Conveying, promoting, and supporting positive attitudes toward infection control

▪ Reporting relevant information to the hospital infection control committee, e.g., problems with implementing specific control measures

▪ Initiating and presenting proposals regarding infection control to the committee

▪ Carrying out an infection control education program for staff

▪ Collecting and analyzing data regarding nosocomial infections among clients and staff

▪ Teaching clients, support persons, and staff specific protective measures for clients

▪ Investigating unusual occurrences of infection

▪ Consulting with staff regarding infection control

▪ Coordinating the hospital program with the community

▪ Acting as the hospital liaison to public health agencies

Chapter Highlights

▪ Microorganisms are everywhere. Most are harmless and some are beneficial; however, many can cause infection in susceptible persons.

▪ Effective control of infectious disease is an inter-national, national, community, and individual responsibility.

▪ Asepsis is the freedom from infection or infectious material.

▪ Medical aseptic practices limit the number, growth, and spread of microorganisms.

▪ Surgical aseptic practices keep an area or objects free of all microorganisms.

▪ An infection can develop if the six links in the chain of infection—infectious agent, reservoir, portal of exit, mode of transmission, portal of entry, and susceptible host—are not interrupted.

▪ Aseptic practices can be used to break any of the six links in the chain of infection.

▪ Humans have both nonspecific and specific defenses that combat infectious agents.

▪ Intact skin and mucous membranes are the body's first line of defense against microorganisms.

▪ Some normal body flora release bacteriocins and antibiotic-like substances that inhibit microbial growth and destroy foreign bacteria.

▪ Some body secretions (e.g., saliva and tears) contain enzymes that act as antibacterial agents.

▪ The inflammatory response limits physical, chemical, and microbial injury and promotes repair of injured tissue.

▪ The immune defense responds to specific antigens; it is mediated either by antibodies produced by lymphoid B cells circulating in blood serum or by lymphoid T cells residing in cells of the lymphoid system.

▪ Both B cells and T cells are memory cells that defend against invasions by the same antigen.

▪ Immunity is the specific resistance of the body to infectious agents and may be natural or acquired.

▪ Acquired immunity is active or passive and in either case may be naturally or artificially induced.

▪ Especially at risk of acquiring an infection are the very young or old; those with poor nutritional status, a deficiency of serum immunoglobulins, multiple stressors, insufficient immunizations, or an existing disease process; and those receiving certain medical therapies.

▪ The incidence of nosocomial infections is significant. Major sites for these infections are the respiratory and urinary tracts, the bloodstream, and surgical or open wounds.

▪ Factors that contribute to nosocomial infections are invasive procedures, medical therapies, the existence of a large number of susceptible persons, inappropriate use of antibiotics, and insufficient hand washing after client contact and after contact with body substances.

▪ Preventing infections in healthy or ill persons and preventing the spread of microorganisms from infected clients to others are major nursing functions.

▪ The nurse must be knowledgeable about sources and modes of transmission of microorganisms.

▪ Microorganisms are invisible, and nurses have an ethical obligation to ensure that appropriate aseptic measures are taken to protect clients, support persons, and health personnel, including themselves.

▪ Selected References

Aspinall, M. J. October 1978. Scoring against nosocomial infections. *American Journal of Nursing* 78:1704–7.

Axnick, K. J., and Yarbrough, M., editors. 1984. *Infection control: An integrated approach.* St. Louis: C. V. Mosby Co.

Benenson, A. S., editor. 1985. *Control of communicable diseases in man.* 14th ed. An official report of the American Public Health Association. Washington, D.C.: The American Public Health Association.

Berger, S. A., editor: 1982. *Clinical manual of infectious diseases.* Menlo Park, Calif.: Addison-Wesley Publishing Co.

Brandt, S. L., and Benner, P. March 1980. Infection control in hospitals: What are the challenges? *American Journal of Nursing* 80:432–34.

Brem, A. M., and Torok, E. M. December 1979. Nosocomial infections in the elderly. *Hospital Topics* 57:10, 40–43.

Byrne, J. C.; Saxton, D. F.; Pelikan, P. K.; and Nugent, P. M. 1986. *Laboratory tests: Implications for nursing care.* Menlo Park, Calif.: Addison-Wesley Publishing Co.

Carroll, M. March/April 1984. Infection control in long-term care. *Geriatric Nursing* 5:100–103.

Centers for Disease Control. 1980. "Antiseptics, handwashing and handwashing facilities." In *Guidelines for the prevention and control of nosocomial infections.* Atlanta: Centers for Disease Control.

———. 1987. Recommendations for prevention of HIV transmission in health-care settings. *Morbidity and Mortality Weekly Report* (suppl) 36:3s–18s.

Garner, J. S., and Favero, M. S. 1985. *Guideline for handwashing and hospital environmental control 1985.* Washington, D.C.: U.S. Government Printing Office.

Garner, J. S., and Simmons, B. P. July/August 1983. CDC guidelines for isolation precautions in hospitals. *Infection Control* 4:245–325. Special Supplements.

Hargiss, C. O., and Larson, E. December 1981. Infection control: How to collect specimens and evaluate results. *American Journal of Nursing* 81:2166–74.

Jackson, M. M.; Lynch, P.; McPherson, D. C.; et al. 1987. Why not treat all body substances as infectious? *American Journal of Nursing* 87:1137–39.

Jones, I. April 1985. You can drive back infection . . . if you know where to make your stand. *Nursing 85* 15:50–52.

Kneedler, J. A., and Dodge, G. H. 1983. *Perioperative patient care: The nursing perspective.* Boston: Blackwell Scientific Publications.

Kolff, C. A., and Sanchez, R. 1979. *Handbook for infectious disease management.* Menlo Park, Calif.: Addison-Wesley Publishing Co.

Larson, E. March/April 1982: Persistent carriage of gram negative bacteria on the hands. *Nursing Research* 31:121–22.

LeMaitre, G. D., and Finnegan, J. A. 1980. *The patient in surgery: A guide for nurses.* 4th ed. Philadelphia: W. B. Saunders Co.

Losos, J., and Trotman, M. May/June 1984. Estimated economic burden of nosocomial infection. *Canadian Journal of Public Health* 75:248–50.

Maki, D. G.; Alvarado, C.; Hassemer, C. 1986. Double-bagging of items from isolation rooms is unnecessary as an infection control measure: A comparative study of surface contamination with single- and double-bagging. *Infection Control* 7:535–37.

Mallison, G. F., and Standard, P. G. 1974. Safe storage times for sterile packs. *Hospitals* 48(20):77–78, 80.

Meers, P. D. March 10, 1982. Infection in hospitals. *Nursing Times* 16:146.

Mott, S. R.; Fazekas, N. F.; James, S. R. 1985. *Nursing Care of Children and Families.* Menlo Park, Calif.: Addison-Wesley Publishing Co.

Moree, N. A., and Garner, J. S. (consultant). February 1984. New infection control guidelines. *American Journal of Nursing* 84:210–11.

Nadolny, M. D. March 1980. What does the infection control nurse do? *American Journal of Nursing* 80:430–1.

Norton, C. F. 1986. *Microbiology.* 2d ed. Reading, Mass.: Addison-Wesley Publishing Co.

Parent, B. December 1985. Moral, ethical, and legal aspects of infection control. *American Journal of Infection Control* 13:278–80.

Pickering, L. K., and DuPont, H. L. 1986. *Infectious diseases of children and adults: A step-by-step approach to diagnosis and treatment.* Menlo Park, Calif.: Addison-Wesley Publishing Co.

Setia, U.; Serventi, I.; and Lorenzo, P. April 1985. Nosocomial infection among patients in a long-term care facility: Spectrum, prevalence, and risk factors. *American Journal of Infection Control* 13:57–62.

Simmons, B. P. August 1983. CDC guidelines for the prevention and control of nosocomial infections. Guidelines for prevention of surgical wound infections. *American Journal of Infection Control* 11.133–41.

Spradley, B. W. 1981. *Community health nursing.* Boston: Little, Brown and Co.

Stark, J. L., and Hunt, V. January 1985. Don't let nosocomial infections get your patients down. *Nursing 85* 15:10–11.

Taylor, L. J. J. January 19, 1978. An evaluation of handwashing techniques—2. *Nursing Times* 74:108–110.

Weissman, I. L.; Hood, L. E.; and Wood, W. B. 1978. *Essential concepts in immunology.* Menlo Park, Calif.: Benjamin/Cummings Publishing Co.

Whaley, L. F., and Wong, D. L. 1987. *Nursing care of infants and children.* 3d ed. St. Louis: The C.V. Mosby Co.

William, A. R. October 1985. Cost-effective application of the Centers for Disease Control guideline for handwashing and hospital environmental control. *American Journal of Infection Control.* 13:218–23.

Williams, P., and Bierer, B. March/April 1984. Wash your hands! *Geriatric Nursing* 5:103–4.

Williams, W. W. July/August 1983. CDC guideline for infection control in hospital personnel. *Infection Control* 4:326–49.

———. February 1984. CDC guidelines for the prevention and control of nosocomial infections: Guideline for infection control in hospital personnel. *American Journal of Infection Control* 12:34–57.

CHAPTER 24

Providing a Safe Environment

OBJECTIVES

Identify clients at risk of physical injury.

Give examples of nursing diagnoses for clients at risk of accidental injury.

Describe nursing responsibilities regarding fires.

Identify precautions to prevent falls of hospitalized clients.

Describe legal implications of restraining clients.

State guidelines for selecting and applying restraints.

Describe measures to minimize noise.

List precautions to prevent exposure to radiation.

List causes and signs of three kinds of sensory disturbances.

Identify clients most at risk of sensory disturbances.

State nursing diagnoses pertaining to sensory disturbances.

Explain nursing interventions to adjust environmental stimuli.

Describe interventions that promote functioning of existing senses.

Identify interventions that help the client adapt to altered sensory function.

List outcome criteria for evaluating selected strategies for preventing injury and disease.

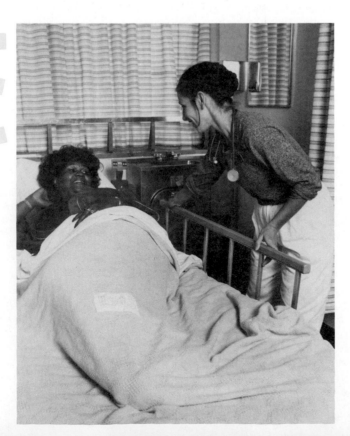

Assessing Clients at Risk for Injury/Disease

The ability of people to protect themselves from injury and disease is affected by a number of factors, such as age, life-style, sensory perception, awareness, mobility, emotional state, ability to communicate, history of previous accidents, and safety knowledge. Nurses need to assess each of these factors when they plan care or teach clients to protect themselves.

Through knowledge and accurate assessment of the environment, people learn to protect themselves from many injuries. Children walking to school learn to stop before crossing the street and wait for oncoming traffic. They also learn not to touch a hot stove. For the very young, learning about the environment is essential. Only through knowledge and experience do children learn what is potentially harmful.

Elderly people also can have special problems protecting themselves from injury. Often the balance of elderly people is impaired by their flexed posture, which places their center of gravity forward. Once balance is lost, it is not readily regained. An elderly person may need to learn to stand up slowly, thus avoiding the fall that can result from a quick, sudden movement. Slowness of movement and diminished sensual acuity also contribute to the likelihood of injury. Elderly persons may neither see nor hear an oncoming car. They may not see a footstool. They may also be unable to pull themselves out of a bathtub safely.

Life-style factors that place people at risk are: unsafe work environments, where workers are in danger from machinery, industrial belts and pulleys, and chemicals; residence in neighborhoods with high crime rates; access to guns and ammunition; insufficient income to buy safety equipment or make necessary repairs; and access to illicit drugs, which may also be contaminated by harmful additives. Risk-taking behavior is a factor in accidents. For example, some people disregard safety recommendations by driving automobiles at high speeds and refusing to wear seat belts in automobiles, headgear on motorcycles, or flotation jackets in boats.

Accurate sensory perception of environmental stimuli is vital to safety. These stimuli, which are received by sensory receptors of the body, travel through the nerves to the central nervous system. In a reflex action, such as jerking the hand away from a hot object, some of the impulses travel directly to motor neurons, which then convey the impulses to the muscles that cause the sudden, quick withdrawing of the hand. At the same time, other sensory impulses travel to the cerebral cortex; and the person, now aware of the stimulus, initiates further impulses that result in voluntary muscle movement. Impairment of any of these areas—the sensory receptors, sensory pathways, the internuncial neurons that transmit the impulse from the sensory pathways to the motor pathways, the motor pathways, or the cerebral cortex—can diminish ability to respond normally to environmental stimuli.

People with impaired touch perception, hearing, taste, smell, and vision are highly susceptible to injury. A person who does not see well may trip over a toy or not see a signal cord at a hospital bed unit. Deaf persons do not hear a siren in traffic, and persons with impaired olfactory sense may not smell burning food or escaping gas. Paralysis and other neurologic impairments diminish touch perceptions. A paralyzed person may not feel a burn from a burning hot-water bottle, and a person whose sense of taste is impaired may not detect contaminated food.

Some neurologic diseases cause changes in kinesthetic sense and tactile perceptions. Disease of the inner ear, for example, can cause loss of kinesthetic sense. Spinal cord injuries and cerebrovascular accidents cause paralysis and loss of tactile perception. Certain problems create sensations that do not arise from normal external or internal stimuli. For example, a client who has a disease of the auditory nerve may hear sounds that correspond to no external stimulus. Hallucinations (perceptions of external stimuli in the absence of such stimuli) can result, for example, from a disease process or hallucinogenic drugs. Illusions are misinterpretations of external stimuli. For example, a person may interpret a shadow cast by a lamp as a person.

Awareness is the ability to perceive environmental stimuli and body reactions and to respond appropriately through thought and action. The normal, alert person can assimilate many kinds of information at one time, perceives reality accurately, and acts on those perceptions. Part of this process is separating necessary stimuli from extraneous ones and reaching logical conclusions by correlating information. Most people do this with little or no awareness of the mental processes involved. Occasionally, people exhibit abnormalities of thought; they may become absent-minded or lose their sense of direction. Often these episodes are due to intense concentration on one subject to the exclusion of others.

Illness and age can affect **consciousness** (the awareness of environment, self, and others), as can hospitalization. Mildly confused hospitalized clients may momentarily forget they are not at home, wander from their rooms, misplace personal belongings, and so forth. Severely confused (disoriented) persons may not know family members or may think the nurse is a relative. Such persons may act atypically: Confused, usually docile people may become combative with nurses and others. Severely confused people do not know where they are or what time of day or day of the week it is. Clients with **impaired awareness** include: persons lacking in sleep, unconscious or semiconscious persons, disoriented persons, (i.e., those who may not understand where they are or what to do to help themselves), persons who perceive stimuli that do not exist, and persons whose judgment is altered by medications, such as narcotics, tranquilizers, hypnotics, and sedatives.

Persons who have impaired **mobility** due to paralysis, muscle weakness, and poor balance or coordination are obviously prone to injury. Clients with spinal cord injury and paralysis of both legs may be unable to move even when they perceive discomfort. Hemiplegic clients or clients with leg casts often have poor balance and fall easily. Clients weakened by illness or surgery are not always fully aware of their condition. It is not uncommon for clients to believe themselves able to walk and fall while trying.

Extreme emotional states can alter ability to perceive environmental hazards. The acutely anxious or angry person has reduced perceptual awareness. Depressed persons may think and react to environmental stimuli more slowly than usual. People worried about their own or loved ones' illnesses are less aware than usual of potential dangers in the environment, such as a street curb or an oncoming automobile.

People with diminished ability to receive and convey information are also at risk for injury and/or disease. Aphasic clients, people with language barriers, and those unable to read are among them. For example, the person unable to interpret the sign "No smoking-oxygen in use" may cause a fire.

It is helpful to know if a client has a previous history of accidents. It has been recognized for some time that some people are accident prone. Predisposition to accidents is thought to have an emotional basis. One theory is that emotional tension impairs a person's perceptions and judgments, thus making that person more likely to have an accident. Some propose that accidents may fulfill masochistic and hostile needs or fulfill desires to be cared for by others.

Information is crucial to safety. Clients in hospitals and other unfamiliar environments frequently need specific safety information. Lack of knowledge about unfamiliar equipment, such as oxygen tanks, intravenous tubing, and hot packs, is a potential hazard. Nurses need to teach clients what safety precautions to take when oxygen is in use and how to maintain intravenous infusions.

Nursing Diagnoses for Clients at Risk for Injury/Disease

Examples of nursing diagnoses for clients at risk for physical injury and with health problems reflecting sensory alterations are shown in the accompanying box. Nurses formulate diagnoses from the assessment data obtained for each client. After deriving pertinent causative factors from the data base, nurses plan individualized interventions for the client.

Planning Care to Prevent Client Injury/Disease

The nurse planning health protective measures must consider the age, knowledge, and sensory deficits of the client. The nursing care plan should include two aspects: educating clients about preventive actions and modifying the environment to make it safe. The latter can

involve not only arranging the environment but also limiting the environment in some ways.

The overall client goal is to prevent injury and illness by helping the client to identify hazards and to take related safety measures. Outcome criteria are discussed later in this chapter. See the section on evaluation.

Health protection strategies are designed to protect both individuals and the general population. These strategies prevent dental disease, infectious diseases, and injury resulting from common accidents such as falls, poisoning, suffocation, burns, and electric shock. Other health protection strategies include water supply protection—through chlorination, pollution control, and control of animals that carry diseases—and public health policies such as food sanitation and pasteurization of milk.

Education is a major factor in preventing accidents and infectious disease. It is directed toward helping people identify potential hazards and changing their health practices and habits accordingly. The environment contains many hazards, both seen and unseen. The automobile is an obvious hazard. Microorganisms and radiation are unseen hazards.

The need for a safe environment is a national, community, and individual concern. Nurses are voicing their thoughts individually and collectively about such issues as air and water pollution and the safety of foods, cosmetics, and medications. The need for safety on the highways is underscored by newspaper reports of morbidity and mortality from automobile accidents. Increasingly, governments are being pressed to take action and legislate in these areas to make the environment safer. In addition, people are also becoming aware of safety hazards in their communities. Regulations to control the speed of boats on lakes used for swimming, local ordinances curbing the burning of refuse, and stricter

NURSING DIAGNOSIS

Potential for Injury and Sensory Disturbances

- Potential for falling related to impaired balance associated with decreased gross muscle coordination

- Potential for burns related to decreased temperature and tactile sensation associated with paralysis

- Potential for trauma related to failure to use headgear when cycling

- Potential for injury related to exposure to dangerous machines, lack of awareness of environmental hazards

- Sensory-perceptual alteration: temporary visual deficit related to postoperative bandages/eye shields

- Sensory-perceptual alteration: auditory deficit related to aging

- Sensory-perceptual alteration: taste deficit related to radiation therapy

- Sensory-perceptual alteration: sensory overload related to hospitalization

local regulation of industrial pollution are all indications of increasing awareness of the need for safety in the environment.

Traditionally, nurses have thought of safety in relation to a client's immediate environment, and this awareness is no less important today in spite of the broader focus on human protection. A primary concern of nurses is awareness of what constitutes a safe environment for a particular person and how this environment can be achieved. The blind person may need railings; the crawling baby, a protective gate at the head of the stairs; and the elderly person, secure footing and an uncluttered floor. Nurses thus focus attention on preventing accidents and injury as well as on assisting the injured.

To provide a safe environment, it may be necessary for the nurse and/or client to modify the environment. Older clients with sensory deficits are particularly susceptible to injury. As a result, they may require assistance from nurses in taking precautions to prevent accidents. A client with loss of vision may require assistance walking. A nurse should stand on the client's nondominant side about one step ahead of the client. A blind person should grasp the nurse's arm with his nondominant arm. In addition, nurses can make the environment safe by:

■ Arranging furniture and other objects so the client will not trip over them and explaining the location of furniture

■ Leaving bedside articles as the client arranges them and within easy reach.

The client whose level of consciousness is altered also requires special protection. Side rails to prevent falls, appropriate positioning in bed, appropriate lighting, and reduced noise level are all common measures nurses employ to ensure client safety. If the client is unconscious, necessary nursing interventions include bathing, giving skin care, feeding, and meeting elimination needs. If the client is disoriented but conscious, the nurse may need to give instructions on how to perform these activities. Unless the person is totally incapacitated, it is preferable to foster independence and feelings of self-worth by helping the individual care for himself or herself than to give complete care to a passive client.

Implementing Strategies in Response to Specific Hazards/Conditions

The nurse should be prepared to act in emergency and recurring situations to protect clients. Common hazards/conditions include: fire, scalds and burns, using restraints, noise, and radiation.

Fire is a constant danger in homes and hospitals. Common causes of hospital fires are smoking in bed and faulty electrical equipment. Hospital fires are particularly hazardous to clients who are incapacitated and unable to leave the building without assistance. Many health care agencies have instituted no-smoking policies both to decrease the chances of fire as well as to promote employee health.

A fire can burn only if three elements are present: sufficient heat to start the fire, a combustible material, and sufficient oxygen to support the fire. To prevent fires, the nurse controls the environment to ensure that the three essential elements are not simultaneously present.

Health care agencies usually follow established procedures in an emergency or during a fire. Nurses need to become familiar with the practices of their employing agency. When a fire occurs, the nurse has two major goals:

1. To protect clients from injury
2. To contain and put out the fire

General protective practices to meet these goals include:

■ Making sure the telephone numbers of emergency services are displayed on all telephones

■ Knowing the location of fire exits

■ Knowing the location and types of fire extinguishers and learning to operate them

■ Learning the agency's fire drill or fire evacuation procedure

■ Keeping access to firehoses clear at all times

■ Keeping hallways free of unnecessary furniture and equipment

■ Posting signs on elevator doors so that people will know to use the stairs in the event of fire

■ Making sure the location of fire exits is clearly marked.

In the event of fire, nurses follow the guidelines in the accompanying box.

There are a number of methods of carrying persons from the scene of a fire. Generally, nurses use these carries when they cannot wheel out bedridden clients in their beds or transfer them out on stretchers. Non-nursing hospital personnel (e.g., maintenance, housekeeping, and dietary staff) may assist with evacuating clients and should receive inservice education on using these carries.

■ *Swing carry.* The swing is a two-person carry used for heavy clients. The client, in a sitting position, places the arms around each nurse's shoulders. Each nurse holds the client's wrists, which are over each nurse's shoulders, to support the client. The nurses then reaches behind the client and grasp each other's shoulder or upper arm. The nurses then release the client's wrists, reach under the client's thighs, and grasp each other's wrists. They lift and carry the client in this sitting position. See Figure 24–1. This carry is sometimes referred to as the two-handed seat, in which a hand-forearm interlock is used. A variation is the four-handed seat, used for clients who are able to sit up with less support. See Figure 24–2.

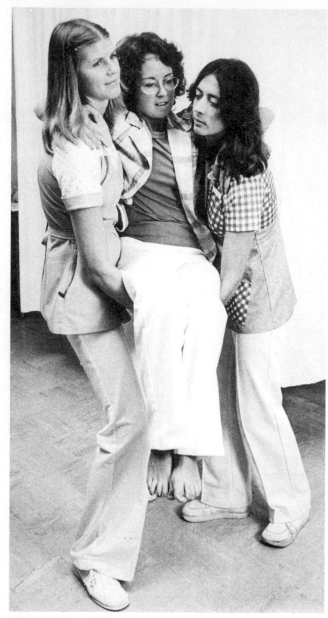

Figure 24—1   The swing carry

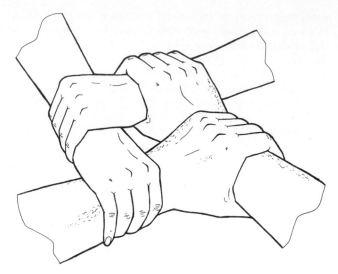

Figure 24—2   Position of the hands for a four-handed seat

stance for balance, the nurse then draws the client onto the nurse's hips so that the client's abdomen is over the nurse's hips. See Figure 24—4.

■ *Piggy-back carry.* This carry is used for clients who are conscious and have some strength to help. The client sits at the edge of the bed. The nurse stands in front of the client with her or his back toward the client. The client reaches over the nurse's shoulders and clasps his or her hands in front of the nurse while the nurse grasps the backs of the client's legs above the knees. With this carry, the nurse can support the client's weight more easily than with the pack strap carry. See Figure 24—5.

■ *Cradle carry.* The cradle carry is used for children or adults who are light in weight. The nurse lifts the

■ *Pack strap carry.* The pack strap is a one-person carry. The nurse faces the seated client and grasps the wrists. The nurse's right hand grasps the client's left wrist; the left hand grasps the client's right wrist. The nurse then pivots and slips under one of the client's arms so that the nurse's back is to the client and the client's arms are crossed in front of the nurse. The nurse assumes a broad stance, one leg in front of the other, and rolls the client onto her or his back. See Figure 24—3.

■ *Hip carry.* The client lies laterally at the side of the bed facing the nurse. The nurse faces the head of the bed. The nurse places the arm nearest the client over the client's back and under the lower axilla. The nurse then turns away from the client and places the second arm around and under the thighs. Assuming a broad

GUIDELINES

Fire

1. Evacuate clients who are in immediate danger. Direct ambulatory clients to a safe area or enlist their help in moving clients in wheelchairs. Evacuate non-ambulatory clients, who can be moved in a stretcher or bed, carried, or dragged on sheets and blankets.
2. Activate the fire alarm if one is nearby.
3. Notify the hospital switchboard of the location of the fire.
4. If the fire is small, use the fire extinguisher on the fire.
5. Close windows and doors in the area of the fire to reduce ventilation.
6. Turn off oxygen and any electrical appliances in the vicinity of the fire.
7. Clear fire exits, if necessary.
8. Contain smoke as necessary by placing damp cloths or blankets around the outside edges of doors.
9. Protect clients from smoke inhalation by giving them wet washcloths through which to breathe.

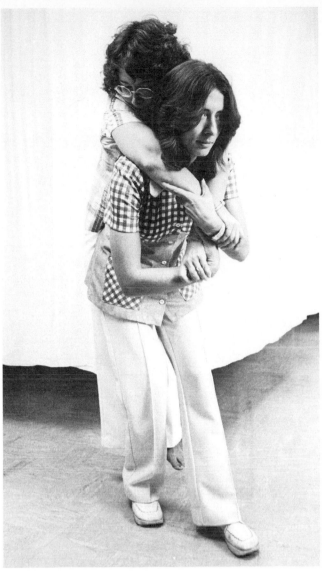

Figure 24—3 The pack strap carry

client by placing one arm beneath the person's knees and the other around the back. See Figure 24–6.

▪ *Three-person carry.* See the instructions for lifting a client between a bed and a stretcher, Chapter 36. Particular attention to the risks of fire injuries needs to be taken when caring for older clients. Impaired skin sensitivity to temperature makes the older adult more prone to burns. Impaired ability to smell may prevent the older person from sensing a fire.

In health care agencies, the risk of scalds and burns is greater for clients with impaired skin sensitivity to temperature. Scalds can occur from overly hot bath water or from overly hot moist dressings. Heat lamps can cause burns. (The therapeutic application of heat is discussed in Chapter 45.) It is important for the nurse to assess how well clients can protect themselves and what special precautions, if any, need to be taken.

Falls are common among the ill or injured, who are

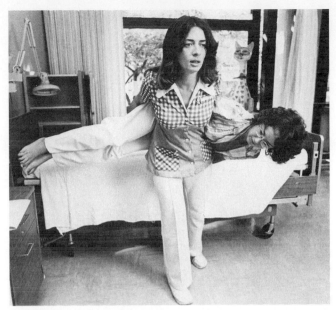

Figure 24—4 The hip carry

weakened and frequently lose their balance. To prevent falls and self-inflicted injury of hospitalized clients, the nurse should consider the guidelines in the accompanying box.

GUIDELINES

Falls

▪ Orient clients on admission to their surroundings and explain the call system.

▪ Carefully assess the client's ability to ambulate and transfer; provide walking aids and assistance as required.

▪ Closely supervise the clients at risk for falls during the first few days, especially at night.

▪ Encourage the client to use call bell to request assistance; ensure that the bell is within easy reach.

▪ Place bedside tables and overbed tables near the bed or chair so that clients do not overreach and consequently lose their balance.

▪ **Always keep hospital beds in the low position when not providing care so that clients can move in or out of bed easily.**

▪ Encourage clients to use grab bars mounted in toilet and bathing areas and railings along corridors.

▪ Make sure nonskid bath mats are available in tubs and showers.

▪ Encourage the client to wear nonskid footwear.

▪ Keep the environment tidy, especially keeping **light** cords from underfoot and furniture out of the way.

▪ Attach **side rails** to the bed of confused, sedated, restless, and unconscious clients, and keep the **rails in place** when the client is unattended.

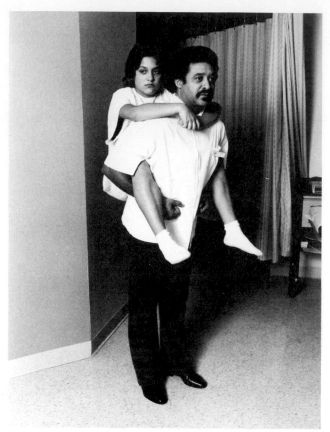

Figure 24—5   The piggy-back carry

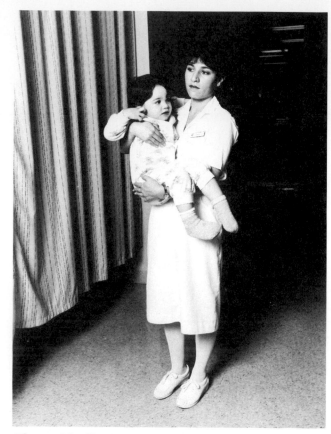

Figure 24—6   The cradle carry

Seventy-five percent of all fatal falls in the United States involve people 65 or older (Louis 1983, p. 142). Planning to prevent such falls should include consideration of the client's visual acuity, depth perception, ability to accommodate to light changes, ability to distinguish colors, hearing loss, posture, gait, decreased tactile sensitivity, physical disorders that impair mobility or cause dizziness, and the effects of prescribed medications. Most injuries of older adults are due to falls, burns, and pedestrian and automobile accidents. See the accompanying box for specific guidelines to minimize potential hazards in the hospital setting and for suggestions for client teaching prior to discharge.

Restraints are protective devices used to limit the physical activity of the client or a part of the body. They are applied to safeguard the client against injury, e.g., from falling, or to prevent movements that would disrupt therapy to a limb connected to tubes or appliances. Since people tend to resist restraint of any kind and consider it a violation of their right to move about freely, nurses need to ensure that clients understand the reason for using a restraint. Because restraints restrict an individual's ability to move freely, their use has legal implications. Many institutions require a doctor's order for the application of restraints. Clients need to know that it is a protective device and understand why the body part has to be kept relatively still.

Restrained clients often become restless and anxious as a result of the loss of self-control. Nurses may need to remain with the restrained client and speak quietly to give reassurance and allay distress. In some settings, the decision to use a restraint is made by the nurse; in others, it must be made by a physician. Often a nurse can apply a restraint in an emergency; however, the physician must order subsequent use of the restraint. It is important for nurses to know their agency's policies and the state or provincial laws about restraining clients.

The nurse must document the type of restraint used, the exact times the restraint was applied and removed, the client's behavior before and with the restraint, care given while the restraint was applied, and notification of the physician. It is important to explain the need for the restraint both to the client and to support persons; the nurse also should document the substance of these explanations.

Restraints are used in a number of situations to limit a client's movement. Some of these are:

■ To prevent a client (e.g., an elderly confused person) from falling out of bed or out of a chair

■ To remind clients to restrict movement (e.g., restraining an arm while an intravenous medication is infusing)

■ To prevent confused clients or children from harm-

GUIDELINES

Accident Prevention for the Older Adult

Preventing Falls

- Make sure all rooms, hallways, and stairwells are adequately lit.

- Have an easily accessible light switch next to the bed.

- Leave a night light on in the hallway or bathroom.

- Get out of bed slowly, i.e., sit before standing and stand briefly before walking, to prevent dizziness from orthostatic hypotension.

- Install grab bars in the bathroom near the toilet and tub.

- Make sure rugs and carpets are firmly attached to floors and stairs.

- Make sure that electrical cords are secured against baseboards to prevent tripping.

- Keep indoor and outdoor walkways and stairs in good repair.

- Install sturdy slip-resistant hand railings along stairs.

Preventing Burns

- Check the temperature of bath water and heating pads.

- Run cold water before and after hot water.

- Lower thermostats of water heaters to provide warm rather than very hot water.

- Avoid smoking in bed or when sleepy.

- Install smoke alarms.

- Place a hand fire extinguisher in a convenient area of the home, e.g., the kitchen.

- Smother kitchen grease fires with a large lid or baking soda.

- Avoid wearing loose-fitting clothing when cooking.

- Do not overload electrical circuits and keep electrical appliances in good repair.

- Keep passageways to outside doors unobstructed.

Preventing Pedestrian Accidents

- Wear reflective or light-colored clothing at night.

- Cross streets at intersections with cross walks and traffic lights when possible; do not cross major streets in the middle of the block.

- Be sure to look both ways before stepping from the curb.

Preventing Automobile Accidents

- Have regular eye examinations to assess vision, acquire appropriate refractive corrections, and detect other problems early.

- Wear good-quality gray or green sunglasses during daytime driving to reduce glare.

- Keep car windows clean and windshield wipers in good condition.

- Place mirrors on both sides of the car and always check rearview and side mirrors before changing lanes.

- Always look behind your vehicle for people or obstacles before backing up.

- Avoid smoking when driving, especially at night. Smoke can reduce visibility.

- Follow your physician's restrictions, if any, about when and where to drive.

- Learn the effects of prescribed medications on driving ability.

- Do not drink and drive.

- Stop periodically to stretch your muscles and rest your eyes.

- Leave car windows partially open and set the radio and fans low so that you can hear sirens and horns.

- Have your ability to drive periodically reevaluated.

- Keep your automobile in good repair and keep headlights, tail lights, and turn signals clean so they are visible to others.

---

ing themselves (e.g., by pulling out urinary catheters or pulling off surgical dressings)

- To prevent clients from harming others through aggressive actions (e.g., placing mitts on clients who hit out at others)

There are a number of kinds of restraints. Among the most common in use in health care settings are the jacket restraint, the belt restraint, the mitt or hand restraint, limb restraints, elbow restraints, mummy restraints, and crib nets. While **jacket restraints** vary, they are all essentially sleeveless jackets (vests) with straps (tails) that can be tied to the bed frame under the mattress or to the legs of a chair. The jacket may be put on with the ties at the front or at the back, depend-

ing on the type. See Figure 24–7. These body restraints are used for confused or sedated clients to prevent them from falling out of a bed or chair.

Belt or safety strap body restraints are used to ensure the safety of all clients who are being moved on stretchers or in wheelchairs. They may also be used for certain clients lying in bed or sitting in a chair. A **mitt or hand restraint** is used to prevent confused clients from using their hands or fingers to scratch and injure themselves. For example, a confused client may need to be prevented from pulling at intravenous tubing or a head bandage following brain surgery. Hand or mitt restraints allow the client to be ambulatory and/or to move the arm freely rather than be confined to a bed or a chair.

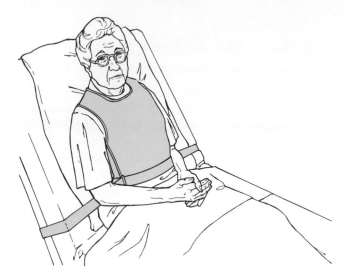

Figure 24–7   Poncho-type jacket restraint

Mitt restraints are commercially available. See Figure 24–8. Hand restraints can also be made using large dressings and stockinette. The nurse asks the client to grasp a small pad, so that the hand assumes a natural position. The client's wrist is padded with large dressings to prevent skin abrasions, and all skin surfaces are carefully separated, also to prevent abrasions. The nurse then places two large dressings over the hand, one from side to side and the other from the ventral surface to the dorsal surface. The dressings are secured with gauze bandage and adhesive tape. Stockinette is then put over the hand and secured just above the wrist pad with adhesive tape. Mittens need to be removed at least once in 24 hours to permit the client to wash and exercise the hands. If the client reports discomfort, the nurse needs to take off the mitten and check the circulation to the hand.

Limb restraints, generally made of cloth, may be used to immobilize a limb, primarily for therapeutic reasons (e.g., to maintain an intravenous infusion). Some

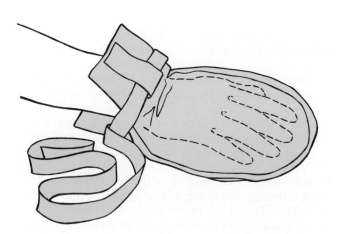

Figure 24–8   A commercially-made mitt restraint

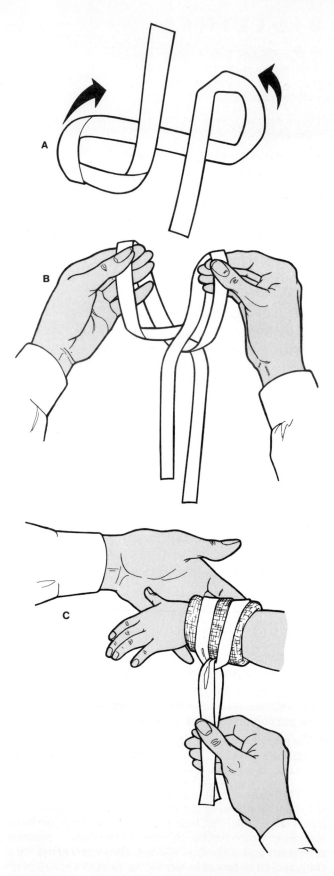

Figure 24–9   To make a clove hitch restraint: **A,** make a figure-eight; **B,** pick up the loops; **C,** put the padded limb through the loops and secure the free ends by tying them to a stationary part of the bed, crib, wheelchair, etc.

commercially prepared restraints are available. A clove hitch limb restraint can also be improvised using padded dressings and gauze. See Figure 24–9.

Elbow restraints are used to prevent infants or small children from flexing their elbows to touch or scratch a surgical incision or skin lesion, e.g., eczema. See Figure 24–10. This restraint consists of a piece of material with pockets into which plastic or wooden tongue depressors are inserted to provide rigidity. After the restraint is applied, it is sometimes pinned to the child's shirt to prevent it from sliding down the arm.

The **mummy restraint** is a special folding of a blanket or sheet around the child to prevent movement during a procedure such as gastric washing, eye irrigation, or collection of a blood specimen. A **crib net** is simply a net placed over the top of a crib to prevent active young children from climbing out of the crib. At the same time, it allows them freedom to move about in the crib.

When using restraints, the nurse may find the guidelines in the accompanying box helpful.

Excessive noise is a health hazard that can cause hearing loss, depending on the overall level of noise, the frequency range of the noise, and the duration of exposure and individual susceptibility. Sound levels above 120 decibels (units of loudness) are painful and may cause hearing damage even if a person is exposed for only a short period. Exposure to 85 to 95 decibels for several hours a day can lead to progressive or permanent hearing loss. Noise levels below 85 decibels usually do not affect hearing.

Tolerance of noise is largely individual. The rural dweller may find the city noisy, whereas the city dweller may be oblivious to urban sounds. Adults often find teenager's music uncomfortably loud. Noise has psychosocial effects, such as feelings of annoyance, disrupted sleep and relaxation, and interruption of thought and conversation patterns. Noise can also interfere with job performance and safety.

The ill and injured are frequently sensitive to noises that normally would not disturb them. Loud voices, the clatter of dishes, and even a nearby television can disturb clients, some of whom react angrily. Physiologic effects of noise include:

■ Increased heart and respiratory rates

■ Increased muscular activity

■ Nausea

■ If the noise is sufficiently loud, hearing loss

Noise can be minimized in several ways. Acoustic tile on ceilings, walls, and floors as well as drapes and carpeting absorb sound. Background music can mask noise and have a calming effect on some people. It is important for nurses to minimize noise in the hospital setting and to encourage clients to protect their hearing as much as possible.

Radiation as a health hazard is a recent source of concern. Nurses are concerned specifically with those radioactive materials used in diagnostic and therapeutic practices. Radiation injury can occur from overexposure or from exposure to radiation that treats specific tissues and at the same time injures other tissues.

Radioactive materials are used in diagnostic procedures such as radiography, fluoroscopy, and nuclear medicine. In nuclear medicine, radioactive isotopes that

GUIDELINES

Restraints

■ Assure the client and the client's support persons that the restraint is temporary and protective. A restraint must never be applied as punishment for any behavior or merely for the nurse's convenience.

■ Apply the restraint in such a way that the client can move as freely as possible without defeating the purpose of the restraint.

■ Ensure that limb restraints are applied securely but not so tightly that they impede blood circulation to any body area or extremity.

■ Pad bony prominences (e.g., wrists and ankles) before applying a restraint over them. The movement of a restraint without padding over such prominences can quickly abrade the skin.

■ Always tie a limb restraint with a knot, e.g., a clove hitch that will not tighten when pulled.

■ Tie the ends of a body restraint to the part of the bed that moves when the head is elevated. Never tie the ends to a side rail or to the fixed frame of the bed if the bed position is to be changed.

■ Assess the restrained client every hour or more frequently as needed. Some facilities have specific forms to be used to record ongoing assessment.

■ Remove most limb restraints at least every 4 hours, and provide range-of-motion (ROM) exercises (see Chapter 35) and skin care (see Chapter 34).

■ For elderly clients, remove restraints more often, e.g., every 2 hours, to maintain blood circulation and mobility of the joints.

■ When a restraint is temporarily removed, do not leave the client unattended.

■ Immediately report to the responsible nurse and record on the client's chart any persistent reddened or broken skin areas under the restraint.

■ At the first indication of cyanosis or pallor, coldness of a skin area, or a client's complaint of a tingling sensation, pain, or numbness, loosen the restraint and exercise the limb.

■ Apply a restraint so that it can be released quickly in case of an emergency and with the body part in a normal anatomic position.

■ Provide emotional support verbally and through touch.

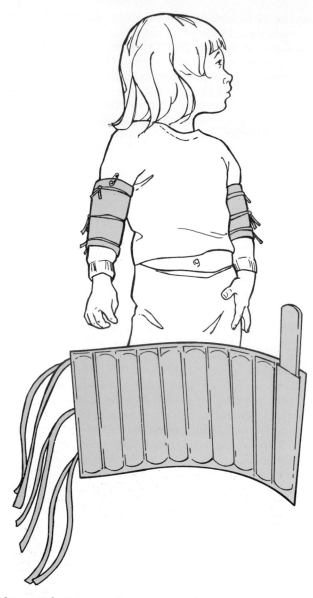

Figure 24—10 An elbow restraint for a young child

have an affinity for specific tissues are given by mouth or intravenously. Isotopes of these elements are used:

- Calcium, which has an affinity for bones
- Iodine, which is attracted to the thyroid gland
- Phosphorus, which is attracted to blood

Radioactive materials are provided in sealed sources and unsealed liquid sources. For example, cobalt implants are sealed; iodine 131 and phosphorus 32 are unsealed liquids. Principles governing the degree of exposure to radiation are as follows:

- The longer the time in the presence of radiation, the greater the exposure.
- The closer a person is to the radioactive source, the greater the exposure.

- The more extensive the use of lead and other radiation shields, the greater the protection against radiation.

Often nurses help care for clients treated or diagnosed with radioactive substances. The client diagnosed through radiography or fluoroscopy generally receives minimal exposure, and few precautions are necessary. The nurse restraining a small child during radiography needs to wear a lead apron. Clients with radioactive implants are a source of radiation to the immediate environment. The nurse who is in close contact with such clients also needs to wear a lead apron.

It is important to deal safely with radioactive body discharges. Nurses wear rubber gloves and in some instances may place excreta in containers for special disposal. It is also important that the nurse's gloved hands be washed well before and after the gloves are removed and that contaminated materials be placed in a special container for disposal.

Hospitals in which radioactive materials are used usually have a radioisotope committee. This committee establishes policies and procedures to be used in the care of clients who receive radioactive materials. It is important that nurses be cognizant of these policies.

One important aspect of caring for clients receiving radiation treatment is making sure they understand the treatment and the precautions they need to take. Often such clients are restricted to bed or to a confined area to protect others. These clients need emotional support to deal with the precautions and will likely accept treatments and precautions better when they know what will happen, when, and why.

Evaluating the Effectiveness of Selected Strategies

After implementing measures to prevent or correct injuries, disease, and hazards, the nurse evaluates the effectiveness of those measures. To do so, the nurse refers back to the goals selected and compares the client's current status (reassessment) to specified outcome criteria indicating that the goals had been met. Examples of outcome criteria for clients with potential for injury and sensory disturbance are shown in the accompanying box.

Chapter Highlights

The provision of a safe external environment is a constant concern of the nurse.

Education is a major health protection strategy in preventing accidents and infectious disease.

When planning to meet safety needs of clients, nurses need to consider physical factors in the environment and the psychologic and physiologic state of the individual.

Nursing assessment of the clients at risk includes assessment of age, life-style, sensory-perceptual alterations, level of awareness, mobility, emotional

OUTCOME CRITERIA

Potential for Injury and Sensory Disturbances

The client will:

- Identify potential environmental hazards.
- Identify measures to avoid falls.
- Identify safety adaptations for home health maintenance.
- Implement safety measures to prevent trauma.
- Sleep for 6 hours without awakening.
- Verbalize feelings of well-being.
- Know the day of the week and place when questioned.
- Expresses interest in watching television.
- Read for 1 hour using new glasses.
- Walk safely to the bathroom and back.
- Talk while using hearing aid.

state, language barriers, history of previous accidents, and knowledge and use of safety precautions.

Nursing diagnoses for clients at risk of accidental injury can be categorized as potential for injury.

Nursing diagnoses for clients with sensory disturbances may include visual, auditory, and taste deficits as well as sensory overload.

Nursing intervention must include education in accident prevention and modification of the environment to make it safe.

Nurses must be familiar with the fire procedures in their employing agency.

In the event of a fire, the nurse must protect clients from injury and contain and put out the fire.

Falls are a common cause of injury among the elderly and the ill or injured.

To prevent falls, the nurse must carefully assess older clients' safety needs.

Side rails and handrails protect hospitalized clients from falls; restraints keep clients from falling and from inflicting injuries on themselves and others.

Because restraints restrict a client's basic freedom to move, careful assessment and accurate, complete documentation are important when restraints are used.

Prolonged exposure to excessive noise can produce hearing loss.

In hospitals, radioactive substances are used for both diagnostic and treatment purposes; agency policy should be followed to safeguard clients and staff from inadvertent exposure.

Because of their diminished sensory acuity and balance, elderly people need to make the home safe. They also need education about ways to prevent automobile and pedestrian accidents.

Selected References

Barbieri, E. B. March 1983. Patient falls are not patient accidents. *Journal of Gerontological Nursing* 9:164–73.

Berger, M. E., and Hubner, K. F. August 1983. Hospital hazards: Diagnostic radiation. *American Journal of Nursing.* 83:1155–59.

Burnside, I. M. 1981. Falls: A common problem in the elderly. In Burnside, I. M., editor. *Nursing and the aged.* 2d ed. New York: McGraw-Hill.

Campbell, E. B.; Williams, M. A.; and Mlynarczyk, S. M. February 1986. After the fall: Confusion. *American Journal of Nursing* 86:151–53.

Friedman, F. B. January 1983. Restraints: When all else fails, there still are alternatives. *RN* 46:79–80, 82, 84.

Gray-Vickrey, M. May/June 1984. Education to prevent falls. *Geriatric Nursing* 5:179–83.

Hernandez, M., and Miller, J. March/April 1986. How to reduce falls. *Geriatric Nursing* 7:97–102.

Jackson, M. M.; Dechairo, D. C.; and Gardner, D. F. February 1986. Perceptions and beliefs of nursing and medical personnel about needle-handling practices and needle stick injuries. *American Journal of Infection Control* 14:1–10.

Lee, P. S., and Pash, B. J. February 1983. Preventing patient falls. *Nursing 83* 13:118, 120 (Canadian edition, pp. 14–15).

Louis, M. March 1983. Falls and their causes. *Journal of Gerontological Nursing* 9:142–56.

McLane, A. M. et al. 1986. *Proceedings of Sixth National Conference.* St. Louis. C. V. Mosby Co.

Nursing guidelines for the use of restraints in nonpsychiatric settings. March 1983. *Journal of Gerontological Nursing* 9:180–81.

Riffle, K. L. May/June 1982. Falls: Kinds, causes, and prevention. *Geriatric Nursing* 3:165–69.

Wyatt, D. M. February 1985. Are you prepared for a hospital fire? *Nursing 85* 15:51.

Yarmesch, M., and Sheafor, M. July/August 1984. The decision to restrain. *Geriatric Nursing* 5:242–44.

Promoting Health

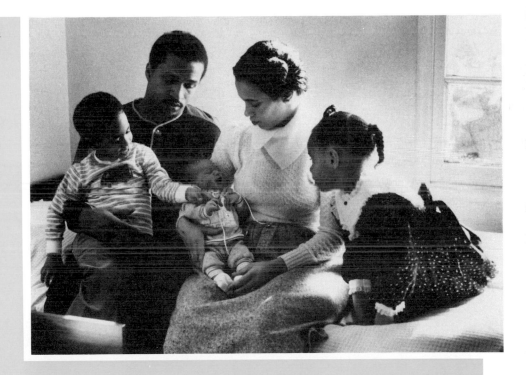

CHAPTER 25

Health Promotion

OBJECTIVES

Describe the concept of health promotion.

Give examples of various types of health promotion programs.

Compare the focus of promoting health to the focus of traditional health care

Identify components of a health promotion assessment.

State types of data to be included in a health history.

Describe ways to assess physical fitness.

List data used to assess nutritional status.

Describe health risk appraisals.

Give the purpose of life-style assessment tools.

Identify steps in the planning stage of health promotion.

List ways of enhancing behavioral change.

Explain modeling and the importance of the nurse as a role model.

Identify desired outcomes of health promotion interventions.

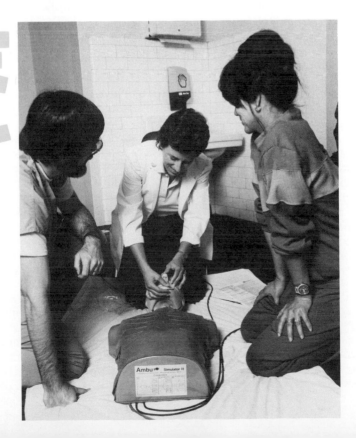

Concept and Scope of Health Promotion

Health promotion is a part of primary health care and prevention. The underlying principles of health promotion are twofold:

1. Regardless of a person's health, the quality of life can be increased.
2. Wellness involves all components of life that affect well-being.

Most health promotion activities or strategies are nonspecific; they are geared toward raising the general level of health and well-being of an individual, family, or community. Activities include stress management, nutrition education, weight control, life-style modification, and organized physical activity programs. Other primary prevention strategies are directed toward the prevention of a specific disease, e.g., using vaccines to produce immunity against communicable diseases such as poliomyelitis. Other specific protection strategies include stop-smoking clinics, purification of public water supplies, and the wearing of helmets by motorcyclists (Moore and Williamson 1984, p. 197).

Health promotion organizations and programs differ from traditional health care centers and programs that focus on illness or specific disease entities and health problems. Opatz (1985, p. 59) outlines the following **types of health promotion programs**:

1. Evaluation/screening programs that provide health risk appraisals and hypertension and multiphasic screenings as well as wellness inventories, fitness and stress evaluations, and diet analyses.
2. Educational/motivation programs to provide health risk appraisal interpretations through health/wellness fairs, wellness lectures, alcohol/drug awareness programs, teaching breast and testicular self-examination, nutrition education, and fitness/weight control.
3. Behavior change (participatory) programs such as aerobic exercise classes, running clubs, stress-management training sessions, smoking-cessation programs, back-strengthening exercise classes, self-care skills programs, blood pressure and pulse monitoring, nutrition modification, weight reduction, and career evaluation and goal-setting programs.
4. Organizational enhancement programs such as those that promote eating healthy foods, air quality management, smoking policies and enforcement, personnel policies (e.g., sick leave), professional development, worksite stress assessments, and employee assistance programs.

Health Assessment

A thorough assessment of the client's health status is basic to health promotion. Components of this assessment may include the health history and physical examination, physical-fitness assessment, nutrition assessment, health risk appraisal, and life-style assessment. As nurses move toward greater autonomy in providing client care, expanded assessment skills are essential to provide the meaningful data needed for health planning.

The **health history and physical examination** provide a means for detecting any existing problems. See Chapter 32 for detailed information about the health history and physical examination. Health histories need to include the following information (Edelman and Mandle 1986, p. 52): demographic data, current and past medical problems, family medical history, surgical and (if appropriate) obstetric history, childhood illnesses, allergies, current medications, psychologic status, social history, environmental background, and review of systems.

During an evaluation of **physical fitness**, the nurse takes girth and skinfold measurements, administers the step test, and assesses strength and endurance of muscles and flexibility of joints. When obtaining **girth measurements,** the nurse measures the girth of the chest, waist, hips, upper arm (biceps), thigh, calf, and ankle. Table 25–1 lists girth measurements.

Skinfold measurements indicate the amount of body fat. To take skinfold measurements, the nurse grasps the skinfold (skin layers and subcutaneous fat) between the thumb and forefinger and measures the skinfold with special calipers. Skinfold sites are the triceps, subscapula, suprailiac, and thigh. For the **step test,** the client steps up and down a 17-inch step for 3 minutes. The following movements constitute one step: left foot up, right foot up, left foot down, right foot down. The rate should be 24 steps per minute for women and 30 steps for men (Getchell 1979, pp. 72–73). After the test, the client sits in a chair while the nurse assesses the pulse rate for 30 seconds at prescribed intervals:

1. 1 to 1 1/2 minutes after the test
2. 2 to 2 1/2 minutes after the test
3. 3 to 3 1/2 minutes after the test

The sum of these three 30-second pulse rates is referred to as the **recovery index.** Normal values for women are 154–170; for men, 149–165 (Getchell 1979, pp. 72–73).

There are several tests of **muscle strength and endurance.** One is performing sit-ups with knees bent (bent-knee sit-ups). Women are asked to do these for 1 minute; men, for 2 minutes. The average rate for women is about 20 to 25 sit-ups per minute; for men, 50 to 60 per 2 minutes (Getchell 1979, p. 56).

Joint flexibility can be assessed quickly by asking the person to touch his or her toes several times. The average touch point is 1 to 3 inches in front of the toes. See Chapter 35 for detailed discussion of joint range of motion.

To assess **nutritional status,** the nurse compares the client's weight to body build and height, measures mid-upper arm circumference to determine muscle mass, observes for signs of malnutrition, and takes a dietary history. Nutrition is discussed in detail in Chapter 39.

A **health risk appraisal** (HRA) is an assessment and educational tool that indicates a client's risk of dis-

Table 25–1 Girth Measurements

	Males	Females
Chest or bust	Same size as hips	Same size as hips
Waist	About 13 to 18 cm less than chest	About 25 cm less than bust
Upper arm	Twice the wrist size	Twice the wrist size
Thigh	20 to 25 cm less than abdomen	15 cm less than abdomen
Calf	18 to 20 cm less than thigh	15 to 18 cm less than thigh
Ankle	15 to 18 cm less than calf	13 to 15 cm less than calf

Source: N.J. Pender, *Health promotion in nursing practice* (Norwalk, Conn.: Appleton-Lange, 1982), p. 87. Used by permission

ease or injury by comparing the client's risk with the mortality risk of his or her age, sex, and racial group. The principle behind risk appraisal is that each person, as a member of a specific group, faces certain quantifiable health hazards and that average risks are applicable to a client if the health professional knows the client's characteristics and the mortality of a large group of cohorts with similar characteristics (Pender 1982, p. 97). An HRA may have from 25 to 300 or more questions. Clients either score their responses themselves or send them to an organization for computer printouts. Scores are often tabulated according to an overall life-style profile, levels of health risk, and life expectancy.

Risk factors may be categorized according to: age, genetic factors, biologic characteristics, personal health habits, life-style, and environment. Clients cannot control some of the risk factors appraised, such as age, sex, and family history; others, such as blood pressure, stress, and cigarette smoking, can be partially or totally controlled.

A client is considered at high risk for developing a specific disease when two or three of the risk factors are at the highest level or four of the risk factors are at the two highest levels. Computer analysis of the client's responses to the questions may be used to predict the person's life expectancy, which may then be compared to the life expectancy of the average person of the client's age, race, and sex. The HRA analysis can also indicate an achievable life expectancy for the client, predicated on the assumption that the client will reduce all possible risk factors.

Life-style assessment focuses on the personal life-style and habits of the client as they affect health. Categories of life-style generally assessed are physical activity, nutritional practices, stress management, and such habits as smoking, alcohol consumption, and drug use. Other categories may also be included. The purposes of using life-style assessment tools are:

1. To provide an opportunity for clients to assess the impact of their present life-style on their health
2. To provide a basis for decisions related to desired behavior and life-style change

Nursing Diagnoses for Health Promotion

Nursing diagnoses related to health promotion often involve potential rather than actual health problems. Examples are shown in the accompanying box.

Planning to Promote Health

Following assessment, the client and nurse have a great deal of information about the client's health status, health risks, life-style, and health beliefs. Health promotion plans need to be developed according to the desires of the client, who decides on goals, priorities, sequencing, methods, and implementation (Black and McDowell 1984, p. 20). The nurse acts as a resource person rather than as an adviser or counselor. She or he provides information when asked, emphasizes the importance of small steps to behavioral change, and reviews the client's goals and plans to make sure they are realistic, measurable, and acceptable to the client.

NURSING DIAGNOSIS

Health Promotion

- Potential alterations in nutrition (more than body requirements) related to sedentary life-style
- Potential alteration in nutrition (less than body requirements) related to inappropriate eating patterns (e.g., unscheduled meals and eating fast foods)
- Ineffective individual coping related to stress and unsatisfactory support system
- Potential alteration in health maintenance related to substance abuse (tobacco)
- Potential alteration in health maintenance related to lack of appropriate immunization
- Potential alteration in health maintenance related to knowledge deficit about parenting
- Potential alteration in health maintenance related to knowledge deficit about breast self-examination
- Potential for injury related to lack of awareness of environmental hazards and acceptance of declining physical capabilities
- Potential alterations in oral mucous membrane related to inadequate oral hygiene
- Diversional activity deficit related to postretirement inactivity
- Impaired social interaction related to self-concept disturbance secondary to obesity
- Impaired adjustment related to alterations in cardiac function requiring change in life-style

Pender (1982, p. 178) outlines **nine steps in the process of health planning**, which is carried out jointly by the nurse and client:

1. *Review and summarize assessment data.* The nurse and client need to consider:
   - Any existing health problems
   - The degree of control the client thinks he or she exerts over his or her health status
   - Level of physical fitness and nutritional status
   - Illnesses for which the client is at risk
   - Current positive health practices
   - Ability to handle stress
   - Information needed to enhance health care practices

   Nonjudgmental awareness of present attitudes, activities, and behaviors is the first step to behavior change.

2. *Identify health care strengths.* Areas of strength, such as flossing teeth daily, eating breakfast daily, and being able to laugh at oneself, need to be acknowledged and supported. Recognition of strengths enhances self-awareness and self-esteem and makes the client aware of what he or she is controlling.

3. *Identify health care goals and areas for improvement.* Interventions necessary to decrease the risk of developing specific diseases are often a concrete starting point for many clients. Interventions for health promotion, a less tangible concept, are often recognized later, as is the concept of high-level wellness.

4. *Identify possible behavior changes.* For each of the selected goals or areas in step 3, determine what specific behavioral changes are needed to bring about the desired outcome. For example, to reduce the risk of cardiovascular disease, the client may decide to:
   - Stop smoking
   - Lose weight
   - Increase activity level
   - Learn to relax
   - Decrease animal fat in diet
   - Discontinue use of oral contraceptives
   - Sleep 7 to 8 hours per night

5. *Assign priorities to behavior changes.* Behavior must be acceptable to the client if it is to be adopted and integrated. From the list of behavior options in step 3, the client selects and assigns priorities to those changes he or she is most willing to try. For example, the client may select increasing activity level, losing weight, and stopping smoking, in that order.

6. *Make a commitment to change behavior.* Motivation to follow through is provided by a positive reinforcement or reward specified in a self-contract or nurse-client contract. Before a contract can be made, the client needs to identify actions that will bring about the desired behavior change. If, for example, the behavior change is to increase activity level, the client may decide to swim for 30 minutes three times a week, walk briskly for 1 hour daily, or engage in some similar activity.

7. *Identify effective reinforcements and rewards.* Rewards tend to provide an incentive for behavior change, more so than individual willpower, provided the reward is meaningful to the client and selected by him or her. Rewards can be objects, experiences, family activities, or praise.

8. *Determine barriers to change.* Some specific barriers to change are:
   - Lack of support from family members
   - Lack of space to carry out a certain activity
   - Inappropriate weather
   - Lack of motivation
   - Fatigue or boredom
   - Strong anxiety
   - Cost of change
   - Inconvenience
   - Lack of time
   - Culture or peer pressure

9. *Develop a schedule for implementing the behavior change.* Time frames may be several weeks or months. Scheduling short-term goals and rewards can offer encouragement to achieve long-term objectives. Clients may need help to be realistic and to deal with one behavior at a time.

Another essential aspect of planning is **identifying support resources available** to the client. These may be community resources, such as a fitness program at a local gymnasium, or educational programs, such as stress management, breast self-examination, nutrition, smoking cessation, and health lectures. The nurse, too, may meet some of the client's educational needs. A major nursing role is to support the client. The nurse can contact the client or be available at specified intervals to review the contract and to assist with problem solving.

Implementing Strategies to Promote Health

Implementing is the "doing" part of behavior change. Although self-responsibility is emphasized for implementing the plans, ongoing support from the nurse, family members, and friends is an essential component of health promotion. The nurse also provides information and educational programs as required, assists the client to make and maintain behavior changes (behavior modification), and is a model of good health behaviors.

Health education programs on a variety of topics can be provided to groups, individuals, or communities. Group programs need to be carefully planned before they are implemented. The decision to establish a health promotion program must be based on the assessed health needs of the people; also, specific health promotion goals must be set. After the program is implemented, program outcomes must be evaluated.

Nurses may offer an abundance of information less formally. To do so, however, nurses need up-to-date knowledge, the ability to assess learning needs, and effective teaching skills. See Chapter 21 for detailed information. For example, nurses often disseminate information about parenting, breast and testicular self-examination, prevention of sexually transmitted disease, nutritional needs, and monitoring blood pressure and pulse rates.

Nurses focus plans on methods of **enhancing behavior changes**. Whether people make and maintain changes to improve health or prevent disease depends on many interrelated factors. Murphy (1982, p. 427) says that the distances between wanting to change, attempting to change, and being able to change can be enormous. She emphasizes this statement by pointing out the difficulty many people have in acquiring regular dental flossing habits. When a client succeeds in making healthy behavior changes because of information the nurse has provided, the nurse feels satisfied and pleased. When, however, the client does not succeed in planned behavioral changes, the nurse tends to feel frustrated and often describes the person as "resistant," "uninterested," "unmotivated," or "noncompliant." Murphy (1982) says that nurses are erroneously inclined to believe:

1. That change will occur simply by bringing unhealthy behavior to the client's attention
2. That when the client does not change, the desire to change is absent

The response of the nurse to lack of change in the client is generally to provide more information or to withdraw from the interaction after concluding that there is no point wasting time on people who do not want to change. Both responses deny the client the opportunity to improve his or her health. By providing more information to the client, the nurse assumes that the client lacks knowledge. If, however, the client has understood the information, repeating or amplifying the information more than likely will annoy the client. The nurse has failed to identify the problem clearly. Withdrawal from clients who have difficulty changing implies that the nurse's health promotion efforts will be directed toward persons who readily and willingly comply. Such people, however, are probably the ones who least need the nurse's help.

To enhance positive behavior changes in clients, the nurse needs to (Murphy 1982, p. 429):

1. Recognize that motivation is the basis of all behavior whether it is healthy or unhealthy, good or bad.
2. Recognize that people are motivated by their needs.
3. Avoid labeling people as unmotivated. The label simply means that the person does not comply with the wishes of the nurse who applies the label.
4. Focus on the sources or factors that motivate the person's behavior rather than on the presence or absence of motivation.
5. Remember that resistance is a normal part of change and a healthy response to a threat.
6. Understand that a client may choose to keep unhealthy habits for many reasons, e.g., culture, lack of knowledge, misconceptions, other activities that interfere with the client's ability to change, or lack of necessary conditions for a change in behavior.

7. Cast aside the idea that the client *must* change. This attitude is not conducive to a helping relationship with the client and does not convey respect for the client. The client who does not change is entitled to the nurse's interest and nonjudgmental response.
8. Measure the nurse's competence in terms of how well the nurse understands the client's needs and implements the client's care rather than by the extent to which a client changes his or her behavior.

Modeling consists of observing the behavior of people who have successfully achieved the goal that the client has set for himself or herself (Pender 1982, p. 216). Modeling is not imitating. Through observing a model, the client acquires ideas for behavior and coping strategies for specific problems. The client is not expected to mimic the sequence of actions or behavior patterns of the model.

The nurse and client should mutually select models with whom the client can identify, since the cultural and ethnic backgrounds of the nurse and client often differ. Models should be frequently available during the early learning and change stages of unfreezing and moving. Models should also be people the client respects.

Nurses should serve as models of wellness. Carlin (1982, p. 48) strongly believes that the philosophy nurses manifest in their lives affects their professional effectiveness more than the philosophy they preach. Nurses, therefore, need to assess their own wellness and initiate changes as required before becoming a model for clients. Clients are more likely to respect and trust the nurse who can tell them what worked for her or him.

Evaluating Health Promotion Strategies

The process of evaluating involves measurement of the client's progress or lack of progress toward goal achievement. Evaluation is a collaborative effort between the nurse and client. Progress or lack of progress is determined by the goals or outcome criteria specified in the client's contract. It may be necessary to reassess, reorder priorities, set new goals, or revise the contract. The outcomes of health promotion are increased levels of health not only among individuals but also among families and communities. The expected outcomes of nursing interventions directed toward promoting health include (Pender 1982, p. 8):

1. Increased levels of health and well-being among individuals, families, and communities
2. Decreased incidence of illness and disability in individuals
3. Increased personal competence to minimize the barriers that prevent personal growth and fulfillment
4. Improvement in the abilities of clients or families to make rational health-related decisions
5. Self-care competence of clients

6. Increased ability of clients to assess personal or family needs for professional health care
7. Judicious use of all types of health care services
8. Greater availability and convenience of health-promoting as opposed to health-damaging options
9. Greater prevalence of health-promoting personal and family life-styles

Chapter Highlights

Health promotion is part of primary health care and prevention.

Health promotion activities are directed toward developing client resources that maintain or enhance well-being.

The goal of health promotion is to raise the client's level of health.

Health promotion programs can be categorized as evaluation/screening programs, educational/motivational programs, behavior change (participatory) programs, and organizational enhancement programs.

A thorough assessment of the client's health status is basic to health promotion.

Health risk or hazard appraisals provide the data that often spur the client to adopt a healthier life-style.

Life-style assessment tools give clients the opportunity to assess the impact of their present life-styles on their health and to make decisions about life-style changes.

To help clients change their life-styles or health behaviors, the nurse provides ongoing support, supplies additional information and education, and explores the motivating sources of the client's behavior.

By acting as models of wellness, nurses show clients what goals to strive for.

Selected References

Alexy, B. September/October 1985. Goal setting and health risk reduction. *Nursing Research* 34:283–88.

Black, A., and McDowell, R. April 1984. Health styles: Moving beyond disease prevention. *The Canadian Nurse* 80:18–20.

Carlin, D. C. March/April 1982. How to assess your wellness—and become a model for your patients. *Nursing Life* 2:48–49.

Chalmers, K., and Farrell, P. July 1985. Lifestyle counselling: The need for diagnostic clarity. *Journal of Advanced Nursing* 10:311–13.

Cox, C. L. May/June 1985. The health self-determinism index. *Nursing Research* 34:177–83.

Edelman, C., and Mandle, C. L. 1986. *Health promotion throughout the life span.* St. Louis: C. V. Mosby Co.

Faber, M. M., and Reinhardt, A. M. 1982. *Promoting health through risk reduction.* New York: Macmillan Co.

Frachel, R. R. June 1984. Health hazard appraisal: Personal and professional implications. *Journal of Nursing Education* 23:265–67.

Getchell, B. 1979. *Physical fitness: A way of life.* 2d ed. New York: John Wiley and Sons.

Moore, P. V., and Williamson, G. C. June 1984. Health promotion: Evolution of a concept. *Nursing Clinics of North America* 19:195–206.

Murphy, M. M. November/December 1982. Why won't they shape up? Resistance to the promotion of health. *Canadian Journal of Public Health* 73:427–30.

Neuman, J.; Sloss, G. S.; and Andersen, S. July/August 1984. Evaluation of a health program. *Geriatric Nursing* 5:234–38.

Opatz, J. P. 1985. *A primer of health promotion: Creating healthy organizational cultures.* Washington, D.C.: Oryn Publications.

Pender, N. J. June 1975. A conceptual model for preventive health behavior. *Nursing Outlook* 23:385–90.

———. 1982. *Health promotion in nursing practice.* Norwalk, Conn.: Appleton-Century-Crofts.

Rosenstock, I. M. 1974. Historical origins of the health belief model. In Becker, M. H., editor. *The health belief model and personal health behavior.* Thorofare, N.J.: Charles B. Slack.

26

Concepts of Growth and Development

OBJECTIVES

Differentiate growth, development, and maturation.

Describe factors that influence growth and development.

Describe the stages of growth and development.

Describe specific growth trends.

Discuss selected theories of psychosocial, cognitive, moral, and spiritual development.

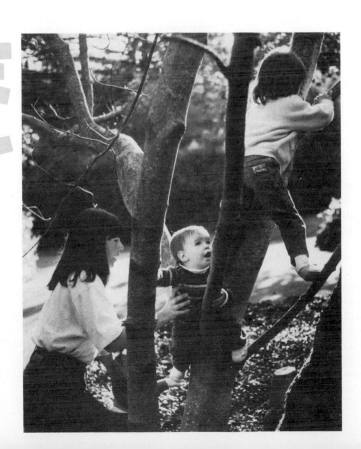

Growth, Development, and Maturation

The terms *growth* and *development* both refer to dynamic processes. Often used interchangeably, these terms have different denotations. **Growth** is physical change and increase in size. Growth can be measured. Indicators of growth include height, weight, bone size, and dentition. **Development** is an increase in the complexity of function and skill progression (Mott et al. 1985, p. 132). It is the capacity and skill of a person to function. Development is the behavioral aspect of growth; for example, a person develops the ability to walk, to talk, and to run. Growth and development are independent, interrelated processes. For example, an infant's muscles, bones, and nervous system must grow to a certain point before the infant can sit up or walk. Growth generally takes place during the first 20 years of life; development continues after that.

Maturation refers to the development of inherited characteristics, such as stature. **Maturation** is the sequence of physical changes that are related to genetic influences (Mott et al. 1985, p. 132). Maturation is independent of the environment, but its timing can be influenced by environmental factors. For example, inadequate nutrition can delay walking and growth.

The rate of a person's growth and development is highly individual; however, the sequence is predictable. **Stages of growth** usually correspond to certain **developmental** changes. See Table 26–1. It is generally accepted that those aspects of growth and development that are not determined genetically are influenced by the environment. Growth and development occur throughout life, although they are more apparent at certain periods, e.g., during adolescence, than at other times.

Factors Influencing Growth and Development

The factors that influence growth and development are both genetic and environmental. Theorists assign different importance to the respective roles of heredity and environment. The genetic inheritance of an individual is established at conception. This genetic inheritance remains unchanged throughout life. **Genetic inheritance** determines such characteristics as sex, physical stature, and race.

Many **environmental factors** affect an individual's growth and development. Some of these are family, religion, climate, culture, school, community, and nutrition. For example, a poorly nourished child is more likely to have infections than a well-fed child is and may not attain his or her full height potential.

Whether one favors heredity, environment, or an interactive approach (i.e., an interrelationship between heredity and environment) to understanding growth and development, some basic principles are commonly accepted. These are summarized in the accompanying box.

Physiologic Growth and Development

Physiologic growth and development refers to an individual's physical size and body functioning. The pattern of physiologic growth is similar for all people. However, growth rates vary during different stages of growth and development. See Table 26–1. For example, the growth rate is very rapid during the prenatal, neonatal, infancy, and adolescent stages. The growth rate slows during childhood, and physical growth is minimal during adulthood. Table 26–2 gives an overview of physiologic growth trends from the prenatal stage to older adulthood.

Psychosocial Development

Psychosocial development refers to the development of personality. It includes feelings, subjective experiences, and interactions with others. **Personality** can be considered as the outward (interpersonal) expression of the inner (intrapersonal) self. It encompasses a person's temperament, feelings, character traits, independence, self-esteem, self-concept, behavior, abil-

PRINCIPLES

Growth and Development

- Growth is a continuous process determined by many factors.
- All humans follow the same pattern of growth and development.
- The sequence of each stage is predictable, although the time of onset, the length of the stage, and the effects of each stage vary with the person.
- Learning can either help or hinder the maturational process, depending on what is learned.
- Each developmental stage has its own characteristics.
- Growth and development occur in a cephalocaudal direction, i.e., starting at the head and moving to the trunk, the legs, and the feet.
- Growth and development occur in a proximal to distal direction, i.e., from the center of the body outward.
- Growth and development become increasingly differentiated (e.g., an infant's initial response to a stimulus involves the total body; a 5-year-old responds more specifically).
- Certain stages of growth and development are more critical than others.

Table 26-1   Stages of Growth and Development

Stage	Age	Significant Characteristics	Nursing Implications
Prenatal	Conception to birth	During 9 months, all significant body systems develop. Inherited factors, maternal health and age are significant.	Help mothers develop strategies to establish a suitable environment for healthy fetal growth.
Neonatal	Birth to 28 days	Behavior is largely reflexive and develops to more purposeful behavior.	Assist parents to identify and meet unmet needs.
Infancy	1 month to 1 year	Physical growth is rapid.	Control the infant's environment so that physical and psychosocial needs are met.
Toddlerhood	1 to 3 years	Motor development permits increased physical autonomy. Psychosocial skills increase.	Safety and risk-taking strategies must be balanced to permit growth.
Preschool	3 to 6 years	The preschooler's world is expanding. New experiences and the preschooler's social role are tried during play. Physical growth is slower.	Provide opportunities for play and social activity.
School age	6 to 12 years	Stage includes the preadolescent period (10 to 12 years). Peer group increasingly influences behavior. Physical, cognitive, and social development increases, and the child has increased competence in communication.	Allow time and energy for the school-age child to pursue hobbies and school activities.
Adolescence	12 to 20 years	Self-concept changes with biologic development. Values are tested. Physical growth accelerates. Stress increases, especially in face of conflicts.	Assist adolescents to develop coping behaviors. Help adolescents develop strategies for resolving conflicts.
Young adulthood	20 to 40 years	A personal life-style develops. Person establishes a relationship with a significant other, a commitment to something, and competence (White, 1975).	Accept adult's chosen life-style and assist with necessary adjustments relating to health. Recognize the person's commitment and the function of competence in life. Support change as necessary for health.
Middle adulthood	40 to 65 years	Life-style changes because of other changes, e.g., children leave home, occupational goals change.	Assist clients to plan for anticipated changes in life, to recognize the risk factors related to health, and to focus on strengths rather than weaknesses.
Older adulthood	65 years and over	Adaptation to changing physical abilities is often necessary. Chronic illness may develop.	Assist clients to cope with loss, e.g., hearing, eyesight, death of loved one. Provide necessary safety measures. Assist clients to maintain peer group interactions.

ity to interact with others, and ability to adapt to life changes. Two commonly recognized theorists who have attempted to explain the psychosocial development of humans are Freud and Erikson.

Freud

Sigmund Freud, whose writings and research were very popular in the 1930s, introduced a number of concepts about development that are still used today. The concepts of the unconscious mind, defense mechanisms, and the id, ego, and superego are Freud's. The **unconscious mind** is the mental life of a person of which the person is unaware. This concept of the unconscious is one of Freud's major contributions to the field of psychiatry. **Defense mechanisms,** or **adaptive mechanisms** as they are more commonly called today, are the result of conflicts between inner impulses and of the anxiety that attends these conflicts. The **id** is the source of instinctive and unconscious urges, which Freud considers chiefly sexual in nature. The id is also the source of all pleasure and gratification. The **ego** is formed by

the person to make effective contact with these social and physical needs. Through the ego, the id impulses are satisfied. The third aspect of the personality, according to Freud, is the **superego.** This is the conscience of the personality, a control on the id. The superego is the source of feelings of guilt, shame, and inhibition. Freud proposed that the underlying motivation to human development is an energy form or life instinct, which he called **libido.**

According to Freud's theory of psychosexual development, the personality develops in five overlapping stages from birth to adulthood. The libido changes its location of emphasis within the body from one stage to another. Therefore, a particular body area has special significance to a client at a particular stage. See Table 26-3. If the individual does not achieve a satisfactory resolution at each stage, the personality becomes fixated at that stage. **Fixation** is immobilization or the inability of the personality to proceed to the next stage because of anxiety.

The first three stages (oral, anal, and phallic) are called the pregenital stages. During the first stage, the

Table 26—2 Growth Trends Throughout Life

Systemic Changes	Prenatal	Neonatal	Infancy	Toddlerhood	Preschool
		Heart and Circulatory System			
During life, the heart is responsive to organ needs and emotional responses.	Heart is formed and begins to beat about third week.		Heart grows more slowly than the rest of the body. ———————		
	Heart rate is approximately 150 beats/min.		Heart rate falls throughout childhood, is 130 beats/min. in infancy.		
		Urinary System			
Development generally parallels the growth of the body. Proportion of body fluids and solids follows pattern related to growth. Proportion of fluid tends to decrease with age.	Fetus is approximately 90% fluid. Urinary system begins in the first month.	Newborn is 70% fluid Renal units are immature. Fluid imbalance occurs readily.	Urinary system is completely developed at end of first year.		
		Gastrointestinal System			
System is responsive to physiologic needs and stress.	Nutrients are supplied through the placental circulation.	Size of stomach increases rapidly during first months. Salivary glands are small.		Stomach size grows ——————— steadily throughout childhood. Salivary glands mature at 2 years.	
			Gastric acidity is low.	Gastric acidity rises in childhood.	
		Senses			
	Senses start to develop at 3 to 6 weeks.	Most senses are well developed at birth.	Eye muscles are fully functioning. Infant perceives simple differences in shape.	Hyperopia increases until eyeball reaches adult size at 8 years.	
		Adipose Tissue			
	Fat accumulates rapidly, peaks at 7 months.	Fat gain increases rapidly during first 6 months.		Fat decreases from age 1 to age 6 or 7. ——————— Tends to be chubby.	
		Lymphoid Tissue			
	Lymphoid tissue begins to grow in ninth month.	Immune system is immature.	System develops rapidly during infancy and childhood. ———————		
		Respiratory System			
	Air sacs in lungs do not contain air; oxygen supplied through maternal circulation.	Starts breathing at birth.			
		Respiratory rate is high in infancy, slows through childhood. ———————			
		Skeletal System			
	70% of head growth occurs before birth.		Trunk grows the most rapidly.		There is a rapid growth spurt.

(continued)

School Age	Adolescence	Young Adulthood	Middle Adulthood	Older Adulthood

Heart and Circulatory System

| | There is a growth spurt during prepuberty. Heart reaches mature size by 16 years. Heart rate is approximately 60 beats/min. | Heart weight remains relatively constant throughout life. Cardiac output decreases 30% to 40% between 25 and 65 years. Cardiac power decreases with age. Capacity to increase rate and strength with physical activity decreases with age. | | |

Urinary System

| | | Adult is 58% fluid. Glomular filtration rate decreases about 47% from age 20 years to 90 years. | | |

Gastrointestinal System

| | Organs have widely varying functional maturity. | Metabolism, enzyme production, HCl production decrease after age 30 years. | | Salivation diminishes. |
| Acidity plateaus at 10 years. | Gastric acidity rises in puberty | | | |

Senses

| | There is a trend toward myopia until 30 years. | | Myopia decreases and hyperopia increases. Lack of normal pain response may occur. | |

Adipose Tissue

| | | There is tendency to gain weight in 50s and 60s. | | Fat stores often lost during 70s. |
| | | From 25 to 75 years fat increases by 16%, and fluid decreases by 8%. | | |

Lymphoid Tissue

| | | Lymphoid tissue mass is smaller in adulthood. | | |
| Immune system is functionally mature. | | | | |

Respiratory System

| | Vital capacity increases with increased stature. | | | Lung tissue becomes more rigid. |

Skeletal System

| Growth slows. Growth spurt in girls starts at about 10 years; in boys, about 13 years. Growth is greater in boys. | | Maximum height is reached by 30s. | Height declines gradually, 1.2 cm every 20 years. | |
| | | | Bone mass begins to decrease from 40 years. | Shortening of spinal column caused by thinning vertebrae. |

(continued)

Table 26–2 continued

Systemic Changes	Prenatal	Neonatal	Infancy	Toddlerhood	Preschool
		Muscular System			
Muscle size varies considerably among individuals.	Muscles begin to assume shape by 2 months.		Muscle size increases rapidly.	Neuromuscular control increases. Abdomen protrudes until abdominal muscles develop.	Muscle size increases slowly.
		Reproductive System			
	Genital organs are formed.	Female sex organs are formed. Male sex organs (testes) are formed but dormant.	System is nonfunctional during childhood. ──────────		
		Nervous System			
	Growth is very rapid.	Temperature regulating system is poorly developed.	Infant has the total number of brain cells by first year. Brain grows rapidly.	Brain cells increase in size and in number and complexity of axons and dendrites.	
		Endocrine System			
		System is immature at birth. Adrenal glands decrease in ─────────────→ size throughout first year.		Adrenal gland size increases during childhood.	
		Integumentary System			
	Hair, skin, and sebaceous glands are fully formed in utero.	Skin contains all structures but is immature in function.		Most children have all deciduous teeth by second year.	Child begins to lose deciduous teeth.
	Lanuga begins to ─────────────→ decrease.				
		Immune System			
		System is immature at birth.			

Sources: Adapted from D. C. Sutterly and G. F. Donnelly, *Perspectives in human development: Nursing throughout the life cycle* (Philadelphia: J. B. Lipppincott Co., 1973); C. Edelman and C. L. Mandle, *Health promotion throughout the lifespan* (St. Louis: C. V. Mosby, 1986); P. Ebersole

mouth is the principal source of pleasure, primarily as a result of eating. Feelings of dependence arise in the oral stage, and they tend, according to Freud, to persist throughout life. A person who is fixated at the oral stage may have difficulty trusting others and may demonstrate such behaviors as nail biting, drug abuse, smoking, overeating, alcoholism, argumentativeness, and overdependency. The *anal stage* occurs when the child is learning toilet training. Fixation at this stage can result in obsessive-compulsive personality traits such as obstinance, stinginess, cruelty, and temper tantrums.

During the *phallic phase,* sexual and aggressive feelings associated with the genitals come into focus. Masturbation offers pleasure at this time, and the child experiences the Oedipus or Electra complex. The **Oedipus complex** refers to the male child's attraction for his mother and his hostile attitudes toward his father. The **Electra complex** is the female child's attraction for her father and her hostility toward her mother. Fixation at the phallic phase can result in such traits as problems with sexual identity and problems with authority.

During the *latency stage,* sexual impulses tend to be repressed. Unresolved conflict at this stage may be reflected in obsessiveness and lack of self-motivation. Following latency come adolescence and the reactivation of the sexual impulses. The person usually displaces these impulses and subsequently passes into the final

School Age	Adolescence	Young Adulthood	Middle Adulthood	Older Adulthood
		Muscular System		
Muscle strength is greater in boys at puberty. →		Muscles reach maximum strength between 20 to 30 years.	Muscle growth continues in proportion to use.	Atrophy and loss of muscle tone.
		Reproductive System		
→ System is mature at puberty with menstruation. At puberty, testes and penis increase in size.			Involution occurs after menopause. Uterus reaches maximum weight at 30 years.	
		Sex drive is active throughout maturity and may subside only during last decade.		
		Nervous System		
→		Brain weight decreases with age. →		
Brain reaches 90% adult				Myelin sheath decreases.
		Endocrine System		
	There is growth spurt of adrenal glands. Basal metabolic rate increases.	Adrenal glands mature with body.		There is a decrease in function of all endocrine glands.
		Integumentary System		
	There is growth spurt of all structures. Hair distribution changes. Sebaceous gland activity increases.	Skin becomes drier with age.		Skin elasticity and moisture decrease.
		Immune System		
System is functionally mature.				Immune system effectiveness possibly declines.

and P. Hess, *Toward healthy aging: Human needs and nursing response* (St. Louis: C. V. Mosby Co., 1985); and C. A. Schuster and S. S. Ashburn, *The process of human development: A holistic approach* (Boston: Little, Brown and Co., 1980).

stage of adult maturity, the *genital stage*. The inability to resolve conflicts during this stage can result in sexual problems.

Erikson

Erik H. Erikson adapted Freud's theory of development. Erikson describes eight stages of development. He expands the work of Freud to include the entire life span, believing that people continue to develop throughout life. In contrast to Freud, Erikson considers the ego to be the core of the personality. See Table 26–4.

Erikson envisions life as a sequence of levels of achievement. Each stage signals a task that must be achieved. The resolution of the task can be complete, partial, or unsuccessful. Erikson believes that the greater the task achievement, the healthier the personality of the person; failure to achieve a task influences the person's ability to achieve the next task. The developmental tasks can be viewed as a series of crises, and successful resolution of these crises is supportive to the person's ego. Failure to resolve the crises is damaging to the ego. After attaining one stage, a person may fall back and need to approach it again.

Erikson's eight stages reflect both positive and negative aspects of the critical life periods. The resolution of the conflicts at each stage enables the person to function effectively in society. Each phase has its developmental task, and the individual must find a balance between, for example, trust versus mistrust (stage 1) or generativity versus stagnation (stage 7).

Table 26–3 Freud's Five Stages of Development

Stage	Age	Characteristics	Implications
Oral	0 to 1 year	Mouth is the center of pleasure.	Feeding produces pleasure and sense of comfort and safety. Feeding should be pleasurable and provided when required.
Anal	2 and 3 years	Anus and rectum are the centers of pleasure.	Controlling and expelling feces provide pleasure and sense of control. Toilet training should be a pleasurable experience, and appropriate praise can result in a personality that is creative and productive.
Phallic	4 and 5 years	The child's genitals are the center of pleasure.	The child identifies with the parent of the opposite sex and later takes on a love relationship outside the family. Encourage identification.
Latency	6 to 12 years	Energy is directed to physical and intellectual activities.	Encourage child with physical and intellectual pursuits.
Genital	13 years and after	Energy is directed toward attaining a mature heterosexual relationship.	Encourage separation from parents, achievement of independence, and making decisions.

Source: Adapted from Patricia H. Miller, *Theories of developmental psychology.* Copyright © 1983. W. H. Freeman and Company.

When using Erikson's developmental framework, nurses should assess client data that indicate positive or negative resolution of each stage. Erikson considers the environment to be highly influential in personality development. Nurses can enhance people's development by being aware of the current developmental stage, by providing opportunities for the individual to resolve his or her developmental task, and by helping the person develop coping skills relative to stressors experienced at that level.

Erikson emphasizes that people must change and adapt their behavior to maintain control over their lives. In his view, no stage in personality development can be bypassed, but people can become fixated at one stage or regress to a previous stage. For example, a middle-aged woman who has never satisfactorily accomplished

Table 26–4 Erikson's Eight Stages of Development

Stage	Age	Central Task	Indicators of Positive Resolution	Indicators of Negative Resolution
Infancy	Birth to 18 months	Trust versus mistrust	Learning to trust others Sense of trust in self	Mistrust, withdrawal, estrangement
Early childhood	18 months to 3 years	Autonomy versus shame and doubt	Self-control without loss of self-esteem Ability to cooperate and to express oneself	Compulsive self-restraint or compliance Willfulness and defiance
Late childhood	3 to 5 years	Initiative versus guilt	Learning the degree to which assertiveness and purpose influence the environment Beginning ability to evaluate one's own behavior	Lack of self-confidence Pessimism, fear of wrongdoing Overcontrol and overrestriction of own activity
School age	6 to 12 years	Industry versus inferiority	Beginning to create, develop, and manipulate Developing sense of competence and perseverance	Loss of hope, sense of being mediocre Withdrawal from school and peers
Adolescence	12 to 20 years	Identity versus role confusion	Coherent sense of self Plans to actualize one's abilities	Confusion, indecisiveness, and inability to find occupational identity
Young adulthood	18 to 25 years	Intimacy versus isolation	Intimate relationship with another person Commitment to work and relationships	Impersonal relationships Avoidance of relationship, career, or life-style commitments
Adulthood	25 to 65 years	Generativity versus stagnation	Creativity, productivity, concern for others	Self-indulgence, self-concern, lack of interests and commitments
Maturity	65 years to death	Integrity versus despair	Acceptance of worth and uniqueness of one's own life Acceptance of death	Sense of loss, contempt for others

Sources: Adapted from E. H. Erikson, *Childhood and society,* 2d ed. (New York: W. W. Norton & Company, 1963). Used by permission of W. W. Norton & Company, Inc. Copyright © 1950, 1963 by W. W. Norton & Company, Inc. Copyright renewed 1978 by Erik H. Erikson.

the task of resolving identity versus role confusion might regress to an earlier stage when stressed by an illness with which she cannot cope.

Cognitive Development

Cognitive development refers to the manner in which people learn to think, reason, and use language. It involves a person's intelligence, perceptional ability, and ability to process information. Cognitive development represents a progression of mental abilities from illogical to logical thinking, from simple to complex problem solving, and from understanding concrete ideas to under-standing abstract concepts. The most widely known cognitive theorist is Jean Piaget (1896–1980). His theory of cognitive development has contributed to other theories, such as Kohlberg's theory of moral development and Fowler's theory of the development of faith, both discussed in this chapter.

According to Piaget, cognitive development is an orderly, sequential process in which a variety of new experiences (stimuli) must exist before intellectual abilities can develop. Piaget's cognitive developmental process is divided into five major phases: the sensori-motor phase, the preconceptual phase, the intuitive phase, the concrete operations phase, and the formal operations phase. Each phase has its own unique characteristics. See Table 26–5.

Table 26–5 Piaget's Phases of Cognitive Development

Phases and Stages	Age	Significant Behavior
Sensorimotor	Birth to 2 years	
Stage 1 Use of reflexes	Birth to 1 month	Most action is reflexive.
Stage 2 Primary circular reaction	1 to 4 months	Perception of events is centered on the body. Objects are extension of self.
Stage 3 Secondary circular reaction	4 to 8 months	Acknowledges the external environment. Actively makes changes in the environment.
Stage 4 Coordination of secondary schemata	8 to 12 months	Can distinguish a goal from a means of attaining it.
Stage 5 Tertiary circular reaction	12 to 18 months	Tries and discovers new goals and ways to attain goals. Rituals are important.
Stage 6 Inventions of new means	18 to 24 months	Interprets the environment by mental image. Uses make-believe and pretend play.
Preconceptual	2 to 4 years	Uses an egocentric approach to accommodate the demands of an environment. Everything is significant and relates to "me." Explores the environment. Language development is rapid. Associates words with objects.
Intuitive thought	4 to 7 years	Egocentric thinking diminishes. Thinks of one idea at a time. Includes others in the environment. Words express thoughts.
Concrete operations	7 to 11 years	Solves concrete problems. Begins to understand relationships such as size. Understands right and left. Cognizant of viewpoints.
Formal operations	11 to 15 years	Uses rational thinking. Reasoning is deductive and futuristic.

Source: Adapted from Jean Piaget, *The Origin of intelligence in children.* (Madison, CT: International Universities Press, Inc.) Copyright © 1966, International Universities Press, Inc.

In each phase, the person uses three primary abilities: assimilation, accommodation, and adaptation. **Assimilation** is the process through which humans encounter and react to new situations by using the mechanisms they already possess. In this way, people acquire new knowledge and skills as well as insights into the world around them. **Accommodation** is a process of change whereby cognitive processes mature sufficiently to allow the person to solve problems that were unsolvable before. This adjustment is possible chiefly because new knowledge has been assimilated. **Adaptation,** or coping behavior, is the ability to handle the demands made by the environment.

Nurses can employ Piaget's theory of cognitive development when developing teaching strategies. For example, a nurse can expect a toddler to be egocentric and literal; therefore, explanations to the toddler should focus on the needs of the toddler rather than on the needs of others. Further, a 13-year-old can be expected to use rational thinking and to reason; therefore, when explaining the need for a medication, a nurse can outline the consequences of taking and not taking the medication, enabling the adolescent to make a rational decision. Nurses must remember, however, that the range of normal cognitive development is very broad, despite the ages arbitrarily associated with each level. When teaching adults, nurses may become aware that some adults are more comfortable with concrete thought and slower to acquire and apply new information than other adults are.

Moral Development

Moral development involves learning what ought to be and what ought to be done. It is more than imprinting parents' rules and virtues or values upon children. The term **moral** means relating to right and wrong. Distinctions need to be made between the terms *morality, moral behavior,* and *moral development.* **Morality** refers to the requirements necessary for people to live together in society; **moral behavior** is the way a person perceives those requirements and responds to them; **moral development** is the pattern of changes in moral behavior with age (White 1975).

Kohlberg

Lawrence Kohlberg suggests three levels of moral development that encompass six stages (Berkowitz and Oser 1985, p. 28). Like Piaget, he focuses on the reasons for the making of a decision, not on the morality of the decision itself. At Kohlberg's first level, called the premoral or preconventional level, children are responsive to cultural rules and labels of good and bad, right and wrong. However, children interpret these in terms of the physical consequences of their actions, i.e., punishment or reward. At the second level, the conventional level, the individual is concerned about maintaining the expectations of the family, group, or nation and sees this as right. The emphasis at this level is conformity and loyalty to one's own expectations as well as society's.

Level three is called the postconventional, autonomous, or principled level. At this level, people make an effort to define valid values and principles without regard to outside authority or to the expectations of others. For additional information about Kohlberg's levels, see Table 26–6.

With reference to Kohlberg's six stages, Munhall writes that stage four, the "law and order" orientation, is the dominant stage of most adults (Munhall 1982, p. 14). It is recognized that there is a difference in action between nurses who act at the conventional level (level II) and those who act at the postconventional or principled level (level III). As conventional thinkers, nurses base perceptions of moral obligations and rights on the maintenance of the social system and loyalty to established institutions and social groups. However, the postconventional nurse understands that societies and social relationships can be arranged in many ways, and that these different ways can maximize or minimize values (Munhall 1982, p. 13). Therefore, the nurse at level III questions authority and follows social norms as long as they support human values.

Gilligan

Carol Gilligan (1982), after more than 10 years research with women subjects, found that women often considered the dilemmas which Kohlberg used in his research to be irrelevant. Women scored consistently lower on Kohlberg's scale of moral development, in spite of the fact they approached moral dilemmas with considerable sophistication. Gilligan believed that most moral frameworks do not include the concepts of caring and responsibility. Yet it is from these frameworks that most research in moral development is done. The result is that emphasis upon individualism and autonomy is central to most moral development theories.

Gilligan believes women see morality in the integrity of relationships and caring, so that the moral problems they encounter are different from those of men. Men consider what is right to be what is just, whereas for women what is right is taking responsibility for others as a self-chosen decision (Gilligan 1982, p. 140).

Gilligan and Murphy, in their studies of postcollege adults, found that these adults began to doubt whether it is possible to construct generalized rules about right and wrong. They found these people evolving a rather new way of thinking in which change and process are primary features of reality. They see contradictions as acceptable and not needing resolution at all costs (Kegan 1982, p. 229).

Spiritual Development

The **spiritual** component of growth and development refers to the relationship individuals understand they have with the universe, and their perceptions about the direction and meaning of life. James Fowler describes the development of faith in people. Fowler believes that faith, or the spiritual dimension, is a force that gives

Table 26-6 Kohlberg's Stages of Moral Development

Level and Stage	Definition	Example
Level I **Preconventional**		
Stage 1: Punishment and obedience orientation	The activity is wrong if one is punished, and the activity is right if one is not punished.	A nurse follows a physician's order so as not to be fired.
Stage 2: Instrumental-relativist orientation	Action is taken to satisfy one's needs.	A client in hospital agrees to stay in bed if the nurse will buy him a newspaper.
Level II **Conventional**		
Stage 3: Interpersonal concordance (good boy, nice girl)	Action is taken to please another and gain approval.	A nurse gives elderly clients in hospital sedatives at bedtime because the night nurse wants all clients to sleep at night.
Stage 4: Law and order orientation	Right behavior is obeying the law and following the rules.	A nurse does not permit a worried client to phone home because hospital rules stipulate no phone calls after 9:00 P.M.
Level III **Postconventional**		
Stage 5: Social contract, legalistic orientation	Standard of behavior is based on adhering to laws that protect the welfare and rights of others. Personal values and opinions are recognized, and violating the rights of others is avoided.	A nurse arranges for an East Indian client to have privacy for prayer each evening.
Stage 6: Universal-ethical principles	Universal moral principles are internalized. Person respects other humans and believes that relationships are based on mutual trust.	A nurse becomes an advocate for a hospitalized client by reporting to the nursing supervisor a conversation in which a physician threatened to withhold assistance unless the client agreed to surgery.

Source: Ronald Duska and Mariaellen Whelan, Adapted from *Moral development: A guide to Piaget and Kohlberg.* Copyright © 1975 by The Missionary Society of St. Paul the Apostle in the State of New York. Used by permission of Paulist Press.

meaning to a person's life. Fowler uses the term *faith* as a form of knowing, a way of being in relation to "an ultimate environment" (Fowler and Keen 1978). To Fowler, **faith** is a relational phenomenon; it is "an active 'mode-of-being-in-relation' to another or others in which we invest commitment, belief, love, risk and hope" (Fowler and Keen 1978). Fowler's stages in the development of faith are given in Table 26-7.

Fowler's theory and developmental stages were influenced by the work of Piaget, Kohlberg, and Erikson. Fowler believes that the development of faith is an interactive process between the person and the environment. In each of Fowler's stages, new patterns of thought, values, and beliefs are added to those already held by the individual; therefore the stages must follow in sequence. Faith stages, according to Fowler, are separate from cognitive stages of Piaget. Faith stages evolve from a combination of knowledge and values.

Chapter Highlights

Growth and development are independent, interrelated processes.

Growth is physical change and increase in size. The pattern of physiologic growth is similar for all people.

Development is an increase in the complexity of function and skill progression.

Maturation refers to the sequence of physical changes that is primarily related to genetic influences.

The rate of a person's growth and development is highly individual, but the sequence of growth and development is predictable.

Heredity and environment are the primary factors influencing growth and development.

Components of growth and development are generally categorized as physiologic, psychosocial, cognitive, moral, and spiritual.

Table 26–7   Fowler's Stages of Spiritual Development

Stage	Age	Description
0. Undifferentiated	0 to 3 years	Infant unable to formulate concepts about self or the environment.
1. Intuitive-projective	4 to 6 years	A combination of images and beliefs given by trusted others, mixed with the child's own experience and imagination.
2. Mythic-literal	7 to 12 years	Private world of fantasy and wonder; symbols refer to something specific; dramatic stories and myths used to communicate spiritual meanings.
3. Synthetic-conventional	Adolescent or adult	World and ultimate environment structured by the expectations and judgments of others; interpersonal focus.
4. Individuating-reflective	After 18 years	Constructing one's own explicit system; high degree of self-consciousness.
5. Paradoxical-consolidative	After 30 years	Awareness of truth from a variety of viewpoints.
6. Universalizing	Maybe never	Becoming an incarnation of the principles of love and justice.

Source: Adapted from J. Fowler and S. Keen, *Life maps: Conversations in the journey of faith* (Waco, Texas: Word Books, 1978); and A. Hollander, *How to help your child have a spiritual life: A parents' guide to inner development* (New York: A and W Publishers, 1980). Used by permission.

■ Each developmental stage has its own characteristics and unique problems.

■ A progression of sequential steps or tasks is proposed in most theories, so that successful achievement of tasks is required in early stages before success can be achieved with later tasks.

■ The nurse's major role in relation to growth and development is to assess the client's growth and development using the standards proposed in these theories, and to plan and implement nursing strategies that will maintain or promote the client's development.

■ Selected References

Berkowitz, M. W., and Oser, F., editors. 1985. *Moral education: Theory and application.* Hillsdale, N.J.: Lawrence Erlbaum.

Bloom, M. 1985. *Life span development: Basis for preventive and interventive helping.* 2d ed. New York: Macmillan Co.

Duska, R., and Whelan, M. 1975. *Moral development: A guide to Piaget and Kohlberg.* New York: Paulist Press.

Ebersole, P., and Hess, P. 1985. *Toward healthy aging: Human needs and nursing response.* 2d ed. St. Louis: C. V. Mosby Co.

Engel, G. L. 1962. *Psychological development in health and disease.* Philadelphia: W. B. Saunders Co.

Erikson, E. H. 1963. *Childhood and society.* 2d ed. New York: W. W. Norton and Co.

———. 1964. *Insight and responsibility: Lectures on the ethical implications of psychoanalytic insight.* New York: W. W. Norton and Co.

———. 1985. *The life cycle completed: A review.* New York: W. W. Norton and Co.

Fowler, J., and Keen, S. 1978. *Life maps: Conversations in the journey of faith.* Waco, Texas: Word Books.

Freud, S. 1961. *The ego and the id and other works* (Vol. 19, James Strachney, translator). London: Hogarth Press and the Institute of Psychoanalysis.

Gilligan, C. 1982. *In a different voice: Psychological theory and women's development.* Cambridge, Mass.: Harvard University Press.

Gress, L. D., and Bahr, R. T. 1984. *The aging person. A holistic approach.* St. Louis: C. V. Mosby Co.

Haber, J.; Leach, A. M.; Schudy, S. M.; and Sideleau, B. F. 1982. *Comprehensive psychiatric nursing.* 2d ed. New York: McGraw-Hill.

Hall, C. S., and Lindzey, G. 1970. *Theories of personality.* 2d ed. New York: John Wiley and Sons.

Havighurst, R. J. 1972. *Developmental tasks and education.* 3d ed. New York: David McKay Co.

Hersh, R. H.; Paolitto, D. P.; and Reimer, J. 1979. *Promoting moral growth from Piaget to Kohlberg.* New York: Longman.

Kegan, R. 1982. *The evolving self: Problem and process in human development.* Cambridge, Mass.: Harvard University Press.

Miller, D. H. 1983. *Theories of developmental psychology.* San Francisco: W. H. Freeman and Co.

Mott, S. R.; Fazekas, N. F.; and James, S. R. 1985. *Nursing care of children and families.* Menlo Park, Calif.: Addison-Wesley Publishing Co.

Munhall, P. L. June 1982. Moral development: A prerequisite. *Journal of Nursing Education* 21:11–15.

Peck, R. 1968. Psychological developments in the second half of life. In Neugarten, B. L. *Middle age and aging.* Chicago: University of Chicago Press.

Peters, R. S. 1981. *Moral development and moral behavior.* London: George Allen and Unwin, Publishers.

Piaget, J. 1963. *Origins of intelligence in children.* New York: W. W. Norton and Co.

Schulman, M., and Mekler, E. 1985. *Bringing up a moral child: A new approach for teaching your child to be kind, just, and responsible.* Reading, Mass.: Addison-Wesley Publishing Co.

Schuster, C. S., and Ashburn, S. S. 1980. *The process of human development: A holistic approach.* Boston: Little, Brown and Co.

Teung, A. G. 1982. *Growth and development: A self-mastery approach.* Norwalk, Conn.: Appleton-Century-Crofts.

Thompson, H. O., and Thompson, J. B. November 1984. Ethic learning to practice ethically synonymous with being a professional. *AORN Journal.* 40:778, 80, 82.

Watson, J. 1979. *Nursing: The philosophy and science of caring.* Boston: Little, Brown and Co.

CHAPTER 27

Infancy Through Adolescence

OBJECTIVES

Identify characteristic tasks at different stages of development during infancy, childhood, and adolescence.

Describe usual physical development throughout infancy, childhood, and adolescence.

Trace psychosocial development according to Erikson through infancy, childhood, and adolescence.

Explain changes in cognitive development according to Piaget throughout infancy, childhood, and adolescence.

Describe moral development according to Kohlberg throughout childhood and adolescence.

Describe spiritual development according to Fowler throughout childhood and adolescence.

Identify essential health promotion and protection activities to meet the needs of infants, toddlers, preschoolers, school-age children, and adolescents.

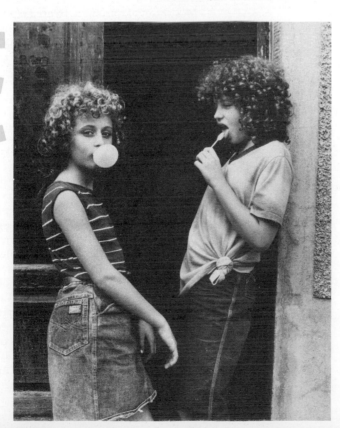

Infancy (Birth to 1 Year)

An infant's basic task is survival, which requires breathing, sleeping, sucking, eating, swallowing, digesting, and eliminating. Duvall (1977) outlines a number of developmental tasks for infants (see the accompanying box).

Physiologic Growth and Development

Infants undergo significant physiologic changes in these areas: weight, height, vital signs, head growth, vision, teeth, and motor development. Infants usually weigh twice their birth weight by 6 months and three times their birth weight by 12 months. By 6 months, they gain another 13.75 cm (5.5 in) of height. By 12 months, they add another 7.5 cm (3 in). Rate of increase in height is largely influenced by the baby's size at birth and by nutrition.

Pulse averages 120 beats per minute between 1 month and 11 months. Respirations are 20 to 40 breaths per minute at 1 year. Temperature at 1 year is 37.7 C (99.7 F). The mean blood pressure at 1 year is 96 mm Hg systolic and 65 mm Hg diastolic.

By 12 months, head circumference has increased about 33% over the birth size. The posterior fontanelle between the parietal bones and the occipital bone closes from 4 to 8 weeks after birth. The anterior fontanelle (between the frontal and parietal bones) closes between 10 and 18 months.

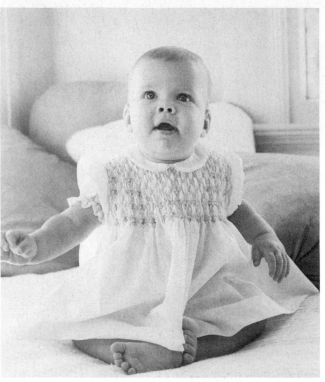

Figure 27–1 An infant sits without support at 6 months of age.

DEVELOPMENTAL TASKS

Infancy

- Establishing oneself as a very dependent being
- Beginning the establishment of self-awareness
- Developing a feeling for affection
- Becoming aware of the alive as against the inanimate, and the familiar as against the unfamiliar
- Developing rudimentary social interaction
- Beginning to adjust to the expectations of others
- Adjusting to adult feeding demands
- Adjusting to adult cleanliness demands
- Adjusting to adult attitudes toward genital manipulation
- Developing physiologic equilibrium
- Developing eye-hand coordination
- Establishing satisfactory rhythms of rest and activity
- Exploring the physical world
- Developing preverbal communication
- Developing verbal communication
- Forming rudimentary concepts

(Duvall 1977, pp. 172–75)

By 3 months, vision develops so that both eyes are coordinated both horizontally and vertically. At 4 months, the infant recognizes familiar objects and follows moving objects. At about 5 to 6 months, the infant's first teeth appear.

Motor development is an area of rapid advancement. By 2 months, infants can raise the head from a prone position, and by 6 months they can sit without support. See Figure 27–1. At 12 months, they can turn the pages of a book, walk with help, and help to dress themselves. See Table 27–1.

Psychosocial Development

According to Erikson, the central crisis at this stage is **trust versus mistrust.** Resolution of this stage determines how the person approaches subsequent developmental stages. An infant first learns trust from the parent or caregiver and then from others in the environment. Parents and caregivers can enhance a sense of trust by consistently responding promptly to an infant's needs and by providing a predictable environment in which routines are established.

Infants have no understanding of waiting and no time frame by which to measure waiting. The initial reaction of an infant to stress is crying, and crying is the infant's way of communicating distress. Infants learn gradually to tolerate stress. Nurses and parents can reduce the stress of an infant by maintaining the infant's routine as much as possible and limiting the number of strangers interacting with the infant.

Table 27–1 Motor and Social Development in Infancy

Age	Motor Development	Social Development
2 months	Lifts head off table when prone Turns from side to back Follows moving object with eyes	Recognizes familiar face Attends to speaking voice Social smile appears
3 months	Actively holds rattle Holds head erect Willfully places objects in mouth	Laughs aloud Shows pleasure in vocalization Smiles in response to mother's face Makes prelanguage vocalizations: coos and babbles
4 months	Holds head steady in sitting position Rolls from back to side and abdomen to back Grasps objects in two hands	Reaches out to people Squeals
5 months	Grasps objects with whole hand Plays with toes Rolls from stomach to back or vice versa	Discriminates between strangers and family Vocalizes displeasure when a desired object is removed Smiles at image in mirror
6 months	Lifts cup by handle Sits without support	Starts to imitate sounds Vocalizes one syllable sounds: *ma ma, da da* Plays peek-a-boo
7 months	Able to bear weight when held in standing position Bangs objects together Grasps toys with one hand	Shows fear of strangers Imitates simple acts
8 months	Feeds self with fingers Pulls toys	Is bashful and nervous with strangers Opens arms to be picked up Responds to *no*
9 months	Creeps and crawls Sucks, chews, and bites objects Handles cup or glass with help Pulls self to standing position Uses pincer grasp with thumb and forefinger	Cries when scolded Complies to simple verbal requests Displays fear of being alone, e.g., going to bed Waves bye-bye
10 months	Sits by falling Picks up objects Pulls self to standing position Stands if holding onto support	Aware of own name Presents toy to another person but will not release it
11 months	Pushes toys Puts objects into container Tries to walk unsupported Tries to hold spoon	Imitates speech sounds
12 months	Hand dominance manifested Walks with help Uses spoon to feed self	Knows own name Shakes head for *no* Does things to attract attention

Source: Adapted from C. Edelman and C. L. Mandle, *Health promotion throughout the life span* (St. Louis: C. V. Mosby Co., 1986), pp. 318–19. Reproduced by permission of the C. V. Mosby Co.

Psychosocial development can be assessed by observing the infant's behavior and by using standardized tests such as the **Denver Developmental Screening Test (DDST).** See Figure 27–2. The DDST is used to screen children from birth to 6 years of age. The test is intended to estimate the abilities of a child compared to those of an average group of children of the same age. The DDST does not provide diagnostic information about a child's problem, does not predict how a child will develop, and should not be used to assign a child to a developmental age group. Four main areas of development are screened: *personal-social, fine motor adaptive, language,* and *gross motor.* For each behavior, an age range is given that indicates whether 25%, 50%, 75%, or 90% of the children perform the task.

DDST manuals, kits, and scoring forms include directions for administering the test. The test is intended to be administered by professionals, such as nurses or psychologists. Usually, the child is asked to perform tasks of increasing difficulty. The child's performance is then scored according to the instructions.

Cognitive Development

Cognitive development involves remembering, thinking, perceiving, abstracting, and generalizing. It results in a logical method of looking at the world and using perceptual and conceptual abilities. *Intelligence,* by contrast, is the ability to learn.

According to Piaget, cognitive development is a result of interaction between an individual and the environment. Piaget refers to the initial period of cognitive development as the sensorimotor phase. See Table 26–5, page 357. This phase has six stages, three of which take place during the first year. From 4 to 8 months, infants

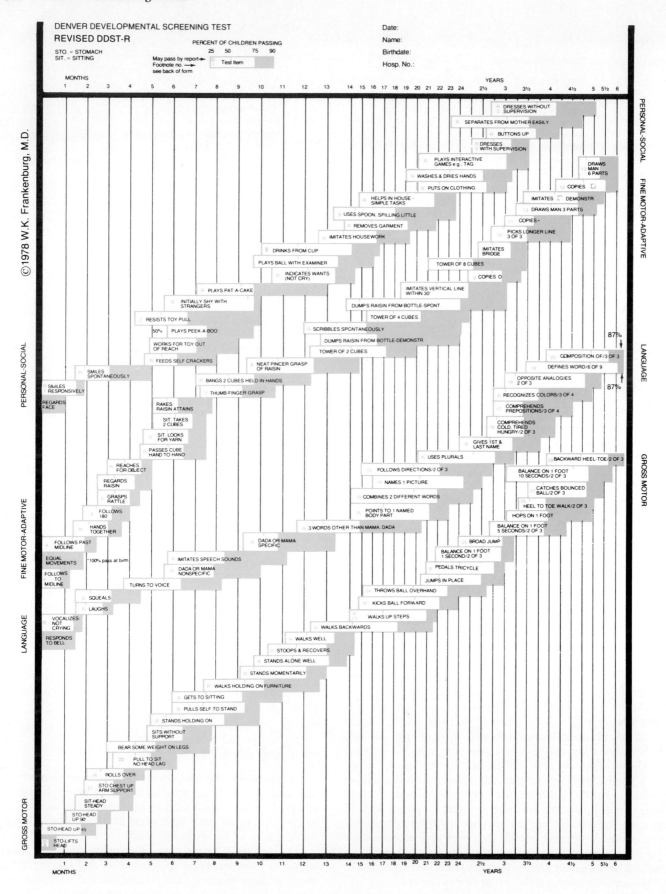

DENVER DEVELOPMENTAL SCREENING TEST
REVISED DDST-R

STO. = STOMACH
SIT. = SITTING

PERCENT OF CHILDREN PASSING
25 50 75 90

May pass by report →
Footnote no. →
see back of form

Date:
Name:
Birthdate:
Hosp. No.:

© 1978 W.K. Frankenburg, M.D.

1. Try to get child to smile by smiling, talking or waving to him. Do not touch him.
2. When child is playing with toy, pull it away from him. Pass if he resists.
3. Child does not have to be able to tie shoes or button in the back.
4. Move yarn slowly in an arc from one side to the other, about 6" above child's face.
   Pass if eyes follow 90° to midline. (Past midline; 180°)
5. Pass if child grasps rattle when it is touched to the backs or tips of fingers.
6. Pass if child continues to look where yarn disappeared or tries to see where it went. Yarn
   should be dropped quickly from sight from tester's hand without arm movement.
7. Pass if child picks up raisin with any part of thumb and a finger.
8. Pass if child picks up raisin with the ends of thumb and index finger using an over hand
   approach.

9. Pass any en-   10. Which line is longer?   11. Pass any   12. Have child copy
   closed form.   (Not bigger.) Turn   crossing   first. If failed,
   Fail continuous   paper upside down and   lines.   demonstrate
   round motions.   repeat. (3/3 or 5/6)

When giving items 9, 11 and 12, do not name the forms. Do not demonstrate 9 and 11.

13. When scoring, each pair (2 arms, 2 legs, etc.) counts as one part.
14. Point to picture and have child name it. (No credit is given for sounds only.)

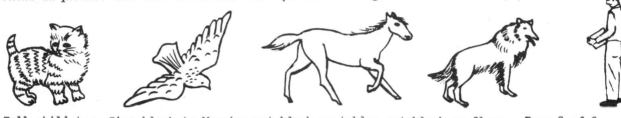

15. Tell child to: Give block to Mommie; put block on table; put block on floor. Pass 2 of 3.
    (Do not help child by pointing, moving head or eyes.)
16. Ask child: What do you do when you are cold? ..hungry? ..tired? Pass 2 of 3.
17. Tell child to: Put block <u>on</u> table; <u>under</u> table; <u>in front</u> of chair, <u>behind</u> chair.
    Pass 3 of 4. (Do not help child by pointing, moving head or eyes.)
18. Ask child: If fire is hot, ice is ?; Mother is a woman, Dad is a ?; a horse is big, a
    mouse is ?. Pass 2 of 3.
19. Ask child: What is a ball? ..lake? ..desk? ..house? ..banana? ..curtain? ..ceiling?
    ..hedge? ..pavement? Pass if defined in terms of use, shape, what it is made of or general
    category (such as banana is fruit, not just yellow). Pass 6 of 9.
20. Ask child: What is a spoon made of? ..a shoe made of? ..a door made of? (No other objects
    may be substituted.) Pass 3 of 3.
21. When placed on stomach, child lifts chest off table with support of forearms and/or hands.
22. When child is on back, grasp his hands and pull him to sitting. Pass if head does not hang back.
23. Child may use wall or rail only, not person. May not crawl.
24. Child must throw ball overhand 3 feet to within arm's reach of tester.
25. Child must perform standing broad jump over width of test sheet. (8-1/2 inches)
26. Tell child to walk forward, ⚬⚬⚬⚬⚬➔   heel within 1 inch of toe.
    Tester may demonstrate. Child must walk 4 consecutive steps, 2 out of 3 trials.
27. Bounce ball to child who should stand 3 feet away from tester. Child must catch ball with
    hands, not arms, 2 out of 3 trials.
28. Tell child to walk backward, ◀─⚬⚬⚬⚬⚬   toe within 1 inch of heel.
    Tester may demonstrate. Child must walk 4 consecutive steps, 2 out of 3 trials.

<u>DATE AND BEHAVIORAL OBSERVATIONS</u> (how child feels at time of test, relation to tester, attention
span, verbal behavior, self-confidence, etc,):

Figure 27–2 The Revised Denver Developmental Screening Test form and instructions. (Reprinted with permission of
W. K. Frankenburg, University of Colorado Medical Center.)

begin to have perceptual recognition. By 6 months, they respond to new stimuli, and they remember certain objects and look for them for a short time. By 12 months, infants have a concept of both space and time. They experiment to reach a goal, such as a toy on a chair.

An infant's cognitive development also proceeds from reflexive ability of the newborn to using one or two actions to attain a goal by the age of 1 year. Nurses can encourage an infant's cognitive development by providing a variety of sensory and motor stimuli. In addition, nurses can help parents understand an infant's future needs and what and how an infant communicates.

▪ Moral Development

Infants associate right and wrong with pleasure and pain. What gives them pleasure is right, since they are too young to reason otherwise. When infants receive abundant positive responses from the parent such as smiles, caresses, and voice tones of approval in these early months, they learn that certain behaviors are wrong or good and that pain or pleasure is the consequence. In later months and years, the child can tell easily and quickly by changes in parental facial expressions and voice tones that his or her behavior is either approved or disapproved. The less pleasure and more frustration the infant experiences in interactions with parents, the more important other sources of pleasure become. The child is then liable to risk parental anger and do things he or she likes and desires even though others disapprove.

▪ Health Promotion and Protection

During the first year, the infant's physical, psychosocial, and cognitive growth proceed at a rapid pace. The nurse's role is largely teaching parents or caregivers what the infant's needs are, how the infant communicates them, and how to meet them. To support rapid growth, food and fluid are extremely important during this stage. The key to infant nutrition is providing sufficient calories for growth but not so many that the infant becomes obese.

Infants usually receive only liquid nourishment until about 4 months of age, when solid foods are introduced. The nutritional needs of infants are initially met by breast milk or formula. The *fluid needs* of infants are proportionately greater than those of adults due to a higher metabolic rate, immature kidneys, and greater water losses through the skin and the lungs. The last is largely due to rapid respiration. Therefore, fluid balance is a critical factor. See Chapter 39 for additional information on nutrition.

Infants have immature temperature regulating systems: they perspire minimally, and shivering starts at a lower temperature than it does in adults; therefore, they lose more heat before shivering begins. In addition, because the infant's body surface area is very large in relation to body mass, the body also loses heat readily (Guyton 1986, p. 1003). Parents and caregivers must be aware of an infant's response to changes in environ-

mental temperatures. Infants must be dressed warmly in cold environments and lightly in hot ones.

Infants are nose-breathers until about 3 to 4 months of age, when they learn to breathe through their mouths. Therefore, an occluded nasal passage is a serious problem in a young infant. In the event of nasal congestion, parents and nurses should use a bulb syringe to remove mucus and keep the air passages patent.

Infants usually cannot control the elimination of urine or feces during the first year. Control is not established until the neuromuscular systems are sufficiently developed. Infants normally excrete 250 to 500 ml per day in increasing amounts during the first year. An infant may urinate as often as 20 times a day. A young infant will pass many stools in 24 hours, often after a feeding. Stools are usually soft, frequent, and even liquid because water is not well absorbed in the large intestine. It is important to keep infants clean and dry to prevent skin irritation.

Infants have longer periods of wakefulness than neonates do. Newborns usually sleep 17 hours daily, but periods of wakefulness gradually increase by the end of the first months. By 4 months, most infants sleep through the night and establish a pattern of daytime naps that varies among individuals. They generally awaken early in the morning, however. At the end of the first year, an infant usually takes one or two naps per day and sleeps about 14 of every 24 hours.

Accidents are the leading cause of morbidity and mortality among infants. Drowning, poisoning, suffocation, and falls are the most common accidents. For example, an unwatched baby may roll off a table; thus infants need careful watching even during ordinary activities. Parents often require assistance in identifying potential dangers in the home, and nurses in hospitals need to be actively involved in accident prevention.

Immunizations are needed to protect infants from the microorganisms causing diphtheria, pertussis, and tetanus. Immunization is provided in a combined diphtheria, tetanus toxoids, and pertussis (DTP) vaccine. Infants also require the orally administered poliomyelitis vaccine. Measles-rubella vaccine or a combined measles-mumps-rubella vaccine is recommended at age 1 year, as well as a tuberculin test to determine exposure to the tuberculosis bacillus. In some areas, smallpox vaccine is also given between the third and twelfth months.

Security needs of the infant are related to the development of trust. The parents or primary caregivers are usually the first people an infant trusts. Erikson believes the development of trust is basic to successful resolution of all other developmental crises. See Table 26–4, page 356.

An environment with a variety of sights, sounds, smells, tastes, and textures stimulates an infant's development. Speech development is enhanced by stimuli. Initially the infant coos, laughs, and imitates sounds. By 1 year, an infant usually can name some objects in the environment. See Table 27–1.

A young infant is not aware of his or her sex. Freud refers to this stage of psychosexual developmental as the oral phase. The parents' attitudes toward the sex of the child can affect their relationship with the infant. For example, parents who hoped for a girl but had a boy may find attachment and engrossment more difficult. Close *bonding* with parents or a caregiver is essential for healthy psychosocial development. This attachment is demonstrated by behaviors such as providing loving care, handling, stroking, and cuddling.

Infants who fail to establish a loving, responsive relationship with an adult often fail to develop normally. The disturbed parent-child relationship can result in the *failure-to-thrive syndrome.* The infants show delayed development without any physical cause. Another problem that can result from a disturbed parent-infant relationship is infant or child abuse. Abusing parents were often abused themselves as children.

Toddlers (1 to 3 Years)

Toddlers develop from having no voluntary control to being able both to walk and speak. They also learn to control their bladder and bowels, and they acquire all kinds of information about their environment. *Developmental tasks* for the toddler are shown in the accompanying box.

Physical Development

Toddlers are usually chubby with relatively short legs and a large head. See Figure 27–3. The face appears small in comparison to the skull; but as the toddler grows, the face seems to grow from under the skull and appears better proportioned.

Toddlers gain about 2 kg (5 lb) between 1 year and 2 years, weighing approximately four times their birth weight at age 2, and gain about 1 to 2 kg (2 to 5 lb) between 2 and 3 years. The 3-year-old weighs about 13.6 kg (30 lb). A toddler's height can be measured as height or length. Height is measured while the toddler stands, and length is measured while the toddler is in a recumbent position. Although the measurements differ only slightly, nurses must specify which measurement is used

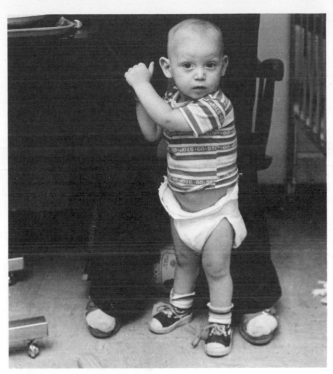

Figure 27–3 The toddler appears chubby with relatively short legs and a large head.

to avoid confusion. Between ages 1 and 2 years the average growth in height is 10 to 12 cm (4 to 5 in) and between ages 2 to 3 years it slows to 6 to 8 cm (2 1/2 to 3 1/2 in).

Toddlers are likely to have between 16 and 20 (all) of their deciduous teeth at 2 years of age. It is also during this period that the permanent teeth, with the exception of the second and third molars, begin to calcify. Visual acuity is fairly well established by 1 year; however, it is continually refined until the age of 6 years, when it becomes 20/20. Full binocular vision is usually established by 1 year. The senses of hearing, taste, smell, and touch become increasingly developed and associated with each other. Touch is a very important sense to the toddler. He or she is often soothed by tactile sensations. When toddlers are hospitalized or ill, it is often the nurse's function to cuddle, hold, or rock them.

Toddlers have a pronounced *lumbar lordosis* and a *protruding abdomen.* The abdominal muscles develop gradually as the toddler grows, and the abdomen flattens. *Fine muscle coordination* and *gross motor skills* improve during toddlerhood. At the age of 18 months, babies can pick up small beads and place them in a receptacle. They can also hold a spoon and a cup and walk upstairs with assistance. They will probably crawl down the stairs.

At 2 years, toddlers can hold a spoon and put it into the mouth correctly. They are able to run; their gait is steady; and they can balance on one foot and ride a tricycle. By 3 years, most children are toilet trained, although they still may have the occasional accident when playing or during the night.

DEVELOPMENTAL TASKS

Toddler (1 to 3 Years)

Erikson's stage: Autonomy vs. shame and doubt

- Achieving physiologic stability
- Learning to become physically independent while remaining emotionally dependent
- Expanding verbal communication
- Learning to control the elimination of body wastes
- Learning to coordinate large muscles and small muscles

Psychosocial Development

According to Freud, the ages of 2 and 3 years represent the *anal phase* of development, when the rectum and anus are the especially significant areas of the body. Erikson sees the period from 18 months to 3 years as the time when the central developmental task is autonomy versus shame and doubt. Nurses can assist parents and caregivers to help a toddler's development by suggesting the activities summarized in the accompanying box.

Toddlers begin to develop their sense of autonomy by asserting themselves with the frequent use of the word *no.* They are often frustrated by restraints to their behavior; between ages 1 and 3 children may have temper tantrums. However, they slowly gain control over their emotions, usually with the guidance of their parents.

The period of the development of a sense of autonomy (1 to 3 years) is a time of expanding social contacts. Toddlers are curious and ask many questions. Children at this age are often creative, although the products of this activity may not be perfect.

Common responses to stress are separation anxiety and regression. For example, toddlers who are stressed may become highly anxious when separated from their parents and admitted to hospital. Regression or reverting to an earlier developmental stage may be indicated by bed wetting or using baby talk. Nurses can assist parents by helping them understand that this behavior is normal and indicates that the toddler is trying to establish his or her position in the family. Toddlers assert their independence by saying no or by dawdling.

Most children learn to imitate words in the second year, when sufficient cortical maturity has taken place. By 2 years, they usually can arrange several words into a sentence. Three-year-olds speak almost constantly. They imitate adults and can express feelings, thoughts, desires, and problems in words.

Cognitive Development

According to Piaget, the toddler completes the fifth and sixth stages of the *sensorimotor phase* and starts the *preconceptual phase* at about 2 years of age. See Table 26–5 on page 357. In the fifth stage, the toddler solves problems by a trial-and-error process. By stage 6, toddlers can solve problems mentally. For example, when given a new toy, the toddler will not immediately handle the toy to see how it works but will look at it carefully to think about how it works.

During Piaget's preconceptual phase, toddlers develop considerable cognitive and intellectual skills. They learn about the sequence of time. They have some symbolic thought; for example, a chair may represent a place of safety, while a blanket may symbolize comfort. Concepts start to form in late toddlerhood. A concept develops when the child learns words to represent classes of objects or thoughts. An example of a concrete concept is *table,* representing a number of articles of furniture, which are all different but all tables.

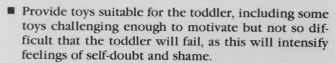

GUIDELINES

Fostering the Toddler's Development

- Provide toys suitable for the toddler, including some toys challenging enough to motivate but not so difficult that the toddler will fail, as this will intensify feelings of self-doubt and shame.

- Make positive suggestions rather than commands. Avoid an emotional climate of negativism, blame, and punishment.

- Give the toddler choices, all of which are safe; however, limit number to two or three.

- When toddler has a temper tantrum, make sure the child is safe and then leave.

- Help the toddler to develop inner control by setting and enforcing consistent, reasonable limits.

- Praise the toddler's accomplishments.

Moral Development

According to Kohlberg, the first level of moral development is the preconventional when children respond to labels of "good" or "bad" (see Table 26–6, page 359). During the second year of life, children begin to know that some activities elicit affection and approval. They also recognize that certain rituals, such as repeating phrases from prayers, also elicit approval. This provides children with feelings of security. By 2 years of age, toddlers are learning what attitudes their parents hold about moral matters.

Spiritual Development

According to Fowler, the toddler's stage of spiritual development is undifferentiated (see Table 26–7, page 360). Toddlers may be aware of some religious practices, but they are primarily involved in learning knowledge and emotional reactions rather than establishing spiritual beliefs. A toddler may repeat short prayers at bedtime, conforming to a ritual, because praise and affection result. This parental response enhances the toddler's sense of security.

Health Promotion and Protection

During their second and third years, toddlers require preventive health care. The American Academy of Pediatrics recommends regular health care visits during this period at 18, 21, 24, 30, and 36 months of age (American Academy of Pediatrics 1972). Assessment guidelines for growth and development of the toddler are shown in the accompanying box. Parents need reassurance that there are wide ranges of "normal" standards.

GUIDELINES

Assessing Toddlers

Does the toddler:

- Indicate physical development within normal range?
- Eat and drink appropriately?
- Feed self?
- Start to develop bowel and bladder control?
- Exhibit physical skills appropriate for his or her age?
- Express likes and dislikes or exhibit any other autonomous behavior?
- Imitate simple words and arrange several words into a sentence?
- Venture away from the mother?
- Begin to play and communicate with children and others outside the immediate family?
- Display curiosity and ask many questions?
- Imitate religious rituals of the family?

Providing adequate nutrition for a toddler can be a challenge. The daily caloric requirement may be only 1000 to 1500 kcal because of their slowed growth rate as compared to the rate of physical growth during the first year, but developing independence may be exhibited through the toddler's refusal of certain foods. Meals should be short because of the toddler's brief attention span and environmental distractions.

Because of a maturing gastrointestinal tract, toddlers can eat most foods and adjust to three meals each day. In addition, by age 3, when most of the deciduous teeth have emerged, the toddler is able to bite and chew adult table food. Toddler's manipulative skills are sufficiently well developed for them to learn how to feed themselves. Before the age of 20 months, most toddlers require help with glasses and cups because their wrist control is limited.

Parents and caregivers should be taught about nutritional needs of the toddler, eating patterns, and sizes of servings. (See Chapter 39 for further information.) A hospitalized toddler may regress for a period of time and want to be fed. Toddlers often display their liking of rituals by eating foods in a certain order, cutting foods a specific way, or accompanying certain foods with a particular drink. Entering hospital can disrupt a toddler's rituals and affect eating; therefore, nurses should consult with the parents to adapt to the toddler's food habits whenever possible.

The toddler is less likely to have fluid imbalances than the infant. Toddlers' gastrointestinal function is more mature, and the percent of fluid body weight is lower. A healthy toddler needs about 100 to 125 ml of liquid per kilogram of body weight per day (Smith et al. 1982, p. 211).

During the toddler's second or third year, bowel control becomes possible as the muscles and nervous system mature. Feces are firmer as a result of a more mature large intestine and increased fluid absorption from the intestinal contents into the bloodstream. Stools are less frequent than during infancy, and timing of defecation is evident.

Control of urinary elimination may also be achieved during toddlerhood. The bladder grows larger, with the average bladder of a 2-year-old holding about 80 ml (2 3/4 oz) of urine (Schuster and Ashburn 1980, p. 234). Increasingly, the toddler can remain dry during the day, thus facilitating toilet training. The urethra of female toddlers is less than 2 cm (0.8 in) long, predisposing them to urinary infections.

Total urinary control at night may not be achieved until preschool years. Toddlers admitted to hospital may regress in toilet training due to the stress of illness and hospitalization, the change in routine, and the unfamiliar environment, e.g., an unfamiliar potty chair. Nurses should consult with parents about the words a toddler uses to indicate the need to void or defecate and the routine used at home. Because of the possibility of urinary infections as well as skin irritation, toddlers should be kept clean and dry.

The sleep requirements of toddlers decrease to 10 to 14 hours per day. Most toddlers still need an afternoon nap, but the need for midmorning naps gradually decreases. Some toddlers have nightmares and need to be comforted and helped to differentiate between dreams and reality. Favorite toys can give toddlers a feeling of security, particularly at night.

As with infants, accidents are a leading cause of morbidity and mortality of toddlers. Drowning, poisoning, suffocation, and falls are the most common accidents. For example, a toddler may swallow liquid household cleaners if they are left in reach. Precautions need to be taken to keep medicines, cleaners, and the like out of the reach of toddlers. Parents may need to learn to lock cupboards or to place dangerous substances out of reach.

Immunizations continue to be an important aspect of safety. The toddler's immune system is now functioning and producing antibodies in response to various microorganisms in the environment. At 15 months, toddlers should receive rubeola, rubella, and mumps (MMR) vaccine; at 18 months, diphtheria, tetanus toxoids, and pertussis (DTP) vaccine as well as oral attenuated poliomyelitis virus (OPV) vaccine.

During early childhood, body temperature appears to be more *labile* than it is later, hence toddlers are likely to have very high fevers, e.g., 40 C (104 F), due to infections. The toddler, however, can respond to changes to the environmental temperature far better than the infant can, largely because of the growth and maturation of the blood capillaries. In response to changing temperatures, the toddler's body can increase or decrease the blood flow to surface capillaries, thereby increasing or decreasing heat loss (Guyton 1986, p. 854). A toddler with an infection or fever should be closely monitored for extreme fluctuations, which should be reported immediately to a nurse or physician.

Parents' attitudes toward the sex of the toddler influence both skills and attitudes. Parents usually encourage more independent behavior in boys; therefore, boys often venture farther and explore more than girls do. Boys are usually expected to achieve more than girls do. By 2 years, toddlers can categorize others as boys or girls and often have some awareness of physical differences.

Nurses can assist parents to understand the sexuality of their child and to be comfortable with their own sexual identities. In this way, parents can demonstrate affection and easily answer their child's questions. Parents need to learn that play can often help children learn adult roles.

Toddlers still need a close, loving relationship with their parents. Abandonment is their greatest fear. Although they like to explore, they always need the security of having a significant person nearby. Toddlers can be loving and cuddly one moment and energetic, exploring, and self-absorbed the next. Nurses may need to explain to parents the toddler's need for approval and attention.

The toddler is vaguely aware of self. As the sense of autonomy develops, the toddler is increasingly aware of the *physical self* and of *emotions*. The child does need some limits on activities for safety. Toddlers develop feelings of self-worth as a result of how others appraise their behavior. Children who constantly get negative feedback see themselves as bad. This perception is the basis of a negative self-concept.

Parents can provide a safe environment in which the toddler can practice skills such as playing or running. They also need to give toddlers positive input so that they develop a positive and emotionally healthy self-image. With a healthy sense of self-esteem and security, the toddler is able to deal with periodic failures later in life without damaging his or her self-esteem.

Preschoolers (4 and 5 Years)

During this period, physical growth slows, but control of the body and coordination increase greatly. The preschooler's world gets larger as he or she meets relatives, friends, and neighbors. Developmental tasks for the preschooler are shown in the accompanying box.

Physical Development

By the time children are 4 or 5 years old, they appear taller and thinner than toddlers because children tend to grow more in height than in weight. The preschooler's brain reaches almost its adult size by 5 years. The extremities of the body grow more quickly than the body trunk, making the child's body appear somewhat out of proportion. The posture of preschoolers gradually changes as the pelvis is straightened and the abdominal muscles become stronger. Thus the preschooler appears slender with erect posture. Weight gain in preschool children is generally slow. By 5 years, they have

---

DEVELOPMENTAL TASKS

Preschooler (4 and 5 Years)

Erikson's stage: Initiative versus guilt

- Learning sex differences and developing sex modesty
- Learning to give affection and to share affection
- Beginning to interact with age-mates
- Relating emotionally to parents, siblings, and others
- Learning to identify with male and female adult roles
- Learning simple concepts about the social and physical world
- Learning to distinguish right and wrong, being obedient, and developing a conscience

---

added only another 3 to 5 kg (7 to 12 lb) to their 3-year-old weight, increasing it to somewhere between 18.1 and 20.4 kg (40 and 45 lb). Preschool children grow about 5 to 6.25 cm (2.0 to 2.5 in) each year. Thus by 5 years of age, they double the birth length and measure 100 cm (40 in).

Preschool children are generally *hyperopic* (*farsighted*). As the eye grows in length, it becomes *emmetropic* (*refracting light normally*). If the eyes become too long, the child becomes *myopic* (*nearsighted*).

By 5 years of age, children are able to wash their hands and face and brush their teeth. They are self-conscious about exposing their body and go to the bathroom without telling others. Typically, preschool children run with increasing skill each year. By 5 years of age, they run skillfully and can jump three steps. Preschoolers can balance on their toes and dress themselves without assistance.

Psychosocial Development

Erikson writes that the major developmental crisis of the preschooler is *initiative versus guilt*. See Table 26–4 on page 356. Preschoolers must solve problems in accordance with their consciences. Their personalities develop. Erikson views the crises at this time as important for the development of the individual's *self-concept*.

Parents and caregivers can enhance the development of the preschoolers by praising effort at new activities and providing opportunities to repeat new activities until they are mastered. According to Erikson, preschoolers must learn what they can do. As a result, preschoolers imitate behavior, and their imagination and creativity become lively. Preschoolers also become increasingly aware of themselves. They play with their bodies largely out of curiosity. They know where the body begins and ends as well as the correct names for the different parts. By 5 years of age, they are able to draw a person including all the features. Preschoolers also learn about their feelings; they know the words *cry, sad, laugh* and the feelings related to them. They also begin to learn how to control their feelings and behavior.

The preschooler uses the same types of *coping mechanisms* in response to stress as the toddler does, although protest behavior (kicking, screaming) is less likely to occur in the older preschooler. Preschoolers usually have greater ability to verbalize stress. During the preschool years, four *adaptive mechanisms* are learned: identification, introjection, imagination, and repression.

Identification occurs when the child perceives the self as similar to another person and behaves like that person. For example, a boy may internalize the attitudes and gender behavior of his father. **Introjection** is similar to identification. It is the assimilation of the attributes of others. When preschoolers observe their parents, they assimilate many of their values and attitudes.

Imagination is an important part of preschoolers' life. The preschooler has an active imagination and fantasizes in play; for example, a chair becomes a beautiful throne to a girl, and she is the ruler. **Repression** is removing experiences, thoughts, and impulses from awareness. The preschooler generally represses thoughts related to the Oedipus or Electra complex.

By 4 years of age, children tend to believe that what they know is right. They tend to be dogmatic in their *speech*. Four-year-olds love nonsense words such as *jump-jump* and can string them together, much to an adult's exasperation. At 4, children are aggressive in their speech and capable of long conversations, often mixing fact and fiction.

By 5 years of age, speaking skills are well developed. Children use words purposefully and ask questions to acquire information. They do not merely practice speaking as 3- and 4-year-olds do, but speak as a means of social interaction. Exaggeration is common among 4- and 5-year-olds.

Preschool children gradually emerge as social beings. At the age of 3 or 4, they learn to play with a small number of their peers. They gradually learn to play with more people as they grow older. Preschoolers participate more in the family than they did previously; however, they also start to play with their peers. In associations with neighbors, family guests, and babysitters, too, they learn about relationships.

The phase of close emotional relationship with both parents changes to the phase Freud referred to as the *Electra* or *Oedipus* complexes (Engel 1962, pp. 90–104). At this time, the child focuses feelings of love chiefly on the parent of the opposite sex, and the parent of the same sex may be the object of some hostile feelings. The child begins to develop sexual interests and becomes interested in clothes and hair styles.

Cognitive Development

The preschooler's cognitive development, according to Piaget, is the phase of intuitive thought. The child is still egocentric, but egocentrism gradually subsides as he or she encounters wider experiences. Preschoolers learn through trial and error, and they think of only one idea at a time. They do not understand relationships such as those between mother and father or sister and brother. Children start to form concepts in late toddlerhood or the early preschool years. Preschoolers become concerned about death as something inevitable, but they do not explain it. They also associate death with others rather than themselves.

Most children at the age of 5 years can count pennies; however, the opportunity to spend money usually does not occur until they attend school. Reading skills also start to develop at this age. Young children like fairy tales and books about animals and other children.

Moral Development

Preschoolers are capable of prosocial behavior, i.e., any action that a person takes to benefit someone else. See Figure 27–4. The term *prosocial* indicates sharing, helping, protecting, giving aid, befriending, showing affection, and giving encouragement (Schulman and Mekler 1985, p. 232).

At this stage of development, preschoolers do not have fully formed consciences; however, they do develop some internal controls. Moral behavior is largely learned by modeling, initially after parents and later after sig-

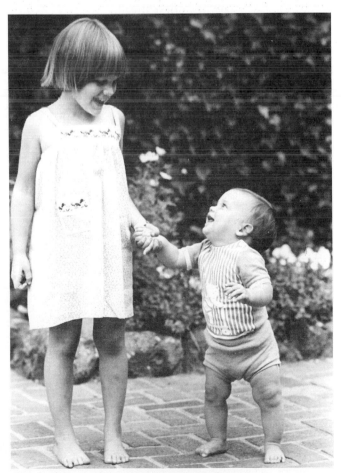

Figure 27–4   Preschoolers are capable of deriving pleasure from helping and encouraging others.

nificant others. The preschooler usually behaves well in social settings.

Children who perceive their parents as strict may become resentful or overly obedient. Preschoolers usually control their behavior because they want love and approval from their parents. Moral behavior to a preschooler may mean taking turns at play or sharing. Nurses can assist parents by discussing moral development and encouraging parents to give preschoolers recognition for actions such as sharing. It is also important for parents to answer a preschooler's "why" questions and discuss values with them.

Spiritual Development

Many preschoolers enroll in Sunday school or faith-oriented classes. The preschooler usually enjoys the social interaction of these classes. According to Fowler, children between the ages of 4 to 6 years are at the intuitive-projective stage of spiritual development. See Table 26–7 on page 360.

Faith at this stage is primarily a result of the teaching of significant others, e.g., parents and teachers. Children learn to imitate religious behavior, e.g., bowing the head in prayer, although they do not understand the meaning of the behavior. Preschoolers require simple explanations, like those in picture books, of spiritual matters. Children at this age use their imaginations to envision such ideas as angels or the devil.

Health Promotion and Protection

Health promotion and protection during the preschool years center on accident prevention, nutrition, dental care, play, and guidance. Therefore, the nurse's role is largely related to detecting children at risk and

counseling children and their parents about health. Assessment guidelines for growth and development of the preschooler are shown in the accompanying box.

Preschool children's nutritional needs include milk and a balanced diet of fruit, vegetables, bread, cereals, and meat or fish daily. Children eat much like adults except that they need smaller quantities. Generally, a preschooler's age is a good guide to the size of a serving: 4-year-olds eat 4 Tbsp servings of foods from each group at each meal; 5-year-olds eat 5 Tbsp servings.

Preschoolers also require sufficient protein for the growth of new tissues. A child who weighs 13.6 kg (30 lb) requires 37 g of protein daily as well as 30 mg of vitamin C. The latter is found in fruits, fruit juices, and some vegetables. One medium orange contains 55 mg of vitamin C.

Preschool children also require snacks, usually in the morning, afternoon, and evening. A snack might be a glass of milk and a sandwich. They usually eat one food at a time and often dislike coarse-textured and strong-tasting foods. Nurses caring for hospitalized or ill children need to be aware of children's special nutritional requirements.

The preschooler's elimination control should be complete at this age. The bladder capacity is between 600 to 750 ml. With a change of environment, e.g., due to hospitalization, the preschooler may be incontinent. Incontinence is usually very distressing to the child. Nurses can assist hospitalized preschoolers by learning about their elimination habits at home and continuing these as much as possible. If a preschooler has an "accident," he or she should not be punished or ridiculed.

Accidents continue to be the major cause of mortality among preschool children. These children are active and often clumsy and are therefore susceptible to injury. Accidents can be prevented in two ways: control of the environment and education of the child. Parents may need to learn to control the environment, for instance, by keeping matches out of the child's reach, teaching the child to put toys away when they are not being used, and safeguarding swimming pools and other potentially dangerous areas. The education of the preschooler may involve learning how to cross streets, what traffic signals mean, and how to ride a bicycle safely.

Preschoolers who have not yet been immunized may need to be so before they can enter school. Regular dental examinations are essential at this age; caries develop quickly in young children. Examinations usually are initiated at about 2 1/2 years. It has been estimated that 80% of children have some tooth decay. Deciduous teeth guide the entrance of permanent teeth; therefore, the abnormal placement or loss of deciduous teeth can cause the misalignment of permanent teeth. Dental care also involves teaching children to brush after each meal and before retiring.

Preschoolers spend most of the day playing. *Play* serves a number of purposes:

1. Children learn to cooperate with others.
2. Focus changes from family to peers.
3. Children develop strength and coordination.
4. Abundant energy is dispersed.

GUIDELINES

Assessing the Preschooler

Does the preschooler:

▪ Indicate physical development within a normal range?

▪ Possess physical skills appropriate for the age?

▪ Demonstrate that he or she is toilet trained?

▪ Perform simple hygiene measures and dress and undress self?

▪ Play cooperatively with peers?

▪ Display imagination and creativity?

▪ Exhibit appropriate emotional expressions in different situations?

▪ Understand right and wrong, and respond to others' expectations about behavior?

▪ Ask questions and exhibit increasing vocabulary?

▪ Appear eager to do things and to please others?

▪ Identify with people of own sex?

5. Children have an avenue to express initiative and imagination.

Play is also fun. Preschoolers take it seriously but express joy and pleasure during play. Play at this age is loosely organized. Preschoolers who are hospitalized can frequently have play time included in their nursing plans.

Preschoolers are very much aware of their *sexual identity*. They often imitate sexual stereotypes. Because boys are traditionally permitted to take more risks than girls, they have a higher incidence of accidents. In contemporary American society, boys and girls participate in many of the same activities.

Preschoolers are aware of the two sexes and identify with the correct sex. They are very curious about others' bodies and sexual function. Questions about others' bodies should be answered simply and truthfully.

Guidance and discipline for preschoolers should be consistent and fair. Through guidance, they gain a sense of security and the feeling that their parents care about them. It is important that parents follow through with a punishment once it is imposed; a child confined to his or her room for 1 hour should stay the full hour. In a hospital setting, nurses often must provide the guidance normally given by parents.

The preschooler emerges from toddlerhood with a sense of self, which he or she continues to develop and refine. The successful accomplishment of tasks builds *self-esteem*. Acceptance in new social roles, e.g., brother, son, or daughter, also enhances self-esteem.

School-Age Children (6 to 12 Years)

The school-age period starts when children are about 6 years of age, when the deciduous teeth are shed. This period includes the preadolescent (prepuberty) period. It ends at about 12 years, with the onset of puberty. Puberty is the age when the reproductive organs become functional and secondary sex characteristics develop. Because the average age of onset of puberty is 10 for girls and 12 for boys, some people define the school-age years as 6 to 10 for girls and 6 to 12 for boys. Skills learned during this stage are particularly important in relation to work later in life and willingness to try new tasks. In general, the period from 6 to 12 years is one of rapid and dramatic change. The developmental tasks of this period are shown in the accompanying box.

▪ Physical Development

School-age children at 7 years gain weight rapidly and thus appear less thin than previously. Individual differences due to genetic influences and environment are generally obvious at this time. At 6 years, boys tend to weigh about 21 kg (46 lb), about 1 kg (2 lb) more than girls. The weight gain of school children from 6 to 12 years of age averages about 3.2 kg (7 lb) per year, but the major weight gains occur from age 10 to 12 for boys and from age 9 to 12 for girls. By 12 years of age, boys

DEVELOPMENTAL TASKS

School Age Children (6 to 12 Years)

Erikson's stage: Industry versus inferiority

- Building a wholesome attitude toward oneself
- Developing and refining skills in the use of small muscles
- Learning to form friendships with peers
- Learning to give as much love as one receives
- Learning appropriate behaviors for the masculine and feminine role and identifying with contemporaries of the same sex
- Learning to use language to exchange ideas or to influence listeners
- Learning more rules and developing a beginning scale of values, inner moral control, and respect for moral rules

and girls weigh on the average 40 to 42 kg (88 to 95 lb); girls are usually heavier. At 6 years, both boys and girls are about the same height, 115 cm (46 in). They are about 150 cm (60 in) by 12 years. Before puberty, children of both sexes have a growth spurt, girls between 10 and 12 years and boys between 12 and 14 years. Thus, girls may well be taller than boys at 12 years, although the boys are usually stronger.

The extremities tend to grow more quickly than the trunk; thus school-age children's bodies appear somewhat ill-proportioned. By 6 years, the thoracic curvature starts to develop, and the lordosis disappears. Full adult posture is not assumed, however, until after the complete development of the skeletal musculature during the adolescent period.

The depth and distance perception of children 6 to 8 years of age is accurate. By age 6, children have full binocular vision: The eye muscles are well developed and coordinated, and both eyes can focus on one object at the same time. Because the shape of the eye changes during growth, the farsightedness of the preschool years gradually changes to 20/20 vision during the school-age years; 20/20 vision is usually well established between 9 and 11 years of age. In later childhood, myopia is not uncommon; that is, the child is able to see clearly only objects that are close. This problem is generally corrected by eyeglasses.

Permanent teeth start to appear between 6 and 7 years of age, and dental caries also can appear. Thus regular dental checkups are needed. By age 13 or 14, children have most of their permanent teeth with the exception of their third molars (wisdom teeth), which erupt between 17 and 24 years of age.

Very little change takes place in the reproductive and endocrine systems until the prepuberty period. During **prepuberty**, endocrine functions slowly increase. This change in endocrine function can result in increased perspiration and more active sebaceous glands. As a result, acne may develop, particularly on the face, neck, and back.

During the middle years (6 to 10), children perfect their muscular skills and coordination. By 9 years, most children are becoming skilled in games of interest, such as football or baseball. These skills are often associated with school, and many of them are learned there. By 9 years most children have sufficient fine motor control for such activities as building models or sewing.

Psychosocial Development

According to Erikson, the central task of school-age children is *industry versus inferiority*. At this time children begin to create and develop a sense of competence and perseverance. School-age children are motivated by activities that provide a sense of worth. They concentrate on mastering skills that will help them function in the adult world. Although children of this age work hard to succeed, they are always faced with the possibility of failure, which can lead to a sense of inferiority. If children have been successful in previous stages, they are motivated to be industrious and to cooperate with others toward a common goal (Erikson 1963).

Parents and caregivers can assist school-age children to develop psychosocially by:

1. Recognizing success and providing praise for achievements
2. Guiding the child to perform tasks in which he or she is likely to succeed
3. Guiding the child to complete the task
4. Teaching the child how to get along with peers by collaborating, compromising, cooperating, and competing
5. Teaching the child how to get along with adults

In school, children have the restraints of the school system imposed on their behavior and learn to develop controls. Children compare their skills with those of their peers in a number of areas, including motor development, social development, and language. This comparison assists in the development of self-concept. Schoolchildren can sometimes be cruel in their honesty, and teachers often need to intercede to assist children who have limitations.

The schoolchild develops a number of adaptive mechanisms. Four of these are regression, malingering, rationalization, and ritualistic behavior. **Regression** is returning to a form of behavior that was suitable at an earlier age. For example, the child who is anxious about starting school may start bedwetting at night or perhaps revert to baby talk. **Malingering** is a familiar mechanism to schoolchildren. It is pretending to be ill rather than facing something unpleasant; the child who feels sick the morning before a test may be malingering. **Rationalization** is an attempt to justify behavior by logical reason and explanation. A girl who does not make the swimming team may rationalize to her parents by saying she really did not try because she doesn't want swimming to interfere with her piano lessons. **Ritualistic behavior** is demonstrated by schoolchildren in many settings. For example, a child may walk down the

sidewalk without stepping on a crack. Clubs and gangs often have rituals of membership. These rituals become very important to schoolchildren even though they usually do not persist for a long time. For example, the boy who must have a shower every morning may forget this ritual after a few weeks.

Cognitive Development

According to Piaget, the ages 7 to 11 years mark the phase of *concrete operations*. See Table 26–5, page 357. During this stage, the child changes from egocentric interactions to cooperative interactions. See Figure 27–5. School-age children also develop an increased understanding of concepts that are associated with specific objects, for example, environmental conservation or wildlife preservation. Children at this time develop logical reasoning from intuitive reasoning. For example, they learn to add and subtract to obtain an answer to a problem. Children learn about cause-and-effect relationships at this age; e.g., they know that a stone will not float because it is heavier than water.

Money is a concept that gains meaning for children when they start school. By the time they are 7 or 8 years old, children usually know the value of most coins. The concept of time is also learned at this age. By 6 years of age, children enter school; the schedule in school helps them to learn time periods, but it is not until 9 or 10 years of age that children are able to understand the long periods of time in the past. Knowing the time of day and the day of the week are relatively easy for children because they relate time to routine activities. For example, a girl may go to school Monday through Friday, play on Saturday, go to Sunday school on Sunday morning, and go out with her father Sunday afternoon. Children are beginning to read a clock by the time they are 6 years old.

Later in childhood reading skills are usually well developed, and what a child reads is largely influenced by the family. By 9 years of age, most children are self-motivated. They compete with themselves, and they like to plan in advance. By 12 years, they are motivated by inner drive rather than by competition with peers. They like to talk, to discuss different subjects, and to debate.

Moral Development

Some school-age children are at Kohlberg's stage 1 of the *preconventional level* (punishment and obedience); i.e., they act to avoid being punished. Some school-age children, however, are at stage 2 (*instrumental-relativist orientation*). These children do things to benefit themselves. Fairness, e.g., everyone getting a fair share or chance, becomes important. Later in childhood, most children progress to the *conventional* level. This level has two stages: Stage 3 is the "good boy-nice girl" stage, and stage 4 is the *law and order orientation*. See Table 26–6 on page 359. Children usually reach the conventional level between the ages of 10 and 13. The child shifts from the concrete interests of individuals to the interests of groups. The motivation for moral action

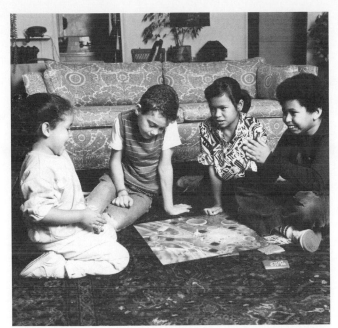

Figure 27–5 The expanding cognitive skills of school-age children enable cooperative interactions of an increasingly complex nature.

at this stage is to live up to what significant others think of the child (Hersh et al. 1979, pp. 71–74).

■ Spiritual Development

According to Fowler, the school-age child is at stage 2 in spiritual development, the *mythical-literal* stage. School-age children learn to distinguish fantasy from fact. Spiritual facts are those beliefs that are accepted by a religious group, whereas fantasy is thoughts and images formed in the child's mind. Parents and the minister, rabbi, or priest help the child distinguish fact from fantasy. These people still influence the child more than peers in spiritual matters.

When the child does not understand events such as the creation of the world, he or she uses fantasy to explain them. The school-age child needs to have concepts such as prayer presented in concrete terms. For example, the child thinks of God as having human qualities, e.g., as a kind old man or a person who punishes when behavior does not meet His standards.

School-age children may ask many questions about God and religion in these years and will generally believe that God is good and always present to help. Just before puberty, children become aware that their prayers are not always answered and become disappointed. At this age, some children reject religion, while others continue to accept it. This decision is largely influenced by the parents. If a child continues religious training, the child is ready to apply reason rather than blind belief in most situations.

■ Health Promotion and Protection

The school-age child understands what health and illness are even though his ideas may differ from those of adults. Wood found that school-age children believed

illness was caused by germs, self, or an outside force, e.g., the rain or an accident (Wood 1983, pp. 103–4). School-age children are usually taught preventive health practices such as dental hygiene and good nutrition by their parents. Assessment guidelines for growth and development of the school-aged child are shown in the accompanying box.

Nutrition continues to be a high priority for growing children. Most school-age children require a balanced diet including 2400 kcal per day. School-age children eat four or five times a day, including a snack after school. Children need a protein-rich food at breakfast to sustain the prolonged physical and mental effort required at school. Studies reveal that children who eat well-balanced breakfasts have better attitudes and school records than those who skip breakfast (Pipes 1981, p. 173). Undernourished children become fatigued easily and face a greater risk of infection, resulting in frequent absences from school.

Nurses may need to counsel children and their parents about preventing obesity. Obesity in school-age children tends to result in decreased activity as well as psychosocial problems. Obese children may be ridiculed by their peers and discriminated against by peers and adults. Such behavior reinforces an already low self-esteem. Counseling should include:

1. Reviewing the child's eating habits, including snacks
2. Altering meal content
3. Using rewards other than food
4. Encouraging regular exercise

Fluid requirements of school-age children vary according to age, activity level, and environmental temperatures. The average healthy 10-year-old schoolchild requires about 2000 to 2500 ml of fluid daily or about

GUIDELINES

Assessing the School-Age Child

Does the school-age child:

- Indicate physical development within normal range?
- Possess coordinated fine motor skills?
- Read, write, and manipulate numbers?
- Develop a concept of money and its value?
- Apply himself or herself to given physical or mental tasks?
- Begin to solve problems?
- Interact well with parents?
- Interact well with peers?
- Become less dependent on family and venture away from them?
- Control strong and impulsive feelings?
- Begin to understand the importance of sharing with family and peers?
- Like to help others?
- Think of self as likeable and healthy?

70 to 85 ml of fluid per kilogram of body weight per day (Pipes 1981, p. 73).

The respiratory and circulatory systems grow as the child grows. The child's gas exchange becomes more efficient, and vital capacity continues to increase. The heart is still small in proportion to the rest of the body and continues to grow slowly. Since the heart must supply the circulatory needs of the body, sustained physical activity is not desirable because of the strain on the heart. The heart reaches its adult size at puberty.

By the time children attend school, they are learning to think before they act. They often prefer adult equipment to toys. They want to be active with other children in such activities as bicycling, hiking, swimming, and boating. Nurses need to teach children and their parents guidelines for safety. The accompanying box provides some suggestions.

During the school-age years, children need boosters for those immunizations given in infancy. Generally, they are given against tetanus, diphtheria, and poliomyelitis. Local health departments have their own recommended schedules, which are revised regularly in light of medical advances. Some physicians recommend that girls receive the rubella vaccine before puberty to prevent the possibility of rubella during pregnancy and subsequent congenital defects. Boys need to be protected against mumps, thus preventing subsequent sterility, which can occur as a result of contracting mumps later in life.

Regular dental checkups every 6 months are required during these years. Permanent teeth begin to appear about 7 years and are usually all in place except for the third molars (wisdom teeth) by 12 years of age. Nurses may need to teach children and their parents about regular dental hygiene.

Play continues to be a source of stimulation to school-age children. They have more friends than preschoolers. In early school years, they like to playact familiar roles, such as police officer or teacher. By the age of 9 or 10 years, they become more interested in games of skill, such as football or baseball. Boys and girls of this age frequently separate for play activities and form preadolescent gangs. Membership in the gang is strictly regulated. Often membership in a gang or club is predicated on a skill, such as tying knots, or a ritual, such as making

a finger bleed without acknowledging pain. At this age, most children have a best friend, usually someone of the same sex; the child shares feelings, thoughts, and activities with the friend.

The sexual identity of school-age children changes during these years. Both boys and girls are independent and dependent. Sex education should begin for both sexes at this time. Children have many questions, which should be answered truthfully and simply to meet the child's needs. It is also important not to give the child too much information at one time. Parents should be as comfortable as possible giving this information.

During the school-age years, the child learns to identify with the parent of the same sex and learns the behaviors associated with the role of that parent. At this time, the child probably has some conflict with siblings, although this conflict is less severe than it is for the preschooler. The school-age child may resent a new baby, although this is less likely than in preschool years. School-age children may resent the freedom given older brothers and sisters. Parents who compare siblings' accomplishments and talents can cause resentment and rivalry.

School-age children begin to enjoy other adults as well as their parents. They want approval from their parents and other significant adults, e.g., teachers. Schoolchildren can discuss matters of discipline with their parents. They may need several alternative courses of action and probably more guidance than discipline. It is important not to embarrass children by disciplining them in front of others. Children also may be confused if a parent provides two messages at once. For example, when a father tells his son that he should not lie, but then tells a lie in front of the child, the child receives two messages.

The schoolchild's self-concept continues to mature. Children recognize similarities and differences between themselves and others. The school-age child compares self with others and obtains *feedback* from teachers and peers. The child who is successful and receives recognition for his or her efforts feels competent and in control of self and of the environment. Children who feel unaccepted by their peers or who receive negative feedback and little recognition can feel inferior and worthless.

GUIDELINES

Safety (School-Age Children)

- Teach school-age children safe ways to use the stove, garden tools, and other equipment.
- Teach them traffic rules for bicycling.
- Teach them safety rules for swimming, boating, skateboarding, and other recreations.
- Supervise them when they use saws, electrical appliances and tools, and other potentially dangerous equipment.
- Teach them not to play with fireworks, gunpowder, and firearms.

Adolescence

Adolescence is a critical period in development. Its length is culturally determined to some extent. In North America, adolescence is longer than in some cultures, extending to 18 to 21 years of age. **Adolescence** is the period during which the person becomes physically and psychologically mature and acquires a personal identity. At the end of adolescence, the person is ready to enter adulthood and assume its responsibilities.

Puberty is the first stage of adolescence in which sexual organs begin to grow and mature. **Menarche** (onset of menstruation) begins in girls. **Ejaculation** (expulsion of semen) occurs in boys. For girls, puberty normally starts between 10 and 14 years; for boys, between 12 and 16 years. In late adolescence, young people are involved mostly with planning their future and economic independence. Developmental tasks that should be met by the end of adolescence are shown in the accompanying box.

Physical Development

During puberty, growth is markedly accelerated compared to the slow, steady growth of the child. This period, marked by sudden and dramatic physical changes, is referred to as the adolescent growth spurt. In boys, the growth spurt usually begins between ages 12 and 16; in girls, it begins earlier, usually between ages 10 and 14. Because the growth spurt begins earlier in girls, many girls surpass boys in height at this time.

Physical growth continues throughout adolescence. Growth is fastest for boys at about 14 years, and the maximum height is often reached at about 18 or 19 years. Some men add another 1 or 2 cm to their height during their 20s, as the vertebral column gradually continues to grow. During the period of 10 to 18 years of age, the average American male doubles his weight, gaining about 30 kg (67 lb) and grows about 34 cm (13 1/2 in) (Suitor and Hunter 1980, p. 95). The fastest rate of growth in girls occurs at about age 12; they reach their maximum heights at about 15 to 16 years. During ages 10 to 18, the average American female gains about 22 kg (49 lb) and grows about 24 cm (9 in) (Suitor and Hunter 1980, p. 95).

The eccrine and apocrine glands increase their secretions and become fully functional during puberty. The **eccrine glands,** found over most of the body, produce sweat. The **apocrine glands** develop in the axillae, anal and genital areas, and external auditory canals, and around the umbilicus and the areola of the breasts. Apocrine sweat is released onto the skin in response to emotional stimuli only.

Sebaceous glands also become active under the influence of androgens in both males and females. The sebaceous glands, which secrete **sebum,** become most active on the face, neck, shoulders, upper back, chest, and genitals. When these glands become plugged and inflamed, the result is *acne,* a condition common in adolescence. Noninflammatory acne appears as open and closed whiteheads and blackheads. Inflammatory acne appears as inflamed skin together with pustules and papules. A **pustule** is a visible collection of pus within the epidermis. A **papule** is a superficial, circumscribed elevation of the skin. Inflammatory acne may cause scarring. Thorough cleansing of the skin is important in the treatment of acne. A well-balanced diet and avoidance of fatigue, stress, and excessive perspiration are also desirable.

During puberty, both primary and secondary sex characteristics develop. **Primary sexual characteristics** relate to the organs necessary for reproduction, such as the testes, penis, vagina, and uterus. **Secondary sexual characteristics** differentiate the male from the female but do not relate directly to reproduction. Examples are pubic hair growth, breast development, and voice changes.

DEVELOPMENTAL TASKS

Adolescents

Erikson's stage: Self-identity versus role confusion

- Accepting changing body size, shape, and function in relation to others and understanding the meaning of sexual and physical maturity.

- Achieving a socially accepted and satisfying masculine or feminine role and recognizing the distinctions and similarities in each.

- Achieving new and more adult relationships with peers of both sexes.

- Selecting and preparing for an occupation and economic independence.

- Desiring and achieving socially responsible behavior.

- Developing a workable set of values, ideals, and standards as a guide for behavior.

The first noticeable sign that puberty has begun in males is usually the appearance of pubic hair. The milestone of male puberty is considered to be the first ejaculation, which commonly occurs at about 14 years of age. Fertility follows several months later. Sexual maturity is achieved by age 18.

Often the first noticeable sign of puberty in females is the appearance of the **breast bud,** although the appearance of hair along the labia may precede this. The milestone of female puberty is the menarche, which occurs about 2 years after the breast bud appears. At first, menstrual periods are scanty and irregular and may occur without ovulation. Ovulation is usually established 1 to 2 years after menarche. Female internal reproductive organs reach adult size about age 18 to 20.

Psychosocial Development

According to Erikson (1963, p. 261), the adolescent seeks answers to "Who am I?" and "What am I to be?" The psychosocial task of the adolescent is the establishment of identity. The danger of this stage is role confusion. The inability to settle on an occupational identity commonly disturbs the adolescent. Less commonly, doubts arise about sexual identity. Because of the adolescent's dramatic body changes, the development of a stable identity is difficult. Erikson says that adolescents help one another through this identity crises by forming cliques and a separate youth culture. These cliques exclude all those who are "different" in skin color, cultural background, aspects of dress, gestures, and tastes.

Adolescents are usually concerned about their bodies, their appearances, and their physical abilities. Hair styling, skin care, and clothes become very important. In-groupers of an adolescent clique can be excessively clannish and cruel in excluding out-groupers; this intolerance is a temporary defense against identity confusion (Erikson 1963, p. 236).

In their search for a new identity, adolescents have to refight the battles of many of the previous stages of development. The task of developing trust in self and others is again encountered when the adolescent looks for ideal persons whom he or she can trust and with whom he or she can prove trustworthy. Development of autonomy is restaged in the adolescent's search for ways to express his or her right to choose freely. The search for an occupational role that allows expression of an autonomous, freely chosen direction is one example. Free choice and autonomy present conflicts to the adolescent. Conflict arises between behaving well in the eyes of the parents and behaving in a manner that may expose them to the ridicule of their peers. The sense of initiative is also restaged. The adolescent has unlimited imagination and ambition and aspires to great accomplishments. The sense of industry is reenacted when the adolescent chooses a career. The extent to which these tasks were achieved earlier influences the adolescent's ability to achieve a healthy self-concept and self-identity.

The adolescent needs to establish a self-concept that accepts both personal strengths and weaknesses. Adolescents need to learn to build on their strengths and not be preoccupied by such defects as acne. They gain self-concepts largely from the impressions that others have of them. If others accept defects—e.g., a lost finger—adolescents accept those defects more readily.

Although sexual identification begins at about 3 or 4 years of age, it is a significant part of adolescence. The adolescent male strives to achieve a masculine sexual identity; the adolescent female, a feminine sexual identity. Because sex roles are becoming less defined in North American society, adopting masculine and feminine roles is increasingly confusing to today's adolescent. Job and family roles are less traditional and sex-specific. In forming a sexual identity, adolescents first fantasize the male or female role and then enact various aspects of that imagined role. In response to their own feelings and that of others, aspects of the role are either adopted or rejected. Later, adolescents begin to establish intimacy with a partner or partners. This intimacy lays the groundwork for the commitments of adulthood. Sexual experimentation is not part of true intimacy, but once intimacy is achieved, sexual activity is included.

Adolescents are sexually active and may engage in masturbation as well as heterosexual and homosexual activity. Homosexual activity during adolescence is not necessarily an indicator of sexual preference, since both gay and nongay adolescents may experiment sexually with persons of the same and opposite sex.

About the age of 15 years, many adolescents gradually draw away from the family and gain independence. This need for independence and the need for family support sometimes create conflict within the adolescent and between the adolescent and the family. The young person may appear hostile or depressed at times during this painful process. At this age, adolescents prefer to be with their peers rather than their parents and may seek advice from adults other than their parents. Parents sometimes are bewildered by this stage of development; instead of reducing controls, they increase them, which causes the adolescent to rebel.

Adolescents also have to resolve their ambivalent feelings toward the parent of the opposite sex. As part of resolution, adolescents may develop brief crushes on adults outside the family—teachers or neighbors, for example. Adolescents sometimes adopt some of the attributes of the adults with whom they are infatuated. This modeling can be helpful in the maturing process.

Some of the discord in the family at this time is due to the generation gap. The values of the adolescent may differ from those of the parents. This difference may be difficult for the parents to understand and accept. Adolescents still need guidance from their parents, although they appear neither to want it nor to need it. However, adolescents need to know that their parents care about them and that their parents still want to help them. Restrictions and guidance need to be presented in a manner that makes adolescents feel loved. They need consistency in guidance and fewer restrictions than previously. They should have the independence they can handle yet know that their parents will assist them when they need help.

During adolescence, peer groups assume great importance. See Figure 27–6. The peer group has a number of functions. It provides a sense of belonging, pride, social learning, and sexual roles. Most peer groups have well-defined, sex-specific modes of acceptable behavior. In adolescence, the peer groups change with

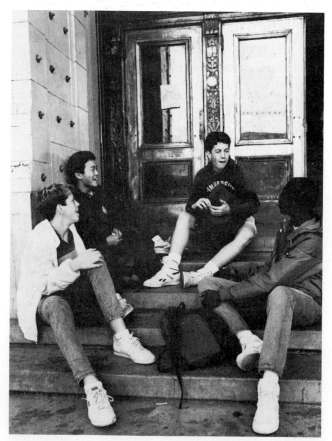

Figure 27–6 Adolescent peer group relationships enhance a sense of belonging, self-esteem, and self-identity.

age. They start as single-sex groups, evolve to mixed groups, and finally narrow to couples who share activities.

Not all adolescents are heterosexual. For homosexuals, adolescence is a difficult time. Because peer acceptance is crucial to self-acceptance, lesbian and gay adolescents usually conform to the heterosexual codes and behaviors of their peer groups even though these do not feel natural or correct. Conforming may exact a great personal cost. Adolescents who choose to be openly gay or lesbian face not only the ostracism of their peers but also the misunderstanding and hostility of parents, teachers, and other important adults.

Cognitive Development

Cognitive abilities mature during adolescence. Between the ages of 11 and 15, the adolescent begins Piaget's *formal operations stage* of cognitive development. The main feature of this stage is that people can think beyond the present and beyond the world of reality. Adolescents are highly imaginative and idealistic. They consider things that do not exist but that might be and consider ways things could be or ought to be. This type of thinking requires logic, organization, and consistency.

The adolescent becomes more informed about the world and environment. Adolescents use new information to solve everyday problems and can communicate with adults on most subjects. The adolescent's capacity to absorb and use knowledge is great. Adolescents usually select their own areas for learning; they explore interests from which they may evolve a career plan. Study habits and learning skills developed in adolescence are used throughout life.

Moral Development

According to Kohlberg, the young adolescent is usually at the *conventional level* of moral development. Most still accept the Golden Rule and want to abide by social order to existing laws. Adolescents examine their values, standards, and morals. They may discard the values they have adopted from parents in favor of values they consider more suitable.

When adolescents move into the *postconventional* or *principled level,* they start to question the rules and laws of society. Right thinking and right action become a matter of personal values and opinions, which may conflict with societal laws. Adolescents consider the possibility of rationally changing the law and emphasize individual rights. Not all adolescents or even adults proceed to this postconventional level. See Kohlberg's stages of moral development in Table 26–6 on page 359.

Spiritual Development

According to Fowler, the adolescent or young adult reaches the *synthetic-conventional stage* of spiritual development (see Table 26–7 on page 360). As adolescents encounter different groups in society, they are exposed to a wide variety of opinions, beliefs, and behaviors regarding religious matters. The adolescent may reconcile the differences in one of the following ways:

1. Deciding any differences are wrong
2. Compartmentalizing the differences (For example, a friend may not be able to go to dances on Friday evenings because of religious observances, but the friend can share activities on other days.)
3. Obtaining advice from a significant other, e.g., a parent or a minister

Often the adolescent believes that various religious beliefs and practices have more similarities than differences. At this stage, the adolescent's focus is on interpersonal rather than conceptual matters. Nursing activities relative to this stage of spiritual development include:

1. Presenting an open, accepting attitude to adolescents' questions and statements regarding spiritual matters and their implications to health.
2. Arranging for the adolescent to see a member of his or her religious faith if this is desired. An adolescent may want to talk with members of his or her church peer group for support.
3. Providing a comfortable environment in which the adolescent can practice the rituals of his or her faith.

Health Promotion and Protection

Assessment guidelines for growth and development of the adolescent are shown in the accompanying box.

Adolescents have increased nutritional needs to support growth. A boy between the ages of 11 and 14 needs 60 kcal per kilogram of body weight per day, decreasing to 42 kcal per kilogram by age 15 to 18. A girl between the ages of 10 and 14 needs 48 kcal per kilogram of body weight per day, thereafter decreasing to 39 kcal per kilogram per day (Howard and Herbold 1982, pp. 280–81). The need for protein, calcium, and vitamin D increases during adolescence. Even when

GUIDELINES

Assessing Adolescents

Does the adolescent:

- Indicate physical and sexual development consistent with standards?
- Interact well with parents, peers, siblings, and persons in authority?
- Like himself or herself?
- Make educational or career plans?
- Have a set of moral values to guide behavior?
- Consider factors contributing to religious beliefs and practices?
- Seek help from appropriate persons about his or her problems?
- Exhibit healthy life-style practices?

adolescents eat nutritionally balanced meals and meet their needs for specific nutrients, they may still require extra calories, particularly young males who are active in sports. This need prompts frequent snacking of high-calorie foods such as cookies, doughnuts, and soft drinks. Parents and nurses can promote better lifelong eating habits by encouraging teenagers to eat healthful snacks. Common problems related to nutrition and self-esteem among adolescents include obesity, anorexia nervosa, and bulimia.

Obesity is a common problem of the preadolescent period and continues to be a problem in the adolescent period. It is estimated that 10 to 16% of people between the ages of 10 and 19 years are obese. Obese adolescents are frequently discriminated against in many ways. They are usually rejected by their peers, badgered by their parents, and ridiculed on television and in the movies. Many feel ugly and socially unacceptable. Depression is not unusual among obese adolescents. Treatment of obesity in this age group includes education on nutrition as well as assessment of psychosocial problems that may produce overeating.

Under social pressure to be slim, some adolescents severely limit their food intake to a level significantly below that required to meet the demands of normal growth. **Anorexia nervosa** is a severe psychophysiologic condition usually seen in adolescent girls and young women. It is characterized by a prolonged inability or refusal to eat and rapid weight loss in persons who believe they are fat even though they are emaciated. Anorexics may also induce vomiting and use laxatives and diuretics to remain thin. This illness is most effectively treated in the early stages by psychotherapy that also involves the parents. Hospitalization may be necessary when the effects of starvation become life-threatening.

An increasing problem among teenagers, **bulimia** is an uncontrollable compulsion to consume enormous amounts of food and then expel it by self-induced vomiting or by taking laxatives. For example, the afflicted person may consume a whole cake, a dozen doughnuts, and a half dozen apple turnovers before inducing vomiting. After prolonged periods of alternately gorging and vomiting, the person no longer needs to induce vomiting; it becomes an uncontrollable reflex. Voluntary organizations are established in some regions to assist individuals with bulimia.

Most adolescents require 8 to 10 hours of *sleep* each night to prevent undue fatigue and susceptibility to infections. A change in sleep pattern is common in adolescence. Children who once were early risers begin to sleep late in the mornings and occasionally take afternoon naps. The reason for daytime sleeping is not fully understood, but it is possibly a result of physical maturity and reduced nocturnal sleep. During adolescence boys begin to experience **nocturnal emissions** (orgasm and emission of semen during sleep), known as "wet dreams," several times each month. Boys need to be informed about this normal development to prevent embarrassment and fear.

Adolescents want to know about sex but are often uneasy discussing sexual concerns with their parents. Accurate information needs to be provided by the family, schools, and nurses. One study of 417 high school students assessed what teenagers believed their needs were and what knowledge they already possessed. Most of the students had obtained their first information about sex from friends or from reading while in grade school. The family and school were the other major sources of information (Inman 1975, pp. 217–19).

Major sexual problems of adolescents are unplanned pregnancies, sexually transmitted diseases, and dysmenorrhea. **Unplanned pregnancies** during adolescence are not uncommon. Adolescents need education about sexuality, sexual actions and consequences, the individual's right to make a decision about ways to express himself or herself sexually, and contraceptive measures. The incidence of abortion is notable among this group, and those who choose to carry their pregnancies to term have unique needs and problems. Adolescents are high-risk mothers, physiologically and emotionally. Rearing a child as an unwed single parent or placing a child for adoption can precipitate an emotional crisis.

Sexually transmitted diseases (STDs) are the most common bacterial infections among adolescents. STDs, formerly called venereal diseases, include syphilis, gonorrhea, genital warts, genital herpes virus type 2, chlamydial urethritis or nongonococcal urethritis (NGU), *Trichomonas* and *Candida* infections, and acquired immune deficiency syndrome (AIDS). *Trichomonas* and *Candida* infections can also be acquired nonsexually. Because the term sexually transmitted disease elicits feelings of guilt, shame, and fear, adolescents frequently do not seek medical help as early as they should. Adolescents need education about these diseases, preventive measures, and early treatment. Table 27–2 lists common signs of STDs for which teenagers should seek medical care.

Dysmenorrhea (painful menstruation) is prevalent among adolescent females and causes much short-term absenteeism. Cramping, lower abdominal pain radiating to the back and upper thighs, nausea, vomiting, diarrhea, and headaches may occur for a few hours up to 3 days. Dysmenorrhea results from powerful uterine contractions, which cause ischemia and in turn cramping pain. Dysmenorrhea is associated with the release of prostaglandins through the activity of progesterone. Traditional treatments for the symptoms of dysmenorrhea have been bed rest, administration of simple analgesics such as aspirin, application of heat to the abdomen, and certain exercises. Today, treatment with antiprostaglandins such as ibuprofen (Motrin or Advil) and naproxen (Naprosyn) helps many. These drugs, however, should be administered under medical supervision and have potentially toxic effects. Aspirin itself is a mild antiprostaglandin. More recently, nondrug approaches, such as biofeedback, are being used.

The adolescent needs to be safeguarded from accidents and injury. Accidents are the leading cause of death and injury among adolescents. Motor-vehicle accidents and sports injuries are the most common accidents. Obtaining a driver's license is an important event in the life of an adolescent, but the privilege is not always wisely handled. Head injuries and fractures are frequent outcomes of automobile and motorcycle accidents. Adoles-

Table 27–2 Clinical Signs of Sexually Transmitted Diseases

Disease	Male	Female
Gonorrhea	Painful urination; urethritis with watery white discharge, which may become purulent.	May be asymptomatic; or vaginal discharge, pain, and urinary frequency.
Syphilis	Chancre, usually on glans penis, which is painless and heals in 4 to 6 weeks; secondary symptoms—skin eruptions, low-grade fever, inflammation of lymph glands—in 6 weeks to 6 months after chancre heals.	Chancre on cervix or other genital areas, which heals in 4 to 6 weeks; symptoms same as for male.
Genital warts (condyloma acuminatum)	Single lesions or clusters of lesions growing beneath or on the foreskin, at external meatus, or on the glans penis. On dry skin areas, lesions are hard and yellow-gray. On moist areas, lesions are pink or red and soft with a cauliflowerlike appearance.	Lesions appear at the bottom part of the vaginal opening, on the perineum, the vaginal lips, inner walls of the vagina, and the cervix.
Herpes genitalis (*Herpes simplex* of the genitals)	Primary herpes involves the presence of painful sores or large, discrete vesicles that last for weeks; vesicles rupture. Recurrent herpes is itchy rather than painful; it lasts for a few hours to 10 days.	Same as for males.
Chlamydial urethritis	Urinary frequency; watery, mucoid urethral discharge.	Commonly a carrier; vaginal discharge, dysuria, urinary frequency.
Trichomonas vaginalis	Slight itching; moisture on tip of penis; slight, early morning urethral discharge. Many males are asymptomatic.	Itching and redness of vulva and skin inside thighs; copious watery, frothy vaginal discharge.
Candida albicans	Itching, irritation, discharge, plaque of cheesy material under foreskin.	Red and excoriated vulva; intense itching of vaginal and vulvar tissues; thick, white, cheesy or curdlike discharge.
Acquired immune deficiency syndrome (AIDS)	Symptoms can appear anytime from several months to several years after acquiring the virus. The person has reduced immunity to other diseases. Symptoms include any of the following, for which there is no other explanation: persistent heavy night sweats; extreme fatigue; severe weight loss; enlarged lymph glands in neck, axillae, or groin; persistent diarrhea; skin rashes; blurred vision or chronic headache; harsh dry cough; thick gray-white coating on tongue or throat.	

cents need appropriate instruction about the safe handling of motor vehicles. Parents often need guidance in setting limits on the use of motor vehicles by their teenage children. Limits should be negotiated by the parents and the teenager and periodically reviewed and revised according to the teenager's safety record. Teenagers may use driving as an outlet for stress, as a way to assert independence, or as a way to impress peers. When setting limits on automobile use, parents need to assess the teenager's level of responsibility, common sense, and ability to resist peer pressure. The age of the teenager alone does not determine readiness to handle this responsibility.

Adolescents are at risk for sports injuries because their coordination skills are not fully developed. However, sports activities are important to the adolescent's self-esteem and overall development. In addition to providing beneficial exercise, sports activities enhance social and personal development. They help the adolescent experience competition, teamwork, and conflict resolution. The nurse can help adolescents prevent sports injuries by encouraging:

1. The use of proper safety equipment
2. Appropriate physical examinations before participating in sports
3. Enforcement of regulations that prevent an injured player from further participation in sports activities until a physician advises it.

Faced with dramatic changes in body structure and function and greater expectations to assume responsibilities, many adolescents experience temporary difficulty in developing a positive self-image. Adolescents who are accepted, loved, and valued by family and peers generally tend to gain confidence and feel good about themselves. Adolescents who have difficulty forming relationships or who are perceived by peers as too different and not included in adolescent cliques may develop less favorable self-images and have low self-esteem. Teenagers with physical handicaps or illnesses are particularly vulnerable to peer rejection. Nurses and educators can promote peer understanding and acceptance by discussing the individual's specific problems with the peer group. Establishing groups of peers who have similar problems can provide an opportunity for the individual to develop close relationships with others and feel valued and accepted.

Common teenage problems related to self-esteem and self-concept include drug abuse, suicide, and homicide, although they can also be considered protection needs. **Drug and substance abuse,** including alcohol abuse, is on the rise among teenagers, especially among those with emotional problems. Many adolescents take drugs to have a new experience, to feel they belong to the group and thus relieve loneliness, or to prove they are courageous. This experimental use of drugs is a one-time or infrequent occurrence. Some teenagers, however, use drugs regularly. Compulsive users become dependent on drugs. Some drugs abused by teenagers are alcohol, glue and similar substances, barbiturates and amphetamines, hallucinogens, marijuana, and cocaine. Adolescent health promotion programs provided by nurses should include the following information:

1. The underlying reasons for drug use and more positive coping mechanisms to deal with stress
2. The hazards of drug misuse and abuse
3. Responsible ways to make decisions about drug use before experimentation and ways to handle peer pressure

The nurse should also be alert for signs that a teenager is misusing drugs. Some of these are a drop in school achievement, mood swings, sleepiness or fatigue, and personality changes, such as withdrawal or boisterous behavior.

Suicide and homicide are two of the leading causes of death among teenagers. Adolescent males are more likely to commit suicide than adolescent females, and blacks are more likely to commit homicide than whites. Suicides by firearms, drugs, and automobile exhaust gases are the most common. Most suicidal persons give verbal or behavioral warnings prior to suicide, and certain tendencies or behaviors are suspect. For example, most people who commit suicide have made previous attempts, are severely depressed, and are at odds with themselves and those close to them. Such individuals need to be referred to professional help. Health promotion programs for adolescents need to include information about suicide, alternatives to suicide, and ways to deal with a peer who might be suicidal.

Homicide is more common among the poor than other economic classes, and both killers and their victims are more likely to be men than women. Often homicide is associated with alcohol abuse and occurs most frequently at night and on weekends. Factors influencing the high homicide rate include economic deprivation, family breakup, and the availability of firearms, which are the most frequently used weapons. Cutting or stabbing tools are the next most frequently used weapons.

Chapter Highlights

Infants from 1 month to 1 year reveal marked growth in size and stature with appropriate nutrition and care: birth weight is doubled by 6 months and tripled by 12 months.

During infancy, motor development is notable; at 3 months, infants can raise their heads from the prone position, at 6 months, they can sit unsupported, and at 12 months, they can stand momentarily and walk with help.

Continuing, sensitive, loving, and consistent attention to the infant's needs must be maintained to develop a sense of trust and security.

The nurse can assess the psychosocial and motor development of infants by using the Denver Developmental Screening Test and similar tests.

To promote and protect the health of the infant, caregivers must provide appropriate nutrition, maintain body temperature, ensure adequate rest and sleep, protect the infant from accidents, immunize the infant, and teach parents to give appropriate stimulation and love.

When infants' needs are met and they receive positive feedback for their achievements, they begin to develop a sense of pride, sense of self, and self-esteem.

Early childhood spans the period from 1 to 6 years and is subdivided into two groups: the toddler group, ages 1 to 3, and the preschool group, ages 4 and 5.

During childhood, dramatic changes occur in physical, psychologic, and cognitive development; the child moves from being a dependent person to becoming an independent person entering school.

As the nervous system develops, body systems mature to the point where the child can control his or her body, achieve finer muscle control, and perform all the activities of daily living, such as washing and dressing.

The child also develops a unique personality and way of behaving.

From age 2 onward, peers play an important role during play.

Investigation of sexual differences among peers is common during childhood.

Critical to psychosocial development during childhood is the development of a sense of autonomy and initiative.

By the end of early childhood, the child has reached the phase of intuitive thought in cognitive development, has developed some internal moral controls, and is at the undifferentiated level of spiritual development.

The school-age period of development begins at age 6 and ends with the onset of puberty.

School-age children perfect their muscular skills and coordination and develop a sense of competence, perseverance, and self-worth.

During emotional development, school-age children face the conflict of industry versus inferiority.

Peers are very important to school-age children; same-sex friendships develop.

School-age children begin to understand relationships and change from being egocentric to having cooperative interactions; according to Piaget, they are in the concrete operations phase of cognitive development.

Most school-age children progress to the conventional level of moral development and to the mythical-literal stage of spiritual development.

Adolescence is a critical period of development extending from the onset of puberty to age 18 or 21.

Rapid growth in height, development of secondary sexual characteristics, sexual maturity, and increasing independence from the family are major landmarks of adolescence.

- The dramatic physical changes of early adolescence require major adjustments in body image.
- Peer groups assume great importance during adolescence; they provide a sense of belonging and self-esteem and facilitate the development of a positive self-concept.
- Late adolescence is a more stable stage, during which the adolescent is mostly involved with planning a future and economic independence.
- Adolescents between the ages of 11 to 15 begin the formal operations stage of cognitive development; they are able to think logically, rationally, and futuristically and can conceptualize things as they could be rather than as they are.
- The adolescent is at Kohlberg's conventional level of moral development, and some proceed to the postconventional or principled level.
- Adolescents are at Fowler's synthetic-conventional stage of spiritual development.
- The nurse plays a major role in assessing the growth and development of children and adolescents.
- Because accidents are the leading cause of morbidity and mortality among toddlers, preschoolers, and school-age children, parental guidance about accident prevention is essential.
- Major problems of adolescents that require primary preventive interventions are obesity, anorexia nervosa, bulimia, sexually transmitted disease, unplanned pregnancy, motor vehicle accidents, sports injuries, drug abuse, and suicide.

Selected References

Adams, B. N. June 1983. Adolescent health care: Needs, priorities, and services. *Nursing Clinics of North America* 18:237–48.

Clark, A. L. 1981. *Culture and childrearing.* Philadelphia: F. A. Davis Co.

Duvall, E. M. 1977. *Marriage and family development.* 5th ed. New York: J. B. Lippincott.

Edelman, C., and Mandle, C. L. 1986. *Health promotion throughout the life span.* St. Louis: C. V. Mosby Co.

Endres, J. B., and Rockwell, R. E. 1980. *Food, nutrition, and the young child.* St. Louis: C. V. Mosby Co.

Engel, G. L. 1962. *Psychological development in health and disease.* Philadelphia: W. B. Saunders Co.

Erikson, E. H. 1963. *Childhood and society.* 2d ed. New York: W. W. Norton and Co.

Fong, B. C., and Resnick, M. R. 1980. *The child: Development through adolescence.* Menlo Park, Calif.: Benjamin/Cummings Publishing Co.

Gedan, S. October 1974. Abortion counseling with adolescents. *American Journal of Nursing* 74:1856–58.

Griffith-Kenney, J. 1986. *Contemporary women's health: A nursing advocacy approach.* Menlo Park, Calif.: Addison-Wesley Publishing Co.

Guyton, A. C. 1986. *Textbook of medical physiology.* 7th ed. Philadelphia: W. B. Saunders Co.

Haber, J.; Leach, A. M.; Schudy, S. M.; and Sideleau, B. F. 1982. *Comprehensive psychiatric nursing.* 2d ed. New York: McGraw-Hill.

Hall, C. S., and Lindzey, G. 1970. *Theories of personality.* 2d ed. New York: John Wiley and Sons.

Havighurst, R. J. 1952. *Developmental tasks and education.* 2d ed. New York: David McKay Co.

Hersh, R. H.; Paolitto, D. P.; and Reimer, J. 1979. *Promoting moral growth from Piaget to Kohlberg.* New York: Longman.

Hogan, R. 1985. *Human sexuality: A nursing perspective.* 2d ed. Norwalk, Conn.: Appleton-Century-Crofts.

Howard, R. M., and Herbold, N. H. 1982. *Nutrition in clinical care.* New York: McGraw-Hill.

Inman, M. 1975. What teen-agers want in sex education. Reprinted in O'Connor, A. B., editor. *Contemporary nursing series: Nursing of children and adolescents.* New York: American Journal of Nursing Co.

Klaus, M. H., and Kennell, J. H. 1983. *Bonding: The beginnings of parent-infant attachment.* St. Louis: C. V. Mosby Co.

Maccoby, E. E., and Jacklin, C. N. 1985. The psychology of sex differences (summary and commentary). In Bloom, M., editor. *Life span development: Bases for preventive and interventive helping.* 2d ed. New York: Macmillan.

Mott, S. R.; Fazekas, N. F.; and James, S. R. 1985. *Nursing care of children and families: A holistic approach.* Menlo Park, Calif.: Addison-Wesley Publishing Co.

Murray, R. B., and Zentner, J. P. 1985. *Nursing assessment and health promotion through the life span.* 3d ed. Englewood Cliffs, N.J.: Prentice-Hall.

Nelms, B. C. November/December 1981. What is a normal adolescent? *American Journal of Maternal Child Nursing* 6:402–5.

Piaget, J. 1963. *Origins of intelligence in children.* New York: W. W. Norton and Co.

Pipes, P. L. 1981. *Nutrition in infancy and childhood.* St. Louis: C. V. Mosby Co.

Schulman, M., and Mekler, E. 1985. *Bringing up a moral child: A new approach for teaching your child to be kind, just, and responsible.* Reading, Mass.: Addison-Wesley Publishing Co.

Schuster, C. S., and Ashburn, S. S. 1980. *The process of human development: A holistic approach.* Boston: Little, Brown and Co.

Smith, M. J.; Goodman, J. A.; Ramsey, N. L.; and Pasternack, S. B. 1982. *Child and family: Concepts of nursing practice.* New York: McGraw-Hill.

Suitor, C. W., and Hunter, M. F. 1980. *Nutrition: Principles and application in health promotion.* Philadelphia: J. B. Lippincott Co.

Wood, S. P. March/April 1983. School-aged children's perceptions of the cause of illness. *Pediatric Nursing* 9:101–4.

CHAPTER 28

Young Adulthood Through Middle Adulthood

O B J E C T I V E S

Describe physical changes that occur from young adulthood through middle adulthood.

Explain psychosocial development of young and middle-aged adults according to Erikson.

Describe cognitive development of young and middle-aged adults according to Piaget.

Explain moral development of young and middle-aged adults according to Kohlberg.

Describe spiritual development of young and middle-aged adults according to Fowler.

Identify common health hazards of young and middle-aged adults.

Describe nursing implications related to the common health hazards identified.

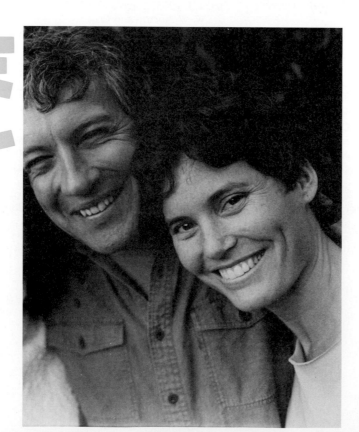

Adulthood and Maturity

The age at which a person is considered an adult depends on how adulthood is described. Legally, a person in the United States can vote at 18 years. The legal age for alcohol consumption outside the home varies among states from 18 years to 21 years. Another criterion of adulthood is financial independence, which is also highly variable. Some adolescents support themselves as early as 16 years of age, usually because of family circumstances. By contrast, some adults are financially dependent on their families for many years, as, for example, during prolonged education.

Adulthood may also be indicated by moving away from home and establishing one's own living arrangements. Yet this independence is also highly variable. Some adolescents leave home perhaps because of family problems, whereas some people in their 20s remain at home. The latter is not unusual during periods of economic depression.

Maturity is the state of maximal function and integration or a state of being fully developed. Maturity in the adult can be described by the following:

1. The individual has developed a system of internal and external behavior controls that are acceptable on the adult level.
2. The individual has developed a value-judgment system that enables him or her to live acceptably in a social group.

Mature people have a number of traits. Kaluger and Kaluger (1979, pp. 372–74) describe a mature person as one whose behavior reflects a balance of intellectual insight, emotion, and imagination. The person learns to live with problems that cannot be solved and looks for solutions to problems that can be solved. Mature people have some knowledge of the requirements for living in society, take responsibility for their own behavior, and do not expect others to make decisions for them.

Young Adults

The adult phase of development encompasses the years from the end of adolescence to death. Because the developmental tasks of young adults differ from those of older adults, adulthood is often divided in three phases—young adulthood, middle adulthood, and late adulthood. In this book young adults are defined as people 20 to 40 years old; middle-aged adults, as 40 to 65; and older adults (those in late adulthood), over 65.

During young adulthood, people have a number of developmental tasks. They become independent of their families, establish careers, often establish a close relationship with a significant other, and decide whether to have children. The young adult is typically a busy person who faces many challenges. See the accompanying box for a summary of young adults' developmental tasks.

DEVELOPMENTAL TASKS

Young Adults

Erikson's stage: Intimacy versus isolation

- Select a life partner
- Choose an occupation or career
- Establish independence from parents and financial self-sufficiency
- Establish intimate relationships
- Establish a social network
- Form a personal philosophy and ethical structure

Physical Development

Persons in their early 20s are in their prime years physically. The musculoskeletal system is well developed and coordinated. This is the period when athletic endeavors reach their peak. Indeed, after 40 years, most athletes are considered old.

All other systems of the body are also functioning at peak efficiency. The circulatory system is well developed. Pregnant women, for example, are able to provide additional blood supplies to the placenta. The reproductive system is fully developed. The woman's menstrual cycle is regular, and sexual organs are sufficiently mature to cope with childbearing. The man's sexual maturity, reached in adolescence, remains at a peak so that the sexual urge remains high throughout this phase. In summary, physical change is minimal during this phase; psychosocial development, by contrast, is great.

Psychosocial Development

According to Erikson, the central task of the young adult is *intimacy versus isolation*. Young adults are viewed as developing an intimate, lasting relationship with another person or a cause, institution, or creative effort (Erikson 1963, p. 263). The basic strength that evolves from this relationship is love; the outcome of negative resolution is exclusivity (Erikson 1982, p. 33).

Young adults face a number of new experiences and changes in life-style. They must make decisions for themselves, and many of the decisions made now influence the person's life-style in years to come. The expectations of the young adult are often taken for granted, since they are well defined in most cultures. **Choices** must be made about education and employment, whether to marry or remain single, starting a home, and rearing children. **Social responsibilities** include forming new friendships and assuming some community activities.

Occupational choice and education are largely inseparable. Education influences occupational opportunities; conversely, an occupation, once chosen, can determine the education needed and sought. Education enhances employment opportunities, enriches leisure time, and ensures economic survival. In the past, more young men than young women were encouraged to pursue advanced education, particularly college education. Education was deemed unnecessary for women who traditionally assumed the roles of wife and mother. This notion has changed as the role of women has changed. Many women now choose to assume active careers and civic roles in society.

Remaining single is becoming the life-style of more and more young adults. Many people choose to remain single, perhaps to pursue an education and then to have the freedom to pursue their chosen vocations. Some unmarried individuals choose to live with another person of the opposite or same sex and share living arrangements and certain expenses. Some unmarried people are gay or lesbian and live with or are involved with a partner to whom they are committed.

Nurses should not assume that an unmarried person has no partner. Discrete, sensitive, and unprejudiced questioning of a client can often elicit information about a friend or support person who is especially significant to the client. Because single adults may live alone or with other adults who are employed, problems can arise when single persons are ill. Finding someone to drive them to a hospital or to help with shopping and meals during recuperation can be major challenges. A support system for a single adult may take more organization than the support system of a married person.

Deciding on a life partner is a difficult task. It is in many ways more complex and confusing than other tasks required of the young adult. In North America, there is emphasis on falling in love as a basis for mate selection. However, the multiple aspects of love make it difficult for some people to recognize and to know the meaning of love. Numerous definitions of love are available in literature, but the one important aspect of love is that it is lasting. Love survives times of frustration, strained relationships, and sadness, as well as times of happiness and achievement. It evolves out of interaction and requires adjustments and readjustments of the personalities of the people involved. There is a desire to do all one can to make the other person's life meaningful. In contrast, infatuation is sexually stimulating and exciting, but it is too shallow to nurture total personal growth of either partner and lasts only a short time.

Cognitive Development

Piaget believes that cognitive structures are complete during the *formal operations period*, from roughly 11 to 15 years. From that time, formal operations (for example, generating hypotheses) characterize thinking throughout adulthood and are applied to more areas. Egocentrism continues to decline; however, according to Piaget, these changes do not involve a change in the structure of thought, only a change in its content and stability (Miller 1983, pp. 62–65).

Moral Development

Young adults who have mastered the previous stages of Kohlberg's theory of moral development now enter the *postconventional level.* See Table 26–6 on page 359. At this time, the person is able to separate self from the expectations and rules of others and to define morality in terms of personal principles. When individuals perceive a conflict between society's rules or laws, they judge according to their own principles. For example, a person may intentionally break the law and join a protest group to stop hunters from killing wild animals, believing that the principle of conservation of wildlife justifies the protest action. This type of reasoning is called **principled reasoning.**

Spiritual Development

According to Fowler, the individual enters the individuating-reflective period sometime after 18 years of age. During this period, the individual focuses on reality. A 27-year-old adult may ask philosophic questions regarding spirituality and may be self-conscious about spiritual matters.

Health Promotion and Protection

To promote and protect health, the nurse must first obtain a baseline assessment of the young adult. Assessment guidelines for growth and development of the young adult are shown in the accompanying box.

Common health hazards during young adulthood include accidents, infections, suicide and homicide, drug abuse, obesity, and hypertension. The risks of breast and testicular cancers occurring also become noticeable during this phase of life, and young adults need to learn to perform self-examinations to promote early identification.

▪ **Accidents.** Accidents are a leading cause of death among people 15 to 24 years old. Alcohol consumption is associated with about 60% of these fatalities. Nursing has a preventive function in this regard, to work toward changing attitudes that allow people to drive recklessly

GUIDELINES

Assessing Young Adults

Does the young adult:

- Feel independent from parents?
- Have a realistic self-concept?
- Like self and the direction in which life is going?
- Interact well with family and friends?
- Have an enriching intimate relationship?
- Have a meaningful social life?
- Have a well-established career or occupation?
- Demonstrate emotional, social, and economic responsibility for own life?
- Have a set of values that guides behavior?
- Have a healthy life-style?

and while intoxicated. This can be implemented through client teaching and by participation in community activities. As citizens, nurses may work with others through interested groups or as individuals to lobby elected officials to enact safety legislation. See Chapter 2.

■ **Infections.** Sexually transmitted diseases (STD) such as genital herpes, syphilis, and gonorrhea are the most common **infections** in young adults. Nursing functions are largely educational. The use of condoms greatly reduces the transfer of infectious microorganisms from one partner to another. Knowledge about the symptoms of these diseases can help the client obtain early treatment. In dealing with clients with STD, the nurse must be nonjudgmental and accepting of the client's life-style and treat any information obtained as confidential.

Upper respiratory tract infections also occur frequently in young adults. Nursing function is largely preventive: reducing the individual's susceptibility by supporting body defenses through adequate nutrition, rest, liquids, and exercise. Part of prevention is reducing susceptibility by teaching the dangers of alcohol, cigarettes, and contaminants. When ill, the young adult should be encouraged to obtain medical treatment rather than risk chronic respiratory problems later in life.

■ **Suicide and Homicide.** **Suicide** is the third leading cause of death among teenagers and young adults. **Homicide** accounts for 10% of all deaths among teenagers and young adults: 7% of all deaths among whites and nearly 30% among blacks in this age group (U.S. DHHS 1984, p. 19). Measures to prevent suicide include (Murray and Zentner 1985, p. 460):

1. Educating the public about the early signs of suicide
2. Establishing significant relationships for high-risk people
3. Encouraging young adults to participate in social activities, thus preventing isolation

Nursing counseling services and crisis facilities can often assist young adults at times of high stress to make important decisions and constructive adaptations to their environments, thereby decreasing the incidence of suicide and homicide.

■ **Substance Abuse.** **Substance abuse** is a major threat to the health of young adults. Alcohol, marijuana, amphetamines, and cocaine, for example, can bring about feelings of well-being that may be highly valued by people with adjustment problems. Prolonged use can lead to physical and psychologic dependency and subsequent health problems. For example, drug abuse during pregnancy can lead to fetal damage. Prolonged use of alcohol can lead to such diseases as cirrhosis of the liver and cancer of the esophagus.

Nursing strategies related to substance abuse include teaching about the complications of their use, changing individual attitudes toward drug and alcohol abuse, and counseling regarding problems that lead to abuse. Smoking is another type of substance abuse that can lead to

GUIDELINES

Discouraging Smoking

- Serve as a role model by not smoking
- Provide educational information regarding the dangers of smoking
- Help make smoking socially unacceptable, e.g., by posting "no smoking" signs in client lounges and offices
- Suggest resources, e.g., hypnosis, life-style training, and behavior modification, to clients who desire to stop smoking.

such diseases as cancer of the lung and cardiovascular disease. Guidelines for nurses to discourage client smoking and provided in the accompanying box.

■ **Obesity.** **Obesity** arises as a problem during the young adult years because physical growth is completed during adolescence or early adulthood and most people require fewer calories. Caloric needs are highly individual, depending primarily on the physical activity of the individual, the climate, and body size. Young adults usually lead busy lives, and fast foods may make up much of their diets. Nurses can counsel clients about the need for a balanced, nourishing diet that includes fruits and vegetables. In response to heightened awareness of nutrition, many fast food restaurants are now providing lower-fat items. Similarly, companies that produce microwave entrees are responding to this demand. Exercise should also be encouraged, because people who exercise are less likely to overeat.

■ **Hypertension.** **High blood pressure** is a major cause of illness in young adults. In the United States, 13 to 17% of whites and 26 to 28% of blacks age 20 and older have both high blood pressure and weight problems (Edelman and Mandle 1986, p. 491). Nursing strategies to prevent and treat hypertension are largely educational. Clients must reduce the intake of foods that are high in cholesterol, fat, and salt. Supportive counseling and positive reinforcement are strategies that promote compliance. See Chapter 21.

■ **Cancer.** Of all cancers among women, **cancer of the breast** is the most frequent cause of death. The peak incidence of breast cancer is during middle age. However, the young woman needs to form the habit of examining the breasts regularly. The effectiveness of treatment increases significantly the earlier a breast lump is discovered.

Breast self-examination (BSE) should be conducted once a month. A regular time is best, such as immediately following menstrual flow or on the first day of the month. Women who examine themselves regularly become familiar with the shape and texture of their breasts. Any changes should be reported immediately to a nurse practitioner or physician for diagnosis. Before beginning to teach BSE to a client, the nurse needs to identify the client's attitudes toward this procedure. Some women are reluctant to conduct BSE because they fear what they might find. The nurse needs to explore these fears with the client. Women often offer these reasons for avoiding BSE: "I don't have time" and "I just don't think of doing it." The nurse also needs to explore these reasons with the client with particular reference to her self-esteem (see Chapter 14) and her need to spend time on herself.

Another reason for not conducting BSE is a reluctance to handle the breasts. Manipulation may be associated with fondling and masturbation. This reason often goes unexpressed among older women and some religious and cultural groups. Changing such attitudes frequently requires in-depth counseling as well as accurate information about BSE. A woman may accept information only after attitudes have changed.

BSE has three stages: the first takes place in the bath or shower; the second takes place while the client sits in front of a mirror; and the third takes place while the client lies down. During a bath or shower, the woman checks for any lumps or thickenings by moving flat fingers over every part of each breast. Fingers glide easily over wet skin. The right hand is used to examine the left breast, and the left hand is used to examine the right breast.

In the second stage, the woman sits before a mirror with hands first at the sides and then clasped over the head. Each breast is observed in both positions for:

▪ Indentations, rippling, puckering, or dimpling

▪ Asymmetry of the nipples; e.g., a nipple pulled to one side

▪ Discoloration

▪ Discharge from the nipple

▪ Any change in the size or shape of the breasts

Dimpling can be caused by scar tissue formation or a lesion. See Figure 28–1. Show the client how to accentuate any retraction by raising her arms above her head, pushing her hands together with elbows flexed (see Figure 28–2, A), or pressing her hands down on her hips (see Figure 28–2, B).

The client conducts the last part of the examination while lying in bed and palpating the breasts. Instruct the client to palpate the breast using the guidelines shown in the accompanying box.

Testicular cancer accounts for approximately 1% of all the cancer in men and often occurs in men in their early 30s (Crooks and Baur 1983, p. 129). It is most commonly found on the anterior and lateral surfaces of the testes. See Figure 28–4. This cancer is often serious and requires extensive surgery if discovered in the later stages. In the early stages, the cancer is asymptomatic except for a mass within the testicle. The lump often feels hard and bumpy and can usually be differentiated from tissue around it. The client may also experience a feeling of heaviness in the scrotum.

Testicular self-examination should be conducted monthly. The client can examine the testicles while he sits, stands, or lies down. A good time for this

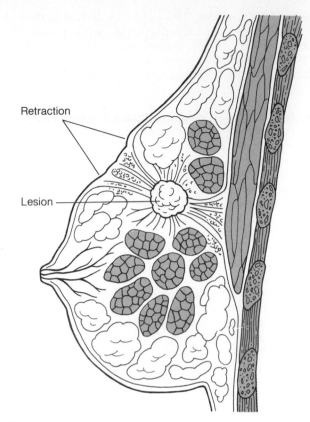

Figure 28–1 A breast lesion can cause retraction or dimpling of breast tissue.

GUIDELINES

Breast Self-Examination

1. To examine the right breast, place a pillow or folded towel under the right shoulder and the right hand behind the head. This position distributes breast tissue more evenly on the breast.
2. With the left hand:
   ▪ Press the palmar surfaces of the middle three fingers on the skin surface, starting in the upper lateral quadrant, i.e., the outermost top of the breast.
   ▪ Use a gentle rotating motion to press the breast tissue against the chest wall.
   ▪ Palpate from the periphery to the areola.
   ▪ Move the peripheral starting point around the breast clockwise. See Figure 28–3.
   ▪ Finally, squeeze the nipple of each breast gently between the thumb and index finger. Note any clear or bloody discharge.
3. Repeat the above for the left breast with a pillow under the left shoulder and the left hand behind the head.
4. Report a lump or nipple discharge to the physician immediately. A ridge of firm tissue in the curve of each breast is normal.

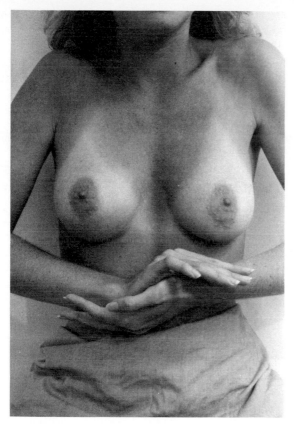
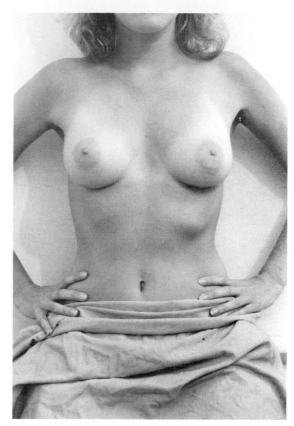

Figure 28—2 Retraction of breast tissue can be accentuated by **A,** pressing the hands together, or

B, pressing the hands down on the hips.

exploration is after a hot bath or shower since the heat causes the scrotal skin to relax and the testes to descend. Guidelines for testicular self-examination are found in the accompanying box.

Like BSE, the topic of testicular self-examination makes many nurses and clients uncomfortable. Factors such as the relative ages of the nurse and client, culture, and prior experiences influence the interpersonal relationship between the nurse and client and likewise the discussion. The nurse who approaches the topic in a matter-of-fact manner and focuses on the health promotion aspects of testicular self-examination is likely to have a successful teaching-learning session. See Chapters 20 and 21 for specific communication and teaching strategies.

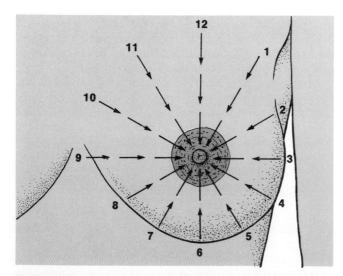

Figure 28—3 The clockwise palpation method for breast self-examination ensures that all parts of the breast are examined.

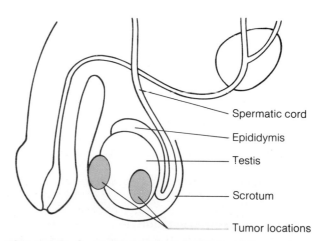

Spermatic cord

Epididymis

Testis

Scrotum

Tumor locations

Figure 28—4 Common tumor locations of the testes

GUIDELINES

Testicular Self-Examination

Instruct the man to:

1. Examine the testicles monthly, one at a time.
2. Use the fingertips to probe the surface gently, as if examining an egg for imperfections. The surface should be smooth and fairly firm.
3. Using the thumb and fingers of both hands and placing one hand under the scrotum, and the other over the scrotum, palpate the testicle. It normally feels rubbery, smooth, and free of lumps.
4. After palpating both testicles, compare the weights of the testicles.
5. Then palpate the epididymis, which is at the top of the testicle and extends behind it. It should feel soft and slightly tender.
6. Last, locate the spermatic cord, which ascends from the epididymis behind the testicle. It normally feels firm and smooth (Murray and Wilcox 1978, p. 2074).

Middle-Aged Adults

The middle years, from 40 to 65, have been called the years of stability and consolidation. For most people, it is a time when children have grown and moved away or are moving away from home. Thus, partners generally have more time for and with each other and time to pursue interests they may have deferred for years. Middle adulthood has a number of broad developmental tasks. See the accompanying box.

Physical Development

A number of changes take place during the middle years. At 40, most adults can function as effectively as they did in their 20s. However, during ages 40 to 65, physical changes do take place. Some of these are as follows:

▪ Gray hair appears.
▪ Crease lines appear at the lateral aspects of the eyes (laugh lines).

DEVELOPMENTAL TASKS

Middle-Aged Adults

Erikson's stage: Generativity vs. stagnation

▪ Accepting the changes of middle age
▪ Investing in a new generation
▪ Adjusting to the needs of aging parents
▪ Reevaluating life's goals and accomplishments

▪ Fatty tissue is redistributed in men and women; men tend to develop fat on their abdomens, and women also deposit fat around the middle of the body.

▪ Energy is more slowly recovered and more quickly expended. Vigor and endurance start to deplete at about 40 years.

▪ Hearing acuity decreases and sight diminishes; reading glasses or bifocals may be needed.

▪ Skeletal muscle bulk decreases at about 60 years.

▪ General slowing of metabolism results in weight gain.

▪ Hormonal changes take place in both men and women.

Both men and women experience decreasing hormonal production during the middle years. The **menopause** refers to the so-called change of life in women, when menstruation ceases. The **climacteric** (andropause) refers to the change of life in men, when sexual activity decreases. The menopause usually occurs anywhere between ages 40 and 55. The average is about 47 years. At this time, the ovaries decrease in activity until ovulation ceases. A number of menstrual patterns can signal the menopause. Four of these are:

1. Periods remain regular, but menstrual flow decreases.
2. Periods occur irregularly, and some periods are missed.
3. Menstrual flow ceases abruptly.
4. Menstrual flow occurs irregularly, with irregular amount of menses.

During menopause, the ovaries decrease in size, and the uterus becomes smaller and firmer. Progesterone is not produced, and the estrogen levels fall. Although the pituitary gland continues to produce the luteinizing hormone (LH) and the follicle-stimulating hormone (FSH), the ovaries do not respond. As a result of the lack of feedback, the pituitary gland increases the production of the gonadotropins, in particular FSH. This disturbed endocrine balance accounts for some of the symptoms of the menopause. Common symptoms are hot flashes, chilliness, a tendency of the breasts to become smaller and flabby, and a tendency to become obese. Insomnia and headaches occur with relative frequency. Psychologically, the menopause can be an anxiety-producing time, especially if the ability to bear children is an integral part of the woman's self-concept.

In men, there is not a change comparable to the menopause in women. Androgen levels decrease very slowly; however, men can father children even in late life. The psychologic problems that men experience are generally related to the fear of getting old and to retirement, boredom, and finances.

Psychosocial Development

Until recently, the developmental tasks of middle-aged adults have received little attention. Erik Erikson (1963, p. 266) viewed the developmental choice of the middle-aged adult as *generativity versus stagnation*. **Generativity** is defined as the concern for establishing and guiding the next generation. In other words, there is concern about providing for the welfare of humankind that is equal to the concern of providing for self. People in their 20s and 30s tend to be self- and family-centered. In middle age, the self seems more altruistic, and concepts of service to others and love and compassion gain prominence. These concepts motivate charitable and altruistic actions, such as church work, social work, political work, community fund-raising drives, and cultural endeavors.

Marriage partners have more time for companionship and recreation; thus, marriage can be more satisfying in the middle years of life. There is time to work together in volunteer activities. There is time for one partner to go out for lunch and for the other to go fishing. Generative middle-aged persons are able to feel a sense of comfort in their life-style and receive gratification from charitable endeavors.

Erikson believes that persons who are unable to expand their interests at this time and who do not assume the responsibility of middle age suffer a sense of boredom and impoverishment, i.e., stagnation. These persons have difficulty accepting their aging bodies and become withdrawn and isolated. They are preoccupied with self and unable to give to others. Some may regress to younger patterns of behavior, e.g., adolescent behavior.

At this time, adults usually face a number of adjustments in relation to their relationships and activities. Husbands and wives generally have more time for leisure activities. Relationships with families change. Children move away and marry and have children of their own. Parents are elderly and often have additional needs. Thus people in their 40s and 50s often find themselves grandparents, enjoying their grandchildren but having few responsibilities for them, and at the same time assisting with the care of their own elderly parents. At this time people often face the death of a parent and as a result come to terms with their own aging and inevitable death.

Robert Peck (1968) believes that although physical capabilities and functions decrease with old age, mental and social capacities tend to increase in the latter part of life. Peck recognizes four sets of developmental challenges during middle age:

1. The person values wisdom over physical strength and attractiveness.
2. Socialization replaces sexuality in male-female relationships; the middle-aged person sees people of the opposite sex as companions and individuals.
3. Experience is used more as a guideline than as a rigid rule for thought and behavior.
4. The person redirects emotional investment to new people, roles, and activities as previous ones become unsatisfactory or change; e.g., as children leave home, parents die, or friends move (Peck 1968).

For adults who are career oriented, the middle adult years often represent the peak professional and occupational performance. Adults have many experiences behind them, which, together with intellectual skills, permit them to be effective in many areas, such as financial and career endeavors.

Retirement plans are also essential for middle-aged people. It is important that feelings about retirement be considered and that thought be given to ways in which increased leisure time is used. Middle-aged people who plan ahead for the financial needs of retirement and establish new ways to keep active often adapt to the retirement situation more effectively than those who do not.

The middle-aged person looks older and feels older. People usually accept the fact that they are aging; however, a few try to defy the years by their dress and even their actions. Some men and women have extramarital affairs and marry younger partners. A new freedom to be independent and follow one's individual interests arises. Prior to this period, the marriage partner or lover and other persons were crucial to a definition of self. Now the middle-aged person does not make comparisons with others, no longer fears aging or death, relaxes his or her sense of competitiveness, and enjoys the independence and freedom of middle age. Other people's opinions become less important, and the earlier habit of trying to please everyone is overcome. The person establishes ethical and moral standards that are independent of the standards of others. The focus shifts from inner self and being to outer self and doing. Religious and philosophical concerns become important.

In middle age, the interests set aside in favor of family and career can be renewed and developed. Hobbies such as photography, collecting antiques, or painting may develop into serious work. Some people who deferred education now pursue it or take refresher and other courses to keep abreast of changes. Some women enter the work force. Many middle-aged people feel a mixture of excitement and fear about these new undertakings.

Gail Sheehy (1977) suggests that the transition into middle life is as critical as adolescence. She outlines characteristics of the midlife crisis and calls the decade between the ages of 35 to 45 the "deadline decade." According to Sheehy, most women pass through the midlife crisis between 35 and 40; most men, between 40 and 45. This crisis occurs when a person recognizes he or she has reached the halfway mark of life. Although people of these ages are reaching their prime, there is a beginning recognition that time is at a premium and that life is finite. Youthfulness and physical strength can no longer be taken for granted. Some characteristics of the midlife crisis include:

- Feeling bored, burdened, restless, and unappreciated
- Dissatisfaction with the way one's life has developed
- Ambivalence and uncertainty about the future
- Dismay about signs of aging
- Fear that time will be insufficient to accomplish goals
- Feelings of self-doubt
- Need to search for self, i.e., establish a true identity
- Worry about health
- Feelings of sadness, loneliness, or depression

Sheehy (1977, p. 44) describes this midlife crisis as an "inner crossroads" or "footbridge" leading to the second half of life. It is an "authenticity" crisis in which people face the discrepancy between their youthful ambitions and their actual attainment. To overcome this crisis, people need to reexamine their purposes and reevaluate ways to use their abilities and energies from now on. In Sheehy's words, it is a time when people ask, "Why am I doing all this? What do I really believe in? Is this all there is?" The parts of self that have been previously suppressed now need to be expressed. Both men and women in midlife crises sense a feeling of urgency and perhaps despair when they look at those options they have set aside and realize that aging and ill health may soon hinder such opportunities.

▪ Cognitive Development

The middle-aged adult's cognitive and intellectual abilities change very little. Cognitive processes include reaction time, memory, perception, learning, problem solving, and creativity. According to Murray and Zentner, reaction time during the middle years stays much the same or begins diminishing during the later part of the middle years. Memory and problem solving are maintained through middle adulthood. Learning continues and can be enhanced by increased motivation at this time in life. Middle-aged adults are able to carry out all the strategies of Piaget's phase of *formal operations*. The middle-aged person can "reflect on the past and current experience and can imagine, anticipate, plan and hope" (Murray and Zentner 1985, pp. 515–17).

▪ Moral Development

According to Kohlberg, the adult can move beyond the *conventional level* to the *postconventional level*. Kohlberg believes that extensive experience of personal moral choice and responsibility is required before people can reach the postconventional level. Kohlberg found that few of his subjects achieved the highest level of moral reasoning. To move from stage 4, a *law and order orientation*, to stage 5, a *social contract orientation*, requires that the individual move to a stage in which rights of others take precedence. People in stage 5 take steps to support another's rights.

▪ Spiritual Development

Not all adults progress through Fowler's stages to the fifth, called the *paradoxical-consolidative stage*. At this stage, the individual can view "truth" from a number of viewpoints. Fowler's fifth stage corresponds to Kohlberg's fifth stage of moral development. Fowler believes that only some individuals after the age of 30 years reach this stage.

In middle age, people tend to be less dogmatic about religious beliefs, and religion often offers more comfort to the middle-aged person than it did previously. People in this age group often rely on spiritual beliefs to help them deal with illness, death, and tragedy.

GUIDELINES

Assessing Middle-Aged Adults

Does the middle-aged adult:

- Accept aging body?
- Feel comfortable with and respect self?
- Adjust to increasing independence of children?
- Adjust to increasing dependence of parents?
- Enjoy new freedom to be independent?
- Feel a sense of comfort in his or her career and lifestyle?
- Interact well and share companionable activities with life partner?
- Expand or renew previous interests?
- Pursue charitable and altruistic activities?
- Consider plans for retirement?
- Have a meaningful philosophy of life?
- Follow preventive health care practices?

▪ Health Promotion and Protection

Assessment guidelines for growth and development of the middle-aged adult are shown in the accompanying box.

Common health hazards during middle adulthood include obesity, chronic diseases, substance abuse, and cancer.

▪ Obesity. **Obesity,** which remains a problem in middle age, is associated with such disorders as diabetes and cardiovascular problems. Weight tends to increase with age. Decreased metabolism together with decreased activity mean a decreased need for calories. For each decade after 25 years, there should be a 7.5% reduction in total calories consumed (Williams 1981, p. 474). Nurses often need to counsel people in this age group to prevent or reduce obesity by reducing caloric intake and increasing exercise, which together help the client attain and maintain weight loss (Overfield 1980, p. 26).

▪ Chronic Disease. A **chronic disease** is a condition that lasts for longer than 3 months (Edelman and Mandle 1986, p. 526). Chronic diseases common in middle age are heart disease, osteoarthritis, cancer, pulmonary disease, glaucoma, and diabetes. The nurse can assist clients by advising regular screening for these diseases and encouraging the individual to attain and maintain an optimum level of health.

▪ Substance Abuse. Heavy **smoking** increases the risk of pulmonary cancer, cardiovascular disease, and chronic obstructive lung disease. See the guidelines suggested earlier in the chapter. The **excessive use of**

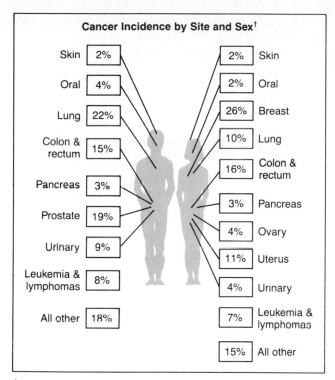

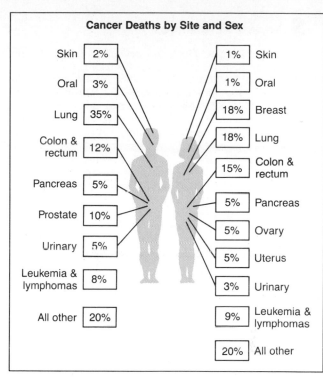

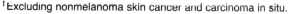

†Excluding nonmelanoma skin cancer and carcinoma in situ.

Figure 28–5 Estimates of cancer incidence and deaths by site and sex, 1985. *Source:* American Cancer Society, *Cancer facts and figures* (New York: American Cancer Society, 1985). Courtesy American Cancer Society.

alcohol is a multifaceted problem for the individual and society. Use of the drug is part of the life-style of many middle-aged Americans and Canadians. Excessive use can result in unemployment, disrupted homes, accidents, and diseases. It is estimated that four million people in the United States are dependent on alcohol and can be considered alcoholics. Nurses can help clients by providing information about the dangers of excessive alcohol use, by helping the individual clarify values about health, and by referring the client to special groups such as Alcoholics Anonymous.

■ **Cancer.** Cancer accounts for considerable mortality and morbidity in both men and women. It is the second leading cause of death among people between the ages of 25 and 64 in the United States. The patterns of cancer types and incidences for men and women have changed over the past several decades. Over one-third of the deaths due to cancer occur between the ages of 35 to 64. Men have a higher incidence of cancer of the lung and bladder than women. In women, breast cancer is highest in incidence, followed by cancer of the colon and rectum, uterus, and lung. See Figure 28–5.

■ Chapter Highlights

■ An adult reaches maturity when he or she has developed a system of internal and external controls and a value-judgment system that enables the person to live acceptably within a social group.

■ The mature person takes responsibility for his or her own behavior and does not expect others to make his or her decisions.

■ The young adult is in essentially a stable period physically but psychosocial change is great.

■ Cognitive development continues throughout adulthood.

■ Some young adults enter Kohlberg's postconventional level of moral development and develop principled reasoning.

■ Spiritual development of young adults continues into Fowler's paradoxical-consolidative stage; young adults often feel self-conscious about spiritual matters.

■ Hazards to the health of young adults include accidents, sexually transmitted diseases, suicide and homicide, substance abuse, obesity, and hypertension.

■ Nurses can assist clients to decrease the impact of these hazards.

■ The middle-aged adult needs to adjust to an aging body, the increasing dependence of parents, and the increasing independence of children; however, new independent interests can be pursued.

■ Both middle-aged men and women enter a midlife crisis in which they need to reexamine their purpose and reevaluate ways to use their energies and abilities.

■ Common health hazards of middle-aged adults include obesity, chronic diseases, substance abuse, and cancer.

■ Positive health practices can protect and promote health.

▪ Selected References

Crooks, R., and Baur, K. 1987. *Our sexuality.* 3rd ed. Menlo Park, Calif: Benjamin/Cummings Publishing Co.

Edelman, C., and Mandle, C. L. 1986. *Health promotion throughout the life span.* St. Louis: C. V. Mosby Co.

Erikson, E. H. 1963. *Childhood and society.* 2d ed. New York: W. W. Norton and Co.

————. 1982. *The life cycle completed: A review.* New York: W. W. Norton and Co.

Kaluger, G., and Kaluger, M. F. 1979. *Human development: The life span.* 2d ed. St. Louis: C. V. Mosby Co.

Miller, P. H. 1983. *Theories of developmental psychology.* San Francisco: W. H. Freeman and Co.

Murray, B. L. S., and Wilcox, L. J. December 1978. Testicular self-examination. *American Journal of Nursing* 78:2074–75.

Murray, R. B., and Zentner, J. P. 1985. *Nursing assessment and health promotion throughout the life span.* 3d ed. Englewood Cliffs, N.J.: Prentice-Hall.

National Academy of Sciences. 1980. *Recommended dietary allowances.* 9th ed. Washington, D.C.: National Academy Press.

Overfield, T. September/October 1980. Obesity: Prevention is easier than cure. *Nurse Practitioner* 5:25–26, 33, 62.

Peck, R. 1968. Psychological developments in the second half of life. In Neugarten, B. L., editor. *Middle age and aging.* Chicago: University of Chicago Press.

Sheehy, G. 1977. *Passages: Predictable crises of adult life.* New York: E. P. Dutton and Co.

U.S. Department of Health and Human Services. December 20, 1984. *Monthly vital statistics report.* Hyattsville, Md.: National Center for Health Statistics.

Williams, S. R. 1981. *Nutrition and diet therapy.* 4th ed. St. Louis: C. V. Mosby Co.

CHAPTER 29

Late Adulthood

OBJECTIVES

Describe the physical changes that occur from middle adulthood through old age.

Explain essential aspects of psychosocial changes.

Describe essential aspects of cognitive changes.

Explain essential aspects of moral development.

Explain essential aspects of spiritual development.

Identify common health hazards and problems affecting elderly adults.

Discuss nursing implications related to the health hazards and problems.

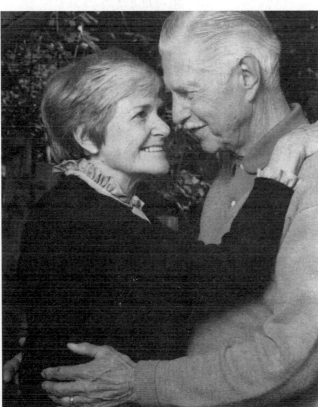

Late Adulthood

Late adulthood, for the purposes of this book, is the years after 65. Sometimes it is referred to as **senescence** or old age. Because of advances in medical and related sciences and health promotion and protection, an increasing number of people are living to an advanced age. In 1960, life expectancy at birth was about 70 years, i.e., the average person born in 1960 could expect to live about 70 years. By 1983, life expectancy had increased to 75 years (U.S. DHHS 1985, p. 1). Because of increasing life expectancy, it may be helpful to divide late adulthood into two periods: 65–75 years, the "young-old," and 75 years and older, the "old-old."

Gerontology is the study of all aspects of aging. **Geriatric nursing** is practice involving the diseases of aging. **Gerontologic nursing** deals with the scientific study and care of the elderly.

The person reaching late adulthood must accomplish a number of broad developmental tasks. These are listed in the accompanying box. Nurses may expect to note a continuum of responses to these tasks, depending upon the individual. For example, a "young-old" person may not be retired. This does not mean that person is having difficulty achieving developmental tasks.

Physical Changes Associated with Aging

As the person ages, a number of physical changes occur; some are visible, some are not. See Table 29–1 for a summary of the normal physiologic changes associated with aging.

Physical Appearance

Obvious changes occur in the **integument** (skin, hair, nails) with age. These changes include wrinkles, dryness, loss of fullness, itching, and baldness or thinning and graying of hair. The skin also becomes paler and blotchy and loses its elasticity. Fingernails and toenails become thickened and brittle, and in women over 60 years, facial hair increases.

Skin changes accompany progressive losses of underlying adipose and muscle tissue and loss of elastic

DEVELOPMENTAL TASKS

Older Adults

Erikson's stage: Integrity versus despair

- Accepting diminishing abilities and limitations
- Adjusting to retirement
- Adjusting to reorganized life patterns
- Accepting loss and death with serenity

fiber. Initially adipose tissue is redistributed from the extremities to the hips and abdomen in middle age. Generalized loss of adipose tissue progresses along with muscle atrophy, creating a wrinkled and wasted appearance. Bony prominences become visible, a double chin develops, and lower eyelids appear puffy. In elderly women, the breasts become smaller and may sag, if large and pendulous, causing chafing where the skin surfaces touch. Loss of subcutaneous fat also decreases the elderly person's tolerance of cold.

Itching increases due to dryness of the skin and deterioration of the nerve fibers and sensory endings. Decreased blood flow to the skin causes pallor and blotchiness. Baldness is thought to be due to decreased blood flow to the skin. The loss of hair color is due to a decrease in the number of functioning pigment-producing cells.

The way people respond to skin and hair changes varies with the individual, the cultures, and, sometimes, the age of the person. For example, one person may feel distinguished with gray hair, while another may feel embarrassed by it. Most women dislike their facial hair because hirsute women do not conform to the feminine cultural ideal of North Americans.

Nursing interventions in this area include teaching the client how to protect the skin from bruising and injury. Inspect the skin regularly for damage and changes in pigmentation. Some skin lesions can reflect circulatory, neurologic, hormone, or metabolic problems. Skin lesions can be premalignant or malignant, and the client needs to be referred to a physician. **Premalignant** (precancerous) means possessing the potential of becoming malignant. **Malignant** means possessing the tendency to grow and invade other tissues. Elderly people with dry skin should bathe less often than before and decrease or eliminate the use of soap, which dries the skin.

Body temperature is lower in the elderly adult due to a decrease in the metabolic rate. It is not uncommon for an elderly adult to have a temperature of 35 C (95 F), particularly in the early morning when the body's metabolism is low. This fact has implications for nurses assessing the elderly adult for fever. For example, a temperature of 37.5 C (99.5 F) can represent a marked fever in some elderly people, although it represents only a mild fever in most young adults. It is important that the normal temperature of each individual person be known as a baseline for assessing changes.

One of the body's normal compensating reactions to a fall in heat production is the contraction of the surface blood vessels and shivering. Because elderly adults have a diminished shivering reflex and do not produce as much body heat from metabolic processes, they tolerate prolonged exposure to cold poorly. At the other extreme, the body compensates for higher temperatures by slowing down muscular activity to produce less heat and by dilating surface blood vessels and sweating to increase losses of body heat. Older people, however, often have sluggish sweating and circulatory mechanisms and therefore cannot cope with heat as well as younger people. For example, they do not tolerate working in moderately high temperatures for prolonged periods. It is therefore important for the elderly adult

Table 29–1   Normal Physiologic Aging

1. Decreased immune system function, which may be related to the increased incidence of infection, cancer, and autoimmune diseases
2. Decreased production of saliva
3. Decreased production of hydrochloric acid and pepsin in the stomach
4. Decrease in kidney mass; 33 to 50% decrease in the number of nephrons
5. Decreased concentrating and diluting ability of the kidney
6. Gradual decline in male reproduction
7. Cessation of ovum production at menopause
8. Slowing of motor neuron transmission
9. Decline in the function of the autonomic nervous system
10. Progressive decrease in sleep stages 3 and 4 (deep sleep)
11. Decline in the visual fields of the eye and hearing ability
12. Decline in sensitivity to the four tastes—salt, sweet, sour, and bitter—after age 50
13. Progressive increase in threshold for deep pain after age 60
14. Decreased ability of the body to adapt to stress

Source: E. C. Gioiella and C. W. Bevil, *Nursing care of the aging client: Promoting healthy adaptation* (Norwalk, Conn.: Appleton-Century-Crofts, 1985). Used by permission.

to have a constant, comfortable environmental temperature. Nurses often need to provide extra clothes to elderly persons who feel cold in rooms with a "normal" temperature.

Musculoskeletal Changes

Slight loss in overall stature occurs with age due to atrophy of the discs between the spinal vertebrae. This can be exaggerated by muscular weakness, resulting in a stooping posture and **kyphosis** (humpback of the upper spine). **Osteoporosis,** a decrease in bone density, along with increased brittleness of bone, makes the elderly adult prone to serious fractures, some of which are spontaneous. Since the incidence of osteoporosis is higher in elderly women, the effects of the menopause on the skeleton are being investigated. Causes of osteoporosis are thought to be lack of activity and inadequate calcium intake or inability to metabolize calcium.

Some degenerative joint changes occur, which make movement stiffer and more restricted. Stiffness is aggravated by inactivity; for example, if persons sit too long, their joints become stiff and they have difficulty standing and walking. Although these skeletal changes do restrict the activity of the elderly adult, prevention of severe disability is possible. Nursing interventions should include counseling clients to take adequate exercise and include adequate amounts of protein and calcium in the diet.

With aging there is a **gradual reduction in the speed and power of skeletal or voluntary muscle contractions.** The capacity for sustained muscular effort is also decreased. Great individual differences in muscular efficiency are apparent throughout life. Exercise

can strengthen weakened muscles, and up to about age 50 the skeletal muscles can increase in bulk and density. After that time, there is a steady decrease in muscle fibers, ultimately leading to the typical wasted appearance of the very old person. Thus, elderly adults often complain about their lack of strength and how quickly they tire. Activities can still be carried out, but at a slower pace. Often balance is impaired with age. Prolonged muscular efforts may be sustained by older people provided they take judicious rest pauses and avoid capacity or peak performance.

The effects of age on the smooth or involuntary muscles such as the stomach, the colon, the respiratory tubes, and the bladder are small in contrast to the effects on the skeletal muscles, with the exception of the blood vessels. These muscles function relatively normally until late senescence.

Nurses can advise clients about safety measures, such as using hand rails to prevent falls, removing small rugs to prevent slips, and putting away items over which an elderly person could trip. Clients may also need to learn to limit their activity to a level they tolerate well.

Sensory Deficits

Changes in **vision** associated with aging include the obvious physical changes around the eye such as the shrunken appearance of the eyes due to loss of orbital fat, the slowed blink reflex, and the looseness of the eyelids, particularly the lower lid, because of poorer muscle tone. Other changes result in loss of visual acuity, less power of accommodation to darkness and dim light, loss of peripheral vision, and difficulty in discriminating similar colors. The degenerative change in the eyes leading to the relative inflexibility of the lens is called **presbyopia.**

As the lens of the eye ages, it becomes more opaque and less elastic. By the age of 80 all elderly people have some lens opacity (**cataracts**) that reduces visual acuity. Surgical removal of cataracts is common at this age. Accompanying this are changes in the ciliary muscles, which control the shape of the lens. These changes reduce the power of the lens to adjust to near and far vision. It is thought that changes in the nervous system play a part in reducing the diameter of the pupil, thereby restricting the amount of light entering the eye. This slows the reaction time to decreases in light or illumination, a problem compounded at night with driving. Reduced blood supply due to arteriosclerosis can diminish retinal function. Reduced peripheral vision also is thought to be a result of arteriosclerosis.

Many older adults require eyeglasses for close work. It is not uncommon for elderly people to buy inexpensive magnifying eyeglasses from department stores. Nurses should encourage older adults to have routine eye examinations by a physician and to use appropriate eyeglasses. Many places now offer free eye examinations and eyeglasses to elderly people.

Hearing loss associated with aging is called **presbycusis.** Presbycusis comes about through changes in the structure of the inner ear: changes in nerve tissues in the inner ear and a thickening of the eardrum. Gradual loss of hearing is usual among the aging and more common among men than women, perhaps because men are more frequently in noisy work environments. Hearing loss is usually greater in the left ear than the right and greater in the higher frequencies than the lower. Thus, older adults with hearing loss usually hear speakers with low, distinct voices best. The elderly may have more difficulty compensating for hearing loss than the young, who pay closer attention to the lip movements of the speaker. Nurses can assist older people who are hard of hearing by the following measures:

1. Speaking more loudly and in a lower tone
2. Speaking slowly and sometimes using alternative words
3. Using facial expressions that convey moods and feelings, thus helping comprehension
4. Encouraging clients to use hearing aids when appropriate
5. Speaking clearly and facing the person, but not shouting
6. Not covering the face or mouth while talking to an elderly person
7. Assisting the person to learn ways to ask others to repeat their words or speak more clearly

Older persons have a poorer sense of **taste and smell** and are less stimulated by food than the young. The number of taste buds in the tongue grows smaller, and the olfactory bulb (responsible for smell perception) at the base of the brain atrophies. Changes in the **voice** occur throughout life as a result of hardening and decreased elasticity of the laryngeal cartilages. These processes are completed by middle age. With age, the laryngeal muscles atrophy, and the vocal cords slacken. The voice becomes higher pitched, less powerful, and restricted in range. These changes are generally unnoticed unless greater demands on capacity, such as singing or public speaking, are made. Noticeable changes, such as slower speech and eventual slurring, are the result of central nervous system changes rather than local mechanisms.

Cardiopulmonary Changes

Respiratory efficiency is reduced with age. The person inhales a smaller volume of air due to the musculoskeletal changes in the chest wall that reduce the size of the chest. There is a greater volume of residual air left in the lungs after expiration and a decreased capacity to cough efficiently because of weaker expiratory muscles. Mucous secretions tend to collect more readily in the respiratory tree due to decreased ciliary activity. Thus, susceptibility to respiratory infections is notable in elderly adults.

Dyspnea (difficulty in breathing) occurs frequently with increased activity, such as running for a bus or carrying heavy parcels up stairs. This dyspnea occurs in response to an oxygen debt in the muscles. Intense exercise is followed by short, heavy, rapid breathing, which is an attempt to repay this oxygen debt in the muscles. Although this response is normal, it occurs more quickly in the aged because delivery and diffusion of oxygen to tissues are often diminished by changes in both respiratory and vascular tissues. Nursing interventions include teaching the client deep breathing and coughing (see Chapters 42 and 46) and prompt treatment at the first sign of a respiratory infection. Also, the client needs to learn how to control activities so as not to become dypsneic (short of breath).

The working capacity of the **heart** is diminished with age. This is particularly evident when increased demands are made on the heart muscles, such as during periods of exercise or emotional stress. The valves of the heart tend to become harder and less pliable, resulting in reduced filling and emptying abilities. In addition, the pumping action of the heart is reduced due to changes in the coronary (cardiac) arteries, which supply progressively smaller amounts of blood to the heart muscle. These changes are evidenced by shortness of breath on exertion and pooling of blood in the systemic veins.

Changes in the **arteries** occur concurrently. The elasticity of smaller arteries is reduced by the thickening of their walls and increased calcium deposits in the muscular layer. Reduced arterial elasticity often results in diminished blood supply to, for instance, the legs and the brain, resulting in pain on exertion in the calf muscles and dizziness, respectively.

Blood pressure measurements often indicate increases in both systolic and diastolic pressures, partly as a result of the inelasticity of the systemic arteries. Variations in the **pulse** rate of the aged also occur. A rate of 70 to 80 beats per minute is quite usual. Nursing interventions include teaching the client to move more slowly so as to avoid dyspnea and cardiac discomfort. Encourage clients to seek medical advice if they experience dyspnea or chest pain.

Changes in Digestion

The **digestive system** is significantly less impaired by aging than other body systems are. Previously mentioned was the diminished ability to taste and smell, which contributes in part to a lack of appetite. Gradual decreases in digestive enzymes occur; examples are ptyalin in salivary secretions, which converts starch; pepsin and trypsin, which digest protein; and lipase, a fat-splitting enzyme. Yet digestive functioning and absorption of food are relatively unimpaired. The common complaints of heartburn, gas, and indigestion are largely due to other disease processes or to dietary excesses, such as highly spiced or fried foods.

Changes in Elimination

Constipation is also a common complaint of older people. However, the aging process has little if any effect on the bowels, which retain their ability to function normally. Thus, constipation is usually a result of poor fluid intake, inadequate roughage in the diet, and insufficient exercise.

The excretory function of the kidney diminishes with age, but usually not significantly below normal levels unless a disease process intervenes. Blood flow can be reduced by arteriosclerotic changes, impairing renal function. With age, the number of functioning nephrons (the basic functional units of the kidney) is reduced to some degree, thus impairing the kidney's filtering abilities.

More noticeable changes are those related to the bladder. Complaints of **urinary urgency** and **frequency** are common. In men, these changes are often due to an enlarged prostate gland; in women, to weakened muscles supporting the bladder or weakness of the urethral sphincter. The capacity of the bladder and its ability to empty completely diminish with age. This explains the need for elderly adults to arise during the night to void (nocturnal frequency) and the retention of residual urine, predisposing the elderly adult to bladder infections.

■ Changes in Reproductive Organs

In men, **degenerative changes** in the gonads are very gradual. The testes can produce sperm well into old age, although there is a gradual decrease in the number of sperm produced. In women the degenerative changes in the ovaries are noticed by the cessation of menses in middle age, during the menopause. Changes in the gonads of elderly women result from **diminished secretion of the ovarian hormones.** Some changes, such as the shrinking of the uterus and ovaries, go unnoticed. Other changes are obvious. The breasts atrophy, and lubricating vaginal secretions are reduced. Reduced natural lubrication is the cause of painful intercourse, which often necessitates the use of lubricating jellies.

Sexual drives persist into the 70s, 80s, and 90s, provided health is good and there is an available and interested partner. However, **sexual activity** does become less frequent with age. Sometimes a chronic cardiac or respiratory illness saps sexual energy. Nurses may need to teach a couple to adjust the time and technique of sexual activity to accommodate such factors as fatigue and arthritic joints.

■ Neurologic Changes

The person's reaction time is slowed with age because of the diminished conduction speed of nerve fibers. Reaction time can be delayed further by decreased muscle tone as a result of diminished physical activity. Elderly people compensate for this reaction difference by being exceptionally cautious, for instance, in their driving habits, which exasperate some impatient young drivers. Because sensory nerve endings in the skin also change with age, old people are less sensitive to touch, and safety precautions are necessary, for example, when a hot-water bottle is applied.

Experts do not agree whether the brain decreases in weight with age, although it is thought that the brain may lose about 10 to 12% of its mass by very old age

(Gioiella and Bevil 1985, p. 76). It is believed, however, that there is a progressive loss of neurons with age. Neurofibrillary tangles have also been found in the hippocampal cortex, the area of the brain concerned with memory. A **neurofibrillary tangle** is an abnormal mass of fibrillar material found in the cytoplasm. Neuritic plaques are also found in the aging brain. A **neuritic plaque** is a structure composed of amyloid material surrounded by abnormal neural structures. Neurofibrillary tangles and neuritic plaques could account for some of the functional changes found in normal aging people.

Elderly people can be taught to take precautions because of their slower reaction times, and they can learn to assist their memories, for example, by writing lists. Nurses may also need to teach aging people how to protect themselves from burns because they often have a diminished perception of heat.

One of the most tragic conditions to strike the elderly is **Alzheimer's disease,** a progressive degenerative disorder that affects more than 2.5 million Americans. Characterized by **dementia,** the deterioration of intellectual capacity, it is the fifth leading cause of total disability in the United States and the fourth leading cause of death among the elderly. Each year 120,000 Americans die from Alzheimer's disease. Experts predict that in the next century, it will be the leading cause of death (Schneider and Emr 1985).

The cause of Alzheimer's disease is unknown; however, in late 1986, researchers identified an abnormal protein, A-68, that appears in the brain of victims and also in the spinal fluid of living persons thought to have the disease. While it is not known whether A-68 is a causative factor, the protein is unique to the disease. Depending on further studies, a routine laboratory test could be developed that would make possible early and accurate diagnosis. Until such a test is developed, definitive diagnosis can only be made at autopsy. Such a test would not only aid in diagnosing the dementia when it is still reversible, but it would also identify those persons who are misdiagnosed as having Alzheimer's disease. These are persons whose apparent confusion and memory loss may be due to depression, malnutrition, or other treatable disorder.

No means of prevention or treatment is yet available. In late 1986, however, early results of a study showed some success with the drug **tetrahydroaminoacridine** (THA) in helping to restore some cognitive function (Davis and Mohs 1986). Further drug trials are underway. The federal government spends $36 million annually on research related to Alzheimer's disease; the care of Alzheimer's clients costs $28 billion annually. Neither of these figures, however, reflects the cost in human terms to persons affected and their families. Witnessing the steady deterioration of a loved one and trying to cope with the increasing disability can have devastating effects on family members, particularly an aging spouse. Thus a large part of the nurse's role is to teach and role model the following concepts for families (Gioiella and Bevil 1985): structured environment; safety; activity; respite; and support. In addition, the nurse can perform important counseling, advocacy, and referral functions.

Psychosocial Development

A number of theories explain psychosocial aging. According to **disengagement theory,** aging involves mutual withdrawal (disengagement) between the older person and others in the elderly person's environment. This withdrawal relieves the elderly person of some of society's pressures and gradually reduces the number of people with whom the elderly person interacts. According to **activity theory,** the best way to age is to stay active physically and mentally, and according to **continuity theory,** people maintain their values, habits, and behavior in old age. A person who is accustomed to having people around will continue to do so, and the person who prefers not to be involved with others will more likely disengage. This theory accounts for the great variety of behavior seen in older adults. Elderly people must adapt to many psychosocial changes, for example, the death of a life partner, retirement, or reduced income.

Erikson

According to Erikson, the developmental task at this time is *ego integrity versus self-despair.* (See Table 26–4 on page 356.) People who attain ego integrity view life with a sense of wholeness and derive satisfaction from past accomplishments. They view death as an acceptable completion of life.

According to Erikson, people who develop integrity accept "one's one and only life cycle" (Erikson 1963, p. 263). By contrast, people who despair often believe they have made poor choices during life and wish they could live life over. Robert Butler sees integrity as bringing serenity and wisdom, and despair as resulting in the inability to accept one's fate. Despair gives rise to feelings of frustration, discouragement, and a sense that one's life has been worthless (Butler 1963, p. 65).

Peck

Acknowledging that the "young-old" and the "old-old" differ not only in physical characteristics but also in psychosocial responses, many people have difficulty with Erikson's singular developmental task. Peck proposes three developmental tasks during old age, in contrast to Erikson's one (integrity versus despair). Peck (1955) believes that the older person must accomplish these three tasks:

1. *Ego differentiation versus work-role preoccupation.* An adult's identity and feelings of worth are highly dependent on his or her work role. Upon retirement, some people experience feelings of worthlessness unless their sense of identity is derived from a number of roles so that one such role can replace the work role or occupation as a source of self-esteem. For example, a man who likes gardening or golf can obtain ego rewards from those activities, replacing rewards formerly obtained from his occupation.

2. *Body transcendence versus body preoccupation.* This task calls for the individual to adjust to decreasing physical capacities and at the same time maintain feelings of well-being. Preoccupation with declining body function reduces happiness and satisfaction with life.

3. *Ego transcendence versus ego preoccupation.* Ego transcendence is the acceptance without fear of one's death as inevitable. This acceptance includes being actively involved in one's own future beyond death. Ego preoccupation, by contrast, results in holding on to life and a preoccupation with self-gratification.

Kart and associates explain how the tasks described by Peck should ideally be enacted. First, elderly people must establish new activities so that the loss of accustomed roles is less keenly felt. Second, they must select activities compatible with the physical limitations of old age. Third, individuals may make contributions that extend beyond their own lifetimes, thereby providing a meaning for life (Kart et al. 1978, p. 180).

Today, a majority of the people over 65 are unemployed. Most industries and professions make retirement mandatory, although this policy is currently being questioned. Some who are self-employed continue to work as long as they are healthy. Work offers these people a better income, a sense of self-worth, and the chance to continue long-established routines. Some older adults need to work for economic reasons.

Retirement

Retirement can be a time when projects or recreational activities deferred for a long time can be pursued. Older retired people are no longer governed by an alarm clock and can get up when they please. The enjoyment of staying up later is another luxury. Few elderly people, however, spend much time resting or sleeping. Being accustomed to activity most of their lives, most elderly find many outlets: jobs, community projects, volunteer services, intellectual or recreational pursuits, or hobbies such as stamp collecting or fishing. Travel opportunities are expanding.

The life-style of later years is to a large degree formulated in youth. This fact was recognized by Robert Browning: "Grow old along with me! / The best is yet to be, / The last of life, for which the first was made." People who attempt suddenly to refocus and enrich their lives at retirement usually have difficulty. Those who learned early in life to live well-balanced and fulfilling lives are generally more successful in retirement. The woman who has been concerned only with the accomplishments of her children or the man who has been concerned only with the paycheck and his job status can be left with a feeling of emptiness when children leave and the job no longer exists. The later years can foster a sense of integrity and continuity, or they can be years of despair.

Economic Factors

The **financial needs** of elderly people vary considerably. Though most need less money for clothing, entertainment, and work, and although some own their homes outright, costs continue to rise, making it difficult for some to manage. Food and medical costs alone are often a financial burden. When older people speak about their greatest need, often it is not happiness or health, but money. Money allows them to be independent and look after themselves.

Nurses should be aware of the costs of health care. For example, while assisting a client to plan a diet, the nurse must consider which foods the client can afford to buy. In addition, the supplies used in a client's care should be as economical as possible.

According to a Chinese saying, the house with an old grandparent harbors a jewel. However, in North American society, most aging people live apart. Most think it unwise to live with married sons and daughters, since overcrowded, tense situations can arise. It is also difficult for some elderly people to assume a new role while living with their children—relinquishing the authority they had, allowing their children to be independent.

Nurses must be sensitive to the stress that the presence of an elderly person in the home of a child may cause for all family members, including the older person. An ill elderly person often requires considerable care, and the primary caregiver may be one of the family. This living arrangement can often involve adjustments in life-style for all concerned. Nurses can assist people in their adjustments and at the same time be supportive and caring.

Living in a Nursing Home

Only a small percentage of elderly adults live in nursing homes. However, an increasing number of nursing home residents are over the age of 85 years (U.S. DHHS 1985, p. 11). These lodgings vary in many ways and offer varying degrees of independence to the residents. All provide meals but vary in giving other services, such as assistance with hygiene and dressing, physical therapy or exercise, recreational activities, transportation services, and medical and nursing supervision.

Nurses in hospitals should find out whether a client is being discharged to a nursing home or to home. Many nursing homes provide nursing services to clients and require appropriate information to provide for continuity of care. Clients returning home, however, may require the assistance of a home care nurse.

Loss and Grieving

Well-adjusted aging couples usually thrive on companionship. Many couples rely increasingly on their mates for this company and may have few outside friends. Great bonds of affection and closeness can develop during this period of aging together and nurturing each other. When a **mate dies**, the remaining partner inevitably experiences feelings of loss, emptiness, and loneliness. Many are capable and manage to live alone; however, reliance on younger family members increases as age advances and ill health occurs. Some widows and widowers remarry, particularly the latter, because widowers are less inclined than widows to maintain a household.

Women face bereavement and solitude more often than men, since women usually live longer. The brevity of life is constantly reinforced by the death of friends. It is a time when one's life is reviewed with happiness or regret. Feelings of serenity or guilt and inadequacy can arise. Independence established prior to loss of a mate makes this adjustment period easier. A person who has some meaningful friendships, economic security, ongoing interests in the community, or private hobbies and a peaceful philosophy of life copes more easily with bereavement. Successful relationships with children and grandchildren are also of inestimable value. Facing death is discussed in Chapter 19.

Nurses can sometimes help clients who are alone a great deal to adjust their living arrangements or lifestyle so that they have more companionship. Moving to a retirement home that has other people in similar circumstances and organized social activities is one example. Many communities provide social centers for the elderly, for example, drop-in centers or community centers that offer day trips for seniors. Nurses can refer clients to services and encourage them to obtain companionship.

Cognitive Development

Piaget's phases of cognitive development end with the formal operations phase. However, there is currently considerable research on cognitive abilities and aging. Researchers generally believe that there is *minimal change in intellectual capacity* of the healthy aging person (Gress and Bahr 1984, p. 72). Intellectual capacity includes perception, cognitive ability, and learning. **Perception,** or the ability to interpret the environment, depends on the acuteness of the senses. If the aging person's senses are impaired, the ability to perceive the environment and react appropriately is diminished. Perceptual capacity may be affected by changes in the nervous system as well.

Cognitive ability, or the ability to know, is related to perceptual ability. An older man, for example, may know that he will be retiring next year but be unable to plan for retirement. He cannot accept the knowledge psychologically because his work provides his sense of worth, self-esteem, and identity. Memory is also a component of intellectual capacity and is closely related to learning. **Memory,** or the ability to retain information, is of two types: short-term or primary memory and long-term or secondary memory.

According to Gress and Bahr, *primary memory* is affected minimally by aging as long as the person perceives the information adequately and need not reorganize it mentally, i.e., need not reintegrate it to fit changing circumstances. *Secondary memory,* however, has been found to decline with aging. The ability to recall declines because aging diminishes the ability to retrieve information from storage in the brain. The reason for this decline may be that the central nervous system functions more slowly or because the search within the brain is longer. The belief that elderly people have intact long-term memories is not supported by research (Gioiella and Bevil 1985, p. 38).

Moral Development

According to Kohlberg, moral development is completed in the early adult years. Most old people stay at Kohlberg's *conventional level* of moral development (see Table 26–6 on page 359), and some are at the *preconventional level.* An elderly person at the preconventional level obeys rules to avoid pain and the displeasure of others. At stage 1, a person defines good and bad in relation to self, whereas an older person at stage 2 may act to meet another's needs as well as his or her own. Elderly people at the conventional level follow society's rules of conduct in response to the expectations of others. They value conformity, loyalty, and social order (Edelman and Mandle 1986, p. 548).

Rybash, Roodin, and Hoyer studied the kinds of moral problems elderly people face. These researchers found that the moral concerns of the elderly are more interpersonal than social or legalistic. For example, an elderly man is more likely to be concerned with the moral problems involving a member of his family than with the moral problems posed by his occupation or a friend's extramarital affair (Rybash et al. 1983, p. 258).

Spiritual Development

Murray and Zentner (1985, p. 584) write that the elderly person with a mature religious outlook strives to incorporate views of theology and religious action into thinking. Elderly people can contemplate new religious and philosophical views and try to understand ideas missed previously or interpreted differently. The elderly person also derives a sense of worth by sharing experiences or views. In contrast, the elderly person who has not matured spiritually may feel impoverishment or despair as the drive for economic and professional success wanes.

The older person's knowledge becomes wisdom, an inner resource for dealing with both positive and negative life experiences. Spiritual development adds joy and meaning to life in later years (Gress and Bahr 1984, p. 85). According to Fowler and Keen (1978), some people enter the sixth stage of spiritual development, *universalizing*. See Table 26–7 on page 360. People whose

spiritual development reaches this level think and act in a way that exemplifies love and justice.

Health Promotion and Protection

Guidelines for assessment of growth and development of the elderly adult are shown in the accompanying box.

Areas of concern for the older adult include safety, nutrition, elimination, exercise and rest, sexuality, independence, respect, and isolation. Chronic health problems, such as altered thought processes, hypertension, cancer, and arthritis, are also common in old age.

Safety

Accident prevention is a major concern for elderly people. Because vision is limited, reflexes are slowed, and bones are brittle, climbing stairs, driving a car, and even walking require caution. Safety precautions for older adults are discussed in Chapter 24. Driving, particularly night driving, requires caution because accommodation of the eye to light is impaired and peripheral vision is diminished. Older persons need to learn to turn the head before changing lanes and should not rely on side vision, for example, when crossing a street. Driving in fog or other hazardous conditions should be avoided.

Fires are a hazard for the elderly person with a failing memory. The older person may forget that the iron or stove is left on or may not extinguish a cigarette completely. Because of reduced sensitivity to pain and heat, care must be taken to prevent burns when the person bathes or uses heating devices. Elderly people do not tolerate cold well and need warm clothing and often a blanket over their extremities. At night, woolen socks are safer for cold feet than hot-water bottles.

Because older clients who take analgesics or seda-

GUIDELINES

Assessing Older Adults

Does the older adult:

■ Enjoy retirement?

■ Have a social network of friends and support persons?

■ View life as worthwhile?

■ Have high self-esteem?

■ Have the abilities to care for self or to secure appropriate help?

■ Gain support from value system or spiritual philosophy?

■ Adapt life-style to diminishing energy and ability?

■ Cope constructively with loss?

tives may become lethargic or confused, they should be monitored regularly and closely. Other measures should be used whenever possible. For example, if an elderly client who lives at home cannot sleep at night without a sedative, a nurse should assess the sleeping environment for noise and light. A light snack before bedtime, e.g., warm milk and a cookie, or soothing music may help the client to sleep. Nurses can help elderly clients make the home environment safe. Specific hazards can be identified and corrected; e.g., stair handrails can be installed. The nurse teaches the importance of taking only prescribed medications and contacting a health professional at the first indication of intolerance to them.

Nutrition

Elderly adults need well-balanced diets. However, smaller servings with fewer calories are appropriate because of the reduction in metabolic rate and exercise. A diet high in protein, moderate in carbohydrates, and low in fat is recommended. **Malnutrition** is not uncommon in elderly people because many have bad teeth, many cannot afford the cost of food (particularly protein), and many eat alone. Also, appetite can be reduced by a dulled sense of taste and smell. In addition, some elderly people's diets are deficient in iron and vitamins A, C, and B. Many older adults have poor teeth or wear **dentures** and therefore may have difficulties masticating food. Foods that require extensive chewing, such as meat and fresh vegetables or fruit, may as a result be avoided, leading to nutritional deficiencies. Nurses need to determine whether the client's nutritional status is adequate and if not, why not. Perhaps artificial teeth need adjusting or the client needs help shopping.

Elimination

Constipation is not infrequent among the elderly. A cup of hot water or tea taken at a regular hour in the morning is helpful for some. For most, an assessment of fluid intake, exercise, and diet will help in deciding on a remedy. Adequate roughage in the diet, adequate exercise, and six to eight glasses of fluid daily are essential preventive measures for constipation.

Many older people learn to deal with nocturnal frequency by restricting their fluid intake in the latter part of the evening, particularly those fluids that stimulate voiding, such as coffee or alcohol. Many older men require prostatic surgery to relieve increasing urinary frequency throughout the day, and some women require vaginal surgery for cystoceles or rectoceles. A **cystocele** is a protrusion of the urinary bladder through the vaginal wall. A **rectocele** is the protrusion of part of the rectum through the vaginal wall. Both of these conditions produce pressure and reduce bladder capacity, thereby creating urinary urgency and frequency.

Nursing interventions to promote regular elimination patterns include encouraging the client to drink an adequate amount of fluid, e.g., 3000 ml per day if health permits. Also advise the client to seek medical advice at the first sign of an infection, urinary frequency, or urinary retention. See Chapters 40 and 41 for specific information on fecal and urinary elimination.

Activity

A regular program of moderate exercise is recommended for elderly adults. Walking, golfing, gardening, bowling, and bicycling are common activities. These can be performed at a leisurely pace. It is important that exercise not be too strenuous and that rest periods be taken as needed. Rapid breathing and accelerated heartbeat should disappear within a few minutes after exercise; exercise should refresh rather than fatigue. People who are too disabled to engage in active exercise can implement a program of isometric exercises to maintain joint mobility and muscle tone. Exercise is also essential to maintain bone calcification. See Chapter 35.

Older people require more rest than before because they tire more easily. Often sleep habits change. Naps taken frequently throughout the day can cause difficulty sleeping at night. Measures to promote rest are discussed in Chapter 37. Moderate exercise often helps the client to sleep at night.

Sexuality

Certain aspects of sexuality persist into later life. Grooming as part of sexual identity is one. For instance, a woman might care greatly about her appearance, e.g., her clothes or her hair. A man, too, might place great value on a neat appearance, close shave, and trimmed hair.

An important aspect of sexual relations is intimacy. The closeness and love manifested as sexuality can provide a sense of belonging and worth. The loss of a partner is a crisis for the older person. Sometimes the survivor feels that it will be impossible to be close to another person. With time, however, a new significant relationship can be formed, although it may differ from the previous relationship. The elderly often find companionship and affection in seniors centers and volunteer societies. Nurses can provide information about such agencies. Nurses may also need to teach clients about the physical sexual changes that take place with advanced age. See Chapter 15.

Self-Esteem

Most elderly people thrive on independence. It is important to them to be able to look after themselves even if they have to struggle to do so. Although it may be difficult for younger family members to watch the oldster completing tasks in a slow, determined way, the aging need this sense of accomplishment. Children might notice that the aging father or mother with failing vision cannot keep the kitchen as clean as before. The aging father and mother may be slower and less meticulous in carpentry tasks or gardening. To maintain the elderly adult's sense of self-respect, nurses and family members need to encourage them to do as much as possible for themselves. Many young people err in thinking that they are helpful to older people when they take over for them and do the job much faster and more efficiently.

Some older people who are ill appear to enjoy the dependent role of being waited on and attended to. Nurses need to show an interest in such people as persons and set realistic, achievable goals. Praise and recognition for each accomplishment, no matter how small, are important. Success at getting out of bed independently or feeding oneself, if recognized by the nurse, can encourage people to achieve more and more. Some people may be afraid that they are not going to get better; others may feel that dependence brings them more recognition and importance. The nurse needs to understand each person's feelings and concerns before helping the older person toward independence. If clients know, for example, that an increasing level of wellness is possible and that the nurse will pay as much attention to them when they attempt tasks independently as when they are dependent, they probably will feel better about their progress.

Aging people need to be recognized for their unique individual characteristics. It can be difficult to recognize these differences, since elderly people have less energy than the young to show how they are different. Perhaps this is one reason elderly people tend to talk about past accomplishments, jobs, deeds, and experiences.

Nurses need to acknowledge the elderly client's ability to think, reason, and make decisions. Most elderly people are willing to listen to suggestions and advice, but they do not want to be ordered around. The nurse can support a decision by an elderly client even if eventually the decision is reversed because of failing health.

Older people appreciate thoughtfulness, consideration, and acceptance of their waning abilities. For example, having dinner out in a well-lighted restaurant or not expecting grandmother to babysit for too many hours, if at all, are actions that recognize the diminishing vision and energy of older people. The values and standards held by older people need to be accepted, whether they are related to ethical, religious, or household matters. For example, it is wise to respect an older person's decision to hang the laundry outside rather than to use a dryer, or to cook on a wood stove.

Chronic Health Problems

Chronic health problems, such as impaired vision or hearing, osteoporosis, hypertension, and depression, must be monitored and treated. Perhaps the elderly person needs assistance and encouragement to seek health care. Programs in the community are directed toward early detection of illness, services (e.g., dietary counseling, eye care, foot care, and routine medical care) and activities that encourage exercise and social interaction to help prevent social isolation.

Nurses can assist elderly people to maintain maximum independent function. Elderly clients can learn new skills to help them function as fully as possible within any limitations. In some cases, episodes of acute illness or injury, e.g., influenza, burns, and falls, can be prevented.

Chapter Highlights

The life expectancy of North Americans is increasing.

Certain physical changes in most body systems are associated with aging.

Psychosocial theories about aging include the disengagement, activity, and continuity theories.

The elderly person usually has to adjust to many psychosocial changes.

There is minimal change in the intellectual abilities of the healthy elderly person.

The moral concerns of elderly people tend to be interpersonal rather than social or legalistic.

Spiritual maturity can provide the elderly person with inner resources for dealing with life experiences.

Selected References

Boettcher, E. G. March 1985. Linking the aged to support systems: Aging. *Journal of Gerontological Nursing* 11:27–33.

Butler, R. 1963. The life review: An interpretation of reminiscence in the aged. *Psychiatry* 26:65.

Butler, R. N., and Lewis, M. I. 1981. *Aging and mental health.* 3d ed. St. Louis: C. V. Mosby Co.

Carnevali, D. L., and Patrick, M., editors. 1986. *Nursing management for the elderly.* 2d ed. Philadelphia: J. B. Lippincott.

Chang, B.; Uman, G.; Linn, L.; Ware, J.; and Kane, R. January/February 1985. Adherence to health care regimens among elderly women. *Nursing Research* 34(1):27–31.

Clites, J. August 1984. Maximizing memory retention in the aged. *Journal of Gerontological Nursing* 10:34–35, 38–39.

Cutler, N. R., and Narang, P. K. May-June, 1985. Drug therapies (Alzheimer's disease). *Geriatric Nursing* 6:160–163.

Davis, K. L., and Mohs, R. C. November 13, 1986. Cholinergic drugs in Alzheimer's disease. *New England Journal of Medicine* 315:1286.

Ebersole, P., and Hess, P. 1985. *Toward healthy aging: Human needs and nursing response.* 2d ed. St. Louis: C. V. Mosby Co.

Edelman, C., and Mandle, C. L. 1986. *Health promotion throughout the life span.* St. Louis: C. V. Mosby Co.

Eliopoullos, C. 1987. *Gerontological Nursing.* 2d ed. Philadelphia: J. P. Lippincott.

Erikson, E. H. 1963. *Childhood and society.* 2d ed. New York: W. W. Norton and Co.

Ferguson, D., and Beck, C. September/October 1983. H.A.L.F.—A tool to assess elder abuse within the family. *Geriatric Nursing* 4:301–4.

Fowler, J., and Keen, S. 1978, 1985. *Life maps: Conversations in the journey of faith.* Waco, Texas: Word Books.

Gioiella, E. C., and Bevil, C. W. 1985. *Nursing care of the aging client: Promoting healthy adaptation.* Norwalk, Conn.: Appleton-Century-Crofts.

Gress, L. D., and Bahr, R. T. 1984. *The aging person: A holistic perspective.* St. Louis: C. V. Mosby Co.

Hirst, S. P., and Metcalf, B. J. February 1984. Promoting self-esteem. *Journal of Gerontological Nursing* 10:72–77.

Kart, C. S.; Metress, E. S.; and Metress, J. F. 1978. *Aging and health: Biologic and social perspectives.* Menlo Park, Calif.: Addison-Wesley Publishing Co.

King, F. E.; Figge, J.; and Harpman, P. January 1986. The elderly coping at home: A study of continuity of nursing care. *Journal of Advanced Nursing* 11:41–46.

Kohlberg, L. 1971. *Recent research in moral development.* New York: Holt, Rinehart and Winston.

Maslow, A. 1970. *Religions, values, and peak-experiences.* New York: Viking Press.

Murray, R. B., and Zentner, J. P. 1985. *Nursing assessment and health promotion through the life span.* 3d ed. Englewood Cliffs, N.J.: Prentice-Hall.

Peck, R. 1955. Psychological developments in the second half of life. In Anderson, J., editor. *Psychological aspects of aging.* Washington, D.C.: American Psychological Association.

Phillips, L., and Rempusheski, V. May/June 1985. A decision-making model for diagnosing and intervening in elder abuse and neglect. *Nursing Research* 34(3):134–39.

Powell, L., and Courtice, K. 1983. *Alzheimer's disease: A guide for families.* Reading, MA: Addison-Wesley.

Prehn, R. A., et al. January 1984. Can you assess the total population? . . . Assessing the elderly. *Journal of Gerontological Nursing* 10:8–13.

Ravish, T. October 1985. Prevent social isolation before it starts. *Journal of Gerontological Nursing* 11:10–13.

Rybash, J. M.; Roodin, P. A.; and Hoyer, W. J. 1983. Expressions of moral thought in later adulthood. *Gerontologist* 23:254–59.

Schneider, E. L., and Emr, M. May-June, 1985. Alzheimer's disease: Research highlights. *Geriatric Nursing* 6:135–138.

Stevens-Long, J. 1984. *Adult life developmental processes.* 2d ed. Palo Alto, Calif.: Mayfield Publishing Co.

Tavon E. January/February 1984. Tips to trigger memory. *Geriatric Nursing* 5:26–27.

United States Department of Health and Human Services. August 1985. *Charting the nation's health trends since 1960.* DHHS Pub. no. (PHS) 85–1251. Hyattsville, Md.: Public Health Service.

CHAPTER 30

The Family

Janice Denehy

OBJECTIVES

Differentiate between the traditional definition of the family and the broader definition needed to describe today's families.

Describe the roles and functions of the family.

Describe selected forms of families in society today.

List the information included in a family health appraisal.

Discuss the importance of assessing family health beliefs.

Identify family communication patterns.

Discuss the effects of cultural heritage on health beliefs and practices.

Describe how family function is altered by the illness of a family member.

Discuss coping strategies used by families.

Describe the impact of death upon a family.

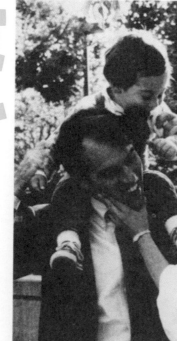
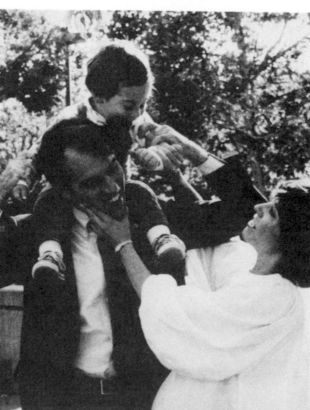

Roles and Functions of the Family

Definitions of *family* are as numerous and different as the many forms of family seen in today's society. There has been a resurgence of interest in the family unit and its impact on the health, values, and productivity of individual family members. In the nursing profession, this interest in the family as a unit has been expressed by the emergence of **family-centered nursing:** nursing that considers the health of the family as a unit in addition to the health of individual family members.

Membership in a family has a tremendous influence on the individual through genetic endowment, ethnicity, and the development of personal, social, moral, and cultural values. Nurses must consider the family's influence on the individual as they assess, diagnose, plan, implement, and evaluate nursing care.

When one envisions a family, the first image that comes to mind is a mother and father—the husband and wife—and their children, usually a boy and a girl. A family of parents and their offspring is known as the **nuclear family.** The relatives of nuclear families, such as grandparents or aunts and uncles, comprise the **extended family.** In some families, members of the extended family live with the nuclear family. Such multigenerational families were more common during the last century but are still seen today in many cultures as well as in many North American homes. Although members of the extended family may live in different areas, they are a frequent source of support and companionship for the family.

The **family** is frequently defined as two or more persons who are related through marriage, blood, birth, or adoption (Duvall 1977). Although this definition characterizes a large number of families, it does not adequately describe the membership of many families today. In many family groups, there are no legal or blood relationships among members. As the structure of the family has become more diverse, it has been necessary to define the family more broadly to encompass the wide variety of family forms seen in today's society. To provide flexibility in the study of families, Friedman (1981, p. 8) defines the **family** as follows: "A family is composed of people (two or more) who are emotionally involved with each other and live in close geographical proximity." Emotional involvement is demonstrated through caring and a commitment to a common purpose.

The family is the basic unit of society. Its major roles are to protect and socialize its members. Among the many functions it serves, of prime importance is the role the family plays in providing emotional support and security to its members through love, acceptance, concern, and nurturing. This affective (emotional) component holds families together, gives family members a sense of belonging, and develops a sense of kinship.

In addition to providing an emotionally safe environment for members to thrive and grow, the family is also a basic unit of physical protection and safety. This is accomplished by meeting the basic needs of its members: food, clothing, and shelter. Provision of a physically safe environment requires knowledge, skills, and economic resources.

In modern society, the economic resources needed by the family are secured by adult members through employment or government programs. The family also protects the physical health of its members by providing adequate nutrition and health care services. Nutritional and life-style practices of the family not only influence the health of family members but also directly affect the developing health attitudes and life-style practices of children.

In addition to providing an environment conducive to physical growth and health, the family creates an atmosphere that influences the cognitive and psychosocial growth of its members. Children and adults in healthy, functional families receive support, understanding, and encouragement as they progress through predictable developmental stages, as they move in or out of the family unit, and as they establish new family units. In families where members are physically and emotionally nurtured, individuals are challenged to achieve their potential in the family unit. As individual needs are met, family members are able to reach out to others in the family and the community, and to society.

The family is a major educator of its members. Parents are often called a child's first teachers. This early learning plays an influential part in the development of a child's attitudes about family, education, health, work, and recreation. These attitudes persist throughout their lives. In addition, families play a major role in the transmission of religious, cultural, and societal values. As the family socializes its new members to the expectations of home, community, and society, it provides a place of warmth, acceptance, and nurturing that insulates its members from the demands of society.

The family is a place of roots, refuge, and rejuvenation. It is a small network where members communicate and work together, delegating roles and responsibilities with a shared purpose: the protection and growth of its members. Through the experiences of family life, the individual learns to participate in and contribute productively to society.

The Family in Today's Society

It is difficult to describe the family of today except as uniquely diverse. Improvements in health care have led to healthier people living longer and more productive lives. The development of reliable contraceptives and the legalization of abortion have resulted in greater control in the planning of families. Today's economic realities, coupled with liberation ideology, have moved many women out of the home and into the workplace, changing traditional family roles. Higher divorce rates and the acceptance of children born to unmarried mothers have led to a dramatic increase in the number of single-parent families. Individuals are also grouping together to form new family units based on sexual preference or economic need.

Traditional Families

The **traditional family** is often viewed as an autonomous unit in which both parents reside in the home with their children, the mother assuming the nurturing role and the father providing the necessary economic resources. The traditional family is still very much a part of North American culture, but it is no longer the predominant family form. Although members of the extended family are not likely to live with traditional nuclear families, they remain an important source of information, support, and security. Contact with members of the extended family is vital to mobile families in times of stress or crisis because contact gives a sense of stability in a complex, impersonal society.

In the modern family, changes are occurring in traditional role patterns. Today's fathers are more involved with their children and family life. Many attend prenatal classes and witness the birth of their infants. In addition, fathers are more involved with household chores as role stereotypes are challenged, even though wives continue to perform a large portion of the housework. Likewise, females are less bound by traditional role patterns in today's society.

Two-Career Families

In **two-career families,** both the husband and wife are employed. Such families have been steadily increasing since the 1960s. The reasons for this trend are many, including the increased educational and career opportunities available to women, a desired increase in standard of living, and economic necessity. Many two-career families are young couples without children who desire to complete and use their education. Other working couples postpone childbearing until they are financially secure, have paid debts, and have purchased some of life's extras. Two-career families may also be parents who have launched their children and find they have many healthy, productive years to spend in the marketplace prior to retirement.

It is estimated that 60 to 70% of working women have children in the home, many of whom are preschoolers. When both parents work, the roles each partner plays are variable. Many husbands become more involved in the care of children and the management of household chores. Time and personal energy constraints also may lead to reevaluation of family activities and goals. Attention must be given to maintaining the husband-wife relationship and individual interests amidst the pressures of juggling family and career commitments.

The increased number of working parents has created a need for quality, affordable child care. Finding such child care is one of the greatest stresses faced by today's working parents. Many children spend part of each working day in daycare homes or child-care centers that may expose them at a young age to a host of people with a wide range of ideas and values.

Once children reach school age, parents find that few resources for after-school child care are available. Many school-age children come home to empty houses or apartments to care for themselves. These **latchkey children,** as they are called because they carry their own house key, may become bored or frightened as they wait for the parents to return from work (McClellan 1984). Parents and professionals are realizing the importance of preparing these children with information about safety and household management to reduce their anxiety and help them make the most of these hours alone. Children of working parents are growing up with new family role models, which will no doubt have an effect on the families of tomorrow.

Single-Parent Families

Today it is estimated that over 50% of North American children live in a **single-parent family**—a home headed by one parent—sometime during their childhood. There are many reasons for single parenthood, including death of a spouse, separation, divorce, birth of a child to an unmarried woman, or adoption of a child by a single man or woman. Single parents frequently express concern about child care, adequate financial resources, social isolation, and lack of adult companionship. Single parents who work outside the home experience fatigue and role overload in managing growing children, household tasks, and a job. At times, these concerns seem to occupy their entire lives, leaving little time for personal or recreational activities.

Nearly 90% of single-parent families are headed by a female. Because these women are often young and poorly prepared for the job market, many single-parent families live with financial strain or poverty. In homes where a divorce has occurred, there is frequently a drop in the standard of living. Child support payments may dwindle after the first year and in many cases are never received. When families live with inadequate financial resources, the health of the family is likely to suffer from substandard living conditions, poor nutrition, stress, and inadequate health care services. The self-esteem of the family is impaired because members, particularly the head of the household, find it difficult to raise their standard of living due to stigma or lack of skills, time, and energy. Depression and despair are common among women struggling to raise a family (Duffy 1982); these feelings not only affect the woman but also influence the outlook of growing family members, who learn to view society as hostile, not as a place full of challenges and hope for the future.

Single-parent families need to identify a support system. Members of the extended family or friends who are supportive provide an opportunity for mutual caring and sharing of concerns. Such support networks reduce social isolation and provide opportunities for relaxation and recreation. A support system helps the single parent cope with and reduce stress; in addition, it gives the individual a chance to have fun and regain self-esteem. Referral to appropriate community resources helps the single parent locate child care, take advantage of financial or social programs, and develop job skills through education or job-training programs.

Blended Families

Existing family units who join together to form new family units are known as **blended** or **reconstituted families.** Families with children living with a birth parent and a nonbirth parent are commonly called step families. The blending of two families presents a unique set of challenges to the individuals involved. The joining of two families is often met with hope and anticipation. Each family brings its own history and expectations to the new family constellation. Often expectations for instantaneous adaptation and affection are too high. Children, depending on their ages and past experiences, usually adjust slowly to new patterns of communication and family authority. Family reintegration requires time and effort. Stress occurs as blended families get to know each other, respect differences, and establish new patterns of behavior (Reutter and Strang 1986).

The greatest success in blending families comes when each family member enters the new relationship with realistic expectations and plans to take the time to make the new family unit succeed. Successful parents get along with and enjoy each other, enjoy life, and bring a sense of humor to the challenge of blending the life-styles and values of two families into one.

Adolescent Parents

A disturbing trend is the growing proportion of infants born each year to **adolescent parents.** These young parents, who are still mastering the developmental tasks of childhood, are physically, emotionally, and financially ill prepared to undertake the responsibilities of parenthood. Over 600,000 infants in America are born each year to adolescent mothers (*The Adolescent Family* 1984, p. 1). An increasing number of these mothers are 15 years and younger. A disproportionate number of adolescent births are to members of minority racial or ethnic groups.

Pregnant adolescents are at greater risk for health problems during pregnancy because of poor nutritional status, physiologic immaturity, and lack of prenatal care. They are more likely to deliver premature infants who are, in turn, at greater risk for subsequent health and developmental problems. In addition, adolescent mothers are more likely to give birth to another infant while still in their teens. Today there is a greater acceptance of unmarried parenthood, and fewer pregnant teens feel pressured to marry the father of the infant or to relinquish the infant for adoption.

Adolescent pregnancy frequently interrupts education and may necessitate changes in life goals of many young women. The newly formed family unit is often dependent upon others for physical, emotional, and financial assistance. Support systems are crucial to its success. Parenting skills need to be developed, and the completion of at least a high school education should be encouraged. While helping the new mother understand the needs of her growing infant is an important intervention for nurses, so is assisting the young mother progress through the developmental tasks of adolescence into adulthood.

The children of adolescent parents are at greater risk for health and social problems as they grow up. These children experience more accidents during their preschool years than their peers, are frequently behind in receiving their childhood immunizations, and are more prone to exhibit learning and behavior problems when they enter school. Often raised in poverty, children of adolescent mothers may have few role models to help them break out of the cycle of poverty and subsequent adolescent parenthood.

Cohabiting Families

A current and growing trend in alternate family forms is unrelated individuals or families cohabiting or living under one roof, forming new family units called **cohabiting** or **communal families.** Some individuals join together out of a need for companionship; for example, two widowed adults who share common interests found that living together eliminated previously lonely hours during the evening. Others cohabit to achieve a sense of family or belonging. Many unmarried couples choose to cohabit; some have no desire for a long-term commitment, others wish to test a relationship prior to marriage.

Financial need often leads to the formation of cohabiting families. In these situations, individuals or families share living expenses as well as the responsibilities of household management. Others may cohabit to share services. For example, a single mother moved in with an elderly man who desired to remain in his home but needed help with cooking and cleaning. The single mother was able to provide these services, and she benefited because she and her daughter were now regularly sitting down to nutritious meals, something they rarely experienced previously. An added bonus was the close friendship the elderly man established with her 6-year-old daughter. The formation of cohabiting families illustrates the flexibility and creativity of the family unit in adapting to meet individual challenges and responding to changing societal demands.

Gay and Lesbian Families

Of recent interest is the awareness of the number of homosexual adults in today's society who have formed **gay** and **lesbian families** based on the same goals of caring and commitment seen in heterosexual relationships. While homosexual relationships have been stereotyped as short term and casual, many gay and lesbian relationships are based on long-term mutuality. As the society becomes more educated about homosexuality, it will better understand the complex emotional attachments and affiliation of many homosexual couples and will provide a more accepting atmosphere for these relationships.

Although homosexual marriages are not legally recognized, many homosexual relationships are the basis of new family units. Lesbian women are more likely to live together or cohabit than gay men. Lesbians have fewer sexual partners, are more likely to spend time with their partner, and place a higher value on sexual fidelity than their male counterparts (Williamson 1986). Lesbian women are also more likely to bring children from previous marriages into their partnerships than gay men are. Although many are concerned about the effects of parental homosexuality on the growing child, studies have shown that these children develop sex-role orientations and behaviors similar to children in the general population (Hoeffer 1981). The greatest danger to children reared in gay and lesbian families is the prejudice and ridicule expressed by others in society. For this reason, many homosexual parents keep their sexual preference private to spare their children pain during early childhood, choosing to explain their sexual preference when the children are able to understand homosexuality and emotionally ready to deal with its implications.

Families from Different Cultures

Families from different cultures are an integral part of North America's rich heritage. Each family has values and beliefs (cultural heritage) that are unique to their culture of origin and that shape the family's structure, methods of interaction, health care practices, and coping mechanisms. These factors interact to influence the health of families. Families from different cultures may cluster to form mutual support systems and to preserve their heritage; however, this practice may isolate them from the larger society.

Children in cultural clusters often have greater contact with the world around them than adults; through school, children become more proficient in language and more comfortable with new customs and behaviors. Sometimes children create conflict in the family when they bring home new ideas and values. They want to become part of the culture in which they live and incorporate new practices into existing family customs. In the process, they may reject previously cherished cultural traditions.

Becoming acculturated is a slow, stressful process of learning the language and customs of a new country. Chapter 17 presents information that helps the nurse understand the family traditions, beliefs, and practices of different cultures. This information helps the nurse to provide nursing care that is sensitive to the unique needs of families from different cultural heritages.

Single Adults Living Alone

Although individuals living alone, by definition, are not considered a family unit, in today's society many individuals live by themselves. When society is studied from a family perspective, these individuals are frequently overlooked, yet they represent a significant proportion of the population. Singles may include young, newly emancipated adults who have left the nuclear family and achieved independence. These young adults may have completed their education and entered the job market, becoming self-sufficient and self-supporting. As young adults postpone marriage or choose singleness, living alone is becoming a more prevalent life-style.

On the other end of the age spectrum is the older adult living alone. Having launched their families, many older adults find themselves single through divorce, separation, or death of a spouse. Some older adults remain in their homes, while others find an apartment more suitable to their changing needs. As they age, and depending on their health status and financial resources, some single adults relocate into retirement homes or extended care facilities. Although many older adults live alone, they may have frequent contacts with other family members, especially adult children and grandchildren. As they enter the golden years, their sense of family becomes stronger, and they seek to communicate the history and values of the family to the new generation.

Assessing and Promoting the Health of Families

The importance of family assessment cannot be overemphasized. The information gathered during assessment is the basis for planning and delivering nursing care to family members or to the family as a whole. Numerous family assessment tools are available. The nurse must consider a number of factors in selecting a family assessment tool or in developing a tool that meets the demands of the families served in a particular practice setting. The home care nurse, for instance, may develop a tool to assess the unique needs and problems of a family who has a member with diabetes.

A family assessment tool should be holistic, eliciting information about a wide variety of family characteristics, beliefs, and behaviors. The tool should be understandable and acceptable to both the family and the nurse (Speer and Sachs 1985). In other words, the nurse must use terminology comprehensible to a wide range of clients, and the tool should be quickly and easily administered. The instrument should also yield clinically relevant data about the family—information useful in formulating nursing diagnoses and planning nursing interventions that promote the health of families.

Families experiencing a great deal of stress are at higher risk of developing physical illnesses or mental health problems. Therefore, identifying family members who are experiencing stress is an important part of the family assessment process. People perceive and respond to stress differently, so the nurse needs to assess how each family member perceives and copes with stress. Common areas of stress and assessment of client coping are discussed in Chapter 16.

Health Appraisal

The health appraisal begins with a complete health history. The nurse focuses first on the family unit and then on the individuals in that family. The health history is one of the most effective ways of identifying existing or potential health problems. The history is followed by physical assessment of family members. If further evaluation is indicated, referral is made to the appropriate health care professional. Frequently the physical examination focuses on identifying pathologic conditions or the potential for them rather than on appraisal of health. When the focus is on health, the appraisal includes information on life-style behaviors and health beliefs. The nurse uses data from the health appraisal to formulate a health profile. The health profile provides the data necessary to establish a nursing diagnosis and to plan appropriate nursing interventions to promote optimal health through life-style modification.

Health Beliefs

In addition to appraising health status, the nurse assesses health beliefs and values to gain information useful in planning effective nursing interventions. Health beliefs and values are influenced by culture, family, education, and past experiences with health and illness. Some people feel they have little control over their health status, while others feel that their behaviors have a direct effect on health. To promote health, the nurse must understand the health beliefs of individuals and families and use this information in planning and delivering nursing care.

Health beliefs may reflect a lack of information or misinformation about health or disease. They may also include folklore and practices from different cultures. Because of the many advances in medicine and health care during the last few decades, many clients have outdated information about health, illness, treatment, and prevention. The nurse is frequently in a position to give information or correct misconceptions about health. This function is an important component of the nursing care plan.

Family Communication Patterns

The effectiveness of family communication determines its ability to function as a cooperative, growth-producing unit. Messages are constantly being communicated among family members, both verbally and nonverbally. The information transmitted influences how members work together, fulfill their assigned roles in the family, incorporate family values, and develop skills to function in society. **Intrafamily communication** plays a significant role in the development of self-esteem, which is necessary for the growth of personality.

Families who communicate effectively transmit messages clearly. Members are free to express their feelings without fear of jeopardizing their standing in the family. Family members support one another and have the ability to listen, empathize, and reach out to one another in times of crisis. When the needs of family members are met, they are more able to reach out to meet the needs of others in society.

When patterns of communication among family members are dysfunctional, messages are often communicated unclearly. Verbal communication may be incongruent with nonverbal messages. Power struggles may be evidenced by hostility, anger, or silence. Members may be cautious in expressing their feelings because they cannot predict how others in the family will respond. Many things remain unsaid to preserve family unity and tranquillity. When family communication is impaired, the growth of individual members is stunted. Members often turn to other systems to seek personal validation and gratification.

The nurse needs to observe intrafamily communication patterns closely. Nurses should pay special attention to who does the talking for the family, which members are silent, how disagreements are handled, and how well the members listen to one another and encourage the participation of others. Nonverbal communication is important because it gives valuable clues about what people are feeling.

Family Coping Mechanisms

Family coping mechanisms are the behaviors families use to deal with stress or changes. Coping mechanisms can be viewed as an active method of problem solving developed to meet life's challenges. The coping mechanisms families and individuals develop reflect their individual resourcefulness. Friedman (1981) states that families may use the same coping patterns rather consistently over time or may change their coping strategies when new demands are made on the family. Coping is a basic function that helps the family meet demands imposed both from within and without. The success of a family depends on how well it copes with the stresses it experiences.

Nurses working with families realize the importance of assessing coping mechanisms as a way of determining how families relate to stress. Also important are the resources available to the family. Internal resources, such as knowledge, skills, effective communication patterns, and a sense of mutuality and purpose within the family, assist in the problem-solving process. In addition, external support systems promote coping and adaptation. These external systems may be extended family, friends, religious affiliations, health care professionals, or social services. The development of social support systems is particularly valuable today, when many families, due to stress, mobility, or poverty, are isolated from resources that would help them cope.

Identifying Families at Risk for Health Problems

Risk assessment helps the nurse identify individuals and groups at higher risk than the general population of developing specific health problems, such as stroke, diabetes, and lung cancer. Risk may be related to genetic factors; for example, persons who have a family history of diabetes are at greater risk of developing diabetes than persons with no family history of diabetes. Certain practices also increase the risk of health problems; for instance, cigarette smokers are at greater risk of developing lung cancer than nonsmokers. Environmental factors, such as air pollution or exposure to toxic chemicals, increase the risk of certain health problems.

Risk reduction among individuals and groups identified as at risk poses a special challenge to health care professionals. Once the individuals or groups are identified, the nurse's role is to plan and implement interventions to reduce health risks when possible or to optimize the current health status of those individuals or groups when risks cannot be reduced. The vulnerability of family units to health problems may be based on family developmental level, age of family members, heredity or genetic factors, sociologic factors, and life-style practices. The goal of the nurse is to promote optimal family health and functioning.

▪ **Developmental Factors.** Families at both ends of the age continuum are at risk of developing health problems. Newly formed families who are entering the childbearing and childrearing phases of development experience many changes in roles, responsibilities, and expectations. These changes occur when adult family members are attempting to establish financial security. The many, often conflicting demands on the young family cause stress and fatigue, which may impede growth of family members and the functioning of the group as a unit.

Adolescent mothers, because of their developmental level and lack of knowledge about parenthood, and single-parent families, because of role overload experienced by the head of the household, are more likely to develop health problems. Moreover, the elderly are at risk of developing degenerative and chronic health problems. Because of the emphasis on youth in today's society, many elderly persons feel a lack of purpose and decreased self-esteem. These feelings in turn reduce their motivation to engage in health-promoting behaviors, such as exercise or community and family involvement.

▪ **Hereditary Factors.** Persons born into families with a history of certain diseases, such as diabetes or cardiovascular disease, are at greater risk of developing these conditions. A detailed family health history, including genetically transmitted disorders, is crucial to the identification of persons and families at risk. These data are used not only to monitor the health of individual family members but also to recommend modifications in health practices that potentially reduce the risk, minimize the consequences, or postpone the development of genetically related conditions.

Other family units or family members may be at risk of developing a disease by reason of sex or race. Males, for example, are at greater risk of having cardiovascular disease at an earlier age than females, and females are at greater risk of developing osteoporosis, particularly after menopause. While at times it is difficult to separate genetic factors from cultural factors, certain risk factors seem to be related to race. Some diseases are more prevalent among whites than blacks, and vice versa. Sickle-cell anemia, for example, is a hereditary disease limited to blacks of African descent (McFarlane 1977). Native Americans and Asians seem more susceptible to certain diseases and less susceptible to others than the general population.

▪ **Life-Style Factors.** As the understanding of health and illness increases, it has become clear that many diseases are preventable, the effects of some diseases can be minimized, or the onset of disease can be delayed through life-style modification. Cancer, cardiovascular disease, adult-onset diabetes, and tooth decay are among the life-style diseases. The incidence of lung cancer, for example, would be greatly reduced if people stopped smoking. Proper nutrition, good dental hygiene, and use of fluoride—in the water supply, in toothpaste, as a topical application, or as supplements—have been shown to reduce dental decay or caries, one of America's most prevalent health problems. Automobile accidents, the leading cause of death among adolescents and young adults, are frequently associated with alcohol consumption and increased risk taking.

In addition to health practices and nutrition, other important life-style considerations are exercise, stress management, and rest. Today, health professionals have the knowledge to prevent or minimize the effects of some of the main causes of disease, disability, and death. Too often, there is little consideration of health until sickness occurs. The challenge is to disseminate information about prevention and to motivate families to make life-style changes prior to the onset of illness. Many demands are made on today's family; an important question is: Will people take the time to be responsible for their own health?

▪ **Sociologic Factors.** **Poverty** is a major problem that affects not only the family but also the community and society. Over 35 million people, or nearly one out of every six Americans, live in poverty (Moccia and Mason 1986, p. 20). A disproportionate number of today's poor belong to ethnic or racial minority groups. Poverty is a real concern among the rising number of one-parent families headed by a female, and, as the number of these families increases, poverty will affect a large number of growing children.

Because many poor families do not possess the skills or support systems necessary to break out of the cycle of poverty, it is likely that poverty will continue to escalate rapidly in the future. When ill, the poor are likely to put off seeking services until the illness reaches an advanced state and requires longer or more complex treatment. Even though the Surgeon General has reported that the health of the American people has never been better (U.S. DHEW 1979), it is clear that this progress has not benefited all segments of society, particularly the poor.

▪ Health Promotion in the Family

Today's families are concerned about living healthy, productive, fulfilling lives. The media regularly inform the public that many personal behaviors endanger life and health, yet at the same time they accept advertising revenues from products that do not promote health. Much has been learned about the effects of diet, stress, and exercise on health, but changing long-established preferences and practices is difficult. Substance abuse, particularly of tobacco and alcohol, as well as personal and environmental safety hazards have needlessly decreased the productivity and shortened the lives of many persons.

To make changes that improve its own well-being, the family must be aware of potential health problems and their relationship to life-style practices. Information on how to reduce risks within the context of the family's value system is crucial. Support and encouragement of life-style changes help ensure that these changes are not temporary but become an important health value that influences lifelong health practices. The role of health education is to inform, motivate, and facilitate adoption of healthful life-style practices—activities that promote the well-being of individuals and families.

One of the major goals of **health promotion** is to help families take responsibility for their own health through self-care. **Self-care** is defined as activities individuals perform in their own behalf to maintain health and well-being (Orem 1980). Effective self-care requires knowledge and skills relating to health and illness. It includes knowing how to solve health problems of the family, as well as knowing when to seek outside guidance in meeting health problems. Self-care also encompasses health promotion for the family. Through health promotion, families can realize higher levels of wellness, productivity, self-awareness, and personal growth. For a more comprehensive discussion of health promotion, see Chapter 25.

The Family Experiencing a Health Crisis

Illness of a Family Member

Illness of a family member is a crisis that affects the entire family system. The family is disrupted as members abandon their usual activities and focus their energy on restoring family equilibrium. Roles and responsibilities previously assumed by the ill person are delegated to other family members, or those functions may remain undone during the duration of the illness. The family experiences anxiety because members are concerned about the sick person and the resolution of the illness. This anxiety is compounded by additional responsibilities when there is less time or motivation to complete the normal tasks of daily living.

Many factors determine the impact of illness on the family unit. Among these are:

- The nature of the illness, which can range from minor to life-threatening.
- The duration of the illness, which ranges from short term to long term.
- The residual effects of the illness, including none to permanent disability.

- The meaning of the illness to the family and its significance to family systems.
- The financial impact of the illness, which is influenced by factors such as insurance and ability of the ill member to return to work.
- The effect of the illness on future family functioning. For instance, previous patterns may be restored or new patterns may be established.

The family's ability to deal with the stress of illness depends on the members' coping skills. Families with good communication skills are better able to discuss how they feel about the illness and how it affects family functioning. They can plan for the future and are flexible in adapting these plans as the situation changes. An established **social support network** provides strength, encouragement, and services to the family during the illness. During health crises, families need to realize that it is a strength, not a sign of weakness, to turn to others for support. Nurses can be part of the support system for families, or they can identify other sources of support in the community.

During a crisis, families are often drawn together by a common purpose. In this time of closeness, family members have the opportunity to reaffirm personal and family values and their commitment to one another. Indeed, illness may provide a unique opportunity for family growth.

Intervening in Families Experiencing Illness

Nurses committed to family-centered care involve both the ailing individual and the family in the nursing process. Through their interaction with families, nurses can give support and information. Nurses make sure that not only the individual but also each family member understands the disease, its management, and the effect of these two factors on family functioning. The nurse also assesses the family's readiness and ability to provide continued care and supervision at home when warranted. After carefully planned instruction and practice, families are given an opportunity to demonstrate their ability to provide care under the supportive guidance of the nurse. When the care indicated is beyond the capability of the family, nurses work with families to identify available resources that are socially and financially acceptable (McClelland et al. 1985).

In helping families to reintegrate the ill person into the home, nurses use data gathered during family assessment to identify family resources and deficits. By formulating mutually acceptable goals for reintegration, nurses help families cope with the realities of the illness and the changes it may have brought about, which may include new roles and functions of family members or the need to provide continued medical care to the ill or recovering person. Working together, nurses and families can create environments that restore or reorganize family functioning during illness and throughout the recovery process.

Death of a Family Member

The death of a family member has a profound effect on the family. The structure of the family is altered, and this change may in turn affect how it functions as a unit. Individual members experience a sense of loss. They grieve for the lost person, and they grieve for the family that once was. (See Chapter 19 for a discussion of loss and grieving.) Some of the early stages of grief accompany family disorganization. However, as the family begins to recover, a new sense of normalcy develops, the family reintegrates its roles and functions, and it comes to grips with the reality of the situation. This painful blow takes time to heal. After the death of a member, families may need counseling to deal with their feelings and to talk about the person who died. They may also want to talk about their fears about and hopes for the future. At this time, families often derive comfort from their religious beliefs and their spiritual adviser. Support groups are also available for families experiencing the pain of death. It is often difficult for nurses to deal with grieving families because the nurses also feel the loss and feel inadequate in knowing what to say or do. By understanding the effect death has on families, nurses can help families resolve their grief and move ahead with life.

Chapter Highlights

Families are the basic social unit of society.

The family plays an important role in forming the health beliefs and practices of its members.

Family-centered nursing addresses the health of the family as a unit, as well as the health of family members.

Through family assessment, the nurse identifies health beliefs and practices that influence the wellness of the family.

In working with the wide variety of family forms in today's society, the nurse must be aware of many factors that affect the health of families.

The nurse must examine her or his own values about family, health, illness, and death to be effective in supporting families in crisis.

Nurses can help families realize their potential and their dreams for health and happiness by promoting healthy family functioning.

Selected References

The adolescent family. 1984. Columbus, Ohio: Ross Laboratories.

Duffy, M. A. September/October 1982. When a woman heads a household. *Nursing Outlook* 30:468–73.

Duvall, E. M. 1977. *Marriage and family development.* 5th ed. Philadelphia: J. B. Lippincott Co.

Ebersole, P., and Hess, P. 1981. *Healthy aging.* St. Louis: C.V. Mosby Co.

Edelman, C., and Mandle, C. L. 1986. *Health promotion throughout the lifespan.* St. Louis: C. V. Mosby.

Friedman, M. 1981. *Family nursing: Theory and assessment.* New York: Appleton-Century-Crofts.

Hoeffer, B. 1981. Children's acquisition of sex-role behavior in lesbian-mother families. *American Journal of Orthopsychiatry* 51:536.

Holmes, T., and Rahe, E. 1967. The social readjustment rating scale. *Journal of Psychosomatic Research* 11:213.

Johnson, S. H. 1986. *Nursing assessment and strategies for the family at high risk: High risk parenting.* 2d ed. Philadelphia: J. B. Lippincott Co.

Knafl, K. May 1985. How families manage a pediatric hospitalization. *Western Journal of Nursing Research* 7(2):151–76.

Logan, B. B., and Dawkins, C. E. 1986. *Family-centered nursing in the community.* Menlo Park, Calif.: Addison-Wesley.

Ludder, P., et al. March/April 1983. Caring for children of divorced families. *The American Journal of Maternal Child Nursing* 8:120–30.

McClellan, M. A. May/June 1984. On their own: Latchkey children. *Pediatric Nursing* 10:198–204.

McClelland, E.; Kelly, K.; and Buckwalter, K. 1985. *Continuity of care: Advancing the concept of discharge planning.* Orlando: Grune & Stratton, Inc.

McFarlane, J. December 1977. Sickle cell disorders. *American Journal of Nursing* 77:1948–54.

Moccia, P., and Mason, D. J. January/February 1986. Poverty trends: Implications for nursing. *Nursing Outlook* 34(1):20–24.

Mott, S. R.; Fazekas, N. F.; and James, S. R. 1985. *Nursing care of children and families.* Menlo Park, Calif.: Addison-Wesley Publishing Co.

Orem, D. E. 1980. *Nursing concepts of practice.* 2d ed. New York: McGraw-Hill.

Pender, N. J. 1982. *Health promotion in nursing practice.* New York: Appleton-Century-Crofts.

Reutter, L., and Strang, V. July/August 1986. Yours, mine, and ours: Step-parents and their children. *The American Journal of Maternal/Child Nursing* 2:264–66.

Spector, R. E. 1979. *Cultural diversity in health and illness.* New York: Appleton-Century-Crofts.

Speer, J. J., and Sachs, B. September/October 1985. Selecting the appropriate family assessment tool. *Pediatric Nursing* 11:349–355.

U.S. Department of Health, Education, and Welfare. 1979. *Healthy people: The Surgeon General's report on health promotion and disease prevention.* DHEW publication no. 79-55071.

Williamson, M. 1986. Lesbians. In Griffith-Kinney, J., editor. pp. 278–96. *Contemporary women's health.* Menlo Park, Calif.: Addison-Wesley Publishing Co.

Assessing Health

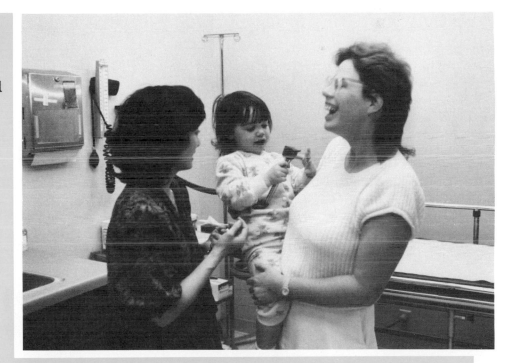

CHAPTER 31

Assessing Vital Signs

OBJECTIVES

Define terms and abbreviations used when measuring body temperature, pulse, respirations, and blood pressure.

Describe five factors influencing the body's heat production.

Identify four ways in which the body loses heat.

Describe the body's temperature-regulating system.

Compare oral, rectal, and axillary methods of measuring body temperature.

Identify situations in which specific methods for measuring body temperature are indicated or contraindicated.

Identify recommended intervals required to obtain accurate temperature readings for each method and for different types of equipment.

Describe selected alterations of body temperature and appropriate nursing care for these alterations.

Identify nine pulse sites commonly used to assess the pulse and state the reasons for their use.

List the characteristics that should be included when assessing pulses.

Explain how to measure the apical pulse.

Describe the mechanics of breathing and the mechanisms that control respirations.

Identify the characteristics that should be included in a respiratory assessment.

Differentiate systolic from diastolic blood pressure.

Describe various methods and sites used to measure blood pressure.

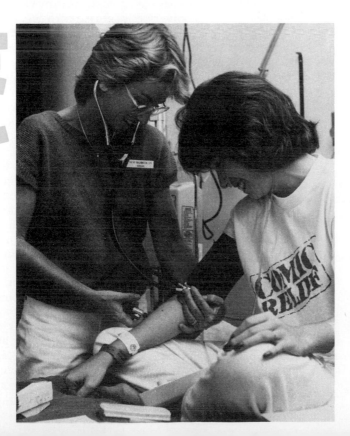

Vital Signs

The **vital signs** are body temperature, pulse, respirations, and blood pressure. These signs, which should be evaluated with reference to the client's present and prior health status as compared to accepted normal values, are used to monitor the functions of the body. Monitoring a client's vital signs should not be an automatic or routine procedure; it should be a conscientious scientific assessment.

When and how often to assess a specific client's vital signs are chiefly nursing judgments depending upon the client's health status. Some agencies or units have policies or protocols about taking clients' vital signs, and physicians may specifically order assessment of a vital sign, e.g., "Blood pressure q2h." Ordered assessments, however, should be considered minimal, and nurses should measure a client's vital signs more often if the current status requires it. Examples of times to assess vital signs are listed in the accompanying box.

Body Temperature

Body temperature is the balance between the heat produced by the body and the heat lost from the body. There are two kinds of body temperature: core temperature and surface temperature. **Core temperature** is the temperature of the deep tissues of the body. It normally remains relatively constant. The **surface temperature,** by contrast, rises and falls in response to the environment (Guyton 1986, p. 849).

The normal core body temperature is not an exact point on a scale but a range of temperatures. When measured orally, the average body temperature of an adult is between 36.7 C (98 F) and 37 C (98.6 F). See Figure 31–1 for the normal ranges of body temperature.

The body continually produces heat as a by-product of metabolism (i.e., all the chemical reactions of the cells of the body). Carbohydrates, fats, and proteins are

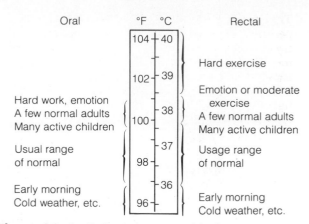

Figure 31–1 Estimated ranges of body temperatures in normal persons. *Source:* From E. F. DuBois, *Fever and the regulation of body temperature* (Springfield, Ill.: Charles C. Thomas, 1948). Courtesy of Charles C. Thomas, Publisher, Springfield, Illinois.

used to synthesize large quantities of adenosine triphosphate (ATP), which in turn is used as source of energy by body cells. However, about 50% of the energy in food becomes heat rather than ATP, and further heat is produced as the food is changed to ATP (Guyton 1986, p. 844). When the amount of heat produced by the body exactly equals the amount of heat lost, the person is in **heat balance.**

A number of factors affect the body's heat production. The most important are:

1. *Basal metabolic rate (BMR).* The BMR is the rate of energy utilization in the body during wakeful and absolute rest. BMRs vary with sex and age. After the age of 2 years, a female's BMR is usually about 5 to 10% less than a male's of the same age and size. The greatest difference between sexes (18 to 27%) occurs during adolescence (Vick 1984, p. 909). Metabolic rates decrease with age. From birth to about 20 years of age, the decline is rapid, after which it slows considerably (Vick 1984, p. 910).

2. *Muscle activity.* Muscle activity, including shivering, can greatly increase metabolic rate. For example, maximum muscle exercise can increase heat production to about 50 times normal (Guyton 1986, p. 845). A person doing heavy work, e.g., mining, can use as much as 6000 to 7000 kcal, or 3.5 times the BMR (Guyton 1986, p. 846).

3. *Thyroxine output.* Increased thyroxine output increases the rate of cellular metabolism throughout the body. This effect is called **chemical thermogenesis:** the stimulation of heat production in the body through increased cellular metabolism.

4. *Epinephrine, norepinephrine, and sympathetic stimulation.* These hormones immediately increase the rate of cellular metabolism in many body tissues. Epinephrine and norepinephrine directly affect liver and muscle cells, thereby increasing cellular activity. Of more importance is sympathetic stimulation of brown fat. When the cells of this fat are stimulated, they produce a large amount of heat.

5. *Increased temperature of body cells (fever).* Fever increases the cellular metabolic rate. Chemical reactions increase an average of about 120% for every 10 C rise in temperature (Guyton 1986, p. 846).

Times To Assess Vital Signs

- When a client has a change in health status or reports symptoms such as feeling hot or faint

- Upon admission to a health care agency

- According to a nursing or medical order

- Before and after surgery or an invasive diagnostic procedure

- Before and after the administration of a medication that could affect the respiratory or cardiovascular systems; for example, before giving a digitalis preparation that affects the heart

- Before and after any nursing intervention, e.g., ambulating a client who has been on bed rest, that could affect any of the vital signs

This means that for every 1 C (0.9 F) rise in temperature, there are about 12% more chemical reactions taking place. Although this mechanism is mediated somewhat by the body's temperature control system (see later in this chapter), the presence of fever acts to increase the body's temperature further.

Heat is lost from the body through radiation, conduction, convection, and vaporization. See Figure 31–2. Sweating, panting, lowering the environmental temperature, and wearing less clothing all promote heat loss. **Radiation** is the transfer of heat from the surface of one object to the surface of another without contact between the two objects. For example, radiation accounts for 60% of the heat lost by a nude person standing in a room at normal room temperature (Guyton 1986, p. 850). Most heat loss through radiation is in the form of infrared rays.

Conduction is the transfer of heat from one molecule to another. Again, a temperature gradient is implied. The heat transfers to a molecule of lower temperature. Conductive transfer cannot take place without contact between the molecules and normally accounts for minimal heat loss except, for example, when a body is immersed in ice water. The amount of heat transferred depends on the temperature difference and the amount and duration of contact.

Convection is the dispersion of heat by air currents. There is usually a small amount of warm air adjacent to the body. This warm air rises and is replaced by cooler air, and so people always lose a small amount of heat through convection. **Vaporization** is continuous evaporation of moisture from the respiratory tract and from the mucosa of the mouth. Vaporization accounts for 20 to 25% of the heat lost from the body (Vick 1984, p. 892). Body sweating increases heat loss by this method, providing that the surrounding air is not saturated (unable to hold more water vapor). Vaporization is a highly variable method of heat loss, depending upon the relative humidity of the surrounding air.

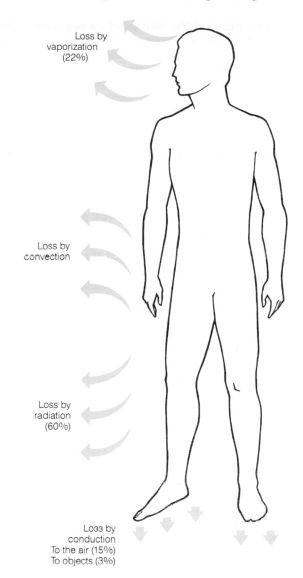

Figure 31–2 Sources of heat loss from the body

▪ **R**egulation of Body Temperature

The system that regulates body temperature has three main parts: sensors in the shell and in the core, an integrator in the hypothalamus, and an effector system that adjusts the production and loss of heat. Most **sensors** or **sensory receptors** are in the skin, which is a major part of the shell. There are fewer receptors in the tongue, respiratory tract, and viscera. The skin has receptors of both cold and warmth; however, far more receptors detect cold than warmth (Guyton 1986, p. 854). Therefore, skin sensors detect cold more efficiently than warmth.

When the skin becomes chilled over the entire body, three physiologic processes take place to increase the body temperature:

1. Shivering increases heat production.
2. Sweating is inhibited to decrease heat loss.
3. Vasoconstriction decreases heat loss.

The receptors in the body's core, i.e., in the abdominal viscera, in the spinal cord, and in or around the large veins, respond only to the body's core temperature, not to the body's surface temperature. They also detect mainly cold rather than warmth. Thermoreceptors in the hypothalamus are likewise sensitive to the core temperature.

The **hypothalamic integrator,** the center that controls the core temperature, is located in the preoptic area of the hypothalamus. Some sensors are sensitive to heat, and some are sensitive to cold. Neurons transmit signals in response to signals from the sensors in the body shell. When the sensors in the hypothalamus detect heat, they send out signals intended to reduce the temperature, i.e., decrease heat production and increase heat loss. When the cold sensors are stimulated, signals are sent out to increase heat production and decrease heat loss.

The signals from the cold-sensitive receptors of the hypothalamus initiate **effectors** such as vasoconstric-

circuit (oral, rectal, or axillary) in models that have separate circuits for each. Place a cover on the probe. Warm up the machine by switching it on, if not kept on.

For an Oral Temperature

3. Determine the time the client last took hot or cold food or fluids or smoked. To obtain an accurate oral temperature reading, it is recommended that nurses allow at least 15 minutes to elapse between a client's intake or smoking and the measurement (Blainey 1974, p. 1861).

4. Place the thermometer or probe at the base of the tongue to the right or left of the frenulum (posterior sublingual pocket). See Figure 31–9.
   Rationale: The thermometer needs to reflect the core temperature of the blood in the larger blood vessels of the posterior pocket.

5. Ask the client to close the lips, not the teeth, around the thermometer.
   Rationale: A client who bites the thermometer can break it and injure the mouth.

6. Leave the thermometer in place according to agency policy.
   Rationale: The nurse must allow sufficient time for the temperature to register. The recommended time is 2 minutes (Baker et al 1984, p. 111) or 3 minutes (Graves and Markarian 1980, p. 323). If an electronic oral thermometer is used, the client holds the thermometer under the tongue 10–20 seconds or until it completes registering.

For a Rectal Temperature

7. Assist the client to assume a lateral position. A newborn may be placed in a lateral or prone position (Axillary temps safer in infants 1978, p. 1081). Provide privacy before folding the bedclothes back to expose the buttocks.
   Rationale: Privacy is essential since exposure of the buttocks embarrasses most people.

8. Place some lubricant on a piece of tissue. Then apply lubricant to the thermometer. For an adult, lubri-

cate 2.5–4 cm (1–1.5 in.) of the bulb end of the thermometer. For an infant, lubricate 1.5–2.5 cm (0.5–1 in.).
Rationale: The lubricant facilitates insertion of the thermometer without irritating the mucous membrane.

9. Don a glove on the dominant hand. With your non-dominant hand, raise the client's upper buttock to expose the anus.

10. Ask the client to take a deep breath, and insert the thermometer into the anus anywhere from 1.5–4 cm (0.5–1.5 in.), depending on the age and size of the client (for example, 1.5 cm for an infant, 4 cm for a large adult). *Do not force insertion of the thermometer.*
    Rationale: Taking a deep breath often relaxes the external sphincter muscle, thus easing insertion. Inability to insert the thermometer into a newborn could indicate the rectum is not patent. The end of the thermometer should not be embedded in feces or the temperature measurement will not be accurate.

11. Hold the thermometer in place for 2 minutes (Nichols 1972, p. 1093) or for the length of time recommended by the agency. For neonates hold the thermometer in place for 5 minutes (Schiffman 1982, p. 276). Hold an electronic thermometer in place for 10–20 seconds.

For an Axilla Temperature

12. Expose the client's axilla. If the axilla is moist, dry it with the towel, using a patting motion.
    Rationale: Friction created by rubbing can raise the temperature of the axilla.

13. Place the thermometer in the client's axilla.

14. Assist the client to place the arm tightly across the chest. See Figure 31–10.
    Rationale: This position keeps the thermometer in place.

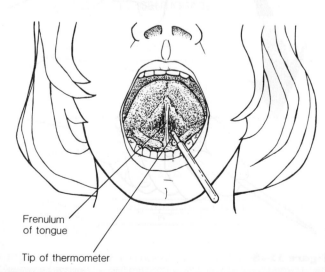

Frenulum of tongue

Tip of thermometer

Figure 31–9

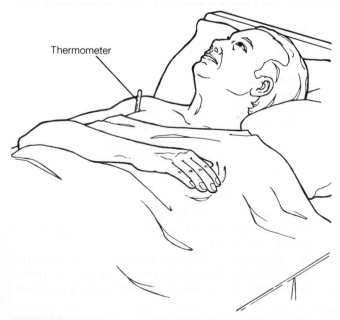

Thermometer

Figure 31–10

15. Leave the thermometer in place for 9 minutes (Nichols et al 1966, p. 310). Remain with the client and hold the thermometer in place if the client is irrational or very young. For infants and children, leave the thermometer in place 5 minutes (Eoff and Joyce 1981, p. 1011).

For All Temperature Sites

16. If using an electronic thermometer:
    a. Read the temperature on the dial or readout.
    b. Remove the thermometer.
    c. Remove and discard the probe cover.

17. If using a mercury thermometer:
    a. Remove the thermometer.
    b. Don a glove if not already worn. Remove the plastic sheath, or wipe the thermometer with a tissue. Start at the end held by you, and wipe in a rotating manner toward the bulb. Discard the tissue. *Rationale:* The thermometer is wiped from the area of least contamination to that of greatest contamination.
    c. Read the temperature. Hold the thermometer at eye level, and rotate it until the mercury column is clearly visible. The upper end of the mercury column registers the client's body temperature. On the Fahrenheit thermometer, each long line reflects 1 degree and each short line 0.2 degree. On the centigrade thermometer, each long line reflects 0.5 degree and each short line 0.1 degree.
    d. Wash the thermometer in tepid, soapy water. Rinse it in cold water, dry it, and store it dry. *Rationale:* Organic material such as mucus must be removed before the thermometer is stored. Organic materials on the thermometer can harbor microorganisms. If a thermometer is disinfected before storage ethyl alcohol 70% is considered effective.
    e. Shake down the thermometer and return it to its container or discard it. Some agencies also have special equipment for spinning down the mercury levels.

18. Assess the client's skin color (eg, pallor, flushing) and the presence of perspiration and "gooseflesh."

19. Determine if the client is thirsty, feeling hot or cold, fatigued, or has any other symptoms of a fever.

20. Record the temperature to the nearest indicated tenth (eg, 98.4 F, 37.1 C) on the book, record, or worksheet. *Rationale:* Recording the temperature immediately ensures it is not forgotten.

▪ Alterations in Body Temperature

According to NANDA, there are currently four accepted diagnostic categories that reflect clients' actual and potential health problems concerning body temperature. These are: alteration in body temperature, hyperthermia, hypothermia, and ineffective thermoregulation. **Alteration in body temperature** is the failure or the risk of failing to maintain body temperature within normal range because of internal factors such as the effects of disease and/or injury to the individual. Although modifying the causative factors is a medical responsibility (i.e., the physician orders measures to modify the internal factor causing the alteration in body temperature), the nurse is responsible for comfort and hydration measures appropriate for the individual client (Carpenito 1987, p. 127).

The remaining three nursing diagnoses reflect changes in body temperature in response to external factors such as the environment. **Hyperthermia** is the risk of sustaining a body temperature greater than 37.8 C (100 F) orally or 38 C (100.5 F) rectally. **Hypothermia** is the risk of sustaining a body temperature below 35 C (95 F) orally or 35.5 degrees C (96 degrees F) rectally. **Ineffective thermoregulation** exists when the client cannot effectively maintain normal body temperatures in the presence of adverse or changing external factors. The major nursing responsibility toward clients with any of these diagnoses related to external factors is modifying or controlling the causative factor or factors. Both hyperthermia and hypothermia, if not treated promptly, can result in medical emergencies; therefore, often the nursing focus is on prevention of these conditions in clients known to be at risk. The diagnoses are often recorded on the nursing care plan as *potential* hyperthermia or *potential* hypothermia (Carpenito 1987, p. 127). Examples of nursing diagnoses for clients with various alterations in body temperature are shown in the accompanying box.

▪ Nursing Assessment

Nursing assessment should include identifying people who are at risk for alterations in body temperature

NURSING DIAGNOSIS

▪ Alterations in Body Temperature

- Alteration in body temperature related to effects of infectious disease (specify disease process)
- Alteration in body temperature related to head trauma
- Hyperthermia related to exposure to an excessively hot environment
- Hyperthermia related to increased metabolic activity and dehydration
- Hyperthermia related to decreased ability to perspire
- Hypothermia related to exposure to a cold environment
- Hypothermia related to excessive evaporation from the skin secondary to consumption of alcohol
- Ineffective thermoregulation related to neonate's limited ability to produce body heat
- Ineffective thermoregulation related to decreased basal metabolism secondary to aging

as well as identifying the clinical signs of specific conditions and the defining characteristics of the likely nursing diagnoses. People at risk of developing **hypothermia** are:

- People who participate in cold-weather sports, e.g., skiing and mountain climbing
- Infants and children whose thermoregulatory systems are immature
- Elderly people who have insufficient food, clothing, or fuel
- People who have neurologic deficits and are unable to identify or respond to cold
- Alcoholics who have extreme heat loss secondary to vasodilation
- "Street people" who lack adequate clothing and shelter

People at risk for **hyperthermia** are those who have an infection or who may acquire an infection, e.g., postsurgical clients. Clients with infections, other disease processes (especially those that may impair thermoregulation, e.g., central nervous system tumors), or head trauma causing increased intracranial pressure are also at risk for alteration in body temperature. Ineffective thermoregulation is particularly likely for neonates, especially premature babies, and for older adults, particularly those with little subcutaneous fat.

Pulse

The **pulse** is a wave of blood created by contraction of the left ventricle of the heart. The heart is a pulsatile pump, and the blood enters the arteries with each heartbeat, causing pressure pulses or pulse waves (Guyton 1986, p. 225). Generally, the pulse wave represents the stroke volume output and the compliance of the arteries. **Stroke volume output** is the amount of blood that enters the arteries with each ventricular contraction. Normally the heart empties about 70% of its volume with each contraction, i.e., about 70 ml of blood in a healthy adult (Guyton 1986, p. 155). **Compliance** of the arteries is the distensibility of the arteries, i.e., their ability to contract and expand. When a person's arteries lose their distensibility, as can happen in old age, greater pressure is required to pump the blood into the arteries.

When an adult is resting, the heart pumps 4 to 6 liters of blood each minute. This volume is called the **cardiac output.** In a healthy person, the pulse reflects the heartbeat, i.e., the pulse rate is the same as the rate of the ventricular contractions of the heart. However, in some types of cardiovascular disease the heartbeat and pulse rates can differ. For example, a client's heart may produce very weak or small pulse waves that are not detectable in a peripheral pulse. In these instances, the nurse should assess the heartbeat *and* the peripheral pulse. See the section on assessing the apical pulse, later

in this chapter. A **peripheral pulse** is a pulse located in the periphery of the body, e.g., in the foot, hand, or neck. The **apical pulse**, in contrast, is a central pulse; i.e., it is located at the apex of the heart.

The pulse rate is regulated by the autonomic nervous system (ANS). Impulses pass through the parasympathetic branch to the sinoatrial node (SA node), which is the pacemaker of the heart. These impulses decrease the heart rate. When body demands indicate a need for an increased heart rate, the impulses of the parasympathetic system are inhibited and the impulses of the sympathetic system increase.

Factors Affecting Pulse Rate

The rate of the pulse is expressed in beats per minute. A pulse rate varies according to a number of factors. The nurse should consider each of the following factors when assessing a client's pulse:

1. *Age.* As age increases, the pulse rate gradually decreases. See Table 31–1 for specific variations in pulse rates from birth to adulthood.
2. *Sex.* After puberty, the average male's pulse rate is slightly lower than the female's.
3. *Exercise.* The pulse rate normally increases with activity. The rate of increase in the professional athlete is often less than in the average person because of greater cardiac size, strength, and efficiency.
4. *Fever.* The pulse rate increases in response to the lowered blood pressure that results from peripheral vasodilation associated with elevated body temperature.
5. *Medications.* Some medications decrease the pulse rate and others increase it. For example, digitalis preparations decrease the heart rate, whereas epinephrine increases it.
6. *Hemorrhage.* Loss of blood from the vascular system (hemorrhage) normally increases pulse rate. The loss of a small amount of blood, e.g., 500 ml, as after a blood donation, results in a temporary adjustment of the heart rate as the body compensates for the lost blood volume. An adult has about 5 liters of blood in his or her system and can lose up to 10% without adverse effects (Vick 1984, p. 346).
7. *Stress.* In response to stress, sympathetic nervous stimulation increases the overall activity of the heart. Stress increases the rate as well as the force of the heartbeat. Emotions such as fear and anxiety as well as the perception of severe pain stimulate the sympathetic system.
8. *Position changes.* When a person assumes a sitting or standing position, blood usually pools in dependent vessels of the venous system. Pooling results in a transient decrease in the venous blood return to the heart and a subsequent reduction in blood pressure. These changes are primarily mediated through the sympathetic nervous system, increasing cardiac rate, force of the ventricular contractions, and tone of the veins and arteries.

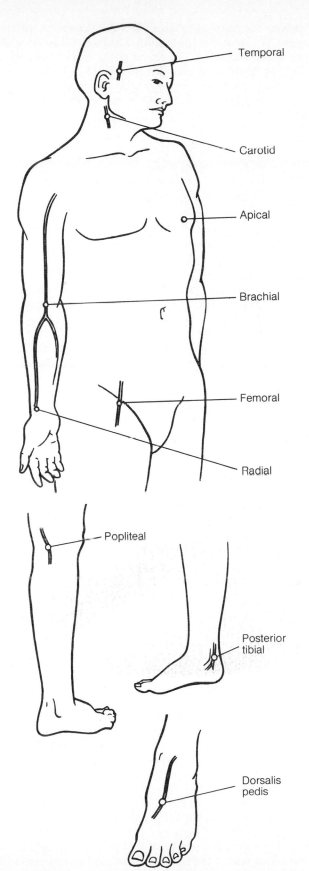

Pulse Sites

Nine of the sites where a pulse is commonly taken (see Figure 31–11) are:

1. *Temporal,* where the temporal artery passes over the temporal bone of the head. The site is superior (above) and lateral to (away from the midline of) the eye.
2. *Carotid,* at the side of the neck below the lobe of the ear, where the carotid artery runs between the trachea and the sternocleidomastoid muscle.
3. *Apical,* at the apex of the heart. In an adult this is located on the left side of the chest, no more than 8 cm (3 in) to the left of the sternum (breastbone) and under the fourth, fifth, or sixth intercostal space (area between the ribs). For a child 7 to 9 years of age, the apical pulse is located between the fourth and fifth intercostal spaces. Before 4 years of age it is left of the midclavicular line (MCL); between 4 and 6 years it is at the MCL. See Figure 31–12.
4. *Brachial,* at the inner aspect of the biceps muscle of the arm or medially in the antecubital space (elbow crease).
5. *Radial,* where the radial artery runs along the radial bone, on the thumb side of the inner aspect of the wrist.
6. *Femoral,* where the femoral artery passes alongside the inguinal ligament.
7. *Popliteal,* where the popliteal artery passes behind the knee. This point is difficult to find, but it can be palpated if the client flexes the knee slightly.
8. *Posterior tibial,* on the medial surface of the ankle where the posterior tibial artery passes behind the medial malleolus.
9. *Pedal (dorsalis pedis),* where the dorsalis pedis artery passes over the bones of the foot. This artery can be palpated by feeling the dorsum (upper surface) of the foot on an imaginary line drawn from the middle of the ankle to the space between the big and second toes.

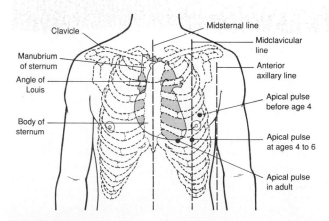

Figure 31–11 Nine sites commonly used for assessing a pulse

Figure 31–12 Locations of the apical pulse for a child under 4 years, a child 4 to 6 years, and an adult

Table 31–3 Reasons for Using Specific Pulse Sites

Pulse Site	Reasons for Use
Radial	Readily accessible and routinely used
Temporal	Used when radial pulse is not accessible
Carotid	Used for infants
	Used in cases of cardiac arrest
	Used to determine circulation to the brain
Apical	Routinely used for infants and children up to 3 years of age
	Used to determine discrepancies with radial pulse
	Used in conjunction with some medications
Brachial	Used to measure blood pressure
	Used during cardiac arrest for infants
Femoral	Used in cases of cardiac arrest
	Used for infants and children
	Used to determine circulation to a leg
Popliteal	Used to determine circulation to the lower leg
	Used to determine leg blood pressure
Posterior tibial	Used to determine circulation to the foot
Pedal	Used to determine circulation to the foot

The reasons for use of each site are given in Table 31–3. The radial site is most commonly used. It is easily found in most people and readily accessible.

Assessing the Pulse

A pulse is commonly assessed by palpation (feeling) or auscultation (hearing). The middle three fingertips are used for palpating all pulse sites except the apex of the heart. A stethoscope is used for assessing apical pulses and fetal heart tones. Increasingly, an ultrasound (Doppler) stethoscope (see Figure 31–13) is being used for pulses that are difficult to assess. The cardiac monitoring machine is another device for assessing the apical pulse. It indicates the rate on a screen or readout graph.

A pulse is normally palpated by applying moderate pressure with the three middle fingers of the hand. The

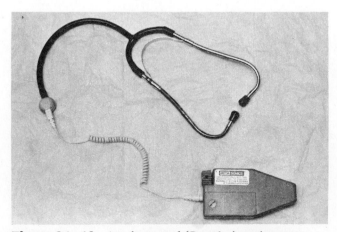

Figure 31–13 An ultrasound (Doppler) stethoscope

pads on the most distal aspects of the finger are the most sensitive areas for detecting a pulse. With excessive pressure, one can obliterate a pulse, whereas with too little pressure, one may not be able to detect it. Before the nurse assesses the pulse, the client should assume a comfortable position. The nurse should also be aware of:

▪ Any medication, e.g., digitalis, that could interfere with the heart rate.

▪ Whether the client has been physically active. If so, wait 10 to 15 minutes until the client has rested and the pulse has slowed to its usual rate.

▪ Any baseline data about the normal heart rate for the client. For example, a physically fit athlete may have a heart rate below 60 beats per minute.

When assessing the pulse, the nurse collects the following data: the rate, rhythm, volume, arterial wall elasticity, and presence or absence of bilateral equality. The **normal pulse rates** are shown in Table 31–1. An excessively fast heart rate, e.g., over 100 beats per minute in an adult, is referred to as **tachycardia.** A heart rate in an adult of 60 beats per minute or less is called **bradycardia.** If a client has either tachycardia or bradycardia, the apical pulse should be assessed.

The **pulse rhythm** is the pattern of the beats and the intervals between the beats. Equal time elapses between beats of a normal pulse. A pulse with an irregular rhythm is referred to as a **dysrhythmia.** It may consist of random, irregular beats or a predictable pattern of irregular beats. When a dysrhythmia is detected, the apical pulse should also be assessed. An electrocardiogram (ECG or EKG) is necessary to define the dysrhythmia further.

Pulse volume, also called the pulse strength or quality, refers to the force of blood with each beat. Usually, pulse volume is the same with each beat. It can range from absent to bounding. A normal pulse can be felt with moderate pressure of the fingers, and it can be obliterated with greater pressure. A forceful or full blood volume that is obliterated only with difficulty is called a *full* or *bounding* pulse. A pulse that is readily obliterated with pressure from the fingers is referred to as *weak, feeble,* or *thready.* A pulse volume is usually measured on a scale of 0 to 4. See Table 31–4.

The **elasticity of the arterial wall** reflects its expansibility or its deformities. A healthy, normal artery feels straight, smooth, soft, and pliable. Elderly people often have inelastic arteries that feel twisted (tortuous) and irregular upon palpation. The elasticity of the arteries may not affect the pulse rate, rhythm, or volume, but it does reflect the status of the client's vascular system.

When assessing a peripheral pulse to determine the adequacy of blood flow to a particular area of the body, the nurse should also assess the corresponding pulse on the other side of the body. This second assessment gives the nurse data with which to compare the pulses. For example, when assessing the blood flow to the right foot, the nurse assesses the right dorsalis pedis pulse and then the left dorsalis pedis pulse. If the client's right and left pulses are the same, the client's dorsalis pedis pulses are **bilaterally equal.**

Peripheral Pulse Assessment

A peripheral pulse, usually the radial pulse, is assessed by palpation for all individuals *except:*

- Newborns and children up to 2 or 3 years. Apical pulses are assessed in these clients.
- Very obese or elderly clients, whose radial pulse may be difficult to palpate. Doppler equipment may be used for these clients, or the apical pulse is assessed.
- Individuals with a heart disease, who require apical pulse assessment.

Table 31–4 Scale for Measuring a Pulse Volume

Scale	Description of Pulse
0	Absent
1	Thready or weak
2	Obliterated with pressure
3	Normal, detected readily
4	Bounding, difficult to obliterate

- Individuals in whom the circulation to a specific body part must be assessed; e.g., following leg surgery the pedal (dorsalis pedis) pulse is assessed.

Procedure 31–2 provides guidelines for assessing peripheral pulses.

PROCEDURE 31–2

Assessing a Peripheral Pulse

Equipment

- A watch with a second hand or indicator to count the pulse rate.
- If a Doppler ultrasound stethoscope (DUS) will be used, the transducer in the DUS probe (a device resembling a small transistor radio), a stethoscope headset, and transmission gel. See Figure 31–13 earlier. Do not use K-Y jelly, which contains probe-damaging salts. The DUS headset has earpieces similar to standard stethoscope earpieces, but it has a long cord attached to a volume-controlled audio unit and an ultrasound transducer. The DUS detects *movement* of red blood cells through a blood vessel. In contrast, the conventional stethoscope amplifies only *sound,* not movement. The DUS can detect blood flow if the blood cells are moving faster than 6 cm per second and at a depth of about 5 cm (Hudson, 1983, p. 55). It cannot detect blood flow in deep vessels or in those underlying bone, such as the vessels in the abdomen, thorax, or skull. The DUS is battery-operated, and batteries need replacement about every 6 months. Many agencies write the date of battery installation on a small adhesive label and attach it to the case as a reminder to replace the battery.

Intervention

1. Assess the client's emotional status and activity level. *Rationale* Emotion and activity, eg, anxiety and exercise, can increase the pulse rate.
2. Select the pulse point. Normally, the radial pulse is taken, unless it cannot be exposed or circulation to another body area is to be assessed.
3. Assist the client to a comfortable resting position. When the radial pulse is assessed, the arm can rest alongside the client with the palm facing down-ward. Or, the forearm can rest at a 90° angle across the chest with the palm downward. For the client who can sit, the forearm can rest across the thigh with the palm of the hand facing downward or inward.
4. a. When palpating the pulse, place three middle fingertips lightly and squarely over the pulse point. See Figure 31–14.
   Rationale Using the thumb is contraindicated because the thumb has a pulse that the nurse could mistake for the client's pulse.
   b. For using a DUS, Hudson (ibid, p. 56) outlines the following steps:

   - Plug the stethoscope headset into one of the two output jacks located next to the volume control. DUS units have jacks for two headpieces and accessory loudspeakers so that another person can listen to the signals.
   - Apply transmission gel either to the probe, at the narrow end of the plastic case housing the transducer, or to the client's skin.

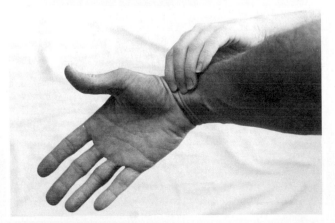

Figure 31–14

Rationale Ultrasound beams do not travel well through air. The gel makes an airtight seal, which promotes optimal ultrasound wave transmission.

- Press the "on" button.
- Hold the probe at a 45° angle against the skin over the pulse site. Use a light pressure, and keep the probe in contact with the skin.
  Rationale Too much pressure can stop the blood flow and obliterate the signal.
- Distinguish between artery and vein sounds. The artery sound (signal) is distinctively pulsating and has a pumping quality. The venous sound is like the wind, is intermittent, and varies with respirations.
  Rationale Both artery and vein sounds are heard simultaneously through the DUS, since major arteries and veins are situated close together throughout the body.
- If you have difficulty hearing arterial sounds, reposition the probe.

5. Count the pulse for 30 seconds and multiply by 2 if the pulse is regular. If it is irregular, count for 1 minute. If taking a client's pulse for the first time or when obtaining baseline data, count the pulse for a full minute.
   Rationale An irregular pulse requires a full minute's count for a correct assessment.

6. Assess the pulse rhythm by noting the pattern of intervals between the beats. A normal pulse has equal time periods between beats. If this is an initial assessment, assess for 1 minute.

7. Assess the pulse volume. A normal pulse can be felt with moderate pressure, and the pressure is equal with each beat. A forceful pulse volume is full; an easily obliterated pulse is weak.

8. To assess the arterial wall, compress the artery firmly and run a finger distal to the heart along the artery. See Figure 31–15. A normal arterial wall is smooth and straight.

9. Document the pulse rate, rhythm, and volume, and the condition of the arterial wall.

Sample Recording

Date	Time	Notes
5/8/89	0900	Pale and listless. Pulse 116, weak and thready. Reported above to Ms N. McNarama. ———————————Sally M. Sahara, NS

10. After using the DUS, remove all the gel from the probe to prevent damage to its surface. Clean the transducer with aqueous solutions.
    Rationale Alcohol or other disinfectants may damage the face of the transducer.

11. Assess the client's skin for color and warmth, eg, assess the color and warmth of a foot after taking a pedal pulse.

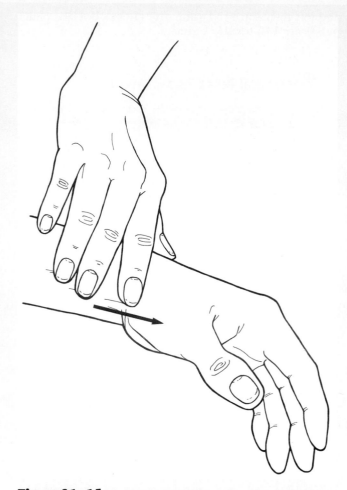

Figure 31–15

Rationale Color and warmth reflect the adequacy of the blood supply to the area.

12. Assess the client for facial pallor and any cyanosis of the lips and nail beds.
    Rationale These can reflect the adequacy of generalized blood flow.

13. Report to the responsible nurse pertinent data such as:
    a. Pale skin color and cool skin temperature.
    b. A pulse rate faster or slower than normal for the client
    c. A full, bounding or weak pulse volume
    d. An irregular pulse rhythm
    e. A tortuous arterial wall

Considerations for the Elderly

The maximal heart rate decreases progressively with age.

The heart of an elderly person is normally less able to respond to the increased demands of physical activity.

Skin color and temperature in an elderly person can reflect circulatory insufficiency (Lewis 1985, pp. 169–72).

The arteries of elderly people are less able to stretch, thereby increasing the pulse wave velocity of the arterial blood (Carnevali and Patrick 1979, p. 57).

▪ **A**pical Pulse Assessment

Assessment of the apical pulse is indicated for clients whose peripheral pulse is irregular as well as for clients with known cardiovascular, pulmonary, and renal dis-eases. It is commonly assessed prior to administering medications which affect heart rate. The apical site is also used to assess the pulse for newborns, infants, and children up to 2–3 years old. Procedure 31–3 presents guidelines for assessing the apical pulse.

P R O C E D U R E 31–3

Assessing an Apical Pulse

Equipment

- A watch with a second hand to time the rate of the apical pulse.
- A stethoscope with a bell-shaped or flat-disc dia-phragm to listen to the heartbeats. See Figure 31–16.
- Antiseptic wipes to clean the earpieces and dia-phragm of the stethoscope if their cleanliness is in doubt. The diaphragm needs to be cleaned and dis-infected if soiled with body substances.
- If using ultrasound, a DUS, probe (transducer), and transmission gel.
- A pacifier if necessary to quiet a newborn or infant.

Intervention

1. Assist an adult or young child to a comfortable supine position with the head of the bed elevated or to a sitting position on a chair, the edge of the bed, or the examination table. Place a baby in a supine posi-tion, and offer a pacifier if the baby is crying or restless.
   Rationale Crying and physical activity increase the pulse rate. For this reason, the nurse also takes the apical pulse rate of infants and small children before assessing body temperature.

2. Expose the area of the chest over the apex of the heart. If the client is in bed, fold the top bedding down to the bottom of the client's rib cage, and roll the gown up toward the neck. If the client is sitting, remove the upper clothing. Untie a hospital gown at the back, and draw it down in front just enough to expose the apical area, or lift the gown up from the bottom and drape it over the client's shoulder.

3. Warm the diaphragm of the stethoscope by holding it in the palm of the hand for a moment.
   Rationale The metal of the diaphragm is usually cold and can startle the client when placed imme-diately on the chest.

4. Insert the earpieces of the stethoscope into your ears. The earpieces may be straight or bent. If they are bent, place them in the direction of the ear canals, slightly forward, to facilitate hearing.

5. Locate the apical impulse; this is the point over the apex of the heart where the apical pulse can be most clearly heard. In 50% of the adult population, the apical impulse can be palpated (Malasanos et al. 1986, p. 347).

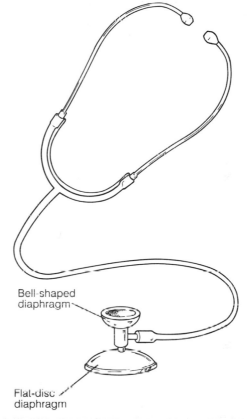

Bell-shaped diaphragm

Flat-disc diaphragm

Figure 31–16 A stethoscope with both bell-shaped and flat-disc diaphragms

a. Palpate the angle of Louis (the angle between the manubrium and the body of the sternum). It is palpated just below the suprasternal notch and is felt as a prominence. See Figure 31–12 earlier.

b. Place your index finger just to the left of the client's sternum and palpate the second intercostal space.

c. Place your middle or next finger in the third intercostal space and continue palpating downward until you locate apical impulse, usually about the fifth intercostal space, if the client is an adult or a child aged 7 years or more. If the client is a young child, palpate downward to the fourth intercostal space.
Rationale The apex of the heart is normally located in the fifth intercostal space, in individuals who are 7 years of age and over; it is in the fourth intercostal space in young children and one or two spaces above the adult apex during infancy (ibid, p. 601).

d. Palpate the apical impulse. For an adult move your index finger laterally along the fifth intercostal space to the MCL. Normally, the apical impulse is palpable at or just medial to the MCL (ibid, p. 347). For a young child move your finger along the fourth intercostal space to a position between the MCL and the anterior axillary line. See Figure 31–12 earlier.

6. Place the diaphragm of the stethoscope over the apical impulse and listen for the normal S_1 and S_2 heart sounds, which are heard as "lub dub." Each lub dub is counted as one heartbeat.

Rationale The heartbeat is normally loudest over the apex of the heart. The two heart sounds are produced by closure of the valves of the heart. The S_1 heart sound, heard as lub, occurs when the atrioentricular valves close after the ventricles have been sufficiently filled. The S_2 heart sound, heard as dub, occurs when the semilunar valves close after the ventricles empty.

7. Count the heartbeats for 30 seconds and multiply by 2 if the rhythm is regular; count the beats for 60 seconds if the rhythm is irregular or if the apical impulse is being taken on an infant or child.

Rationale A 60-second count provides a more accurate assessment of an irregular pulse than a 30-second count.

8. Assess the rhythm of the heartbeat by noting the pattern of intervals between the beats. A normal pulse has equal time periods between beats.

9. Assess the strength (volume) of the heartbeat. Normally, the heartbeats are equal in strength and can be described as strong or weak.

10. Assess the client for skin pallor and cyanosis of the lips or nail beds and for dyspnea and restlessness. Also assess the emotional status of the client.

Rationale Pallor and/or cyanosis and dyspnea can reflect circulatory problems. Emotions such as anxiety can affect the cardiac rate.

11. Document the pulse, noting that it is an apical pulse rate.

Sample Recording

Date	Time	Notes
1/26/89	0900	Apical pulse 56. Beats strong and equal. Digitoxin withheld. Notified Ms S. Santos, RN. ———————— ————————Thomas A. Jones, NS

Respirations

Respiration is the act of breathing; it includes the intake of oxygen and the output of carbon dioxide. Reference is often made to **external respiration** and **internal respiration.** The former refers to the interchange of oxygen and carbon dioxide between the alveoli of the lungs and the pulmonary blood. Internal respiration, by contrast, takes place throughout the body; it is the interchange of these same gases between the circulating blood and the cells of the body tissues.

The term **inhalation** or **inspiration** refers to the intake of air into the lungs. **Exhalation** or **expiration** refers to breathing out or the movement of gases from the lungs to the atmosphere. **Ventilation** is another word that is used to refer to the movement of air in and out of the lungs. **Hyperventilation** refers to very deep, rapid respirations; **hypoventilation** refers to very shallow respirations.

There are basically two types of breathing that nurses observe, **costal** or thoracic breathing and **diaphragmatic** or abdominal breathing. Costal breathing involves chiefly the external intercostal muscles and other accessory muscles, such as the sternocleidomastoid muscles. It can be observed by the movement of the chest upward and outward. By contrast, diaphragmatic breathing chiefly involves the contraction and relaxation of the diaphragm, and it is observed by the movement of the abdomen, which occurs as a result of the diaphragm's contraction and downward movement.

Mechanics of Breathing

Respiration includes the intake of oxygen and the output of carbon dioxide. During **inhalation** the following processes normally occur (see Figure 31–17): The diaphragm contracts (flattens), the ribs move upward and outward, and the sternum moves outward, thus enlarging the thorax and permitting the lungs to expand. During **exhalation** (see Figure 31–18), the diaphragm relaxes (its curvature increases), the ribs move downward and inward, and the sternum moves inward, thus decreasing the size of the thorax as the lungs are compressed. Normal breathing is called **eupnea.** An inspiration normally lasts 1 to 1.5 seconds, and an expiration lasts 2 to 3 seconds.

Control of Respirations

Breathing is normally carried out without effort and automatically. Respiration is controlled by respiratory centers in the brain, sensors, and the mechanisms of response. The **medulla oblongata** contains two respiratory centers; one controls *inspiration* and another controls *expiration.* The **apneustic center** in the **pons** prolongs inspiration when not inhibited by impulses carried by the vagus nerve. The **pneumotaxic center,** in the upper area of the **pons,** receives impulses from other respiratory centers and is thought to "fine tune" the *pattern of breathing* (Vick 1984, p. 449).

Ventilation is regulated by the concentrations of oxygen (O_2), carbon dioxide (CO_2) and hydrogen (H^+)

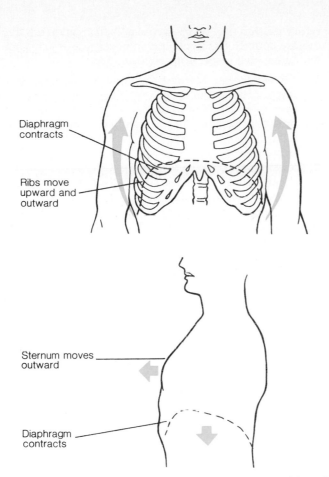

Figure 31–17 Respiratory inhalation: anterior and lateral views

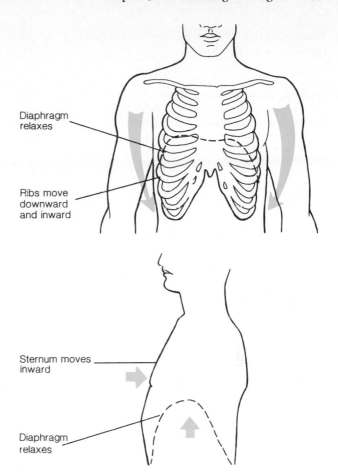

Figure 31–18 Respiratory exhalation: anterior and lateral views

in the arterial blood. Certain **sensors** (also called **chemoreceptors**), located centrally and peripherally, respond to these concentrations. The central sensors are located in the upper medulla, near the medullary respiratory centers. The peripheral sensors are located in the carotid bodies just above the bifurcation of the common carotid arteries. These sensors are stimulated by a decrease in the partial pressure of the oxygen (P_{O_2}) in the arterial blood.

There are **three mechanisms of response:** to CO_2, O_2, and H^+. The **mechanism of response to CO_2** affects alveolar ventilation *directly*. The normal partial pressure of CO_2 (P_{CO_2}) is 40 mm Hg. An increase in the P_{CO_2} stimulates the respiratory centers to increase respirations. A concentration of about 10% CO_2 in the inspired air stimulates ventilation maximally (Vick 1984, p. 451). A decrease in the P_{CO_2} in the alveoli enhances the ventilatory response. Therefore, the **partial pressure of carbon dioxide** (P_{CO_2}) in the arterial blood is the *most important* factor controlling ventilation.

The **peripheral sensors,** mainly in the **carotid bodies,** are sensitive to the *partial pressure of oxygen* in the arterial blood. When the P_{CO_2} falls, the sensors send impulses to the respiratory centers to stimulate breathing. When the P_{CO_2} increases at the same time, ventilation is greatly stimulated.

Changes in the hydrogen ion (H^+) concentration or pH of the blood also affect breathing. The H^+ con-

centration in the arterial blood is sensed by the **peripheral H^+ sensors.** When H^+ concentration is increased, e.g., in respiratory acidosis, respirations are increased. For additional information about breathing, see Chapter 42.

Respiratory Assessment

A client's respirations should be assessed when he or she is at rest because exercise affects respirations, increasing their rate and depth. Anxiety is likely to affect respiratory rate and depth as well. Before assessing a client's respirations, a nurse should be aware of:

- the client's normal breathing pattern
- the influence of the client's health problems on his or her respirations
- any medications or therapies that might affect respirations
- the relationship of the client's respirations to his or her cardiovascular function

The rate, depth, rhythm, and special characteristics of respirations should be assessed.

The respiratory **rate** is normally described in breaths per minute. A healthy adult normally takes between 15 and 20 breaths per minute. For the respiratory rates for

Table 31–5 Major Factors Influencing Respiratory Rate

Factor	Influence
Exercise: increases metabolism	Increase
Stress: readies the body for "fight or flight"	Increase
Environment: increased temperature	Increase
Increased altitude: lower oxygen concentration	Increase
Certain medications, e.g., morphine	Decrease

different age groups, see Table 31–1. Several factors influence respiratory rate. Some factors are listed in Table 31–5.

A number of terms are used to describe respiratory rate. A respiratory rate greater than 24 breaths per minute is called **tachypnea.** A rate of fewer than 10 respirations per minute is described as **bradypnea.** The complete absence of respirations is **apnea,** which is often described by its duration, e.g., 30 seconds of apnea. Prolonged apnea results in death.

The **depth** of a person's respirations can be established by watching the movement of the chest. Respiratory depth is generally described as normal, deep, or shallow. **Deep respirations** are those in which a large volume of air is inhaled and exhaled, inflating most of the lungs. **Shallow respirations** involve the exchange of a small volume of air and often the minimal use of lung tissue. During a normal inspiration and expiration, an adult takes in about 500 ml of air. This volume is called the **tidal volume.**

The capacity of the lungs varies with sex, age, stature, physical development, and body position. Men generally have a greater lung capacity than women of the same age. Variance by age is obvious: Babies have less vital capacity than children, children less than adolescents, and adolescents less than adults. However, elderly people usually have less vital capacity than young adults. Stature affects lung volume: Tall, thin people usually have a greater vital capacity than obese people. The athlete in top condition usually has a vital capacity that is above normal. (**Vital capacity** is the total of the tidal volume plus the inspiratory reserve volume plus the expiratory reserve volume.)

Body position also affects the amount of air that can be inhaled. People in a supine position experience two physiologic processes that suppress respiration: an increase in the volume of the intrathoracic blood and compression of the chest. Consequently, clients in a supine position have poorer lung aeration, which can predispose to the stasis of fluids and subsequent infection. Certain medications also affect the respiratory depth. For example, such barbiturates as secobarbital sodium, when taken in large doses, depress the respiratory centers in the brain, thereby depressing the respiratory rate and depth.

Respiratory **rhythm** or **pattern** refers to the regularity of the expirations and the inspirations. Normally, respirations are evenly spaced. Respiratory rhythm can be described as *regular* or *irregular.* An infant's respi-

ratory rhythm may be less regular than an adult's. Some disease conditions affect a person's respiratory rhythm. Four abnormal respiratory rhythms are:

1. *Cheyne-Stokes.* Marked rhythmic waxing and waning of respirations from very deep to very shallow breathing and temporary apnea (cessation of breathing); common causes include congestive heart failure, increased intracranial pressure, and drug overdose.
2. *Kussmaul's (or hyperventilation).* Increased rate and depth, often exceeding 20 breaths per minute; seen in metabolic acidosis and renal failure.
3. *Apneustic.* Prolonged gasping inspiration followed by a very short, usually inefficient, expiration; associated with central nervous system disorders.
4. *Biot's.* Shallow breaths interrupted by apnea; may be seen in healthy people and in clients with central nervous system disorders.

The **quality** of respiration refers to those aspects of breathing that are different from normal, effortless breathing. Two of these are the amount of effort a client must exert to breathe and the sound of breathing. Usually, breathing does not require noticeable effort; some clients, however, breathe only with decided effort. Difficult breathing is referred to as **dyspnea.** Dyspnea is usually evidenced by the obvious effort of the accessory muscles, such as the sternocleidomastoid, to maintain respirations.

The sound of breathing is also significant. Normal breathing is silent, but a number of abnormal sounds are obvious to the nurse's ear. Wheezing occurs when the airway is constricted; wheezing is usually more apparent on expiration than inspiration. Acute constriction of the trachea produces a harsh crowing sound on inspiration called **stridor.** This usually reflects respiratory distress. **Rales** are bubbling or crackling sounds that are evident with respirations. These sounds occur as a result of the presence of fluid in the lungs and are most clearly heard with a stethoscope. See Chapter 32, pages 456–60, for auscultation and percussion methods used to assess lung sounds. Procedure 31–4 provides guidelines for assessing respirations.

Blood Pressure

Arterial blood pressure is a measure of the pressure exerted by the blood as it pulsates through the arteries. Because the blood moves in waves, there are two blood pressure measures: the **systolic pressure,** which is the pressure of the blood as a result of contraction of the ventricles, i.e., the pressure at the height of the blood wave; and the **diastolic pressure,** which is the pressure when the ventricles are at rest. Diastolic pressure, then, is the lower pressure, present at all times within the arteries. The difference between the diastolic and the systolic pressures is called the **pulse pressure.**

PROCEDURE 31–4

Assessing Respirations

Equipment

- A watch with a second hand or indicator to time the respiratory rate

Intervention

1. Inspect the client's:
   - Skin and mucous membrane color, eg, for cyanosis and/or pallor
   - Position assumed for breathing, eg, whether the client is orthopneic
   - Any change that might indicate cerebral anoxia (decreased oxygen to the brain), eg, anxious behavior, irritability, restlessness, drowsiness, or loss of consciousness
   - If severe respiratory disease is present, specific chest movements, such as intercostal retractions (indrawing between the ribs) and substernal or suprasternal retractions (indrawing below or above the sternum)

2. Determine the client's activity schedule so as to choose a suitable time to monitor the respirations. *Rationale* A client who has been exercising will need to rest for a few minutes to permit the accelerated respiratory rate to return to normal. An infant or child who is crying will have an abnormal respiratory rate and will need quieting before an accurate assessment of the respirations can be made.

3. Place a hand against the client's chest to feel the client's chest movements or place the client's arm across his or her chest and observe the chest movements while supposedly taking the radial pulse.

4. Count the respiratory rate for 30 seconds if the respirations are regular. Count for 60 seconds if they are irregular. An inhalation and an exhalation count as one respiration.

5. Observe the respirations for depth by watching the movement of the chest. During deep respirations a large volume of air is exchanged; during shallow respirations a small volume is exchanged.

6. Observe the respirations for regular or irregular rhythm. Normally, respirations are evenly spaced.

7. Observe the character of respirations—the sound they produce and the effort they require. Normally, respirations are silent and effortless.

8. Report to the responsible nurse:
   a. A respiratory rate significantly above or below the normal range
   b. An irregular respiratory rhythm
   c. An inadequate respiratory depth
   d. An abnormal character of breathing—orthopnea, wheezing, stridor, rales, or rhonchi
   e. Any complaints of dyspnea

9. Document the respiratory rate, depth, rhythm, and character on the appropriate record.

Sample Recording

Date	Time	Notes
6/20/89	0900	R 38 and shallow. Dyspneic when talking. Dr Woo notified. ————————————————————————John P. Brown, NS

Considerations for the Elderly

Elderly people often have an increased rigidity of the thoracic wall and decreased strength of the expiratory muscles. Those factors decrease the ability to cough effectively and increase the likelihood of post-surgical chest infections.

The average blood pressure of a healthy young adult is 120/80 mm Hg. A number of conditions are reflected by changes in blood pressure. The most common is **hypertension,** an abnormally high blood pressure of 140 mm Hg systolic and/or 90 mm Hg diastolic when these are confirmed during a minimum of two consecutive visits by a client (National Heart, Lung, and Blood Institute 1984, p. 1045). **Hypotension,** or an abnormally low blood pressure, is a pressure below 100 mm Hg systolic.

Because blood pressure can vary considerably among individuals, it is important for the nurse to know a specific client's usual blood pressure. For example, if a client's usual blood pressure is 180/100 mm Hg and it is assessed following surgery to be 120/80 mm Hg, this drop in pressure must be reported to the charge nurse or physician. A number of conditions affect blood pressure. Some of these are listed in Table 31–6.

Table 31–6 Selected Conditions Affecting Blood Pressure

Condition	Effect	Cause
Fever	Increase	Increases metabolic rate
Stress	Increase	Increases heart rate
Arteriosclerosis	Increase	Decreases artery compliance
Obesity	Increase	Increases peripheral resistance
Hemorrhage	Decrease	Decreases blood volume
Low hematocrit	Decrease	Decreases blood viscosity
External heat	Decrease	Increases vasodilation and thus decreases peripheral vascular resistance
Exposure to cold	Increase	Causes vasoconstriction and thus increases peripheral vascular resistance

Physiology of Arterial Blood Pressure

The arterial blood pressure is the result of the cardiac output times the resistance the blood encounters while it flows, i.e., the peripheral vascular resistance. A person's blood pressure is directly affected by the *volume* of blood in the systemic circulation. The human body normally has about 5 liters of blood. Of this 5 liters, about 80 to 90% is in the systemic circulation and 10 to 20% is in the pulmonary circulation. Blood flows in the vascular system along a *pressure gradient*. The pressure of the blood in the aorta, for example, is higher than the pressure in the arterioles, and in the arterioles it is higher than in the capillaries. See Figure 31–19.

Cardiac output increases with fever and exercise, and the systolic pressure may increase as a result. However, cardiac output can be decreased as a result of heart disease, and the systolic pressure may then be low. **Peripheral resistance** can increase blood pressure, especially diastolic pressure. Some factors that create resistance in the arterial system are the size of the arterioles and capillaries, the compliance of the arteries, and the viscosity of the blood.

The *size* of the arterioles and the capillaries determines in great part the peripheral resistance to the blood in the body. A **lumen** is a channel within a tube: the smaller the lumen of a vessel, the greater the resistance. Normally, the arterioles are in a state of partial constriction. Increased vasoconstriction raises the blood pressure, whereas decreased vasoconstriction lowers the blood pressure.

The arteries contain smooth muscles that permit them to contract, thus decreasing their **compliance** (distensibility). Arteries normally yield somewhat during systole and retract during diastole. The arteries account for most of the peripheral resistance (Vick 1984, p. 199). The major factor reducing arterial compliance is pathologic change affecting the arterial walls. In old age, the elastic and muscular tissues of the arteries are replaced with fibrous tissue; thus, the arteries lose much of their compliance. The condition is known as **arteriosclerosis.**

Viscosity is a physical property that results from friction of molecules in a fluid. In a viscous (or "thick") fluid, there is a great deal of friction among the molecules as they slide by each other. The blood pressure is higher when the blood is highly viscous, i.e., when the proportion of red blood cells to the blood plasma is high. This ratio is referred to as the **hematocrit.** The viscosity increases markedly when the hematocrit is more than 60 to 65% (Vick 1984, p. 204).

Factors Affecting Blood Pressure

Among the factors influencing blood pressure are age, exercise, stress, race, obesity, sex, medications, and diurnal variations:

- *Age.* In older adults, the diastolic pressure often increases as a result of the reduced compliance of the arteries.

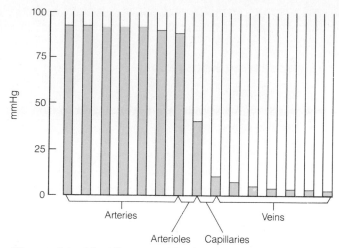

Figure 31–19 The mean blood pressure in the different parts of the vascular system. *Source:* adapted from R. L. Vick, *Contemporary medical physiology* (Menlo Park, Calif.: Addison-Wesley Publishing Co., 1984), p. 198.

- *Exercise.* Physical activity increases both the cardiac output and hence the blood pressure; thus, a rest of 20 to 30 minutes following exercise is indicated before the blood pressure can be reliably assessed.
- *Stress.* Stimulation of the sympathetic nervous system increases cardiac output and vasoconstriction of the arterioles, thus increasing the blood pressure reading; however, severe pain can decrease blood pressure greatly and cause shock by inhibiting the vasomotor center and producing vasodilation.
- *Race.* Black males over 35 years have higher blood pressures than white males of the same age.
- *Obesity.* Pressure is consistently higher in overweight and obese people than in people of normal weight (Overfield 1985, p. 46).
- *Sex.* After puberty, females usually have lower blood pressures than males of the same age; this difference is thought to be due to hormonal variations. After menopause, women generally have higher blood pressures than before.
- *Medications.* Many medications may increase or decrease the blood pressure; nurses should be aware of the specific medications a client is receiving and consider their possible impact when interpreting blood pressure readings.
- *Diurnal variations.* Pressure is usually lowest early in the morning, when the metabolic rate is lowest, then rises throughout the day and peaks in the late afternoon or early evening.

Blood Pressure Assessment

Blood pressure can be assessed directly or indirectly. **Direct (invasive monitoring) measurement** involves the insertion of a catheter into the brachial, radial, or femoral artery. Arterial pressure is represented as wavelike forms displayed on an oscilloscope. Generally, physicians insert the catheters, and nurses monitor the pressure readings. With proper placement, this pressure reading is highly accurate.

There are three **noninvasive methods** of measuring blood pressure **indirectly:** the auscultatory, palpatory, and flush methods. The **auscultatory method** is most commonly used in hospitals, clinics, and homes. Required equipment is a sphygmomanometer, cuff, and a stethoscope. External pressure is applied to a superficial artery, and the nurse reads the pressure from the sphygmomanometer when the blood flow is first heard through a stethoscope. When carried out correctly, the auscultatory method is relatively accurate.

When taking a blood pressure using a stethoscope, the nurse identifies five phases in the series of sounds called **Korotkoff's sounds.** First the nurse pumps the cuff up to about 30 mm Hg above the point where the last sound is heard; that is the point when the blood flow in the artery is stopped. Then the pressure is released slowly (2 to 3 mm Hg per sound), while the nurse observes the pressure readings on the manometer and relates them to the sounds heard through the stethoscope. Five phases occur (American Heart Association 1980, p. 11):

Phase 1. The period initiated by the first faint clear tapping sounds. These sounds gradually become more intense. To ensure that they are not extraneous sounds, the nurse should identify at least two consecutive tapping sounds.
Phase 2. The period during which the sounds have a swishing quality.
Phase 3. The period during which the sounds are crisper and more intense.
Phase 4. The period during which the sounds become muffled and have a soft, blowing quality.
Phase 5. The point where the sounds disappear.

The American Heart Association (AHA) recommends that the systolic pressure be considered the point where the first tapping sound is heard (phase 1). In adults, the diastolic pressure is the point where the sounds become inaudible (phase 5). In children, however, the AHA recommends that diastolic pressure be considered to be the onset of phase 4, where the sounds become muffled. In agencies where the fourth phase is considered the diastolic pressure of adults, three measures are recommended (systolic pressure, diastolic pressure, and phase 5). These may be referred to as systolic, first diastolic, and second diastolic pressures. The phase 5 (second diastolic pressure) reading may be zero; that is, the muffled sounds are heard even when there is no air pressure in the blood pressure cuff. In some instances, muffled sounds are never heard, in which case a dash is inserted where the reading would normally be recorded.

The **palpatory method** is sometimes used when Korotkoff's sounds cannot be heard and electronic equipment to amplify the sounds is not available. Instead of listening for the blood flow sounds, the nurse palpates the pulsations of the artery as the pressure in the cuff is released. The systolic pressure is read from the sphygmomanometer when the first pulsation is felt. A single whiplike vibration, felt in addition to the pulsations, identifies the point at which the pressure in the cuff nears the diastolic pressure (Enselberg 1961, p. 273). This vibration is no longer felt when the cuff pressure is below the diastolic pressure. To palpate the diastolic pressure, the nurse applies light to moderate pressure over the pulse point.

The **flush method** for determining blood pressure is another method used when Korotkoff's sounds cannot be heard by auscultation and electronic equipment is not available. The measurement is determined by a change in skin color when blood flow to an extremity resumes, i.e., when the extremity is no longer extremely pale but becomes reddened (vascular flush). The cuff is applied to the client's arm and the limb is wrapped in a bandage distally to proximally to force venous blood out of and restrict arterial flow into the extremity. The cuff is then inflated and the bandage is removed. The cuff pressure is released, and the nurse reads the pressure from the sphygmomanometer when the extremity flushes. This reading is the **mean blood pressure,** the midway point between the systolic and diastolic pressures. Procedure 31–5 gives guidelines for assessing blood pressure.

PROCEDURE 31–5

Assessing Blood Pressure

The blood pressure is usually assessed in the client's arm using the brachial artery and a standard stethoscope. If the arm is very large or grossly misshapen and the conventional cuff cannot be properly applied, leg or forearm measurements can be taken. To obtain a leg blood pressure, a standard-sized cuff is applied over the lower leg with the distal border of the cuff at the malleoli. Korotkoff's sound are auscultated over the posterior tibial or dorsalis pedis arteries. To obtain a thigh blood pressure, an appropriate-sized cuff is applied to the thigh. Korotkoff's sounds are heard over the popliteal artery. To obtain a forearm blood pressure an appropriate-sized cuff is applied to the forearm 13 cm (5 in.) from the elbow. Korotkoff's sounds then can be heard over the radial artery.

Assessing the blood pressure on a client's thigh is usually indicated:

■ When the blood pressure cannot be measured on either arm, eg, because of burns or other trauma.

■ When the blood pressure in one thigh is to be compared with the blood pressure in the other thigh.

Blood pressure is not measured on a client's arm or thigh in the following situations:

- The shoulder, arm, or hand (or the hip, knee, or ankle) are injured or diseased.
- There is a cast or bulky bandage on any part of the limb.
- The client has had breast or axilla (or hip) surgery on that side.
- The client has an intravenous infusion or a blood transfusion running.
- The client has an arteriovenous fistula (eg, for renal dialysis).

Equipment

- A stethoscope.
  or
  DUS (see Figure 31–13 earlier).
- A blood pressure cuff of the appropriate size (newborn, infant, child, small adult, adult, large adult, thigh).
- A sphygmomanometer.

Intervention

1. Determine the time the client last ate, smoked, or exercised.
   Rationale: For accurate measurements the blood pressure should not be taken within 30 seconds of the above.

For an Arm Blood Pressure

2. Help the client to assume the appropriate position. A sitting position is normally used unless otherwise specified. The arm should be slightly flexed with the palm of the hand facing up and the forearm supported at heart level. Readings in any other position should be specified.
   Rationale: The blood pressure is normally similar in sitting, standing, and lying positions, but it can vary significantly by position in certain persons. There is an increase in the blood pressure when the arm is below heart level and a decrease when it is above heart level.
3. Expose the upper arm.
4. Wrap the deflated cuff evenly around the upper arm so that the center of the bladder is applied directly over the medial aspect of the arm. To take an adult's blood pressure, place the lower border of the cuff about 2.5 cm (1 in.) above the antecubital space. The lower edge can be nearer the antecubital space of an infant.
   Rationale: The bladder inside the cuff must be directly over the artery to be compressed if the reading is to be accurate.
5. If this is the client's initial examination, perform a preliminary palpatory determination of systolic pressure.
   Rationale: The initial estimate tells the nurse the maximal pressure to which the manometer needs to be elevated in subsequent determinations. It also

prevents underestimation of the systolic pressure or overestimation of the diastolic pressure should an auscultatory gap occur. An *auscultatory gap,* which occurs particularly in hypertensive clients, is the temporary disappearance of sounds normally heard over the brachial artery when the cuff pressure is high and then the reappearance of the sounds at a lower level. This temporary disappearance of sounds occurs in the latter part of Phase 1 and Phase 2 and may cover a range of 40 mm Hg.
   a. Palpate the brachial artery with the fingertips. The brachial artery is normally found medially in the antecubital space. See Figure 31–20.
   b. Close the valve on the pump by turning the knob clockwise.
   c. Pump up the cuff until you no longer feel the brachial pulse.
   Rationale: At that pressure the blood cannot flow through the artery.
   d. Note the pressure on the sphygmomanometer at which the pulse is no longer felt.
   Rationale: This gives an estimate of the maximum pressure required to measure the systolic pressure.
   e. Release the pressure completely in the cuff and wait 1–2 minutes before further measurements are made.
   Rationale: A waiting period gives the blood trapped in the veins time to be released.
6. Insert the ear attachments of the stethoscope in your ears so that they tilt slightly forward.
   Rationale: Sounds are heard more clearly when the ear attachments follow the direction of the ear canal.
7. Ensure that the stethoscope hangs freely from the ears to the diaphragm.
   Rationale: Rubbing the stethoscope against an object can obliterate the sounds of the blood within an artery.
8. Place the diaphragm of the stethoscope over the brachial pulse. Use the bell-shaped diaphragm of the stethoscope (see Figure 31–16 earlier). Hold the diaphragm with the thumb and index finger.
9. Pump up the cuff until the sphygmomanometer registers about 30 mm Hg above the point where the brachial pulse disappears.
10. Release the valve on the cuff carefully so that the pressure decreases at the rate of 2–3 mm Hg per second.
    Rationale: If the rate is faster or slower, an error in measurement may occur.
11. As the pressure falls, identify the manometer reading at each of the five phases.
12. Deflate the cuff rapidly and completely and wait 1–2 minutes before making further determinations.
    Rationale: This permits blood trapped in the veins to be released.
13. Repeat steps 9–12 once or twice as necessary to confirm the accuracy of the reading.
14. Remove the cuff from the client's arm.
15. If this is the client's initial examination, repeat the procedure on his or her other arm. The arm found

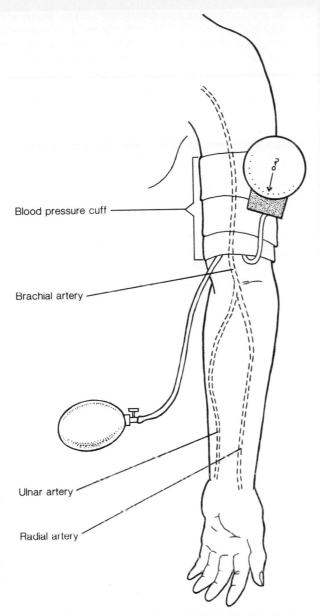

Blood pressure cuff

Brachial artery

Ulnar artery

Radial artery

Figure 31—20

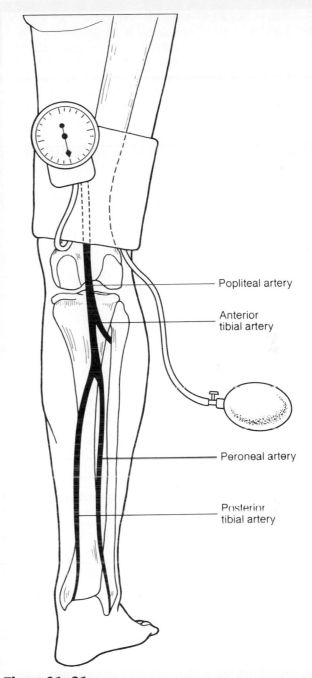

Popliteal artery

Anterior tibial artery

Peroneal artery

Posterior tibial artery

Figure 31—21

to have the higher pressure should be used for subsequent examinations.

16. Assess the client for signs of hypertension (eg), frequent nose bleeds, irritability, ringing in the ears) and assess for signs of hypotension (eg, increased pulse rate, cold clammy skin, dizziness).

17. Document the blood pressure according to agency policy. Record two pressures in the form "130/80" where "130" is the systolic (Phase 1) and "80" is the diastolic (Phase 5) pressure. Record three pressures in the form "130/110/90," where "130" is the systolic, "110" is the first diastolic (Phase 4), and "90" is the second diastolic (Phase 5) pressure. Use the abbreviations *RA* for right arm and *LA* for left arm.

18. Report any significant change in the client's blood pressure to the nurse in charge. Also report findings such as:

a. Systolic blood pressure (of an adult) above 140 mm Hg

b. Diastolic blood pressure (of an adult) above 90 mm Hg

c. Systolic blood pressure (of an adult) below 100 mm Hg

Sample Recording

Date	Time	Notes
8/14/89	1300	BP 130/90 in RA in bed-sitting position. Color pale.
		—Ruth P. O'Shea, SN

For a Thigh Blood Pressure

19. Help the client to assume a prone position. If the client cannot assume this position, measure the blood pressure while he or she is in a supine position with the knee slightly flexed.
Rationale: Slight flexing of the knee will facilitate placing the stethoscope of the popliteal space.

20. Expose the thigh, taking care not to expose the client unduly.

21. Wrap the cuff evenly around the midthigh with the compression bladder over the posterior aspect of the thigh.
Rationale: The bladder must be directly over the artery if the reading is to be accurate.

22. If this is the client's initial examination, perform a preliminary palpatory determination of systolic pressure by palpating the popliteal artery. See Figure 31–21 and step 5 on preceding page.

23. Follow steps 6–13.

24. Remove the cuff from the client's thigh.

25. Follow step 16 above.

26. Record the systolic and diastolic pressures. The systolic pressure in the popliteal artery is usually 10–40 mm Hg higher than that in the brachial artery because of use of a larger bladder; the diastolic pressure is usually the same.

27. Record an adult's pressure readings in the form "RT 130/90," where "RT" is right thigh, "130" is systolic pressure (Phase 1), and "80" is diastolic pressure (Phase 5). Record a child's pressure readings in the form "LT 140/90," where "LT" is left thigh, "140" is systolic pressure and "90" is diastolic pressure (Phase 4). In agencies where the onset of the fourth phase is considered the diastolic pressure of adults, take three readings: Phase 1, Phase 4, and Phase 5. Record the readings in the form "RT 130/100/90."

28. Follow step 18 above.

Considerations for the Elderly

Systolic and diastolic blood pressures increase with age (Carnevali and Patrick 1979, p. 58). In elderly people elasticity of the arteries is decreased—the arteries are more rigid and less yielding to the pressure of the blood. This produces an elevated systolic pressure. Because the walls no longer retract as flexibly with decreased pressure, there is also higher diastolic pressure. Several baseline blood pressure readings should be taken in the elderly person who has an elevated blood pressure.

Exercise and stress tend to raise the blood pressure more in the elderly than in younger people, and it takes longer to return to normal.

Common Errors in Assessing Blood Pressure

The importance of the accuracy of blood pressure assessments cannot be overemphasized. Many judgments about a client's health are made as a result of his or her blood pressure. It is an important indicator of the client's condition and is used extensively as a basis for nursing interventions. Mitchell and Van Meter found a mean difference of 7 mm Hg or less for recordings of systolic, diastolic phase 4, and diastolic phase 5 pressures as taken by nursing personnel and the investigators. There was also a difference of greater than 10 mm Hg in 37 to 46% of the readings. Nursing personnel consistently recorded higher readings than the investigators (Mitchell and Van Meter 1971, p. 352). Two possible reasons for the blood pressure errors are haste on the part of the nurse and subconscious bias. For example, a nurse may be influenced by the client's previous blood pressure measurements or diagnosis and "hear" a value consonant with the practitioner's expectations. An example of such a bias is "digit preference," a predilection for pressures ending with zero, e.g., 130 systolic, 70 diastolic, more often than would be expected (AHA 1980, p. 21). Some reasons for erroneous blood pressure readings are given in Table 31–7.

Table 31–7 Sources of Error in Blood Pressure Assessment

Error	Effect
Bladder cuff too narrow	Erroneously high
Bladder cuff too wide	Erroneously low
Arm unsupported	Erroneously high
Insufficient rest before the assessment	Erroneously high
Repeating assessment too quickly	Erroneously high systolic or low diastolic readings
Cuff wrapped too loosely or unevenly	Erroneously high
Deflating cuff too quickly	Erroneously low systolic and high diastolic readings
Deflating cuff too slowly	Erroneously high
Failure to use the same arm consistently	Inconsistent measurements
Arm above level of the heart	Erroneously low
Assessing immediately after a meal or while client smokes or has pain	Erroneously high
Failure to identify auscultatory gap	Erroneously low

Chapter Highlights

▪ Vital signs reflect changes in body function that otherwise might not be observed.

▪ Vital signs are assessed when a client is admitted to a health care agency to establish baseline data and when there is a change or possibility of a change in the client's condition.

▪ Data obtained from vital signs measurements are used to plan and implement appropriate nursing interventions.

Vital signs measurements are also used to evaluate a client's response to nursing interventions or prescribed medical therapy.

Knowledge of the normal ranges of vital signs and of the factors that regulate and influence vital signs helps the nurse interpret the measurements that deviate from normal.

Body temperature is the balance between heat produced by the body and heat lost from the body.

Heat is produced by the body's metabolic processes, which can be accelerated by muscle activity, thyroxine output, and stimulation of the sympathetic nervous system.

Heat is lost from the body by radiation, conduction, convection, and vaporization.

Knowledge of factors affecting heat production and heat loss helps the nurse to implement appropriate interventions when the client has a fever, hypothermia, or other related disorders, such as heat stroke.

Pulse rate and volume reflect the stroke volume output, the compliance of the client's arteries, and the adequacy of blood flow.

Normally, a peripheral pulse reflects the client's heartbeat, but it may differ from the heartbeat in clients with certain cardiovascular diseases; in these instances, the nurse takes an apical pulse and compares it to the peripheral pulse.

Respirations are normally quiet, effortless, and automatic and are assessed by observing respiratory movements.

Blood pressure reflects cardiac output and peripheral vascular resistance; peripheral vascular resistance varies according to the size of the arterioles and capillaries, compliance of the arteries, and blood viscosity.

Various sites and methods can be used to assess vital signs.

The nurse selects the site and method that is safe for the client and that will provide the most accurate measurement possible.

The most accurate values are obtained when the client is at rest and comfortable.

Change in one vital sign can trigger changes in other vital signs.

Suggested Readings

American Heart Association. 1980. *Recommendations for human blood pressure determination by sphygmomanometers.* Pub No. 70-019-B, 80-100M, 9-81-100M. American Heart Association.

Axillary temps safer in infants. June 1978. (Medical Highlights.) *American Journal of Nursing* 78:1081.

Baker, N. C.; Cerone, S. B.; Gaze, N.; and Knapp, T. R. March/April 1984. The effect of thermometer and length of time inserted on oral temperature measurements of afebrile subjects. *Nursing Research* 33:109–11.

Blainey, C. G. October 1974. Site selection in taking body temperature. *American Journal of Nursing* 74:1859–61.

Carpenito, L.J. 1987. *Nursing Diagnosis.* 2nd ed. Philadelphia: J.B. Lippincott Co.

Carnevali, D. L. and Patrick, M., editors. 1979. *Nursing management for the elderly.* Philadelphia: J. B. Lippincott Co.

Creative Care Unit. June 1977. Turnabout: Rectal temperatures for postcoronary patients. *American Journal of Nursing* 77:997.

Enselberg, C. D. 1961. Measurement of diastolic blood pressure by palpation. *New England Journal of Medicine* 265:272–74.

Eoff, M. J., and Joyce, B. May 1981. Temperature measurement in children. *American Journal of Nursing* 81:1010–11.

Erickson, R. May/June 1980. Oral temperature differences in relation to thermometer and technique. *Nursing Research* 29.157–64.

Graas, S. October 1974. Thermometer sites and oxygen. *American Journal of Nursing* 74:1862–63.

Graves, R. D., and Markarian, M. F. September/October 1980. Three-minute intervals when using an oral mercury-in-glass thermometer without J-temperature sheaths. *Nursing Research* 29:323–24.

Guyton, A. C. 1986. *Textbook of medical physiology.* 7th ed. Philadelphia: W. B. Saunders Co.

Hasler, M. E., and Cohen, J. A. September/October 1982. The effect of oxygen administration on temperature assessment. *Nursing Research* 31:265–68.

Hudson, B. May 1983. Sharpen your vascular skills with the Doppler ultrasound stethoscope. *Nursing 83* 13:55–57.

Kolanowski, A., and Gunter, L. September/October 1981. Hypothermia in the elderly. *Geriatric Nursing* 2:362–65.

Lewis, C. B. 1985. Aging: The health care challenge. Philadelphia: F. A. Davis Co.

Malasanos, L.; Barkauskas, V.; Moss, M.; and Stoltenberg-Allen, K. 1986. *Health Assessment.* 3rd ed. St. Louis: The C. V. Mosby Co.

Mitchell, P. W., and Van Meter, M. J. July/August 1971. Reproducibility of blood pressure recorded on patients' records by nursing personnel. *Nursing Research* 20:348–52.

National Heart, Lung, and Blood Institute. May 1984. *The 1984 report of the Joint National Committee on Detection, Evaluation, and Treatment of High Blood Pressure.* U.S. Department of Health and Human Services, Public Health Service, National Institutes of Health. Reprinted in *Archives of Internal Medicine* 144:1045–57.

Nichols, G. A., et al. Fall 1966. Oral, axillary, and rectal temperature determinations and relationships. *Nursing Research* 15:307–10.

Olds, S. B.; London, M. L.; and Ladewig, P. A. 1988. *Maternal-newborn nursing: A family-centered approach.* 3rd ed. Menlo Park, Calif.: Addison-Wesley Publishing Co.

Overfield, T. 1985. *Biologic variation in health and illness.* Menlo Park, Calif.: Addison-Wesley Publishing Co.

Schiffman, R. F. September/October 1982. Temperature monitoring in the neonate: A comparison of axillary and rectal temperatures. *Nursing Research* 31:274–77.

Vick, R. L. 1984. *Contemporary medical physiology.* Menlo Park, Calif.: Addison-Wesley Publishing Co.

CHAPTER 32

Assessing Health Status

OBJECTIVES

Define terms associated with health assessment.

Identify purposes of physical health assessment.

Compare and contrast the four modes of physical assessment.

Identify the various steps in selected assessment procedures.

Describe suggested sequencing to conduct a physical health assessment in an orderly fashion.

Explain the significance of selected physical findings.

Identify expected outcomes of health assessment.

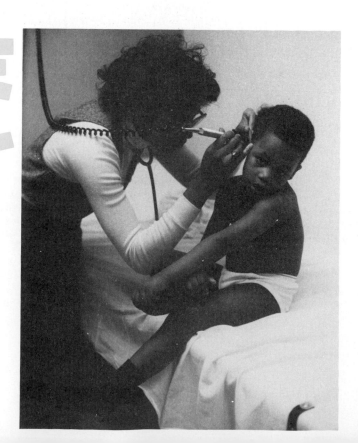

Physical Health Examination

Assessment of a client's health status encompasses both physical and psychosocial aspects. This chapter focuses primarily on the essential aspects of a basic physical assessment. A complete **physical assessment** is often conducted from the head to the toes; however, the procedure can vary in many ways according to the age of the individual, the severity of the illness, the preferences of the nurse, and the agency's priorities and procedures. Regardless of what sequence is used, the client's energy and time need to be considered. The physical assessment should therefore be conducted in a systematic and efficient manner that requires the fewest position changes for the client.

Purposes

Purposes of the physical health examination include:

1. To obtain baseline data about the client's functional abilities
2. To supplement, confirm, or refute data obtained in the nursing history
3. To obtain data that will help the nurse establish nursing diagnoses and plan the client's care
4. To evaluate the physiologic outcomes of health care and thus the progress of a client's health problem

Preparation of the Client

Most people need an explanation about the physical health examination. The nurse should explain when and where the examination will take place, why it is necessary, who will conduct it, and what will happen during the examination. Children need explanations that address their concerns (e.g., that most examinations are not painful, how the child can assist, whether a parent can accompany the child, and that a nurse will be there to help). Special circumstances—for instance, the need to go to a different room or assume a special position—should be explained. (See Table 32–1 for suggested positioning and precautions.) The client should also be told that appropriate draping will be provided so that his or her body will not be unnecessarily exposed. No special preparation is required when the examination is part of the nurse's assessment at the beginning of each shift.

Table 32–1   Client Positions and Body Areas Examined

Position	Description	Areas Examined	Cautions
Dorsal recumbent	Back-lying position with knees flexed and hips externally rotated; small pillow under the head	Head and neck, axillae, anterior thorax, lungs, breasts, heart, abdomen, extremities, peripheral pulses, vital signs, and vagina	May be difficult for elderly clients to assume
Horizontal recumbent	Back-lying position with legs extended; small pillow under the head	Head, neck, axillae, anterior thorax, lungs, breasts, heart, extremities, peripheral pulses	Not used for abdominal assessment because of the increased tension of abdominal muscles
Dorsal (supine)	Back-lying position without a pillow	As for horizontal recumbent	Tolerated poorly by clients with cardiovascular and respiratory problems
Sitting	A seated position, back unsupported and legs hanging freely	Head, neck, posterior and anterior thorax, lungs, breasts, axillae, heart, vital signs, upper and lower extremities, reflexes	Elderly and weak clients may require support
Lithotomy	Back-lying position with feet supported in stirrups	Female genitals, rectum, and female genital reproductive tract	May be difficult and tiring for elderly people
Genupectoral	Kneeling position with body at a 90° angle to hips	Rectum	Uncomfortable position tolerated poorly by clients who have respiratory problems
Sims's	Side-lying position with lowermost arm behind the body and uppermost leg flexed (See Chapter 38)	Rectum, vagina	Difficult for the elderly and people with limited joint movement
Prone	Face-lying position, with or without a small pillow	Posterior thorax, hip movement	Often not tolerated by the elderly and people with cardiovascular and respiratory problems

Most clients should empty their bladders before the examination. This helps them feel more relaxed and facilitates palpation of the abdomen and pubic area. Since an empty rectum facilitates rectal examination, the client should be encouraged to defecate before a complete physical examination. If a urinalysis is required, the urine should be collected in a container for that purpose. Enemas or medications may be required before special examinations such as sigmoidoscopy. Special procedures and examinations are discussed in Chapter 33.

Physical Assessment

The four methods or modes of physical assessment (inspection, palpation, percussion, and auscultation) are discussed in Chapter 8. Most data about the client's general appearance and behavior are obtained during the nursing assessment or nursing health history (see Chapter 8).

General Appearance and Behavior

The general appearance and behavior of an individual must be assessed in terms of culture, educational level, socioeconomic status, and current circumstances. An individual who has recently experienced a personal loss may appropriately appear depressed. Points to consider when observing the client's **general appearance** include:

- *Sex and race*. This information is useful in interpreting findings that suggest increased risk for known conditions.
- *Body build, height, and weight in relation to the client's age, life-style, and health*. Note whether the client is excessively thin, obese, or muscular.
- *Posture and gait*. Note whether the client
  — is relaxed or tense
  — has an erect, slouched, or bent posture
  — has coordinated or uncoordinated movements or tremors
- *Hygiene and grooming*. Relate findings to the person's activities prior to the assessment.
- *Dress*. Note whether dress is appropriate to age, life-style, climate, socioeconomic status, culture, current circumstances.
- *Body and breath odor*. Note these in relation to activity level.
- *Signs of distress*. Posture, behavior, and facial expression (e.g., wincing or labored breathing) can reflect distress.
- *Obvious signs*. Note obvious signs of health or illness.
- *Attitude*. Attitude is reflected in appearance, speech, and behavior; note whether the client is cooperative, withdrawn, negative, or hostile.
- *Affect* (the emotional state as it appears to others) and *mood* (the emotional state as described by the individual). Assess whether client's responses are appropriate or inappropriate to the circumstances.
- *Speech*. Listen for quantity (amount of speech and the pace of talking), quality (loudness, clarity, and inflection), and organization (coherence of thought, overgeneralization, and vagueness).
- *Thought processes*. Listen for relevance and organization of the thoughts.

The **level of consciousness** or state of awareness is often determined at the beginning of the physical examination. Ask the client to state his or her name, the day or date, tell where he or she is, and give the reason for hospitalization or for seeking assistance. Record the client's ability to provide this information. For clients who are unable to speak, describe their specific responses to verbal and physical stimuli.

Skin, Hair, and Nails

During a health examination, the skin, hair, scalp, and nails are checked. The entire skin surface may be assessed at one time, or it may be assessed as the nurse assesses the various aspects of the body. Assessment of the skin usually involves *inspection* and *palpation*. In some instances, the nurse may also need to use her or his olfactory sense to detect unusual skin odors; these are usually most evident in the skin folds or in the axillae. Pungent body odor is frequently related to poor hygiene, excessive perspiration (**hyperhidrosis**), or foul-smelling perspiration (**bromhidrosis**).

Nursing history data relative to the skin are outlined in the accompanying box.

The skin should be assessed for color, uniformity of color, moisture, surface temperature, vascularity and edema, pigmented areas, turgor and elasticity, texture and thickness, and the presence of lesions.

Skin **color** should be assessed in areas that have not

NURSING HISTORY

Skin

Determine:

- Presence of pain or itching
- Presence and spread of any lesions, bruises, abrasions, pigmented spots
- Previous experience with skin problems
- Associated clinical signs
- Family history
- Presence of problems in other family members
- Related systemic conditions
- Use of medications, lotions, home remedies
- Relative dryness or moisture of the skin
- History of easy bruising
- Possible relation of a problem to season of year, stress, occupation, medications, recent travel, housing, personal contact, etc.
- Any recent contact with allergens, e.g., metal paint

been exposed to the sun. Normal skin pigmentation varies from light to deep brown, ruddy pink to light pink, or yellow overtones to olive. Abnormal findings include **pallor** (absence of normal skin color reflected in a whitish-gray tinge resulting from decreased blood flow to the peripheral blood vessels or from decreased hemoglobin in the blood), **cyanosis** (bluish tinge to the skin, caused by decreased oxyhemoglobin binding in the blood or by decreased oxygenation of the blood), and **jaundice** (a yellow or green hue to the skin, occurring when tissue bilirubin is increased).

Pallor may be difficult to detect in clients with dark skin. In these clients, pallor is most readily seen in the buccal mucosa. Pallor in people with light skins may also be evident in the face, the conjunctiva of the eyes, and the nails. Cyanosis is most evident in the nail beds, lips, and buccal mucosa. In adults, jaundice may first be evident in the sclera of the eyes and then in the mucous membranes and the skin. Nurses should take care not to confuse jaundice with the normal yellow pigmentation in the sclera of a dark-skinned or black client.

The **color** of the **skin** is generally **uniform** over the body except in areas exposed to the sun. Dark-skinned clients have areas of lighter pigmentation, such as the palms, lips, and nail beds. Areas of hyperpigmentation (increased pigmentation) and hypopigmentation (decreased pigmentation) may also occur. An example of hyperpigmentation in a defined area is a birthmark; an example of hypopigmentation is vitiligo. **Vitiligo,** seen as patches of hypopigmented skin, is caused by the destruction of melanocytes in the area.

Skin moisture is assessed visually and by palpation. Moisture refers both to wetness and oiliness. The skin folds and axillae are normally moist. The moisture varies according to environmental temperature and humidity, muscular activity, and body temperature. Skin is often dry when environmental temperature and humidity are low and often moist when they are elevated. The elderly often have dry skin. Excessive oiliness may occur during adolescence.

The **skin temperature,** assessed by palpation, depends on the peripheral vascular circulation to the skin, which can reflect the client's cardiovascular status. Normally, a person's skin temperature is relatively uniform over the body. When skin temperature is higher or lower in one area, the nurse should palpate the corresponding area on the other side of the body to gain comparative data. Skin temperature should always be assessed when there is concern about the blood circulation to a body part.

Vascularity refers to the blood circulation to the skin. Abnormal vascularity can be seen by the presence of petechiae or bruises, for example. **Petechiae** are pinpoint red spots in the skin. **Edema** is the presence of excess interstitial fluid. An area of edema appears swollen, shiny, and taut. The location, color, temperature, and shape of edematous skin, and the degree to which it remains indented when pressed by a finger, should be assessed. See the accompanying box for a scale describing degrees of edema. Edema is most often an indication of impaired venous circulation and in some cases reflects cardiac dysfunction or vein abnormalities.

ASSESSMENT

Scale for Describing Edema

- ▪ 1+ Barely detectable
- ▪ 2+ Indentation of less than 5 mm
- ▪ 3+ Indentation of 5 to 10 mm
- ▪ 4+ Indentation of more than 10 mm

Turgor means fullness or elasticity. Skin or tissue turgor refers to the normal skin fullness, or the capacity of the skin and underlying tissue to return to their prior condition after being lifted and pinched. If skin turgor is poor, e.g., in a dehydrated client, the skin returns to its original shape slowly, remaining pinched or "tented" after it is released. Loss of skin turgor is often related to advanced age, when the skin becomes lax and wrinkled.

Although there is some variation in the **texture** of normal skin, it is usually smooth, soft, and flexible. Skin can become dry and rough as a result of certain diseases, such as hypothyroidism. The **thickness** of the skin is widely variable: thicker in areas that are exposed to pressure, friction, or other types of irritation. The skin is often thickest on the soles of the feet and the palms of the hands.

Normally, the skin does not have lesions. The nurse who observes any lesions is responsible for describing them accurately, including distribution and location, size, contour, and consistency. Table 32–2 lists some common skin lesions.

Hair grows on the whole body surface except on the palms of the hands, the soles of the feet, the dorsal surfaces of terminal phalanges, and parts of the genitals (the inner surface of the labia and inner surface of the prepuce of the glans penis). The visible part of a hair is called the hair shaft. The root is in a tube known as a hair follicle. The arrector pili muscles are attached to the hair follicles. See Figure 32–1. When these contract, the skin assumes a gooseflesh appearance. Sebaceous glands, which secrete sebum, grow from the walls of hair follicles. Sebum is produced in greater quantities on the scalp and the face than elsewhere on the body.

Normal, natural hair is black, brown, red, yellow, or shades of these colors. Hair fibers vary in shape—they may be straight, spiral, wavy, or helical. This variation makes the texture of the hair straight, wavy, kinky, or woolly. Hair also varies from fine to coarse. Black-skinned people often have thicker, drier, curlier hair than white-skinned people.

Normal hair has resilience and is evenly distributed. People with severe protein deficiency (kwashiorkor) have faded hair colors that appear reddish or bleached and coarse, dry hair texture. Some therapies for cancer cause **alopecia** (baldness), and some disease conditions affect the coarseness of hair. The box on page 446 provides guidelines for assessing hair.

The **nail plate** is normally colorless and composed of epithelial cells. Covering the base of the nail plate is the posterior nail fold; the lateral borders are covered by the lateral nail folds. The nail bed is highly vascular,

Table 32–2   Skin Lesions

Type of Lesion	Description	Examples
Primary		
Macula	A flat, circumscribed area of color with no elevation of its surface; 1 mm to several cm	Freckles, flat nevi
Papule	A circumscribed solid elevation of skin; less than 1 cm	Warts, acne, pimples, flat nevi
Nodule	A solid mass extending deeper into dermis than a papule	Pigmented nevi
Tumor	A solid mass larger than a nodule	Epitheliomas
Cyst	An encapsulated, fluid-filled mass in dermis or subcutaneous tissue	Epidermoid cysts
Wheal	A relatively reddened, flat, localized collection of edema fluid	Mosquito bites, hives
Vesicle	A circumscribed elevation containing serous fluid or blood	Herpes, chickenpox
Bulla	A larger fluid-filled vesicle	Second-degree burns
Pustule	A vesicle or bulla filled with pus	Acne vulgaris
Secondary		
Scale	Thickened epidermal cells that flake off	Dandruff
Fissure	A linear crack	Athlete's foot
Erosion	Loss of epidermis that does not extend deeper	Abrasions
Atrophy	A decrease in the volume of epidermis	Striae
Scar	A formation of connective tissue	Keloid
Ulcer	An excavation extending into the dermis or below	Stasis ulcer
Crust	Dried serum on the skin surface	Infected dermatitis

ASSESSMENT

Hair

Determine:

- The evenness of growth over the scalp and, in particular, any patchy loss of hair.
- Texture, i.e., whether it is coarse or silky.
- Oiliness, i.e., whether it is dry or greasy.
- Thickness or thinness.
- Presence of infections or infestations on the scalp, including flaking, sores, lice, nits (louse eggs), and ringworm.
- Presence on the body. **Hirsutism** is the presence of unusually dark, thick hair on the body. It has little significance in men but should be noted in children and women, since it may be associated with endocrine imbalances.

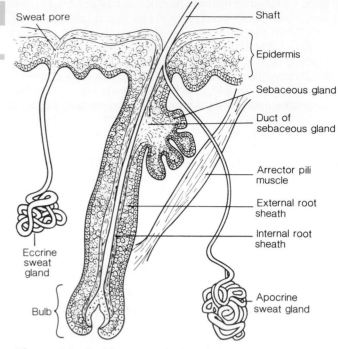

Figure 32–1   The parts of a hair follicle

which accounts for its pink color. However, the nail bed is not associated with nail growth or nail formation. At the base of the nail is a semilunar whitish area called the *lunula*; this is part of the underlying tissue from which the nail develops. The lunula is usually prominent on the thumb. See Figure 32–2. Normally, the nail plate has longitudinal ridges that often become more prominent with age.

Nails should be inspected for nail plate shape, angle between the nail and the nail bed, nail texture, nail bed color, and the intactness of the tissues around the nails. The **nail plate** is normally a convex curve. The nail

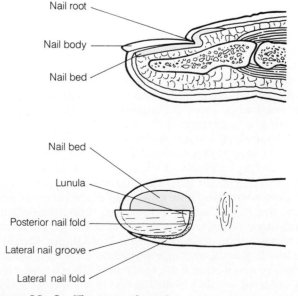

Figure 32–2   The parts of a nail

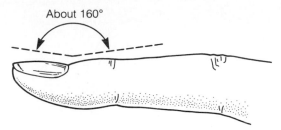

Figure 32—3   A normal nail, showing the convex shape and a nail plate angle of about 160°

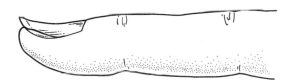

Figure 32—4   A spoon-shaped nail

plate **angle** is normally 160°. See Figure 32–3. One nail abnormality is the spoon shape. Here, the nail curves upward from the nail bed. See Figure 32–4. This condition is called **koilonychia** and may be seen in clients with iron-deficiency anemia. **Clubbing** is a condition in which the nail plate angle is 180° or greater. It may be caused by long-term oxygen lack and is seen in the elderly. See Figure 32–5.

Nail **texture** is normally smooth. Excessively thick nails can appear in the elderly, and excessively thin nails or the presence of grooves or furrows can reflect prolonged iron-deficiency anemia. *Beau's lines* are horizontal depressions in the nail that can result from injury or severe illness. See Figure 32–6. The nail bed color in Caucasians is pink; in blacks, brown or black pigmentation in longitudinal streaks or along the edge of the nail may normally be present. A bluish or purplish tint to the nail bed may reflect cyanosis, and pallor may reflect poor arterial circulation.

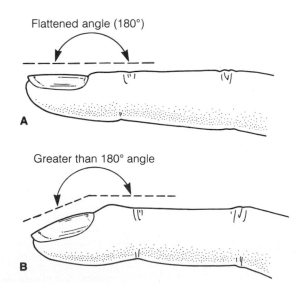

Figure 32—5   **A,** Early and **B,** late clubbing

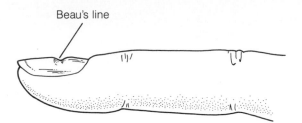

Figure 32—6   Beau's line on a nail

A **blanch test** can be carried out to test the capillary refill, i.e., peripheral circulation. Normal nail bed capillaries blanch when pressed but quickly turn pink (in Caucasians) or their usual color when pressure is released. In dark-skinned people, the nail may be pigmented along the edges or in lines along the nail, and the rate of return of nail bed color may be more significant than the color. A slow rate of capillary refill may indicate circulatory problems.

■ Head and Neck

During an examination of the head and neck, the nurse often uses inspection and palpation simultaneously, as well as auscultation. The nurse examines the head, face, neck muscles, trachea, thyroid gland, and lymph nodes. Areas to be included in the nursing history are shown in the accompanying box. Required equipment includes a good light source, a glass of water, and a stethoscope.

There is a large range of normal shapes of skulls. Inspect the **head** at all angles for size, shape, and symmetry. Areas of the head are named from underlying bones: frontal, parietal, occipital, mastoid process, mandible, maxilla, and zygomatic. See Figure 32–7. Note

N U R S I N G   H I S T O R Y

■ Head and Neck

Determine:

- Any past problems with lumps or bumps, neck pain, stiffness, itching, scaling, or dandruff
- Any history of loss of consciousness, dizziness, seizures, headache, facial pain, or injury
- The cause of any lumps and time elapsed since the lumps occurred
- Duration of any other problem
- Any known cause of problem
- Associated symptoms, treatment, and recurrences
- Any previous diagnosis of thyroid problem, including whether thyroid was over- or underfunctioning, what tests were taken, what the test results were, whether and what medications were ordered, what amounts were taken, whether still being taken, and whether other treatments (e.g., surgery, radiation) were provided

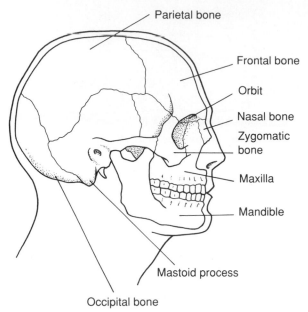

Parietal bone

Frontal bone

Orbit

Nasal bone

Zygomatic bone

Maxilla

Mandible

Mastoid process

Occipital bone

Figure 32–7   The bones of the head

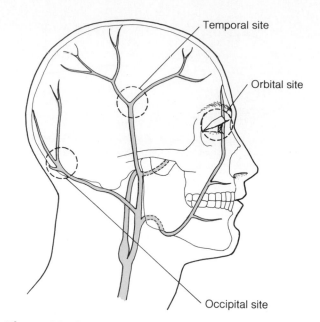

Temporal site

Orbital site

Occipital site

Figure 32–8   Auscultation sites for bruits

particularly areas of local trauma, lumps or bumps, and overall size. In adults, a large head may result from **osteitis deformans** (Paget's disease, a disorder in which bony thickness increases) or **acromegaly** (a disorder caused by excessive secretion of growth hormone). Auscultate over the occipital, temporal, and orbital regions for *bruits,* audible pulsations. See Figure 32–8.

Inspect the **facial skin** for color, the hair distribution and condition, and the facial structures (eyebrows, eyes, nose, mouth, and ears) for size and symmetry. Many disorders cause a change in facial shape or condition. Kidney or cardiac disease can cause edema of the eyelids. Thyroid overactivity (hyperthyroidism) can cause protrusion of the eyeballs with elevation of the upper eyelids, resulting in a startled or staring expression. Thyroid underactivity (hypothyroidism or myxedema) can cause a dry, puffy face with dry skin and coarse features, referred to as **myxedema facies,** and thinning of scalp hair and eyebrows. **Cushing's syndrome,** a disorder in which there is increased adrenal hormone production, can cause a round face with reddened cheeks, referred to as "moon face," and excessive hair growth on the upper lips, chin, and sideburn areas. Intake of synthetic adrenal hormones also produces these changes. Prolonged illness, starvation, and dehydration can result in sunken eyes, cheeks, and temples.

Ask the client to elevate the eyebrows, frown or lower the eyebrows, close the eyes tightly, puff the cheeks, and smile and show the teeth. These movements determine the function of the muscles of facial expression and the seventh cranial (facial) nerve. Sensation of the face, supplied by the fifth cranial (trigeminal) nerve, is tested as part of the neurologic examination, discussed later in this chapter.

Have the client hold his or her head erect, and inspect the **neck muscles** (sternocleidomastoid and trapezius) for abnormal swellings or masses. Each sternocleido-

mastoid muscle extends from the upper sternum and the medial third of the clavicle to the mastoid process of the temporal bone behind the ear. See Figure 32–9. These muscles turn and laterally flex the head. Each trapezius muscle extends from the occipital bone of the skull to the lateral third of the clavicle. These muscles draw the head to the side and back, elevate the chin, and elevate the shoulders to shrug them. Areas of the neck are defined by the sternocleidomastoid muscles,

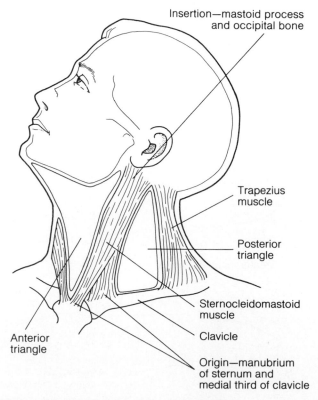

Insertion—mastoid process and occipital bone

Trapezius muscle

Posterior triangle

Sternocleidomastoid muscle

Clavicle

Origin—manubrium of sternum and medial third of clavicle

Anterior triangle

Figure 32–9   Major muscles of the neck

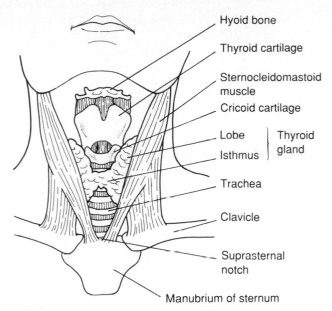

Hyoid bone
Thyroid cartilage
Sternocleidomastoid muscle
Cricoid cartilage
Lobe } Thyroid gland
Isthmus
Trachea
Clavicle
Suprasternal notch
Manubrium of sternum

Figure 32–10 Structures of the neck

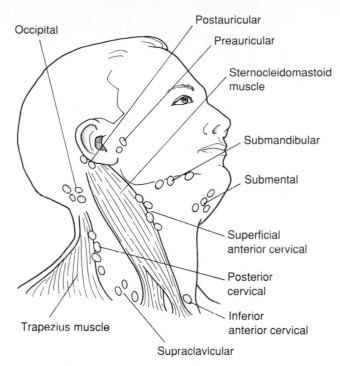

Occipital
Postauricular
Preauricular
Sternocleidomastoid muscle
Submandibular
Submental
Superficial anterior cervical
Posterior cervical
Inferior anterior cervical
Trapezius muscle
Supraclavicular

Figure 32–11 Lymph nodes of the neck

which divide each side of the neck into two triangles: the anterior and posterior triangles.

The trachea, thyroid gland, anterior cervical nodes, and carotid artery lie within the anterior triangle (the carotid artery runs parallel and anterior to the sternocleidomastoid muscle); the posterior lymph nodes lie within the posterior triangle. See Figure 32–10. Physical assessment of these structures is not usually performed by a beginning student.

Several **lymph nodes** or centers in the head collect lymph from the head, ears, nose, cheeks, and lips. Nodes in the neck that collect lymph from the head and neck structures are grouped serially and referred to as chains. See Figure 32–11 and Table 32–3. The deep cervical chain is not shown in Figure 32–11, since it lies beneath the sternocleidomastoid muscle. Complete physical assessment, performed by an advanced practitioner, includes palation of the lymph nodes.

Table 32–3 Lymph Nodes of the Head and Neck

Node Center	Location	Area Drained
Head		
Occipital	At the posterior base of the skull	The occipital region of the scalp and the deep structures of the back of the neck
Postauricular (mastoid)	Behind the auricle of the ear over or in front of the mastoid process	The parietal region of the head and part of the ear
Preauricular	In front of the tragus of the ear	The forehead and upper face
Floor of mouth		
Submandibular (submaxillary)	Along the medial border of the lower jaw, halfway between the angle of the jaw and the chin	The chin, upper lip, cheek, nose, teeth, eyelids, part of the tongue and of the floor of the mouth
Submental	Behind the tip of the mandible, in the midline, under the chin	The anterior third of the tongue, gums, and floor of the mouth
Neck		
Superficial (anterior) cervical chain	Along and anterior to the sternocleidomastoid muscle	The skin and neck
Posterior cervical chain	Along the anterior aspect of the trapezius muscle	The posterior and lateral regions of the neck, occiput, and mastoid
Deep cervical chain	Under the sternocleidomastoid muscle	The larynx, thyroid gland, trachea, and upper part of the esophagus
Supraclavicular	Above the clavicle, in the angle between the clavicle and the sternocleidomastoid muscle	The lateral regions of the neck and lungs

NURSING HISTORY

Eyes

Determine:

- When the client last visited an ophthalmologist
- Whether there is a family history of diabetes; hypertension; blood dyscrasia; or eye disease, injury, or surgery
- Whether the client is currently taking eye medications
- Whether the client wears contact lenses or eyeglasses
- What hygienic practices the client uses for corrective lenses
- Whether there are current symptoms of eye problems, such as changes in visual acuity, blurring of vision, tearing, spots or floaters, photophobia, burning, itching, pain, diplopia, flashing lights, or halos around lights

Eyes and Vision

Many people consider vision the most important sense, since it allows them to interact freely with their environment and enjoy the beauty of life around them. To maintain optimum vision, people need to have their eyes examined throughout life. It is recommended that people under age 40 have their eyes tested every 3 to 5 years, or more frequently if there is a family history of diabetes, hypertension, blood dyscrasia, or eye disease (e.g., glaucoma). After age 40, an eye examination is recommended every 2 years to rule out the possibility of glaucoma.

An eye assessment should be carried out as part of the client's initial physical examination; periodic reassessments need to be made for long-term care clients. Examination of the eyes includes assessment of visual acuity, ocular movement, visual fields, external structures, and the fundus. Most eye assessment procedures involve inspection. Consideration is also given to developmental changes and to individual hygienic practices, if the client wears contact lenses or an artificial eye. Nursing history data taken in conjunction with assessment of the eyes are shown in the accompanying box. For the anatomic structures of the eye, see Figures 32–12 and 32–13.

Normal visual acuity (assessed by use of a Snellen chart—see Figure 32–14) is usually present by 6 years of age. **Loss of visual acuity** occurs in elderly people as the lens of the eye ages, becomes more opaque, and loses elasticity. Other changes include loss of ability of the iris to accommodate to darkness and dim light, loss of peripheral vision, and difficulty in distinguishing similar colors.

Many people wear eyeglasses or contact lenses to correct common **refractive errors of the lens** of the eye. These errors include **myopia** (nearsightedness), **hyperopia** (farsightedness), and **presbyopia** (loss of elasticity of the lens and thus loss of ability to see close

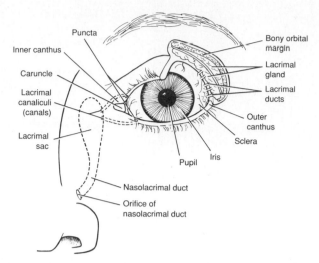

Figure 32–12 The left eye showing the external structures and the lacrimal apparatus

objects). Presbyopia begins at about 45 years of age. People notice that they have difficulty reading newsprint. Often two corrective lenses (bifocals) are required—one for near vision or reading, and the other for far vision. **Astigmatism,** an uneven curvature of the cornea that prevents horizontal and vertical rays from focusing on the retina, is a common problem that may occur in conjunction with myopia and hyperopia.

Common **inflammatory visual problems** that nurses may encounter in clients include conjunctivitis.

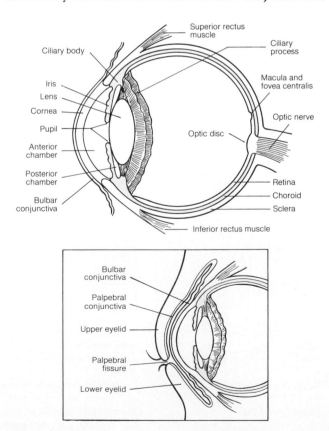

Figure 32–13 Anatomic structures of the right eye, lateral view

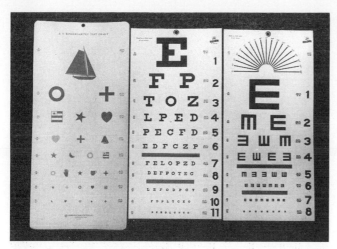

Figure 32–14 Three types of eye charts: the preschool children's chart (left), Snellen standard chart (center), and Snellen E chart (right)

dacryocystitis, hordeolum, iritis, and contusions or hematomas of the eyelids and surrounding structures. **Conjunctivitis** (inflammation of the bulbar and palpebral conjunctiva) may result from foreign bodies, chemicals, allergenic agents, bacteria, or viruses. Redness, itching, tearing, and mucopurulent discharge occur. After sleep, the eyelids may be encrusted and matted together. **Dacryocystitis** (inflammation of the lacrimal sac) is manifested by tearing and a discharge from the nasolacrimal duct. **Hordeolum** (sty) is a redness, swelling, and tenderness of the hair follicle and glands that empty at the edge of the eyelids. **Iritis** (inflammation of the iris) may be caused by local or systemic infections and results in pain, tearing, and **photophobia** (sensitivity to light). **Contusions** or **hematomas** are "black eyes" resulting from injury.

Cataracts tend to occur in those over 65 years old. This opacity of the lens or its capsule, which blocks light rays, is frequently corrected by surgery. Cataracts may also occur in infants due to a malformation of the lens if the mother contracted rubella in the first trimester of pregnancy. **Glaucoma** (a disturbance in the circulation of aqueous fluid, which causes an increase in intraocular pressure) is the most frequent cause of blindness in people over 40. It can be controlled if diagnosed early. Danger signs of glaucoma include blurred or foggy vision, loss of peripheral vision, difficulty focusing on close objects, difficulty adjusting to dark rooms, and seeing rainbow-colored rings around lights.

The **corneal light reflex test** may be performed to determine eye alignment. Darken the room and ask the client to stare straight ahead. Shine a penlight on the bridge of the client's nose and observe the light reflection in both corneas. Light reflection is normally situated in the same spot on both eyes.

Assess the **external eye structures** by having the client sit at eye level directly in front of you and inspect the **eyebrows** for hair distribution and alignment, skin quality, and movement. Ask the client to raise and lower the eyebrows. Note loss of hair, and scaling or flakiness of the skin. Inspect the **eyelashes** for evenness of dis-

tribution and direction of curl. Normally, eyelashes are equally distributed and curled slightly outward. Inward turning of the eyelashes occurs with inversion of the eyelid.

Inspect the **eyelids** for surface characteristics, (e.g., skin quality and texture), position, ability to close, ability to blink, and frequency of blinking. Eyelids that lie at or below the pupil margin are referred to as **ptosis** and are usually associated with aging, edema from drug allergy or systemic disease (e.g., kidney disease), congenital lid muscle dysfunction, neuromuscular disease (e.g., myasthenia gravis), and third cranial nerve impairment. Eversion, an outturning of the eyelid, is called **ectropion;** inversion, an inturning of the lid, is called **entropion.** These abnormalities are often associated with scarring injuries or the aging process.

The **conjunctiva** should be transparent, although capillaries are sometimes evident. The **sclera** should appear white or slightly yellow in blacks. Sclera that appear jaundiced, excessively pale, or reddened are not normal and may indicate biliary obstruction; anemia; or damage by mechanical, clinical, allergenic, or bacterial agents. Any lesions or nodules must also be reported.

ASSESSMENT

Pupils

1. Ask the client to look straight ahead.
2. Inspect the pupils for color, shape, and symmetry of size. Pupil charts are available in some agencies. See Figure 32–15 for variations in pupil diameters in millimeters.
3. Assess each pupil's direct and consensual reaction to light to determine the function of the second (oculomotor) and third (trochlear) cranial nerves.

   a. Partially darken the room.
   b. Ask the client to look straight ahead.
   c. Using a penlight and approaching from the side, shine a light on the pupil.
   d. Observe the response of the illuminated pupil. It should constrict (direct response).
   e. Again shine the light on the pupil, and observe the response of the other pupil. It should also constrict (consensual response).

4. Assess each pupil's reaction to accommodation.

   a. Hold an object (a penlight or pencil) about 10 cm (4 in) from the bridge of the client's nose.
   b. Ask the client to look first at the top of the object and then at a distant object (e.g., the far wall) behind the penlight. Alternate the gaze from the near to the far object.
   c. Observe the pupil response. The pupils should constrict when looking at the near object and dilate when looking at the far object.
   d. Next move the penlight or pencil toward the client's nose. The pupils should converge.

5. To record normal assessment of the pupils, use the abbreviation PERRLA (pupils equally round and react to light and accommodation).

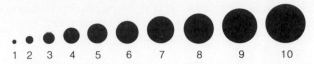

Figure 32–15 Variations in pupil diameters in millimeters

Normally, the **cornea** is transparent, shiny, and smooth. Details of the iris are visible. In older people, a thin, grayish-white ring around the margin, called **arcus senilis,** may be evident. Arcus senilis in clients under age 40 is abnormal. An opaque or uneven surface of the cornea may be the result of trauma or an abrasion.

Pupils are normally black, are equal in size (about 3 to 7 mm in diameter), and have round, smooth borders. Cloudy pupils are often indicative of cataracts. Enlarged pupils (**mydriasis**) may indicate injury, glaucoma, or be the result of certain drugs (e.g., atropine). Constricted pupils (**miosis**) may indicate an inflammation of the iris or be the result of such drugs as morphine or pilocarpine. Unequal pupils (**anisocoria**) may result from of a central nervous system disorder; however, slight variations may be normal. Steps in assessing the pupil are shown in the accompanying box. The iris is normally flat and round. A bulging toward the cornea can indicate increased intraocular pressure.

Ears and Hearing

Assessment of the ear includes direct inspection and palpation of the external ear, inspection of the remaining parts of the ear by an otoscope, and determination of auditory acuity. The ear is usually assessed during an initial physical examination; periodic reassessments may be necessary for long-term clients or those with hearing problems.

Nursing history data to be obtained during assessment of the ear are shown in the accompanying box.

Audiometric evaluations to assess hearing at various decibels levels are recommended for the elderly. A common hearing deficit in aging clients is inability to hear high-frequency sounds, such as *f, s, sh,* and *ph*. Because

NURSING HISTORY

Ears

Determine:

▪ Family history of hearing problems or loss

▪ Recent complaints of ear problems such as pain, itching, discharge, tinnitus (ringing in the ears)

▪ Any hearing difficulty, its onset, factors contributing to it, and its interference with activities of daily living

▪ Use of a corrective hearing device, duration of use, and supplier

▪ Medication history, especially if there are complaints of ringing in the ears

▪ Presence of high noise levels in the work environment

NURSING HISTORY

Nose and Sinuses

Determine:

▪ Whether the client has history of allergies, difficulty breathing through the nose, sinus infections, injuries to nose or face, or nosebleeds

▪ Whether the client takes any medications

▪ Whether the client has experienced any changes in sense of smell

of this hearing deficit, older people may sometimes display inappropriate or confused behaviors. This neurosensory hearing deficit is not alleviated by the use of a hearing aid.

Gross hearing acuity can be assessed by the client's response to voice tones, i.e., normal voice tones and whispered voice tones, and the ticking of a watch. First note generally how well the client hears your voice. If the client has difficulty, assess the client's response to the whispered voice. Requesting that the nurse repeat words or statements, leaning toward the speaker, turning the head, cupping the ears, and speaking in a loud or unvaried tone of voice all suggest hearing problems.

Tuning fork tests are used by advanced practitioners to assess whether the client's hearing loss is a conduction, sensorineural, or mixed problem. **Conduction hearing loss** is the result of interrupted transmission of sound waves through the outer and middle ear structures. Possible causes are a tear in the tympanic membrane or an obstruction, due to swelling or other causes, in the auditory canal. **Sensorineural hearing loss** is the result of damage to the inner ear, the auditory nerve, or the hearing center in the brain. **Mixed hearing loss** is a combination of conduction and sensorineural loss.

Nose and Sinuses

A nurse can inspect the nasal passages very simply with a flashlight. However, for a more thorough assessment, the advanced practitioner uses a **nasal speculum,** a lighted instrument that facilitates examination of the nasal chambers. The accompanying box lists data to obtain during the nursing history.

Normally, the nares are patent; the external nose is symmetrical, straight, and not tender; and there is no discharge. Air should move freely as the client breathes through his or her nares. The sinuses are normally nontender. Transillumination of the sinuses can reveal the presence of air or fluid. Since the sinuses contain air, they appear darker when fluid is present.

Mouth

Assessment of an individual's mouth includes examination of its physical characteristics, consideration of developmental changes, and determination of the per-

Table 32—4 Assessment Data: Mouth

Structure	Normal Findings	Abnormal Findings	Possible Health Problems
Lips	Uniform pink color (darker in Mediterranean groups and blacks, e.g., bluish hue) Soft, moist, smooth texture Symmetry of contour Ability to purse lips	Pallor Bluish discoloration Blisters Generalized swelling Localized swelling Fissures, crusts, scales Inability to purse lips	Anemia Cyanosis Herpes simplex Allergic reaction Trauma Excessive moisture; nutritional deficiency; fluid deficit Facial nerve damage
Inner lips and buccal mucosa	Uniform pink color (brown freckled pigmentation in blacks) Moist, smooth, soft and elastic texture (drier oral mucosa in elderly due to decreased salivation)	Pallor White patches (leukoplakia) Excessive dryness Mucosal cysts Irritations Abrasions Ulcerations, nodules	Anemia Early oral cancer; heavy smoking and drinking Dehydration Glandular irritation Infections; ill-fitting dentures Trauma Possible carcinoma
Teeth	32 adult teeth Smooth, white tooth enamel	Missing teeth, bridges, full or partial dentures Dental caries Discoloration of enamel	Trauma; dental disease Poor oral hygiene Excessive use of tobacco; certain medications (e.g., iron)
Gums	Pink color (bluish or dark patches in blacks) Moist, firm texture No retraction (pulling away from the teeth)	Excessive redness Spongy texture, bleeding, tenderness Receding atrophied gums Swelling that partially covers the teeth	Ill-fitting dentures; periodontal disease Periodontal disease Normal aging process Dilantin therapy; leukemia
Tongue	Central position Pink color (some brown pigmentation on tongue borders in blacks), moist, slightly rough, thin whitish coating Moves freely Smooth tongue base with prominent veins	Deviated from center Dry, furry Smooth and red Nodes, ulcerations, discolorations, restricted mobility Varicosities (tiny bluish-black or purple swollen areas)	Damage to hypoglossal (12th cranial) nerve Fluid deficit Iron, vitamin B_{12}, or vitamin B_3 deficiency Possible carcinoma Normal aging process
Palates	Light pink, smooth, soft palate Lighter pink hard palate, more irregular texture	Discolorations Palates the same color Irritations	Jaundice Anemia Ill-fitting dentures
Uvula	Positioned in midline of soft palate	Deviation to one side Immobility	Tumor; trauma Damage to trigeminal (fifth cranial) nerve or vagus (tenth cranial) nerve
Oropharynx and tonsils	Pink and smooth posterior wall Tonsils pink and normal size	Reddened, lesions, plaques Tonsillar crypts inflamed, filled with exudate, swollen	Pharyngitis Tonsillitis

son's hygienic practices. Oral assessment should be carried out as part of the client's initial assessment. Periodic reassessments need to be made for long-term-care clients. Physical examination of the mouth includes inspection and palpation techniques. The status of the lips, mucous membranes, teeth, gingiva (gums), tongue, palates, and uvula (see Figure 32–16) is assessed. See the accompanying box for data to be obtained during nursing history. Table 32–4 summarizes significant assessment findings.

▪ Thorax, Lungs, and Breasts

Assessing the thorax and lungs is essential when analyzing the client's aeration status. Changes in the respiratory system can come about slowly or quickly. In clients with chronic obstructive pulmonary disease (COPD), changes are frequently gradual; however, in clients who are acutely ill, e.g., those who have a pneumothorax (accumulation of gas or fluid in the pleural cavity), changes occur quickly, and death can result if

NURSING HISTORY

Mouth

Determine:

- Routine pattern of dental care
- The date of the last visit to the dentist
- Length of time ulcers or other lesions have been present
- The presence of dentures and any associated discomfort
- Any medications the client is receiving

immediate action is not taken. For information about the mechanics of breathing see Chapter 42.

To assess a client's **thorax,** the nurse uses the examination techniques of inspection and palpation. Before beginning the assessment, the nurse should identify a number of imaginary lines on the client's chest. These lines help the nurse to locate underlying organs and to record assessment findings. See Figures 32–17, 32–18, and 32–19 for these chest landmarks. The **midsternal line** is a vertical line running through the center of the sternum. The **midclavicular lines** (right or left) are vertical lines from the midpoints of the clavicles. The **anterior axillary lines** (right or left) are vertical lines from the anterior axillary folds. Figure 32–18 shows the three imaginary lines of the lateral chest. The **posterior axillary line** is a vertical line from the posterior axillary fold. The **midaxillary line** is a vertical line from the apex of the axilla. The anterior axillary line is described above. Figure 32–19 shows the posterior chest landmarks. The **vertebral line** is a vertical line along the spinous processes. The **scapular lines** (right or left) are vertical lines from the inferior angles of the scapulae.

The client's **posture** is important to note. Some people with chronic respiratory problems tend to bend

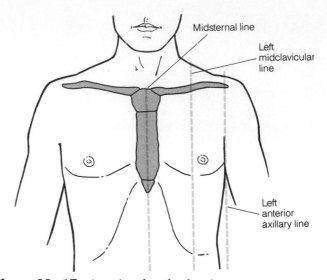

Figure 32–17 Anterior chest landmarks

forward or even prop their arms on a support to elevate their clavicles. This posture is an attempt to expand the chest fully and thus breathe with less effort. In the **infant,** the thorax is rounded; that is, the diameter from the front to the back (**anteroposterior diameter**) is equal to the **transverse diameter.** It is also cylindrical, having a nearly equal diameter at the top and the base. When a **child** reaches 6 years, the anteroposterior diameter has decreased in proportion to the transverse one. In **adults,** the thorax is oval. Its anteroposterior diameter is two times smaller than its transverse diameter. See Figure 32–20. The overall shape of the thorax is elliptical; i.e., its diameter is smaller at the top than at the base. In the **elderly,** kyphosis and osteoporosis alter the size of the chest cavity as the ribs move downward and forward.

The **shape** of the chest is assessed from the front, sides, and back. There are several deformities of the chest. See Figure 32–21. **Pigeon chest** (pectus cari-

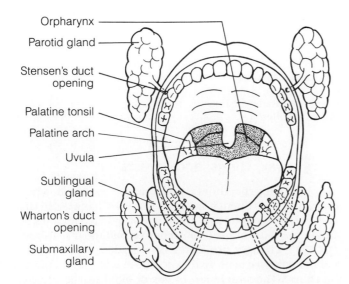

Figure 32–16 Anatomic structures of the mouth

Orpharynx
Parotid gland
Stensen's duct opening
Palatine tonsil
Palatine arch
Uvula
Sublingual gland
Wharton's duct opening
Submaxillary gland

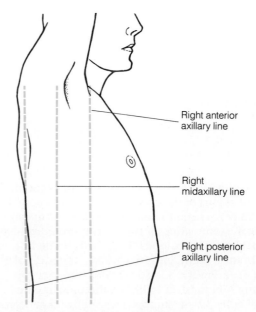

Right anterior axillary line

Right midaxillary line

Right posterior axillary line

Figure 32–18 Lateral chest landmarks

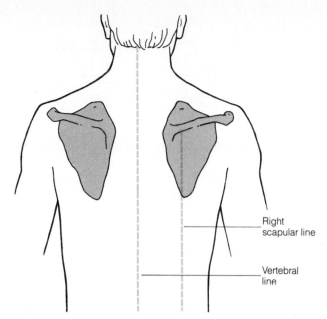

Figure 32–19 Posterior chest landmarks

A. Normal infant

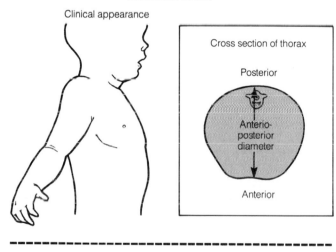

B. Normal adult

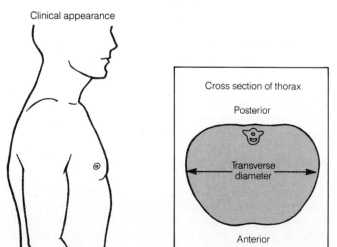

Figure 32–20 Configurations of the thorax showing anteroposterior and transverse diameters: **A,** infant; **B,** adult

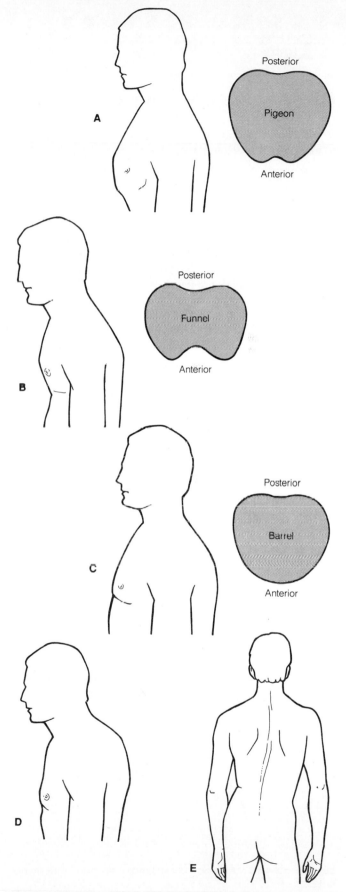

Figure 32–21 Chest shapes: **A,** pigeon chest; **B,** funnel chest; **C,** barrel chest; **D,** kyphosis; **E,** scoliosis

NURSING HISTORY

Lungs

Determine:

- Family history of illness, including cancer, allergies, tuberculosis
- Life-style, including smoking and occupational hazards, e.g., inhaling fumes
- Any medications the client is currently taking
- Current problems, e.g., swelling, cough, wheezing, pain

natum), a permanent deformity, may be caused by rickets. Pigeon chest is characterized by a narrow transverse diameter, an increased anteroposterior diameter, and a protruding sternum. A **funnel chest** (pectus excavatum), a congenital defect, is the opposite of pigeon chest in that the sternum is depressed, narrowing the anteroposterior diameter. Because the sternum points posteriorly in clients with a funnel chest, abnormal pressure on the heart may result in altered function. A **barrel chest,** in which the ratio of the anteroposterior to lateral diameter is 1 to 1, is seen in clients with thoracic **kyphosis** (excessive convex curvature of the thoracic spine) and **emphysema** (chronic pulmonary condition in which the air sacs, or alveoli, are dilated and distended).

The nurse notes spinal deformities, such as kyphosis or **scoliosis** (lateral deviation of the spine), during examination of the thorax. In addition, the nurse looks for changes in the exterior chest wall, such as bulges caused by cardiac enlargement or neoplasms. Depressions in the chest may be the result of the surgical removal of some ribs. The chest muscles should also be palpated to detect tenderness and the presence of masses.

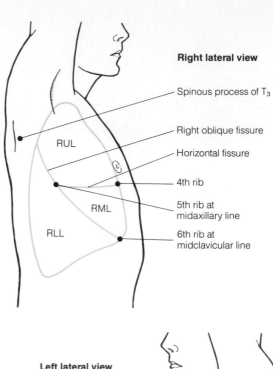

Right lateral view

- Spinous process of T₃
- Right oblique fissure
- Horizontal fissure
- 4th rib
- 5th rib at midaxillary line
- 6th rib at midclavicular line

RUL
RML
RLL

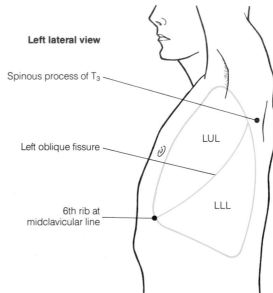

Left lateral view

- Spinous process of T₃
- Left oblique fissure
- 6th rib at midclavicular line

LUL
LLL

Figure 32–23 Lateral chest landmarks and underlying lungs

During a **lung examination,** the client needs to assume a sitting position. See the accompanying box for data to be obtained during a nursing history. First the nurse should identify the landmarks on the chest under which the various lobes of the lung lie. Figure 32–22 is an anterior view of the chest and underlying lungs. Each lung is first divided into the upper and lower lobes by an oblique fissure that runs from the level of the spinous process of the third thoracic vertebra to the level of the sixth rib at the midclavicular line. The right lung is further divided by a minor fissure into the right upper lobe (RUL) and right middle lobe (RML). This fissure runs anteriorly from the right midaxillary line at the level of the fifth rib to the level of the fourth rib. The lateral views show the three lobes of the right lung and the two lobes of the left lung. See Figure 32–23. The pos-

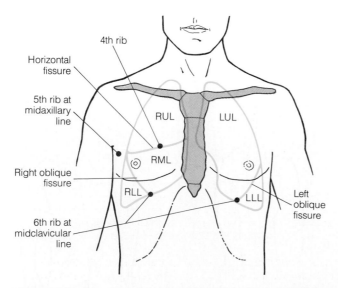

- 4th rib
- Horizontal fissure
- 5th rib at midaxillary line
- Right oblique fissure
- 6th rib at midclavicular line
- RUL
- LUL
- RML
- RLL
- LLL
- Left oblique fissure

Figure 32–22 Anterior chest landmarks and underlying lungs

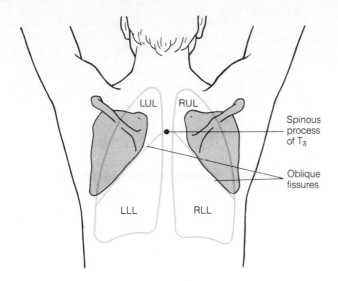

terior view shows the upper and lower lobes of each lung. See Figure 32–24. These abbreviations are commonly used by nurses conducting lung assessments:

- T₃   Third thoracic vertebra
- RUL   Right upper lobe
- RML   Right middle lobe
- RLL   Right lower lobe
- LUL   Left upper lobe
- LLL   Left lower lobe

Procedure 32–1 provides guidelines for assessing clients' lungs.

Figure 32–24   Posterior chest landmarks and underlying lungs

PROCEDURE 32–1

Assessing the Lungs

Equipment

1. A stethoscope
2. A plumb line (a line or string with a weight at one end)
3. A marking pencil

Intervention

See Table 32–5 for normal and abnormal findings.

1. Assess the rate, depth, and type of respirations. See Chapter 31, page 435.

Palpation

2. Palpate the posterior chest for respiratory excursion (expansion). Place the palms of both hands over the lower thorax with the thumbs adjacent to the spine and the fingers stretched laterally. See Figure 32–25. Ask the client to take a deep breath while you observe the movement of your hands and any lag in movement.
   Rationale: When the client takes a deep breath, the nurse's thumbs should move apart an equal distance and at the same time, reflecting chest expansion.

3. Palpate the anterior chest as in step 2, placing the palms of both hands on the lower thorax with the fingers laterally along the lower rib cage and the thumbs along the costal margins.

4. Palpate the lungs for vocal (tactile) **fremitus,** the vibration felt through the chest wall when the client speaks.
   a. Place the palms of your hands on the posterior chest near the apex of the lungs, position *A* in Figure 32–26.
   b. Ask the client to repeat words such as "blue moon" or "one, two, three."

c. Repeat steps a and b with the hands moving sequentially to the base of the lungs, through positions *B–E* in Figure 32–26.
d. Compare the fremitus on both lungs and between the apex and the base of each lung. Increased fremitus occurs with consolidated lung tissue as in pneumonia, and decreased or absent fremitus occurs in pneumothorax.

5. Repeat steps 4a–d for the anterior chest. See Figure 32–27, positions *A–E.*
   Rationale: The vibrations from speaking are normally transmitted through the chest wall. They are felt most clearly at the apex of the lungs. Low-pitched voices of males are more readily palpated than the higher pitches of females.

Table 32–5   Assessment Data: Lungs

Normal Findings	Abnormal Findings
Respiratory rate 16–20/min and regular (adult)	Increased or decreased rate Irregular pattern Retraction or bulding of intercostal muscles
Respiratory excursion is full and symmetrical	Impairment in movement
Vocal fremitus is symmetric bilaterally	Decreased or increased fremitus
Percussion notes resonant except over liver, heart, sternum, scapula, and stomach	Asymmetry in percussion Areas of dullness Areas of hyperresonance
Auscultated vesicular breath sounds (see Table 32–7)	Auscultated adventitious breath sounds (see Table 32–8)

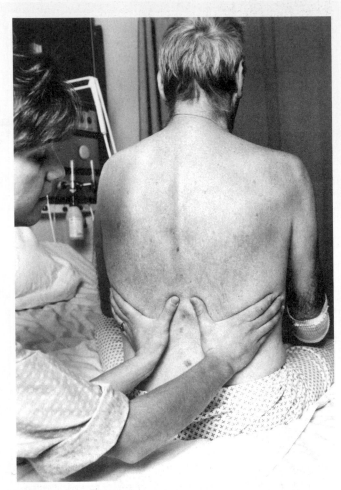

Figure 32—25

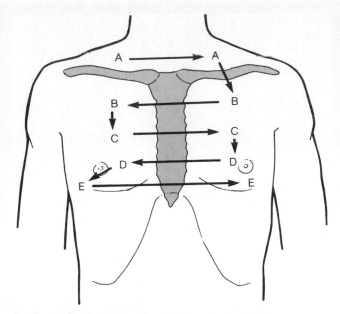

Figure 32—27

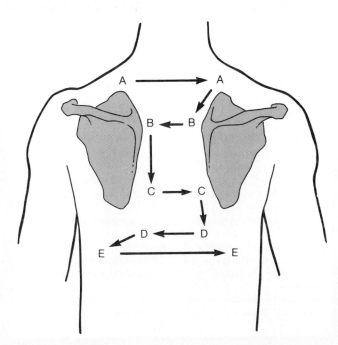

Figure 32—26

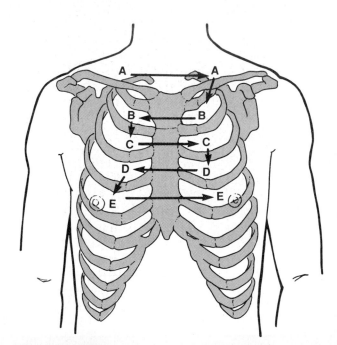

Figure 32—28

Percussion

6. Percuss the anterior surface of the chest. See the description of percussion in Chapter 8.

a. Percuss in the intercostal spaces in a systematic sequence, beginning above the clavicles in the supraclavicular space, and proceeding downward to the diaphragm. See Figure 32—28.

Rationale: Percussion on a rib normally elicits dullness. The lowest point where resonance can normally be detected is at the diaphragm, i.e., at the level of the eighth to tenth rib.

b. Compare one side of the chest with the other.

Table 32—6   Percussion Sounds

Sound	Intensity	Pitch	Duration	Quality	Example of Location
Flatness	Soft	High	Short	Extremely dull	Muscle, bone
Dullness	Medium	Medium	Moderate	Thudlike	Liver, heart
Resonance	Loud	Low	Long	Hollow	Lung
Hyperresonance	Very loud	Very low	Very long	Booming	Emphysematous lung
Tympany	Loud	High (distinguished mainly by musical timbre)	Moderate	Musical	Stomach filled with gas (air)

For each percussion, note the intensity, pitch, and duration. See Table 32–6.

7. Percuss the lateral chest wall, starting at the axilla and working down to the tenth rib. Percuss every few inches. Repeat for the other side.

8. Percuss the posterior chest wall while the client leans forward, neck flexed. Start at the apex of each lung and proceed downward to the diaphragm. See Figure 32–29.
   Rationale: Percussion sounds are loudest where the chest wall is thinnest. For normal percussion sounds, see Figure 32–30.

9. Determine the excursion (movement) of the diaphragm.
   a. Ask the client to take a deep breath and hold it.
   Rationale: On inspiration, the diaphragm normally moves downward.
   b. Percuss downward on one side of the posterior chest until dullness is produced.
   Rationale: The dullness indicates the level of the diaphragm.
   c. With a marking pencil place a mark on the skin at the level of dullness.
   d. Ask the client to expel the breath completely and hold it.

Rationale: Upon expiration, the diaphragm normally moves upward.
e. Percuss as in step b for the level of dullness
Rationale: The level normally is above the inspiratory level, because the lungs have deflated.
f. Mark the level of dullness on the skin.

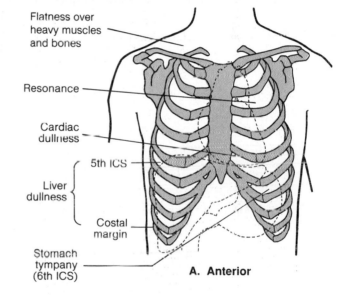

A. Anterior

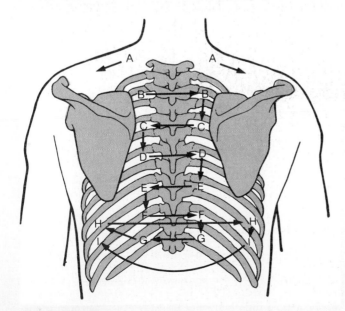

Figure 32—29

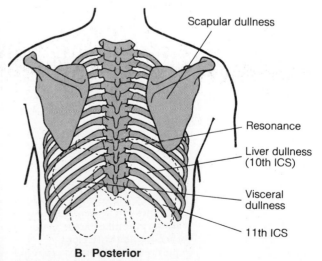

B. Posterior

Figure 32—30   Normal percussion sounds: **A,** anterior; **B,** posterior

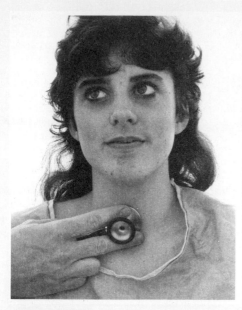

Figure 32–31

g. Measure the distance between the two marks.
Rationale: Normal excursion is 3 to 5 cm (1 to 2 in) in females and 5 to 6 cm (2 to 2.3 in) in males.
h. Repeat steps a–g on the other side of the posterior chest.

Auscultation

10. To auscultate the lungs, use the flat-disc diaphragm of the stethoscope.
Rationale: The flat diaphragm best transmits high-pitched sounds, e.g., breath sounds.
a. Facing the client, place the diaphragm firmly against the skin starting over the trachea. See Figure 32–31.
b. Ask the client to breathe normally.
c. Proceed in the sequence shown in Figure 32–28, earlier, first auscultating over the bronchi between the sternum and the clavicles, then following the same sequence as for percussion.
d. Listen for normal and adventitious breath sounds at each point on the chest. See Tables 32–7 and 32–8.
Rationale: Breath sounds occur as a result of the movement of the air through the trachea, bronchi, and alveoli.
e. Repeat for the lateral chest and the posterior chest. Follow the percussion sequence described in steps 7–8 and shown in Figure 32–29.

11. When abnormal breath or percussion sounds—bronchophony, whispered pectoriloquy (exaggerated bronchophony), and egophony—are discovered, carry out further investigation.
Rationale: Fluid or consolidated tissue transmits vibrations of the spoken or whispered voice through the chest wall.
a. Bronchophony and whispered pectoriloquy. Using a stethoscope, listen to the chest, using the sequence described for assessing vocal fremitus. See Figures 32–26 and 32–27, earlier. Have the client softly repeat "one, two, three."
Rationale: With tissue consolidation, the words may be clearly heard in the periphery of the lung.
b. Egophony. Listen to the chest while the client repeats the sound of a long *e,* as in "she."
Rationale: Fluid in the lungs alters the sound from an *e* to an *ay,* as in "say," when heard through the stethoscope.

Table 32–7   Normal Breath Sounds

Type	Description	Location	Characteristics
Vesicular	Soft, low-pitched, "gentle sighing"	Over bronchioles and alveoli; best heard at base of lungs	Best heard on inspiration
Bronchial (tracheal)	Moderately high-pitched, "harsh"	Over trachea; not normally heard over lung tissue	Louder than vesicular sounds; long inspiratory phase and short expiratory phase
Bronchovesicular	Moderate intensity	Over bronchioles lateral to the sternum at the first and second intercostal spaces and between the scapulae	Equal inspiratory and expiratory phases

---

Table 32–8   Adventitious Breath Sounds

Name	Description	Characteristics
Rales	Fine crackling sounds; alveolar rales are high-pitched; bronchial rales are lower-pitched	Best heard on inspiration
Rhonchi	Coarse, gurgling, harsh, louder sounds as air passes through bronchi filled with fluid	Best heard on expiration
Wheeze	Squeaky musical sounds often indicative of bronchial constriction	Best heard on expiration
Friction (pleural rub)	Rubbing of the pulmonary and visceral pleura; grating sound	Best heard over the lower anterior and lateral chest

▪ Breasts

The breasts of men, women, and children should be examined. Men and children have some glandular tissue beneath each nipple, while mature women have glandular tissue throughout the breast. Each breast is observed for size, shape, and position, and then the two breasts are compared according to these criteria. Size varies according to age, heredity, endocrine functions, and amount of adipose tissue. See the accompanying box for data to be obtained during a nursing history.

Breasts must also be palpated for masses. Women today are encouraged to palpate their own breasts regularly. During a breast examination, the nipples are observed for discharge, crusting, edema, retraction, and disease. Although retraction is not necessarily indicative of any disease process, it needs to be noted.

The axillae are usually examined for enlarged lymph nodes, infections, and bulges. To palpate the axillae, the nurse helps the client relax the arm, perhaps by resting it on a table. The nurse presses the fingers as far up toward the apex of the axilla as possible and brings them downward, pressing against the chest wall. Nodes in the central area of the axilla and toward the thorax may be palpated in this manner. The central nodes are the most readily palpable. If the thoracic nodes are palpable and/or either group of nodes feels enlarged, this finding is reported. The procedure is then repeated on the other axilla. Procedure 32–2 provides guidelines for breast assessment.

PROCEDURE 32–2

Assessing the Breasts

Intervention

See Table 32–9 for normal and abnormal findings and possible health problems.

1. Ask the client to assume a sitting position, and assess the breasts.
   a. Inspect the size, shape, and symmetry of the breasts. Breasts are normally round and fairly symmetric, and may be described as small, medium, or large.
   b. Inspect the skin for lesions, increased vascular patterns, edema, and "pig skin" or a pitted appearance. *Rationale:* Pitting of the skin can be the result of lymphatic edema.
   c. Inspect the color of the areolae. They are normally darker in brunettes and pregnant women than in fair-haired women.
   d. Inspect the breasts and nipples for any dimpling or retraction, which can be the result of scar tissue formation or can be caused by the presence of a lesion. See Figure 32–32. In front of a mirror, show the client how to accentuate any retraction by raising her arms above her head, pushing her hands together with elbows flexed (see Figure 32–33), or pressing her hands down on her hips (see Figure 32–34).
   e. Inspect the nipples for any discharge, ulceration, inversion, crusting, or scaling. Note the position of the nipples. Both nipples normally point in the same direction.
2. Inspect the axilla and clavicular areas for any swelling or redness.
3. Palpate around the nipple to check for discharge. If discharge is present, strip the breast by compressing the breast tissue between the thumb and index finger while moving the fingers toward the nipple. Strip one lobe at a time to identify the source of the discharge.
   a. Observe any discharge for amount, color, consistency, and odor.
   b. Note any tenderness upon palpation.
4. Palpate the clavicular and axillary regions while the client is sitting, arms at her sides.

Table 32–9 Assessment Data: Breasts

Normal Findings	Abnormal Findings	Possible Health Problems
Rounded shape; small, medium, or large size	Change in breast size; swellings	Inflammation
Symmetric	Marked asymmetry	
Skin smooth, intact	Dimpling, redness, vascularities, edema	
	Retraction	Scarring, carcinoma
Nipples everted, no discharge or lesions	Nipples inverted, crusting, ulcers, cracks, discharge	Inflammation; abscess; malignancy
No swelling in axillae	Swelling, tenderness in axillae	Malignancy
		Tumor, abscess
No tenderness, masses, or nodules on palpation	Tenderness, masses, or nodules (note location, client's position, size, mobility, consistency, surface, tenderness, and shape)	

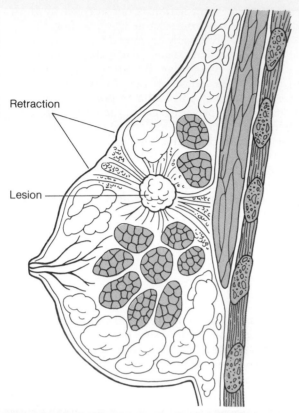

Figure 32–32 Breast tissue and a lesion that causes retraction of the skin

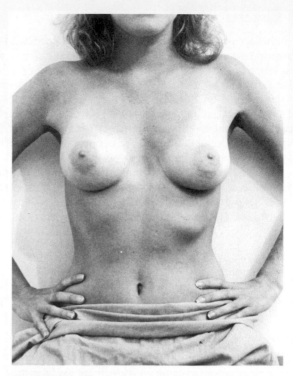

Figure 32–34

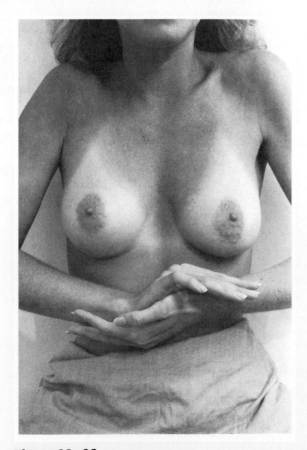

Figure 32–33

Rationale: These areas contain lymph nodes that drain the breasts. See Figure 32–35.

5. Lightly palpate each breast. A bimanual technique is often preferred, particularly for large breasts. The nondominant hand is placed under the breast, and the dominant hand palpates the breast.
   Rationale: A bimanual technique can be most effective in detecting small deep masses.
   a. Press the palmar surfaces of the middle three fingers on the skin surface starting in the upper lateral quadrant.
   b. Use a gentle rotary motion pressing the breast tissue against the other hand (bimanual) or against the chest wall.
   c. Palpate from the periphery to the areola.
   d. Move your peripheral starting point around the breast clockwise. See Figure 32–36.

6. Record the following data about any masses:
   a. *Location:* the exact location relative to the clock (as in Figure 32–36) and the distance from the nipple in centimeters.
   b. *Client's position:* whether the arms were raised or lowered, the client was sitting or supine.
   Rationale: The position can change the perceived location of the mass.
   c. *Size:* the length, width, and thickness of the mass in centimeters. If you are unable to determine the discrete edges, record this fact.
   d. *Mobility:* whether the mass is movable or fixed. If it is fixed, determine whether it is firmly or moderately fixed, if possible.
   e. *Consistency:* whether the mass is hard or soft.
   f. *Surface:* whether the surface is smooth or irregular.

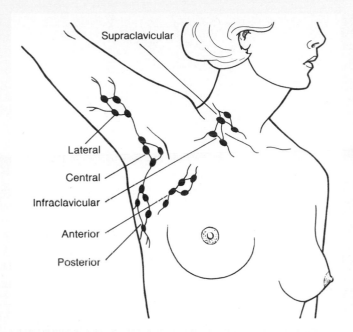

Figure 32–35

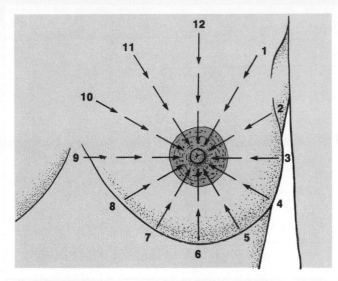

Figure 32–36

g. *Tenderness:* whether the palpation is painful to the client.

h. *Shape:* whether the mass is round, discoid, regular, or irregular.

NURSING HISTORY

Breasts

Determine:

▪ In both males and females, past history of breast masses, nipple discharge, areolar rash, breast pain, and tenderness.

▪ Relation of pain or tenderness, if experienced, to the menstrual cycle.

▪ Family history of breast cancer, particularly of the client's mother, sister, aunt, or grandmother before menopause.

▪ Age at menarche, at menopause, and at time of first pregnancy; there is a higher incidence of breast cancer among women who had an early menarche (before age 13), who had a late menopause (after age 50), and who had the first child after age 35.

▪ Racial background. Incidence of breast cancer is higher among white women than among Japanese or Chinese women.

▪ Frequency of breast self-examination, technique used,

7. Repeat steps 5–6 for the other breast.

8. Assist the client to a supine position, with a small pillow or towel under the shoulder of the side to be palpated. Repeat steps 5–6 for each breast. *Rationale:* Slightly raising the shoulder helps spread the breast tissue over the chest wall, facilitating palpation.

and time performed in relation to the menstrual cycle (see breast self-examination in Chapter 25).

▪ Normal breast changes for young adolescent females (see Chapter 24).

▪ Breast enlargement in young adolescent males; 50% of young adolescent males have enlargement of one or both breasts due to the hormonal changes of puberty. It is usually resolved in 1 or 2 years but is abnormal in adult males.

▪ Breast changes in pregnant women. Normal changes include tingling or tenderness, enlargement, prominent veins, and erect nipples. In later pregnancy, the aerolae darken and a thick yellowish fluid can be extracted from the nipples.

▪ Normal decreasing breast size and firmness in menopausal women.

▪ Currently prescribed medications. Oral contraceptions, digitalis, diuretics, and steroids can alter hormone balance and cause nipple discharge. Estrogens may cause cystic breast changes.

Heart

Heart function can be assessed to a large degree by findings in the history, by symptoms such as shortness of breath, by the client's general appearance (e.g., cyanosis and edema of the legs suggest impaired function), and by pulse rate, rhythm, and quality. Direct examination of the heart, however, offers more specific information, including the heart sounds, the heart size, and findings such as lifts, heaves, or murmurs.

Nurses assess heart functions through observations (inspection), palpation, and auscultation, in that sequence.

NURSING HISTORY

Heart

Determine:

- Family history (include age of onset) of heart disease, high cholesterol levels, high blood pressure, stroke, obesity, congenital heart disease, and rheumatic fever
- Client's past history of heart problems, e.g., rheumatic fever, heart murmur, heart attack, or heart failure
- Life-style habits (e.g., smoking, alcohol intake, eating habits, exercise patterns, and areas and degree of stress perceived) that place the client at risk of cardiac disease
- Present symptoms (e.g., fatigue, dyspnea, orthopnea, edema, cough, chest pain, palpitations, syncope, hypertension, or wheezing) indicative of heart disease
- Presence of diseases (e.g., obesity, diabetes, lung disease, endocrine disorders) that affect the heart

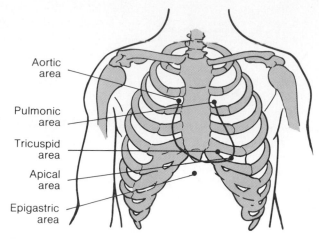

Figure 32–37 Anatomic sites of the precordium

Auscultation is more meaningful when other data are obtained first. The heart is usually assessed during an initial physical examination; periodic reassessments may be necessary for long-term or at-risk clients or those with cardiac problems. Nursing history data taken in conjunction with physical assessment are shown in the accompanying box.

To perform **cardiac assessment,** the nurse must first determine the exact location of the client's heart. In the average adult, most of the heart lies behind and to the left of the sternum. A small portion (the right atrium) extends to the right of the sternum. The upper portion of the heart (both atria), referred to as its **base,** lies toward the back. The lower portion (the ventricles), referred to as its **apex,** points forward. The apex of the left ventricle actually touches the anterior chest wall at or medial to the left midclavicular line (MCL) and at or near the fifth left intercostal space (LICS), which is slightly below the left nipple. See Figure 31–12 on page xxx. This point where the apex touches the anterior chest wall is known as the **point of maximal impulse** (PMI).

The **precordium,** the area of the chest overlying the heart, is inspected and palpated simultaneously for the presence of abnormal pulsations or lifts or heaves. The terms *lift* and *heave,* often used interchangeably, refer to a rising along the sternal border with each heartbeat. A lift occurs when cardiac action is very forceful (overactive). It should be confirmed by palpation with the palm of the hand. Enlargement or overactivity of the left ventricle produces a heave lateral to the apex, while enlargement of the right ventricle produces a heave at or near the sternum. The precordium is inspected in a systematic manner at the following anatomic sites: **aortic** area, **pulmonic** area, **tricuspid** (or right ventricular) area, **apical** (or mitral) area, and **epigastric** area. See Figure 32–37. All pulsations are described by their location in an intercostal space and their distance from the midsternal, midclavicular, or axillary line.

An apical impulse can be seen in about 50% of the adult population and is palpable in most people. The apical impulse is a good index of cardiac size. If the heart is enlarged, this impulse is lateral to the MCL and may be lower. Record the distance between the apex and the MCL in centimeters. If the apical beat cannot be observed, the apex may be located by palpation, but not always. If you have difficulty locating the PMI, have the client roll onto the left side, thus moving the apex closer to the chest wall. Normally, no lifts or heaves are visible or palpable in this area. Diffuse lifts or heaves lateral to the apex indicate enlargement or overactivity of the left ventricle. Abdominal aortic pulsations are normally felt in the epigastric area; however, bounding pulsations are abnormal.

Several heart sounds can be heard by **auscultation.** Only the first and second heart sounds (S_1 and S_2) will be emphasized in this book. The normal first two heart sounds are produced by closure of the valves of the heart. The **first heart sound (S_1)** occurs when the atrioventricular (A-V) valves close. These valves close when the ventricles have been sufficiently filled. Although the right and left A-V valves do not close simultaneously, the closures occur closely enough to be heard as one sound (S_1), a dull, low-pitched sound described as "**lub.**" After the ventricles empty their blood into the aorta and pulmonary arteries, the semilunar valves close, producing the **second heart sound (S_2),** described as "**dub.**" S_2 has a higher pitch than S_1 and is also shorter. These two sounds, S_1 and S_2 ("**lub-dub**"), occur within 1 second or less, depending on the heart rate.

Auscultation is performed systematically, starting at the aortic area, then moving to the pulmonic, the tricuspid, and the apical. See Figure 32–37, earlier. Auscultation need not be limited to these areas, however. First locate these areas, and then move the stethoscope to find the most audible sounds for each particular client. The two heart sounds are audible anywhere on the precordial area, but they are best heard over these areas. Each area is associated with the closure of heart valves: the **aortic** area with the aortic valve (inside the aorta as it arises from the left ventricle); the **pulmonic** area with the pulmonic valve (inside the pulmonary artery as it arises from the right ventricle); the **tricuspid** area with the tricuspid valve (between the right atrium and ventricle); and the **apical (mitral)** area with the mitral valve (between the left atrium and ventricle).

Associated with these sounds are systole and diastole. **Systole** is the period in which the ventricles are contracted. It begins with the first heart sound and ends at the second heart sound. Systole is usually shorter than diastole. **Diastole** is the period in which the ventricles are relaxed. It starts with the second sound and ends at the subsequent first sound. Normally no sounds are audible during these periods. See Figure 32–38. The experienced nurse, however, may perceive extra heart sounds (S_3 and S_4) during diastole. Both sounds are low in pitch and heard best at the apical site, with the bell of the stethoscope, and with the client lying on the left side. S_3 occurs early in diastole right after S_2 and sounds like "**lub-dub-*ee***" (S_1, S_2, S_3) or "**Ken-tuc-*ky*.**" It often disappears when the client sits up. S_3 is normal in children and young adults. In older adults it may indicate heart failure. S_4 is rarely heard in normal clients. It occurs near the very end of diastole just before S_1 and creates the sound of "***dee*-lub-dub**" (S_4, S_1, S_2) or "***Ten*-nes-see.**" S_4 may be heard in many elderly clients and can

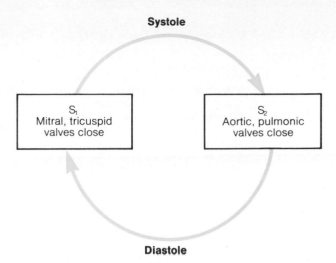

Figure 32–38 Relationship of heart sounds to systole and diastole

be a sign of hypertension. Normal heart sounds are summarized in Table 32–10. See Procedure 32–3 for the steps of heart auscultation.

PROCEDURE 32–3

Auscultating the Heart

Equipment

A stethoscope with a bell-shaped and flat-disc diaphragm. The bell transmits lower-pitched sounds best, while the flat disc transmits higher-pitched sounds best.

Intervention

1. Eliminate all sources of room noise.
   Rationale: Heart sounds are of low intensity, and other noise lowers the nurse's ability to hear them.
2. Assist the client to a supine position with head elevated 30° to 45°, and stand at the client's right side. Later reexamine the heart while the client is in the upright sitting position.
   Rationale: Certain sounds are more audible in certain positions.
3. Auscultate the heart in the following manner using both the flat-disc diaphragm and the bell to listen to all areas. See Table 32–10 for descriptions of normal heart sounds. See Table 32–11 for normal and abnormal findings. In every area of auscultation, both S_1 and S_2 need to be distinguished. When auscultating, concentrate on one particular sound at a time in each area; the first heart sound, followed by sys-

Table 32–10 Assessment Data: Normal Heart Sounds

Sound or Phase	Description	Area			
		Aortic	Pulmonic	Tricuspid	Apical
S_1	Dull, low-pitched, and longer than S_2; sounds like "lub"	Less intensity than S_2	Less intensity than S_2	Louder than or equal to S_2	Louder than or equal to S_2
S_2	High-pitched, snappy, and shorter than S_1; creates sound of "dub"	Louder than S_1	Louder than S_1; abnormal if louder than the aortic S_2 in adults over 40	Less intensity than or equal to S_1	Less intensity than or equal to S_1
Systole	Normally silent interval between S_1 and S_2				
Diastole	Normally silent interval between S_2 and next S_1				

Table 32–11 Assessment Data: Heart Auscultation

Auscultation Sound	Normal Findings	Abnormal Findings	Possible Health Problem
S₁	Usually heard at all sites	Increaed or decreased intensity	
	Usually louder at apical area	Varying intensity with different beats	Complete heart block
S₂	Usually heard at all sites	Increased intensity at aortic area	Arterial hypertension
	Usually louder at base of heart	Increased intensity at pulmonic area	Pulmonary hypertension
Systole	Silent interval	Sharp-sounding ejection clicks	Valvular deformities
	Slightly shorter duration than diastole at normal heart rate (60 to 90 beats/min)		
Diastole	Silent interval	S₃ in older adults	Heart failure
	Slightly longer duration than systole at normal heart rates		
	S₃ in children and young adults		
	S₄ in older adults		

tole, then the second heart sound, then diastole. Systole and diastole are normally silent intervals.

a. Locate and auscultate the aortic area (see Figure 32–37), using the flat diaphragm and bell attachment of the stethoscope. Listen for both sounds and for systole and diastole. S₂ is loudest in this area, louder than S₁.
Rationale: The higher-pitched sounds of S₁ and S₂ are transmitted better through the flat diaphragm of the stethoscope. The lower-pitched sounds of S₃ and S₄ are best transmitted through the bell of the stethoscope.

b. Locate and auscultate the pulmonic area as in step a. S₂ is normally louder than S₁ in this area.

c. Compare the loudness of S₂ between the aortic and pulmonic areas.
Rationale: The loudness of S₂ in the pulmonic area relates to the blood pressure in the pulmonary artery, while the loudness of S₂ in the aortic area relates to the arterial blood pressure in the systemic circulation. Thus, when the pulmonary artery pressure increases, e.g., in clients with some chronic obstructive lung diseases, the loudness of pulmonic S₂ also increases. In contrast, the aortic S₂ is louder than normal in clients with hypertensive disease. When the pulmonic S₂ is louder than the aortic S₂ in adults over age 40, the finding is abnormal.

d. Locate and auscultate the tricuspid area as in step a. S₂ is normally louder than or equal to S₁ in this area.

e. Locate and auscultate the apical (mitral) area as in step a. S₂ is normally louder than or equal to S₁ in this area.

f. Assess the heart rate and rhythm at the apical area as described in Chapter 31 on page 431. Note irregularities in rhythm, and note murmurs. **Murmurs** result when blood flow becomes turbulent within the heart due to valve defects or abnormal openings between the compartments of the heart. Not all murmurs indicate cardiac disease. Murmurs are described in terms of their location of maximum intensity, quality (e.g., loud, harsh, rumbling), and timing in relation to the phases of the cardiac cycle. Diastolic murmurs are usually considered abnormal. Murmurs relating to the valves are usually heard over the valvular areas. To increase your ability to hear an S₃ sound or a mitral murmur, have the client lie on the left side. Using the bell of your stethoscope, listen carefully in and around the apical area.

g. Record your assessment findings. Describe the intensity or loudness of the sounds as normal, absent, diminished, or accentuated, and the quality of sounds as sharp, full, booming, or snapping.

▪ Peripheral Vascular System

Assessment of the peripheral vascular system includes measurement of the blood pressure; palpation of peripheral pulses; inspection, palpation, and auscultation of the carotid pulse; inspection of the jugular and peripheral veins; and inspection of the skin and tissues to determine perfusion to the extremities. Certain aspects of peripheral vascular assessment are often incorporated into other parts of the assessment procedure. For example, blood pressure is usually measured at the beginning of the physical examination (see the section on assessing blood pressure in Chapter 31). Nursing history data taken in conjunction with assessment of the peripheral vascular system are shown in the accompanying box.

Pulse sites and pulse assessments are described in Chapter 31. Figure 32–39 illustrates the sites for palpating the peripheral pulses. To assess the client's peripheral pulses:

1. Palpate the peripheral pulses (except the carotid pulse) on both sides of the client's body simultaneously and systematically to determine the symmetry of pulse volume; inequality may indicate arterial disease.

2. If you have difficulty palpating some peripheral pulses, use a Doppler ultrasound probe.

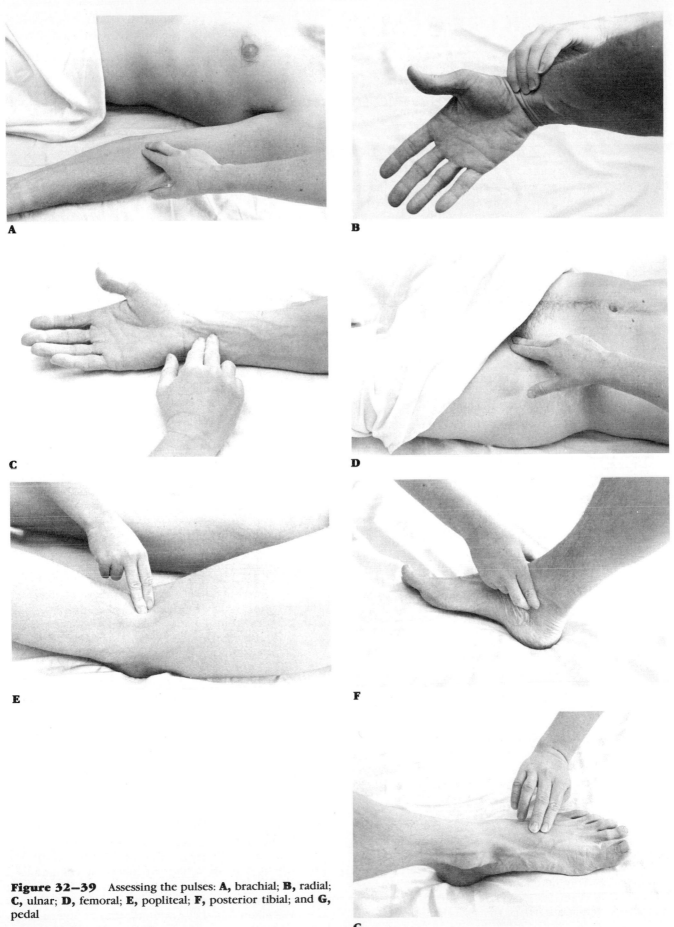

Figure 32–39 Assessing the pulses: **A,** brachial; **B,** radial;
C, ulnar; **D,** femoral; **E,** popliteal; **F,** posterior tibial; and **G,**
pedal

NURSING HISTORY

Peripheral Vascular System

Determine:

- Past history of heart disorders, phlebitis, varicosities, arterial disease, and hypertension

- Life-style, specifically exercise patterns, activity patterns and tolerance, smoking habits, and use of alcohol

- Presence of signs indicative of peripheral vascular disease in one or more extremities, such as pain or cramping, numbness, tingling, burning, edema, enlarged or bulging veins, and changes in temperature and color

- The relation of pain or cramping to activity and the effectiveness of rest in relieving them.

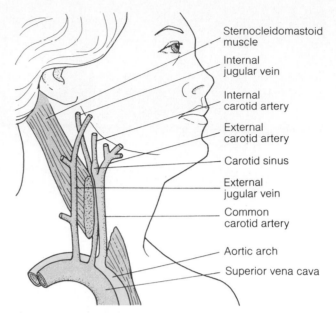

Figure 32–40 Arteries and veins of the right side of the neck

Note whether each pulse volume is absent; weak, thready, or decreased; normal; or increased and bounding. **Normal findings** are symmetric pulse volumes and easily palpable full pulsations. A scale for grading pulse volumes is shown in the accompanying box. Asymmetric volumes indicate **impaired circulation;** absent pulsations indicate **arterial spasm** or **occlusion.** Decreased, weak, thready pulsations indicate **impaired cardiac output,** and increased pulse volumes may indicate **hypertension, high cardiac output,** or **circulatory overload.**

The **carotid arteries** supply oxygenated blood to the head and neck. See Figure 32–40. Since they are the only source of blood to the brain, prolonged occlusion of one of these arteries can result in serious brain damage. The carotid pulses correlate with central aortic pressure, thus reflecting cardiac function better than the peripheral pulses. When cardiac output is diminished, the peripheral pulses may be difficult or impossible to feel, but the carotid pulse should be felt easily.

With the client in a sitting position, inspect the carotid arteries for obvious pulsations; sometimes a wave

ASSESSMENT

Scale for Grading Pulse Volumes

0   No pulse.
1   Pulse is thready, weak, and difficult to palpate; it may fade in and out and is easily obliterated with pressure.
2   Pulse is difficult to palpate and may be obliterated with pressure; thus, light palpation is necessary. Once located, pulse is stronger than scale 1 pulse.
3   Pulse is easily palpable, does not fade in and out, and is not easily obliterated by pressure (normal pulse).
4   Pulse is strong or bounding, easily palpated, and not obliterated with pressure; in some cases, e.g., in cases of aortic regurgitation, scale 4 pulse may indicate disease (Miller 1978, p. 1674).

can be seen. **Extreme caution is required when palpating the carotid artery. Generally, carotid artery palpation is done only by highly experienced practitioners on clients who have specific cardiac conditions.** Only one carotid artery is palpated at a time to ensure adequate cerebral blood flow through the other and thus prevent possible cerebral ischemia. The examiner avoids exerting too much pressure and massaging the area, since pressure can occlude the artery and carotid sinus massage can precipitate bradycardia. The **carotid sinus** is a small dilation at the beginning of the internal carotid artery just above the bifurcation of the common carotid artery, in the upper third of the neck.

Normally, carotid pulse volumes are symmetric, full, and thrusting. The thrusting quality remains the same when the client inhales or exhales, turns the head, and changes from a sitting to a supine position. The arterial wall normally feels elastic. Asymmetric volumes or decreased pulsations may indicate **carotid artery stenosis** or **thrombosis,** or **inadequate left cardiac output.** Thickened, hard, rigid, beaded, inelastic walls are indicative of **arteriosclerosis.**

To auscultate the carotid artery, turn the client's head slightly away from the side being examined to facilitate placement of the stethoscope. Auscultate the carotid artery on one side and then the other. Listen for the presence of a **bruit** (a blowing or swishing sound) created by turbulence of blood flow due either to a narrowed arterial lumen (a common development in older people) or to a condition, such as anemia or hyperthyroidism, that elevates cardiac output. Normally no sound is heard by auscultation. If a bruit is heard, gentle palpation of the artery is indicated to determine the presence of a thrill, which frequently accompanies a bruit. A **thrill** is a vibrating sensation like the purring of a cat or water running through a hose. It, too, indicates turbulent blood flow due to arterial obstruction.

Table 32-12 Clinical Signs of Adequate and Inadequate Tissue Perfusion

Assessment Criterion	Normal Findings	Abnormal Findings	Possible Health Problem
Skin color	Pink	Cyanotic	Venous insufficiency
		Pallor that increases with limb elevation	Arterial insufficiency
		Dusky red color when limb lowered	Arterial insufficiency
		Brown pigmentation around ankles	Arterial insufficiency
Skin temperature	Skin not excessively warm or cold	Skin cool	Arterial insufficiency
Edema	Absent	Marked edema	Venous insufficiency
		Mild or absent	Arterial insufficiency
Skin texture	Skin resilient, moist	Skin thin and shiny or thick, waxy, shiny, and fragile, with reduced hair and ulceration	Venous or arterial insufficiency
Arterial adequacy test	Original color returns in 10 seconds; veins in feet or hands fill in about 15 seconds	Delayed color return or mottled appearance; delayed venous filling; marked redness of arms or legs	Arterial insufficiency
Capillary refill test	Immediate return of color	Delayed return of color	Arterial insufficiency
Peripheral pulse	Easily palpable	No pulse, decreased or absent	Arterial insufficiency

The **jugular veins** drain blood from the head and neck directly into the superior vena cava and right side of the heart. See Figure 32–40. The external jugular veins are superficial and may be visible above the clavicle. The internal jugular veins lie deeper along the carotid artery and may transmit pulsations onto the skin of the neck. Normally, external neck veins are distended and visible when a person lies down; they are flat and not as visible when a person stands up, since gravity encourages venous drainage. By inspecting the jugular veins for pulsations and distention, the nurse can assess the adequacy of function of the right side of the heart and venous pressure. Bilateral jugular vein distention (JVD) may indicate right-sided heart failure. Unilateral distention may be caused by local obstruction.

Peripheral veins in the arms and legs are inspected for the presence and/or appearance of superficial veins when limbs are dependent and when limbs are elevated. When the limb is dependent, distention and nodular bulges in the calf veins are common, especially in older people. Distended veins in the anteromedial part of the thigh and/or lower leg or in the posterolateral part of the calf from the knee to the ankle are abnormal. When the legs are elevated, the veins normally collapse.

The nurse also assesses the peripheral leg veins for signs of phlebitis by inspecting the calves for redness and swelling over vein sites and palpating the calves for firmness or tension of the muscles, the presence of edema over the dorsum of the foot, and areas of localized warmth. Palpation augments inspection findings, particularly when the client is highly pigmented and redness may not be visible. Next, gently push the client's calves from side to side to test for tenderness and firmly dorsiflex the client's foot while supporting the entire leg extension or have the person stand or walk. If forceful dorsiflexion of the foot produces pain in the calf muscles (positive **Homans's sign**), a deep phlebitis of the leg may be present.

As part of an overall head-to-toe assessment, nurses commonly test capillary refill by squeezing a client's fingernail and toenail between their fingers with enough pressure to cause blanching. After releasing the pressure, the nurse observes how quickly normal color returns. Color normally returns immediately. Delayed capillary refill indicates inadequate peripheral perfusion. See Table 32–12 for clinical signs of adequate and inadequate tissue perfusion.

▪ Abdomen

Description of abdominal findings is facilitated by two commonly used methods of subdivision: **quadrants** (see Figure 32–41) and **nine regions** (see Figure 32–42). Specific organs or parts of organs lie in each abdominal quadrant and/or region. See Tables 32–13 and 32–14.

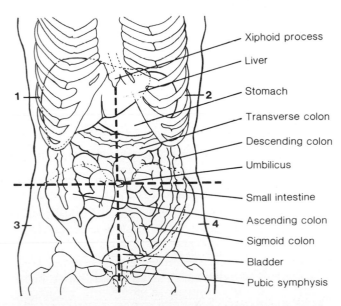

Xiphoid process
Liver
Stomach
Transverse colon
Descending colon
Umbilicus
Small intestine
Ascending colon
Sigmoid colon
Bladder
Pubic symphysis

Figure 32–41 The four abdominal regions and the underlying organs: **1,** right upper quadrant; **2,** left upper quadrant; **3,** right lower quadrant; **4,** left lower quadrant

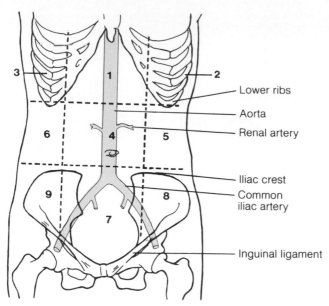

Figure 32—42 The nine abdominal regions: **1,** epigastric; **2, 3,** left and right hypochondriac; **4,** umbilical; **5, 6,** left and right lumbar; **7,** suprapubic; **8, 9,** left and right inguinal or iliac

Assessment of the abdomen involves all four methods of examination (inspection, palpation, auscultation, and percussion). Of these, beginning practitioners usually perform only inspection and auscultation. If abnormalities are detected, the beginner consults a more experienced practitioner, who may perform palpation and percussion. Several body organs are assessed during the abdominal examination: the stomach, intestines, liver, spleen, kidneys, and, if it is distended or enlarged, the bladder. Pertinent data to be obtained from the nursing history are summarized in the accompanying box.

NURSING HISTORY

Abdomen

Determine:

- Incidence of abdominal pain, its location, onset, sequence, and chronology
- Its quality (description)
- Its frequency
- Associated symptoms, e.g., nausea, vomiting, diarrhea
- Bowel habits
- Incidence of constipation or diarrhea (have client describe what he or she means by these terms)
- Change in appetite, food intolerance, and foods ingested in last 24 hours
- Specific signs and symptoms, e.g., heartburn, flatulence and/or belching, difficulty swallowing, hematemesis, blood or mucus in stools, and aggravating and alleviating factors
- Previous problems and treatment, e.g., stomach ulcer, gallbladder surgery, history of jaundice

Table 32—13   Organs in the Four Abdominal Quadrants

Upper right quadrant	*Upper left quadrant*
Liver	Left lobe of liver
Gallbladder	Stomach
Duodenum	Spleen
Head of pancreas	Upper lobe of left kidney
Right adrenal gland	Pancreas
Upper lobe of right kidney	Left adrenal gland
Hepatic flexure of colon	Splenic flexure of colon
Section of ascending colon	Section of transverse colon
Section of transverse colon	Section of descending colon
Lower right quadrant	*Lower left quadrant*
Lower lobe of right kidney	Lower lobe of left kidney
Cecum	Sigmoid colon
Appendix	Section of descending colon
Section of ascending colon	Left ovary
Right ovary	Left fallopian tube
Right fallopian tube	Left ureter
Right ureter	Left spermatic cord
Right spermatic cord	Part of uterus (if enlarged)
Part of uterus (if enlarged)	

Midline

Uterus
Bladder

When assessing the abdomen, inspection is done first, followed by auscultation, palpation, and/or percussion. Auscultation is done before palpation and percussion, since movement or stimulation of the bowel caused by palpation and percussion can increase bowel motility and thus heighten bowel sounds, creating false results.

To facilitate validity of observations and enhance client comfort, have the client has urinate before beginning the assessment. Assist the client to a supine position with the arms placed comfortably at the sides. Place small pillows beneath the knees and the head. This position and an empty bladder prevent tension in the abdominal muscles. By contrast, the abdominal muscles tense when the client is sitting or supine with knees and arms extended and with hands clasped behind the head.

Ensure that the room is warm, and expose only the client's abdomen from chest line to the pubic area to avoid chilling and shivering, which can tense the abdominal muscles. Direct the examining light over the abdomen, and inspect the abdominal surface, with your head only slightly higher than the client's abdomen. Assessment guidelines are summarized in the accompanying box.

Abdominal contour (described as flat, rounded, or scaphoid) is the profile line from the rib margin to the pubic bone viewed by the examiner at a right angle to the umbilicus when the client is supine. A **flat** contour lies in an approximately horizontal plane from the rib cage to the pubic area; **rounded** contour is convex to the horizontal plane; and **scaphoid** is concave to the horizontal plane. After instructing the client to take a deep breath and to hold it, inspect the abdominal contour again. A deep breath forces the diaphragm downward, thus decreasing the size of the abdominal cavity

Table 32—14 Organs in the Nine Abdominal Regions

Right hypochondriac	*Epigastric*	*Left hypochondriac*
Right lobe of liver	Aorta	Stomach
Gallbladder	Pyloric end of	Spleen
Part of duodenum	stomach	Tail of pancreas
Hepatic flexure of	Part of duodenum	Splenic flexure of
colon	Pancreas	colon
Upper half of	Part of liver	Upper half of left
right kidney		kidney
Suprarenal gland		Suprarenal gland
Right lumbar	*Umbilical*	*Left lumbar*
Ascending colon	Omentum	Descending colon
Lower half of	Mesentery	Lower half of left
right kidney	Lower part of	kidney
Part of duodenum	duodenum	Part of jejunum
and jejunum	Part of jejunum	and ileum
	and ileum	
Right inguinal	*Hypogastric (pubic)*	*Left inguinal*
Cecum	Ileum	Sigmoid colon
Appendix	Bladder (if	Left ureter
Lower end of	enlarged)	Left spermatic
ileum	Uterus (if	cord
Right ureter	enlarged)	Left ovary
Right spermatic		
cord		
Right ovary		

and making masses such as an enlarged liver or spleen more obvious.

After inspecting the abdomen, listen for the presence or absence of two abdominal sounds: bowel or peristaltic sounds caused by gas and food moving along the intestines, and vascular sounds. In the pregnant woman, fetal heart sounds are also assessed. The stethoscope diaphragms and the nurse's hands should be warmed prior to auscultation, since cold hands and a cold stethoscope may cause the client to contract the abdominal muscles, and these contractions may be heard during auscultation.

ASSESSMENT

Abdomen

Determine:

- Surface characteristics
- Distention
- Masses
- Visible peristaltic waves or pulsations
- Movements with respiration
- Abdominal and umbilical contours
- Presence of scars or rashes
- Presence or absence of bowel sounds
- Presence or absence of bruits

Applying light pressure with the stethoscope, use the flat-disc diaphragm to listen to the abdominal intestinal sounds (which are relatively high-pitched) and the bell-shaped diaphragm to detect arterial and venous sounds (which are lower-pitched). Place the flat diaphragm of the stethoscope in each of the four quadrants of the abdomen and listen for active bowel sounds—irregular, gurgling noises occurring about every 5 to 20 seconds. The duration of a single sound may range from less than a second to more than several seconds. The frequency of sounds relates to the state of digestion or the presence of food in the gastrointestinal tract. Shortly after or long after eating, bowel sounds may be normally increased. They are loudest when a meal is long overdue. Four to 7 hours after a meal, bowel sounds may be heard continuously over the ileocecal valve area, while the digestive contents from the small intestine empty through the valve into the large intestine. Normal bowel sounds are described as **audible.** Alterations in sounds are described as **absent** or **hypoactive,** i.e., extremely soft and infrequent (e.g., one per minute), and **hyperactive** or increased (**borborygmi**), i.e., high-pitched, loud, rushing sounds that occur frequently (e.g., every 3 seconds). If bowel sounds appear to be absent, listen for 3 to 5 minutes before concluding that they are absent. Because bowel sounds are so irregular, a longer time and more sites are used to confirm absence of sounds.

After listening for bowel sounds, place the bell of the stethoscope over the aorta, renal arteries, and iliac arteries, and listen for arterial sounds (**bruits**). Place the bell of the stethoscope over the periumbilical (around the umbilicus) region and listen for a venous hum, rarely heard in the abdomen. At the various auscultating sites, especially above the liver and spleen, listen for peritoneal friction rubs that sound like two pieces of leather rubbing together. The liver and spleen have large surface areas in contact with the peritoneum; thus they are most frequently the beginning sites for friction rubs. Table 32—15 provides an overview of normal and abnormal abdominal assessment findings.

Rectum and Anus

Nursing history data taken in conjunction with assessment of the rectum and anus are shown in the accompanying box. Completeness of assessment of the rectum and anus depends on the needs and problems of the individual client. In many practice settings, the nurse performs only inspection of the anus.

Genitals and Reproductive Tract

During assessment of male adolescents, it is most important to establish the descent of the testicles into the scrotum; undescended testes are noted. Assessment of adolescent girls is limited to an inspection of the external genitals unless the girl is sexually active. If so, a Papanicolaou test (Pap test) is advised once a year to detect cancer of the cervix and uterus. If the adolescent is sexually active and has an increased or abnormal vagi-

Table 32–15 Assessment Data: Abdomen

Method and Structure	Normal Findings	Abnormal Findings
	Inspection	
Abdomen	Smooth, soft; flat, rounded, or scaphoid contour	Tense, glistening skin Distention Visible peristalsis Visible midline pulsations
	Symmetric contour	Asymmetric contour, e.g., localized protrusions around umbilicus, around inguinal ligaments, or near scars
	Silver-white striae or surgical scars	Purple striae
	Unblemished skin	Rash or other skin lesions
	After deep breath, smooth, even, symmetrical movements	After deep breath, bulges or masses appear After deep breath, abdominal movement is restricted
	After raising head and shoulders, little or no midline bulge	After raising head and shoulders, marked ridge or bulge
	Auscultation	
Abdomen	Audible bowel sounds	Absent or hypoactive bowel sounds Hyperactive bowel sounds
	Absence of arterial bruits	Loud bruit over aortic area Bruit over renal or iliac arteries
	Absence of venous hum	Medium-pitched hum in perioumbilical region Friction rub
	Percussion	
Abdomen	Predominantly tympanic percussion sound; suprapubic dullness over distended bladder	Dullness in localized area
Liver	Span of 6–12 cm at midclavicular line and 4–8 cm at midsternal line	Span exceeding 12 cm at midclavicular line and 8 cm at midsternal line Midsternal line span is equal to midclavicular line span Lower liver border displaced inferiorly Lower liver border displaced superiorly
Spleen	Span of about 7 cm at left midaxially line between sixth and tenth ribs	Span exceeds 7 cm
Shifting dullness test		Change in first and second demarcation lines (between tympany and dullness)
Fist percussion	No tenderness of liver or kidney	Tenderness of liver Tenderness of kidney
	Palpation	
Light abdominal	No tenderness; relaxed abdomen with smooth, consistent tension	Tenderness and hypersensitivity Superficial masses Localized areas of increased tension
Deep abdominal	Tenderness may be present near xiphoid process, over cecum, and over sigmoid colon	Generalized or localized areas of tenderness Mobile or fixed masses
Liver	May not be palpable Border feels smooth	Enlarged but smooth and not tender Smooth but tender Nodular Hard
Spleen	Not palpable	Palpated
Kidney	Neither kidney palpable Pole of right kidney palpable, feels smooth and firm	Either or both kidneys palpable Enlarged, hard, tender, or nodular
Bladder	Not palpable	Distended and palpable as smooth, round, tense mass

nal discharge, specimens should be taken to check for sexually transmitted disease.

In **adult females,** complete examination of the genitals and reproductive tract includes assessment of the inguinal lymph nodes, external genitals, vagina and cervix, uterus, ovaries, and cervix. The accompanying box contains data to be collected during a nursing history. Completeness of the assessment of the genitals and reproductive tract depends on the needs and problems of the individual client. In most practice settings, nurses perform only inspection of the external genitals.

Begin an inspection of the external female genitals

NURSING HISTORY

Rectum and Anus

Determine:

- History of diarrhea, constipation, rectal bleeding, black or tarry stools, rectal pain, itching, or spasm
- Current clinical signs of bowel or rectal disorders, such as abdominal pain or tenderness, excessive flatulence, abdominal distention or cramping, painful defecation, bleeding, and diarrhea
- Use of laxatives, including the type and frequency of use
- Currently prescribed medications, specifically those that cause constipation (e.g., codeine) or black, tarry stools (e.g., iron or Pepto-Bismol)
- Recent changes in defecation patterns and stool consistency and shape, e.g., alternating constipation and diarrhea
- Dietary patterns particularly as they relate to colorectal cancer (Low-fiber diets, high intake of fats, and red meats are thought to be related to carcinogenic changes in the gastrointestinal tract.)
- Family history of inflammatory or carcinogenic bowel disease

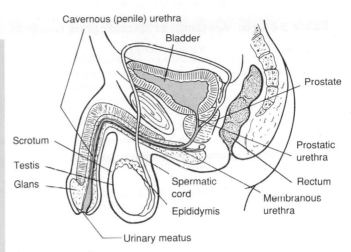

Figure 32–43

by observing the distribution and amount of pubic hair. There are wide variations. Generally, the pubic hair of menstruating adults is kinky; after menopause, it is thinner and straighter. Inspect the skin in the pubic area for lice, lesions, erythema, leukoplakia, fissures, and excoriations. Separate the labia majora, and inspect the interior of the labia majora and the labia minora as well. Observe the clitoris for size and lesions. The normal clitoris is about 0.5 cm (0.2 in) in diameter. Note any signs of inflammation around the urethral meatus.

In **adult males,** complete examination should include assessment of the external genitals, the presence of any hernias, and the prostate gland. As with females, nurses performing routine assessment of clients usually assess only the external genitals. The male reproductive and urinary systems (see Figure 32–43) share the urethra, which is the passageway for both urine and semen. Therefore, in physical assessment of the male, these two systems are frequently assessed together. The accompanying box contains a list of data to be collected during a nursing history.

Begin an assessment of the external male genitals by observing the amount and pattern of the pubic hair. There are wide variations among people, and only very thin hair or absence of hair should be reported. The normal pattern is triangular, often spreading up the abdomen. Inspect the skin covering the penis and scrotum for excoriations, ulcers, and lesions. Inspect the size of the penis. Variations are normal, and only an extreme variation is probably significant.

Retract the foreskin or have the client do this. The foreskin should retract readily. A small amount of thick white smegma is normally seen between the glans and the foreskin. Locate the site of the urethral meatus, which is normally at the tip of the penis. Variations in its location are: **hypospadius,** on the underside of the penile shaft, and **epispadius,** on the upper side of the penile shaft. Inspect the urethral meatus and the glans for ulcers, scars, nodules, inflammation, and discharge. Compress the glans slightly to open the urethral meatus to inspect

NURSING HISTORY

Female Genitals

Determine:

- Age of onset of menstruation, last menstrual period (LMP), regularity of cycle, duration, amount of daily flow, and presence of painful menstruation
- Incidence of pain during intercourse
- Vaginal discharge
- Number of pregnancies, number of live births, labor or delivery complications
- Frequency, urgency, frequency of urination at night, blood in urine, painful urination, incontinence
- History of sexually transmitted disease, past and present

NURSING HISTORY

Male Genitals

Determine:

- Usual fluid intake and output, voiding patterns and any changes, bladder control, urinary incontinence, frequency, urgency, or abdominal pain
- Any symptoms of sexually transmitted disease
- Any swellings that could indicate presence of hernia
- Family history of nephritis, malignancy of the prostate, or malignancy of the kidney.

Table 32—21 Joint Movement (*continued*)

Instruction*	Movement	Normal Range
Bend wrist toward the fifth finger side while palm faces upward.	Ulnar flexion,	30 to 50°
Repeat all motions, using other hand.	Adduction	
Hand and finger joints		
Make a fist of one hand.	Flexion	90°
Straighten fingers of one hand.	Extension	90°
Bend fingers of hand back as far as possible	Hyperextension	30°
Spread fingers of one hand apart as far as pssible.	Abduction	20°
Bring fingers together from abducted position.	Adduction	20°
Repeat all motions, using other hand and fingers.		
Thumb joint		
Move thumb across the palm of hand toward fifth finger.	Flexion	90°
With palm uppermost, move thumb away from palm toward self.	Extension	90°
Move thumb as far as possible to the side.	Abduction	30°
Move thumb from abducted position toward hand.	Adduction	30°
Touch the tip of each finger with thumb of same hand.	Opposition	
Repeat all motions, using other thumb.		
Hip joint		
Move leg forward with knee:	Flexion	
▪ straight		90°
▪ bent		120°
Move leg from flexed position back to other leg.	Extension	90 to 120°
Move leg back behind the body.	Hyperextension	30 to 50°
Move leg out to the side as far as possible.	Abduction	45 to 50°
Move leg from abducted position back to other leg and in front of it as far as possible.	Adduction	20 to 30° beyond second leg
Move leg backward, up, to the side, and down, making a circle.	Circumduction	360°
Turn foot and leg inward toward other leg as far as possible	Internal rotation	90°
Turn foot and leg outward from other leg as far as possible.	External rotation	90°
Repeat all motions, using other leg.		
Knee joint		
Bend leg as far as possible bringing heel toward back of thigh.	Flexion	120 to 130°
Straighten leg from flexed position.	Extension	12 to 130°
Straighten knee beyond extended position.	Hyperextension	0 to 10°
Repeat all motions, using other knee.		
Ankle joint		
Point toes of foot downard as far as possible.	Extension (plantar flexion)	45 to 50°
From normal ankle position point toes of foot upward as far as possible.	Flexion (dorsiflexion)	20°
Repeat both motions, using other knee.		
Foot and toe joints		
Turn sole of foot to the side as far as possible.	Eversion	5°
Turn sole of foot from normal position toward other foot.	Inversion	5°
Curve toes downward.	Flexion	35 to 65°
Straighten toes.	Extension	35 to 65°
Spread toes apart as far as possible.	Abduction	0 to 15°
Bring toes together from abducted position.	Adduction	0 to 15°
Repeat all motions, using other foot.		
Vertebral joints		
Bend trunk toward toes.	Flexion	70 to 90°
Straighten trunk from flexed position.	Extension	70 to 90°
Bend trunk backward as far as possible.	Hyperextension	20 to 30°
Bend trunk to the right side as far as possible and then to the left side.	Lateral flexion	35° from the midline to each side
Turn the upper part of body as far as possible to the right and then to the left.	Rotation	30 to 45° from the midline to each side

*For illustrations of each movement and the muscles involved, see Chapter 35.

Neurologic System

The nervous system integrates all other body systems, but it also depends on the appropriate functioning of peripheral organs from which it receives internal and external environmental stimuli. A thorough neurologic examination may take 1 to 3 hours; however, routine screening tests are usually done first. If the result of these tests are questionable, then more extensive evaluations are made.

Examination of the neurologic system is not usually performed by the beginning student. It includes assessment of the cranial nerves, the proprioception and cerebellar function, the motor system, the sensory system, reflexes, mental status, and levels of consciousness. For the specific functions and assessment methods of each cranial nerve, see Table 32–22. The nurse needs to be aware of these functions to detect abnormalities. (The names and order of the cranial nerves can be recalled by remembering this sentence: "On old Olympus's treeless top, a Finn and German viewed a hop." The first letter of each word in the phrase is the same as the first letter of the names of the cranial nerves.) Table 32–23 summarizes assessment data related to proprioception and cerebellar functioning. Nursing history data are shown in the accompanying box.

Sensory functions include touch, pain, vibration, position, temperature, and tactile discrimination. The first three are routinely tested in a few locations. Vibration is tested at the wrists, elbows, knees, and ankles. Generally the face, arms, legs, hands, and feet are tested for touch and pain, although all parts of the body can be tested. If the client complains of numbness, peculiar sensations, or paralysis, sensation should be checked more carefully over flexor and extensor surfaces of limbs. Abnormality of touch or pain should then be mapped out clearly by examining responses in the area about every 2 cm (1 in). This is a lengthy procedure. A more detailed neurologic examination includes position sense, temperature sense, and tactile discrimination.

To assess the client's response to painful stimuli, ask the client to close his or her eyes and to say "sharp," "dull," or "don't know" when the sharp or dull end of the safety pin or needle is felt. Alternately use the sharp and dull end of the sterile pin or needle to lightly prick designated anatomic areas at random, e.g., hand, forearm, foot, lower leg, abdomen. The face is not tested in this manner. Alternating the sharp and dull ends of the instrument more accurately evaluates the client's response. A sterile safety pin or needle is used to avoid the risk of infection. Allow at least 2 seconds between each test to prevent summation effects of stimuli, i.e., several successive stimuli perceived as one stimulus. Note areas of reduced, heightened, or absent sensation, and map them out for recording purposes. If pain sensation is dulled or lost, assess temperature sensation in these areas. When sensations of pain are dulled, temperature sense is usually also impaired because distribution of these nerves over the body is similar.

Temperature sensation is not routinely tested if pain sensation is found to be within normal limits. If pain sensation is not normal or is absent, testing sensitivity to temperature may prove more reliable. Touch skin areas with test tubes filled with hot or cold water. Have the client respond by saying "hot," "cold," or "don't know."

A **reflex** is an automatic response of the body to a stimulus. It is not voluntarily learned or conscious. The deep tendon reflex (DTR) is activated when a tendon is stimulated (tapped) and its associated muscle contracts. The quality of a reflex response varies among individ-

NURSING HISTORY

Neurologic System

Determine:

▪ History of loss of consciousness, convulsions, fainting, tingling or numbness, tremors or tics, clumsiness, paralysis, limps, loss of memory, speech impairments, disorientation, mood swings, nervousness, anxiety, phobias, or depression

▪ Onset of above symptoms, cause, treatment, and outcomes of the treatment

▪ Current signs of the above

▪ Changes in vision, hearing, smell, taste, or touch

▪ Current symptoms, e.g., numbness and tingling, paresthesia, dizziness, falling, uncontrolled muscle movements, tics, tremors, or speech changes

▪ Decrease in memory

▪ Muscle weakness or paralysis

uals and by age. As a person ages and the nervous system gradually deteriorates, reflex responses become less intense.

Reflexes are tested using a percussion hammer. The response is described on a scale of 0 to +4. See the accompanying box for a scale describing reflex responses. Experience is necessary to determine appropriate scoring for an individual. It is important to compare one side of the body with the other when assessing reflexes to evaluate the symmetry of response. Several reflexes are normally tested during a physical examination. These are the biceps reflex, triceps reflex, bradioradialis reflex, patellar reflex, Achilles reflex, and the plantar reflex.

The **plantar** (or **Babinski**) reflex is a superficial reflex that is easily evaluated. Using a moderately sharp object (e.g., the handle of the percussion hammer, a key, or the dull end of a pin or applicator stick), the examiner strokes the lateral border of the sole of the client's foot, starting at the heel, continuing to the ball of the foot, and then proceeding across the ball of the foot toward the big toe. See Figure 32–45. Normally, all five toes bend downward; this reaction is **negative Babinski**. In an abnormal response, **positive Babinski**, the toes spread outward and the big toe moves upward. Positive Babin-

ASSESSMENT

Scale for Grading Reflex Responses

▪ 0 No reflex response

▪ +1 Minimal activity (hypoactive)

▪ +2 Normal response

▪ +3 More active than normal

▪ +4 Maximum activity (hyperactive)

Table 32–22 Cranial Nerve Functions and Assessment Methods

Cranial Nerve	Name	Type	Function	Assessment Methods
1	Olfactory	Sensory	Smell	Ask client to close eyes and identify different mild aromas, such as coffee, tobacco, vanilla, oil of cloves, peanut butter, orange, lemon, lime, chocolate.
II	Optic	Sensory	Vision and visual fields	Ask client to read Snellen chart; check visual fields by confrontation; and conduct an ophthalmoscopic examination.
III	Oculomotor	Motor	Extraocular eye movement (EOM); movement of sphincter of pupil; movement of ciliary muscles of lens	Assess directions of gaze and pupil reaction.
IV	Trochlear	Motor	EOM, specifically moves eyeball downward and laterally	Assess directions of gaze.
V	Trigeminal			
	Ophthalmic branch	Sensory	Sensation of cornea, skin of face, and nasal mucosa	While client looks upward, lightly touch lateral sclera of eye to elicit blink reflex; to test light sensation, have client close eyes, wipe a wisp of cotton over client's forehead and paranasal sinuses; to test deep sensation, use alternating blunt and sharp ends of a safety pin over same areas.
	Maxillary branch	Sensory	Sensation of skin of face and anterior oral cavity (tongue and teeth)	Assess skin sensation as for ophthalmic branch above.
	Mandibular branch	Motor and sensory	Muscles of mastification; sensation of skin of face	Ask client to clench teeth.
VI	Abducents	Motor	EOM; moves eyeball laterally	Assess directions of gaze.
VII	Facial	Motor and sensory	Facial expression; taste (anterior two thirds of tongue)	Ask client to smile, raise the eyebrows, frown, puff out cheeks, close eyes tightly; ask client to identify various tastes placed on tip and sides of tongue: sugar (sweet), salt, lemon juice (sour), and quinine (bitter); identify areas of taste.
VIII	Auditory			
	Vestibular branch	Sensory	Equilibrium	Assessment methods for cerebellar functions.
	Cochlear branch	Sensory	Hearing	Assess client's ability to hear spoken word and vibrations of tuning fork.
IX	Glossopharyngeal	Motor and sensory	Swallowing ability and gag reflex, tongue movement, taste (posterior tongue)	Use tongue blade on posterior tongue while client says "ah" to elicit gag reflex; apply tastes on posterior tongue for identification; ask client to move tongue from side to side and up and down.
X	Vagus	Motor and sensory	Sensation of pharynx and larynx; swallowing; vocal cord movement	Assessed with cranial nerve IX; assess client's speech for hoarseness.
XI	Accessory	Motor	Head movement; shrugging of shoulders	Ask client to shrug shoulders against resistance from your hands and turn head to side against resistance from your hand (repeat for other side).
XII	Hypoglossal	Motor	Protrusion of tongue	Ask client to protrude tongue at midline, then move it side to side.

Table 32—23   Assessment Data: Proprioception and Cerebellum

Test	Normal Findings	Abnormal Findings
Gross motor function and balance		
Walking gait	Has upright posture and steady gait with opposing arm swing; walks unaided maintaining balance	Has poor posture and unsteady, irregular, staggering gait with wide stance; bends legs only from hips; has rigid or no arm movements
Romberg test	May sway slightly but is able to maintain upright posture and foot stance	Cannot maintain foot stance; moves the feet apart to maintain stance
Standing on one foot with eyes closed	Maintains stance for at least 5 seconds	Cannot maintain stance for 5 seconds
Heel-toe walking	Maintains heel-toe walking along a straight line	Assumes a wider foot gait to stay upright
Toe or heel walking	Able to walk several steps on toes or heels	Cannot maintain balance on toes or heels
Hopping in place	Has adequate muscle strength to hop on one foot	Cannot hop or maintain single leg balance
Knee bends	Has adequate balance and muscle strength to perform knee bends	Does not have adequate balance or muscle strength to perform knee bends
Fine motor function: upper extremities		
Finger-to-nose test	Repeatedly and rhythmically touches the nose	Misses the nose or gives lazy response
Alternating supination and pronation of hands on knees	Can alternately supinate and pronate hands at rapid pace	Performs with slow, clumsy movements and irregular timing, has difficulty alternating from supination to pronation
Finger to nose and to examiner's finger	Performs with coordination and rapidity	Misses the finger and moves slowly
Fingers to fingers	As above	Moves slowly and is unable to touch fingers consistently
Fingers to thumb (same hand)	Rapidly touches each finger to thumb with each hand	Cannot coordinate this fine discrete movement with either one or both hands
Patting and polishing the examiner's hand	Performs these maneuvers smoothly and rapidly	Performs with clumsy movements and irregular timing
Fine motor function: lower extremities		
Heel down opposite shin	Demonstrates bilateral equal coordination	Has tremors, is awkward, heel moves off shin
Toe or ball of foot to examiner's finger	Moves smoothly, with coordination	Misses the examiner's finger, is unable to coordinate movement
Figure-eight	Can perform this test	Unable to perform the test

ski is normal in infants but abnormal after the child ambulates.

Any defects in or loss of the power to express oneself by speech, writing, or signs or to comprehend spoken or written language due to disease or injury of the cerebral cortex is called **aphasia.** Aphasias can be categorized as sensory or receptive aphasia and motor or expressive aphasia. **Sensory/receptive** aphasia is the loss of the ability to comprehend written or spoken words. Two types of sensory aphasia are **auditory** or **acoustic** aphasia, in which clients have difficulty understanding what is being said even though they hear the sounds, and **visual** aphasia, in which clients cannot read words even though they can see them.

Motor/expressive aphasia involves loss of the power to express oneself by writing, making signs, or speaking. Clients may find that even though they can recall words, they have lost the ability to combine speech sounds into words. The most common aphasias involve partial sensory and motor losses. Because speech is a complex act involving the tongue, mouth, palate, larynx, respiratory system, and cerebrum, the nurse must keep in mind that

disturbances of speech may or may not relate to the nervous system.

Various types of aphasia are reflected in characteristic speech patterns. A pattern of repeating the same response as different questions are asked (**perseveration**) is common in all forms of aphasia. The speech of clients with auditory receptive aphasia is abundant and appropriately expressive but contains many incorrect words (**paraphasia**). Clients with motor aphasia have painfully slow speech, poor articulation, and a tendency to delete prepositions and pronouns (Kneisl and Ames 1986, p. 171).

As the nurse takes the nursing history, the client's responses to questions about dates, places, and persons indicate whether a more detailed assessment is required during neurologic assessment. The client's **orientation to time, place, and person** is determined by tactful questioning. Orientation is easily assessed by asking the client the city and state of residence, time of day, date, day of the week, duration of illness, and names of family members. More direct questioning may be necessary for some people, e.g., "Where are you now?" "What day is

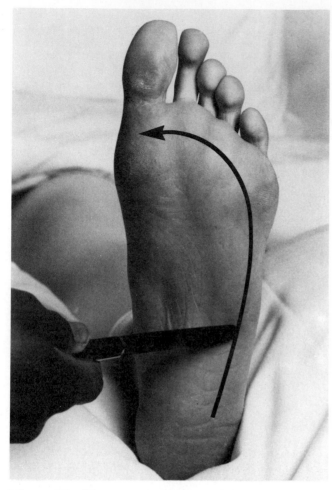

Figure 32–45 Assessing the plantar (Babinski) reflex

it today?" "What is your name?" Listen for lapses in memory. First, ask the client about difficulty with memory. If problems are apparent, three categories of memory are tested: immediate recall, recent memory, and remote memory.

Chapter Highlights

- The physical health examination is conducted to assess the function and integrity of the client's body parts.
- The health assessment is conducted in a systematic manner that requires the fewest position changes for the client.
- Data obtained in the physical health examination supplement, confirm, or refute data obtained during the nursing history.
- Nursing history data help the nurse focus on specific aspects of the physical health examination.
- Data obtained in the physical health examination help the nurse establish nursing diagnoses, plan the client's care, and evaluate the outcomes of nursing care.
- Initial assessment findings provide baseline data about the client's functional abilities against which subsequent assessment findings are compared.

- Skills in inspection, palpation, percussion, and auscultation are required for the physical health examination; these skills are used in that order throughout the examination except during abdominal assessment, when auscultation follows inspection.
- Knowledge of the normal structure and function of body parts and systems is an essential requisite to conducting physical assessment.

Selected References

Bates, B. 1987. *A guide to physical examination.* 4th ed. Philadelphia: J. B. Lippincott Co.

Bellack, J. P., and Bamford, P. A. 1984. *Nursing assessment: A multidimensional approach.* Monterey, Calif.: Wadsworth Health Sciences Division.

Bowers, A. C., and Thompson, J. M. 1988. *Clinical manual of health assessment.* 3d ed. St. Louis. C. V. Mosby Co.

Gillies, D. A., and Alyn, I. B. 1976. *Patient assessment and management by the nurse practitioner.* Philadelphia: W. B. Saunders Co.

Grimes, J., and Iannopollo, E. 1982. *Health assessment in nursing practice.* Monterey, Calif.: Wadsworth Health Sciences Division.

Hagerty, B. K. 1984. *Psychiatric-mental health assessment.* St. Louis: C. V. Mosby Co.

Hudson, M. F. November 1983. Safeguard your elderly patient's health through accurate physical assessment. *Nursing 83* 13:58–61, 63–64.

Humbrecht, B., and VanParys, E. April 1982. From assessment to intervention: How to use heart and breath sounds as part of your nursing care plan. *Nursing 82* 12:34–41.

King, P. A. October 1980. Foot problems and assessment. *Geriatric Nursing* 1:182–86.

Kneisl, C. R., and Ames, S. W. 1986. *Adult health nursing: A biopsychosocial approach.* Menlo Park, Calif.: Addison-Wesley Publishing Co.

Malasanos, L.; Barkauskas, V.; Moss, M.; and Stoltenberg-Allen, K. 1986. *Health assessment.* 3d ed. St. Louis: C. V. Mosby Co.

Miller, K. M. October 1978. Assessing peripheral perfusion. *American Journal of Nursing* 78:1673–74.

Peterson, F. Y. November 1983. Assessing peripheral vascular disease at the bedside. *American Journal of Nursing ???*

Roach, L. B. November 1972. Color changes in dark skins. *Nursing 72* 2:19–22.

Saul, L. December 1983. Heart sounds and common murmurs. *American Journal of Nursing* 83:1679–89.

Smith, C. E. April 1984. Assessment under pressure: When your patient says "my chest hurts." *Nursing 84* 14:34–39.

———. December 1984. With good assessment skills you can construct a solid framework for patient care. *Nursing 84* 14:26–31.

Taylor, D. L. January 1985. Clinical applications: Assessing heart sounds. *Nursing 85* 15:51–53.

———. March 1985. Clinical applications: Assessing breath sounds. *Nursing 85* 15:60–62.

Visich, M. A. November 1981. Knowing what you hear: A guide to assessing breath and heart sounds. *Nursing 84* 14:34–39.

Westra, B. May 1984. Assessment under pressure: When your patient says "I can't breathe." *Nursing 84* 14:34–39.

White, J. H., and Schroeder, M. A. March 1981. When your client has a weight problem: Nursing assessment. *American Journal of Nursing* 81:550–52.

CHAPTER 33

Assisting with Special Procedures

OBJECTIVES

Define terms related to selected special procedures used in diagnosing and treating clients.

Describe the purposes and sequencing of selected procedures.

Identify assessment data required for specific procedures.

Identify education needs of clients about to have certain tests and treatments.

Outline measures to prepare the client physically for specific procedures.

Identify the nursing responsibilities during selected procedures.

Describe guidelines for evaluating and recording client responses after special procedures.

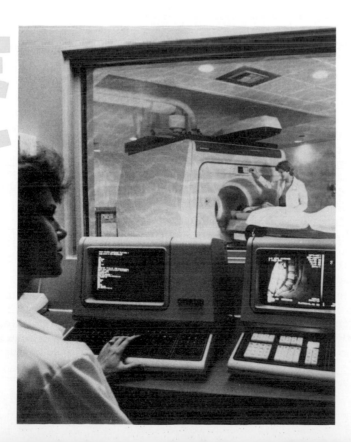

General Nursing Guidelines

In this technological society, health care practioners frequently use highly specialized procedures and diagnostic equipment to better assess the health status of clients. This chapter focuses on providing information about some of the more commonly used special procedures to enable the nurse to:

1. Better prepare clients for these procedures
2. Skillfully care for clients during these procedures
3. Competently evaluate client responses after these procedures

Tests and treatments are frightening to many people. People may fear pain, the results of tests, or their reactions to either the pain or the findings of a test. Fear of the unknown increases these misgivings. It is important for nurses to be aware of the needs of clients and their support persons and to help them meet these needs by preparing clients **psychologically** as well as physically.

The client and, very often, the support persons need explanations of why a test or treatment is necessary and what it will entail. The explanation needs to be adjusted to the client's needs. A small child requires a different explanation than a curious adult. Some persons want to know every detail, but others need only a general explanation. It is important that the nurse be honest with the client; if the client will feel sharp pain during the test, it is better to say so than not to mention it.

Often clients want to know where the test will take place, who will do it, how long it will last, and when the results will be available. The last question is often associated with fear. The nurse can base answers on knowledge of the test and on experience. An honest answer (e.g., "I don't know, but I'll try to find that out for you") is more psychologically supportive than an ambiguous answer (e.g., "Well, we'll see about that") or a condesending one ("Now, don't you worry about that at all").

It is usually the nurse's responsibility to assemble the **equipment** for tests and treatments carried out at a hospitalized client's bedside or in an adjacent clinical treatment room. It is also a nursing responsibility to maintain the sterility of sterile equipment. When a client goes to another area for the procedure, that department assumes responsibility for assembling the equipment.

Before any procedure, nurses should obtain information that can be used as **baseline data for assessment** during and following the procedure. Before a lumbar puncture, for example, it is important to record the client's vital signs (temperature, pulse, blood pressure) as well as any client complaints of headache or neurologic signs, e.g., tingling in the feet or legs. These clinical signs will be assessed after the lumbar puncture. In addition, signs that the client's life is threatened (e.g., falling blood pressure; irregular, weak pulse; or dyspnea) must be reported to the physician before the procedure.

If a client appears unduly anxious about the procedure, the nurse should intervene and attempt to relieve the anxiety. Often repeated explanations of what the physician has said to the client, clarification of certain aspects of the procedure, or validation of the client's feelings may reduce anxiety. Report unrelieved anxiety to the physician, who may give additional information and reassurance and in some instances order a tranquilizer or other medication.

During the treatment or test, the nurse needs to continue to **assess** the client and **provide** emotional support. The nurse should be sensitive to signs of distress, such as pallor, profuse sweating, accelerated pulse, or signs of nausea or acute pain. Any distress needs to be reported immediately to the physician conducting the procedure. The nurse can support the client by providing information, for instance: "It will be about only 2 minutes more," "The needle is all the way in now," or "You won't feel any additional discomfort." Sometimes the nurse can distract the client by asking questions; however, some clients do not respond well to this tactic.

Specimens obtained during a procedure should be appropriately labeled. Hospital specimens usually are marked with the client's name, identification number, and date. Some specimens require special care if not sent directly to the laboratory. Some urine specimens are refrigerated, and some fecal specimens are kept warm to keep microorganisms alive.

The nurse **reassesses** the client **after** any test or treatment. The interval between assessments depends on the client's condition and the procedure performed. Even if there are no adverse reactions, in many instances clients should be assessed immediately after the procedure and 30 minutes thereafter. Data obtained during the assessments are compared with the baseline data to **evaluate** any changes in the client's health status. After a procedure, the nurse assists the client to a prescribed or comfortable position. For example, after a lumbar puncture, the client must assume a dorsal recumbent position.

Support persons need to be told when a procedure is completed and when they can see the client or take the ambulatory client home. It is usually best to remove equipment before support persons enter the treatment room because many people find long needles and similar equipment disquieting. The ambulatory client who is returning home after the procedure should receive written directions for any follow-up measures. People are often anxious and preoccupied at these times and find it difficult to remember verbal directions.

Examinations Involving Electric Impulses

A number of machines measure and record electric impulses. The **electrocardiograph** receives impulses from the heart; the **electroencephalograph,** from the brain. These machines have electrodes that are sensitive to electric activity, which is recorded graphically. The graphic reading can also be shown on an oscilloscope screen.

▪ Electrocardiography

An **electrocardiogram** (**ECG** or **EKG**) is a graph of electric impulses from the heart. The heart muscle is **polarized** or charged when it is at rest. When the muscle cells of the ventricles and the atria contract, they **depolarize** or lose their charge. During a resting stage, they regain their electric charge or **repolarize.** Cardiac depolarization and repolarization are recorded on an EKG. Figure 33–1 shows a normal EKG and indicates the intervals of depolarization and repolarization. The **P wave** arises when the impulse from the SA node causes the atria to contract or depolarize. The **QRS complex** occurs with contraction and depolarization of the ventricles. The **T wave** represents the resting or repolarization of the ventricles.

Repolarization of the atria occurs during the QRS segment of the graph; it is normally not seen on an EKG. The EKG is produced on finely lined paper. The horizontal lines represent the voltage of the electric impulse, and the vertical lines represent time. See Figure 33–2. The graph waves can be abnormal in size, position, and form when cardiac disease exists.

Electrocardiography is painless and usually takes about 10 minutes, although newer computerized electrocardiograph machines are much quicker. Some physicians order an EKG as part of routine physical examinations of clients over age 40. No special preparation is required before the test unless the physician so specifies, e.g., "exercise strenuously for 5 minutes just prior to EKG." If the client is critically ill, the heart may be monitored continually. For such clients, a **cardiac monitor** is used. This machine shows cardiac waves on an oscilloscope.

Before the EKG is taken, the nurse assesses the client's vital signs (body temperature, pulse, respirations, and blood pressure) for baseline data, if not already available. The nurse also determines whether the client has had an EKG before and explains the procedure, as the client requires. The client may be anxious, not about the test, which is painless, but about the results, which might indicate a problem with the heart.

Following the procedure, the nurse assesses the client's response to the test, including reported discomfort, pulse, respirations, and blood pressure. The nurse then records on the client's chart the time the EKG was carried out, the person who performed it, and the client's response. If the client is particularly anxious about the test, the nurse notifies the physician so that the results can be explained as soon as possible.

▪ Electroencephalography

Electroencephalograms (**EEGs**) are recordings of electric activity in the brain. Electroencephalographs have leads to electrodes that attach to the client's scalp with paste or small needles. The client lies in a dorsal recumbent position in a darkened room. The client may be asked to hyperventilate, and readings may also be taken while the client sleeps. If performed on a sleeping client, the test may take 2 hours; otherwise it lasts no more than 1 hour. The test is normally painless, although the client may feel occasional pinpricks if needle electrodes are used in the scalp.

Preparation for an EEG varies. Some agencies advise that, on the day of the test, the client not take stimulants such as coffee or depressants such as alcohol. Usually the client takes no medications prior to the test, and the nurse shampoos the client's hair, which should be free of hair spray, hair creams, and the like.

In some instances, serial EEGs are ordered by the physician. These would be taken at 12- or 24-hour intervals to detect possible changes in brain activity in brain-injured clients. Hospital policy and/or legal requirements may influence the number and sequencing of serial EEGs being performed prior to discontinuing life-support systems.

▪ Examinations Involving Visual Inspection

Visual inspection or direct visualization techniques involve the use of special instruments called **endoscopes,** through which interior parts of the body can be seen. Originally, endoscopes were straight, rigid, metal tubes. Today, most endoscopes are fiberoptic; i.e., they are flexible, easily maneuvered, brightly lighted tubes. These fiberoptic endoscopes or fiberscopes make examination easier to perform and more comfortable for the

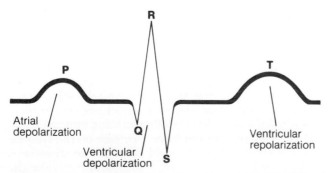

Figure 33–1 Schematic of a normal electrocardiogram

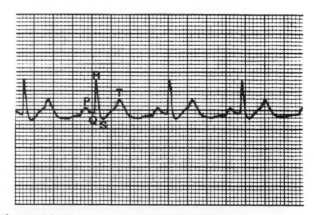

Figure 33–2 A normal electrocardiogram

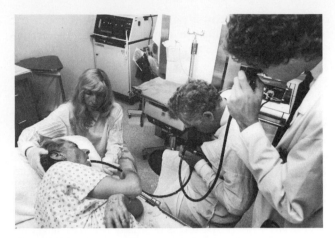

Figure 33–3 An endoscopic procedure in progress

client. Some endoscopes are equipped with a camera that takes color photographs, which can be studied following the examination; others allow the attachment of a second eyepiece (see Figure 33–3) so that another diagnostician or student can observe the procedure simultaneously.

Endoscopes and the examinations performed with them assume their names from the body part to be examined. For example, a broncho**scope** is used to visualize the bronchi of the lungs, and the examination is called a broncho**scopy.** Endoscopic examinations are usually performed in surgery or special treatment rooms. They generally take about 30 to 60 minutes to complete. See Table 33–1 for nursing responsibilities before, during, and after each type of endoscopic examination.

Examinations Involving Removal of Body Fluids and Tissues

Certain body fluids and tissues can help physicians diagnose disease. Table 33–2 lists some common procedures for removing body fluids and tissues. The procedures are normally performed by a physician at the bedside, in an examining room, or sometimes in the emergency department of a hospital. All the procedures involve inserting an instrument, often a needle, through the skin and withdrawing some fluid or tissue. The fluid or tissue is usually placed in a special container and sent to the laboratory for examination. During each procedure, the nurse's responsibility is to assist the physician as requested (maintaining sterile technique) and to support the client verbally, describing the steps of the procedure if the physician does not do so.

High Tech Studies

With the technological advances of the twentieth century and those anticipated in the twenty-first century, more and more health assessment can be per-

formed with relatively minimal discomfort to clients. This section highlights some of the more commonly performed technological procedures.

Roentgenography

Roentgen rays (x rays) are part of the spectrum of electromagnetic radiation. They travel at the speed of light and have considerably shorter wavelengths than light or radio waves. This distinctive property enables radiation to penetrate organs and tissues according to their thickness and density. High-voltage x rays have shorter wavelengths and produce a more penetrating (harder) radiation; low-voltage x rays have longer wavelengths and produce a more easily absorbable (softer) radiation. X rays that are not absorbed pass through the tissue to form an image on the photographic film (a plain, or static, radiograph) or on a fluorescent screen (fluoroscopy).

It is the differential absorption of x rays by the various tissues that makes roentgenography diagnostically useful. **Bones,** which are dense, permit fewer x rays to pass through to the film, so they appear as light areas. The **soft tissues** surrounding bone are less dense, so they appear darker on the film. **Natural contrasts** in density also occur between blood-filled cardiovascular structures and air-filled lung areas. Such natural contrasts, however, do not occur in the abdomen or between the soft tissue structures of the extremities. Thus, **contrast agents** must be introduced for certain body parts, e.g., the digestive tract and blood vessels, to show on the film.

Contrast materials (solids, liquids, or gaseous substances) must absorb either more or fewer x rays than the surrounding tissues. Commonly used contrast agents are compounds of iodine, barium, air, and carbon dioxide. Iodine and barium absorb more x rays than soft tissues; air and carbon dioxide absorb fewer. Contrast materials are introduced into the body in four ways to view specific organs:

1. Orally or rectally for the digestive tract (esophagus, stomach, intestines) and gallbladder. See Figure 33–4.
2. Intravenously for the blood vessels, bile ducts, and kidneys.
3. Into the subarachnoid space for the spine and the ventricles of the brain.
4. Through a nasotracheal tube or bronchoscope for the bronchial tree. (This method is used infrequently now, since the advent of fiberoptic bronchoscopy, which has increased the area available to direct visual examination.)

Radiography of the gastrointestinal tract often involves fluoroscopy as well as a radiographic examination. **Fluoroscopy** is an examination during which x rays are used to visualize body structures on a screen. A fluoroscope is a machine for examining internal structures by viewing the shadows they cast on the fluorescent screen after x rays travel through the structures. For example, a physician uses fluoroscopy to view the

Table 33–1   Nursing Interventions for Endoscopic Examinations

Examination	Preprocedure	During Procedure	Postprocedure
Laryngoscopy or bronchoscopy	Explain the procedure and clarify concerns of the client. Explain that a local spray or gargle will be given or that some medications will be injected through a needle in the vein, that the client will rest the teeth against a small plastic mouthpiece, that the procedure is painless but some pressure may be felt. Explain that the test will take about 30–60 minutes. Assess vital signs, sputum, and character of respirations for baseline data. Remove dentures, necklaces, earrings, hairpins, and combs. Ensure good oral hygiene. Ensure nothing by mouth 6 to 8 hours beforehand. Confirm that the client is not allergic to any medications that will be given. Administer analgesic, sedative, antianxiety agent, and medication to dry secretions, if ordered.	Assist the physician as required, e.g., to hold the head piece or to move the client's head. Monitor the client's pulse and respirations. Support the client using touch and verbal communication.	1. Monitor vital signs every 30 minutes during the recovery period and compare results to baseline data. 2. Withhold fluids until the gag reflex is restored and the client is conscious. 3. Position the client as ordered or indicated. Place the unconscious client in the lateral position so that secretions are not aspirated. 4. Inspect the client's sputum for blood caused by tissue damage. 5. Observe the client for signs of dyspnea, stridor, and shortness of breath, which may result from laryngeal edema or laryngospasm. 6. Provide ice chips and warm saline gargles or throat lozenges and administer ordered analgesics as required for throat discomfort. 7. Advise the client to contact the physician if client has persistent difficulty with breathing, blood in sputum, fever, or pain.
Esophagoscopy, gastroscopy, and duodenoscopy	As above for bronchoscopy, with the exception of assessing sputum. Explain that the client may feel pressure in the stomach as the tube is moved about and fullness or bloating, like that after eating a large meal.	As above for bronchoscopy. Administer oral simethicone (Mylicon) before test if ordered; it decreases air bubbles in the stomach. If atropine is given intravenously to reduce gastrointestinal spasm, carefully monitor the client's pulse rate. Atropine increases the heart rate.	1. Follow steps 1 to 3 and 6, as for bronchoscopy. 2. Inspect emesis for blood and test it for occult blood if agency practice indicates. 3. Advise the client to contact the physician if client has persistent difficulty swallowing, pain, fever, blood in vomitus, or black stools.
Cystoscopy	Assess vital signs, frequency of urination, dysuria, amount and consistency of urine for baseline data. Administer enema if ordered. A clear bowel is necessary if x-ray films are planned. Ensure nothing by mouth for 6 to 8 hours or only IV fluids if general anesthetic is being given. Ensure appropriate fluid intake, if ordered, for the client having a local anesthetic to ensure an adequate flow of urine for the collection of specimens. Administer sedative and medication to dry secretions, if ordered.	Support the client emotionally. Monitor vital signs. Label specimens, if taken, appropriately. Assist the physician as requested.	1. Monitor vital signs, urination, and urine and compare with baseline data. 2. Position the unconscious client appropriately (as above for bronchoscopy). 3. Inspect the client's urine for blood and report bright red bleeding. 4. Report inability to urinate by 8 hours. 5. Encourage increased fluid intake to decrease irritation of urinary tissue. 6. If dyes were used in the procedure, warn the client that the urine may be an unusual color.

(continued)

some urine in the bladder to enable better visualization. Inform the client to void 4 hours before the procedure and then not to void until after the procedure. If this is difficult for the client, 2 hours without voiding may be acceptable if the client drinks several glasses of fluid before the examination. The client also needs to know that:

1. Mineral oil or water-soluble jelly will be spread over the skin. The oil prevents air from becoming trapped between the probe and the skin and facilitates acoustic contact.
2. The procedure is painless. The client will merely feel the probe moving over the skin.
3. He or she will be asked to change positions on the table to allow visualization of the organ from different angles.
4. During a scan of upper abdominal organs, the client may be asked periodically to inhale deeply and hold the breath for a few seconds. Inspiration displaces upper abdominal organs downward.

Chapter Highlights

- Tests and treatments are frightening for many people; they may fear pain, the findings of the tests, or their reactions to either the pain or the findings.
- The nurse must identify the concerns of the client and provide information and support to alleviate concern.
- Baseline assessment data are collected before the test and compared with the client's responses during and after the test.

- During the procedure, the nurse, if present, is usually the client's primary support person.
- The nurse is responsible for ensuring that specimens taken during the procedure are appropriately labeled, handled, and transported to the laboratory for study.
- Knowledge of the procedure and complications that may arise helps the nurse provide necessary interventions following the procedure to ensure the recovery and safety of the client.

Selected References

Byrne, C. J.; Saxton, D. F.; Pelikan, P. K.; and Nugent, P. M. 1986. *Laboratory tests: Implications for nursing care.* 2d ed. Menlo Park, Calif.: Addison-Wesley Publishing Co.

Contrast radiography fact sheet: Update your knowledge of these contrast radiography studies. August 1984. *Nursing 84* 14:22–23.

Guyton, A. C. 1986. *Textbook of medical physiology.* 7th ed. Philadelphia: W. B. Saunders Co.

Haughey, C. April 1981. Understanding ultrasonography. *Nursing 81* 11:36–40.

Mammography Guidelines. 1983. Background statement and update of cancer related check-up guidelines for breast cancer detection in asymptomatic women age 40 to 49. *Cancer* 33:255.

The Nurses' Reference Library. 1986. *Diagnostics.* 2nd ed. Springhouse, Pa.: Intermed Communications.

Questions and answers about the CT scan exam: Patient education aid. April 15, 1985. *Patient Care* 19:185.

Schuster, P., and Jones, S. November 1982. Preparing the patient for a barium enema: A comparison of nurse and patient opinions. *Journal of Advanced Nursing* 7:523–27.

Supporting Health

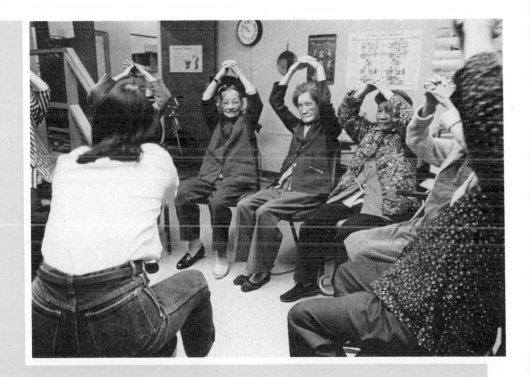

34

Personal Hygiene

OBJECTIVES

Describe kinds of hygienic care nurses provide to clients.

Identify factors influencing personal hygiene.

Identify normal and abnormal findings obtained during inspection and palpation of the skin, feet, nails, mouth, hair, eyes, ears, and nose.

Describe variations in the appearance of the skin, nails, and mucous membranes of light-skinned and dark-skinned clients.

Identify common problems of the skin, feet, nails, mouth, hair, eyes, ears, and nose and formulate related nursing diagnoses.

Describe guidelines for planning and implementing nursing interventions for the skin, feet, nails, mouth, hair, eyes, ears, and nose.

List outcome criteria to evaluate for selected nursing diagnoses.

Identify the purposes of bathing.

Describe various types of baths.

Describe steps in perineal and genital care.

Explain five techniques used in back rubs.

Explain specific ways in which nurses help hospitalized clients with oral hygiene.

Identify steps in inserting and removing contact lenses and artificial eyes.

Describe steps in inserting and removing hearing aids.

Identify safety and comfort measures underlying bed-making procedures.

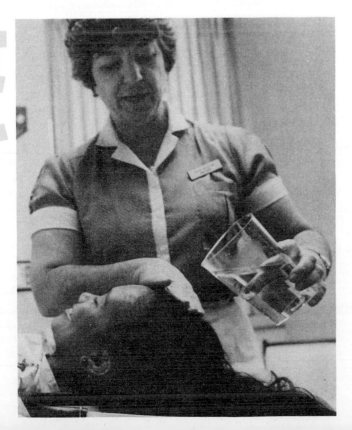

Hygienic Care and Concepts

Hygiene is the science of health and its maintenance. Personal hygiene is the self-care by which people maintain health. Hygiene is a highly personal matter determined by individual values and practices. It is influenced by cultural, social, familial, and individual factors, as well as by the person's knowledge of health and hygiene and perceptions of personal comfort and needs.

When people are ill, hygienic practices frequently become secondary to other functions, such as breathing, which in health are taken for granted. One sign that a formerly ill or depressed client is feeling better is an interest in shaving, hair care, or makeup. Hygiene involves care of the skin, hair, nails, teeth, oral and nasal cavities, eyes, ears, and perineal and genital areas. The purposes of hygiene are summarized in the accompanying box.

People who are very ill often are unable or lack the energy to bathe or brush their teeth, for example. They require assistance to carry out many hygienic activities. It is important for nurses to know exactly how much a client can safely do and how much assistance is required. Clients may require care after urinating or defecating, after vomiting, and whenever they become soiled, e.g., from wound drainage or from profuse perspiration. Nurses must keep the hygiene needs of clients in mind and assist them whenever indicated.

General Guidelines for Care of the Skin

The **normal** skin of a healthy person has transient microorganisms that are not usually harmful. Adults usually have some resident micrococci, bacteria of the genera *Corynebacterium* and *Propionibacterium,* and a genus of fungi, *Pityrosporon.* Children also have gram-positive, spore-forming rods and *Neisseria* bacteria. Transient microorganisms vary considerably from one person to another. They do not maintain themselves on the skin.

In **adolescence,** the sebaceous glands increase in activity as a result of increased levels of hormones

Purposes of Hygiene

Promotes cleanliness, e.g., removes transient microorganisms and body secretions and excretions.
Provides comfort and relaxation, refreshes the client, and relaxes tired, tense muscles.
Improves self-image by improving appearance and eliminating offensive odors.
Conditions skin, e.g., a warm bath causes peripheral vasodilation and thus increases the blood circulation to the skin.

Functions of the Skin

Regulates body temperature.
Protects underlying tissues from drying and injury by preventing the passage of microorganisms. The skin and mucous membrane are considered the body's **first line of defense.**
Secretes sebum, which has antibacterial and antifungal properties.
Transmits sensations through nerve receptors, which are sensitive to pain, temperature, touch, and pressure.

(androgens). This is thought to be one factor responsible for the development of acne, a common skin problem of adolescents. The **older adult** also experiences skin changes. The skin tends to be thinner, drier, somewhat inelastic, and thus subject to fine wrinkling. This process begins any time after age 40. The elderly person's skin typically shows wrinkles, sagging, pigmentations, and keratotic spots, usually on areas exposed to the sun. The skin is less resilient; i.e., when pinched, it returns to place more slowly than the skin of a younger person does. The major functions of the skin are summarized in the accompanying box.

Sudoriferous (sweat) glands are on all body surfaces except the lips and parts of the genitals. The body has from two to five million, which are all present at birth. They are most numerous on the palms of the hands and the soles of the feet. Sweat glands are classified as apocrine and eccrine. The **apocrine glands,** located in the axillae and pubic areas, are of little use. Bacteria act upon the sweat produced by these glands, causing odor. The **eccrine glands** are important physiologically. The sweat they produce cools the body through evaporation. Sweat is made up of water, sodium, potassium, chloride, glucose, urea, and lactate. Guidelines for skin care are summarized in the accompanying box.

Clients at Risk

A number of conditions place **clients at risk** for developing skin impairments. When bathing these clients, the nurse should be especially observant in noting any reddened areas (which might indicate increased pressure over a bony prominence) or blanched areas (indicative of inadequate circulation to the skin tissues). Some common conditions associated with increased incidence of impaired skin integrity are:

▪ *Alterations in nutritional status.* For instance, **emaciation** (a wasted appearance due to extreme weight loss) and insufficient protein intake increase the individual's susceptibility to skin breakdown.

▪ *Immobility.* When position cannot be altered, e.g., if the person is paralyzed or unconscious, or when it is not altered for prolonged periods (1 or 2 hours), blood circulation, which carries essential nutrients to the skin, is reduced.

GUIDELINES

Skin Care

An intact, healthy skin is the body's first line of defense.

The degree to which the skin protects the underlying tissues from injury depends on the general health of the cells, the amount of subcutaneous tissue, and the dryness of the skin.

Moisture in contact with the skin for a period of time can result in increased bacterial growth and irritation.

Body odors are caused by resident skin bacteria acting on body secretions.

Skin sensitivity to irritation and injury varies among individuals and in accordance with their health.

Agents used for skin care have selective actions and purposes. Commonly used agents are described in Table 34–1.

- *Altered hydration.* In dehydrated individuals, the skin becomes excessively dry, and skin turgor is diminished. Both conditions make the skin less resistant to injury.

- *Altered sensation.* Altered sensation reduces a person's ability to discern injurious heat and cold and to feel the tingling (pins and needles) that signals loss of circulation.

- *Presence of secretions or excretions on the skin.* An accumulation of secretions or excretions is irritating to the skin and harbors microorganisms, increasing the risk of infection and impaired skin integrity.

- *Mechanical devices.* Devices such as restraints, casts, or braces create pressure or a shearing force that can alter skin integrity considerably.

Table 34–1 Agents Commonly Used on the Skin

Type	Description
Soap	Lowers surface tension, and thus helps in cleaning. Some soaps contain antibacterial agents, which can change the natural flora of the skin.
Detergent	Used instead of soap for cleaning. Some people who are allergic to soaps may not be allergic to detergents, and vice versa.
Bath oil	Used in bath water; provides an oily film on the skin that softens and prevents chapping.
Skin cream, lotion	Provides a film on the skin that prevents evaporation and therefore chapping.
Powder	Can be used to absorb water and prevent friction. For example, powder under the breasts can prevent skin irritation. Some powders are antibacterial.
Deodorant	Masks or diminishes body odors.
Antiperspirant	Reduces the amount of perspiration.

- *Altered venous circulation.* Stasis of venous blood in the lower extremities (associated with varicose veins) can cause **stasis dermatitis** (inflammation of the skin) on the feet and around the ankles, characterized by redness, dryness, itching, and swelling. Ultimately, skin tissues become **ischemic** (deficient of blood) and **necrotic** (dying), and ulcerations form.

Assessment data indicate whether or not a client has an actual or potential alteration in skin integrity. Examples of nursing diagnoses related to skin problems are shown in the accompanying box. Common skin problems are outlined in Table 34–2.

When planning to assist a client with personal hygiene, the nurse considers the client's personal preferences, health, and limitations; the best time to give care; and the equipment, facilities, and personnel available. Clients' personal preferences—about when and how they bathe, for example—should be followed as long as they are compatible with such factors as clients' health and the equipment available. Nurses need to provide whatever assistance the client requires because of individual limitations. The nurse may provide help directly or delegate this task to other nursing personnel. In some instances, clients say they can perform activities, e.g., shaving, that they should not or cannot do. A man who is accustomed to being clean shaven may feel unkempt when whiskers grow on his face. Moreover, after 2–3 days of whisker growth, the skin of the face can become irritated. Clients who are able to shave themselves should be assisted as needed (e.g., by obtaining equipment or assisting the client to the sink). Clients who are unable to shave themselves may have a family member or friend shave them, or the nurse may do so with either an electric or safety razor. Planning also involves establishing outcome criteria to gauge attainment of established goals and resolution of the client's health problem. For suggestions of outcome criteria for clients with skin problems, see the accompanying box.

Bathing Clients

Bathing has a number of functions. The skin continuously secretes sebum and perspiration, which have protective functions: Sebum prevents dryness, and perspiration makes the skin slightly acid, thus discouraging bacterial growth. Accumulation of sebum, perspiration, and dead skin cells, however, can be injurious or disadvantageous. Excessive perspiration interacts with bacteria on the skin, causing body odor, considered offensive in some cultures.

Overaccumulation of sebum on the skin can be irritating in itself, since it promotes the growth of bacteria. Large numbers of bacteria on the skin can cause problems, particularly when the skin integrity is interrupted, for example, by a cut. Dead skin cells also harbor bacteria. Bathing, then, removes accumulated oil, perspiration, dead skin cells, and some bacteria. Excessive bathing, however, can interfere with the intended lubricating effect of the sebum, causing dryness of the skin.

NURSING DIAGNOSIS

Skin Problems

- Potential impairment of skin integrity related to edema

- Potential impairment of skin integrity related to emaciation

- Potential impairment of skin integrity related to peripheral vascular alterations

- Potential impairment of skin integrity related to radiation

- Potential impairment of skin integrity related to urinary incontinence

- Potential impairment of skin integrity related to imposed immobility

- Potential impairment of skin integrity related to reduced sensation in lower extremities

- Potential impairment of skin integrity related to wound drainage

- Actual impairment of skin integrity (decubitus ulcer) related to immobility

- Actual impairment of skin integrity (dry, cracked skin) related to fever and dehydration

- Actual impairment of skin integrity related to pruritus and scratching

- Actual impairment of skin integrity (stasis ulcer of left leg) related to impaired venous circulation

This is an important consideration for people who produce limited sebum.

In addition to cleaning the skin, bathing also stimulates circulation. A warm or hot bath dilates superficial arterioles, bringing more blood and nourishment to the skin. Vigorous rubbing has the same effect. Rubbing with long smooth strokes from the distal to proximal parts of extremities (from the point farthest from the body to the point closest) is particularly effective in facilitating venous blood flow.

Bathing also produces a sense of well-being. It is refreshing and relaxing and frequently improves morale, appearance, and self-respect. Some people take a morning shower for its refreshing, stimulating effect. Others prefer an evening bath because it is relaxing. These effects are more evident when a person is ill. For example, it is not uncommon for clients who have had a restless or sleepless night to feel relaxed, comfortable, and sleepy after a morning bath.

Bathing offers an excellent opportunity for the nurse to assess ill clients. The nurse can observe the condition of the client's skin and physical conditions such as sacral edema or rashes. While assisting a client with a bath, the nurse can also assess the client's psychosocial needs, e.g., orientation to time and ability to cope with the illness. Learning needs, such as a diabetic client's need to learn foot care, can also be assessed.

There are generally **two categories of baths** given to clients: cleaning and therapeutic. **Cleaning** baths are given chiefly for general hygienic purposes, whereas **therapeutic** baths are given for a specific physical effect, such as to soothe irritated skin or to treat an area (e.g., the perineum). Cleaning baths include:

- *Complete bed bath.* The nurse washes the entire body of a dependent client in bed.

- *Self-help bed bath.* A client confined to bed is able to bathe himself or herself with help from the nurse, e.g., in washing the back and perhaps the feet.

- *Partial bath (abbreviated bath).* Only the parts of the client's body that might cause discomfort or odor, if neglected, are washed: the face, hands, axillae, perineal area, and back. Omitted are the arms, chest, abdomen, legs, and feet. The nurse provides this care for dependent clients and assists self-sufficient clients confined to bed by washing their backs. Some ambulatory clients prefer to take a partial bath at the sink. The nurse can assist them by washing their backs.

- *Tub bath.* Tub baths are preferred to bed baths, since washing and rinsing are easier in a tub. Tubs are also used for therapeutic baths. The amount of assistance offered by the nurse depends on the abilities of the client. Many agencies have specially designed tubs for dependent clients. These tubs greatly reduce the work of the nurse in lifting clients in and out of the tub.

- *Shower.* Many ambulatory clients are able to use shower facilities and require only minimal assistance from the nurse.

OUTCOME CRITERIA

Skin

The client will:

- Have intact, pink, smooth, soft, and hydrated skin

- Have good tissue turgor

- Have warm skin

- Experience less discomfort

- Describe factors, when known, that contribute to skin alterations

- Demonstrate evidence of healing (e.g., reduced size of impairment or amount of drainage)

- Describe hygienic and other interventions to maintain skin integrity

- Describe interventions to prevent specific skin problems

- Express positive statements about sense of well-being

- Participate in prescribed treatment plan to promote wound healing

Table 34–2 Common Skin Problems

Problem and Appearance	Nursing Implications
Abrasion Superficial layers of the skin are scraped or rubbed away. Area is reddened and may have localized bleeding or serous weeping.	1. Prone to infection; therefore, wound should be kept clean and dry. 2. Do not wear rings or jewelry when providing care to avoid causing abrasions to clients. 3. Lift, do not pull, a client across a bed. See Chapter 38.
Excessive dryness Skin can appear flaky and rough.	1. Prone to infection if the skin cracks; therefore, provide lotions to moisturize the skin and prevent cracking. 2. Bathe client less frequently and use no soap or limit use of nonirritating soap. Rinse skin thoroughly because soap can be irritating and drying. 3. Encourage increased fluid intake if health permits to prevent dehydration.
Ammonia dermatitis (diaper rash) Caused by skin bacteria reacting with urea in the urine. The skin becomes reddened and is sore.	1. Keep skin dry and clean by applying protective ointments containing zinc oxide to areas at risk, e.g., buttocks and perineum. 2. Treat by exposing area to the warmth of a 40-watt gooseneck lamp, placed 30 cm (12 inches) away for 30 minutes, three times a day. This warmth helps to dry the rash. 3. Boil an infant's diapers or wash them with an antibacterial detergent to prevent infection. Rinse diapers well, because detergent is irritating to an infant's skin.
Acne Inflammatory condition with papules and pustules.	1. Keep the skin clean to prevent secondary infection. 2. Treatment varies widely.
Erythema Redness associated with a variety of conditions: e.g., rashes, exposure to sun, elevated body temperature.	1. Wash area carefully to remove excess microorganisms. 2. Apply antiseptic spray or lotion to prevent itching, promote healing, and prevent skin breakdown.
Hirsutism Excessive hair on a person's body and face, particularly in women.	1. Remove unwanted hair by using depilatories, shaving, electrolysis, or tweezing. 2. Enhance client's self-concept. See Chapter 48.

A therapeutic bath is usually ordered by a physician. Medications may be placed in the water. A therapeutic bath is generally taken in a tub one-third or one-half full, about 114 liters (30 gal). The client remains in the bath for a designated time, often 20 to 30 minutes. If the client's back, chest, and arms are to be treated, these areas need to be immersed in the solution. The bath temperature is generally included in the order; 37.7 to 46 C (100 to 115 F) may be ordered for adults, and 40.5 C (105 F) is usually ordered for infants. See Table 34–3 for types of therapeutic baths. Procedure 34–1 provides guidelines for bathing clients.

Table 34–3 Types of Therapeutic Baths

Bath Solution	Directions	Uses
Saline	4 ml (1 tsp) sodium chloride (NaCl) to 500 ml (1 pt) water.	Has a cooling effect. Cleans. Decreases skin irritation.
Oatmeal or Aveeno	720 ml (3 cups) cooked oatmeal in a cheesecloth bag. Tie the bag securely and twirl it in the tub until the water is opalescent.	Soothes skin irritations. Softens and lubricates dry, scaly skin.
Cornstarch	0.45 kg (1 lb) cornstarch in sufficient cold water to dissolve it; then add boiling water until the mixture is thick. Add to the tub water.	Soothes skin irritation.
Sodium bicarbonate	4 ml (1 tsp) sodium bicarbonate to 500 ml (1 pt) water, or 120–360 ml (4–12 oz) to 120 liters (30 gal).	Has a cooling effect. Relieves skin irritation.
Potassium permanganate ($KMnO_4$)	Available in tablets, which are crushed, dissolved in a little water, and added to the bath.	Cleans and disinfects. Treats infected skin areas.

who is unconscious and unable to blink can develop corneal abrasions from lack of tears for lubrication. Clients with impaired judgment, e.g., due to psychiatric illness or substance abuse, may develop eye damage from prolonged lens wearing.

Artificial eyes are usually made of glass or plastic. Some are permanently implanted; others are removed regularly for cleaning. Most clients who wear a removable artificial eye follow their own care regimen. Even for an unconscious client, daily removal and cleaning are not necessary. If the nurse notices problems, e.g., redness of the surrounding tissues, drainage from the eye socket, or crusting on the eyelashes, or if the client is scheduled for surgery, the nurse must remove the eye from the socket; clean the eye, the socket, and the surrounding tissues; and then reinsert the eye. Clients whose mobility is impaired by injury or paralysis may also require assistance. In addition, the nurse must determine the client's routine eye care practices so that these can be followed. Some clients may remove and clean the eye and socket daily.

To remove an artificial eye, the nurse dons clean gloves and uses the dominant thumb to pull the client's lower eyelid down over the infraorbital bone, exerting slight pressure below the eyelid to overcome the suction. See Figure 34–12. An alternate method is to compress a small rubber bulb and apply the tip directly to the eye. As the nurse gradually releases the finger pressure on the bulb, the suction of the bulb counteracts the suction holding the eye in the socket and draws the eye out of the socket.

The eye is cleaned with normal saline. If the eye is not to be reinserted, the nurse places it in a container filled with water or saline solution, closes the lid, labels the container with the client's name and room number, and places it in the drawer of the bedside table. The nurse should also clean the socket and tissues around the eye with soft gauze or cotton wipes and normal saline or warm tap water. After inspecting these tissues, the nurse must report and record any abnormal findings. To re-insert the eye, the nurse uses the thumb and index finger of one hand to retract the eyelids, exerting pressure on the supraorbital and infraorbital bones. Holding the eye between the thumb and index fingers of the other hand, the nurse slips the eye gently into the socket. See Figure 34–13.

People may need to be encouraged to avoid home remedies for eye problems. Eye irritations or injuries at any age need to be treated medically and immediately. If dirt or dust gets into the eyes, copious cleaning with clean, tepid water can be used as an emergency treatment. Nurses may need to reinforce **good visual hygiene measures** to prevent eyestrain and protect vision. Among them are use of adequate lighting for reading and appropriate use of glasses when prescribed. Shatterproof lenses are recommended. Middle-aged and older adults

OUTCOME CRITERIA

Eyes

The client will:

- Have clear conjunctiva and white sclera without inflammation
- Have reduced secretions on eyelids
- Experience no tearing
- Experience no eye discomfort
- Express positive feelings about appearance with eye prostheses
- Demonstrate appropriate methods of caring for contact lenses
- Describe interventions to prevent eye injury and infection

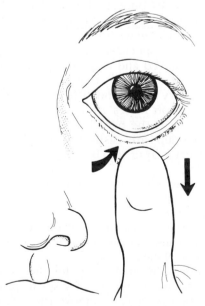

Figure 34–12 When removing an artificial eye, the nurse, wearing a glove, retracts the lower eyelid and exerts slight pressure below the eyelid.

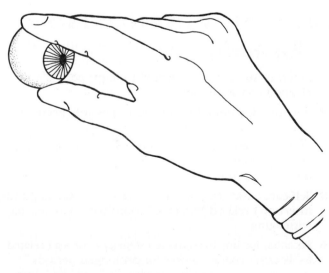

Figure 34–13 An artificial eye is held between the thumb and index finger for insertion.

may need to be reminded of the importance of regular eye examinations to detect **glaucoma** or **cataracts.** Examples of outcome criteria to gauge the achievement of client goals or the effectiveness of nursing intervention are shown in the accompanying box.

▪ Ears

Normal **ears** require minimal hygiene. Clients who have excessive **cerumen** (earwax) and dependent clients who have hearing aids may require assistance from the nurse. While bathing the client, the nurse inspects external ear structures for signs of inflammation, excessive drainage, discomfort, or other obvious abnormalities. If a client wears a hearing aid, the nurse determines:

1. When and where the hearing aid was obtained and from whom
2. How the client maintains and cleans the hearing aid
3. Whether the client experiences problems with the hearing aid
4. What ear problems, if any, the client experiences

Nursing diagnoses related to ear problems are shown in the accompanying box.

The auricles of the ear are cleaned during the bed bath. The nurse or client must remove excessive cerumen that is visible or that causes discomfort or hearing difficulty. Visible cerumen may be loosened and removed by retracting the auricle downward. If this measure is ineffective, irrigation is necessary (see the section on otic irrigation in Chapter 44). Clients need to be advised never to use bobby pins, toothpicks, or cotton-tipped applicators to remove earwax. Bobby pins and toothpicks can injure the ear canal and rupture the tympanic membrane; cotton-tipped applicators can cause wax to become impacted within the canal.

A **hearing aid** is a battery-powered, sound-amplifying device used by hearing-impaired persons. It consists of a microphone that picks up sound and converts it to electric energy, an amplifier that magnifies the electric energy electronically, a receiver that converts the amplified energy back to sound energy, and an earmold that directs the sound into the ear. There are several types of hearing aids:

NURSING DIAGNOSIS

Ear Problems

▪ Potential for injury related to methods used to remove cerumen

▪ Potential for infection related to ineffective practices for cleaning of hearing aid

▪ Potential for impaired verbal communication related to refusal to wear hearing aid

▪ Self-care deficit (hearing aid removal, cleaning, and inserting) related to neuromuscular impairment

▪ Potential for disturbance in self-concept associated with need to wear hearing aid

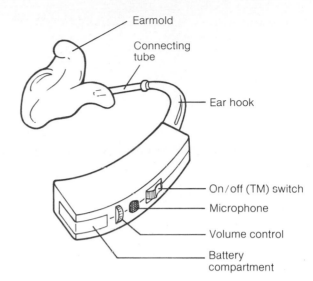

Figure 34–14 A behind-the-ear hearing aid

▪ *Behind-the-ear aid.* This is the most widely used type, since it fits snugly over the ear. The hearing aid case, which holds the microphone, amplifier, and receiver, is attached to the earmold by a plastic tube. See Figure 34–14.

▪ *In-the-ear aid.* This one-piece aid is the most compact hearing aid. All its components are housed in the earmold. See Figure 34–15.

▪ *Eyeglasses aid.* This is similar to the behind-the-ear aid except that the components are housed in the temple of the eyeglasses. A hearing aid can be in one or both temples of the glasses. See Figure 34–16.

▪ *Body hearing aid.* This pocket-sized aid, used for more severe hearing losses, clips onto an undergarment, shirt pocket, or harness carrier supplied by the manufacturer. See Figure 34–17. The case, containing the microphone and amplifier, is connected by a cord to the receiver, which snaps into the earpiece.

To ensure proper functioning, the wearer must handle the hearing aid appropriately during insertion and removal, clean the earmold regularly, and replace dead batteries. Although most clients can look after their hearing aids themselves, some debilitated clients may require assistance. Hearing aids must be removed before surgery.

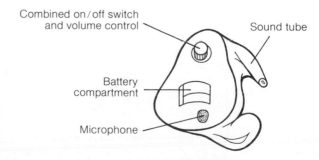

Figure 34–15 An in-the-ear hearing aid

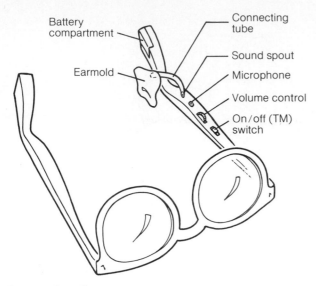

Figure 34–16 An eyeglasses hearing aid

Examples of outcome criteria to gauge the achievement of client goals or the effectiveness of nursing interventions are shown in the accompanying box.

■ Nose

Nurses usually need not provide special care for the **nose** because clients can ordinarily clear nasal secretions by blowing into a soft tissue. However, clients with tubes that exit from the nares or those whose excessive secretions impair breathing may require special assistance.

When a client has a nasogastric tube or any tube exiting from the nares, the nurse inspects the nares, particularly the surfaces in contact with the tube, for signs of inflammation, tenderness, bleeding, and sloughing. Pressure and movement of these tubes can cause

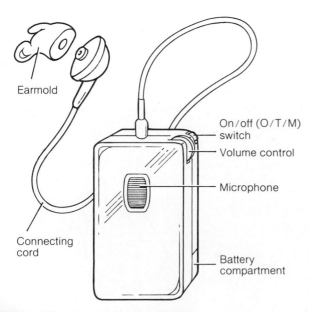

Figure 34–17 A body hearing aid

tissue irritation and damage. Nursing diagnoses related to nose problems are shown in the accompanying box. Excessive nasal secretions can be removed by inserting a cotton-tipped applicator moistened with water or normal saline or by applying suction. A cotton-tipped applicator should not be inserted beyond the length of the cotton tip. Suctioning of the nares is discussed in Chapter 42.

The nares of clients with nasal tubes should be cleaned with a moistened, cotton-tipped applicator to prevent the accumulation of secretions around the tubing. The tape that anchors the tube should be changed when it becomes moist to prevent maceration of the skin and mucous membrane. Methods of taping tubes to minimize their movement are discussed in Chapter 46. Outcome criteria for problems related to the nose are shown in the accompanying box.

■ Supporting a Hygienic Environment

Ill persons are frequently confined to bed, sometimes for weeks or months. The bed then becomes an important piece of furniture, and the client's ability to rest and sleep depends on how comfortable he or she feels in bed. A hospital bed has characteristics particularly suited to people who are in bed continuously or for a long time.

Hospital beds can be adjusted to a variety of positions (see the discussion later in this chapter). Some hospitals use gatch beds. When the gatches, or joints,

OUTCOME CRITERIA

Nose

The client will:

- Have intact nasal mucous membranes
- Have pink nasal mucosa with clear watery discharge
- Experience no tenderness
- Have patent nares

are flexed, the client is raised to a sitting position with the knees elevated. The cranks that operate the gatches are usually at the bottom or side of the bed. When not in use, manual cranks are left in the retracted position under the bed. Otherwise, people walking by the bed might easily hit their legs against the cranks. Increasingly, most hospitals are purchasing beds with electric motors to operate the gatches. The motor is activated by pressing a button or moving a small lever, located either at the side of the bed or on a small panel separate from the bed but attached to it by a cable.

Hospital beds are usually 66 cm (26 in) high and 0.9 m (3 ft) wide, narrower than the usual bed, so that the nurse can reach the client from either side of the bed without undue stretching. The length is usually 1.9 m (6.5 ft). Some beds can be extended in length, if required. Long-term care facilities for ambulatory clients usually have low beds to facilitate movement in and out of bed. Most hospital beds have "high" and "low" positions that can be adjusted either mechanically by a crank at the center of the foot of the bed or electrically by a button or lever on the same panel as the gatch controls. The high position permits the nurse to reach the client without undue stretching or stooping. The low position allows the client to step easily to the floor.

Most **mattresses** used in hospitals have innersprings, which give even support to the body. When changing a bed, nurses need to note any unevenness of the mattress surface, which might indicate a broken spring. Mattresses are usually covered with a water-repellent material that resists soiling and can be cleaned easily. Most mattresses have handles on the sides called lugs by which the mattress can be removed.

Foam rubber **egg crate mattresses** are also used in hospitals. They provide support and have the advantage of relieving pressure on the body's bony prominences, such as the heels. Foam mattresses are particularly helpful for clients confined to bed for a long time. Another option is the **air mattress** (also called an **alternating pressure mattress**), which is attached to a motor that lowers or raises the air pressure inside the mattress.

The **water mattress** is a plastic bag filled with water. This mattress employs the principle of weight displacement. If the body displaces 9 kg (20 lb) of water, there is 9 kg less pressure on the weight-bearing areas. The surfaces of air and water mattresses must be intact so that the air or water will not escape. It is therefore inadvisable to use pins on the sheets covering these mattresses. Special mattresses are placed atop the standard bed mattress, although the water mattress may be placed on the base springs.

Side rails, or safety sides, are used on both hospital beds and stretchers. They are of various shapes and sizes and are usually made of metal. Devices to raise and lower them differ. Often one or two knobs are pulled to release the side and permit it to be moved. When side rails are being used, it is important that the nurse **never** leave the bedside while the rail is lowered. Some side rails have two positions: up and down. Others have three: high, intermediate, and low. The down and low positions are employed when a side rail is not needed. With some models, the bed foundation must be raised before the side rail can be put in the low position; otherwise, the side rail might hit the floor and be damaged. The intermediate position is used when the bed is in the low position and the nurse is present. The up or high side rail position is used when a client is in bed and requires protection from falling.

A **footboard** is a flat panel, often made of wood or plastic, placed at the foot of a bed. It serves three purposes:

1. To provide support for the client's feet and maintain a natural foot position while the client is in bed. See Figure 34–18.
2. To keep the top bed covers off the client's feet, relieving the pressure of the weight of the covers.
3. To make the foot comfortable (for example, when a client has a painful foot).

Without the support of a footboard, a client's feet drop from their normal right angle to the legs and assume a plantar flexion position with the toes pointing toward the foot of the bed. See Figure 34–19. Prolonged assumption of this position results in permanent shortening of the muscles and tendons at the back of the legs. When that happens, the client is unable to stand flat-footed on the floor, and walking is seriously impaired.

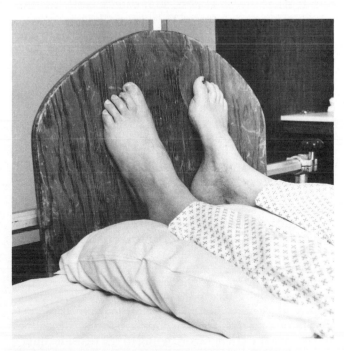

Figure 34–18 A footboard maintains dorsiflexion

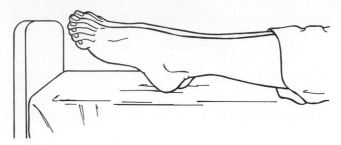

Figure 34–19 Feet in plantar flexion

A **bed cradle,** sometimes called an Anderson frame, is a device designed to keep the top bedclothes off the feet, legs, and even abdomen of a client. The bedclothes are arranged over the device and may be pinned in place. There are several types of bed cradles. One of the most common is a curved metal rod that fits over the bed. Part of the cradle fits under the mattress, and small metal brackets press down on each side of the mattress to keep the cradle in place. The frame of some cradles extends over only half of the bed, above only one leg.

Intravenous rods (poles, stands, standards), usually made of metal, support intravenous (IV) infusion containers while fluid is being administered to a client. These rods were traditionally freestanding on the floor beside the bed. Now, intravenous rods are often attached to the hospital beds. Some hospital units have overhead hanging rods on a track for IVs.

A small table placed beside the bed frequently has a drawer for the client's personal articles and below that a cupboard containing a washbasin, soap dish and soap, mouthwash container, and emesis or kidney basin. Some **bedside tables** also have a place for a bedpan or urinal and a rod at the back for washcloths and towels. The **overbed table** stands on the floor but fits over the client's bed. It is usually on casters, so it can be easily moved. It can be raised or lowered to suit the client, usually by turning a handle at the side. Some overbed tables have a mirror and a small compartment for personal articles beneath the table top. Overbed tables are often used for the client's meal tray. A client who can assume a sitting position in bed can eat from that table in relative comfort. Nurses also use these tables for necessary supplies for treatments.

Most bed units have **chairs** for client and visitor use. Hospital bed units generally contain a **locker** or **closet** for the storage of clothes. These facilities are usually larger in a long-term care unit than in an acute care setting. Some units also have a chest of drawers or other drawer space for clothing.

Each bed unit has one or more **lights.** At the head of the bed, there is often a movable light with an extendable neck. Some rooms have overhead lights as well. Bed units also have a signal light. When a client pulls a switch or presses a button, a light goes on at the nurses' station. Clients generally turn on their signal lights when they require assistance. Some acute hospitals are equipped with intercoms that permit a nurse at the nursing station to talk with the client before going to the bedside. Intercom signal lights can also be turned off from the nurse's

station. Nursing units generally have subdued night lighting.

Hospitals vary in the equipment provided as part of the bed unit. Long-term care facilities may have very little additional equipment; an acute care facility may have several commonly used devices built into each unit. Three types of equipment are often installed on the wall at the head of the bed: a **suction outlet** for several kinds of suction, an **oxygen outlet** for most oxygen equipment, and a **sphygmomanometer** to measure the client's blood pressure.

Some long-term care agencies also permit clients to have **personal** equipment, such as a television, a chair, and lamps, at the bedside. A number of specialized beds are manufactured to meet the individualized needs of clients and may be ordered by the physician as part of the prescribed regimen. Among these are the Stryker wedge frame, the CircOlectric bed, and the Clinitron bed. The Stryker wedge frame, which is manually operated by the nurse, turns the client laterally through the side-lying position. The CircOlectric bed, which is operated electrically by the nurse using a push button, rotates the client vertically through the standing position. The Clinitron bed is similar in principle to the flotation and air mattresses. It is especially useful for clients extensive burns, arthritis, and pressure sores who require position changes that cannot be effectively managed in the standard bed.

■ Bed Positions

When the bed is in the **flat** position, the mattress is completely horizontal. Pillows may or may not be used. **Fowler's** position is a semisitting (head of the bed is raised to at least 45°) bed position frequently used in hospitals. It gives clients relief from the lying positions and is convenient for eating and reading. In **Trendelenburg's** position, the head of the bed is lowered and the foot of the bed is elevated in a straight incline. See Figure 34–20. If the foundation cannot be raised mechanically, this position may be obtained by placing blocks or special pins under the foot of the bed. The blocks are often referred to as shock blocks, because this position was used some years ago for clients in shock. It is now con-

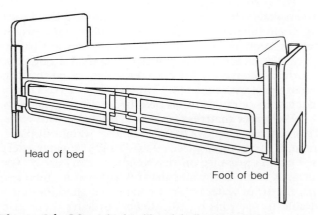

Head of bed

Foot of bed

Figure 34–20 A bed in Trendelenburg's position

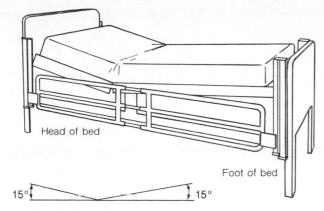

Figure 34—21   A bed in contour position

traindicated for clients suffering from head injuries, respiratory distress, chest injuries, or shock. Currently it is used for some postural drainage.

Reverse Trendelenburg's position is a straight tilt in the opposite direction: The head of the bed is elevated, and the foot of the bed is lowered. Sometimes the legs at the head of the bed are raised by blocks or by pins if the foundation cannot be raised mechanically. This position may be used for clients experiencing problems with arterial circulation to the legs.

In the **contour** bed position, both the head and foot of the bed are elevated about 15°. See Figure 34—21. It is necessary to raise both the knee and the foot sections of some hospital beds to obtain this position. For the **hyperextension** bed position, both the head and the foot sections are lowered 15°. See Figure 34—22. This position is sometimes used for clients with spinal fractures. It should be used only with specific orders and continuous nursing assessment of the client is important. Not all hospital beds can be adjusted to this position.

■ Making Beds

Nurses need to be able to prepare hospital beds in different ways for specific purposes. In most instances, beds are made after the client receives certain care and

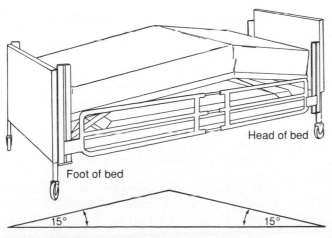

Figure 34—22   A bed in hyperextension position

when beds are unoccupied. At times, however, nurses need to make an occupied bed or prepare a bed for a client who is having surgery.

Regardless of what type of bed equipment is available, whether the bed is occupied or unoccupied, or the purpose for which the bed is being prepared, certain guidelines pertain to all bed making. These are summarized in the accompanying box.

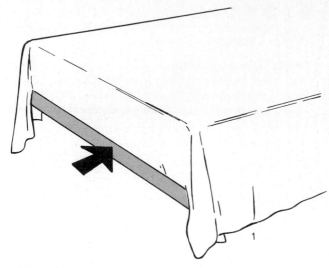

Figure 34–23

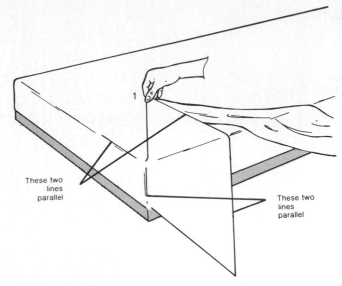

These two lines parallel

These two lines parallel

Figure 34–24

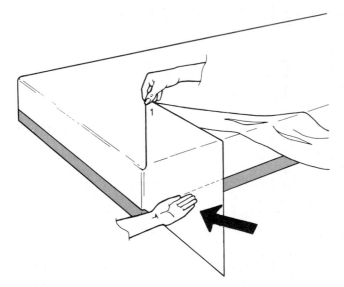

Figure 34–25

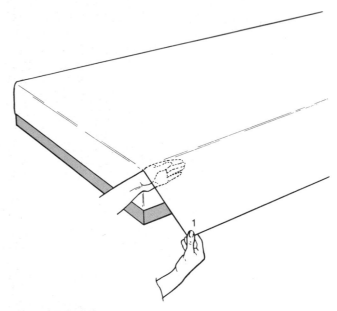

Figure 34–26

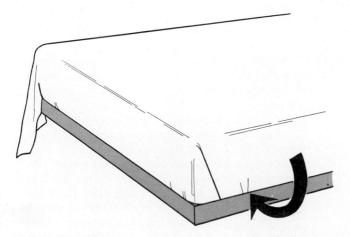

Figure 34–27

An **unoccupied bed** can be either closed or open. Generally the top covers of an open bed are folded back (**open bed**) to make it easier for a client to get in. Open and closed beds are made the same way, except that the top sheet, blanket, and bedspread of a **closed** bed are drawn up to the top of the bed and under the pillows.

Procedure 34–5 explains how to change an unoccupied bed.

Hospital beds are often changed after bed baths. The linen can be collected before the bath. Nurses in some hospitals do not change all the linen unless it is soiled. Check the policy at each clinical agency.

PROCEDURE 34–5

Changing an Unoccupied Bed

Equipment

- A mattress pad, if used. Some agencies do not use pads, so check agency practice. Some mattress pads are attached to the bed by elastic or ties at the corners. Some lie freely on the mattress.

- Two large sheets. Fitted sheets, which do not require mitering, are being used increasingly in hospitals.

- A cloth drawsheet (optional) to protect the bottom sheet from soiling or to help lift or move the client.

- One blanket.

- One bedspread.

- Waterproof pads (optional) to place under the client at points where drainage is expected.

- Two pillowcases for the two head pillows. Additional pillowcases may be needed if additional pillows are used.

- Portable linen hamper for the soiled linen, if available.

Intervention

1. Place the fresh linen on the client's chair or overbed table; do not use another client's bed.
   Rationale It is important to prevent cross-contamination (the movement of microorganisms from one client to another) via soiled linen.

2. Make sure that this is an appropriate and convenient time for the client to be out of bed.

3. Assess the client's health status to determine that he or she can safely get out of bed. In some hospitals it is necessary to have a written order if the client has been in bed continuously.

4. Assess the client's pulse, respirations, and present health status if the client's health indicates.

5. Assist the client to a comfortable chair.

Stripping the Bed

6. Starting at the head of the bed, on the side nearer the clean linen, loosen the bedding, including the foundation, moving down the bed, working around the foot, and moving up to the other side of the head. Remove the call signal, if it is attached to the linen.

7. Return to the first side.

8. Remove the pillowcases, if soiled, and place the pillows on the bedside chair near the foot of the bed. The bedside chair can be used to hold bedding that can be reused.

9. Using both hands, grasp the top edge of the spread, one hand at the center, the other at the mattress edge. Fold it in half by bringing the top edge even with the bottom edge.

Rationale Linens folded this way are readily reapplied to the bed later. If the spread is soiled, place it in the linen hamper, if the agency has portable linen hampers that can be taken to the bed unit. If the agency has a central disposal chute for linen, tuck in the soiled spread at the foot of the bed, and collect all the soiled linen here to take to the chute. Take care to prevent soiled bed linen from touching your uniform or the clean linen.
Rationale The uniform can become soiled and transmit microorganisms to other clients.

10. If the spread is not soiled, pick it up carefully by grasping it at the center of the middle fold and the bottom edges. See Figure 34–28.
    Rationale It is useful to fold the spread in such a way that it can be readily reapplied.

11. Lay the spread over the back of the bedside chair if it is to be reused.

12. Repeat steps 9–11, first for the blanket and then for the top sheet.

13. Remove waterproof pad and discard if soiled.

14. Pick up the cotton drawsheet at the center of the top and bottom edges, and lay it over the back of the bedside chair or, if soiled, discard it in the hamper.

15. Repeat steps 9–11 for the bottom sheet, if it is to be changed.

16. Grasp the mattress lugs and, using good body mechanics, move the mattress up to the head of the bed. If there are no lugs, grasp the lower edge of the mattress. See Figure 34–29.

Head of bed

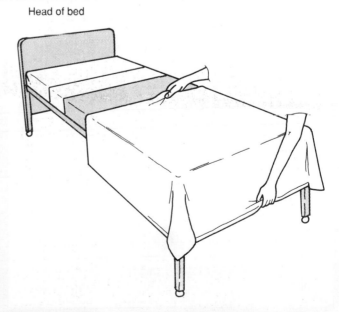

Figure 34–28

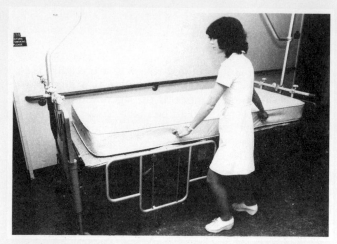

Figure 34—29

Making the Bed

17. Standing at the same side of the bed as the linen supply, place the mattress pad on the bed.

18. Smooth the mattress pad so that it is free of wrinkles.
Rationale Wrinkles can irritate the client's skin and feel uncomfortable.

19. Working from the foot of the bed, place the bottom sheet, folded into four layers, on the bed so that the vertical center fold of the sheet is at the center line of the mattress and the bottom edge of the sheet extends about 2.5 cm (1 in.) over the end of the mattress.
Rationale Unless a contour sheet is used, the sheet is not tucked in at the foot of the bed so that it can be changed without removing the top bedcovers. Make sure that the hem of the sheet is facing down.
Rationale The hem edge can be irritating to the client's skin. Open the sheet across the bottom of the bed, and then pull the top layer up to the top of the bed so that the sheet is fully spread. (Agency practice may vary on methods of folding and spreading sheets on beds. This is one common method. In some agencies the sheet is spread over only one side of the bed at a time.)

20. Move to the head of the bed on the same side. Tuck the excess sheet under the mattress at the near side of the head of the bed. If a contour sheet is used, fit it under the corner of the mattress.

21. Miter the sheet at the top corner on that side, and tuck the sheet under the mattress side, working from the head of the bed to the foot.

22. Lay the cloth drawsheet on the bed, folded in half, with the center fold at the center line of the bed. Fanfold the uppermost half of the drawsheet at the center of the bed. Place the top edge of the drawsheet 30–37 cm (12–15 in.) from the head of the bed.

23. Tuck in the drawsheet on the near side.

24. Place waterproof pad, if needed, on bed where the client's buttocks will be.

25. Move to the opposite side of the bed.

26. Starting at the head of the bed, tuck the excess bottom sheet under the head of the mattress.

27. Pulling the sheet firmly, miter the side corner at the head of the bed or fit a contour sheet under the mattress corner.

28. Tuck in the bottom sheet, working toward the foot of the bed. Pull the sheet firmly so that there are no wrinkles in it.

29. Pull the cotton drawsheet firmly and tuck it in at the side.

30. Return to the first side of the bed. The foundation of the bed is now complete.

31. Place the top sheet on the bed so that the vertical center fold is at the center line of the bed, the top edge is even with the top edge of the mattress, and the hems of the sheet will be facing up when unfolded.
Rationale With the hems facing up, the edges of the sheet will not rub against the client's skin.

32. Spread the sheet over the bed as described in step 19 or according to agency practice.

33. Tuck in the sheet at the bottom of the bed on the near half (optional).

34. Make either a vertical or a horizontal toe pleat in the sheet:
 a. *Vertical toe pleat:* Standing at the foot of the bed, make a fold in the sheet 5–10 cm (2–4 in.), perpendicular to the foot of the bed. See Figure 34–30. Tuck in the end of the sheet at the foot of the bed. See Figure 34–31.
 b. *Horizontal toe pleat:* Make a fold in the sheet 5–10 cm (2–4 in.), across the bed, 15–20 cm (6–8 in.) from the foot. Tuck in the sheet at the foot. See Figure 34–32.
 Rationale A toe pleat provides additional room for the client's feet. It is an optional comfort measure. Additional toe space can also be provided by loos-

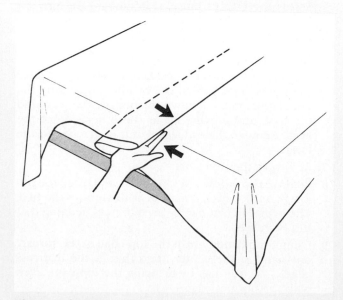

Figure 34—30

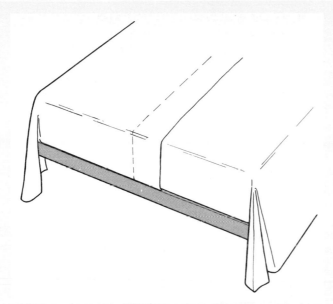

Figure 34–31

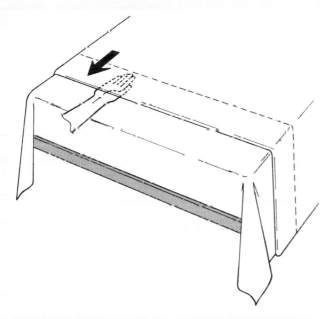

Figure 34–32

ening the top covers around the feet after the client is in bed.

35. Place the blanket on the bed so that the top edge is about 15 cm (6 in.) from the head of the bed and the center fold is at the center of the bed.
Rationale This allows a cuff of sheet to be folded over the blanket and spread.

36. Tuck in the blanket at the foot of the bed on the near side. Make a toe pleat if needed. See step 34.

37. Put the bedspread on the bed so that the center fold is at the center of the bed and the top edge extends about 2.5 cm (1 in.) beyond the blanket. Tuck the top edge of the spread under the top edge of the blanket.

38. Fold the top of the top sheet down over the spread, providing a cuff of about 15 cm (6 in.). Smooth the

spread, working from the top to the foot of the bed.
Rationale The cuff of sheet protects the client's face from rubbing against the blanket or bedspread, thus preventing skin irritation.

39. Tuck in the spread at the foot of the bed on the near side.

40. Miter the bottom corner of the bed, using all three layers of linen (top sheet, blanket, and spread). See Technique 12–3. Leave the sides of the top sheet, blanket, and spread hanging freely.
Rationale Mitering makes the corner of the bed-clothes secure even though they are left hanging freely to permit easy access by the client.

41. Walk around the foot of the bed to the far side, pulling the blanket and spread over the bed. Work toward the head of the bed on the second side.

42. Fold the remainder of the spread under the top of the blanket. Fold the remainder of the top sheet over the spread to make a cuff.

43. Going to the foot of the bed, tuck in the top sheet, blanket, and spread at the bottom of the bed on the second side. Maintain the toe pleat if one was made.

44. Miter this corner as in step 40.

45. Moving to the first side of the bed, put clean pillowcases on the pillows:
    a. Grasp the closed end of the pillowcase at the center with one hand.
    b. Gather up the sides of the pillowcase, and place them over the hand grasping the case. Then grasp the center of one short side of the pillow through the pillowcase. See Figure 34–33.
    c. With the free hand, pull the pillowcase over the pillow.
    d. Adjust the pillowcase so that the pillow fits into the corners of the case and the seams are straight.

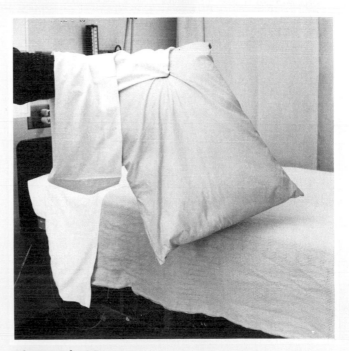

Figure 34–33

Rationale A smoothly fitting pillowcase is more comfortable than a wrinkled one.

46. Place the pillows at the head of the bed in the center, with the open ends of the pillowcases facing away from the door of the room.
Rationale This provides a neat appearance.

47. Attach the signal cord so that the client can conveniently use it. Some cords have clamps that attach to the sheet or pillowcase. Others are attached by a safety pin.

48. If the bed is currently being used by a client, either fold back the top covers at one side or fanfold them down to the center of the bed.
Rationale This makes it easier for the client to get into the bed.

49. Put the bedside table and the overbed table in order so that they are available to the client.

50. Leave the bed in the high position if the client is returning by stretcher or place in the low position if client is returning to bed after being up.

51. Document assessment data. Bed making is not normally recorded.

When changing an occupied bed, the nurse must work quickly and disturb the client as little as possible. Guidelines for changing an occupied bed are listed in the accompanying box.

A **surgical** bed is made for clients who are having surgical or diagnostics procedures that require use of an anesthetic agent. See Chapter 46 for information about how to prepare a surgical bed.

GUIDELINES

Changing an Occupied Bed

1. Maintain the client in good body alignment. Never move or position a client in a manner that is contraindicated by his or her health. Obtain help if necessary to ensure safety.

2. Move the client gently and smoothly. Rough handling can cause the client discomfort and abrade the skin.

3. Throughout the procedure, explain what you plan to do before you do it. Use terms that the client can understand.

4. Use the bed-making time, like the bed bath time, to assess and meet the client's needs.

5. Leave the top sheet over the client (the top sheet can remain over the client if it is being discarded and if it will provide sufficient warmth) *or* replace it with a bath blanket as follows:
   ▪ Spread the bath blanket over the top sheet.
   ▪ Ask the client to hold the top edge of the blanket.
   ▪ Reaching under the blanket from the side, grasp the top edge of the sheet and draw it down to the foot of the bed, leaving the blanket in place.
   ▪ Remove the sheet from the bed and place it in the soiled linen hamper.

6. Assist the client to turn on his or her side facing away from the side where the clean linen is. Raise the side rail nearest the client.

7. Loosen the foundation linen on the side of the bed near the linen supply. Fanfold the drawsheet and the bottom sheet at the center of the bed, as close to the client as possible.

8. Smooth the mattress pad, if it is to be retained. If not, fanfold it, and place a new pad on the bed, with the center fold at the center of the bed and the uppermost half fanfolded at the center.

9. Place the new bottom sheet on the bed and vertically fanfold the half to be used on the far side of the bed at the center.

10. Place the clean drawsheet on the bed with the center fold at the center of the bed. The drawsheet should extend from midway down the client's back to midway down the thighs. Fanfold the uppermost half vertically at the center of the bed and tuck the near side edge under the side of the mattress.

11. Assist the client to roll over toward you onto the clean side of the bed. The client rolls over the fanfolded linen at the center of the bed.

12. Move the pillows to the clean side for the client's use. Raise the side rail before leaving the side of the bed.

13. Move to the other side of the bed and lower the side rail.

14. Remove the used linen and place in the portable hamper.

15. Smooth out the mattress cover to remove any wrinkles. Unfold the fanfolded bottom sheet from the center of the bed.

16. Facing the side of the bed, use both hands to pull the bottom sheet so that it is smooth, and tuck the excess under the side of the mattress. See Figure 34–34.

17. Unfold the drawsheet fanfolded at the center of the bed, and pull it tightly with both hands. Pull the sheet in three sections:
    ▪ Face the side of the bed to pull the middle section.
    ▪ Face the far top corner to pull the bottom section.
    ▪ Face the far bottom corner to pull the top section.

18. Tuck the excess drawsheet under the side of the mattress.

19. Reposition the pillows at the center of the bed.

20. Assist the client to the center of the bed. Determine what position the client requires or prefers, and assist him or her to that position.

21. Raise the side rails and place the bed in the low position before leaving the bedside.

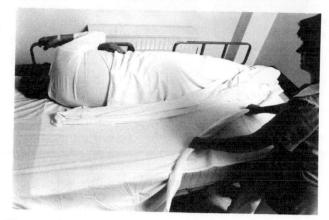

Figure 34–34

Chapter Highlights

Clients' hygiene is influenced to a large degree by their sociocultural background.

When people become ill, hygiene is often of secondary importance to vital body needs, such as breathing and rest.

When a client cannot meet his or her hygiene needs, the nurse usually assumes them.

The major functions of the skin are to help regulate body temperature, to protect underlying tissues, to secrete sebum, to contain nerve receptors that act in sensory perception.

While assisting a client with hygiene measures, the nurse has an opportunity to assess the client's health.

While planning hygiene care, the nurse must take the client's preferences into consideration.

The back rub is an essential part of hygiene care for clients confined to bed.

Nurses provide perineal-genital care for clients who are unable to do so for themselves.

Nurses can often teach clients how to prevent foot problems.

Oral hygiene should include daily dental flossing and mechanical brushing of the teeth.

Nurses provide special oral care to clients who are helpless, e.g., unconscious, and who have oral problems.

Hair care includes daily combing and brushing and regular shampooing.

Nurses may need to assist helpless clients with their artificial eyes, eyeglasses, and contact lenses.

The deaf client may require nursing assistance with his or her hearing aid.

Changing beds is a part of maintaining hygiene.

It is important to keep beds clean and comfortable for clients.

Selected References

Bates, B. 1987. *A guide to physical examination.* 4th ed. Philadelphia: J. B. Lippincott Co.

Bowers, A. C., and Thompson, J. M. 1988. *Clinical manual of health assessment.* 3d ed. St. Louis: C. V. Mosby Co.

Eliopoulos, C., editor. 1984. *Health assessment of the older adult.* Menlo Park, Calif.: Addison-Wesley Publishing Co.

Holder, L. April 1982. Hearing aids: Handle with care. *Nursing 82* 12:64–67.

Martin, B. J., and Reeb, R. M. November/December 1982. Oral health during pregnancy: A neglected nursing area. *American Journal of Maternal and Child Nursing* 7:391–92.

Norman, S. April 1982. The pupil check. *American Journal of Nursing* 82:588–91.

Osguthorpe, N. C. October 1984. If your patient has contact lenses. *American Journal of Nursing* 84:1255–56.

Roach, L. B. January 1977. Color changes in dark skin. *Nursing 77* 7:48–51.

Schaeffer, A. M. May/June 1982. Nursing measures to maintain foot health. *Geriatric Nursing* 3:182–83.

Smiler, I. May/June 1982. Foot problems of elderly diabetics. *Geriatric Nursing* 3:177–81.

Todd, B. March/April 1982. Drugs and the elderly: Dry mouth—causes and cures. *Geriatric Nursing* 3(2):122–23.

Wells, R., and Trostle, K. January 1984. Creative hairwashing techniques for immobilized patients. *Nursing 84* 14:47–51.

Zucnick, M. M. May 1975. Care of an artificial eye. *American Journal of Nursing* 75:835.

Disuse osteoporosis is a result of lack of weight-bearing, decreased muscular activity, and complex endocrine and metabolic disturbances that accompany bed rest. During immobility, increased amounts of calcium are extracted from the bone, resulting in a significant decrease in bone mass. Studies demonstrate that bone **demineralization** starts in the second or third day of immobilization; there is measurable calcium loss from bone after 2 weeks of bed rest (Mitchell and Laustau 1981, p. 355). The bone becomes porous and brittle and can fracture easily. Demineralization occurs regardless of the amount of calcium in the person's diet.

Fibrosis (an increase in the amount of fibrous connective tissue) and **ankylosis** (fixation) of joint structures occur whenever joints are not moved normally. The flexor muscles of an immobilized person, because they are strong, often remain contracted for long periods, and the weaker extensors are not used. In turn, the fibrous muscle tissue that covers the joint is gradually replaced by connective tissue, and the joint becomes increasingly stiff and painful.

The problem may be exacerbated by the deposition of excessive amounts of calcium in the soft tissues around the joint. In time, the joint may become irreversibly deformed and ankylosed, and the muscles that cover the joint may permanently shorten into a **contracture.** The most common are flexion contractures of the lower extremities: hips, knees, and the plantar flexors of the ankles. The position that the client most consistently assumes in bed and wheelchair is mirrored when the person eventually is able to stand and walk. The result is a stooped "wheelchair" posture. The client's heels cannot rest flat on the floor, making ambulation difficult or impossible.

Cardiovascular

Prolonged immobility weakens the **cardiovascular system,** which cannot respond adequately to meet the demands placed on it. Decreased mobility creates an imbalance in the autonomic nervous system, resulting in a preponderance of sympathetic activity over cholinergic activity that increases heart rate. Resting heart rate increases approximately 0.5 beats/minute per each day of immobilization (Kottke et al. 1982, p. 210).

In a mobile, active person with a slow heart rate, the diastolic phase of the cardiac cycle is longer than the systolic phase. Since blood flow through coronary vessels occurs primarily during the diastolic phase, there is sufficient time for adequate blood flow through the coronary arteries. During immobility, however, the rapid heart rate reduces diastolic pressure, coronary blood flow, stroke volume, and the capacity of the heart to respond to any metabolic demands above basal levels. Due to this diminished cardiac reserve, the immobilized person may experience tachycardia and angina with even minimal exertion. Bedfast clients tend to use the **Valsalva maneuver,** during which the person takes a deep breath and strains against a closed glottis as he or she turns and moves about in bed. The Valsalva maneuver markedly increases intrathoracic pressure, which is followed by a marked increase in the volume of blood within the heart and possible arrhythmias when the glottis is again opened. When the heart has marginal reserves, the client may have difficulty coping with this additional stress.

Orthostatic (postural) hypotension is a common sequel of immobilization. Due to sympathetic nervous system activity, automatic vasoconstriction occurs in the blood vessels in the lower half of the body when a mobile person changes from a horizontal to a vertical posture. Vasoconstriction prevents pooling of the blood in the legs and effectively maintains central blood pressure to ensure adequate perfusion of the heart and brain. During prolonged immobility, this reflex becomes dormant. When the immobilized person attempts to sit or stand, this reconstricting mechanism fails to function properly in spite of increased adrenaline output. The blood pools in the lower extremities, and central blood pressure drops. Cerebral perfusion is seriously compromised, and the person feels dizzy or lightheaded and may even faint. This sequence is usually accompanied by a sudden and marked increase in heart rate, the body's effort to protect the brain from an inadequate blood supply.

The skeletal muscles of an active person contract with each movement, compressing the blood vessels in those muscles and helping to pump the blood back to the heart against gravity. The tiny valves in the leg veins, which remain constricted, aid in venous return to the heart by preventing backward flow of blood and pooling. In an immobilized person, the skeletal muscles do not contract sufficiently, and the muscles atrophy. The skeletal muscles can no longer assist in pumping blood back to the heart against gravity. Blood pools in the leg veins, causing vasodilation and engorgement. The valves in the veins can no longer work effectively to prevent backward flow of blood and pooling (see Figure 35–3). This phenomenon is known as **incompetent valves.**

As the blood continues to pool in the veins, its greater volume increases venous blood pressure, which can become much higher than that exerted by the tissues surrounding the vessel. When the venous pressure is sufficiently great, some of the serous part of the blood is forced out of the blood vessel into the interstitial spaces surrounding the vessel, causing **edema.** Edema is most common in parts of the body positioned below heart level and maintained in that position. It is most likely to occur around the sacrum or heels of a client who sits up in bed or in the feet and lower legs of a client who sits on the side of the bed. Edema further impedes venous return of blood to the heart, causing more pooling and more edema. Edematous tissue is uncomfortable and more susceptible to injury than normal tissue.

Three factors, known as **Virchow's triad,** collectively predispose a client to the formation of a **thrombophlebitis** (a clot that is loosely attached to an inflamed vein wall). These are impaired venous return to the heart, hypercoagulability of the blood, and injury to a vessel wall. Although prolonged immobility has not clearly been shown to slow **venous return** in most persons, it is a significant factor in the **immobile elderly**

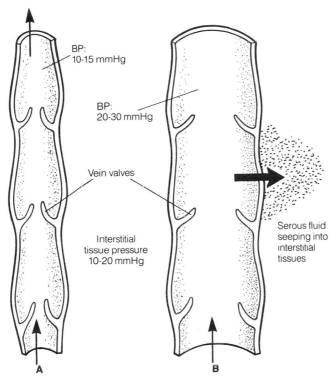

Figure 35–3 Leg veins: **A**, in a mobile person; **B**, in an immobilized person

who are paralyzed, have heart disease, or have had recent surgery (Kottke et al. 1982, p. 969; Patrick et al. 1986, p. 623). **Hypercoagulability** due to a disturbance in the clotting mechanism or to decreased blood volume may be a factor in immobilized persons as it is in post-operative clients. **Injury to vein walls** can occur as a result of atherosclerotic plaque formation due to aging or sustained pressure against a leg due to improper body alignment and immobility.

A thrombus is particularly dangerous if it breaks loose from the vein wall to enter the general circulation as an **embolus.** At least 15% of deep vein thrombi do migrate (Fahey 1984, p. 36). Large emboli that enter the pulmonary circulation may occlude the vessels that supply the lungs and cause an infarcted (dead) area of the lung. If the infarcted area is large, pulmonary function may be seriously compromised, or death may ensue. Emboli traveling to the coronary vessels or brain can produce a similarly dangerous outcome.

■ Respiratory

An upright, mobile person has no impediments against the chest wall to restrict respiratory movement. During normal activity, the person periodically sighs, maximally inhaling or forcefully exhaling to expand the alveoli fully and allow effective gaseous exchange. Mucus, normally present in the respiratory tract, is loosened by movement and removed from the bronchi by ciliary action and coughing.

In a recumbent, immobilized client, ventilation of the lungs is passively altered. The rigid bed presses against the body and curtails chest movement. The abdominal

organs push against the diaphragm, further restricting chest movement and making it difficult to expand the lungs fully. An immobilized, recumbent person rarely sighs, partly because overall muscle atrophy also affects the respiratory muscles and partly because there is no need to do so without the stimulus of activity. Without these periodic stretching movements, the cartilaginous intercostal joints may become fixed in an expiratory phase of respiration, further restricting the potential for maximal ventilation (Kottke et al. 1982, p. 970). These changes produce shallow respirations and reduce vital capacity significantly. An immobilized, paralyzed client can lose as much as 25 to 50% of normal vital capacity (Kottke et al. 1982, p. 970).

Blood flow through the lungs is also passively altered by the client's horizontal position, due primarily to the effects of gravity. The dependent parts of the lung, tightly sandwiched between the bed with the body's weight on top, expand less effectively with each respiration. These dependent areas are least effectively ventilated, yet blood tends to pool there. The result is reduced gaseous exchange. Poor oxygenation and retention of carbon dioxide in the blood can, if allowed to continue, predispose the person to respiratory acidosis, a potentially lethal disorder. See Figure 35–4.

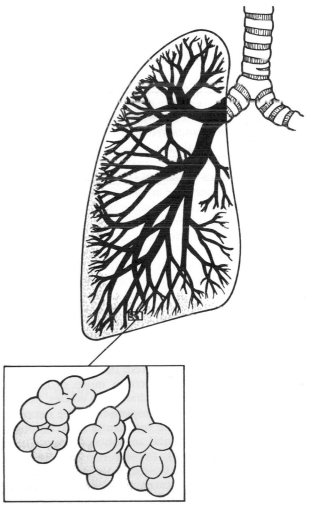

Figure 35–4 Pooling of secretions in the lungs of an immobilized person

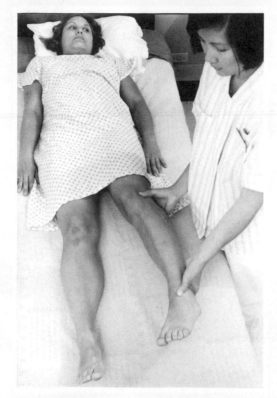

Figure 35–27

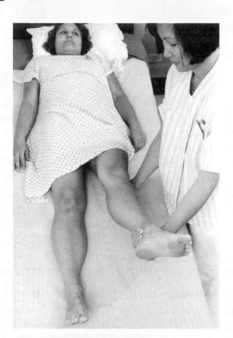

Figure 35–28

Place one hand over the arch of the foot to push the foot away from the leg. Place the fingers of the other hand under the toes, to bend the toes upward (see Figure 35–32), and then over the toes, to push the toes downward (see Figure 35–33).

Neck Movement

Remove the client's pillow.

19. *Flex and extend the neck:* Place the palm of one hand under the client's head and the palm of the

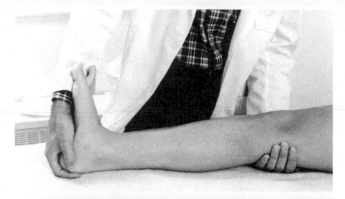

Figure 35–29

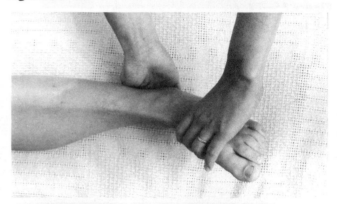

Figure 35–30

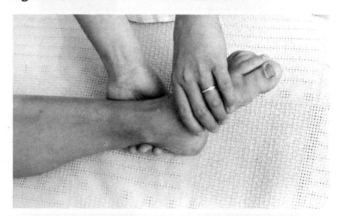

Figure 35–31

other hand on the client's chin. Move the head forward until the chin rests on the chest, then back to the resting supine position without the head pillow. See Figure 35–34.

20. *Laterally flex the neck:* Place the heels of the hands on each side of the client's cheeks. Move the top of the head to the right and to the left. See Figure 35–35.

Hyperextension Movements

21. Assist the client to a prone or lateral position on the side of the bed nearest the nurse.

22. *Hyperextend the shoulder:* Place one hand on the shoulder to keep it from lifting off the bed and the other under the client's elbow. Pull the upper arm up and backward. See Figure 35–36.

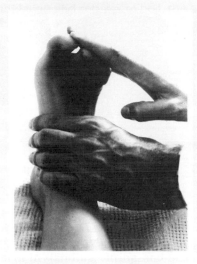

Figure 35–32

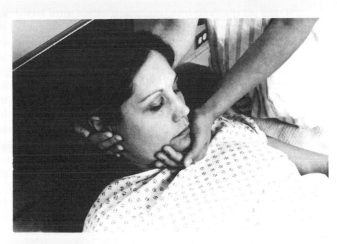

Figure 35–34

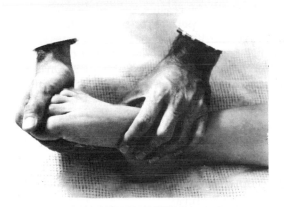

Figure 35–33

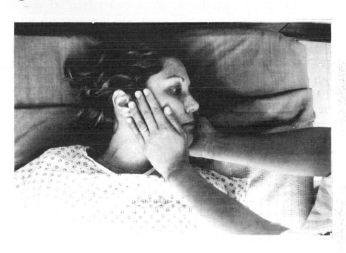

23. *Hyperextend the hip:* Place one hand on the hip to stabilize it and keep it from lifting off the bed. With the other arm and hand, cradle the lower leg in the forearm, and cup the knee joint with the hand. Move the leg backward from the hip joint. See Figure 35–37 on page 552.

24. *Hyperextend the neck:* Remove the pillow. With the client's face down, place one hand on the forehead and the other on the back of the skull. Move the head backward. See Figure 35–38 on page 552.

Following the Exercises

25. Assess the client's pulse and endurance of the exercise.

26. Report to the nurse in charge any unexpected problems or notable changes in the client's movements, eg, rigidity or contractures.

27. Document the exercises and your assessments.

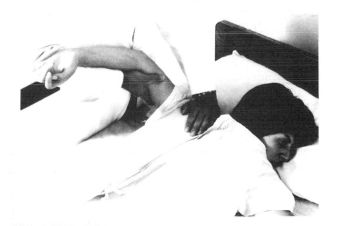

Figure 35–36

Considerations for the Elderly

For elderly clients it is not essential to achieve full range of motion in all joints. Instead, emphasize achieving a sufficient range of motion to carry out ADL, such as walking, dressing, combing hair, showering, and preparing a meal.

Sample Recording

Date	Time	Notes
6/14/89	1100	Passive exercises provided to R leg and foot. Full ROM in hip, knee, and ankle. ————————————Sally S. Ames, NS

Chapter Highlights

▪ Immobility affects almost every body organ and system adversely; complications include psychosocial problems.

▪ Factors influencing mobility include life-style, disease process or injury, understanding of health and physical fitness, motivation, attitudes toward health, and age.

▪ Pressure sores are thought to be the result of pressure, friction, and shearing forces.

▪ Clients at risk of developing pressure sores include the poorly nourished, the elderly, and people with superficial sensory loss, motor paralysis, or disturbances in autonomic nervous system function.

▪ Nursing interventions can help prevent and heal complications associated with immobility.

Selected References

Ahmed, M. C. December 1980. Special report: Choosing the best method to manage pressure ulcers. *Nurses' Drug Alert* 4(15):113–20.

Bassett, C.; McClamrock, E.; and Schmelzer, M. March/April 1982. A 10-week exercise program for senior citizens. *Geriatric Nursing* 3:103–5.

Baum, L. March 1985. Heed the early warning signs of peripheral vascular disease. *Nursing 85* 15:50–58.

Beller, L. C., and Neunaber, K. L. April 1986. The "simple" Valsalva. *American Journal of Nursing* 86:398–99.

Berecek, K. March 1975. Treatment of decubitus ulcers. *Nursing Clinics of North America* 10:171–210.

Blom, M. F. March/April 1985. Dramatic decrease in decubitus ulcers. *Geriatric Nursing* 6:84–87.

Brower, P., and Hicks, D. July 1972. Maintaining muscle function in patients on bedrest. *American Journal of Nursing* 72:1250–53.

Byrne, N., and Feld, M. April 1984. Preventing and treating decubitus ulcers. *Nursing 84* 14:55–57.

Downs, F. March 1974. Bed rest and sensory disturbances. *American Journal of Nursing* 74:434–38.

Fahey, V. March 1984. An in-depth look at deep-vein thrombosis. *Nursing 84* 14:35–41.

Gordon, M. January 1976. Assessing activity tolerance. *American Journal of Nursing* 76:72–75.

Guyton, A. C. 1986. *Textbook of medical physiology.* 7th ed. Philadelphia: W. B. Saunders Co.

Hogan, L., and Beland, I. July 1976. Cervical neck syndrome. *American Journal of Nursing* 76:1104–7.

Howard-Kurzuk, G.; Simpson, L.; and Palmeri, A. 1985. Decubitus ulcer care: A comparative study. *Western Journal of Nursing Research* 7(1):58–79.

Judd, C. O. July/August 1981. The prevention and treatment of pressure sores. *Canadian Nurse* 77:32–33.

Kerr, J. C.; Stinson, S. M.; and Shannon, M. L. July/August 1981. Pressure sores: Distinguishing fact from fiction. *Canadian Nurse* 77:23–28.

Kottke, F. G.; Stillwell, G. K.; and Lehmann, J. F., editors. 1982. *Krusen's handbook of physical medicine and rehabilitation.* 3d ed. Philadelphia: W. B. Saunders Co.

Lane, L. D., and Gaffney, F. A. June 1985. Overcautious use of the bedpan. *American Journal of Nursing* 85:642–44.

Lindan, O.; Greenway, R. M.; and Piazza, J. M. 1965. Pressure distribution on the surface of the human body; evaluation in lying and sitting positions using a bed of springs and nails. *Archives of Physical Medicine and Rehabilitation* 46:378–85.

Lowthian, P. January 20, 1982. A review of pressure sore pathogenesis. *Nursing Times* 78:117–21.

Mitchell, P. H., and Laustau, A. 1981. *Concepts basic to nursing.* 3d ed. New York: McGraw-Hill.

Morley, M. H. July/August 1981. Sixteen steps to better decubitus ulcer care. *Canadian Nurse* 77:29–31.

Norton, D. February 13, 1975. Research and the problem of pressure sores. *Nursing Mirror* 140:65–67.

Patrick, M. I., et al., editors. 1986. *Medical-surgical nursing: Pathophysiological concepts.* Philadelphia: J. B. Lippincott Co.

Peterson, F. November 1983. Assessing peripheral vascular disease. *American Journal of Nursing* 83:1549–51.

Reeder, J. M. November 1984. Help your disabled patient be more independent. *Nursing 84* 14:43.

Robertson, D., and Robertson, R. February 1985. Orthostatic hypotension: Diagnosis and therapy. *Modern Concepts of Cardiovascular Disease* 54:1–14.

Rodts, M. F. May 1983. An orthopedic assessment you can do in 15 minutes. *Nursing 83* 13:65–73.

Shannon, M. L. October 1984. Five famous fallacies about pressure sores. *Nursing 84* 14:34–41.

Smith, S. E. 1978. Prostaglandins. *Nursing Times* 74(6):231–33.

Wade, D. July 1982. Teaching patients to live with chronic orthostatic hypotension. *Nursing 82* 12:64–65.

Walker, J. M., et al. June 1984. Active mobility of the extremities in older subjects. *Physical Therapy* 64:919–23.

36

Body Mechanics, Ambulation, and Alignment

OBJECTIVES

Identify the importance for both clients and nurses of using good body mechanics.

Describe the importance of good body alignment for clients and nurses.

Describe how musculoskeletal function and voluntary and involuntary muscle and reflex activity affect movement.

Identify factors that influence body mechanics, ambulation, and alignment.

Identify occupational groups at risk of back injury.

Describe ways to prevent back injury.

Identify structural abnormalities that affect body mechanics and ambulation.

Identify ways to determine the client's capabilities and limitations for movement.

Identify criteria used to assess a client's gait.

Describe assessment criteria for the alignment of adults in standing, sitting, and various bed-lying positions.

State nursing diagnoses for clients with alignment and ambulation problems.

Describe nursing interventions to maintain, promote, or restore normal body mechanics, alignment, and ambulation.

Describe how to move and turn a client in bed and to transfer a client from a bed to a chair or stretcher.

Identify special assessments and interventions for clients with casts and in traction.

State outcome criteria for evaluating client responses to nursing interventions.

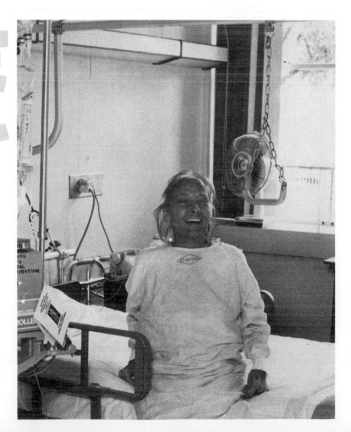

Concepts and Principles of Body Mechanics and Alignment

Using good body mechanics promotes musculoskeletal functioning, reduces the energy required to move and maintain balance, and decreases the risks of injury. **Body alignment** is the geometric arrangement of body parts in relation to each other. Good alignment promotes optimal balance and maximal body function in whatever position the client assumes. Proper body alignment enhances lung expansion and promotes efficient circulatory, renal, and gastrointestinal functions. Conversely, poor body alignment detracts from a pleasing appearance and affects an individual's health adversely.

A person's posture is one criterion for assessing his or her general health, physical fitness, and attractiveness. Posture reflects the mood, self-esteem, and personality of an individual. People often define their health status by their ability to move about, maintain their independence, and feel useful. When movement is impaired, the client may feel helpless and dependent on others. Body alignment and balance for independent movement require integrated functioning of the musculoskeletal and nervous systems and are dependent upon adequate muscle tone, coordinated movements of opposing muscle groups, and neuromuscular reflexes.

A person maintains balance as long as the **line of gravity** (an imaginary vertical line) passes through the **center of gravity** (the point at which all of the mass of an object is centered) and the **base of support** (the foundation on which an object rests). The broader the base of support and the lower the center of gravity, the greater the stability and balance. Whenever the line of gravity and the center of gravity lie outside the base of support, the body is unbalanced and unstable.

The center of gravity of a standing adult is located slightly anterior to the upper part of the sacrum. The base of support is just over the instep of the foot. Standing posture can be unstable because of a narrow base of support, a high center of gravity, and a constantly shifting line of gravity. For greatest balance and stability, a standing adult must center body weight symmetrically along the line of gravity. The base of support is easily widened by spreading the feet farther apart. The center of gravity is readily lowered by flexing the hips and knees until a squatting position is achieved.

In a well-aligned standing person, the center of gravity remains fairly stable, slightly anterior to the upper sacrum. When the person moves, however, the center of gravity shifts continuously in the direction of the moving body parts. Balance depends on the interrelationship of the center of gravity, the line of gravity, and the base of support. When a person moves, the closer the line of gravity is to the center of the base of support, the greater his or her stability. See Figure 36—1, A. Conversely, the closer the line of gravity is to the edge of the base of support, the more precarious the balance. See Figure 36—1, B. If the line of gravity falls outside the base of support, the person falls, See Figure 36—1, C.

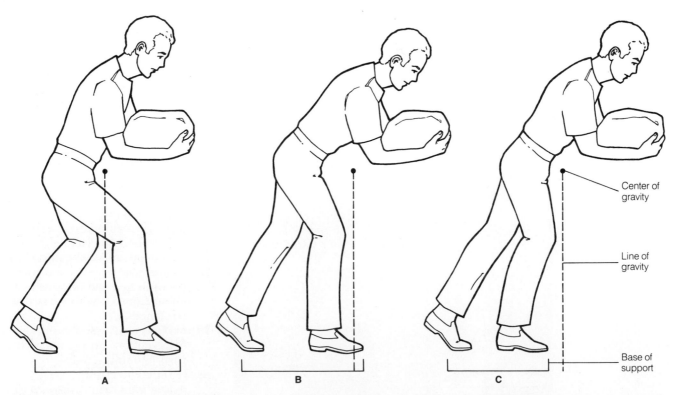

Center of
gravity

Line of
gravity

Base of
support

A   B   C

Figure 36—1 Balance is maintained when the line of gravity falls close to the base of support (**A**), is precarious when the line of gravity falls at the edge of the base of support (**B**), and cannot be maintained when the line of gravity falls outside the base of support (**C**).

When a person lifts or carries an object, the weight of the object becomes part of the person's body weight. This weight alters the person's center of gravity, which is displaced in the direction of the added weight. To counteract this potential imbalance, body parts move in a direction away from the weight. In this way, the center of gravity is maintained over the same point in the base of support. See Figure 36–2. Guidelines for moving objects are summarized in the accompanying box.

The heavier an object and the greater the friction against the surface beneath it, the greater the force required to move the object. Friction (see Table 36–1 for definitions of concepts applicable when moving clients) can be reduced by sliding the object on a smooth, clean, dry, firm surface, in contrast to a rough, wet, or soiled surface. To reduce friction when moving (sliding) a client up in bed, for example, the nurse provides a smooth, dry, firm bed foundation. Pulling creates less friction than pushing, since the nurse must pull at an upward angle that reduces friction between the client and the bed (Broer and Zernicke 1979, pp. 228–30).

GUIDELINES

For Moving Objects

When pushing an object, enlarge the base of support by moving the front foot forward.

When pulling an object, enlarge the base of support by either moving the rear leg back when facing the object, or moving the front foot forward when facing away from the object.

It is easier and safer to pull an object toward you than to push it away, because you exert more control of the object's movement when pulling it.

Move an object on a level surface when possible, since it requires less energy than moving that same object up an inclined surface against the pull of gravity.

Slide an object along a surface rather than lifting the object, since lifting requires moving the weight of the object against the pull of gravity.

Rolling, turning, and pivoting require much less energy expenditure than lifting does.

Friction can be further avoided by rolling, rather than pushing or pulling, the person.

Because of inertia, one must use more force to put an object into motion than to keep it in motion. The heavier the object, the greater the force required to put it into motion. To move an object efficiently, one applies force directly toward or against the object's center of gravity and in the direction in which the movement is to occur. A person can use his or her body weight in a rocking motion to apply additional force or leverage, thus counteracting the object's inertia and reducing the energy required to start the pulling, pushing, or lifting movement (Broer and Zernicke 1979, pp. 74–75).

When the nurse lifts objects, the resisting force or weight is held in the hands or on the forearms, the fulcrum is the elbow, and the force is applied by contrac-

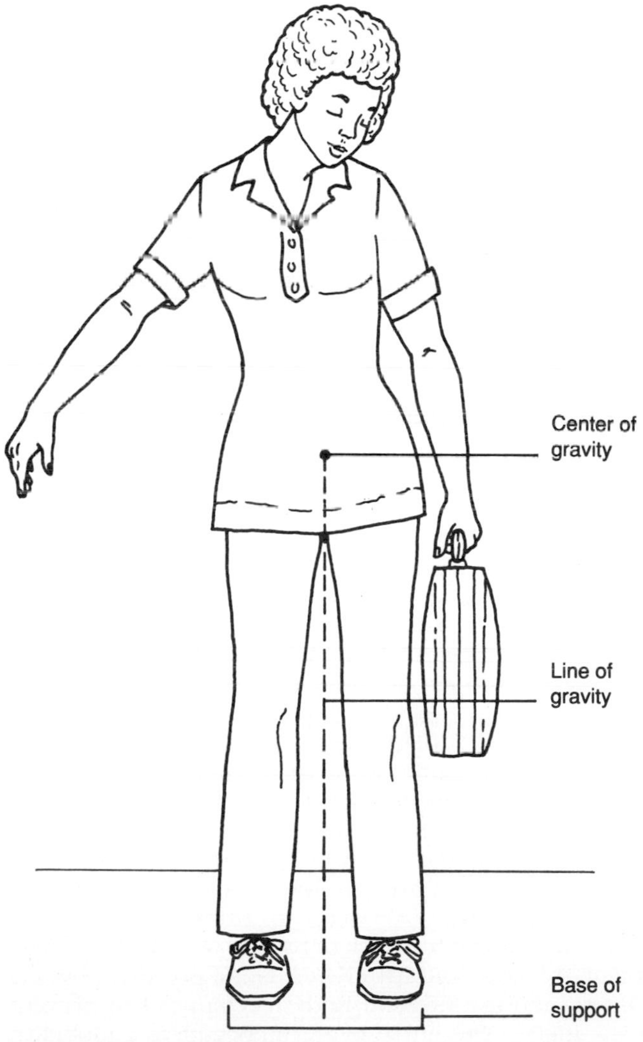

Center of gravity

Line of gravity

Base of support

Figure 36–2 Body parts move in the direction opposite the weight to compensate for it and maintain the center of gravity over the base of support.

Table 36–1 Concepts Applicable to Moving Clients

Concept	Definition
Friction	Force that opposes the motion of an object as it is slid across the surface of another object.
Force	The energy or power required to accomplish movement.
Inertia	The tendency of an object at rest to remain at rest and an object in motion to remain in motion.
Fulcrum	A fixed point (e.g., elbow) about which a lever moves.
Lever (first class)	A rigid piece that transmits or modifies motion or force. When force (energy) is applied to the rigid arm with a fixed point (fulcrum), an object at the other end of the rigid arm can be lifted more easily.

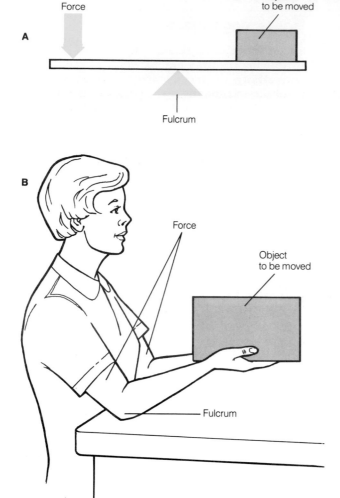

Figure 36–3 **A**, A first class lever; **B**, using the arm as a lever

tion of the biceps (flexor) muscles of the arm. See Figure 36–3. The lifting power is increased when the elbow (fulcrum) is supported on a bed surface or a countertop. People can lift more weight when they use this lever than when they do not (Broer and Zernicke 1979, pp. 80–101). Women's arm muscles have much less strength for lifting than men's (Hayne 1981). The ordinary person can lift only about 20 pounds of weight without danger of back strain when a lever is not used. When the weight to be lifted exceeds 35% of body weight, the lifter must use mechanical devices or seek the assistance of other persons (Owen 1980, p. 896).

Musculoskeletal Function

Muscle tone, the coordinated movements of opposing voluntary muscle groups (the antagonistic, synergistic, and antigravity muscles), and the **neuromuscular reflexes** (including the visual and proprioceptive reflexes) play important roles in producing balanced, smooth, purposeful movement. Moving bones act as levers. The cartilage between bones provides a smooth surface over which the bones glide and absorbs shock from sudden movement or injury. Each skeletal muscle attaches to a stationary bone (the *origin* of the muscle) and to a movable bone (the *insertion* of the muscle). A muscle shortens as it contracts, decreasing the angle between the two bones to which it is attached (flexion). As the muscle relaxes, it lengthens, increasing the angle between the two bones to which it is attached (extension).

Sustained contraction of the extensor muscles to support the upright position against the force of gravity is called **postural tonus.** Postural or **righting reflexes** that stimulate and maintain postural tonus are:

1. Labyrinthine sense.
2. Tonic neck-righting reflexes.
3. Visual or optic reflexes.
4. Proprioceptor or kinesthetic sense.
5. Extensor or antigravity (stretch) reflexes.
6. Plantar reflexes.

Structures in the cerebral cortex, midbrain, brain stem, cerebellum, and spinal cord regulate and control these postural reflexes. This internal regulation enables opposing muscle groups to work together automatically to coordinate the delicate muscle movements required to maintain upright posture, body alignment, and balance. When the flexors contract to bend a joint, the extensors relax; when the extensors contract to straighten a joint, the flexors relax.

The larger muscles of the lower extremities and the muscles of the abdomen and back all produce movement by leverage and synchronized action. The flexors of the legs, and to a lesser degree the leg extensors, are the largest and strongest muscles in the body. Exercise and consistent use of the weaker lumbar muscle groups and the abdominal muscles maintain their tone and strength, and protect them from injury. One can increase overall muscle strength by synchronized use of as many muscle groups as possible during an activity. For instance, when the arms are used in an activity, dividing the work between the arms and legs helps to prevent back strain. Exercise and use increase the mass and strength of skeletal muscles, increasing their capacity for work and protecting them from injury.

Two movements to avoid because of their potential for causing back injury are twisting (rotation) of the lumbarthoracic spine and acute flexion of the back with hips and knees straight. Undesirable twisting of the back can be prevented by squarely facing the direction of movement, whether pushing, pulling, or sliding, and moving the object directly toward or away from one's center of gravity.

Nurses are at high risk of back injuries because they regularly move and lift clients. Good posture, physical fitness, and use of good body mechanics can prevent back injury. The nurse is an important role model in teaching good body mechanics to others. A nurse who uses poor body mechanics in daily activities and whose

Table 36—2 Common Structural Abnormalities Affecting Alignment

Deviation	Description	Cause	Treatment
Scoliosis	Lateral curvature of the spine, which increases during active growth periods	May be secondary to other deformities, such as a discrepancy in leg lengths, or defects of spinal supporting tissues (a functional scoliosis); the most common cause of structural scoliosis is heredity, which produces an idiopathic structural scoliosis, a condition occurring five times more often in females than males, between the ages of 8 and 15	Treatment of underlying cause or application of a brace or cast from occiput to pelvis; surgical fusion of the spinal vertebrae may be necessary
Kyphosis (round-back or humpback)	A fixed flexion deformity of the thoracic spine	Congenital—rickets, tuberculosis of spine	Exercises to extend the thoracic spine; sleeping without a pillow; occasionally bracing or spinal fusion may be required
Lordosis (swayback)	A fixed hyperextension deformity of the lumbar spine	Congenital, most often secondary to other abnormalities such as kyphosis or muscular dystrophy	The underlying disease is treated

back hurts as a result cannot teach health promotion and prevention of disability as effectively as a nurse who uses good body mechanics.

Structural Abnormalities Affecting Alignment

Structural impairments in body alignment are usually caused by congenital abnormalities, developmental abnormalities, or abnormal intrauterine positions. Several common abnormalities are listed in Table 36–2. Functional abnormalities, such as poor posture during

the growing years or improper alignment during illness, can also result in structural abnormalities.

Developmental Variations in Body Alignment

Body alignment or posture changes significantly during growth and with age. An understanding of the normal variations is helpful for the nurse in promoting good posture, in assessing postural faults, and in helping others correct them. Table 36–3 provides a summary of developmental variations.

Table 36—3 Developmental Variations in Body Alignment

Age-Group	Characteristics	Implications
Infants	Usual posture is horizontal rather than upright; abdomen is rounded and prominent; extremities are generally flexed and inwardly rotated; feet are usually inverted, but may be passively everted.	The congenital condition *metatarsus adductus* may be present if inversion of feet occurs in early infancy, especially if the lower legs are straight. Balance is precarious as the older infant learns to stand and walk; may fall backward.
Toddlers	Marked lumbar lordosis and protruding abdomen; slight outward rotation of hips and eversion of feet.	Child commonly widely abducts arms for balance. Growth should produce inward rotation of hips and correct foot eversions.
Preschoolers	Protrusion of abdomen less exaggerated; extremities more proportionate to trunk.	Developing coordination and refining gross motor skills.
School-age children	Legs have straightened and toes point straight ahead. Scoliosis screening should be performed.	Usually have excellent posture; often, best during lifetime.
Adolescents	Significant changes in body proportions and contour; differentiation of male and female characteristics.	Growth spurts may result in awkwardness which may be manifested in posture.
Older adults	Tend to have some contractures of flexor muscles; may show **kyphosis** (humpback) with disappearance of earlier lumbar lordosis; osteoporosis common among older women and may cause compression fractures of the vertebrae, resulting in a forward leaning stooped posture, sometimes called **dowager's hump.**	Deterioration of postural reflexes may require conscious widening of base of support to maintain balance; use of bifocals may result in hyperextension of cervical spine and may cause injury to nearby ligaments and joints.

Table 36—4 Assessing Gait

Normal Findings	Abnormal Findings	Some Associated Conditions
Head is erect, and vertebral column straight	Body is rigid and bent forward.	Parkinsonism
Gaze is straight ahead.	Gaze is toward ground.	Fear of falling
Toes point forward.	Toes are everted.	Flat-footedness
Kneecaps point forward.	Legs are knock-kneed with feet apart (normal until age 3 or 4).	Rickets; congenital bone disorders
	Legs are bowlegged with feet together (normal until age 2 or 2½).	Rickets; congenital bone disorders
Elbows are slightly flexed.	One elbow is flexed and held close to body.	Hemiplegia
Foot is dorsiflexed in swing phase.	One foot is plantar flexed and drags.	Hemiplegia
Arm opposite swing-through foot moves forward at same time.	Arms swing forward and do not swing with steps.	Parkinsonism
Steps are smooth, coordinated, and rhythmic.	Steps are weaving, uncoordinated, and uneven.	Alcohol or barbiturate intoxication; cerebellar disorder
	Steps are short, shuffling, and often on tiptoe.	Parkinsonism
	Gait starts slowly, gradually increases, and may be difficult to stop.	Parkinsonism
	Steps are stiff, jerking, and uncoordinated, with legs held stiffly together.	Spastic paraplegia; multiple sclerosis; spinal cord tumor
	Exaggerated lateral leaning accompanies steps.	Hip disorder

need. The nurse must be sensitive to the client's need to function as independently as he or she can yet provide assistance when the client needs it. Clients who are not very mobile and can help themselves only minimally may also have low energy levels. They are at high

NURSING DIAGNOSIS

Alignment and Gait

- Alteration in comfort related to kyphosis
- Alteration in comfort related to impaired standing alignment secondary to pregnancy
- Fear of falling related to unsteady gait and muscle weakness
- Impaired physical mobility related to long leg cast
- Impaired physical mobility related to musculoskeletal spasms in lower extremities
- Impaired physical mobility related to painful, inflamed joints
- Knowledge deficit (body mechanics) of unknown etiology
- Potential for injury from falling related to altered judgment and drowsiness associated with medication (Elavil)
- Potential for injury related to difficulty with alignment and balance associated with neurologic impairment and muscle weakness
- Potential for injury related to unsteady gait
- Self-care deficit specifically related to impaired physical mobility

risk of developing contractures and other complications of immobility outlined in Chapter 35. These persons are totally dependent on caregivers and must be instructed to achieve and maintain correct body alignment.

Most clients require some nursing guidance and assistance to learn about, achieve, and maintain proper alignment. All nurses have the responsibility to use proper body mechanics to prevent back injury to themselves and their clients. A serious back injury could prevent a nurse from participating in the full range of nursing activities. As a role model, the nurse continuously teaches clients through the body mechanics she or he uses. The nurse is expected to protect the client from harm, anticipating safety risks and protecting the client from unsafe practices. The more vulnerable the client, the greater the nurse's responsibility to protect him or her from harm (Cushing 1985, p. 138).

The nurse should also plan to teach clients applicable skills. For example, a postoperative cataract client needs to learn to squat rather than stoop to avoid increased intraocular pressure. Similarly, a client with a back injury needs to learn how to get out of bed safely and comfortably, a client with an injured leg needs to learn how to transfer from bed to wheelchair safely, and a client with a newly acquired walker needs to learn how to use it safely. Nurses often teach family members or caregivers in the home safe moving, lifting, and transfer techniques. Nurses who practice in hospitals and nursing homes have a responsibility to teach nursing assistants how to protect their backs from injury as they move, lift, and transfer clients.

Providing proper body mechanics and ambulatory care to clients is almost always an independent nursing function. Although certain activity orders are medically prescribed, the physician rarely writes specific directions to indicate how the order is to be accomplished. The physician usually orders specific body positions only after surgery, anesthesia, or trauma involving the nervous and musculoskeletal systems. The client's current "activity order" contains data essential for planning nursing interventions for body alignment. All clients should have an activity order written by their physician when they are admitted to the agency for care. Examples of common activity orders are shown in the accompanying box.

Implementing Preventive Strategies and Treatment Interventions

As noted earlier, many problems concerning alignment, body mechanics, and ambulation are preventable and/or treatable. A frequent postural problem in the **standing** client is a forward thrusting of the neck, which produces a stooped position (see Figure 36–5, B). Slight flexion contractures of the neck, preventing appropriate neck extension, are common by late adolescence and are usually due to poor posture. If the client has a flexion contracture of the cervical spine, the nurse should make every effort to prevent further contractures and, if possible, to reduce the contracture already present.

Another frequent postural problem in the standing client is an exaggerated curvature, or lordosis, of the lumbar spine (see Figure 36–5, B). The lordosis is usually accompanied by an abnormally protruding abdomen. Conscientious use of the pelvic tilt, shown in Figure 36–5, A, flattens the abdomen and prevents lordosis of the lumbar spine. Exercises to strengthen and protect the back muscles that support the lumbar spine and the abdominal muscles help prevent or reduce postural lordosis. Persons with a history of back problems should follow an exercise program prescribed by a physician. Any program of exercise should be started slowly and intensified gradually.

Flexion of the hip and knee straightens the lumbar spine and reduces lordosis. Clients should avoid prolonged standing; when prolonged standing is unavoidable, the client should elevate one foot onto a support to straighten the spine. Periodically changing the foot that is elevated prevents undue strain to one side of the spinal column at the expense of the other (Ishmael and Shorbe 1969, p. 7).

General exercise promotes good standing alignment. Walking and swimming, which maintain overall muscle tone, are especially useful. Conscientious and continuous awareness of and effort to improve posture in everyday activities are important in achieving and maintaining good posture. To put forth this effort, the client must be motivated; motivation is, in turn, usually dependent on self-image. The nurse who practices good postural habits can be a significant role model and motivator. No amount of verbal instruction and encouragement will influence clients to use good posture as strongly as the example of a nurse who "practices what she or he preaches" (Memmer 1974c, p. 28).

Nursing interventions to promote good sitting alignment apply whether the client is sitting in a chair, in a wheelchair, or on the side of the bed. When the client is **sitting**, alignment problems frequently affect not only the back, but also the top extremities. Alignment problems are often due to the size and shape of the object on which the person is sitting (e.g., the chair or wheelchair may simply not fit the person). A chair seat that is too high creates undue pressure against the thighs, especially in the popliteal area behind the knees, since the lower legs and feet are unsupported. Prolonged pressure can damage the delicate nerves and blood vessels in the popliteal area. A firm footrest of an appropriate height improves alignment and comfort.

A chair seat that is too low causes no alignment problems of the back but, unless the thighs are supported, exerts undue pressure on the ischial tuberosities, due to the narrow base of support for the trunk. If too low, the seat may be difficult to get into and, especially, out of. Pillows placed on the chair seat support the thighs and improve alignment. A chair seat that is too deep produces undue flexion of the thoracolumbar spine. The weight of the body does not rest on the ischial tuberosities, and the lower back is not supported properly by the chair back. This position can be quite uncomfortable. Pillows placed between the chair back and the person's back improve alignment.

If the chair back is too low or if there is no chair back, there is no effect on alignment, but most persons find that a chair back supports the spinal column and prevents fatigue. In all instances, proper alignment in the sitting client is best promoted by a chair seat that allows the knees to be slightly higher than the hips and supports the full length of the thighs and by a chair back that supports the entire back.

Moving, Turning, and Positioning Clients

When the client is not able to move independently or assist with moving, the **preferred** method is to use two or more nurses to move or turn the client. When positioning clients in bed, there are a number of things

---

Examples of Activity Orders

▪ BR (bed rest) or CBR (complete bed rest). This order indicates that the client is not to get out of bed for any reason.

▪ BRP (bathroom privileges). This order indicates that the client is not to get out of bed except to urinate or defecate.

▪ Up ad lib. This order indicates that the client may be in and out of bed as he or she wishes.

▪ HOB 30 continuously. This order indicates that the head of the bed is to be elevated 30° (in Fowler's position) both day and night.

In the **prone position,** the client lies on his or her abdomen with the legs extended and the head turned to one side. The hips are not flexed. Both children and adults frequently sleep in this position, sometimes with one or both arms flexed over their heads. See Figure 36–9. This position has several advantages. It is the only bed position that allows full extension of the hip and knee joints. When used periodically, the prone position helps to prevent flexion contractures of the hips and knees, thereby counteracting a problem caused by all other bed positions. The prone position also promotes drainage from the mouth and is especially useful for clients recovering from surgery of the mouth or throat.

The prone position poses some distinct disadvantages. The pull of gravity on the trunk produces a marked lordosis in most persons, and the neck is rotated laterally to a significant degree. For this reason, many orthopedists do not recommend this position, especially for persons with problems of the cervical or lumbar spine (Ishmael 1969, p. 9). This position also causes plantar flexion. Some clients with cardiac or respiratory problems find the prone position confining and suffocating, since chest expansion is inhibited during respirations. The prone position should be used only when the client's back is properly aligned, only for short periods, and only for persons with no evidence of spinal abnormalities.

PROCEDURE 36–3

Supporting a Client in Prone Position

Equipment

▪ Three pillows

Intervention

Figure 36–9 shows the outcome of the following steps.

1. Assist the client to a prone position.
2. Turn the client's head to one side and either omit the pillow entirely or place a small pillow under the head (unless contraindicated, eg, if the pillow will impede the drainage of mucus) to align the head with the trunk. Avoid placing the pillow under the shoulders.
   Rationale: The absence of a pillow prevents flexion of the neck laterally. A pillow placed under the shoulders increases lumbar lordosis.
3. Place a small pillow or roll under the abdomen in the space between the diaphragm (or the breasts of a woman) and the iliac crests.
   Rationale: This pillow prevents hyperextension of the lumbar curvature, difficulty breathing, and pressure on some women's breasts. Supports placed too high impede respirations. Supports placed too low can increase lumbar lordosis and pressure on bony prominences.
4. Place a pillow under the lower legs from below the knees to just above the ankles, or position the client on the bed so that the feet extend in a normal anatomic position over the lower edge of the mattress. There should be no pressure on the toes.

Rationale: The pillow raises the toes off the bed surface, flexes the knees slightly for comfort, and prevents excessive pressure on the patellae. It also reduces plantar flexion.

Critical Elements of Supporting a Client in Prone Position

▪ Support the client appropriately to prevent
▪ Acute flexion or hyperextension of the neck.
▪ Hyperextension of the lumbar curvature.
▪ Pressure on a woman's breasts.
▪ Plantar flexion.
▪ Omit the pillow under the head if drainage of mouth secretions is to be encouraged.
▪ Place abdominal supports at or below the level of the diaphragm to enable appropriate chest expansion.
▪ Assess pressure areas of particular concern in the prone position:

Toes.

Knees.

Genitalia (men).

Breasts (women).

Acromial processes of shoulders.

Cheek and ear.

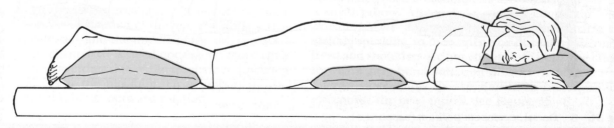

Figure 36–9 Prone position (supported)

In the **lateral** or **side-lying position,** the person lies on one side of the body. See Figure 36–10. By having the client flex the top hip and knee and placing this leg in front of the body, a wider, triangular base of support is created, and greater stability is achieved. The greater the flexion on the top hip and knee, the greater the stability and balance in this position.

This flexion reduces lordosis and promotes good back alignment. For this reason, the lateral position is good for resting and sleeping clients. The lateral position helps to relieve pressure on the sacrum and heels in persons who sit for much of the day or who are confined to bed and rest in Fowler's or dorsal recumbent positions much of the time. In the lateral position, most of the body's weight is borne by the lateral aspect of the lower scapula, the lateral aspect of the ilium, and the greater trochanter of the femur. Persons who have sensory or motor deficits on one side of the body usually find that lying on the uninvolved side is more comfortable.

In the **Sims'** or **semiprone position,** the client assumes a posture halfway between the lateral and the prone positions. In Sims' position, the client's lower arm is positioned behind him or her, and the upper arm is flexed at the shoulder and the elbow. Both legs are flexed in front of the client. The upper leg is more acutely flexed at both the hip and the knee than the lower one is.

Sims' position is occasionally used for unconscious clients because it facilitates drainage from the mouth. It is also used for paralyzed (paraplegic or hemiplegic) clients because it reduces pressure over the sacrum and greater trochanter of the hip. It is often used for clients receiving enemas and occasionally for clients undergoing examinations or treatments of the perineal area. Many people, especially pregnant women, find Sims' position comfortable for sleeping. Persons with sensory or motor deficits on one side of the body usually find that lying on the uninvolved side is more comfortable.

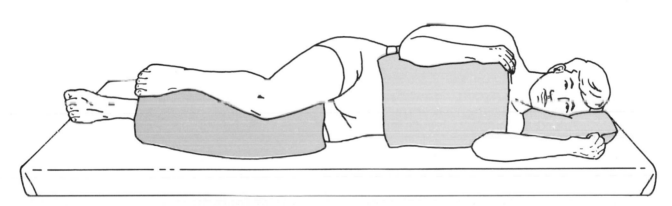

Figure 36–10   Lateral position (supported)

PROCEDURE 36-4

Supporting a Client in Sims' Position

Equipment
- Three small pillows
- Sandbag or rolled towel

Intervention

Figure 36–11 shows the outcome of the following steps.

1. Turn the client as for a prone position.
2. Place a small pillow under the client's head, unless drainage from the mouth is being encouraged.

Rationale: This pillow prevents lateral flexion of the neck and cushions the cranial and facial bones and the ear. It is contraindicated if drainage of mucus is required. Too large a pillow produces an uncomfortable lateral flexion of the neck.

3. Place the lower arm behind and away from the client's body in a position that is comfortable and does not disrupt circulation.
Rationale: This position prevents damage to nerves and blood vessels in the axillae.

4. Position the upper shoulder so that it is abducted slightly from the body and the shoulder and elbow

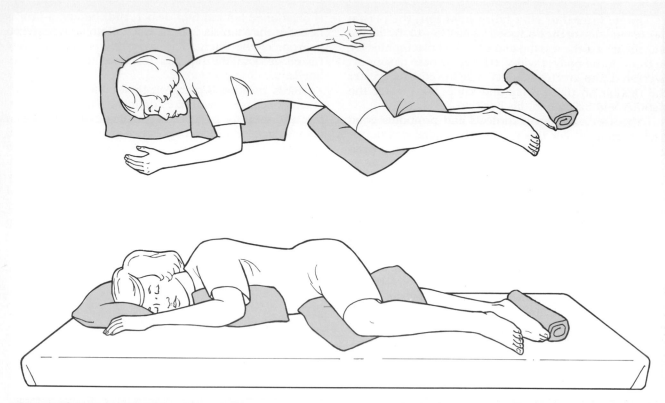

Figure 36–11 Sims' position (supported)

are flexed. Use a pillow to support the space between the chest and abdomen and the upper arm and bed. *Rationale:* This position prevents internal shoulder rotation and adduction and maintains alignment of the upper trunk.

5. Use a pillow to support the space between abdomen and pelvis and the upper thigh and bed.
Rationale: This position prevents internal rotation and adduction of the hip and also reduces lumbar lordosis.

6. Ensure that the two shoulders are aligned in the same plane as the two hips. If not, pull one shoulder or hip forward or backward until all four joints are aligned in the same plane.
Rationale: Proper alignment prevents twisting of the spine.

7. Place a support device, eg, a sandbag or rolled towel, against the lower foot.
Rationale: This device may prevent foot drop. Efforts to correct plantar flexion in this position, however, are usually unsuccessful.

Critical Elements of Supporting a Client in Sims' Position

- Support the client appropriately to prevent
- Lateral flexion of the neck, unless drainage from the mouth is being encouraged.
- Disruption of circulation to the arm placed behind.
- Internal shoulder rotation and adduction of the upper arm.
- Internal rotation and adduction of the hip, and lumbar lordosis.
- Twisting of the spine.
- Assess pressure areas of particular concern in Sims' position:
- Side of the skull (temporal and parietal bones and the ear).
- Acromial process of lowermost clavicle.
- Lowermost anterior superior iliac spine.
- Lowermost greater trochanter of the femur.
- Lateral aspect of undermost knee.
- Medial aspect of uppermost knee.
- Lateral malleolus of undermost ankle.
- Medial malleolus of uppermost ankle.
- Medial aspect (epicondyle) of uppermost elbow.
- Omit the head pillow if drainage of mouth secretions is to be encouraged.
- Position the lower arm appropriately so that circulation is maintained.

Transferring Clients Between a Bed and a Stretcher

The stretcher, or gurney, is used to transfer supine clients from one location to another. Whenever the client is capable of accomplishing the transfer from bed to stretcher independently, either by lifting onto it or by rolling onto it, the client should be encouraged to do so. Procedure 36–5 describes guidelines for transferring clients between a bed and a stretcher. See also the accompanying box for safety tips when using stretchers.

PROCEDURE 36–5

Transferring a Client Between a Bed and a Stretcher

Equipment
- A stretcher
- A roller bar (optional)

Intervention

1. In preparation for the transfer, lower the head of the bed until it is flat or as low as the client can tolerate.

2. Raise the bed so that it is slightly higher than the surface of the stretcher. Ensure that the wheels on the bed are locked.
   Rationale: Moving down an incline is easier and requires less effort.

3. Pull the drawsheet out from both sides of the bed and roll it as close to the client's sides as possible.

4. Pull the client to the edge of the bed where the stretcher will be positioned.

5. Cover the client with a sheet or bath blanket.

6. Place the stretcher parallel to the bed, next to the client, and lock its wheels.

7. Fill the gap that exists between the bed and the stretcher loosely with bath blankets.

8. All nurses press their bodies tightly against the stretcher to prevent its movement, roll the pull sheet tightly against the client, flex their hips, and pull the client on the pull sheet directly toward themselves and onto the stretcher. Ask the client to flex the neck during the move, if possible, and place arms across the chest to prevent injury to these body parts.

Rationale: Keeping their bodies against the stretcher prevents its movement. Better control over client movement is achieved when the pull sheet is tightly rolled against the client. Also, pulling downward is easier and requires less force than pulling along a flat surface.

9. Make the client comfortable, unlock the stretcher wheels, and move the stretcher away from the bed.

10. Immediately raise the stretcher side rails and/or fasten the safety straps across the client.
    Rationale: Because the stretcher is high and narrow, the client is in danger of falling unless these safety precautions are taken.

Variation: Using a Roller Bar During the Transfer

A roller bar is a metal frame covered with longitudinal rollers. The bar is placed over the gap between the bed and the stretcher. The client is pulled on a pull sheet onto the roller bars and rolled easily onto the stretcher.

Critical Elements of Transferring a Client Between a Bed and a Stretcher

See critical elements for Technique 13–1 on page 225. In addition:

- Lock the wheels of the bed and the stretcher before the client transfers in or out of them.

- Fasten safety straps across the client on a stretcher, and raise the side rails.

- Push a stretcher from the end with the stationary wheels, and the end where the client's head is positioned.

- When entering an elevator, maneuver the stretcher so that the client's head goes in first.

Assisting Clients to a Sitting Position in Bed

A client may need assistance to raise the head and shoulders while pillows are rearranged or for back care. If the client needs to rise to a sitting position in bed, the easiest way to do so is simply to raise the head of the bed to the desired height. If the client is not in a hospital bed that can be raised mechanically, the nurse may need to assist the client.

When the client needs assistance, the nurse first asks the client to place the arms at the sides with the palms of the hands ready to push against the surface of the bed. Client assistance provides additional power during the movement and reduces the potential for strain and injury to the nurse's back. The nurse faces the center of the head of the bed and assumes a broad stance at the side of the bed beside the client's buttocks. The nurse places the foot farthest from the bed forward and

GUIDELINES

Safe Use of Stretchers

Never leave a client unattended on a stretcher unless the wheels are locked and the side rails are raised on both sides of the stretcher and/or the safety straps are securely fastened across the client.

Always push the stretcher from the end above the client's head. This position protects the client's head in the event of a collision.

When using a stretcher with two swivel wheels and two stationary wheels, always position the client's head at the end with the stationary wheels. The stretcher is more easily maneuvered when pushed from the end with the stationary wheels.

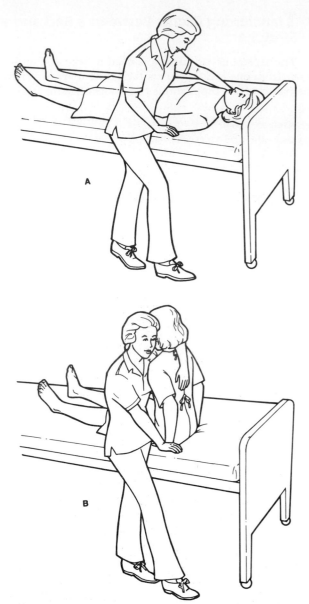

puts her or his weight on this foot. Facing the head of the bed at the angle in which the movement will occur prevents twisting of the spine. The nurse then places the hand nearest the client over the client's far shoulder to rest between the client's shoulder blades. This hand position enables the nurse to pull the client's upper body directly toward the nurse. The nurse places the other hand on the edge of the surface of the bed near the client's shoulder and uses it to support and push during the lift. See Figure 36–12, *A*.

During the move, the motions of the nurse and client are coordinated. On the nurse's signal, both nurse and client lift simultaneously. The nurse lifts by pulling with the arm and hand over the client's shoulder, pushing on the bed surface with the other hand, and shifting her or his weight from the forward to the back foot in a rocking motion. The client simultaneously pushes with his or her hands and arms. See Figure 36–12, *B*. The backward rocking movement increases the lifting force. The nurse avoids spinal twisting by pulling the weight of the client's upper body directly toward the nurse's center of gravity and in the direction of the movement. Pushing with the muscles of one arm while pulling with the muscles of the other arm distributes the work load and increases lifting power. The client's pushing motion provides additional power for the lift.

Figure 36—12 Assisting a client to a sitting position in bed

Source: Adapted from A.J. Bilger and E. H. Greene, editors, *Winters protective body mechanics* (New York: Springer Publishing Co., 1973), p. 35.

Wheelchair Safety Guidelines

Wheelchairs, like stretchers, are unstable and can predispose the client to falls and injury. Always lock the brakes on both wheels of the wheelchair when the client transfers in or out of it. Use seat belts that fasten behind the wheelchair to protect confused clients from falls. Back the wheelchair into or out of an elevator, rear large wheels first. When on an incline, place your body between the wheelchair and the bottom of the incline. Procedure 36–6 describes suggested ways of transferring a client between a bed and a wheelchair.

PROCEDURE 36–6

Transferring a Client Between a Bed and a Wheelchair

This procedure can be used to transfer a client between the bed and a wheelchair or chair, the bed and the commode, and a wheelchair and the toilet. There are numerous variations of this transfer technique; several are described in this procedure. Transfer belts provide the greatest safety. See Figure 36–13. This belt has a handle that allows the nurse to control movement of the client during the transfer.

Intervention

1. Assist the client to a sitting position on the side of the bed.

2. Assist the client to put on a bathrobe and nonskid slippers or shoes.

3. Place a transfer belt snugly around the client's waist. Check to be certain that the belt is securely fastened.

4. Lower the bed to its lowest position so that the client's feet rest flat on the floor. Lock the wheels of the bed.

5. Assess the client for orthostatic hypotension prior to moving him or her from the bed.

6. Place the wheelchair at a right angle to the bed and as close to the bed as possible, as shown in Figure 36–14. Lock the wheels of the wheelchair and raise the foot plates.

7. Ask the client to move forward to sit on the edge of the bed, lean forward slightly from the hips, place the foot of the stronger leg beneath the edge of the bed, and put the other foot forward.

   Rationale: These actions bring the client's center of gravity closer to the nurse's and more directly over the client's base of support as the weight is shifted forward during the transfer. By placing the stronger foot and leg in this way, the client can use the stronger leg muscles to stand and power the movement. A broader base of support makes the client more stable during the transfer.

8. Ask the client to place his or her hands on the bed surface or on the nurse's shoulders and to push on the hands while standing. The client should not grasp the nurse's neck for support because doing so can injure the nurse.

   Rationale: Use of the client's arm muscles provides additional force for the movement and reduces the potential for strain on the nurse's back.

9. Stand directly in front of the client. Incline the trunk forward from the hips. Flex the hips, knees, and ankles. Assume a broad stance, placing one foot forward and one back. Mirror the placement of the client's feet, if possible.

   Rationale: The broad stance provides balance. Flexing the joints of the lower extremities lowers the center of gravity, increases stability, and ensures

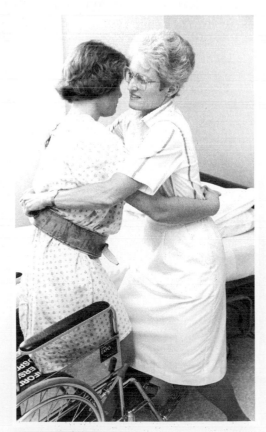

Figure 36–13

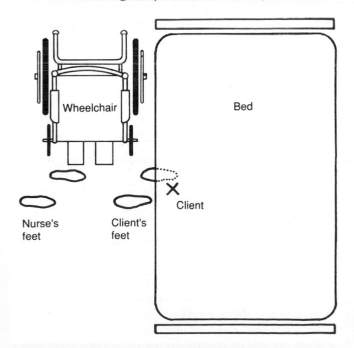

Wheelchair

Bed

Nurse's feet

Client's feet

Client

Figure 36–14

use of the large leg muscles during movement. Facing the client in the direction of the movement prevents twisting of the spine. The complementary placement of the feet helps to prevent loss of balance during the transfer.

10. Encircle the client's waist with your arms and grasp the transfer belt at the client's back. Your thumbs should point down as you grasp the belt.
Rationale: The belt provides a secure handle for holding onto the client and controlling the movement. The downward placement of the thumbs prevents potential wrist injury as the nurse lifts (Leinweber 1978, p. 2080). By encircling the client in this manner, the nurse keeps the client from tilting backward during the transfer.

11. Tighten your gluteal, abdominal, leg, and arm muscles.
Rationale: Isometric contraction of stabilizing muscles helps to prevent musculoskeletal strain and injury.

12. To assist the client to stand: (a) Have the client push with the back foot, rock to the forward foot, extend the joints of the lower extremities, and push or pull up with the hands while (b) the nurse pushes with the forward foot, rocks to the back foot, extends the joints of the lower extremities, and pulls the client into a standing position.
Rationale: The broad stance promotes stability for both nurse and client. Client assistance provides additional power for movement and reduces the potential for strain and injury to the nurse's back. Pulling the client directly toward the nurse's center of gravity prevents spinal twisting.

13. Support the client in an upright standing position for a few moments. Then, both client and nurse pivot or take a few steps together toward the wheelchair. Ask the client to back up to the wheelchair, placing the legs against the seat.
Rationale: Standing upright for a few moments extends the joints and provides an opportunity to ensure that the client is all right before moving away from the bed. Having the client place the legs against the wheelchair seat minimizes the risk of the client's falling when sitting down.

14. Ask the client
   a. to place the foot of the stronger leg slightly behind the other
   b. to keep the other foot, with the weight upon it, forward
   c. to place both hands on the wheelchair arms or on the nurse's shoulders
   Rationale: See rationale for steps 7 and 8.

15. Stand directly in front of the client. Place one foot forward and one back. Tighten your grasp on the transfer belt.
Rationale: See rationale for steps 9 and 10.

16. Tighten your gluteal, abdominal, leg, and arm muscles.
Rationale: See rationale for step 11.

17. To assist the client to sit: (a) Have the client shift body weight by rocking to the back foot, lower the body onto the edge of the wheelchair seat by flex-

ing the joints of the legs and arms, and place some body weight on the arms while (b) the nurse shifts her or his body weight by rocking to the forward foot and flexes the hips and knees to lower and guide the client onto the wheelchair seat.
Rationale: See rationale for step 12.

18. Ask the client to push back into the wheelchair seat and apply a seat belt as needed.
Rationale: Sitting well back on the seat provides a broader base of support and greater stability and minimizes the risk of falling from the wheelchair. A wheelchair can topple forward when the client sits on the edge of the seat and leans far forward.

19. Lower the foot plates and place the client's feet on them.

Variation: Transferring Without a Belt

For clients who need minimal assistance, the nurse places the hands against the side of the client's upper chest (not at the axillae) during the transfer. See Figure 36–15. For clients who require more assistance, the nurse reaches through the client's axillae and places the hands on the client's scapulae during the transfer. Avoid placing hands or pressure *on* the axillae, especially for clients who have upper extremity paralysis or paresis. The other steps are the same as described previously.

Variation: Transferring with a Belt and Two Nurses

When the client is able to stand, the nurses position themselves on both sides of the client, facing the same

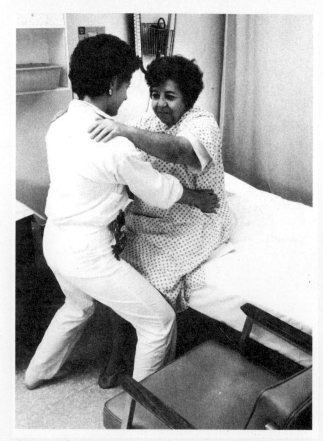

Figure 36–15

direction as the client. The nurses flex their hips, knees, and ankles; grasp the client's transfer belt with the hand closest to the client; and with the other hand support the client's elbows. Coordinating their efforts, all three stand simultaneously, pivot, and move to the wheelchair where the process is reversed to lower the client onto the wheelchair seat.

Variation: Transferring a Client with an Injured Lower Extremity

When the client has an injured lower extremity, movement should always occur toward the client's unaffected (strong) side. For example, if the client's right leg is injured and he or she is sitting on the edge of the bed preparing to transfer to a wheelchair, the nurse positions the wheelchair on the client's left side so that the client can use the left leg most effectively and safely.

Variation: Using a Sliding Board

Clients who cannot stand can use a sliding board to move without nursing assistance. This method not only promotes the client's sense of independence but preserves the nurse's energy. See Figure 36–16.

Variation: Using a Roller Bar During the Transfer

A roller bar is a metal frame covered with longitudinal rollers. The bar is placed over the gap between the bed

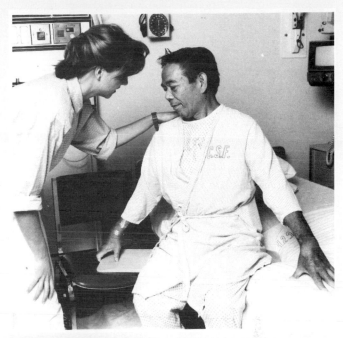

Figure 36–16

and the stretcher. The client is pulled on a pull sheet onto the roller bars and rolled easily onto the stretcher.

Mechanical lifters are used primarily for clients who cannot help themselves or who are too heavy for others to lift safely. Transfers may be made between the bed and a wheelchair, the bed and the bathtub, and the bed and a stretcher. Various types of mechanical lifters are used to lift and move clients. It is important that nurses be familiar with the model used and the practices that accompany use. The general principles of alignment and body mechanics apply when using these devices for transfers. See the clinical agency's procedure manual for specific instructions.

Assisting Clients to Ambulate

Most people who are ill require only a brief period of rest before they begin to walk and gradually increase their activity. The more physically fit the person is before becoming ill or immobilized, the sooner the person returns to health.

Even 1 or 2 days of bed rest can make a person feel weak, unsteady, and shaky when first getting out of bed. A client who has had surgery, is elderly, or has been immobilized for a longer time will feel more pronounced weakness. The potential problems of immobility (see Chapter 35) are far less likely to occur when clients become ambulatory as soon as possible. The nurse can assist clients to prepare for ambulation by helping them become as independent as possible while in bed. Nurses should encourage clients to perform activities of daily living, maintain good body alignment, perform orthostatic tension stimulating exercises, and carry out active range-of-motion exercises to the maximum degree

possible yet within the limitations imposed by their illness and recovery program.

Clients who have been in bed for long periods often need a plan of muscle tone exercises to strengthen the muscles used for walking before attempting to walk. One of the most important muscle groups is the quadriceps femoris, which extends the knee and flexes the thigh. This group is also important for elevating the legs, e.g., for walking upstairs. To strengthen these muscles, the client consciously tenses them, drawing the kneecap upward and inward. The client pushes the popliteal space behind the knee against the bed surface, raising the heels off the bed surface. See Figure 36–17. On the count of 1, the muscles are tensed; they are held during the counts of 2, 3, 4; and they are relaxed at the count of 5. The exercise should be done within the client's tolerance,

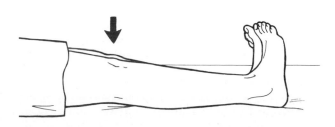

Figure 36–17 Tensing the quadriceps femoris before ambulation

GUIDELINES

Ambulation

- Carefully assess the client for signs and symptoms of orthostatic hypotension (dizziness, lightheadedness, or a sudden increase in heart rate) prior to leaving the bedside and periodically during the ambulatory experience.

- Have the client wear comfortable shoes with nonskid soles.

- Remain physically close to the client in case assistance is needed.

- If the client can ambulate independently, encourage the client to do so but walk beside him or her.

- If the client is slightly weak and unstable, use a transfer or walking belt. Make sure the belt is pulled snugly around the client's waist and fastened securely. Grasp the belt at the client's back and walk behind and slightly to one side of the client. See Figure 36–18.

- If it is the client's first time out of bed following surgery, injury, or an extended period of immobility or if the client is quite weak or unstable, have an assistant follow the nurse and client with a wheelchair in the event that it is needed quickly.

- If the client is moderately weak and unstable, interlock your forearm with the client's closest forearm and walk on the client's weaker side. Encourage the client to press his or her forearm against your hip or waist for stability if desired. In addition, have the client wear a transfer or walking belt so that you can quickly grab the belt and prevent a fall if he or she feels faint.

- If the client is very weak and unstable, place your near arm around the client's waist and with your other arm support the client's near arm at the elbow. Walk on the client's stronger side. Again, have the client wear a transfer or walking belt in case of an emergency.

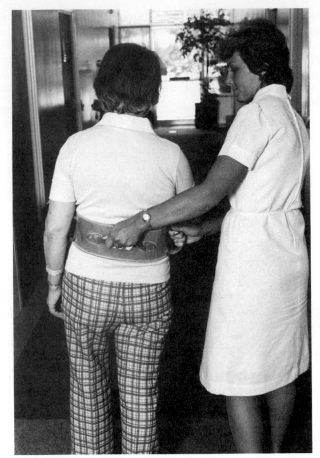

Figure 36–18 A walking belt

i.e., without fatiguing the muscles. Carried out several times an hour during waking hours, this simple exercise significantly strengthens the muscles used for walking. When the client is ready to ambulate, the nurse follows the guidelines in the accompanying box to ensure client safety and facilitate ambulation.

If a client begins to experience the signs and symptoms of orthostatic hypotension or extreme weakness, he or she should be quickly assisted into a chair and helped to lower his or her head between the knees. The nurse must stay with the client. If the client faints while in this position, he or she could fall, head first, out of the chair. When the client feels better, he or she can be wheeled back to bed.

If a chair is not close by, the client should be assisted to a horizontal position on the floor before fainting occurs, since a vertical position may increase feelings of faintness. Clients who do faint or start to fall and cannot regain their strength or balance usually drop straight downward or pitch slightly forward due to the momen-

tum of ambulating; thus, the head, hips, and knees are most vulnerable to injury. In this situation, a nurse assumes a broad stance with one foot in front of the other and brings the client backward so that he or she is supported by the nurse's body. The nurse then allows the client to slide down the nurse's leg and lowers the client gently to the floor, making sure that the client's head does not hit any objects. See Figure 36–19. The nurse's broad stance widens the base of support for stability. Placing one foot behind the other allows the nurse to rock backward and use the femoral muscles when supporting the client's weight and lowering his or her center of gravity, thus preventing back strain. Bringing the client's weight backward against the nurse's body allows gradual movement to the floor without injury to the client.

Mechanical Aids for Walking

Canes, walkers, and crutches are three commonly used mechanical aids for walking. Three types of **canes** are used today: the simple straight-legged cane; the tripod or crab cane, which has three feet; and the quad cane, which has four feet and provides the most support. See Figure 36–20. Cane tips should have rubber caps to improve traction and prevent slipping. The standard cane is 91 cm (36 in) long; some aluminum canes can be adjusted from 56 to 97 cm (22 to 38 in). Clients may use either one or two canes, depending on how much

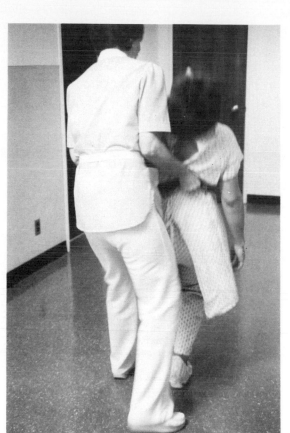

Figure 36—19 A client who has fainted is lowered to the floor.

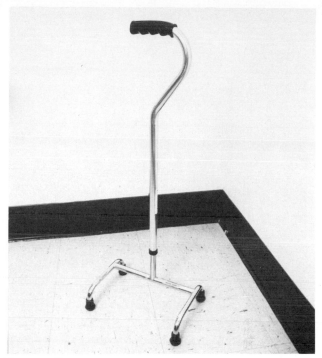

Figure 36—20 A quad cane

support they require. The accompanying box provides guidelines for clients using canes.

The client should hold a cane with the hand on the stronger side of the body to provide maximum support and appropriate body alignment when walking. The tip of the cane is positioned about 15 cm (6 in) to the side and 15 cm (6 in) in front of the near foot so that the elbow is slightly flexed.

Walkers are mechanical devices for ambulatory clients who need more support than a cane provides. There are many types of walkers of different shapes and sizes, with devices suited to individual needs. The standard type is made of polished aluminum. It has four legs with rubber tips and plastic hand grips. See Figure 36—21. Many walkers have adjustable legs. The standard walker needs to be picked up to be used. The client therefore requires partial strength in both hands and wrists, strong elbow extensors, such as the triceps brachii, and strong shoulder depressors, such as the pectoralis minor. The client also needs the ability to bear at least partial weight on both legs.

Four-wheeled models of walkers (roller walkers) do not need to be picked up to be moved, but they are less stable than the standard walker. They are used by clients who are too weak or unstable to pick up and move the walker with each step. Some roller walkers have a seat at the back so that the client can sit down to rest when desired. The nurse may need to adjust the height of a client's walker so that the hand bar is just below the

client's waist and the client's elbows are slightly flexed. This position helps the client assume a more normal stance. A walker that is too low causes the client to stoop; one that is too high makes the client stretch and reach. The accompanying box provides guidelines for using walkers.

Crutches may be a temporary need for some people and a permanent one for others. Crutches should

GUIDELINES

Using Canes

For maximum support, the client:

- Moves the cane forward about 30 cm (1 ft), or a distance that is comfortable while the body weight is borne by both legs
- Then moves the affected (weak) leg forward to the cane while the weight is borne by the cane and stronger leg
- Next, moves the unaffected (stronger) leg forward ahead of the cane and weak leg while the weight is borne by the cane and weak leg
- Repeats steps 1—3. This pattern of moving provides at least two points of support on the floor at all times.

As the client becomes stronger and requires less support, the client can:

- Move the cane and weak leg forward at the same time, while the weight is borne by the stronger leg
- Move the stronger leg forward, while the weight is borne by the cane and the weak leg

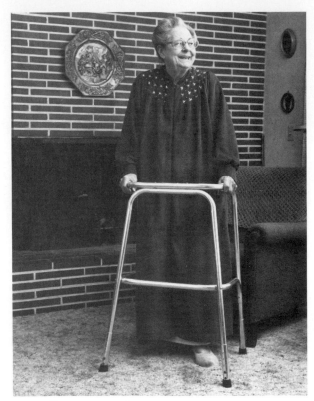

Figure 36-21 A walker permits this woman to ambulate independently and safely.

enable a person to ambulate independently; therefore, it is important to learn to use them properly. There are several kinds of crutches. The most frequently used are the *underarm* or *axillary crutch* with hand bars and the *Lofstrand crutch,* which extends only to the forearm. The underarm crutch can be extended. It has double uprights, an underarm bar, and a hand bar. See Figure 36-22, *A.* The Lofstrand crutch is a single adjustable tube of aluminum to which are attached a curved piece of steel, a rubber-covered hand bar, and a metal forearm

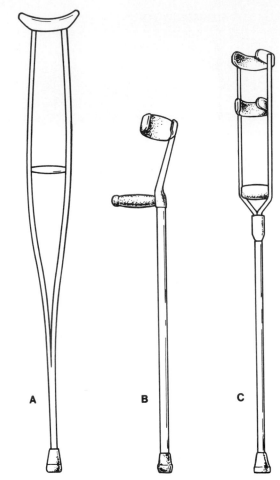

Figure 36-22 Three types of crutches: **A**, axillary; **B**, Lofstrand; **C**, Canadian (elbow extensor)

cuff. See Figure 36-22, *B.* This type of crutch is most useful as a substitute for a cane. The metal cuff around the forearm and the metal bar stabilize the wrists and thus make walking safer and easier. The person can release the hand bar to use his or her hand, and the metal cuff will hold the crutch in place, while a cane would fall.

The *Canadian* or *elbow extensor crutch* is like the Lofstrand in that it is made of a single tube of aluminum with lateral attachments, a hand bar, and a cuff for the forearm, but it also has a cuff for the upper arm. See Figure 36-22, *C.* This crutch is usually used by clients who require support for weak extensor muscles of the forearm and trunk (e.g., weak triceps brachii). All crutches have suction tips, usually made of rubber, which help to prevent the crutches from slipping on a floor surface. Suggested guidelines for using crutches are summarized in the accompanying box.

In crutch walking, the client's weight is borne by the muscles of the shoulder girdle and the upper extremities. Five major muscle groups are used: the flexor muscles of the arms (e.g., the pectoralis major and brachialis), the extensor muscles of the forearms (e.g., the triceps brachii), the finger and thumb flexors (e.g., the flexor pollicis brevis), the muscles that dorsiflex the wrists (e.g., the flexor carpi radialis), and the shoulder girdle depressors and the downward rotators (e.g.,

GUIDELINES

Using Walkers

For maximum support, the client:

■ Moves the walker ahead about 15 cm (6 in) while body weight is borne by both legs

■ Moves the right foot up to the walker while body weight is borne by the left leg and both arms

■ Moves the left foot up to the right foot while body weight is borne by the right leg and both arms

If one leg is weaker than the other, the client:

■ Moves the walker and the weak leg ahead together about 15 cm (6 in) while the weight is borne by the stronger leg

■ Moves the stronger leg ahead while the weight is borne by the affected leg and both arms

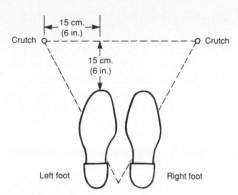

Figure 36–23 The tripod position

the pectoralis minor). Before beginning crutch walking, the client should exercise to develop and strengthen these muscle groups.

The proper standing position with crutches is called the **tripod (triangle) position.** See Figure 36–23. The crutches are placed about 15 cm (6 in) in front of the feet and out laterally about 15 cm (6 in), creating a wide base of support. The feet are slightly apart. A tall person requires a wider base than a short person. Hips and knees are extended, the back is straight, and the head is held straight and high. There should be no hunch to the shoulders and thus no weight borne by the axillae. The palms are positioned lateral to the feet, and the elbows are extended sufficiently to allow weight bearing on the hands. If the client is unsteady, the nurse places a walking belt around the client's waist and grasps the belt from above, not from below. A fall can be prevented more effectively if the belt is held from above.

The **four-point alternate gait** is the most elementary and safest gait, providing at least three points of support at each time. Clients can use it when walking in crowds because it does not require much space. To use this gait, the client needs to be able to bear weight on both legs. See Figure 36–24 (reading from bottom to top). The client:

1. Moves the right crutch ahead a suitable distance, e.g., 10 to 15 cm (4 to 6 in)

GUIDELINES

Crutches

- The weight of the body should be borne by the arms rather than the axillae. Pressure on the axillae can injure the radial nerve and eventually cause crutch palsy, a **paresis** (weakness of the muscles) of the forearm, wrist, and hand.

- The client should maintain erect posture to prevent strain on muscles and joints and to maintain balance.

- Each step taken with crutches should be a comfortable distance for the client. It is wise to start with a small rather than a large step.

- Crutch tips should be inspected regularly and replaced if worn and should be kept dry to maintain their surface friction.

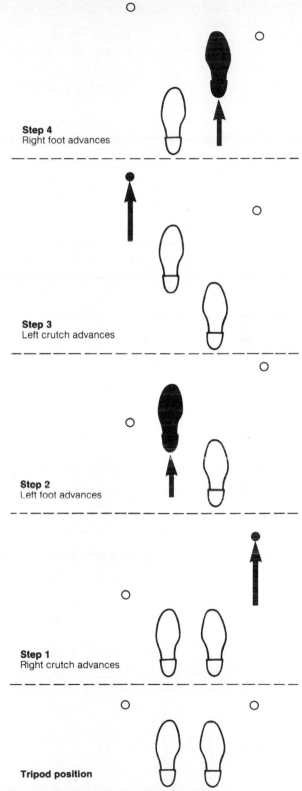

Step 4
Right foot advances

Step 3
Left crutch advances

Step 2
Left foot advances

Step 1
Right crutch advances

Tripod position

Figure 36–24 The four-point alternate gait

2. Moves the left front foot forward, preferably to the level of the left crutch
3. Moves the left crutch forward
4. Moves the right foot forward

To use the **three-point gait,** the client must be able to bear his or her entire weight on the unaffected leg. The two crutches and the unaffected leg bear weight alternately. See Figure 36–25 (reading from bottom to top). The client:

1. Moves both crutches and the weaker leg forward
2. Moves the stronger leg forward

Chairs that have armrests and are secure or braced against a wall are essential for clients using crutches. To assist the client in sitting down, the nurse instructs the client to:

1. Stand with the back of the unaffected leg centered against the chair. The chair helps support the client during the next steps.
2. Transfer the crutches to the hand on the affected side, hold the crutches by the hand bars and grasp the arm of the chair with the hand on the unaffected side. This allows the client to support the body weight on the arms and the unaffected leg.
3. Lean forward, flex the knees and hips, and lower into the chair.

When assisting a client in getting out of a chair, the nurse instructs the client to:

1. Move forward to the edge of the chair and place the unaffected leg slightly under or at the edge of the chair. This position helps the client stand up from the chair and achieve balance, since the unaffected leg is supported against the edge of the chair.
2. Grasp the crutches by the hand bars in the hand on the affected side, and grasp the arm of the chair by the hand on the unaffected side. The body weight is placed on the crutches and the hand on the armrest to support the unaffected leg when the client rises to stand.
3. Push down on the crutches and the chair armrest while elevating his or her body out of the chair.
4. Assume the tripod position before moving.

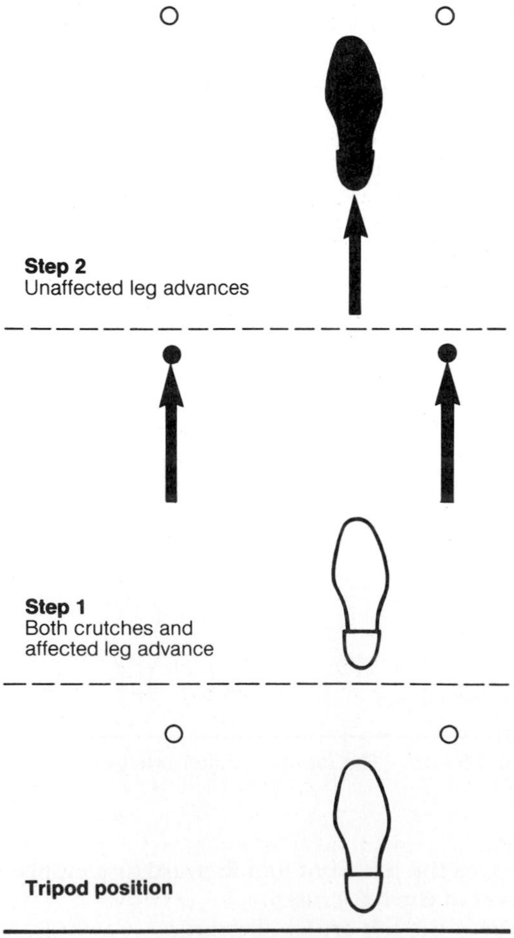

To teach the client how to go up stairs, the nurse stands behind the client and slightly to the affected side and instructs the client to:

1. Assume the tripod position at the bottom of the stairs.
2. Transfer the body weight to the crutches and move the unaffected leg onto the step. See Figure 36–26.
3. Transfer the body weight to the unaffected leg on the step and move the crutches and affected leg up to the step. The affected leg is always supported by the crutches.
4. Repeat steps 2 and 3 until the client reaches the top of the stairs.

To show the client how to go down stairs, the nurse stands one step below the client on the affected side and instructs the client to:

1. Assume the tripod position at the top of the stairs.

Step 2
Unaffected leg advances

Step 1
Both crutches and
affected leg advance

Tripod position

Figure 36–25 The three-point crutch gait

ASSESSMENT

Neurovascular Checks for Clients with Casts

Check the skin for:

Color. Pallor or cyanosis may indicate circulatory impairment.

Temperature. Excessive coldness can indicate circulatory impairment; excessive warmth may reflect inflammation and possibly infection.

Swelling. Some is expected during the early period and is not a differential symptom of circulatory impairment; the development of swelling several days after application should be reported to the physician.

Paresthesia. Decreased sensation may indicate neurovascular impairment.

Capillary refill. Compress the nail of the thumb or large toe for a few seconds until it blanches and then noting the time elapsed until return of blood flow after release of pressure. Normally, the capillaries refill immediately. A sluggish return may indicate venous congestion or arterial insufficiency.

Distal pulse. Palpate the affected extremity and compare it to the symmetric pulse of the unaffected extremity for equality. This check is not always possible because the cast may cover the pulse point.

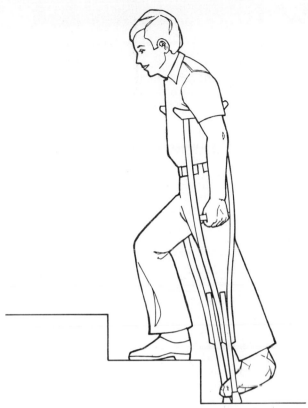

Figure 36–26 When climbing stairs, the client places weight on the crutches while moving the unaffected leg onto a step.

2. Shift the body weight to the unaffected leg and move the crutches and affected leg down onto the next step. See Figure 36–27.
3. Transfer the body weight to the crutches, and move the unaffected leg to that step. The affected leg is always supported by the crutches.
4. Repeat steps 2 and 3 until the client reaches the bottom of the stairs.

▪ Maintaining Alignment of Clients with Casts and in Traction

Clients with orthopedic problems may require medical intervention through the application of casts or traction to achieve proper alignment. The nurse is primarily responsibile for maintaining that alignment, assessing neurovascular functioning, maintaining the integrity of client's skin surfaces, and preventing complications of immobility (e.g., by exercising the joints above and below the cast). Additionally, the nurse should intervene to reduce swelling (see Chapter 16), prevent infection (see Chapter 23), and control pain (Chapter 38).

▪ Caring for Clients with Casts. Neurovascular assessment of affected limbs is a priority of care for clients with casts, especially during the first 24 to 48 hours after application. Rapid swelling under a cast can cause neurovascular injury. Preventive nursing measures, frequent assessment, and prompt intervention when needed contribute to satisfactory client healing. The nurse

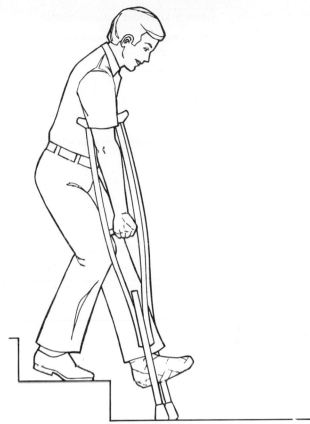

Figure 36–27 When descending stairs, the client places weight on the crutches while moving the unaffected leg onto a step.

should assess the affected extremity, distal to the application of the cast, for nerve or circulatory impairments every 30 minutes for several hours after application and then every 3–4 hours until there are no signs and symptoms of impairment. The nurse assesses the extremity by comparing it to the unaffected limb. The accompanying box provides guidelines for neurovascular assessment.

Neurologic integrity is assessed by evaluating the client's motor ability and sensation. See Table 36–6 for nerve function assessment guidelines. Inability to perform motor function tests suggests possible compression of a nerve and potential paralysis. Common affected nerves are the peroneal, tibial, radial, median, and ulnar nerves. See Figure 36–28. When the nurse assesses sensation, all fingers and toes must be checked, since they are innervated by different nerves. Lack of sensation may indicate impaired function of the associated nerves. If pain is present, note particularly whether the pain is persistent or occurs over a bony prominence. See Table 36–7 for common pressure points associated with various casts.

▪ Caring for Clients in Traction. Traction is applied by a device that immobilizes a part of the body. Clients in traction are often confined to bed for weeks or even months. Nursing care, therefore, involves giving assistance with ADLs, maintaining proper alignment, and preventing problems such as pressure sores. Traction can be either continuous or intermittent. Continuous

Table 36—6 Nerve Function Assessments

Nerve	Motor Function Tests	Sensory Function Tests
Radial	Instruct client to hyperextend thumb or wrist and straighten all four fingers.	Prick web space between thumb and index finger.
Median	Instruct client to oppose thumb and little finger and flex wrist.	Prick distal fat pad of index finger.
Ulnar	Instruct client to abduct all fingers.	Prick fat pad at distal end of small finger.
Peroneal	Instruct client to dorsiflex ankle and extend toes.	Prick web between great toe and second toe or lateral surface of great toe and medial surface of second toe.
Tibial	Instruct client to plantar flex ankle and flex toes.	Prick medial and lateral surfaces of sole of foot.

Sources: J. Farrell: *Illustrated Guide to Orthopedic Nursing,* 2nd ed. (Lippincott, 1982), p. 66; P. L. Swearingen: *The Addison-Wesley Photo-Atlas of Nursing Procedures* (Addison-Wesley, 1984), pp. 519–521.

Table 36—7 Common Cast Pressure Areas

Type of Cast	Common Pressure Areas
Short arm cast	Radial styloid Ulnar styloid Joint at base of thumb
Hanging arm cast	Radial styloid Ulnar styloid Olecranon Lateral epicondyle
Short leg cast	Heel Achilles tendon Malleolus
Long leg cast	Heel Achilles tendon Malleolus Popliteal artery behind knee Peroneal nerve at side of knee
Hip spica	As above for long leg cast Sacrum Iliac crests

traction (skeletal or skin) should be applied and released by a physician, and a physician should be responsible for handling the affected part when it is not in traction. Intermittent traction (nonadhesive skin traction) can be applied and released by nurses implementing the prescribed orders of the physician. Table 36—8 summarizes types of traction that are commonly used and the related nursing responsibilities.

Evaluating Client Responses and Nursing Actions

The principles of body mechanics and ambulation, used previously as assessment criteria, are also used as outcome criteria to evaluate the effectiveness of the nurse's interventions in moving and transferring clients. The quality of anyone's body mechanics in daily activities is evaluated according to how well the person conforms to the principles of body mechanics and prevents back injury. The quality of anyone's ambulation is evaluated according to how well he or she conforms to the principles of ambulation and achieves stability in gait without falling. Examples of outcome criteria to measure the client's goal achievement and the effectiveness of nursing interventions are shown in the box on page 590.

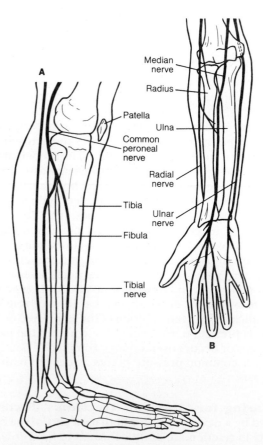

Figure 36—28 The peroneal and tibial nerves (**A**) and the radial, median, and ulnar nerves (**B**) can be injured by prolonged compression in a cylindrical cast.

Table 36–8 Specific Tractions: Uses and Nursing Interventions

Traction	Uses	Key Considerations	Nursing Interventions
Buck's extension	Prior to surgery for fractured femur Knee and hip contractures Disease processes of knee and hip	Bandages applied too tightly can cause: ■ Constriction of circulation in the extremity. Symptoms: numbness and coldness. ■ Pressure on and possible damage to peroneal nerve. Symptoms: tingling or pain of anterior aspect of lower leg and dorsal surface of foot; foot inversion and inability to extend toes. Pressure areas: skin over the tibia, if bandage slips; popliteal space; hamstring tendon; heels.	Provide regular back care, especially for the buttocks, because client is confined to a back-lying position. Two nurses may be required to place and remove a bedpan if client has pain or is obese. Because traction is often temporary, exercises generally restricted to turning (e.g., for back care), deep breathing, coughing, and foot movement.
Russell traction	Fractured femur Knee and hip contractures	See Buck's extension, first consideration. Pressure areas: popliteal space, due to sling; sole of foot, due to footplate.	Provide regular back care. Place and remove bedpan from the unaffected side. Teach exercises in preparation for crutch walking. Provide regular skin care of the leg, foot, and back. Teach exercises in preparation for crutch walking.
Thomas leg splint and Pearson attachment	Fractured femur Pre- or postoperative immobilization	Pressure areas: The groin (adductor muscle and ischial area), from ring; popliteal space; Achilles tendon; heel; peroneal nerve, if splint and Pearson attachment slip to one side.	Provide regular skin care of the leg, foot, and back. Teach exercises in preparation for crutch walking.
Pelvic belt (girdle) traction	Lower back pain	Belt will slip if too loose or incorrectly applied, causing uneven pull. Pressure areas: iliac crests, back.	Teach exercises to move extremities through full range of motion. Teach exercises to strengthen back muscles. Evaluate back pain: type, relief, etc.
Cervical head halter traction	Cervical injuries ("whiplash")	Pressure areas: chin, occiput of the head, ears, mandible.	Provide regular skin care, e.g., every two hours. Keep the chin dry, using alcohol or cornstarch. Closely monitor food and fluid intake to ensure adequate diet, since eating and chewing are often difficult. A soft diet may be easier for client to take. Assess for neck discomfort and for numbness and tingling in arms and hands.
Halo-thoracic vest traction	Thoracic and cervical spine injuries	Head pin migration (anchoring pin shifts in position), resulting in misalignment and loosening of halo. Discomfort from metal objects striking the metal traction rods. Conduction of sound through skull bones is discomforting, so care should be taken to avoid hitting rods with metallic objects. Pressure areas: where jacket edges touch the skin.	Meticulous pin site care with hydrogen peroxide and water in equal amounts needs to be given at least twice a day. Povidone-iodine is not used (may corrode pins). Some agencies advocate use of antibiotic ointment after cleaning with hydrogen peroxide. Infection at pin site is evidenced by increased drainage, inflammation, elevated body temperature, and headache. Encourage deep breathing and coughing exercises q.4h., and auscultate chest sounds periodically. Incentive spirometry can be used also. (Respiratory complications from the vest and from decreased mobility can occur.)

(continued)

Traction	Uses	Key Considerations	Nursing Interventions
			Open or remove vest daily to inspect the skin and provide skin care. At other times, inspect and massage skin around vest edges at least q.4h. Change or clean the sheepskin lining at least weekly.
			Assess for neurologic impairment of upper extremities due to the thoracic disorder. Check client's hand grasps and sensation in fingers and hands q.4h. for first few days, then daily.
			Assess for cranial nerve impingement by the pins and traction forces.
Side-arm traction	Fracture of the humerus Contractures or fracture of the elbow	Muscle stiffness due to maintenance of one position. Pressure areas: soft tissues near shoulder; anterior surface of elbow joint, due to bandages.	Do a neurovascular assessment of the arm and hand. Provide regular skin care of the back, arm, and hand. Encourage regular range-of-motion exercises for the unaffected extremities to prevent thrombophlebitis.

OUTCOME CRITERIA

Body Mechanics and Ambulation

The client will demonstrate use of good body mechanics when lifting and pulling objects, by:

■ Using a wide base of support when moving objects

■ Enlarging his or her base of support by placing feet appropriately in the direction in which the movement occurs

■ Keeping objects to be moved close to his or her body (center of gravity)

■ Pushing, pulling, rolling, or sliding objects rather than lifting them whenever possible

■ Avoiding twisting the spine by pushing or pulling objects directly away from or toward the body and squarely facing the direction of movement

■ Squatting rather than stooping to pick up heavy objects from the floor and using large muscle groups of the body

■ Using his or her body weight to counteract the weight of the object when pushing or pulling objects

■ Tensing stabilizing muscles before moving objects

■ Maintaining muscle mass and strength through exercise

■ Identifying factors contributing to back strain

■ Experiencing no back pain or muscle fatigue

■ Standing erect when walking

■ Using a walker to move independently from the bed to the nursing station three times a day

■ Demonstrating correct use of four-point (or three-point) crutch gait

■ Demonstrating correct methods of getting into and out of a chair and ascending and descending stairs with crutches

Chapter Highlights

■ Maintaining good body alignment, using good body mechanics, and promoting ambulation are essential for good body functioning and for preventing injury to body structures, discomfort, and fatigue.

■ The nurse acts as a role model and teacher of good body alignment and body mechanics.

■ Factors influencing body alignment, body mechanics, and ambulation include general health, nutrition, emotions, environment, life-style, attitudes and values, level of understanding, and neuromuscular or skeletal impairments.

■ The nurse identifies nursing diagnoses and goals related to impairments or potential impairments in body alignment and ambulation.

■ The principles of body alignment and the guidelines for positioning clients help the nurse to plan individualized interventions.

■ Assessment of body mechanics and ambulation includes identification of the client's capabilities and limitations for movement, use of body mechanics, and gait.

■ Nursing diagnoses related to the client's body mechanics and gait may include impaired physical mobility, potential for injury, fear, self-care deficit, and knowledge deficit.

■ The nurse uses assessment data and nursing diagnoses to identify goals for care and design an individualized plan of nursing interventions.

■ Overall client goals include improved use of proper body mechanics in work and in daily life, restored or improved ambulatory capability, and prevention of back injuries and falls.

■ Assistance from others or the use of mechanical lifting aids is essential when clients are too heavy for the nurse to move or lift safely.

■ Ambulating techniques that facilitate normal walking gait yet provide the support needed are most effective.

The nurse can assist clients to prepare for ambulation by helping them become as independent as possible while in bed and encouraging them to perform orthostatic tension.

Safety precautions and use of appropriate body mechanics are essential whenever assisting others to move to prevent client injury from falls and to prevent back strain of the nurse.

Clients with casts and traction require nursing vigilance regarding neurovascular assessment and maintenance of skin integrity.

Selected References

Broer, M. R., and Zernicke, R. F. 1979. *Efficiency of human movement.* 4th ed. Philadelphia: W. B. Saunders Co.

Byrne, C. J.; Saxton, D. F.; Pelikarn, P. K.; and Nugent, P. M. 1986. *Laboratory tests: Implications for nursing care.* 2d ed. Menlo Park, Calif.: Addison-Wesley Publishing Co.

Campbell, E. B.; Williams, M. A.; and Mlynarczyk, S. M. February 1986. After the fall—confusion. *American Journal of Nursing* 86:151–54.

Cushing, M. February 1985. First, anticipate the harm. *American Journal of Nursing* 85:137–38.

Donaldson, W. F., and Hoover, N. W. 1982. *The American Medical Association book of back care.* New York: Random House.

Drapeau, J. September 1975. Getting back into good posture: How to ease your lumbar aches. *Nursing 75* 5:63–65.

Eliopoulos, C., editor. 1984. *Health assessment of the older adult.* Menlo Park, Calif.: Addison-Wesley Publishing Co.

Foss, G. May 1973. Use your head and save your back: Body mechanics. *Nursing 73* 3:25–32.

———. January/February 1984. Nonenvironmental causes of falls in a nursing home. *Geriatric Medicine Currents.* Ross Laboratories.

Gates, S. May 1988. On-the-job back exercises. *American Journal of Nursing* 88:656–59.

Harber, P., et al. July 1985. Occupational low-back pain in hospital nurses. *Journal of Occupational Medicine* 27:518–24.

Hayne, C. R. August 1981. Manual transport of loads by women. *Physiotherapy* 67:226–31.

Hogan, L., and Beland, I. July 1976. Cervical neck syndrome. *American Journal of Nursing* 76:1104–7.

Hogue, C. March 1982. Injury in late life. Part I: Epidemiology. *American Geriatric Society* 30: 183–89.

Hoover, S. December 1973. Job-related back injuries in a hospital. *American Journal of Nursing* 73:2078–79.

Ishmael, W., and Shorbe, H. 1969. *Care of the back.* 2d ed. Philadelphia: J. B. Lippincott Co.

Kottke, F.; Stillwell, G.; and Lehmann, J., editors. 1982. *Krusen's handbook of physical medicine and rehabilitation.* 3d ed. Philadelphia: W. B. Saunders Co.

Lee, P. S., and Pash, B. J. February 1983. Preventing patient falls. *Nursing 83* 13:118–20.

Leinweber, E. December 1978. Belts to make moves smoother. *American Journal of Nursing* 78:2080–81.

Marino, N. M. April 1985. After the fall: An analysis. *American Journal of Nursing* 95:362.

Memmer, M. K. 1974a. *Body Mechanics.* Los Angeles: Intercampus Nursing Project, California State University and College System.

———. 1974b. *Introduction to alignment, body mechanics, and exercise.* Los Angeles: Intercampus Nursing Project, California State University and College System.

———. 1974c. *Posture and alignment.* Los Angeles: The Intercampus Nursing Project, California State University and College System.

Owen, B. D. May 1980. How to avoid that aching back. *American Journal of Nursing* 80:894–97.

Witte, N. S. November 1979. Why the elderly fall. *American Journal of Nursing* 79:1950–52.

Rest and Sleep

OBJECTIVES

Identity conditions necessary to promote rest.

Identify factors influencing rest and sleep.

Identify characteristics of NREM and REM sleep.

Identify four stages of NREM sleep.

Describe information that helps the nurse assess sleep habits.

Identify factors contributing to selected sleep disorders.

Identify clinical signs and symptoms indicative of insufficient rest and sleep.

Identify developmental variations in rest and sleep patterns.

Define terms related to common rest and sleep disorders.

Identify three types of insomnia.

Identify interventions that promote sleep and rest.

Identify interventions that restore appropriate sleep and rest patterns for selected disorders.

Describe outcome criteria for evaluating a client's response to nursing interventions to promote sleep and rest.

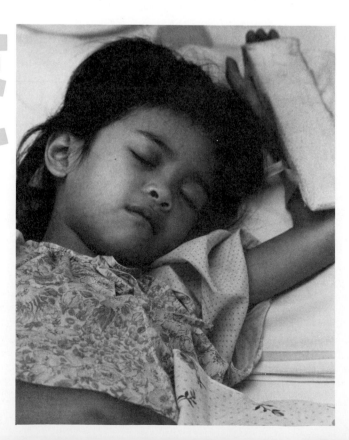

Purposes of Rest and Sleep

Rest and sleep are essential for health. During sleep, the body repairs itself for the next day. People who are ill frequently require more rest and sleep than they normally do. Often, debilitated people expend unusual amounts of energy just to regain health or maintain the activities of daily living. As a result, such people experience increased and frequent fatigue and thus need more rest and sleep than usual. In addition, the ill person's normal sleep schedule is usually altered, and nursing intervention may be needed to promote the required sleep.

Rest implies calmness, relaxation without emotional stress, and freedom from anxiety. Therefore, rest does not always imply inactivity; in fact, some people find some activities restful. For example, a student studying for examinations may find it restful to walk in the fresh air. The meaning of rest and the need for rest vary among individuals. To assess the client's need for rest and to evaluate how effectively this need is met, nurses need to consider conditions that promote rest.

To rest, clients need to feel that their personal lives are under control and that they are receiving competent health care. By providing competent care, the nurse gives peace of mind and allows the client to relax. A nurse often can promote rest by listening carefully to clients' personal concerns and alleviating them when possible. For example, a man taken to an emergency ward may be unable to relax until a nurse telephones his wife to inform her.

Even when the person comes prepared for hospitalization, the nurse must consider the client's personal concerns and worries. For example, if a client admitted for elective diagnostic cystoscopy is also recovering successfully from a fractured hip and routinely walks prescribed distances each day, the client may worry that recovery from the fracture will be slowed by this interruption in exercise. Many clients experience discomfort or anxiety when well-established routines are interrupted. The routine might be reading oneself to sleep, drinking hot milk each evening, or following certain religious practices. Children often have security rituals before sleeping. Clients hospitalized for long periods may need the routine of sleeping in on a Saturday or Sunday morning or scheduled daily quiet or privacy. Most people need some time to themselves.

Rest may be impossible for clients who do not feel accepted. Clients need to feel acceptable to themselves and to others. Grooming is often one important aspect of self-acceptance. Women may be concerned about the growth of hair on their legs or the need for a shampoo or manicure; men may be concerned about an untrimmed beard or mustache. The nurse needs to be sensitive to these aspects of care and attend to them. Acceptance by the staff is also important to the client. Acceptance can be conveyed, for instance, by recognizing client limitations, client progress, and individual differences.

A client's understanding of what is happening is another condition essential for rest. The unknown generates varying degrees of anxiety and interferes with rest. The nurse can help by offering explanations about diagnostic tests, surgery, agency policies or routines, and the client's progress. When information is given freely, clients do not feel the tension associated with having to ask questions.

Irritation and discomfort have both physical and emotional aspects. Generally, the nurse can easily detect physical discomforts, such as pain, insufficient supports for body positions, damp bedclothes, and loud noise. Emotional discomforts include having too many or too few visitors, feeling a lack of privacy, being hurried, having to wait long periods, being alone, or being concerned about the life problems of self or others.

Purposeful activity can be relaxing and often provides a sense of self-worth. The grandparent who knits a scarf for a grandchild, the person who helps make the bed, the adolescent who makes a wallet for her father, or the child who makes a toy puppet generally have a sense of contentment and accomplishment. Such activity often promotes rest throughout the day and undisturbed sleep at night.

Clients who feel isolated and helpless may not be able to rest properly. Friends and family members can promote rest by helping the client with daily tasks and difficult decisions. Nurses can help by anticipating and meeting clients' needs. Knowing that the call bell will be answered, for example, can be exceedingly important to a client. Also, the support and understanding of the nurse can help clients facing major decisions. Although such decisions are the client's alone, nurses can be instrumental in helping the client clarify issues (e.g., by offering additional information about referral agencies or by helping the client to express feelings).

Sleep, a basic physiologic need, is defined as a state of unconsciousness from which a person can be aroused by appropriate sensory or other stimuli (Guyton 1986, p. 670). Sleep is characterized by minimal physical activity, variable levels of consciousness, changes in the body's physiologic processes, and decreased responsiveness to external stimuli (Hayter 1980, p. 457). Energy is conserved during sleep. With relaxation of the skeletal muscles, energy is redirected to essential cellular activities.

Functions of Sleep

Sleep is restorative. During sleep, stress on the pulmonary, cardiovascular, nervous, endocrine, and excretory systems decreases. For example, the normal heart rate of a healthy adult decreases from a rate of 70 to 80 beats per minute during wakefulness to 60 or fewer beats per minute during sleep. In addition, sympathetic activity decreases and parasympathetic activity occasionally increases (Guyton 1986, p. 674). Other body changes during sleep are shown in the accompanying box.

Sleep is believed to mediate stress, anxiety, and tension and to help the person regain energy for concentrating, coping, and maintaining interest in daily activities. Sleep does not appear to be necessary to recharge

Physiologic Changes During Sleep

- Arterial blood pressure falls.
- Pulse rate decreases.
- Peripheral blood vessels dilate.
- Activity of the gastrointestinal tract occasionally increases.
- Skeletal muscles relax.
- Basal metabolic rate decreases 10 to 30% (Guyton 1986, p. 674)

Table 37–1   Characteristics of REM and NREM Sleep

REM	NREM
Active dreaming	Dreamlessness
Sleeper more difficult to arouse than during NREM (slow-wave) sleep	Profound restfulness
Muscle tone depressed	Decreased blood pressure
Heart rate and respiratory rate often irregular	Decreased respiratory rate
Irregular movements—in particular, rapid eye movements	Decreased metabolic rate; slow and rolling eye movements

energy lost during the day. If that were the case, the relative durations of wakefulness and sleep would remain constant, and they do not. For example, when people are deliberately kept awake for 3 to 10 days, they sleep for less than a day after the enforced wakefulness. Conversely, when people are immobilized for long periods, they still sleep and apparently need to.

There are two kinds of sleep: **REM** (rapid eye movement) **sleep** and **NREM** (non-REM slow-wave) **sleep.** REM sleep is not a passive state but a relatively active state; thus, REM sleep is also referred to as **paradoxical sleep.** The characteristics of REM and NREM sleep are compared in Table 37–1. The sympathetic nervous system dominates during REM sleep. REM sleep is thought to restore a person mentally for learning, psychologic adaptation, and memory (Hayter 1980, p. 458). During REM sleep, the sleeper reviews the day's events and processes and stores the information. The sleeper gains perspective on problems and may resolve some problems. Thus, there is wisdom in the traditional advice to "sleep on" a problem or big decision. NREM sleep is also referred to as deep, restful sleep or slow-wave sleep, because the brain waves of a sleeper during NREM sleep are slower than the alpha and beta waves of a person who is awake or alert.

An **electroencephalogram** (**EEG**) graphically represents brain activity on an oscilloscope. This pattern can be printed out for permanent recording. Electrodes are placed on various parts of the client's scalp. The electrodes transmit electric energy from the cerebral cortex to pens that record the fluctuations in energy (**brain waves**) on graph paper. Each pen of the electroencephalograph corresponds to an electrode, moving up when the electric charge is negative and down when it is positive. See Figure 37–1.

Control of sleep is centered in two specialized areas of the brain stem: the reticular activating system (RAS) and the bulbar synchronizing region (BSR) in the medulla. There are two theories about sleep, the passive theory and the active theory. The passive theory holds that the RAS brain simply becomes fatigued and therefore becomes inactive. The active theory, which is more widely accepted today, proposes some sort of center or centers that cause sleep by inhibiting other parts of the brain (Guyton 1986, p. 672).

The two systems, RAS and BSR, are thought to activate and then suppress the brain centers intermittently,

resulting in cycles of sleep. The RAS is associated with the body's state of alertness and receives sensory input, i.e., auditory, visual, pain, and tactile stimuli. These sensory stimuli maintain a person's sense of wakefulness and alertness. During sleep the body sends fewer stimuli from the cerebral cortex or the peripheral sensory receptors to the RAS. The person awakens from sleep when there is an increase in such stimuli. There is less known about the BSR; however, it is known that its activity increases with sleep. NREM (slow-wave) sleep is generally divided into four stages:

Stage I. This is the stage of very light sleep. The brain waves are of low voltage, though broken periodically by *sleep spindles* (short, spindle-shaped bursts of alpha waves). The person feels drowsy and relaxed, the eyes roll from side to side, and the heart and respiratory rates drop slightly. The sleeper can be readily awakened during this stage.

Stage II. Stage II is the stage of light sleep during which body processes continue to slow down. The eyes

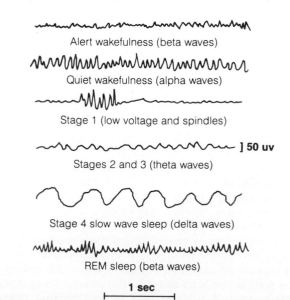

Alert wakefulness (beta waves)

Quiet wakefulness (alpha waves)

Stage 1 (low voltage and spindles)

] 50 uv

Stages 2 and 3 (theta waves)

Stage 4 slow wave sleep (delta waves)

REM sleep (beta waves)

1 sec

Figure 37–1   Characteristic brain waves during waking, the four stages of NREM sleep, and REM sleep. *Source:* From A. C. Guyton, *Textbook of medical physiology,* 7th ed. (Philadelphia: W. B. Saunders Co., 1986), p. 671. Used by permission.

are generally still, the heart and respiratory rates decrease slightly, and body temperature falls. The brain waves during stages II and III are theta waves. Stage II lasts only about 10 to 15 minutes.

Stage III. During stage III, the heart and respiratory rates as well as other body processes slow further, due to domination of the parasympathetic nervous system. The sleeper becomes more difficult to arouse. The brain waves become more regular. Slow delta waves are added to the stage II theta wave pattern.

Stage IV. Stage IV signals deep sleep, during which delta waves predominate and become even slower. The sleeper's heart and respiratory rates drop 20 to 30% below those exhibited during waking hours. The sleeper is very relaxed, rarely moves, and is difficult to arouse. Stage IV is thought to restore the body physically. Physical exercise 2 hours before bedtime promotes stage IV sleep (Hayter 1980, p. 457).

The usual sleeper experiences four to six cycles of sleep during 7 to 8 hours. Each cycle lasts about 90 minutes. See Figure 37–2. A sleeper passes from stage I NREM sleep through stages II and III to stage IV in about 20 to 30 minutes. Stage IV may last about 30 minutes. The process is then reversed, and the sleeper ascends through stages III and II, after which REM sleep occurs. REM sleep completes the first cycle, and the cycle then repeats. The sleeper who is awakened during any stage must begin anew at stage I NREM sleep and proceed through all the stages to REM sleep.

The duration of NREM stages and REM sleep varies throughout the 8-hour sleep period. As the night progresses, the sleeper becomes less tired and spends less time in stages III and IV of NREM sleep. REM sleep increases, and dreams tend to lengthen. See Figure 37–2. If the sleeper is very tired, REM cycles are often short (e.g., 5 minutes instead of 20) during the early portion

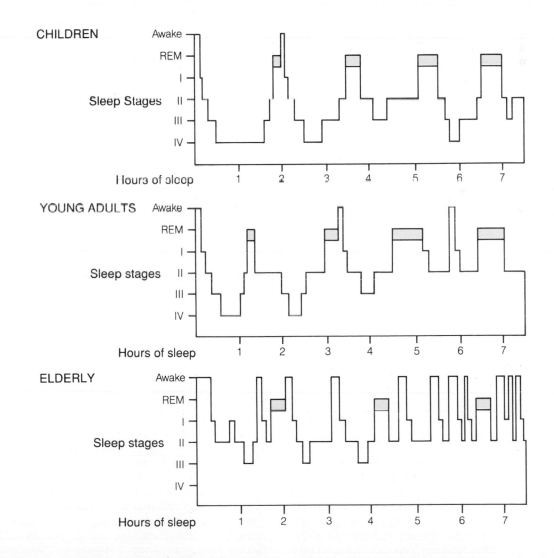

Figure 37–2 Normal sleep cycles of children, young adults, and elderly adults. The sleep of children and young adults shows early preponderance of NREM Stages III and IV, progressive lengthening of the first three REM periods, and infrequent awakenings. In elderly adults there is little or no NREM Stage IV sleep, REM periods are fairly uniform in length, and awakenings are frequent and often lengthy. *Source:* A. Kales, Sleep and dreams: Recent research in clinical aspects, *Annals of Internal Medicine,* May 1968, 68:1078. Reprinted with permission.

of sleep. Before sleep ends, periods of near wakefulness occur, and stages I and II NREM sleep and REM sleep predominate.

Sleep Requirements

The amount of sleep individuals require decreases not only with age but also as the growth rate decreases. See Table 37–2. Young adults' need for sleep is largely determined by such factors as emotional and physical health, amount of activity, pregnancy, and personality. Although most young adults require 7 to 8 hours, it is also normal for adults to sleep less than 6 hours or more than 9. Sometimes young adults find their sleep disturbed by young children. Sleeping a few hours at a time produces the same effect as sleeping less, even if the total time is the same. Stage IV sleep is most often disturbed, and the sleeper obtains little REM sleep. Middle-age adults normally sleep on an average of 7 hours a day and get more NREM (deep and restful) sleep than young adults. The 90-minute REM cycle remains relatively constant; however, there is a marked decrease in the amount of stage IV sleep.

People 60 and older take longer to go to sleep and tend to awaken earlier. Older adults also experience changes in sleep patterns. The amount of stage IV sleep decreases by about 15 to 30% (Hayter 1980, p. 460). Elderly people awaken more often during the night—six times per night at age 60 compared to once a night in young adulthood (Hayter 1980, p. 460). It is also believed that women's sleep patterns change about 10 years later than men's.

Factors Affecting Sleep

Both the quality and the quantity of sleep are affected by several factors. *Quality of sleep* means the individual's ability to stay asleep and to get appropriate amounts of REM and non-REM sleep. Sleep stages can be differentiated and measured only in a laboratory. *Quantity of sleep* is the total time the individual sleeps. Some of the most common factors that affect sleep adversely are illness, environment, exercise, fatigue, psychologic stress, medications, alcohol and stimulants, and nutrition. See Table 37–3.

Illness increases sleep requirements and disturbs the normal rhythm of sleep and wakefulness. People deprived of REM sleep subsequently spend more sleep time than normal in this stage. Pain also can affect sleep, either preventing sleep or awakening the sleeper. Respiratory conditions can disturb an individual's sleep. Shortness of breath often makes sleep difficult, and people frequently need to lie in bed with two or more pillows elevating their heads and chest to ease breathing. In addition, people who have nasal congestion or sinus drainage may have trouble breathing and hence difficulty sleeping.

Table 37–2	**Sleep Patterns According to Age**
Developmental Level	Normal Sleep Pattern
Newborn	Sleeps 14 to 18 hours a day Regular breathing, little body movement 50% REM sleep Sleep cycles last 45 to 60 minutes each
Infant	Sleeps 12 to 14 hours a day 20 to 30% REM sleep May sleep through the night
Toddler	Sleeps about 11 to 12 hours a day 25% REM sleep Sleeps during the night and takes daytime naps
Preschooler	Sleeps about 11 hours a day 20% REM sleep
School-age child	Sleeps about 10 hours a day 18.5% REM sleep
Adolescent	Sleeps about 8.5 hours a day 20% REM sleep
Young adult	Most sleep 7 to 8 hours a day 20 to 25% REM sleep
Middle-age adult	Sleeps about 7 hours a day About 20% REM sleep May have insomnia
Elderly adult	Sleeps about 6 hours a day 20 to 25% REM sleep May have insomnia

Adapted from L. Malasanos, V. Barkauskas, M. Moss, and K. Stoltenberg-Allen, *Health assessment,* 3d ed. (St. Louis: C. V. Mosby Co., 1986).

People who have gastric or duodenal ulcers may find their sleep disturbed because of pain, often a result of the increased gastric secretions that occur during REM sleep. Certain endocrine disturbances can also affect sleep. Hyperthyroidism lengthens presleep time, often making it difficult for a client to fall asleep. Hypothyroidism, in contrast, decreases stage IV sleep. The need to urinate during the night (enuresis) also disrupts sleep, and people who awaken at night to urinate sometimes have difficulty getting back to sleep.

Environment can promote or hinder sleep. People usually become accustomed to the sleeping environment in their home, and any change (e.g., in the noise level) can inhibit sleep. People often become accustomed to certain noises, lights, etc., and the absence of these or the presence of unfamiliar stimuli can keep them from sleeping. A nurse may hear a client say, "I can't sleep here; it is too quiet," or "I can't sleep because of the bell that rings every hour."

The effect of **exercise** on sleeping may vary. It is generally believed that a person who exercises during the day is more likely to sleep well at night and that a person who exercises just before retiring will have difficulty getting to sleep. **Fatigue** can also affect a person's sleep pattern. The more tired the person is, the shorter the first period of paradoxical (REM) sleep. As the person rests, the REM periods become longer.

Anxiety and other **emotional problems** can disturb sleep. A person preoccupied with personal prob-

Table 37—3   Factors Influencing Sleep

Factor	Effect
Liver failure	Day-night reversal
Encephalitis	Day-night reversal
Hypothyroidism	Decreases NREM stage IV sleep
Antidepressant	Decreases REM sleep
Amphetamine	Decreases REM sleep
Alcohol	Speeds onset of sleep, but decreases REM sleep and disrupts other stages
Depression	Decreases or increases REM sleep
Sedative-hypnotic drug	Suppresses REM sleep and decreases NREM stages III and IV. On withdrawal, causes rebound REM sleep with vivid dreams and increased awakening
Tranquilizer	Interferes with REM sleep
Bedtime snack of protein food	Induces and maintains sleep

lems may be unable to relax sufficiently to get to sleep. **Medications,** especially hypnotics and sedatives, affect the sleep pattern. Hypnotics and barbiturates decrease REM sleep, even though they may increase total sleep time. Amphetamines and antidepressants decrease REM sleep abnormally. Long-term use of amphetamines can produce abnormal behavior, attributable to long-term REM sleep deprivation. A client withdrawing from any of these drugs gets much more REM sleep than usual and as a result may experience upsetting nightmares. Nurses need to be aware of this possibility and give the client support.

People who drink an excessive amount of **alcohol** often find their sleep disturbed. Excessive alcohol disrupts REM sleep, although it may hasten the onset of sleep. While making up for lost REM sleep after some of the effects of the alcohol have worn off, clients often experience nightmares. Tolerance to alcohol also affects sleep; the alcohol-tolerant person may be unable to sleep well and may become irritable as a result.

Nutritional balance can be a factor influencing sleep. Weight loss and weight gain have been found to affect sleep. Crisp and Stonehill (1976, p. 166) found that weight loss is associated with reduced total sleep time as well as broken sleep and earlier awakening. Weight gain, in contrast, was associated with an increase in total sleep time, less broken sleep, and later waking. The amino acid *L-tryptophan* is thought to affect sleep. Dietary L-tryptophan (found in cottage cheese, milk, beef, and canned tuna) may be sleep-inducing, which might explain why warm milk helps some people get to sleep.

Common Sleep Disorders

The two most common sleep disorders are insomnia in adults and parasomnias in children. Less common sleep disorders are hypersomnia, narcolepsy, and sleep apnea.

Insomnia

Insomnia is the inability to obtain adequate quality or quantity of sleep. It is *not* the lack of sleep; in fact, people with insomnia often obtain more sleep than they realize. There are three types of insomnia: inability to fall asleep (initial insomnia), inability to stay asleep because of frequent waking (intermittent insomnia), and early awakening and subsequent inability to return to sleep (terminal insomnia). Terminal insomnia is characteristic of depressed people. Insomniacs do not feel refreshed on arising.

Insomnia can result from physical discomfort but more often is a result of mental overstimulation due to anxiety. People sometimes become anxious because they think they might not be able to sleep. People who become habituated to drugs or who drink large quantities of alcohol are likely to have insomnia. Treatment for insomnia frequently requires the client to develop new behavior patterns that induce sleep. The usefulness of sleeping medications is questionable. Such medications do not deal with the cause of the problem, and their prolonged use creates drug dependencies.

Hypersomnia

Hypersomnia, the opposite of insomnia, is excessive sleep of more than 9 hours at night. The afflicted person often sleeps until noon and takes many naps during the day. Hypersomnia is generally related to psychophysiologic problems, such as psychiatric disorders (depression or anxiety), central nervous system damage, and certain kidney, liver, or metabolic disorders.

Parasomnias

Parasomnias refer to a cluster of disorders that interfere with children's sleep, such as **somnambulism** (sleepwalking), **night terrors** (*pavor nocturnus*), and **nocturnal enuresis** (bed wetting). These disorders often appear together in the same child, run in families, and tend to occur during stages III and IV of NREM sleep. Somnambulism occurs in about 1 to 6% of children between the ages of 5 and 12 years (Malasanos et al. 1986, p. 128). It is normally outgrown without incident. A sleepwalker may not awaken if he or she walks only 3 or 4 minutes; if the walk lasts any longer, then some awakening is usually shown. The main concern is to protect the somnambulist from injury. Usually the sleepwalker can be awakened and quietly led back to bed.

Night terrors are frightening to both parents and children. Children 6 and younger are most often afflicted. After having slept for a few hours, the child bolts upright in bed, shakes and screams, appears pale and terrified, but is difficult to arouse. In contrast to nightmares, night terrors are not remembered the next morning.

Nocturnal enuresis can occur in preadolescent children. Its cause is unknown, although in preschool children it may be due to bladder training that is too severe or too early, or to overtraining. If the child is 3 or 4 years old, environmental factors such as a dark hall may contribute to the child's reluctance to go to the bathroom. In the school-age child, enuresis may be caused by inadequate bladder capacity or jealousy over a new brother or sister. Parents should rule out physical abnormalities first and provide an environment in which the child feels loved. Restricting fluids before bedtime may reduce the incidence of bed wetting but does not address the cause of the problem.

Narcolepsy

Narcolepsy (from the Greek *narco,* meaning "numbness," and *epsis,* meaning "seizure") is a sudden wave of overwhelming sleepiness that occurs during the day; thus it is referred to as a "sleep attack." Its cause is unknown, although it is believed to be a genetic defect of the central nervous system in which the REM period cannot be controlled. In narcoleptic attacks, sleep starts with the REM phase. Even though narcoleptics sleep well at night, they nod off several times a day.

Narcoleptics are often accused of laziness, disinterest in life and work, and even drunkenness. Their handicap, however, is life-threatening in a world fraught with potential hazards. Drug therapy is used with some success to treat narcolepsy. Stimulants such as amphetamines or methylphenidate hydrochloride (Ritalin) prevent attacks; and antidepressants such as imipramine hydrochloride (Tofranil) prevent the muscle weakness and paralysis of cataplexy. Narcoleptics should avoid liquor, which increases drowsiness.

Sleep Apnea

Sleep apnea is the periodic cessation of breathing during sleep. This disorder needs to be assessed by a sleep expert, but it is often suspected when the person has obstructive snoring, excessive daytime sleepiness, and sometimes insomnia. The periods of apnea, which last from 10 seconds to 3 minutes, occur during REM or NREM sleep. Frequency of episodes ranges from 50 to 600 per night. These apneic episodes drain the person of energy and lead to excessive daytime sleepiness.

Sleep apnea profoundly affects a person's work or school performance. In addition, prolonged sleep apnea can cause a sharp rise in blood pressure and may also lead to cardiac arrest. Over time, apneic episodes can cause pulmonary hypertension and subsequent left-sided heart failure.

Assessing Disturbances in Sleep

Sleep assessment should include taking a sleep history, observing any clinical signs of sleep problems, and identifying possible causes or contributing factors.

Sleep History

A sleep history should include questions about a client's usual sleeping habits and any sleep problems. See the accompanying box for the suggested content of a sleep history. Sometimes clients can provide more precise information if they keep a written record for about a week of their sleep pattern and the habits associated with it.

Clinical Assessment

The severity of the signs and symptoms associated with sleep disturbances is related to the length of time the disturbance has existed. Sleep deprivation or prolonged loss of sleep triggers certain biochemical changes in the body. Sleeplessness lowers the seizure threshold. Consequently, people with epilepsy should not go without sleep for prolonged periods. Table 37–4 provides an overview of the signs and symptoms of early and prolonged sleep insufficiency.

Identifying Causal or Contibuting Factors

The causes of sleep disturbance are varied. Sometimes the client will readily identify the cause, e.g., "pain in my leg" or "the man snoring in the next bed." Other times the nurse and client together may be able to identify the causes or contributing factors after reviewing the sleep history. For hospitalized clients, sleep problems are often related to the hospital environment or illness. Assisting the client to sleep in such instances can be challenging to a nurse, often involving schedul-

NURSING HISTORY

Sleep

- Usual times of retiring, falling asleep, and waking
- Number of naps taken during the day, as well as their time and duration
- Whether the client's sleep time varies—for example, because of shift work
- Typical day's activities, with specific reference to exercise and recreation
- Usual sleep habits and environment
- Use of rituals before sleep and special equipment, e.g., pillows
- Whether the client sleeps alone
- Medications used for sleeping, either over-the-counter or prescription drugs
- Intake of stimulants, e.g., caffeinated coffee
- How well the client feels he or she sleeps
- Any difficulty sleeping
- Any changes in the client's sleep pattern

Table 37–4 Clinical Assessment of Sleep Disturbances

Early Signs and Symptoms	Signs of Sleep Deprivation
Complaints of fatigue	Behavior and personality changes, such as aggressiveness, withdrawal, depression
Irritability and restlessness	
Lassitude and apathy	
Darkened areas around the eyes, puffy eyelids, reddened conjunctivae, and burning eyes	Increased restlessness
	Distorted perceptions
	Visual or auditory hallucinations
Marked periods of inattention	Confusion and disorientation as to time and place
Complaints of headache	Impaired coordination
Complaints of nausea	Slurred speech or inappropriate speech and tone

ing activities, administering analgesics, and providing a supportive environment.

Nursing Diagnoses of Sleep Disturbances

After analyzing the assessment data and identifying the nature and suspected etiology of sleep disturbances, the nurse is ready to make a nursing diagnosis of the problem. Examples of nursing diagnoses for clients who have sleep problems are listed in the accompanying box.

Planning Strategies to Prevent and Modify Sleep Disturbances

Planning for sleep disturbances involves establishing client goals, identifying outcome criteria to gauge achievement of the goals (see page 601 for examples), and selecting nursing strategies to meet the established goals. Among these strategies are: reducing environmental distractions and sleep interruptions, increasing daytime activities, identifying age-appropriate interventions, helping to induce sleep, reducing the potential for injury during sleep, and providing teaching and referrals as indicated.

NURSING DIAGNOSIS

Clients with Sleep Problems

- Sleep pattern disturbance related to immobility
- Sleep pattern disturbance related to disturbing roommate
- Sleep pattern disturbance related to pain in left leg
- Sleep pattern disturbance related to fear of surgery

Nursing Implementation of Planned Strategies

Reducing Environmental Distractions and Sleep Interruptions

Environmental distractions are particularly troublesome for hospitalized clients. The noises are unfamiliar, and it is usually impossible to eliminate all sounds. Some interventions that may help are listed in the accompanying box. To reduce sleep interruptions, nurses can schedule activities so that the client has the fewest possible interruptions while resting or sleeping. For example, if a client requires an intramuscular injection during the night, other interventions, such as assessing vital signs or changing position, may be carried out at the same time. Nurses should also avoid waking a sleeping client for unnecessary care, such as to ask if he or she wants a sleeping pill. To reduce the number of times a client needs to void at night, fluid intake after dinner can be limited.

Increasing Daytime Activities

Establishing a schedule of daytime activities can often help clients. This schedule must be appropriate to the client's health status as well as his or her sleep and rest needs. Sometimes clients cannot sleep at night because they sleep too much during the day. If the nurse schedules daytime activities, the client remains awake and may be able to sleep better at night. Or the nurse can arrange for other people to converse with the client or share an activity such as watching television or playing cards. These are often sufficiently stimulating for the client to remain awake during the day.

Age-Appropriate Interventions

Specific nursing interventions should be safe, supportive of healthy sleep patterns and habits, and appropriate to the individual's age. **Newborns and infants** should sleep on a firm mattress covered with thick plastic material that cannot be pulled over the face and cause suffocation. A flat surface provides the best alignment for bone development. Pillows should not be used because they can cause accidental suffocation.

Sleeping infants dislike both darkness and bright light and like to face a dim light. The nurse provides soft lighting directed away from the eyes and ensures that the infant is dry and comfortable. Dry diapers, warm, soft clothing, and a comfortable room temperature promote sleep. Quieting activities before putting the infant to bed (e.g., cuddling or rocking the infant, talking in soothing tones) also promote sleep.

To promote sleep in **toddlers,** the nurse (or parent) should provide consistent bedtime or naptime rituals, firmly adhere to sleeping schedules, and encourage quieting activities before sleep. Giving the child only one

Reducing Environmental Distractions

- Close the door of the client's room.
- Pull curtains around the client's bed.
- Unplug the telephone.
- Provide soft music.
- Reduce or eliminate lighting.
- Provide a night light.
- Decrease the amount and type of stimuli, e.g., staff conversations, television.
- Place the client with a compatible roommate.

toy at bedtime promotes rest and sleep; too many toys are overstimulating. The toddler should never be put to bed as a disciplinary measure.

Measures to promote sleep and rest in **preschoolers** are similar to those for toddlers. Preschoolers show increasing independence during the presleep ritual, but they must be encouraged to express fears, which also increase at this age. The nurse usually can reassure the child by listening to the child's fears and making it clear that nurses will be nearby.

Sometimes preschoolers have difficulty getting to sleep because they are so highly stimulated. Often they need time to settle down before sleep, e.g., a quiet time during which the nurse reads bedtime stories. If a child fears going to sleep, reassurance that others are nearby will help allay fears. Some children feel less afraid when there is a night light in the room.

School-age children require considerable rest; however, they often want to stay up longer than is wise. As children grow, they should have a greater say about when to go to bed. In the hospital environment, it is desirable to place school-age children in separate rooms from younger children to accommodate their different sleeping requirements and patterns. The nurse must sometimes set limits so that hospitalized or ill **adolescents** get enough rest and sleep. Adolescents often need time before sleep to tend to grooming and personal hygiene, which is frequently important to them.

The following measures frequently help promote sleep in older children, adolescents, and **adults**:

- Help the client relax before sleep by providing diversions, pain relief, a clean, comfortable bed, and an odor-free room.
- Provide an environment in which clients feel safe and are assured that help is nearby even when they sleep.
- Provide sufficient covers so that the client does not feel cold. Elderly people often need additional covers because normal body temperature drops as people age.
- Encourage progressive relaxation exercises. These are particularly helpful for persons who have mild or

moderate insomnia. See the relaxation techniques described in Chapter 38.

- Provide a light snack or glass of warm milk before the client sleeps. Milk and most protein foods as well as some vegetables contain an amino acid (L-tryptophan) that is a precursor of the neurotransmitter serotonin. Serotonin is thought to induce and maintain sleep.
- Provide a hypnotic or sedative if it is ordered by the physician and needed by the client. If the client also requires an analgesic, administer the analgesic before the sedative so that he or she feels comfortable when becoming sleepy.
- Assist the client to his or her normal sleeping position if this is possible.
- Give the client a backrub to reduce psychologic stress and promote muscular relaxation.

Helping to Induce Sleep

A number of comfort measures help clients sleep. Many clients are accustomed to bedtime rituals, such as a soothing bath or a glass of milk. Some people read before going to sleep; others like to watch the nighttime news on television. Provided these practices are not contraindicated because of health status, nurses should help clients maintain their habitual practices. Also, encouraging or providing hygienic care, e.g., brushing teeth, and providing a partial bath and a clean bed, promotes sleep.

Reducing the Potential for Injury

Some clients are afraid to go to sleep for fear of rolling off the bed, or they are afraid to walk to the bathroom at night in an unfamiliar environment because of the danger of tripping over furniture. Specific safety measures are listed in the accompanying box.

Safety Measures

- Use night lights.
- Place the bed in the low position.
- Employ side rails if appropriate.
- Place the call bell within easy reach.
- Teach the client on how to obtain assistance.
- Teach the client attached to I.V. or drainage tubing how to move about.
- Ensure that tubing is long enough to permit the client to move.

▪ Health Teaching and Referrals

Health teaching regarding exercise and stress reduction, as appropriate, is important. The nurse can enlist support persons to help a client deal with a sleep problem and teach them interventions to relieve the symptoms (Carpenito 1987, pp. 561–562). When a client requires further teaching or counseling, the nurse should make the appropriate referral.

▪ Evaluating Client Responses to Nursing Interventions

Examples of outcome criteria appropriate for clients with sleep problems are listed in the accompanying box.

▪ Chapter Highlights

▪ During sleep a person's level of consciousness is reduced.

▪ The sleep cycle is controlled by the reticular activating system and the bulbar synchronizing region in the brain stem.

▪ During a normal night's sleep a person has four to six sleep cycles, each with five stages—four stages of NREM sleep and one stage of REM sleep.

▪ NREM (slow-wave) sleep comprises most of a sleep cycle; the ratio of NREM to REM sleep varies with age.

▪ Many factors, including psychologic stress, exercise and fatigue, medications, and alcohol, can affect sleep.

▪ Common sleep disorders include insomnia, hypersomnia, parasomnias, narcolepsy, and sleep apnea.

▪ A sleep history helps the nurse plan interventions to help clients sleep.

▪ People usually develop their own rituals to prepare for sleep.

▪ Pain control and comfort promote sleep.

▪ L-tryptophan, a component of dairy products and meat, may help induce sleep.

OUTCOME CRITERIA

Clients with Sleep Problems

The client will:

▪ Sleep 8 hours without awakening

▪ Have restored strength and the energy to walk unaided to the end of the corridor and back

▪ Describe factors that prevent or inhibit sleep

▪ Describe techniques that induce sleep

▪ Demonstrate a balance of rest and activity appropriate to the client's health status

▪ Selected References

Bahr, R. T. October 1983. Sleep-wake patterns in the aged. *Journal of Gerontological Nursing* 9:534–37, 540–41.

Bellack, J. P., and Bamford, P. A. 1984. *Nursing assessment. A multidimensional approach.* Monterey, Calif.: Wadsworth Health Sciences Div.

Carpenito, L. J. 1987. *Nursing diagnosis. Application to clinical practice.* 2d ed, Philadelphia: J. B. Lippincott Co.

Crisp, A. N., and Stonehill, E. 1976. *Sleep, nutrition and mood.* New York: John Wiley and Sons.

Guyton, A. C. 1986. *Textbook of medical physiology.* 7th ed. Philadelpha: W. B. Saunders Co.

Hayter, J. March/April 1985. To nap or not to nap? *Geriatric Nursing* 6:104–6.

———. July/August 1983. Sleep behaviors of older persons. *Nursing Research* 32:242–46.

———. March 1980. The rhythm of sleep. *American Journal of Nursing* 80:457–61.

Hoch, C., and Reynolds, III, C. January/February 1986. Sleep disturbances and what to do about them. *Geriatric Nursing* 7:24–27.

Malasanos, I.; Barkauskas, V.; Moss, M.; and Stoltenberg-Allen, K. 1986. *Health assessment.* 3d ed. St. Louis: C. V. Mosby Co.

Schirmer, M. S. January 1983. When sleep won't come. *Journal of Gerontological Nursing* 9:16–21.

Walsleben, J. June 1982. Sleep disorders. *American Journal of Nursing* 82:936–40.

Weaver, T., and Millman, R. P. February 1986. Broken sleep. *American Journal of Nursing* 86:146–50.

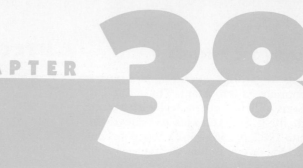

CHAPTER 38

Pain

OBJECTIVES

Identify various types of pain.
Describe pain pathways to the brain.
Identify physiologic manifestations of the response to pain.

Describe subjective and objective data to be collected and analyzed when assessing pain.
Identify examples of possible nursing diagnoses for clients with pain.

List ways of decreasing factors that amplify the pain experience.
Explain methods used to reduce pain intensity.
Identify situations in which relaxation techniques can relieve pain effectively.
Describe selected skin stimulation techniques used to relieve pain.
Identify methods used to control intractable pain.
Describe selected medical interventions to control pain.
State outcome criteria by which to evaluate a client's response to interventions for pain.

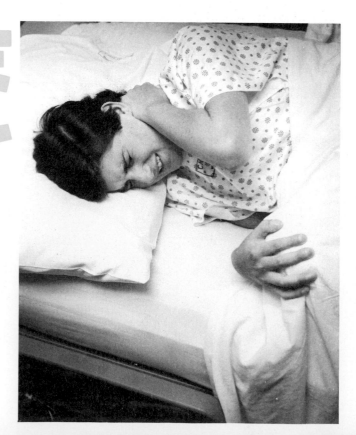

Nature of Pain

Pain is a highly unpleasant and very personal sensation that cannot be shared with others. It is often an important sign that something is physiologically wrong. As such, pain is useful because it prompts the client to seek help for a health problem that might otherwise go unnoticed. McCaffery (1979, p. 11) defines **pain** as "whatever the experiencing person says it is, existing whenever he says it does." Basic to this definition is the caregiver's willingness to believe the client's pain.

Types of Pain

Pain can be described as either acute or chronic. **Acute pain** is generally of relatively short duration, such as the pain of a fracture or abdominal surgery. A client with acute pain normally exhibits one or more of the following clinical signs: increased perspiration, increased cardiac rate or blood pressure, and pallor. Clients may respond to acute pain by crying, moaning, or rubbing the painful area, although the absence of these behaviors does not mean a client is not experiencing pain.

Chronic pain develops more slowly and lasts much longer than acute pain, and sufferers may find it difficult to remember when such pain first started. Often, it is the result of an acute injury which, by all other clinical standards, has healed. Clients with chronic pain may present few if any clinical signs of pain. Some find a way to handle the pain or are so accustomed to it that their reaction is minimal. For others, pain may become the central focus of their lives, influencing all other activities.

Intractable pain is resistant to cure or relief. An example is the pain of arthritis, for which narcotic analgesics are contraindicated because of the long duration of the disease and the risk of addiction. Behavior modification is used in some cases of intractable pain. Behavior that is not pain-oriented is rewarded, and pain-oriented behavior is ignored. The aim of this technique is to change behavior so that the client can live more comfortably and productively.

Guyton (1986, p. 592) classifies pain into two types: acute pain and slow pain. **Acute pain** occurs within 0.1 second of the application of a pain stimulus. The client may describe acute pain as "sharp," "cutting," or "like a needle prick." **Slow pain** begins a second or more after a pain stimulus is applied and increases slowly over a period of seconds or even minutes. Slow pain can be described as "burning," "aching," "throbbing." This type of pain is associated with tissue destruction and can occur, according to Guyton (1986, p. 592), in the skin or in deeper tissues of the body.

Sometimes a client feels pain in an area other than the site of the source of the pain. This is called **referred pain.** Referred pain is the result of a synapse between nerve fibers that carry the pain impulses in the spinal cord and neurons that carry pain impulses from the skin. Thus the individual perceives the pain as originating in the skin or internal tissues. **Radiating pain** is perceived at the source and extends to surrounding or nearby tissues. For example, cardiac pain may be felt radiating to the left shoulder and down the left arm, or the pain from an inflamed appendix may be felt throughout the abdomen.

Phantom pain is actual pain felt in a body part that is no longer present, such as an amputated foot. It can be distinguished from a *phantom sensation,* i.e., feeling that a missing body part is still present. Phantom pain is thought to result from stimulation of a severed dendrite rather than stimulation of the usual receptor. It occurs most frequently in clients who experienced pain before the removal of the body part, especially if that pain was dismissed as not significant.

Perceiving Pain

An individual's **pain threshold** is the amount of pain stimulation a person requires before feeling pain. A person's pain threshold is generally fairly uniform, although it can be dramatically altered by the person's state of consciousness. For instance, an anesthetized client feels no pain; an unconscious client may or may not react to suborbital pressure, that is, pain on the lower aspect of the eye. It is also possible for a person's pain threshold to change. For example, the same stimulus that once produced mild pain can produce intense pain. Such excessive sensitivity to pain is called **hyperalgesia. Pain tolerance** is the maximum amount and duration of pain that an individual is willing to endure. Some clients are unwilling to tolerate even the slightest pain, whereas others are willing to endure severe pain rather than be treated for it.

The skin, certain internal tissues such as the periosteum, the joint surfaces, and the arterial walls have many pain receptors, whereas most other deep tissues have few. The alveoli of the lungs have no pain receptors. A pain receptor, called a **nociceptor,** is stimulated either directly by damage to the receptor cell or secondarily by the release of chemicals such as bradykinin, histamine, prostaglandins, acids, and potassium ions from the damaged tissues. Basically, three types of stimuli excite corresponding types of nociceptors: mechanical, thermal, and chemical. See Table 38–1.

Pain signals are transmitted along two types of fibers: delta type A fibers and type C fibers. Type A fibers transmit the signal relatively quickly, i.e., between 6 and 30 meters per second. It is thought that type A fibers chiefly transmit sharp pain. Type C fibers transmit signals more slowly, i.e., 0.5 to 2 meters per second, and it is believed they transmit burning and aching pain. Therefore, a sudden pain can give a double sensation: a sharp, fast pain sensation followed by a slow burning sensation. The latter tends to become more painful over time (Guyton 1986, p. 594).

Pain fibers enter the spinal cord through the dorsal roots. From there they ascend or descend one or two cord segments to terminate in neurons in the dorsal horns of the gray matter called the *substantia gelatinosa.* Type A fibers terminate in the gray matter of lam-

Table 38–1   Types of Pain Stimuli

Stimulus Type	Physiologic Basis
Mechanical	
1. Trauma to body tissues, e.g., surgery	Tissue damage; direct irritation of the pain receptors; inflammation
2. Alterations in body tissues, e.g., edema	Pressure on pain receptors
3. Blockage of a body duct	Distention of the lumen of the duct
4. Tumor	Pressure on pain receptors; irritation of nerve endings
5. Muscle spasm	Stimulation of pain receptors (also see *Chemical*)
Thermal	
Extreme heat or cold, e.g., burns	Tissue destruction; stimulation of thermosensitive pain receptors
Chemical	
1. Tissue ischemia, e.g., blocked coronary artery	Stimulation of pain receptors because of accumulated lactic acid (and possibly other chemicals, such as bradykinin) in tissues
2. Muscle spasm	Secondary to mechanical stimulation (see above), causing tissue ischemia

inae I and V, type C fibers in that of laminae II and III. Most signals pass through one or more neurons before reaching long-fibered neurons that cross to the opposite side of the cord. The stimulus then passes upward via the anterolateral spinothalamic tract to the brain. See Figure 38–1.

Both the slow and fast fibers are differentiated in the lateral spinothalamic tract. Both types of pain fiber enter the brain stem. About 75 to 90% of all acute, fast pain fibers terminate in the reticular formation of the medulla, pons, and mesencephalon. From there some of the acute fast fibers connect with higher-order neurons, transmitting the pain signals to the thalamus, hypothalamus, and other areas of the diencephalon and cerebrum. See Figure 38–2. Almost all of the slow chronic fibers terminate in the reticular formation. However, some signals are relayed to the thalamus. Because these fibers activate the reticular system, they arouse the entire nervous system, even when a person is asleep (Guyton 1986, p. 596).

There is also a proprioceptive reflex that occurs with the stimulation of pain receptors. Impulses travel along sensory pain fibers to the spinal cord. There they synapse with motor neurons, and the impulses travel back via motor fibers to a muscle near the site of the pain. See Figure 38–3. The muscle then contracts in a protective action. For example, when a person touches a hot stove, the hand reflexively draws back from the heat even before the person is aware of the pain.

Pain perception involves both physiologic and psychosocial factors. Consequently, individuals vary widely in their perception of pain; for instance, some people perceive a cut finger as exceedingly painful, whereas others hardly notice such a cut. **Physiologically,** pain impulses that originate at a nociceptor travel to the spinal cord and up the lateral spinothalamic tract to the reticular formation of the medulla, pons, and mesencephalon. From there some impulses continue to the cerebrum, which makes the individual consciously aware of the location, severity, and type of pain.

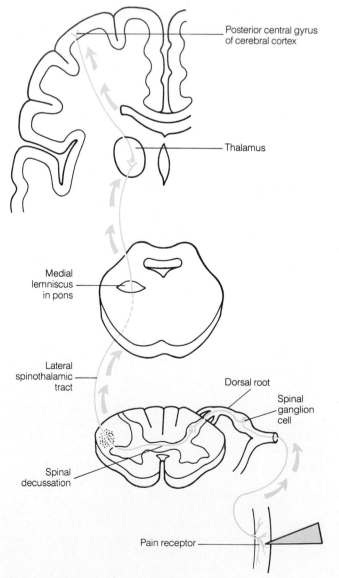

Figure 38–1   Acute pain pathway

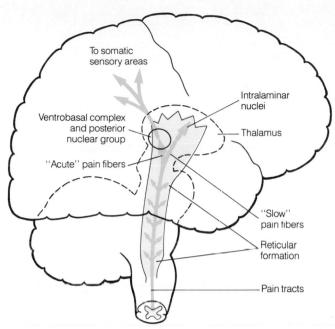

Figure 38–2 Transmission of pain signals to the higher brain centers

impulses along the thick nerve fibers, which carry impulses of heat, cold, touch, etc., the gates close to the pain impulses on the thinner fibers, thus blocking the pain. (Pain impulses are thought to travel along these thinner fibers.) Only when the synaptic gates are open, as when impulses on the pain fibers predominate, does the person feel pain.

The body's response to pain is a complex process rather than a specific action. The **pain response** can be studied by separating it into three stages: activation, rebound, and adaptation. The initial stage, **activation,** begins with the perception of pain. The body assumes a fight-or-flight reaction, initiated by the sympathetic nervous system. See Table 38–2 and Chapter 16 for further information.

During the **rebound** stage, the pain experienced is intense but brief. It is at this stage that the parasympathetic nervous system takes over. Its effects, the opposite of the sympathetic system's, include decreased cardiac rate and decreased blood pressure. When pain is long-lasting, the physiologic response is **adaptation,** i.e., a decreased sympathetic response. Adaptation may be due to endorphins counteracting the pain. The body experiences a general adaptive reaction when the pain

▪ Pain Responses

The stimulation of the reticular formation alerts the person to the pain and motivates the individual to take steps in response. A number of theories attempt to explain how pain is transmitted and perceived physiologically. Three of these are the pattern theory, the specificity theory, and the gate-control theory.

According to the **pattern theory,** pain impulses generated by the nociceptors form a pattern or code that conveys to the central nervous system information that a particular pain is present. A key concept in this theory is that, following tissue injury, circuits established in the spinal interneurons enable the pain to be perceived even though the stimuli that initiated the pain are no longer present. This *reverberating circuit* might explain phantom pain.

The **specificity theory** originated about 200 years ago. This theory assumes that pain travels from a specific nociceptor to a pain center in the brain. Current knowledge sheds light on several limitations of this theory. Research has shown that the nerve fibers that carry pain impulses also carry pressure and temperature sensations (Nursing Now 1985, p. 16). Two other assumptions of this theory conflict with current research findings: it assumes a direct relationship between the intensity of the pain stimulus and the perceived intensity of pain; and it assumes that only one structure in the brain is involved in a pain response.

The **gate-control theory** was first proposed in 1965 by Melzack and Wall. This theory assumes that the synapses in the dorsal horns act as gates that close to keep impulses from reaching the brain or open to permit impulses to ascend to the brain. Melzack and Wall further hypothesize that when there are a great number of

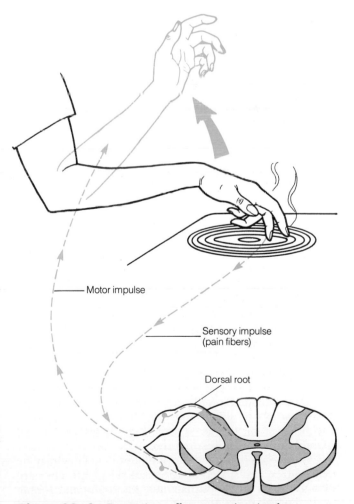

Figure 38–3 Protective reflex to a pain stimulus

Table 38—2 Responses to Pain

Sympatho-Adrenal Responses	Muscular Responses	Emotional Responses
Increased pulse rate	Increased muscle tension or rigidity	Excitement
Increased systolic blood pressure	Writhing	Irritability
Increased respiratory rate	Restlessness	Behavior change
Excessive perspiration	Knees drawn up to abdomen or other unusual postures	Extreme quietness
Nausea and vomiting due to blood flow shift from viscera to muscles of the lungs, heart, and striated body muscles		Groaning
Pallor	Rubbing	Crying
Bronchial dilation	Scratching	Increased alertness
Conversion of stored glycogen to glucose	Immobility	
Release of erythrocytes from the spleen		
Pupil dilation		

lasts for many hours or days. See the section on the general adaptation syndrome, Chapter 16, for current concepts of physiologic reactions to stress.

Changes in body chemistry due to pain influence a person's behavior. The secretion of excessive norepinephrine causes the individual to feel powerful, in control, confident, and excited. However, when norepinephrine is depleted (e.g., when the pain is prolonged) the individual may feel helpless, worthless, and lethargic. Stimulation of the inhibitory system increases the production of serotonin. This reaction is seen in clients after they meditate or take narcotics. The individual feels secure, serene, and safe. Depleted serotonin levels, seen in clients with chronic pain, produce tension, agitation, anxiety, hypersensitivity, and a variety of sleep disorders (Booker 1982, p. 49). Clients with depleted levels of both norepinephrine and serotonin may demonstrate agitated depression. In addition, depression may be aggravated by narcotics, which block the norepinephrine and serotonin receptor sites in the central nervous system (Booker 1982, p. 49).

Endogenous opioids are chemical regulators that may modify pain. Their exact action is still largely theoretical; however, they are thought to bind with opiate receptor sites throughout the body, particularly in the dorsal horn of the spinal cord, thereby inhibiting the production of substances that probably transmit pain impulses and that may also alter pain perception. Certain pain-relief therapies, such as acupuncture, may stimulate the release of endogenous opioids. Three groups of opioids have so far been identified: enkephalins, endorphins, and dynorphins.

Enkephalins are small polypeptides. They combine with opiate receptors in the dorsal horn of the spinal cord and apparently inhibit the release of substance P. **Substance P** is a neurotransmitter that acts to enhance transmission of pain impulses across synapses. Enkephalins are also found outside the spinal cord in the brain stem, limbic system, hypothalamus, adrenal glands, and gastrointestinal tract.

Endorphins are larger polypeptides. They may be synthesized and stored by the pituitary gland. They are also found in the hypothalamus, midbrain, and limbic system of the central nervous system. There are several subgroups of endorphins, including beta-endorphins, which are highly concentrated in the hypothalamus and pituitary gland. The beta-endorphins have been found to be more potent than the enkephalins. **Dynorphins,** only recently discovered, are compounds found in the pituitary gland, hypothalamus, and spinal cord. They seem to have an analgesic effect, one that is 50 times greater than that of the beta-endorphins.

Factors Influencing Pain Perception and Response

Numerous **psychosocial factors** can affect a person's perception of pain. These include past experience, values regarding pain, family expectations, environment, emotions, and a person's culture. **Past experience** can certainly influence a person's present perception of pain. It is known that people who have had previous experience with pain, either their own or that of a significant other, are more threatened by anticipated pain than people who have had no such pain experience (Nursing Now 1985, p. 20). In addition, clients often view interventions in light of past experience. For example, a client who in the past has found certain analgesics to be ineffective is likely to have little faith in their effectiveness in the present. Or, if a client has had prior experience with severe pain, he or she may perceive a present pain as less intense, even though another person with a similar injury might perceive severe pain.

How a client **values** pain can also affect his or her perceptions and responses. A person who views pain as a weakness or a necessary evil may withstand pain well. If benefits are associated with the pain, e.g., absence from a distasteful job or sympathy from a spouse, then the pain will most likely be tolerated well. In contrast, a client who perceives the pain as unnecessary or as a threat to his or her comfort, well-being, or valued lifestyle is likely to tolerate it less well.

Family expectations can affect a person's perceptions of and responses to pain. Family role can affect how a person perceives or responds to pain. For instance, a single mother supporting three children may ignore pain because of her need to stay on the job. The presence of support persons often changes a client's reaction to pain. For example, toddlers tolerate pain more readily when supportive parents or nurses are nearby. Adults, too, handle pain better when supportive, trusted people are present.

An individual's **environment** affects pain perception and response. For instance, the woman entertaining her husband's co-workers at home may have decreased perceptions and responses to the pain while the guests are present; in a hospital, she may perceive the pain as more severe and respond more openly. **Emotions** influence the perception of pain. A person absorbed in playing basketball may be unaware of the pain of an injury until after the game is over. In contrast, a person who is bored or depressed is more likely to think about his or her pain and be more aware of it. Also, a highly anxious client is more likely to have a heightened perception of pain, and a less anxious person will tolerate pain more effectively.

Response to pain is **partly culturally determined;** i.e., the meaning of pain and the expected interventions vary from culture to culture. A number of research studies in the 1950s and 1960s indicate that culture affects a person's tolerance and reaction to pain. Some groups, such as native American Indians and the Chinese, were found to respond stoically to pain. Other groups, such as Italians and Jews, tended to react more expressively (Blaylock 1968, p 270) More recently it has been recognized that although culture has a role to play in a person's perceptions of and reactions to pain, generalizations about an individual client should not be made. A multicultural society influences individuals in many ways, and although a knowledge of cultural orientation to pain can be helpful, each client should be assessed individually.

It is important that nurses recognize the wide variety of learned responses considered appropriate by different cultural groups. For instance, the stoical response to pain is largely accepted in North American society; however, because of the many ethnic groups in North America, nurses will observe a variety of responses to pain, none of which should be judged as good or bad. It is also true that a stoical person probably will not tell the nurse when he or she is in pain, making recognition of nonverbal clues even more important during assessment.

Assessing Clients' Pain

Pain assessment should include a pain history and data collection regarding factors that augment or decrease pain as well as the clinical signs and symptoms of pain. An in-depth initial assessment permits more definitive nursing diagnoses and enables the nurse to plan and implement an individualized plan of care. The client is the most important source of information during pain assessment.

Pain History

By obtaining the client's history of pain experience (including pain location, intensity, and duration), the nurse can establish how long the client has experienced

NURSING HISTORY

Pain

Determine:

- Location
- Intensity
- Quality, e.g., aching, piercing
- Time of onset and duration
- Precipitating factors
- Associated symptoms
- Effect on activities of daily living
- Measures taken to relieve pain
- Analgesics history

the pain; what effects the pain had on normal activity; how the pain occurred, e.g., quickly or slowly; and what events precipitated it. The history should also include a description of measures employed in the past to relieve pain. See the accompanying box for an outline of a pain history. When taking the pain history, the nurse should provide an opportunity for the client to express in his or her own words how the client views the pain and the situation. This will help the nurse understand what the pain means to the client and how the client is coping with it.

Factors That Augment Pain

Many factors can augment pain, including others' disbelief that the client is in pain, misconceptions about pain, fear, fatigue, and monotony. The nurse must convey to the client that she or he is asking questions to understand the pain, *not* to determine if the pain is real. For example: "How does your pain feel now?" or "Tell me how it feels compared to an hour ago." The nurse verbally acknowledges the presence of the pain: "I understand your leg is very painful; how do you feel about the pain?" It is important to listen attentively to what the client says about the pain. If the nurse is honest and sincere and promptly attends to the client's needs, the client is much more likely to know that the nurse does believe he or she is in pain.

Misconceptions about pain and its treatment can intensify the pain. For example, a client whose pain increases in the evening may mistakenly think this is the result of something he ate for dinner. By providing accurate information, a nurse also can reduce many of the client's **fears,** such as a fear of addiction or a fear that he or she will always have pain. Fear of addiction, for example, may interfere with compliance to a medication regimen prescribed to control pain. Nurses, as well as clients, often cling to this misconception.

Fatigue is another factor that can intensify pain. When assessing the client, the nurse needs to identify any relationships that might exist between increased pain and fatigue. If fatigue is identified as a factor contributing to a client's pain, the nurse should help the client develop patterns of activity that provide sufficient rest, including ordered analgesics at bedtime. The nurse intervenes to correct misconceptions and allay fears. Clients may be relieved to know that pain is a stressor and as such can be a cause of fatigue.

Monotony can increase pain, and psychologic factors influence the individual's perception of pain. A person who is anxious, lonely, or bored feels pain more intensely. The person with chronic pain may be especially susceptible to monotony, particularly if he or she has limited usual activities because of the pain.

▪ Clinical Signs and Symptoms

Guidelines for assessment of the clinical signs and symptoms of a client's pain are summarized in the accompanying box. Two simple descriptive scales are shown in Figure 38–4. The client is asked to indicate the scale point that best represents the intensity of his or her pain. It is very important to note and report any change in intensity described by the client, which may indicate a change in the client's pathologic condition. For example, the abrupt cessation of acute abdominal pain may indicate a ruptured appendix.

A client's reports of pain must be considered in relation to the client's ability and need to report. The elderly or confused may distort the intensity of pain; a child may minimize pain to avoid admission to the hospital or unpleasant tests. The pain ruler shown in Figure 38–5 was designed to help clients describe the intensity of their pain.

Certain activities sometimes precede pain; for example, physical exertion may precede chest pain, or abdominal pain may occur after eating. These observations are helpful not only in preventing the pain but also in determining its cause. Environmental factors can increase pain in those who are well or ill. Extreme cold or heat and extremes of humidity can affect some types of pain. For example, sudden exercise on a hot day can cause muscle spasm. Physical and emotional stressors can precipitate pain. Emotional tension frequently brings on a migraine headache. Intense fear or physical exertion can cause angina.

Knowing how activities of daily living are affected by the pain helps the nurse understand the client's perspective on the pain's severity. A number of tools have

0	1	2	3	4	5	6	7	8	9

No pain			Moderate pain					Severe pain

No pain	Mild pain	Moderate pain	Severe pain	Unbearable pain

Figure 38–4 Two simple descriptive pain-intensity scales

GUIDELINES

Assessing Pain

Ask the client about the following:

- Location
- Intensity (e.g., slight, mild, medium, severe, excruciating)
- Quality (e.g., aching, burning, gnawing, piercing, throbbing)
- Time of onset
- Duration
- Precipitating factors

Observe the client's behavioral responses:

- Facial expression (e.g., clenched teeth, biting the lower lip, tightly shut eyes)
- Purposeful body movements (e.g., immobilizing the painful body part, flexing the knees and hips when experiencing abdominal pain)
- Purposeless body movements (e.g., flinging arms about, tossing and turning)
- Rhythmic body movements (e.g., rubbing, tapping, massaging)
- Changes in speech (e.g., rapid speech and elevated pitch may indicate anxiety; slow speech and monotonous tone can signal intense pain)
- Associated symptoms (e.g., vomiting, dizziness, constipation)

been developed to assist the nurse with this assessment, including a scale measuring the effects of pain on daily life. See Table 38–3. The McGill-Melzack Pain Questionnaire (see Figure 38–6) is meant to assess a client's level of pain and the effectiveness of pain interventions.

Table 38–3 Scale for Assessing the Effects of Pain on Daily Life

On a scale of 0 (no pain) to 5 (maximum pain) the client should indicate the areas of life (listed below) currently affected and the severity of the interference. If the client's current level of pain is less than that usually felt, the client should be asked to rate the most pain ever experienced in these areas.

Sleep	Home activities
Appetite	Driving/walking
Concentration	Leisure activities
Work/school	Emotional status (mood, irritability, depression, anxiety)
Interpersonal relationships	
Marital relations/sex	

Source: From E. Matassarin-Jacobs, unpublished presentation, "Pain Assessment," Chicago, Illinois, May 1981.

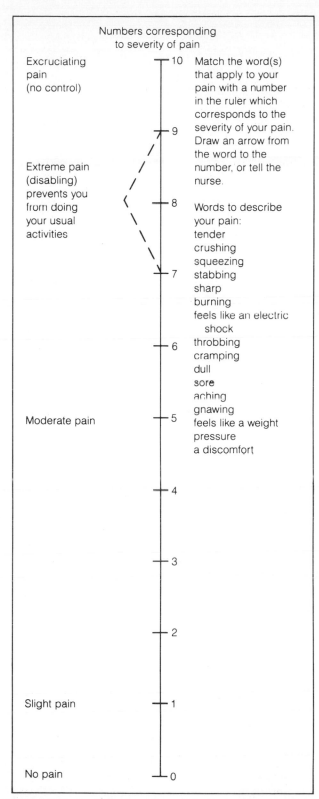

Figure 38–5 The pain ruler. Clients match the words that describe their pain to a number that corresponds to the intensity of their pain. *Source:* F. Bourbonnais, "Pain assessment: Development of a tool for the nurse and the patient," *Journal of Advanced Nursing,* 1981, 6:280. Reprinted with permission of Blackwell Scientific Publications Ltd.

NURSING DIAGNOSIS

Pain

- Altered comfort: acute pain related to fracture of the right hip
- Altered comfort: acute pain related to inflammation at incision site
- Altered comfort: chronic pain related to altered peripheral tissue perfusion secondary to arterial insufficiency
- Altered comfort: chronic pain related to arthritis
- Ineffective denial related to chest pain
- Fatigue related to chronic arthritic pain
- Potential for disuse syndrome related to acute pain in left arm
- Impaired mobility related to pain in right foot
- Self-care deficit related to inability to move arms secondary to pain in shoulder joints

Nursing Diagnoses for Clients with Pain

Currently two diagnostic categories that deal specifically with pain are accepted by NANDA: *Comfort altered: acute pain* (first accepted in 1978 as *Comfort: Alterations in: Pain*) and *Comfort, altered: chronic pain* (accepted in 1986). Additionally, other nursing diagnoses may be appropriate, since pain may interfere with movement or achievement of activities of daily living. Examples of nursing diagnoses for clients experiencing pain are listed in the accompanying box. By identifying the specific kind of pain, the location, and any implications, the nurse becomes better able to plan nursing interventions. For example, if the client is diagnosed as having a self-care deficit related to inability to move the arms secondary to shoulder joint pain, the nurse can help arrange the client's bathing, dressing, and eating practices to accommodate the pain.

Planning to Control Pain

Scheduling measures to prevent pain is far more supportive of the client than trying to deal with pain when the client perceives it. Many postoperative clients need regularly administered analgesics as well as other nursing measures. In this way, the client's pain is anticipated and avoided, and recovery is often hastened. When planning, nurses need to choose pain relief measures appropriate for the client. Heat stimulates serotonin production; cold, norepinephrine production. One of

Figure 38–6 **A**, McGill Pain Questionnaire. The descriptors fall into four major groups: sensory, 1 to 10; affective, 11 to 15; evaluative, 16; and miscellaneous, 17 to 20. The rank value of each descriptor is based on its position in the word set. The sum of the rank values is the pain rating index (PRI). The present pain intensity (PPI) is based on a scale of 0 to 5. **B**, Spacial display of pain descriptors based on intensity ratings by clients. The intensity scale values range from 1 (mild) to 5 (excruciating). *Source:* A and B reprinted with permission from R. Melzack. *Pain measurement and assessment.* (New York: Raven, 1983).

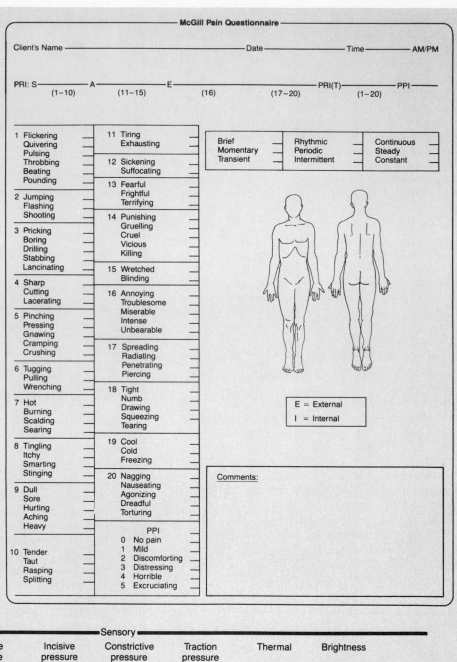

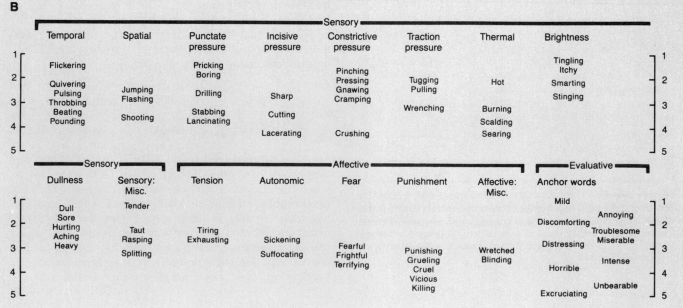

these measures may be appropriate (if it is not contraindicated for other health reasons). The nurse may need a physician's order before applying heat or cold. The accompanying box summarizes guidelines for pain management.

If pain is not relieved within an hour after administration or if the client is in too much pain to perform activities required for recovery (e.g., coughing, deep breathing, and ambulation), the dosage is insufficient. If the client complains of pain before the next dose is scheduled, the interval between doses may be too long. Higher doses are needed to alleviate severe pain than to prevent it. This is particularly true for oral analgesics, which may take 1 hour to act. The client on an inadequate schedule could be in pain a substantially long time before feeling relief. Clients often need to be encouraged to inform nurses before pain becomes too severe.

Clients with certain respiratory diseases are at increased risk of respiratory depression induced by narcotics, and clients with bleeding gastrointestinal ulcers need to avoid aspirin. Those with liver or kidney disease may not metabolize or excrete drugs appropriately. Those with intestinal problems may not absorb oral medications appropriately. Thus, the nurse always need to bear in mind the side effects of analgesics in relation to the client's disease.

Management of Intractable Pain

The management of intractable pain presents a special challenge to nurses working closely with the physician and clinical pharmacist. A physician's order is required to administer the prescribed medications, but the nurse implements the orders and evaluates the client's response. Thus, the client and the nurse assume much of the responsibility for controlling the pain. Drugs commonly used for intractable pain are methadone, Brompton's mixture, and continuous morphine infusion. Patient controlled analgesia (P.C.A.) is gaining popularity as an effective method of pain control.

Methadone is advantageous because it is effective orally, has a long duration of action, has a cumulative effect that can maintain steady analgesic levels, and does not substantially alter mood (Maxwell 1980, p. 1606). **Brompton's mixture,** developed in the 1930s at Brompton's Hospital, London, was originally used as an oral analgesic for postoperative clients. Several different preparations are called Brompton's mixture, since these mixtures are prepared in hospice and hospital pharmacies. The original mixture contained heroin (narcotic analgesic), cocaine (central nervous system stimulant to counteract the sedation and respiratory depression of the narcotic), alcohol (flavor enhancer), and syrup and chloroform water to improve the taste and texture (Gever 1980, p. 57). In many places in North America, morphine or methadone is substituted for heroin, and amphetamine is used in place of cocaine, since cocaine is poorly absorbed and its importation is curtailed. The alcohol component may be ethanol, gin, or brandy. Fruit-flavored syrups are used to improve the flavor. In some hospitals, an antiemetic is also added for its tranquilizing effect.

GUIDELINES

Pain Management

- Try palliative measures (e.g., positioning, massage, applying heat) before administering drugs, or use palliative measures as well as administering analgesics.
- Involve the client and support persons in planning, carrying out, and evaluating the pain-management program.
- Use nonnarcotic analgesics rather than narcotics if the pain is mild to moderate.
- Administer prescribed narcotics for the management of severe pain. Studies show that less than 1 to 3% of clients become addicted, and people stop taking narcotics when pain stops (McCaffery 1980a, p. 38).
- Assess the client's response to analgesics, and note the degree and duration of pain relief and side effects.
- Give analgesics at regular, scheduled intervals around the clock (a.t.c.) rather than as needed (p.r.n.).
- Keep in mind the client's disease process and allergies when administering analgesics.
- Administer analgesics at least 30 minutes before scheduled activities that may result in increased pain (e.g., a complicated dressing change) or would be more effective when pain is controlled (e.g., physical therapy).
- When possible, stay with clients who are in pain unless they prefer to be left alone.

Continuous morphine infusion is used for clients with end-stage terminal illness who are suffering extreme pain, have built up a tolerance to other pain medication, have difficulty taking anything orally, and cannot tolerate repeated injections. This method of pain control provides continuous pain relief, allows the client limited functional capacity, and supports the client's desire to die with dignity (O'Donnell and Papciak 1981, pp. 69–71).

Patient-controlled analgesia (P.C.A.) is a new method of pain control that is useful for clients with severe pain not readily controlled by usual methods of administering analgesics. It employs the use of a programmable intravenous infusion pump to administer intermittent boluses of medication. Its use is not limited to clients with terminal illness; it has been shown effective in controlling various types of pain. For example, one study demonstrated improved pain control in adolescents in sickle-cell crisis (Schechter et al. 1988, p. 719).

The client pushes a button attached to the infusion pump when he or she needs pain medication and a small preset dose of analgesic is administered. After each dose is administered, there is a programmable lockout interval (usually 10–15 minutes) during which the infusion pump cannot be reactivated, allowing time for the medication to take effect before the client receives another dose. There is also a mechanism for programming the maximum amount of medication to be administered within a given time interval (usually 4 hours). Thus, the client typically receives the same amount of medication that would be given on a p.r.n. or a.t.c. schedule (and frequently less), but the client, rather than the nurse, decides when the medication is actually administered.

As with more traditional methods of pain control, the nurse is responsible for frequent assessments of the client and for recording the medication administered. A flow sheet may be used (see Figure 38–7). The nurse is also responsible for setting up and maintaining the infusion pump system and for teaching the client how to operate the system.

Medical Management of Pain

In addition to pharmaceutical measures for pain, there are a number of other treatments for pain which the physician may prescribe. Nursing roles in these therapies vary according to legal standards, institutional policies, physician preferences, and the qualifications of the nurse. Among these therapies are nerve blocks, electric stimulation, acupuncture, hypnosis, surgery, and biofeedback.

A **nerve block** is a chemical interruption of a nerve pathway, effected by injecting a local anesthetic into the nerve. Nerve blocks are widely used during dental work: The injected drug blocks nerve pathways from the painful tooth, thus stopping the transmission of pain impulses to the brain. Nerve blocks are often used to relieve the pain of whiplash injury, low-back disorders, bursitis, and cancer. Sometimes alcohol blocks are used. These, however, destroy nerve fibers and as a result are generally used for peripheral blocks only, since peripheral nerve fibers regenerate.

Electric stimulation is sometimes used to combat certain intractable pain. There are several methods. In **transcutaneous electric stimulation,** electrodes are placed on the surface of the skin over the painful area and over peripheral nerve pathways. In **percutaneous electric stimulation,** needles are inserted near a major peripheral nerve (e.g., the sciatic nerve). In both methods, an electric charge blocks the pain impulse by stimulating the gate-control mechanism. The percutaneous method is used primarily to determine whether a client should consider having a permanent implant inserted.

Acupuncture has been practiced for centuries in China and is receiving increasing attention in North America. It is currently being used selectively in North America to treat chronic pain. The acupuncturist inserts long, slender needles into the body at various sites, which are not necessarily near the body parts to be treated. The needles can be heated, attached to a mild electric current, or twirled continuously with the hand. It is possible that the insertion of the acupuncture needle closes the gate mechanism to pain or stimulates sites near pain fibers leading to the brain, thereby blocking the perception of pain.

Hypnosis has been used to treat psychogenic pain, to achieve anesthesia, and to enhance the effectiveness of medications given for pain aggravated by tension. The susceptible person accepts positive suggestions, which tend to alter perceptions. The success of hypnosis depends to a large degree on the person's openness to suggestion, emotional readiness, and faith in the effectiveness of the hypnosis (*American Journal of Nursing* 1974a, p. 515).

Pain conduction pathways can be interrupted **surgically.** Because this disruption is permanent, surgery is performed only as a last resort, generally for intractable pain. Several surgical procedures may be performed. A **cordotomy** obliterates pain and temperature sensation below the level of the spinothalamic portion of the anterolateral tract severed, and is usually done for pain in the legs and trunk. **Rhizotomy** interrupts the anterior or posterior nerve root between the ganglion and the cord. Interruption of anterior *motor* nerve roots stops spasmodic movements that accompany paraplegia. Interruption of posterior *sensory* nerve roots eliminates pain in areas innervated by that specific nerve root. Rhizotomies are generally performed on cervical nerve roots to alleviate pain of the head and neck from cancer or neuralgia.

In **neurectomy,** peripheral or cranial nerves are interrupted to alleviate localized pain, such as pain in the lower leg or foot arising from a vascular occlusion. In a **sympathectomy,** pathways of the sympathetic division of the autonomic nervous system are severed. This procedure eliminates vasospasm, improves peripheral blood supply, and thus is effective in treating painful vascular disorders such as angina and Raynaud's disease.

Biofeedback is a method of controlling certain physiologic functions by providing information normally unavailable to the individual. In the past, most physiologic processes were considered involuntary. However, it has been discovered that many of these processes are partially subject to voluntary control. Studies show that muscle tension, heart rate, blood flow, and pain, for example, can be controlled voluntarily. The feedback is usually provided through auditory or visual means, e.g., the client sees an electromyogram that shows the electric potential created by the contraction of muscles.

Implementing Nursing Strategies for Relief of Pain

Nursing management of pain consists of both independent and collaborative nursing actions. In general, noninvasive measures may be performed as an independent nursing function, whereas administration of analgesic medications requires a physician's order. However, the decision to administer the prescribed medication is frequently the nurse's, often requiring judgment as to the dose to be given and the time of administration. Similarly, after a medication has been administered, the nurse is responsible for monitoring the effects of the medication (both desired and untoward), whether or not she or he was the one to administer the medication. Providing encouragement to both clients and to their

General Purpose Flow Sheet

Patient Controlled Analgesia

ADDRESSOGRAPH PLATE

DATE	TIME	Amount of Morphine*	Number of Doses*	Vital Signs as ordered by physician				**Comments and/or initials
				H.R.	RR	BP	Temp	
	0200							
	0600							
	0800							
	1000							
	1200							
	1400							
	1600							
	1800							
	2000							
	2200							

* - Record amount of morphine and number of doses administered only since last recording (every 2 hours, days and evenings; every 4 hours nights.

** - Comments optional → record any observations of patient's level of pain, ability to use pump, pump function. You might want to use a pain rating scale such as 0–10, with 0 = no pain and 10 = worst pain could have.

GENERAL PURPOSE FLOW SHEET

Figure 38–7 Patient controlled analgesia flowsheet (Courtesy of University of Virginia Health Sciences Center) *Source:* This form was developed by Catherine J. Webb, M.A., R.N., Pediatric Clinical Nurse Specialist/Assistant Professor, and Debra A. Stergios, M.S.N., R.N., Administrative Head Nurse; Children's Medical Center and School of Nursing at the University of Virginia Health Sciences Center.

support persons is also an independent nursing function that augments all other therapies selected.

Reducing Pain Intensity through Noninvasive Techniques

The intensity of pain can be reduced through a number of techniques, including distraction, relaxation, and cutaneous stimulation. **Distraction** draws the person's attention away from the pain and lessens the perception of pain. In some instances, distraction can make a client completely unaware of pain. For example, a client recovering from surgery may feel no pain while watching a football game on television, yet feel pain again when the game is over.

The effectiveness of distraction to decrease pain can be explained by the gate-control theory. In the spinal cord, the receptor cells receiving the peripheral pain stimuli are inhibited by stimuli from other peripheral nerve fibers carrying different stimuli. Because pain messages are slower than diversional messages, the spinal cord gate, which controls the amount of input to the brain, closes, and the client feels less pain (Cummings 1981, p. 62).

Distraction is most effective when pain is mild or moderate, but intense concentration on other subjects can also relieve acute pain. An example of the latter is an adolescent who feels pain from a fractured foot bone only after she finishes playing a basketball game. Certain distractions, however, (e.g., disturbing stimuli such as loud noises, bright lights, unpleasant odors, or an argumentative visitor), can increase pain perception. There-fore, the nurse needs to reduce disturbing stimuli. Guidelines for using selected distraction techniques are included in the accompanying box.

Relaxation techniques, a specific form of distraction, are effective primarily for chronic pain and thus provide many benefits. Using relaxation techniques enables the client to reduce anxiety related to pain or stress, ease muscle tension pain, dissociate himself or herself from pain, obtain maximum benefits from rest and sleep periods, enhance the effectiveness of other pain therapies, and relieve hopelessness and depression associated with pain. For many years, nurses on maternity units have encouraged women in labor to relax and breathe rhythmically. These techniques, however, can be useful for any client in pain.

Three requisites to relaxation are correct posture, a mind at rest, and a quiet environment. The client must be positioned comfortably, with all body parts supported, joints slightly flexed, and no strain or pull on muscles (e.g., arms and legs should not be crossed). To rest the mind, the client is asked to gaze slowly around the room, e.g., across the ceiling, down the wall, along a window curtain, around the fabric pattern, and back up the wall. This exercise focuses the mind outside of the body (away from the pain) and creates a second center of concentration. To relax the face, the client is encouraged to smile slightly or let the lower jaw sag. Stewart (1976, p. 959) describes one relaxation technique:

1. The client takes a deep breath and fills the lungs with air.
2. The client slowly hisses out the air while letting the body go limp and concentrating on how good this feels.
3. The client breathes in natural rhythm a few times.
4. The client takes another deep breath and releases it slowly, this time letting only the legs and feet go limp. The nurse asks the client to concentrate on how each leg feels (e.g., loose, heavy, and warm).
5. The client repeats step 4, concentrating on the arms, abdomen, back, and other muscle groups.
6. After the client is relaxed, slow, rhythmic breathing is added. Either abdominal or chest breathing may be used. If pain becomes intense, the client can use a more rapid, shallow breathing pattern.

There are several relaxation methods. Some recommend that separate muscle groups (e.g., neck, shoulder, back, arm, leg) be first tensed and then relaxed. After all muscle groups are tensed and relaxed, the whole body is tensed and then relaxed. Others suggest a stretching form of relaxation. The client lies supine, points the toes toward the knees, presses the back of the knees against the mattress or floor, flattens the hollow of the back and neck as much as possible, holds this position for several minutes, and then relaxes completely for several minutes.

Conscious suggestion by the nurse can help relax an anxious, frightened client in pain. It involves skillful use of the voice, body language, and word choice. A calm, soft, but distinct voice makes the client listen and gives a sense of security. Bending near the client, estab-

GUIDELINES

Distraction Techniques

Slow, rhythmic breathing. Instruct the client to stare at an object and inhale slowly through the nose while counting from 1 to 4 and then exhale slowly through the mouth while counting to 4 again. Encourage the client to concentrate on the sensation of breathing and to picture a restful scene. Continue until a rhythmic pattern is established.

Massage and slow, rhythmic breathing. Instruct the client to breathe rhythmically and at the same time massage a painful body part with stroking or circular movements.

Rhythmic singing and tapping. Ask the client to select a well-liked song and concentrate attention on its words and rhythm. Encourage the client to mouth or sing the words and tap a finger or foot. Loud, fast songs are best for intense pain.

Active listening. Have the client listen to music and concentrate on the rhythm by tapping a finger or foot.

Guided imagery. Ask the client to close his or her eyes and imagine and describe something pleasurable. As the client describes the image, ask about the sights, sounds, and smells imagined, encouraging the client to provide details.

lishing eye contact, and placing a hand on the client's shoulder communicate the nurse's concern and calmness to the client. Positive, affirmative words help to convey the suggestion of relaxation to the client.

Cutaneous stimulation of the skin can reduce pain intensity. Again, this is another refinement of distraction, using tactile stimulation to "distract" the client from the pain experience. Guidelines for using specific techniques for cutaneous stimulation are summarized in the accompanying box.

Providing Optimum Relief through Analgesics

Analgesics alter perception and interpretation of pain by depressing the central nervous system at the thalamus and cerebral cortex. Analgesics are more effective when given before the client feels severe pain than when given after the pain is severe. For this reason, analgesics are given at regular intervals, such as every 4 hours (q4h) after surgery.

There are two major classifications of analgesics: narcotic (strong analgesics) and nonnarcotic (mild analgesics). **Narcotic analgesics** include opiate derivatives, such as morphine and codeine. Narcotics relieve pain largely by binding to opiate receptors and activating endogenous pain suppression in the central nervous system. Changes in mood and attitude and feelings of well-being make the person feel more comfortable even though the pain persists. **Nonnarcotic analgesics** include nonsteroidal anti-inflammatory drugs (NSAIDs), aspirin, and acetaminophen. Nonnarcotic analgesics relieve pain by acting on peripheral nerve endings at the injury site and interfering with the prostaglandin system (American Pain Society 1988, p. 817). In addition, several combinations of analgesic drugs are available, e.g., a narcotic and nonnarcotic such as Tylenol #3, which combines acetaminophen with codeine, 30 mg.

A newer type of injectable analgesic is the **narcotic agonist-antagonist.** This type has *agonistic* properties in that it acts like a narcotic and relieves severe pain, but it also has *antagonistic* properties in that it acts against a narcotic. When given to a client who has taken a pure narcotic, these drugs reverse its effects; when given to a narcotic-free client, they have a narcotic effect. Examples are butorphanol (Stadol), nalbuphine (Nubain), and pentazocine (Talwin, Fortal).

When administering analgesics, it is essential that the nurse review the side effects. For example, narcotic analgesics depress respiration and must be used cautiously in clients with respiratory problems. If the client experiences significant respiratory depression (e.g., a drop from 18 to 12) or is overly sedated, the dosage is excessive. *Before* administering narcotics, the nurse needs to assess a client's respiratory rate and level of alertness, for baseline data. The nurse also needs to note other side effects, such as nausea and vomiting. Nonnarcotics such as aspirin may aggravate gastrointestinal bleeding and therefore are contraindicated in clients with peptic ulcers. *After* medicating the client, the nurse records

GUIDELINES

Cutaneous Stimulation

Cold packs slow the conduction of pain impulses to the brain and motor impulses to muscles in the painful area. They provide quicker and longer-lasting pain relief than hot packs (McCaffery 1980d, p. 57). Use cold packs to help relieve headaches, muscle strains, joint pain, muscle spasm, and back pain during childbirth.

Analgesic ointments containing menthol relieve pain, but the analgesic mechanism is unknown. These ointments produce immediate sensations of warmth that last for several hours, and even longer if the body part is wrapped in plastic. They can be used to relieve joint or muscle pain. Moreover, menthol ointment rubbed into the neck, scalp, or forehead sometimes relieves tension headaches, and some cultures (e.g., Filipino) use it on the abdomen to relieve gas pains or on the abdomen or lower back to relieve the pain of labor or delivery (McCaffery 1980d, p. 57).

Counterirritants, such as mustard plasters, flaxseed poultices, and liniments, may be used to relieve the aching joint pain of rheumatoid arthritis and osteoarthritis. Counterirritants are thought to relieve pain by increasing circulation to the painful area.

Contralateral stimulation can be accomplished by stimulating the skin in an area opposite to the painful area (e.g., stimulating the left knee if the pain is in the right knee). The contralateral area may be scratched for itching, massaged for cramps, or treated with cold packs or analgesic ointments. This method is particularly useful when the painful area cannot be touched because it is hypersensitive, inaccessible by a cast or bandages, or when the pain is felt in a missing part (phantom pain) (McCaffery 1980d, p. 57).

the response. Some nurses use pain medication flowsheets for this purpose. See Figure 38–8.

A **placebo** is any form of treatment, e.g., medication or nursing intervention, that produces an effect in the client because of its intent rather than its physical or chemical properties (McCaffery 1982, p. 22). A medication that contains no analgesic properties (e.g., sugar, normal saline, or water) but is intended to relieve pain is a placebo. Years ago, the client who claimed the placebo gave relief was assumed to be malingering or falsely claiming pain. These assumptions have been proved wrong. Placebos do provide pain relief. Thirty-six percent of subjects in a study of 446 clients with severe postoperative pain reported relief after taking a placebo (Goodwin et al. 1982, p. 25). Placebos may help clients return to health and do have a physiologic effect; in some instances they cause the body to release endorphins, which are powerful analgesics (McCaffery 1982, pp. 23–24). It has also been proposed that placebos

Date	Time	Medication	Pain level (0 = no pain; 10 = worst pain imaginable) and ct. comments	Respirations
10/1	12:30 p.m.	- - - - - - - - -	8 "can't stand the pain"	22 (baseline)
	12:55 p.m.	morphine, 5 mg, I.V. push	8	22
	1:00 p.m.	morphine drip, 5 mg in 25 ml to run over 1 hour	7 "beginning to ease somewhat"	18
	1:30 p.m.	- - - - - - - -	7	18
	2:00 p.m.	morphine drip, 5 mg in 25 ml to run over 1 hour	5 (ct. has slept some)	17
	2:30 p.m.	- - - - - - - -	5	20
	3:00 p.m.	morphine drip, 5 mg in 25 ml to run over 1 hour	5 "feel sore"	17
	3:30 p.m.	- - - - - - - -	6 "more cramping and aching"	22
	4:00 p.m.	morphine drip, 7 mg in 25 ml to run over 1 hour	6	22
	4:30 p.m.	- - - - - - - -	4 "pain is easing"	18
	5:00 p.m.	morphine drip, 28 mg in 100 ml to run over 4 hours	3 "much more comfortable" (ct. sleeping intermittently)	18
	9:00 p.m.	morphine drip, 28 mg in 100 ml to run over 4 hours	3	18

Figure 38–8 Pain medication flowsheet *Source:* From L. McGuire and A. Wright, Continuous narcotic infusion. It's not just for cancer patients, *Nursing 84,* December 1984, 14:53. Used by permission. Copyright © 1984, Springhouse Corporation, 1111 Bethlehem Pike, Springhouse, PA 19477.

relieve pain by relieving anxiety or by classic conditioning. In the latter instance the client is conditioned to pain relief and responds positively to the placebo (Nursing Now 1985, p. 95).

Before administering a placebo, nurses must have a physician's order. Just because there are no active chemical ingredients in a placebo does not mean that nurses can administer them independently. It is important that nurses know why a placebo is being given before they give it. Placebos should not be used to punish a "difficult" client. Nor can they be used to prove that a client does not really have pain.

Since it is legal to administer placebos, nurses must also examine their own values relative to the ethics of giving placebos. Nurses have a number of choices. They can deceive the client by giving the placebo and saying it is another medicine. They can refuse to give the placebo. They can inform the client about the placebo and obtain his or her consent to use it. They can set up a double-blind situation, explaining the double blind to the client and requesting his or her consent. Neither the nurse nor the client knows whether a placebo or an active drug is being administered, because both have been packaged identically by the pharmacist. Nurses need to clarify their own feelings about placebos before selecting an option for intervening.

Assisting Support Persons

Support persons often need assistance to respond positively to the client experiencing pain. Nurses can help support persons by giving them accurate information about the pain and by providing opportunities for them to discuss their emotional reactions, which may include anger, fear, frustration, and feelings of inadequacy. Enlisting the aid of support persons in the provision of pain relief to the client, such as massaging the client's back, may diminish their feelings of helplessness and foster a more positive attitude toward the client's pain experience. Support persons also may need the nurse's verbal recognition of their concern and participation in the client's care.

Evaluating Client Responses to Pain Interventions

Examples of outcome criteria for clients experiencing pain are listed in the accompanying box. The specific criteria selected depend on the identified nursing diagnosis and the individual client's condition. More,

OUTCOME CRITERIA

Pain

The client will:

■ State that he or she feels no postoperative pain

■ Carry out deep-breathing exercises and cough without severe pain

■ Walk to the end of the corridor and back without discomfort

■ Perform relaxation exercises as scheduled

perhaps, than in any other area of nursing practice, the client's reassessment is the most reliable evaluation criterion.

Chapter Highlights

Pain is a personal experience.

Pain warns the individual of tissue injury.

The pain experience has three components: pain stimulation, perception, and response.

The pain response has three stages: activation, rebound, and adaptation.

Assessment of a client who is experiencing pain should include a pain history and collection of data about the factors that augment pain and the clinical signs and symptoms of pain.

Nursing diagnoses regarding pain involve the pain itself, the effect of the pain on the client, and a component of the pain experience.

Planning for intervening with a client in pain must include reducing or eliminating factors that intensify pain.

Specific noninvasive techniques can modify pain experience.

Distraction lessens the perception of pain.

Relaxation techniques are helpful in reducing the intensity of chronic pain.

A regular schedule for analgesic administration can help prevent pain.

Evaluating the client's pain therapy includes the response of the client, the changes in the pain, and the client's perceptions of the effectiveness of the therapy.

Suggested Readings

American Journal of Nursing. March 1974a. Hypnotic suggestion. *American Journal of Nursing* 74:515.

———. March 1974b. Chemical and surgical intervention. *American Journal of Nursing* 74:511.

American Pain Society. June 1988. Relieving pain. *American Journal of Nursing* 88:815–831.

Beyerman, K. February 1982. Flawed perceptions about pain. *American Journal of Nursing* 82:302–4.

Blaylock, J. 1968. The psychological and cultural influences on the reaction to pain: A review of literature. *Nursing Forum* 7(3):262–74.

Booker, J. E. March 1982. Pain: It's all in your patient's head (or is it?). *Nursing 82* 12:46–51.

Broome, A. April 16–22, 1986. Coping with pain: Strategies for relief. *Nursing Times* 82:43–44.

Carpenito, L. J. 1987. *Nursing diagnosis application to clinical practice.* 2nd ed. Philadelphia: J. B. Lippincott Co.

Copp, L. A. Summer 1985. Pain coping model and typology *Image: The Journal of Nursing Scholarship.* 17:69–71.

Cummings, D. January 1981. Stopping chronic pain before it starts. *Nursing 81* 11:60–62.

Dernham, P. January/February 1986. Phantom limb pain. *Geriatric Nursing* 7:34–37.

Escobar, P. L. January 1985. Management of chronic pain. *Nurse Practitioner* 10:24–25, 29–30, 32.

Gever, L. N. May 1980. Brompton's mixture. How it relieves pain of terminal cancer. *Nursing 80* 10:57.

Goodwin, J. S.; Goodwin, J. M.; and Vogel, A. V. February 1982. Placebo misuse. *Nursing 82* 12:24–25.

Guyton, A. C. 1986. *Textbook of medical physiology.* 7th ed. Philadelphia: W. B. Saunders Co.

Hamm, B. H., and King, V. Spring 1984. A holistic approach to pain control with geriatric clients ... guided imagery. *Journal of Holistic Nursing* 2:32–37.

McCaffery, M. 1979. *Nursing management of the patient with pain.* 2d ed. Philadelphia: J. B. Lippincott Co.

———. September 1980a. Understanding your patient's pain. *Nursing 80* 10:26–31.

———. October 1980b. Patients shouldn't have to suffer. How to relieve pain with injectable narcotics. *Nursing 80* 10:34–39.

———. November 1980c. How to relieve your patients' pain fast and effectively ... with oral analgesics. *Nursing 80* 10:58–63.

———. December 1980d. Relieving pain with noninvasive techniques. *Nursing 80* 10:55–57.

———. June 1981 When your patient's still in pain don't just do something: Sit there. *Nursing 81* 11:58–61.

———. February 1982. Would you administer placebos for pain? These facts can help you decide. *Nursing 82* 12:22–27.

McGuire, L., and Wright, A. December 1984. Continuous narcotic infusion. It's not just for cancer patients. *Nursing 84* 14:50–55.

Maxwell, M. B. September 1980. How to use methadone for the cancer patient's pain. *American Journal of Nursing* 80:1606–9.

Melzack, R., and Wall, P. D. 1982. *The challenge of pain.* New York: Penguin Books.

———. 19 November 1965. Pain mechanisms: A new theory. *Science* 150:971–79.

———. 1983. *The challenge of pain.* New York: Basic Books.

Nursing Now. 1985. *Pain.* Hicksville, N.Y.: Nursing 85 Books, Springhouse.

O'Donnell, L., and Papciak, B. August 1981. When all else fails: Continuous morphine infusion for controlling intractable pain. *Nursing 81* 11:69–72.

Schechter, N. L.; Berrien, F. B.; and Katz, S. M. May 1988. PCA For adolescents in sickle cell crisis. *American Journal of Nursing* 88:719–22.

Stewart, E. June 1976. To lessen pain: Relaxation and rhythmic breathing. *American Journal of Nursing* 76:958–59.

Warfield, C. A. July 15, 1985. Patient-controlled analgesia. *Hospital Practice* 20:32L, O–P.

West, B. A. February 1981. Understanding endorphins: Our natural pain relief system. *Nursing 81* 11:50–53.

Wilson, R. W., and Elmassian, B. J. April 1981. Endorphins. *American Journal of Nursing* 81:722–25.

CHAPTER 39

Nutrition

OBJECTIVES

Describe nutrition, metabolism, and energy requirements.

Identify functions and food sources of selected nutrients and some clinical signs of deficiency and excess.

Describe the use of daily food group guides.

Identify potential nutritional problems of vegetarians and suggest ways to avoid them.

Describe necessary dietary modifications for older adults.

Identify clinical signs of inadequate nutritional status.

Describe a format for nutritional assessment.

Identify factors that influence a person's eating patterns.

Identify nursing diagnoses and factors contributing to the client's nutritional status.

Identify interventions to stimulate a client's appetite.

Describe ways to assist clients with meals.

Describe some aids that enable self-feeding.

Discuss some special nutritional services available for selected subgroups of the population.

Recognize characteristics of commonly prescribed diets.

Identify nursing responsibilities in administering enteral and parenteral nutrition.

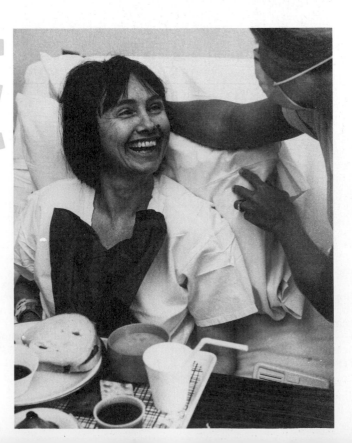

Nutrition and Metabolism

Nutrition is the sum of all the interactions between an organism and the food it consumes (Christian and Greger 1985, p. 4). In other words, nutrition is what a person eats and how the body uses it. People require food or essential nutrients for the growth and maintenance of all body tissues and the normal functioning of all body processes. **Nutrients** are the organic and inorganic chemicals found in foods and required for proper body functioning.

An adequate food intake consists of a balance of essential nutrients: water, carbohydrates, proteins, fats, vitamins, and minerals. Foods differ greatly in their **nutritive value** (the nutrient content of a specified amount of food), and no one food provides all essential nutrients. Nutrients have three major functions (Suitor and Hunter 1980, p. 4): providing energy for body processes and movement, providing structural material for body tissues, and regulating body processes.

The amount of energy that nutrients or foods supply to the body is their caloric value. A **calorie** is a unit of heat energy. A **small calorie** is the amount of heat required to raise the temperature of 1 g of water 1 degree C. A **large calorie (Calorie, kilocalorie [kcal])** is the amount of heat required to raise the temperature of 1 kg of water 1 degree C and is the unit used in nutrition. The energy liberated from each gram of carbohydrate and protein after it is metabolized is about 4 kcal; from each gram of fat, about 9 kcal are liberated through metabolism. The average North American receives approximately 45% of energy from carbohydrates, 40% from fat, and 15% from protein (Guyton 1986, p. 861). In most other parts of the world, people derive far more energy from carbohydrates than from fats and proteins.

Metabolism refers to all cellular chemical reactions that make it possible for body cells to continue living (Guyton 1986, p. 844). The energy in food maintains the basal metabolic rate of the body and provides energy for activities such as running and walking. Metabolic rate is normally expressed in terms of the rate of heat liberated during chemical reactions. The **basal metabolic rate** (BMR) is the rate at which the body metabolizes food to maintain the energy requirements of a person who is awake and at rest.

A person's energy requirements beyond the BMR are influenced by many factors, e.g., age, body size, activity, body temperature, environmental temperature, growth, sex, and emotional state. When energy requirements are completely met by calories taken in as food, people maintain their activity level without weight change. When caloric intake exceeds energy needs, the person gains weight. When caloric intake fails to meet energy requirements, the person burns body fat for energy and loses weight. Energy requirements vary from day to day, reflecting changes in the factors that influence them. For example, illness frequently increases energy requirements because of increased body temperature, increased metabolic rate, and stress.

Essential Nutrients

Essential nutrients include water, carbohydrates, proteins, fats, vitamins, and minerals. The most basic nutrient need is water. Because every cell requires a continuous supply of fuel, the body's most urgent nutritional need, after water, is for nutrients that provide fuel, or energy. The energy-providing nutrients are carbohydrates, fats, and proteins. Hunger impels people to eat enough energy-providing nutrients to satisfy their energy needs, but no clear-cut body signals lead a person to ingest certain vitamins or minerals, both of which are often referred to as **micronutrients.**

■ Carbohydrates

Carbohydrates are composed of the elements carbon, hydrogen, and oxygen and are of two basic kinds: sugars (simple carbohydrates) and starches (complex carbohydrates). The sugars may be **monosaccharides** (single molecules), which include glucose, fructose, and galactose, or **disaccharides** (double molecules), which include sucrose or table sugar (a combination of glucose and fructose), maltose or grain sugar (two glucose molecules), and lactose or milk sugar (a combination of glucose and galactose). Starches are **polysaccharides** because they are composed of branched chains of dozens of molecules of glucose. Nearly all carbohydrates (with the exception of those in milk and milk products, which contain the disaccharide lactose) are derived from plants.

Carbohydrates are also categorized as natural (those found in foods as they come from the earth, e.g., fruits, vegetables, wheat) and refined or processed (those extracted from their natural sources and added to foods, e.g., cookies, candy, cakes, and pies). The natural carbohydrates supply vital nutrients such as protein, vitamins, and minerals and an important nonnutrient, dietary fiber. **Fiber,** a carbohydrate derived from plants, cannot be digested by humans but supplies roughage or bulk to the diet. This bulk not only satisfies appetite but also helps the digestive tract to function effectively and to eliminate wastes. Refined carbohydrates are relatively low in nutrients in relation to the large number of calories they contain and thus are often referred to as empty calories.

The desired end products of carbohydrate digestion are monosaccharides (glucose, fructose, and galactose). Some simple sugars, therefore, require no digestion. Of the three monosaccharides, glucose is by far the most abundant. Major enzymes of carbohydrate metabolism include ptyalin (salivary amylase), pancreatic amylase, and the disaccharidases: maltase, sucrase, and lactase. **Enzymes** are biologic catalysts that speed up chemical reactions. Digestive enzymes, which break down nutrients chemically into smaller compounds by hydrolysis, are categorized according to the types of nutrients on which they act. See Table 39–1.

Table 39—1 ▪ **Actions of Major Digestive Enzymes**

Name	Source	Site of Action	Agents Acted Upon	Resulting Products
Carbohydrate enzymes				
Ptyalin (salivary amylase)	Saliva (secretions from parotid and sub-maxillary glands)	Mouth; some in body of stomach	Starch, e.g., grains, potatoes, legumes	Dextrins, maltose, glucose
Pancreatic amylase	Pancreatic secretions	Small intestine	Starch Dextrins	As above Maltose, glucose
Disaccharidases	Small intestine	Brush border of small intestine	Disaccharides	Monosaccharides
a. Lactase			Lactose in milk	Glucose and galactose
b. Maltase			Maltose in corn syrup	Glucose
c. Sucrase			Sucrose in table sugar, fruits	Glucose and fructose
Protein enzymes				
Pepsin	Peptic cells of stomach; inactive proenzyme pepsinogen is activated to pepsin by hydrochloric acid	Stomach	Large protein molecules	Proteoses, peptones, and large polypeptides
Rennin (in infants only)	Gastric mucosa	Stomach; calcium is necessary for activity	Casein in milk	Coagulated milk
Trypsin	Pancreatic cells; inactive proenzyme trypsinogen activated to trypsin by enterokinase (hormone produced in duodenal wall)	Lumen of small intestine	Whole and partially digested proteins, e.g., proteoses, peptones	Smaller polypeptides and dipeptides
Chymotrypsin	Pancreatic cells; inactive proenzyme chymotrypsinogen is activated to chymotrypsin by trypsin	Lumen of small intestine	Same as trypsin	Same as trypsin; also coagulates milk
Carboxypeptidase	Pancreatic cells; inactive proenzyme procarboxypeptidase is activated to carboxypeptidase by trypsin	Lumen of small intestine	Same as trypsin	Same as trypsin plus some amino acids
Aminopeptidase	Glands in intestinal wall	Brush border of small intestine	Polypeptides	Short chain peptides and amino acids
Dipeptidase	Glands in intestinal wall	Brush border of small intestine	Dipeptides	Amino acids
Fat enzymes				
Pancreatic lipase	Pancreas	Small intestine	Triglycerides, diglycerides	Diglycerides, monoglycerides, fatty acids

In healthy persons, essentially all digested carbohydrate is absorbed by the small intestine. Glucose transport through the cell membrane is augmented by insulin, a hormone secreted by the pancreas. In the absence of insulin, the amount of glucose that diffuses to the cell is far too little to supply normal requirements for energy (with the exception of the liver and brain cells). Glucose metabolism is therefore controlled by the rate at which insulin is available from the pancreas.

Once in the cell, glucose is either used for immediate release of energy or stored in the form of **glyco-gen** (a large polymer of glucose). Although all cells of the body are capable of storing some glycogen, certain cells (liver and muscle) can store large amounts. The process of glycogen formation is called **glycogenesis,** and the breakdown of glycogen to re-form glucose is called **glycogenolysis.** Two hormones activate glycogenolysis: *glucagon* from the alpha cells of the pancreas, and *epinephrine* from the adrenal medulla. Glucagon is secreted when blood glucose concentrations fall to low levels; glucagon stimulates glycogenolysis mainly in the liver. The liver delivers large amounts of glucose into the bloodstream, thus elevating the blood glucose. Epinephrine is released whenever the sympathetic nervous system is stimulated. Epinephrine stimulates glycogenolysis in both liver and muscle cells, thereby releasing energy needed by the body for action during sympathetic stimulation.

When the body's stores of carbohydrates fall below normal, certain quantities of glucose are formed from protein (amino acids) and fat reserves by **gluconeogenesis,** a process that occurs in the liver. Up to 60% of the amino acids in the body's protein can be converted into glucose. Some types of amino acids cannot be converted. During periods of starvation, the body depletes its fat first and later its protein reserves.

▪ Proteins

Proteins are organic substances that upon hydrolysis or digestion yield amino acids (Williams 1981, p. 51). Like carbohydrates, proteins are composed of carbon, hydrogen, and oxygen, but proteins also contain nitrogen. Every cell in the body contains some protein, and about three-quarters of body solids are proteins. The only body substances normally lacking protein are urine and bile.

Proteins can be categorized by chemical structure as simple or compound. **Simple proteins** contain only amino acids or their derivatives, e.g., lactalbumin in milk, serum albumin in blood, keratin in hair and skin, ovoglobulin in egg, gluten in wheat. **Compound proteins** are composites of simple protein and another nonprotein group, e.g., hemoglobin, mucin found in mucous membrane secretions, and purines found in glandular tissue.

Amino acids are categorized as essential or nonessential. **Essential amino acids** are those that cannot be manufactured in the body and must be supplied in their final form as part of the protein ingested in the diet. They are essential for tissue growth and maintenance. Ten essential amino acids are threonine, leucine, isoleucine, valine, lysine, methionine, phenylalanine, tryptophan, histidine, and arginine. Histidine and arginine are necessary during growth but not during adulthood (Brody 1981, p. 36; Williams 1981, p. 53).

Nonessential amino acids are those that the body can manufacture. The body takes apart amino acids derived from the diet and reconstructs new ones from their basic elements (carbohydrates and nitrogen). Nonessential amino acids include glycine, alanine, aspartic acid, glutamic acid, proline, hydroxyproline, cystine, tyrosine, and serine (Williams 1981, p. 53).

Proteins may be complete or incomplete. **Complete proteins** contain all of the essential amino acids plus many nonessential ones. Most animal proteins, including meats, poultry, fish, dairy products, and eggs, are complete proteins. Some animal proteins, however, contain less than the required amount of one or more essential amino acids and therefore alone cannot support continued growth. These proteins are sometimes referred to as partially complete proteins. Examples are some fish, which have small amounts of methionine, and the milk protein casein, which has little arginine.

Incomplete proteins are deficient in one or more essential amino acids (most commonly deficient in lysine, methionine, or tryptophan) and are usually derived from vegetables. If, however, an appropriate mixture of plant proteins is provided in the diet, a balanced ration of essential amino acids can be created. Because protein is not stored, these mixtures must be eaten at the same meal. For example, a combination of corn (low in tryptophan and lysine) and beans (low in methionine) is a complete protein. Such combinations of two or more vegetables are called **complementary proteins.** Another way to take full advantage of vegetable proteins is to eat them with a small amount of animal protein. Examples are spaghetti with cheese, rice with pork, noodles with tuna, and cereal with milk.

Like carbohydrates, protein foods are altered physically by mechanical breakdown in the mouth and mixing with secretions in the stomach and intestine. Complete digestion of proteins to amino acids (the desired end products of protein digestion) could occur in the stomach if protein were held in the stomach longer. However, because the stomach normally empties in a relatively short time, only the beginning stages of protein breakdown are activated by pepsin, the main gastric enzyme specific for protein. Protein breaks down into successively smaller molecules in this sequence: proteins, proteoses, peptones, polypeptides, dipeptides, and finally amino acids.

Amino acids are absorbed from the small intestine directly into the portal blood. They are transported into the cells only by active transport or facilitated diffusion through carrier mechanisms. Soon after entry into the cells, amino acids are converted by intracellular enzymes into cellular protein. Thus, amino acids are not stored in the cells as amino acids but as actual proteins.

An obligatory loss of proteins occurs daily if a person eats no proteins. Thus, to prevent a net loss of protein, a person must ingest at least 20 to 30 g of protein each day (Guyton 1982, p. 544). All body protein is in a dynamic state of breakdown and renewal. Free amino acids present in the liver and plasma comprise an amino acid pool. This pool is a supply of essential and nonessential amino acids that can be used for protein synthesis in any part of the body. The supply of amino acids in the pool is maintained by dietary intake of protein and by catabolism of body proteins.

The state of protein nutrition is usually referred to as **nitrogen balance,** since nitrogen is the element that distinguishes protein from carbohydrate and fat. Almost all nitrogen ingested is in the form of protein. However, most of the nitrogen lost from the body is in the form of nonprotein nitrogen compounds, i.e., the end products of protein catabolism. These end products include urea, creatinine, uric acid, and ammonia salts. The state of nitrogen balance is the net result of intake and loss of nitrogen. When intake of nitrogen equals output, a state of nitrogen balance exists.

Positive nitrogen balance exists when nitrogen input exceeds output; in other words, when the total anabolism of protein and other nitrogenous substances exceeds catabolism and loss. Positive nitrogen balance is desired during periods of growth and tissue replacement. Eating more protein than is necessary to meet body needs does *not* result in an increase in positive nitrogen balance or lean body mass in healthy adults. However, excess protein intake can lead to weight gain (positive caloric balance). Generally, a surplus of nitrogen intake is balanced by increased excretion of nitrogen as urea.

Negative nitrogen balance exists when nitrogen output exceeds intake (when catabolism exceeds anabolism). This state may occur when an inadequate diet is ingested, a person is immobilized, or when a person is exposed to unusual stress as a result of trauma (e.g., surgery or disease).

▪ Fats

Fats are groups of organic substances (fats, oils, waxes, and related compounds) that are greasy and insoluble in water but soluble in alcohol or ether (Williams 1981, p. 34). These organic substances are **lipids.** Fats have the same elements (carbon, hydrogen, and oxygen) as carbohydrates, but the hydrogen content of fats is higher. Fats are actual or potential esters of fatty acids, which are used in metabolism. **Fatty acids** are the basic structural units of fats. **Esters** are compounds of an alcohol and an acid.

Fats can be classified as simple lipids or compound lipids. Simple lipids are known also as **triglycerides,** since they are esters of fatty acids with glycerol in the ratio of three fatty acids to each glycerol base. Compound lipids are various combinations of triglycerides with other components. Three compound lipids important in nutrition are phospholipids, glycolipids, and lipoproteins.

Lipoproteins contain mixtures of triglycerides, phospholipids, cholesterol, and protein. Very low density lipoproteins contain high concentrations of triglycerides and moderate concentrations of phospholipids and cholesterol. Low-density lipoproteins contain few triglycerides but very high concentrations of cholesterol. High-density lipoproteins contain small concentrations of lipids but high concentrations of protein (about 50%). Although cholesterol does not contain fatty acid, it does have many of the physical and chemical properties of other lipids and is capable of forming esters with fatty acids. Large quantities of cholesterol and phospholipids are present in cell membranes and are essential for the structural elements of cells. High blood levels of one or more of the lipids, particularly cholesterol or triglycerides, is called **hyperlipidemia.** Hyperlipidemia puts people at risk of coronary heart disease.

Fatty acids are described as saturated or unsaturated. The degree of saturation is determined by the relative number of hydrogen atoms in the fatty acid. **Saturated** fatty acids are those in which all carbon atoms are filled to capacity (i.e., saturated) with hydrogen. An example of a saturated fatty acid is butyric acid found in butter. **Unsaturated** fatty acids have less hydrogen attached to the available carbon atoms. When several carbon atoms in a fatty acid are not bonded to a hydrogen atom, the fatty acid is **polyunsaturated.** An example of a polyunsaturated fatty acid is linoleic acid found in vegetable oil.

Although chemical digestion of fats begins in the stomach, fats are digested mainly in the small intestine. Enzymes that break down fats include lipase, a pancreatic enzyme, and enteric lipase, an intestinal enzyme. Most chemical digestion is facilitated by pancreatic lipase. See Table 39–1. The desired end products of chemical digestion of fats are monoglycerides, fatty acids, and glycerol.

Some end products of fat digestion (e.g., glycerol and some free fatty acids) are absorbed into the portal blood system and carried to the liver. Other end products (e.g., monoglycerides and cholesterol) are absorbed into the abdominal lacteals and transported through the lymphatic system to the thoracic duct, where they enter the blood through the left subclavian vein. Large quantities of fat are stored in two major tissues: adipose tissue and the liver. Adipose tissue, referred to as the fat depot, stores triglycerides until they are needed for energy. Adipose tissue also has the subsidiary function of providing body insulation. The liver functions in lipid metabolism to degrade fatty acids into smaller compounds that can be used for energy, synthesize triglycerides from carbohydrates and proteins, and synthesize other lipids from fatty acids, such as cholesterol and phospholipids (Guyton 1982, p. 536).

▪ Micronutrients

A **vitamin** is an organic compound that cannot be manufactured by the body and is needed in small quantities to catalyze metabolic processes. Thus, when vitamins are lacking in the diet, metabolic deficits result. Vitamins are generally classified as fat soluble or water soluble. **Fat-soluble** vitamins include A, D, E, and K. **Water-soluble** vitamins include C and the B-complex vitamins: B_1 (thiamine), B_2 (riboflavin), B_3 (niacin or nicotinic acid), B_6 (pyridoxine), B_9 (folic acid), B_{12} (cobalamin), pantothenic acid, and biotin. The body cannot store water-soluble vitamins; thus, people must get a daily supply in the diet. Water-soluble vitamins can be affected by food processing, storage, and preparation. The body can store fat-soluble vitamins, although there is a limit to the amounts of vitamins E and K the body can store. A daily supply of fat-soluble vitamins is therefore not absolutely necessary. Vitamin content is highest in fresh foods that are consumed as soon as possible after harvest. Table 39–2 indicates the usually recommended daily requirement of vitamins, food sources, functions, and signs of deficiencies and excesses.

Minerals are found in organic compounds, as inorganic compounds, and as free ions. Upon oxidation, minerals leave an ash, which can be acid or alkaline. Calcium and phosphorus make up 80% of all the mineral elements in the body. There are two categories of minerals: macrominerals and microminerals. **Macrominerals** are those that people require daily in amounts over 100 mg. They include calcium, phosphorus, sodium, potassium, magnesium, chloride, and sulfur. **Microminerals** are those that people require daily in amounts

Table 39—2   Key Information about Vitamins

Vitamin	RDAs* for Healthy Adults (per day)	Major Food Sources	Major Functions	Signs of Severe Prolonged Deficiency	Signs of Extreme Excess
Water-soluble					
C (ascorbic acid)	35–60 mg	Citrus fruits, cantaloupe, strawberries, tomatoes, potatoes, broccoli, green pepper, spinach	Still under intense study. Thought to aid in metabolism of certain amino acids, aid collagen formation for healing, enhance iron absorption, aid in formation of red blood cells, and maintain integrity of capillary walls.	Scurvy (bleeding gums, loose teeth, skin spots, and bruising); delayed wound healing; impaired immune response	Gastrointestinal upsets, poorer immune response, confounds certain lab tests
B_1 (thiamine)	Females: 1.1 mg; males: 1.5 mg	Pork, liver, whole grains, peas, eggs, milk, peanuts, oatmeal, pasta	Function as coenzymes in metabolism of carbohydrates, fats, amino acids, and alcohol.	Beriberi (nerve changes; sometimes edema, heart failure, muscle weakness)	Unknown
B_2 (riboflavin)	Females: 1–3 mg; males: 1–7 mg	Milk and milk products; eggs; Cheddar cheese, organ meats (liver, heart, kidney); whole grains; green vegetables	As above for thiamine.	Skin lesions, e.g., inflammation and cracking at angles of mouth, dermatitis at angles of nares, keratitis of corneas	Unknown
B_3 (niacin or nicotinic acid)	Females: 14 NE (niacin equivalents; males: 19 NE)	Beef, pork, fish, liver, whole grains, peanuts, green vegetables, dairy products	As above for thiamine.	Pellagra (diarrhea, dermatitis, dementia)	Flushing of face, neck, hands; liver damage
B_6 (pyridoxine)	Females: 2 mg; males: 2.2 mg	High-protein foods (e.g., meat, liver, tuna, poultry, nuts); some vegetables (e.g., green beans, potatoes; bananas)	Protein metabolism, acts in transport of some amino acids across cell membranes, converts tryptophan to niacin.	Nervous and muscular problems, e.g., depression, confusion, weakness, convulsions	Unstable gait, numb feet, poor hand coordination, abnormal brain function
B_9 (folacin or folic acid)	400 µg (microgram)	Green leafy vegetables, broccoli, green beans, whole grains, nuts, orange juice, cottage cheese, peanuts	Maturation of red blood cells; acts as coenzyme in metabolism of certain amino acids and DNA and RNA; essential during growth periods.	Megaloblastic anemia (large, immature red blood cells), gastrointestinal disturbances	None known

(continued)

Table 39–2   Key Information about Vitamins (continued)

Vitamin	RDAs* for Healthy Adults (per day)	Major Food Sources	Major Functions	Signs of Severe Prolonged Deficiency	Signs of Extreme Excess
B₁₂ (cobalamin)	3 µg	Animal products (meats, chicken, fish, eggs, liver, milk)	As above for folacin.	Megaloblastic anemia, pernicious anemia when due to inadequate intrinsic factor, nervous system damage	Unknown
Pantothenic acid	4–7 mg	Widely distributed in foods	Assists in metabolism of carbohydrates and fats.	Fatigue, sleep disturbances, nausea, poor coordination	Unknown
Biotin	100–200 µg	Widely distributed in foods	As above for pantothenic acid.	Fatigue, depression, muscular pain, dermatitis	Unknown
Fat-soluble					
A (retinol, retinoic acid, carotene, palmitate)	Females: 800 RE (retinol equivalents), 4000 IU (international units); males: 1000 RE, 5000 IU	Dark green and deep orange fruits and vegetables: apricots, broccoli, cantaloupe, carrots, pumpkin, winter squash, sweet potatoes, spinach and other dark leafy greens	Still under intense study: known to maintain health and normal functioning of cartilage, bone, and body coverings and linings (e.g., corneas, mucous membrane, skin); is a component of rhodopsin, a colored and light-sensitive substance in retina.	Keratinization of epithelial tissues, opacity of the cornea, night blindness, dry and scaling skin	Damage to liver, kidney, bone, headache, irritability, vomiting, hair loss, blurred vision, yellow skin from carotene
D (cholecalciferol, ergocalciferol)	5 µg or 200 IU	Fortified and full-fat dairy products, egg yolk; synthesized in the skin on exposure to sunlight	Increases calcium absorption from gastrointestinal tract; helps control calcium deposition in bones.	Rickets (bone deformities in children, osteomalacia (bone softening) in adults	Gastrointestinal upset; lethargy; cerebral, cardiovascular, and kidney damage; kidney stones
E (tocopherols: alpha, beta, gamma, and delta)	8–10 mg as alpha tocopherol equivalents	Vegetable oils and their products (e.g., salad dressings, many margarines); peanuts	Antioxidant, i.e., prevents oxygen from combining with other substances (vitamins A and C and polyunsaturated fatty acids) and damaging them; prevents cell membrane damage.	Possible anemia	In anemic children, blood abnormalities may develop

(continued)

Table 39–2   Key Information about Vitamins (continued)

Vitamin	RDAs* for Healthy Adults (per day)	Major Food Sources	Major Functions	Signs of Severe Prolonged Deficiency	Signs of Extreme Excess
K (menadione, phylloquinone)	70–40 μg	Green leafy vegetables (e.g., lettuce, cabbage, spinach, peas, asparagus); meat	Necessary for formation of prothrombin in liver; prothrombin is essential for blood clotting.	Severe bleeding on injury; internal hemorrhage	Liver damage and anemia from high doses of synthetic forms

*RDAs are recommended daily allowances.
Sources: Adapted from National Research Council, Committee on Dietary Allowances, Food and Nutrition Board, *Recommended dietary allowances,* 9th ed. (Washington, D.C.: National Academy of Sciences, 1980) and J. L. Christian and J. L. Greger, *Nutrition for living* (Menlo Park, Calif.: Benjamin/Cummings Publishing Co., 1985).

less than 100 mg. They include iron, zinc, manganese, iodine, fluoride, copper, cobalt, chromium, and selenium.

Common problems associated with the mineral nutrients are iron deficiency resulting in anemia, and osteoporosis resulting from loss of bone calcium. Key information about many essential minerals is shown in Table 39–3. Additional information about major minerals associated with the body's fluid and electrolyte balance is given in Chapter 43.

Standards for a Healthy Diet

Several guides have been developed to provide standards for an adequate or healthy diet that includes all nutrients needed by the average person. These include: daily food group guides, recommended dietary allowances, and vegetarian food guides.

Table 39–3   Key Information about Many Essential Minerals

Mineral	RDA for Healthy Adults	Major Dietary Sources	Major Functions	Signs of Severe, Prolonged Deficiency	Signs of Extreme Excess
Major minerals					
Calcium	800 mg	Milk, cheese, dark green vegetables, legumes	Bone and tooth formation; blood clotting; nerve transmission	Stunted growth; maybe bone loss	Depressed absorption of some other minerals
Phosphorus	800 mg	Milk, cheese, meat, poultry, whole grains	Bone and tooth formation; acid-base balance; component of coenzymes	Weakness; demineralization of bone	Some forms depress absorption of some minerals
Magnesium	Females: 300 mg; males: 350 mg	Whole grains, green leafy vegetables	Component of enzymes	Neurologic disturbances	Neurologic disturbances
Sulfur	(Provided by sulfur amino acids)	Sulfur amino acids in dietary proteins	Component of cartilage, tendon, and proteins; acid-base balance	(Related to protein deficiency)	Excess sulfur amino acid intake leads to poor growth; liver damage
Sodium	1100–3300 mg*	Common salt, soy sauce, cured meats, pickles, canned soups, processed cheese	Body water balance; nerve function	Muscle cramps; reduced appetite	High blood pressure in genetically predisposed individuals
Potassium	1875–5625 mg*	Meats, milk, many fruits and vegetables, whole grains	Body water balance; nerve function	Muscular weakness; paralysis	Muscular weakness; cardiac arrest

(continued)

mended levels, especially if they eat more than the minimum amounts recommended.

In 1979, the USDA modified the Basic Four Food Guide and published the **Hassle-Free Guide.** This plan adds a fifth group to the basic four. The fifth group includes foods high in fats, sugar, and alcohol. Moderation in consumption of these foods is recommended. Critics of this plan say that people may misinterpret the purpose of the fifth group and believe that the foods in the fifth group are being recommended for regular consumption rather than being restricted.

The **SANE Guide,** developed by Christian and Greger (1985, p. 38), is an attempt to build on the strengths of previous guides and add other useful information. SANE is an acronym for Sound Approach to Nutritious Eating. The SANE Guide recommends the same major food groups found in the Basic Four Food and Hassle-Free Guides and the same numbers of daily minimum servings for an adult. The SANE Guide recommends different intakes of milk products by people of different ages. Unique aspects of the SANE Guide are:

■ *Limited extras.* The foods in this additional group are not needed for good nutrition, since they do not contain the essential nutrients in significant amounts. Therefore, they should be used as limited supplements rather than as mainstays of the diet. Many of these foods, e.g., fatty foods, sugary foods, alcoholic beverages, and unenriched baking goods, are high in calories. Examples are salad dressings, cream cheese, bacon, chocolate, sour cream, soy sauce, olives, ketchup, jam, jellies, and cakes. Overweight people should eat fewer of these foods. Other foods in this group are low both in calories and nutrients but contribute water. Examples are tea, coffee, broth, low-calorie soft drinks, and diet gelatin desserts.
■ *Plant sources of protein.* The plant sources are richer in certain nutrients, e.g., magnesium and the B vitamin folacin, than meats are and should be substituted for meat sources several times each week. Plant sources include legumes (e.g., garbanzo, kidney, lima, navy, and pinto beans; soybeans; lentils; and split peas), nuts, seeds, and nut or seed butters.
■ *Serving sizes.* The guide provides suggested servings for representative foods within each group.
■ *Fat, sodium, and sugar content.* The guide indicates the relative content of fat, sodium, and added sugar of certain foods in each group, allowing the user to reduce the amounts of fat, sodium, and added sugar in the diet.
■ *Combination foods.* Directions for including common combination foods, e.g., casseroles and sandwiches, are given. Each ingredient must be identified by group. For example:
— 1 cup spaghetti with meatballs includes: 1 serving meat (2 oz); 1 serving grain (3/4 cup spaghetti); and 1/2 serving vegetable (1/4 cup tomato sauce).
— 1/4 of a 12-inch cheese pizza includes: 1 1/2 servings milk (2 oz cheese); 3 servings grain (pizza dough); 1/2 serving vegetable (1/4 cup vegetables).

Recommended Dietary Allowances

The Committee on Dietary Allowances of the Food and Nutrition Board of the National Academy of Sciences in Washington D.C. publishes lists of recommended dietary allowances (RDAs). RDAs are the levels of intake of essential nutrients that, to the best available scientific knowledge, adequately meet the known nutritional needs of most healthy persons (National Research Council 1980, p. 1). About every 5 years, the findings of recent studies are reviewed, and daily nutrient intake recommendations are updated.

Because a person's actual need for any given nutrient can be influenced by sex, body size, growth, and reproductive status, separate recommendations are made for various subgroups, defined by sex, age, pregnancy, and lactation. Recommended nutrient levels are usually set high enough to include the needs of 97.5% of the people in that group and to allow for some loss of the nutrient as it makes its way through the body. For example, the RDA allows for losses that occur during absorption or conversion from one chemical form to another, when some of the nutrient's activity may be decreased. Factors not taken into account in the RDAs are the effect of illness or injury (increasing the need for nutrients) and the variability among individuals within any given group.

Vegetarian Diets

There are two basic vegetarian diets: those that allow only plant foods and those that include milk, eggs, and dairy products. Some people, not strictly vegetarians, eat fish and poultry but not beef, lamb, or pork; others eat only fresh fruit, juices, and nuts; and still others eat plant foods and dairy products but not eggs. See Table 39–6.

People may become vegetarians for economic, health, religious, ethical, and ecologic reasons. Increased meat prices during the last decade have forced some people to become vegetarians or eat meat infrequently. Some people avoid meat because they believe it is healthy to

Table 39—6 Types of Vegetarian Diets

Kind	Description
Vegans	Strict vegetarians, use no animal or milk products
Lacto-ovo-vegetarians	Drink milk and eat eggs but eat no other products of animals
Lacto-vegetarians	Drink milk but do not eat eggs or other products of animals
Ovo-vegetarians	Eat eggs but do not drink milk or eat other meat products
Pesco-vegetarians	Drink milk, eat eggs and fish but no other meat products
Partial vegetarians (semivegetarians)	Eat chicken and fish but do not eat red meat
Fruitarians	Eat only fresh (raw) fruits, juices, and nuts

do so. They cite as evidence that vegetarians tend to be less obese than others and that blood cholesterol levels of vegetarians tend to be lower, two factors that reduce the probability of heart disease. Some people are vegetarians for ethical reasons: They object to the killing of animals or the way they are raised. People who follow vegetarian diets for ecologic reasons point out the wastefulness of eating animals that consume a large part of the world's supply of grain when this grain could be better used for people.

Vegetarian diets can be nutritionally sound if they include a wide variety of legumes, grains, fruits, vegetables, nuts, milk, and milk products and if proper protein complementation and vitamin-mineral supplementation is provided. Protein intake can be insufficient if complementary protein relationships are not understood and followed. Although plant foods contain amino acids, many do not contain them in sufficient quantity or variety. When *eaten together,* however, certain foods often contain about the right proportions of amino acids. This phenomenon of one food supplementing low levels of amino acids in another is called **protein complementing** or **mutual supplementation.** Examples of foods that contain complementary amino acids are shown in Table 39–7. Generally, legumes (starchy beans, peas,

lentils) have complementary relationships with grains and with nuts and seeds. Protein complementing is of particular importance for growing children and pregnant and lactating women whose protein needs are high.

Because foods of animal origin provide vitamin B_{12}, vegans need to eat other sources of vitamin B_{12}: brewer's yeast, foods fortified with vitamin B_{12}, or a direct vitamin supplement. Iron deficiency is also a possibility if red meat is not eaten because plant sources of iron are not absorbed efficiently. Vegans, therefore, are advised to consume a vitamin-C-rich food with each meal to enhance iron absorption from plant sources, iron-rich foods (e.g., green leafy vegetables, whole grains, raisins, and molasses), and iron-enriched foods. Calcium deficiency is a concern for strict vegetarians. It can be prevented by including soybean milk fortified with calcium, leafy green vegetables, and tofu (soy bean curd) that has added calcium.

A good guide for vegetarians is shown in Table 39–8. It includes four basic food groups: milk group; vegetable protein foods; fruits and vegetables; and breads and cereals. In addition, eggs and fats are advised. Diets such as the fruitarian diet do not provide sufficient amounts of essential nutrients and are not recommended for long-term use.

Table 39–7 Complementary Protein Relationships

Food Groups	Complementary Food Combinations

Legumes	Legumes with rice
	Soybeans with:
	  Rice and wheat
	  Corn and milk
	  Wheat and sesame seeds
	  Peanuts and sesame seeds
	Beans with corn or wheat

Grains	Rice with:
	  Legumes
	  Milk and milk products
	  Brewer's yeast
	Corn with legumes
	Wheat with:
	  Legumes
	  Milk and milk products
	  Peanuts and milk
	  Sesame seeds and soybeans

Vegetables	Lima beans, peas, Brussels sprouts, cauliflower, or broccoli with sesame seeds, Brazil nuts, and mushrooms

Nuts and seeds	Sesame seeds with:
	  Beans
	  Soybeans and wheat
	Peanuts with:
	  Sesame seeds and soybeans
	  Milk and milk products
	  Sunflower seeds
	  Wheat and milk

Source: Adapted from R. B. Howard and N. H. Herbold, *Nutrition in clinical care,* 2d ed. (New York: McGraw-Hill Book Co., 1982), p. 352. Used by permission.

Modifications for Older Adults

Metabolic rates decrease with age and physical activity usually slackens; therefore, elderly people require fewer calories than previously, and some may have an increased need for carbohydrates for fiber and bulk, but most nutrient requirements remain relatively unchanged. Such physical changes as tooth loss and impaired sense of taste and smell may also affect eating habits. Other physical deficiencies that may affect eating habits and nutritional status are (Raab and Raab 1985, p. 24) decreased bile/gastric juice secretion, peristalsis, and glucose tolerance; impaired circulation; and loss of bone density and lean body mass.

In addition, psychosocial factors may contribute to nutritional problems. Some elderly people who live alone do not want to cook for themselves or eat alone. As a result, the person may adopt poor dietary habits and is at risk of malnourishment. Loss of spouse, living alone, anxiety, depression, dependence on others, and lowered income all affect eating habits. Guidelines for the inclusion of high-nutrient foods that are compatible with the diminished chewing and swallowing abilities and other problems of older adults are summarized in the accompanying box.

Factors Influencing Dietary Patterns

Before attempting to assess a client's nutritional status, it is helpful to recognize the factors that affect an individual's eating habits. Some of these are culture, reli-

Table 39—8   Vegetarian Food Guide

Food Group	Recommended Serving per Day	Examples of Foods
Milk group	2 or more servings. One serving is 1 cup or designated equivalent.	Whole, skim, or soy milk; yogurt; cheese (1 oz); cottage cheese (¼ cup); powdered soy milk (4 Tbsp); evaporated milk (½ cup)
Vegetable protein foods	2 or more servings.	Beans, lentils, peas, and garbanzos (1 cup); peanut butter (4 Tbsp); nuts and seeds (1½ Tbsp); tofu (4 oz); dry textured vegetable proteins (20—30 g)
Fruits and vegetables	4 or more servings (include 1 serving vitamin-C—rich foods and 1 or 2 servings carotene-rich foods). One serving is ½ cup cooked vegetables or fruits, ½ cup juice, or 1 cup raw vegetables.	Vitamin-C—rich foods: orange, grapefruit, cabbage, tomatoes, melon, green pepper, strawberries Carotene-rich foods: dark yellow vegetables and fruits and leafy green vegetables
Breads and cereals	4 or more servings. One serving is 1 slice of bread or ½ to ¾ cup cereal or pasta.	Whole wheat or enriched bread; hamburger bun (½); graham crackers (2); Saltines (5); Wheat Thins (8); enriched or whole rice; enriched spaghetti, macaroni, noodles, granola
Other: Eggs and fats	3 or 4 eggs per week, 1 Tbsp oil or soft margarine per day.	

Source: Adapted from I. B. Vhymeister, U. D. Register, and L. M. Sonnenberg, Safe vegetarian diets for children, *Pediatric Clinics of North America,* February 1977, 24(1):207. Used by permission.

gion, economic status, personal preference, emotions, hunger, appetite, satiety, and health. These factors frequently occur in combination.

Culture

Ethnicity often determines food preferences. Traditional foods (e.g., rice for Orientals, pasta for Italians, curry for Indians) are eaten long after other customs are abandoned. Although food patterns vary from region to region and person to person, the examples in the accompanying box illustrate the diversity of food preferences among cultures.

Religion

Religion also affects diet. Some Roman Catholics avoid meat on certain days, and some Protestant faiths prohibit tea, coffee, or alcohol. Both Orthodox Judaism and Islam prohibit pork. Orthodox Jews observe kosher customs, eating certain foods only if they are inspected by a rabbi and prepared according to dietary laws. The nurse must be sensitive to such religious dietary practices.

Economic Status

What, how much, and how often a person eats are frequently affected by economic status. For example, people with limited income, including some elderly people, may not be able to afford beef and fresh vegetables. In contrast, people with higher incomes may purchase more proteins and fats and fewer complex carbohydrates. Regardless of economic status, people may not purchase foods containing essential nutrients. Many other factors, such as personal food preferences, are involved.

Food Preferences by Culture

Chinese	Rice
	Green tea
	Mixtures of fish, pork, or chicken and vegetables (bamboo shoots, broccoli, cabbage, mushrooms, onions, and pea pods)
Italian	Dishes made with pasta
	Bread
	Cheese
	Vegetables such as artichokes, eggplant, greens, tomato, and zucchini
Japanese	Rice
	Green tea
	Raw fish and soy sauce
	Abundance of vegetables
Mexican	Dried beans
	Tortillas made from wheat or corn flour instead of bread
	Tacos, burritos, enchiladas
	Chili peppers, especially in sauces
Polish	Highly salted and seasoned foods
	Sausages; smoked and cured meats
	Noodles, potatoes, dumplings
	Bread
	Coffee with sugar and cream
Puerto Rican	Rice and beans with spicy sauce
	Plantain (vegetable similar in appearance to a large banana)
	Coffee with large amount of milk
Southern black	Pork and chicken
	Dried peas, beans, squash, and greens cooked with fatback or salt pork

(Whitney and Cataldo 1983, pp. 730—31)

GUIDELINES

Nutrition for Older Adults

Reduce fat consumption by drinking low-fat milk, eating more poultry and fish rather than red meats, limiting meat portions to 4 to 6 oz per day, and limiting the intake of added fats, e.g., butter, margarine, and oil-based salad dressings.

Consume desserts such as fresh or canned fruit and puddings made with low-fat milk rather than pies, cookies, cakes, or ice cream.

Make sure that intake of meat, poultry, fish, eggs, and cheese is sufficient, since intakes of these foods are often decreased in the older population.

Because of a lowered glucose tolerance, consume more complex carbohydrates, e.g., breads, cereals, rice, pasta, potatoes, and legumes, rather than sugar-rich foods.

Ensure an intake of at least 800 mg of calcium to prevent bone loss. Milk and milk products, e.g., cheese, yogurt, cream soups, milk puddings, and frozen milk products, are principal sources of calcium. See Table 39–9 for additional calcium-rich foods.

Make sure that intake of vitamin D is sufficient. Vitamin D is essential to maintain calcium homeostasis. To meet vitamin D requirements, include some milk in the diet, since such dairy products as cheese, cottage cheese, and yogurt are not usually fortified with vitamin D. If milk or milk products cannot be tolerated due to a lactose deficiency, supplements should be taken.

Because sodium may be restricted for older adults who have hypertension or other cardiac problems, avoid such foods as canned soups; ketchup; mustard; and salted, smoked, cured, and pickled meats, poultry, and fish. No salt should be added during the cooking of foods.

Due to the increased incidence of gastrointestinal disturbances and chronic diarrhea, the regular aspirin use among some elderly women, and the possible reduction in meat intake, the need for iron may be increased. See Table 39–10 for iron-rich foods.

Difficulties with chewing raw fruits and vegetables may lead to a deficiency in vitamins A and C, minerals, and fiber. Adaptions in food preparation may be necessary. Chop fruits and vegetables finely, shred green leafy vegetables, and select ground meat, poultry, or fish rather than foods that are more difficult to chew.

Consume fiber-rich foods to prevent constipation and minimize use of laxatives. See Table 39–11 for examples of fiber-rich foods. Fiber-rich foods also provide bulk and a feeling of fullness. They are therefore useful in helping people control their appetites and lose weight.

Mealtime is commonly a social activity. When possible, make arrangements to promote appropriate social interaction at meals.

Eat essential foods first and follow with limited foods in moderation afterward.

Having the major meal at noon may decrease difficulty sleeping at night after a heavy meal. Avoid tea, coffee, or other stimulants in the evening.

Peer Groups

Peer groups or other subgroups distinguished by age, sex, occupation, or other interests also influence a person's food choices. For example, certain foods may become "in" with teenagers. Members of any group may change their food choices to align themselves more closely with an influential group member. For example, when a financially successful member of a group of business executives shows a strong preference for decaffeinated coffee, some associates are likely to make similar choices. Sexism may also influence food choices. Some men, for example, may not choose a salad as an entree because they perceive such a choice as feminine.

Personal Preference and Uniqueness

What an individual likes and dislikes significantly affects eating habits. People often carry childhood preferences into adulthood. People develop likes and dislikes based on associations with a typical food. A child who loves to visit his grandparents may love pickled crabapples because they are served in the grandparents' home. Another child who dislikes a very strict aunt grows up to dislike the chicken casserole she often prepares.

Individual likes and dislikes can also be related to familiarity, particularly for children. Children often say they dislike a food before they sample it. Some adults are very adventuresome and eager to try new foods. Others prefer to eat the same foods over and over again. Preferences in the tastes, smells, flavors (blends of taste and smell), textures, temperatures, colors, shapes, and sizes of food influence a person's food choices uniquely. For example, some people may prefer sweet and sour tastes to bitter or salty tastes. Textures play a great role in food preferences. Some people prefer crisp food to limp food, firm to soft, tender to tough, smooth to lumpy, or dry to soggy. Many people like certain combinations of taste and textures.

Life-Style

Certain life-styles are linked to food-related behaviors. People who are always in a hurry probably buy convenience grocery items or eat restaurant meals. People who spend many hours at home may take time to prepare more meals "from scratch." Individual differences also influence life-style patterns. Is the person skilled in cooking? Is the person willing to learn to make new things? Does the person thrive on routine and

Table 39–12   Selected Drug-Nutrient Interactions

Drug	Effect on Nutrition
Acetylsalicylic acid (aspirin)	Decreases serum folate and folacin nutrition
	Increases excretion of vitamin C, thiamine, potassium, amino acids, and glucose
	May cause nausea and gastritis
Antacids containing aluminum or magnesium hydroxide (Maalox)	Decrease absorption of phosphate and vitamin A
	Inactivate thiamine
	May cause deficiency of calcium and vitamin D
Thiazide diuretics (Diuril, HydroDIURIL)	Increase excretion of sodium, potassium, chloride, calcium, magnesium, zinc, and riboflavin
	May cause anorexia, nausea, vomiting, diarrhea, or constipation
Potassium chloride (Kaochlor, K-Lor, Slow-K)	Decreases absorption of vitamin B_{12}
	May cause diarrhea, nausea, or vomiting
	Increases excretion of potassium, magnesium, and calcium
	May cause anorexia, nausea, or vomiting
	Is incompatible with protein hydrolysates
Laxatives	May cause calcium and potassium depletion
	Mineral oil and phenolphthalein (Ex-lax) decrease absorption of vitamins A, D, E, and K
Antihypertensives	Hydralazine (Apresoline) may cause anorexia, vomiting, nausea, and constipation
	Methyldopa (Aldomet) increases need for vitamin B_{12} and folate
	May cause dry mouth, nausea, vomiting, diarrhea, constipation
Antiinflammatory agents	Colchicine decreases absorption of vitamin B_{12}, carotene, fat, lactose, sodium, potassium, protein, and cholesterol
	Prednisone decreases absorption of calcium and phosphorus
Antidepressants	Amitriptyline (Elavil) increases food intake (large amounts may suppress intake)

References: A. B. Natow and J. Heslin, *Nutritional care of the older adult* (New York: Macmillan Publishing Co., 1986), pp. 252–255; and D. Raab and N. Raab, Nutrition and the aging: An overview, *Canadian Nurse,* March 1985, 81:25.

alcohol often leads to protein, thiamine, folacin, niacin, and vitamin B_6 deficiencies as a result of interruptions in the body's normal nutritional processes anywhere from ingestion through excretion.

The effects of drugs on nutrition vary considerably. They may alter appetite, disturb taste perception, or interfere with nutrient absorption or excretion. Nurses need to be aware of the nutritional effects of specific drugs when evaluating a client for nutritional problems. The nursing history interview should include questions about the medications the client is taking. Nutrients can also affect drug utilization. Some nutrients can decrease drug absorption; others enhance absorption. For example, the calcium in milk hinders absorption of the antibiotic tetracycline but enhances the absorption of the antibiotic erythromycin. Selected drug and nutrient interactions are shown in Table 39–12.

Clients at Risk for Nutritional Problems

Some clients are at greater risk for having or developing nutritional problems than most. The nurse needs to identify these clients on the basis of their medical and medication histories. When such an identification is made, the nurse then collects additional data to make a specific nursing diagnosis regarding the client's nutritional status. See the accompanying box for a summary of the risk factors for altered nutrition status.

Assessing Nutritional Status

One method of assessing a client's nutritional status is to follow the "ABCD" approach:

A   Collecting *anthropometric measurements*
B   Looking at *biochemical data*
C   Examining the client for the *clinical signs* of nutritional status
D   Obtaining a *dietary history*

Anthropometric Measurements

Anthropometric measurements are measurements of the size and composition of the body. They include measurements of height, weight, skin folds (fat folds), and arm circumference. The triceps, subscapular, biceps, and suprailiac skin folds can be measured with special calipers. The site most commonly used is the triceps fold. An inadequately nourished person can be underweight, overweight, or obese: in every case his or her caloric intake is not in balance with expenditure of energy. Anthropometric measurements reflect the client's caloric-energy expenditure balance, muscle mass, body fat, and protein reserves.

Biochemical Data

Biochemical measurements can be used to detect subclinical malnutrition. Blood and urine samples are taken to measure a nutrient or a **metabolite** (end product or enzyme) of a nutrient. Blood tests are often ordered in packages referred to as SMAs (simultaneous multiple analysis) followed by a number, e.g., SMA-12 or SMA-18. The number following SMA indicates the number of tests that will be done.

The laboratory studies most commonly used today to assess nutrition include hemoglobin and hematocrit, total lymphocyte count, albumin, transferrin level, blood urea nitrogen (BUN), and creatinine excretion tests. Although less commonly used, other laboratory tests can be performed to assess vitamins, minerals, and trace elements. Because many factors can influence these laboratory tests, it is important to realize that no single test can confirm a nutritional problem.

■ Clinical Signs

Since nutrition affects all parts of the body, physical assessment can assist in identifying nutritional problems. Table 39–13 lists some of the data that can be collected to determine a client's nutritional status.

■ Dietary History

A dietary history generally includes data about the client's usual eating patterns and habits, food preferences and restrictions, daily fluid intake, use of vitamin or mineral supplements, any dietary problems (e.g., difficulty chewing or swallowing), physical activity, health history, and concerns related to food buying and preparation. See Figure 39–1 for a sample nutritional history tool for an adult. Data about the client's medication intake are also important, especially in relation to mealtimes. Many medications are to be taken only before or after meals, so variations from the usual breakfast-lunch-dinner mealtimes need to be documented.

Two commonly used approaches for analyzing the data obtained from the dietary history involve using daily food group guides and food composition tables. Using daily food group guides is a relatively workable

■ Risk Factors for Nutritional Problems

Diet history

Chewing or swallowing difficulties (including ill-fitting dentures, dental caries, and missing teeth)
Inadequate food intake
Restricted or fad diets
No intake for 10 or more days
Intravenous fluids (other than total parenteral nutrition for 10 or more days)

Inadequate food budget
Inadequate food preparation facilities
Inadequate food storage facilities
Physical disabilities
Elderly living and eating alone

Medical history

Overweight
Underweight
Recent weight loss or gain
Recent major illness
Recent major surgery
Surgery of the GI tract
Anorexia
Nausea
Vomiting
Diarrhea
Alcoholism

Cancer
Liver disease
Kidney disease
Diabetes
Thyroid or parathyroid disease
Adrenal disease
Mental disability
Teenage pregnancy
Multiple pregnancies
Pancreatic insufficiency
Radiation therapy

Medication history

Aspirin
Antibiotics
Antacid
Antidepressants
Antihypertensives
Antiinflammatory agents

Antineoplastic agents
Digitalis
Laxatives
Diuretics (thiazides)
Potassium chloride
Vitamin or other nutrient preparations

Table 39–13 Clinical Signs Indicating Nutritional Status

Body Part or System	Normal Signs	Abnormal Signs
Hair	Shiny, neither dry nor oily	Oily, dry, dull, patchy in growth
Skin	Smooth, slightly moist, good turgor	Dry, oily, broken out in rash, scaly, rough, bruised
Eyes	Bright, clear	Dry, reddened
Tongue	Pink, moist	Reddened in patches, swollen
Mucous membranes	Reddish pink, moist	Reddened, dry, cracked
Cardiovascular	Heart rate and blood pressure within normal ranges, heart rhythm regular	Rapid heart rate, elevated blood pressure, irregular heart rhythm
Muscles	Firm, well developed	Poor in tone, soft, underdeveloped
Gastrointestinal	Appetite good, elimination regular and normal	Manifesting anorexia, indigestion, diarrhea, constipation
Neurologic	Reflexes normal, alert, good attention span, emotionally stable	Reflexes decreased, irritable, inattentive, confused, emotionally labile
Vitality	Vigorous, energetic, able to sleep well	Lacking energy, tired, apathetic, sleeping poorly
Weight	Normal for age, build, and height	Overweight, underweight

NUTRITIONAL HISTORY

Name _____

Age _____ Height _____

WEIGHT

Current weight _____

Weight history (obesity, onset, fluctuations) _____

Percentage of
  Overweight _____
  Underweight _____

OTHER ANTHROPOMETRIC DATA

Triceps skin fold measurement _____

Arm muscle circumference _____

EATING PATTERNS AND HABITS

1. Typical day's food intake

Time	Item	Portion
____	_____	_____
____	_____	_____
____	_____	_____
____	_____	_____
____	_____	_____
____	_____	_____
____	_____	_____
____	_____	_____
____	_____	_____
____	_____	_____
____	_____	_____
____	_____	_____
____	_____	_____
____	_____	_____

2. Food likes _____

3. Food dislikes _____

4. Food allergies _____

5. Foods considered harmful or beneficial to health
  Harmful _____

  Beneficial _____

6. Food restrictions
  Special diet _____
  Religious _____
  Cultural _____

7. Fluid intake
  Number of glasses of water per day _____
  Number of cups of tea or coffee per day _____
  Number of soft drinks per day _____
  Amount of alcohol or wine per day _____

8. Use of vitamins
  Kind _____
  Frequency _____

9. Use of minerals (eg, calcium, iron)
  Kind _____
  Frequency _____

10. Perception of diet
  Nutritionally balanced _____
  Not nutritionally balanced _____

DIETARY PROBLEMS

1. Describe appetite (usual, increased, decreased) _____

2. Foods causing indigestion, diarrhea, or gas _____

3. Difficulty following special diet
  Yes _____ No _____
  If yes, how _____

4. Chewing difficulties
  Number of teeth
  Upper _____ Lower _____
  Dentures
  Partial _____
  Complete _____
  Fit of dentures _____

5. Swallowing difficulties _____

6. Usual bowel movements _____

HEALTH HISTORY

1. Physical activity
  Type _____
  Frequency _____

2. Medication intake
  Name _____
  Time _____

3. History of diseases, surgical procedures, or weight problems

	Yes	No
Diabetes	____	____
Heart problems	____	____
Surgery (specify) _____	____	____
Cancer	____	____
Kidney stones	____	____
Gallstones	____	____
Ulcers	____	____
Intestinal disorder	____	____
Allergies other than food (specify) _	____	____
Weight problems	____	____

4. Perception of general health
  Good _____
  Satisfactory _____
  Poor _____

FOOD BUYING AND PREPARATION

1. Ingredients used
  Salt _____
  Soy _____
  MSG _____
  Other _____

2. Methods most used
  Boil _____
  Bake _____
  Fry _____
  Broil _____
  Steam _____
  Other _____

3. Shopping/cooking capabilities
  Is able to shop _____
  Relies on others _____
  Is able to cook _____
  Relies on others _____

4. Living situation
  Number of family members _____
  Lives alone _____

5. Do food costs affect diet?
  Yes _____ No _____
  How? _____

Figure 39—1 A sample dietary history tool

approach for the nurse and provides a quick estimate of the client's nutritional balance. The nurse simply determines whether the client is receiving the daily recommended servings of the four basic food groups.

Dietary analyses using food composition tables provide more specific data about specific nutrient intake. This calculation method takes time. Fortunately, computerized nutrient data bases and diet analysis software have been developed.

Nursing Diagnosis

The nursing diagnostic category for clients with nutritional problems may be broadly stated as alterations in nutrition and further defined as:

■ Less than body requirements or nutritional deficit (insufficient intake)
■ More than body requirements or obesity (excessive intake)

For both of these categories, intake is a relative term that depends on the client's energy expenditures. For example, a person who eats an apparently balanced and adequate diet but who routinely performs rigorous physical activity may have a nutritional deficit. Similarly, a client may have what appears to be a "normal" intake that is, in fact, excessive in light of the person's minimal activity level.

Nutritional Deficit

Nutritional deficit is insufficient intake of one or more nutrients required to meet metabolic needs (Gordon 1982, p. 68). When possible, the nurse should state the specific deficit, e.g., inadequate protein, iron, or vitamin C intake. Indications of nutritional deficits of specific vitamins are outlined in Table 39–2. The following signs may indicate other generalized deficits:

■ Weight 20% or more under the ideal for height and frame
■ Loss of weight with adequate food intake
■ Food intake less than that recommended by food guides or evidence of lack of food
■ Eating difficulties
■ Gastrointestinal signs, such as abdominal pain, cramping, diarrhea, and hyperactive bowel sounds
■ Muscle weakness and reduced energy level
■ Excessive loss of hair
■ Pallor of skin, mucous membranes, and conjunctivae

Obesity

Obesity is the result of calorie intake that exceeds metabolic need. People become obese by eating too much food or eating too many foods of high caloric density. Caloric density describes the number of kilocalories per unit weight of food. Fats and oils have the highest caloric density, whereas vegetables such as celery and lettuce have low densities. Energy expenditure is also a factor in weight control. By increasing activity, the individual increases energy expenditure and often decreases weight.

Obesity is present when the weight is 20% greater than the ideal for height and frame and when triceps skin folds are greater than 15 mm in men and 25 mm in women (Kim and Moritz 1982, p. 300). It is currently one of the most prevalent health problems in North America and is associated with hypertension, cardiovascular diseases, and diabetes. Factors contributing to obesity include:

■ Sedentary habits (low activity level)
■ Inappropriate eating patterns (e.g., eating large amounts of carbohydrates and saturated fats)
■ Depression or anxiety (often accompanied by stressors such as a death in the family or a change in marital or work status)
■ Eating the largest meal at the end of the day

Examples of Nursing Diagnoses

Examples of nursing diagnoses for clients with nutritional problems are shown in the accompanying box.

NURSING DIAGNOSIS

Nutritional Problems

Potential alteration in nutrition: less than body requirements related to lack of knowledge about increased requirements during pregnancy

Potential alteration in nutrition: less than body requirements related to lack of knowledge about necessary requirements for growth

Potential alteration in nutrition: less than body requirements related to lack of knowledge about ways to get essential proteins on vegetarian diets

Potential alteration in nutrition: less than body requirements (iron) related to pregnancy

Alteration in nutrition: less than body requirements related to inability to chew secondary to ill-fitting dentures

Alteration in nutrition: less than body requirements related to inability to procure food associated with financial and transportation problems

Alteration in nutrition related to self-imposed starvation secondary to denial of being underweight and desire to remain slender

Alteration in nutrition: less than body requirements (calcium) related to age and potential osteoporosis

Alteration in nutrition: more than body requirements related to compulsive overeating

Alteration in nutrition: more than body requirements related to excessive intake of carbohydrates and sedentary habits

Planning to Modify Nutritional Problems

When planning measures to meet the client's nutrition needs, the nurse needs to consider the learning needs of the person and plan specific measures to help him or her obtain nourishment. A client may need to learn information about a healthy or newly prescribed therapeutic diet and even new skills for eating. For example, the client with limited ability to move the arms may need to learn to eat with a special long-handled spoon. Planning also involves establishing outcome criteria. For suggestions, see the section on evaluation later in this chapter. The nurse's overall responsibilities in relation to a client's nutrition include maintaining or restoring the client's nutritional status, preventing nutritional problems, and making the client's mealtimes pleasurable.

Implementing Nursing Strategies

Nursing strategies for clients with nutritional problems include both teaching and intervening. Depending on clients' learning needs, specific information concerning a prescribed diet or general counseling on nutrition may be planned. Clients with problems involving the actual intake of nutrients are assisted by nurses to attain the specific nutrients required.

Counseling about Nutrition

Nutrition counseling involves much more than simply providing information. The nurse must help the client integrate diet changes into the client's life-style and provide strategies to motivate the client to change his or her eating habits. Counseling can be likened to the teaching-learning process discussed in Chapter 21. First, a thorough assessment of the client's nutritional status and nutrient intake is necessary. Next, the nurse needs to find out what the client knows about nutrition. At this point, the nurse must assess her or his own knowledge of the client's specific learning needs and, if necessary, obtain the appropriate information or refer the client to an expert on the subject. Then the client and nurse set goals or objectives for learning, plan strategies to achieve the goals, and establish criteria to evaluate achievement of the goals. Because it is the client's responsibility to make the necessary dietary changes and to change his or her behavior, the nurse's role is to support and encourage the client.

Teaching about Special Diets

Assisting clients and support persons with special or therapeutic diets prescribed by the physician is a function shared by the dietitian and the nurse. The di-

etitian informs the client and support persons about the specific foods allowed and not allowed and assists the client with meal planning. The nurse reinforces this instruction, assists the client to make beneficial changes, and evaluates the client's response to the planned changes.

Physicians order special diets for clients who cannot eat the usual foods. A special or therapeutic diet is one in which the amount of food, the kind of food, or the frequency of eating is prescribed. Special diets are used to treat a disease process, e.g., a low-salt diet for high blood pressure; to prepare for a special examination or surgery; and to promote health, e.g., a low-calorie diet for an overweight client.

Some diets are temporary, observed perhaps for one meal or 1 week, but some clients must follow certain diets (e.g., the diabetic diet) for a lifetime. If the diet is long term, the client must not only understand the diet but also develop a healthy, positive attitude toward it. The client needs to know the consequences of choosing not to comply with the prescribed dietary regimen. Progressive hospital diets (e.g., postoperative dietary protocols) are often unique to institutions, and nurses need to be familiar with the diets prescribed in their agencies.

Clients who do not have special needs eat the **regular diet,** whose quantity and content are designed to meet the needs of most clients. In some agencies, the regular diet is referred to as the normal, house, or standard, diet. Some hospitals offer clients a daily menu from which to select their meals for the next day. Other hos-

Soft Diet Foods

Meats and Alternates
Any tender meat, fish, poultry (chopped or shredded)
Chopped meat in cream sauce
Omelet or scrambled egg
Spaghetti sauce with chopped meat over small shaped pasta
Cottage cheese

Vegetables
Rice in cream or cheese sauce
Mashed potatoes
Mashed sweet potatoes
Mashed squash
Mashed potatoes with chopped spinach
Vegetables in cream or cheese sauce
Vegetables pureed with diced vegetables (e.g., carrot or turnip puree with baby peas)
Avocado
Cauliflower

Asparagus tips
Spinach

Fruits
Chunky apple sauce
Ripe banana
Cooked, peeled fresh fruits
Canned fruits

Desserts
Pudding
Custard
Ice cream
Yogurt
Pudding cake
Junket
Gelatin
Sherbet
Soft cake

Cereals and Breads
Cooked cereal
Crustless bread

Liquids
All allowed (except when restricted by physician)

pitals provide standard meals to each client on the general diet. Certain foods (e.g., cabbage, which tends to produce flatus, and highly seasoned and fried foods, which are difficult for some people to digest) are usually omitted from the regular diet.

A variation of the regular diet is the **light diet,** designed for postoperative and other clients who are not ready for the regular diet. Foods in the light diet are plainly cooked. Foods containing large amounts of fat are usually omitted, as are bran and foods containing a great deal of fiber. Not all agencies provide a light diet.

A **soft diet** is easily chewed and digested. It is often ordered for clients who have difficulty chewing and swallowing. It is a lightly seasoned, low-residue (low-fiber) diet. Examples of foods that can be included in a soft or semisoft diet are shown in the accompanying box. The **pureed diet** is a modification of the soft diet. Liquid is added to the food, which is then blended to a semi-solid consistency.

A **full liquid diet** contains only liquids or foods that turn to liquid at room temperature, such as ice cream. Full liquid diets are eaten by clients who have gastrointestinal disturbances or are otherwise unable to tolerate solid or semisolid foods. Full fluid foods are free of cellulose, irritating condiments such as mustard or ketchup, and spices such as black pepper or chili powder. This diet is not recommended for long-term use. Its iron content, protein content, and caloric density are low, and its cholesterol content is high because of the amount of milk offered. Clients who must receive only liquids for longer periods are usually given a nutritionally balanced oral supplement, e.g., Sustacal. The full liquid diet is monotonous and difficult for clients to accept. Planning six or more feedings per day may encourage a more adequate intake.

The **clear liquid diet** is often limited to water, tea, coffee, clear broths, ginger ale or other carbonated beverages, apple juice, and plain gelatin. It does not permit milk. This diet provides the client with fluid and carbohydrate (in the form of sugar), but it does not supply adequate protein, fat, vitamins, minerals, or calories. No more than 600 kcal/day are provided. It is usually a short-term diet (24 to 36 hours) provided for clients after certain surgery or clients in the acute stages of infection, particularly of the gastrointestinal tract. The major objective of this diet is to relieve thirst, prevent dehydration, and minimize stimulation of the gastrointestinal tract. Clear fluids are offered throughout the day as tolerated by the client.

There are many other special diets, sometimes especially devised for individual clients. Details about these diets are provided in nutrition and medical/surgical nursing textbooks. Common special diets are reducing, diabetic, low salt, and allergy diets.

Clients often need assistance adapting special diets to their cultural, religious, ethnic, and economic patterns. Most diets in North America are devised for the Anglo-American taste and omit many otherwise acceptable ethnic foods. Such a diet may be unfamiliar or unpalatable to the ethnic client. Nutritionists and dietitians can often assist nurses to adapt a diet to suit a person's life-style. Another important aspect is adapting a diet to a person's economic status. Often, less costly foods can be substituted for recommended foods, such as powdered milk for fresh milk.

Motivation is highly important for success. If a client does not accept the need for a diet, he or she will probably not adhere to it, and its therapeutic value is lost. A client may understand that sugar in coffee is not allowed on a low-calorie diet but may not understand that bread also contains sugar and is also restricted. An elderly woman may understand that she is not to add salt to foods when cooking but salts her food at the table. This client does not really understand the importance of or the reason for salt restriction.

▪ Stimulating Appetite

Because of accompanying physical illness, unfamiliar food or food the client finds unpalatable, environmental and psychologic factors, and physical discomfort or pain, many hospitalized clients have poor appetites. Lowered food intake of a few days' duration is not often a problem for adults; however, a prolonged decreased food intake leads to weight loss, decreased strength and stamina, and subsequent nutritional problems. Decreased food intake is often accompanied by decreased fluid intake, which may cause fluid and electrolyte problems. See Chapter 42 for further information.

Increasing a person's appetite requires determining the reason for the lack of appetite and then dealing with the problem. Some guidelines for interventions that may improve client's appetites are summarized in the accompanying box.

▪ Assisting Clients with Meals

Because clients are frequently confined to their beds, particularly in acute care settings, most hospitals must

GUIDELINES

▪ Improving Appetite

Relieve illness symptoms that deaden appetite prior to mealtime; e.g., give an analgesic for pain or an antipyretic for a fever or allow rest for fatigue.

Provide familiar food that the person likes. Often the relatives of clients are pleased to bring food from home but may need some guidance about special diet requirements.

Select small portions so as not to discourage the anorexic client.

Avoid unpleasant or uncomfortable treatments immediately before or after a meal.

A tidy, clean environment that is free of unpleasant sights and odors is important. A soiled dressing, a used bedpan, an uncovered irrigation set, or even used dishes can destroy appetite.

Reduce psychologic stress. A lack of understanding of therapy, the anticipation of an operation, and fear of the unknown can cause anorexia. Often, the nurse can help by discussing feelings with the client, giving information and assistance, and allaying fears.

PROCEDURE 39–1

Administering a Tube Feeding

Feedings are usually administered at room temperature unless the order specifies otherwise. The specified amount of solution is warmed in a basin of warm water or left to stand for a while until it reaches room temperature. Continuous feeding should be kept cold (see the discussion of the optional feeding pump later in this section). Excessive heat coagulates feedings of milk and egg, and hot liquids can irritate the mucous membranes. However, excessively cold feedings can reduce the flow of digestive juices by causing vasoconstriction and may cause cramps. Commercially prepared feedings are available in cans and bottles ready for administration. Some containers are designed so that ice chips can be placed in an outer section to keep the formula cooled.

Equipment

- The correct amount of feeding solution ordered by the physician. Check the expiration date on a commercially prepared formula or the preparation date and time if the solution was prepared in the agency. Discard an agency solution that is more than 24 hours old or a commercial formula that has passed the expiration date.

- A 20- to 50-ml syringe with an adapter. The syringe is used to check that the tube is in the stomach.

- An emesis basin to collect the aspirated stomach contents.

- If an intermittent feeding is being given, a bulb syringe. The bulb is removed from the syringe, and the barrel is attached to the tube.
    or
  A burette (calibrated plastic bag) and a drip chamber, which can be attached to the tubing.
    or
  A prefilled bottle with a drip chamber, tubing, and a flow-regulator clamp.

- A measuring container from which to pour the feeding if the syringe or burette method is used.

- Water (60 ml unless otherwise specified) at room temperature to clean the inside of the tube after the feeding.

- Optional: A feeding pump, which can be used with a prefilled tube-feeding set to regulate the exact amount of feeding for the client. See Figure 39–7. The pump is often used to administer the feeding when small-bore tubes are used or when gravity flow is insufficient to instill the feeding. Because the feeding is administered over a long time period, a formula that is warmed can grow microorganisms. It should not hang longer than the manufacturer recommends, eg, 3–4 hours. If it will hang longer, it should be kept cool with ice chips.

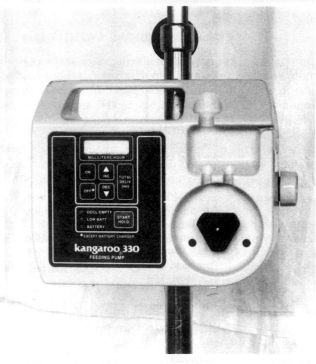

Figure 39–7

Intervention

1. Explain to the client that the feeding should not cause any discomfort, but it may cause a feeling of fullness. For an adult, the usual intermittent feeding takes about 30 minutes; the exact length of time depends largely on the volume of the feeding.

2. Provide privacy for this procedure if the client desires it. Tube feedings are embarrassing to some people.

3. Assist the client to a Fowler's position in bed or a sitting position in a chair, the normal position for eating. If a sitting position is contraindicated, a slightly elevated right side–lying position is acceptable.
   Rationale: These positions enhance the gravitational flow of the solution and prevent aspiration of fluid into the lungs.

4. If the client does not have a tube in place, insert one. Confirm that the tube is in the stomach. Attach the syringe to the open end of the tube, and aspirate stomach contents. Small-bore feeding tubes should not be aspirated. Placement in the duodenum or jejunem is confirmed by X-ray.

5. If the gastric tube is maintained in the client:
   a. Aspirate all the stomach contents and measure the amount prior to administering the feeding.
   Rationale: This is done to evaluate absorption of the last feeding, ie, whether undigested formula of a previous feeding remains.
   b. If 50 ml or more of undigested formula is withdrawn in adults, or 10 ml or more in infants, check

with the nurse in charge before proceeding. The precise amount is usually determined by the physician's order or by agency policy.

Rationale: At some agencies a feeding is withheld when the specified amount or more of formula remains in the stomach. In other agencies, the amount withdrawn is subtracted from the total feeding and that volume (less the undigested portion) is administered slowly.

or

Reinstill the gastric contents into the stomach if this is the agency's or physician's practice. Remove the syringe bulb or plunger, and pour the gastric contents via the syringe into the tube.

Rationale: Removal of the contents could disturb the client's electrolyte balance.

Bulb Syringe Method

6. When using a bulb syringe:

a. Remove the bulb from the syringe, and connect the syringe to a pinched or clamped tube.

Rationale: Pinching or clamping the tube prevents excess air from entering the stomach and causing distention.

b. Add the feeding to the syringe barrel. See Figure 39–8.

c. Permit the feeding to flow in slowly. Raise or lower the syringe to adjust the flow as needed. Pinch or clamp the tubing to stop the flow for a minute if the client experiences discomfort.

Rationale: Quickly administered feedings can cause flatus, crampy pain, and/or reflex vomiting.

d. After the feeding has been administered, instill 60 ml of water through the tube. Be sure to add the water before the feeding solution has drained from the neck of the syringe.

Rationale: Water cleans the lumen of the tube and prevents future blockage. Adding water before the syringe is empty prevents instillation of air into the stomach.

e. Clamp the tube before removing the syringe.

Rationale: Clamping prevents reflux of the feeding.

Burette Method

7. When using a burette:

a. Hang the burette from an infusion pole about 30 cm (12 in.) above the tube's point of insertion into the client.

b. Clamp the tubing, and pour the formula into the burette.

c. Open the clamp, run the formula through the burette tubing, and reclamp the tube.

Rationale: The formula will displace the air in the burette and its tubing, thus preventing the instillation of excess air into the client's stomach.

d. Confirm placement of the tube by withdrawing stomach contents or injecting air through the tube while listening for a rushing sound with a stethoscope placed over the client's stomach.

e. After confirming tube placement, attach the burette tubing to the tube (see Figure 39–9), and regulate the drip by adjusting the clamp.

f. Just before all the formula has run through and

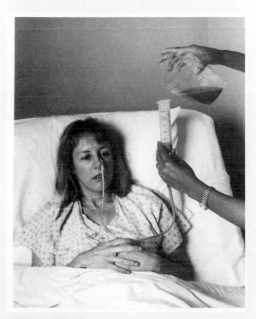

Figure 39–8

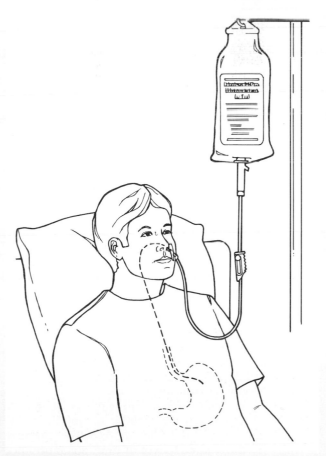

Figure 39–9

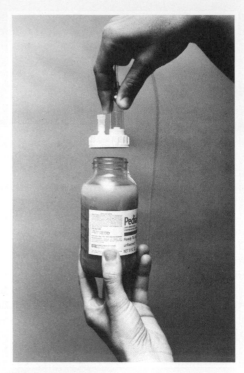

Figure 39–10

the burette is empty, add 60 ml of water to the burette and run it through the nasogastric tube.
Rationale: The water rinses the nasogastric tube and maintains its patency by removing sticky formula that can occlude the tube.
g. Clamp the burette tube before all the water has gone through the tube.
Rationale: Clamping the tube prevents air from entering the stomach.

Prefilled Bottle with Drip Chamber

8. When using a prefilled tube-feeding set:
a. Remove the sealed cap from the container, and replace it with the screw-on cap to which the drip chamber and tubing are attached. See Figure 39–10.
b. Close the clamp on the tubing.
c. Hang the container on an intravenous pole about 30 cm (12 in.) above the tube's insertion point into the client.
Rationale: At this height the formula should run at a safe rate into the stomach.
d. Squeeze the drip chamber to fill it to one-third to one-half of its capacity.
e. Open the tubing clamp, run the formula through the tubing, and reclamp the tube.
Rationale: The formula will displace the air in the tubing, thus preventing the instillation of excess air into the client's stomach.
f. Confirm placement of the tube as in step 7d above. Then attach the feeding set tubing to the tube, and regulate the drip rate to deliver the feeding over the desired length of time. Some prefilled tube-feeding sets can be attached to a feeding pump.

g. Just before all the formula has run through the tubing, clamp the feeding tube and the nasogastric tube and disconnect the two.
h. Using a 50-ml syringe, instill 30–50 ml of water through the nasogastric tube to rinse it.

Continuous-Drip Feeding

9. If the feeding is a continuous-drip tube feeding, discontinue the feeding at least every 6 hours, or as indicated by agency policy, and aspirate and measure the gastric contents. Then flush the tubing with 30–50 ml of water. Small-bore tubes should be flushed but not aspirated.
Rationale: This ensures adequate absorption and verifies correct placement of the tube. If placement of a small bore tube is questionable, a repeat x-ray should be done.

For All Methods

10. After the feeding and tube rinsing, clamp the client's nasogastric tube.
Rationale: Clamping prevents leakage from the tube.
11. Cover the end of the tube with a cap or with gauze held by an elastic band, and pin the tubing to the client's gown. See Figure 39–11.
Rationale: Covering the tube end prevents leakage from the tube.
12. Ask the client to remain sitting upright in Fowler's position or in a slightly elevated right lateral position for at least 30 minutes.

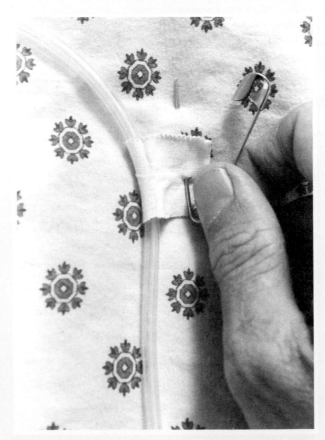

Figure 39–11

Rationale: These positions facilitate digestion. A right lateral position facilitates movement of the feeding from the stomach into the small intestine.

13. If the equipment is to be reused, wash it thoroughly with soap and water so that it is ready for reuse. Change equipment every 24 hours or according to agency policy.

14. Check the agency's policy on the frequency of changing the tubes and the use of smaller-lumen tubes.
Rationale: These measures prevent irritation and erosion of the pharyngeal and esophageal mucous membranes.

15. Document the feeding, including the amount and kind of solution taken, duration of the feeding, and the response of the client. Record the volume of feeding and water administered on the client's intake and output record.

Sample Recording

Date	Time	Notes
6/9/89	1210	350 ml Meritene feeding administered in 30 min. Eructed small amount of flatus. Tolerated feeding $\overline{S}$ emesis. No discomfort noted. ———— Juan S. Ramirez, SN

Carefully assess clients receiving tube feedings for possible problems. Table 39–15 summarizes common problems and suggested corrective measures. All clients should receive supplemental water in addition to the prescribed tube feeding to prevent dehydration.

▪ Gastrostomy or Jejunostomy Feeding.

A **gastrostomy feeding** is the instillation of liquid nourishment through a tube that enters an opening (called a gastrostomy) through the abdominal wall into the stomach. A **jejunostomy feeding** is the instillation of liquid nourishment through a tube that enters a surgical opening (a jejunostomy) through the abdominal wall into the jejunum. These feedings are usually temporary measures. When there is an obstruction in the esophagus, they may become permanent measures, for example, after removal of the esophagus.

Increasingly, **percutaneous endoscopic gastrostomy (PEG)** is being used. This procedure does not require general anesthesia or the use of an operating room. PEG is usually performed in the endoscopy suite, but may also be done in the client's room. Using an endoscope to visualize the inside of the stomach, the physician makes a puncture through the skin and subcutaneous tissues of the abdomen into the stomach and inserts the PEG catheter through the puncture. The catheter has internal and external bumpers and an inflatable retention balloon to maintain placement. Once the opening has healed, replacement tubes can be inserted without the use of endoscopy.

Critical Elements of Administering a Tube Feeding

Before administering the feeding:

▪ Assess the client for feelings of abdominal distention, belching, loose stools, flatus, or pain; bowel sounds; and allergies to foods in the feeding.

▪ Check the expiration date of the feeding.

▪ Warm the feeding to room temperature.

▪ Confirm correct placement of the tube.

▪ Aspirate residual stomach contents, measure the amount, and check about reinstilling it or continuing the feeding.

▪ Remove air from the feeding tubes of burette and prefilled bottles with drip chambers.

▪ Deliver the feeding over the desired length of time.

After the feeding:

▪ Rinse the nasogastric tube with water.

▪ Clamp the nasogastric tube before all of the rinse solution has run through.

▪ Have the client remain in a Fowler's or slightly elevated right lateral position for at least 30 minutes.

Long-term use of PEG feedings is preferable to gastric or small intestine feedings; there are fewer risks of aspiration, and it is psychologically more acceptable. Clients initially receive feedings continuously, but are advanced to intermittent feedings after a few days of uncomplicated continuous feedings. Thus, the feeding tube is not visible except when in use. PEG tubes often have smaller lumens than other types of feeding tubes (except for the small-intestine tubes), and care must be taken to avoid clogging the tube. Use liquid medications when possible. If liquid preparations are not available, finely crush tablets and dissolve with water before inserting; flush with water afterward.

For conventional gastrostomies and jejunostomies, a surgeon inserts a plastic or rubber tube or catheter into either the stomach or the jejunum. The surgical opening is sutured tightly around the tube or catheter to prevent leakage. Care of this opening before it heals requires surgical asepsis. When the incision heals (10 to 14 days), the tube or catheter can be removed and reinserted for each feeding. Between feedings, a prosthesis may be used to close the "ostomy" opening. It consists of a shaft 4 to 6 cm (1 1/2 to 2 in) long, with internal and external flanges and a screw cap.

Gastrostomy and jejunostomy feedings allow the client greater mobility than gastric or duodenal tube feedings and enable the client to feed himself or herself. Similar principles for administration and assessment are appropriate. Guidelines for providing care to clients with gastrostomy and jejunostomy feedings are summarized in the accompanying box.

Table 39–15 Common Problems of Tube Feedings

Factors to Assess to Determine How Client Is Tolerating the Feeding	Possible Causes of Problems	Corrective Measures
Gastrointestinal function		
Vomiting	Feeding too soon after intubation	Allow client to relax and rest after tube is inserted
	Improper location of tip of feeding tube	Repositioning of tube by qualified health professional
	Rapid rate of infusion	Administer slowly
	Excessive volume:	Be sure tube feeding container does not run dry before feeding is completed
	(1) Air	
	(2) Formula	Check with physician regarding number and size of feedings
	Position of client	Position on right side for ½ hr following feeding—reverse Trendelenburg or semi-Fowler's
(Applies to both vomiting and diarrhea)	Food infection or poisoning	Check sanitation of formula and equipment
	Anxiety	Explain procedures; provide reassurance and other needed types of support; provide privacy
Diarrhea	Rapid rate of infusion	Administer slowly—very slowly if formula is cold
	High osmolality of formula or high concentration of formula	Adapt client to formula gradually
	Lactose intolerance	Contact physician regarding change of formula
Constipation	High content of milk in formula	Contact physician regarding:
	Lack of fiber	(1) Change in formula
	Inadequate fluid intake	(2) Laxatives
		(3) Increasing fluid
Fluid and electrolyte balance		
Dehydration	Rapid infusion of carbohydrate → hyperglycemia → osmotic diuresis → dehydration	Administer slowly; exogeneous insulin sometimes needed
	Excess protein and electrolytes in formula	Change formula and/or increase fluid according to physician's orders
	Inadequate fluid intake	
Edema	Excessive sodium in formula	Check with physician about change in formula
Nutritional adequacy		
Undernutrition (gradual weight loss)	Inadequate number of calories to meet energy requirements	Check to see if client is receiving prescribed amount of formula; estimate client's caloric intake
		Check with physician regarding increasing the volume, concentration, or number of feedings given
Overnutrition (gradual gain of undesirable weight)	Excessive caloric intake	Check with physician regarding decreasing the volume, concentration, or number of feedings given
Undernutrition (inadequate intake of protein and/or micronutrients leading to biochemical or clinical signs of deficiency)	Amount of standard formula needed to maintain weight is too low to meet requirements for essential nutrients	Check with physician regarding providing appropriate nutrient supplements

Source: C. W. Suitor and M. F. Hunter, *Nutrition: principles and applications in health promotion,* 2d ed. Philadelphia: J. B. Lippincott Co., 1984.

▪ **Total Parenteral Nutrition.** **Total parenteral nutrition (TPN)** is the intravenous administration of solutions of dextrose, water, fat, proteins, electrolytes, vitamins, and trace elements. TPN provides all needed calories, achieving an anabolic state in clients who are unable to maintain a normal nitrogen balance. Such clients may include those with severe malnutrition, severe burns, bowel disease disorders (e.g., ulcerative colitis or enteric fistula), acute renal failure, hepatic failure, metastatic cancer, or major surgeries after which nothing may be taken by mouth for more than 5 days.

TPN is a mixture of 10 to 50% dextrose in water, amino acids, and special additives such as vitamins (e.g., B complex, C, D, K), minerals (e.g., potassium, sodium, chloride, calcium, phosphate, magnesium), and trace elements (e.g., cobalt, zinc, manganese). Additives are included according to each client's nutritional needs. Fat emulsions may be given to provide essential fatty acids, to correct and/or prevent essential fatty acid deficiency, or to provide extra calories for clients who, for example, have high calorie needs or cannot tolerate glucose as the only calorie source.

Many of the sepsis problems associated with conventional I.V. therapy are also associated with TPN. Moreover, the problems are magnified for a number of reasons. Clients receiving TPN therapy are often critically ill, may be malnourished, and are sometimes immunosuppressed. The solutions used in TPN therapy support the growth of a wide variety of microorganisms.

Infection control is of utmost importance during TPN therapy. The nurse must always observe surgical asepsis (see Chapter 46) when changing solutions, tubing, dressings, and filters. Because TPN solutions are **hypertonic** (highly concentrated in comparison to the solute concentration of blood), they are infused only into high-flow central veins, where they are diluted by the client's blood. This prevents injury to the intimal layer of these blood vessels. Clients receiving TPN are at risk for developing thrombophlebitis and possibly bacteremia.

Typically, TPN solutions are administered through a central I.V. line that rests in the client's superior vena cava. This may be a standard line or a Hickman, Broviac, or other catheter. (See Chapter 43.) The catheter is secured in place by suture, appropriate taping, or both. An antimicrobial ointment and a dressing are then applied over the insertion site.

Because an improperly placed catheter may cause a pneumothorax, the nurse must assess the client for signs of chest pain and labored breathing and auscultate the lungs for abnormal breath sounds. Placement of the catheter is confirmed by x-ray examination. If the catheter is misplaced, the physician will either manipulate it or remove it and insert another catheter. When correct catheter placement is confirmed, the nurse places a secure occlusive dressing over the insertion site and then commences infusion of the TPN solution.

Because TPN solutions are high in glucose, infusions are started gradually to prevent hyperglycemia. The client needs to adapt to TPN therapy by increasing his or her insulin output from the pancreas. For example, an adult client may be given 1 liter (40 ml/hr) of TPN solution the first day, if the infusion is tolerated; the amount may be increased to 2 liters (80 ml/hr) for 24 to 48 hours, and then to 3 liters (120 ml/hr) within 3 to 5 days. When TPN therapy is to be discontinued, the TPN infusion rates are decreased slowly to prevent hyperinsulinemia and hypoglycemia. Weaning a client from TPN may take up to 48 hours but can occur in 6 hours as long as the client receives adequate carbohydrates either orally or intravenously.

Meticulous client assessment is necessary during TPN therapy. The assessment should focus on the client and on the TPN system. The nurse observes the client for signs of thrombosis or thrombophlebitis at the catheter insertion site (e.g., edema or redness) and along the course of the vein (e.g., pain or swelling of the arm, neck, or face). Purulent thrombophlebitis may result in a purulent discharge, which appears at the insertion site with slight pressure. If such signs are observed, the nurse

GUIDELINES

Gastrostomy and Jejunostomy Feedings

Ascultate for bowel sounds prior to each feeding (or every 4–8 hours for continuous feedings) to determine intestinal activity.

Check for residual feedings every 4–6 hours (for continuous feedings) and hold feedings if there is a 2 hour volume. Recheck in 2 hours and restart unless the residual remains large; the physician should be notified if a large residual persists.

Check for residual before each intermittent feeding. Hold if there is more than 150 ml and recheck in 3–4 hours. Notify the physician if a large residual remains at that time.

Inspect the stoma for signs of inflammation or infection; record and report the client's condition.

Change dressings as ordered until the stoma has healed.

Position the client with the head of the bed elevated or in a sitting position for 30–60 minutes after feedings to decrease the risk of aspiration.

Observe for common complications of enteral feedings: aspiration, hyperglycemia, abdominal distention, diarrhea, and fecal impaction. Report findings to physician. Often a change in formula or rate of administration can correct problems.

Teach the client how to administer feedings and when to notify the physician or nurse practitioner concerning problems.

notifies the physician, who may order removal of the catheter and initiation of a heparin infusion at a peripheral vein site. The nurse also observes the client for signs of air embolism (apprehension, dyspnea, tachycardia, chest pain, hypotension, cyanosis, and loss of consciousness). If air embolism is suspected, oxygen is administered and the client is placed on his or her left side with the head lowered. Lowering the head increases intrathoracic pressure, decreasing the flow of air into the vein during inhalation. A left side-lying position helps prevent the air from moving to the pulmonary artery.

The nurse monitors vital signs every 4 hours or more often, depending on the client's health. An elevated temperature is one of the earliest indications of catheter-related sepsis. The TPN tubing is changed every 48 hours or according to agency practice. The TPN infusion line should never be used to take central venous pressure (CVP) measurements or blood samples or to administer other solutions (e.g., "piggy-backing" or directly "pushing" intravenous medications), blood, or blood products. Before administering any TPN solution, the nurse checks its expiration date. Most solutions must be used within 24 hours of preparation, unless they are refrigerated. The infusion flow rate and the laboratory test results are carefully monitored to detect such complications as hyperglycemia or electrolyte imbalance. Use of an infusion pump keeps the infusion rate regular. The nurse monitors the client for hyperglycemia as accord-

CHAPTER 40

Fecal Elimination

OBJECTIVES

Describe the functions of the lower intestinal tract.

Identify factors that influence fecal elimination and patterns of defecation.

Distinguish between normal and abnormal characteristics and constituents of feces.

Describe methods used to assess the intestinal tract.

Differentiate among specific common fecal elimination problems.

Identify common causes and effects of selected fecal elimination problems.

Identify measures that maintain normal fecal elimination patterns.

Relate common interventions to specific fecal elimination problems.

Give reasons for selected nursing interventions.

Describe modifications for clients with ostomies.

State outcome criteria essential for evaluating the client's progress.

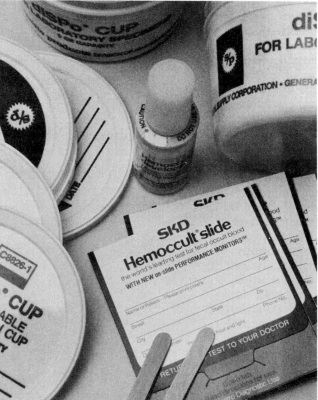

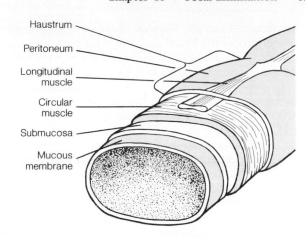

Figure 40–2 The layers of the wall of the large intestine

Physiology of Defecation

Elimination of the waste products of digestion from the body is essential to health. These excreted waste products are referred to as **stool** or **feces.** The large intestine extends from the ileocecal (ileocolic) valve, which lies between the small and large intestines, to the anus. It has seven parts: the cecum; ascending, transverse, and descending colons; sigmoid colon; rectum; and anus or external orifice. See Figure 40–1.

The waste products leaving the stomach through the small intestine and then passing through the ileocecal valve are called **chyme.** Usually about 450 ml of chyme enters the adult cecum each 24 hours. Of this amount only about 100 ml remains for excretion by the time it reaches the rectum; the remainder is reabsorbed into the capillaries of the large intestine.

The contents of the colon normally represent foods ingested over the previous 4 days, although most of the waste products are excreted within 48 hours of ingestion. The large intestine is a muscular tube lined with mucous membrane. See Figure 40–2. The muscle fibers are both circular and longitudinal, thus permitting the intestine to enlarge and contract in both width and length. The longitudinal muscles are shorter than the colon and therefore cause the large intestine to form pouches, or **haustra.**

The colon's main functions are the absorption of water and nutrients, the secretion of mucus to protect the intestinal wall, and fecal elimination. The colon absorbs water and significant amounts of sodium and chloride as food passes along it. The colon also serves a protective function in that it secretes mucus containing large amounts of bicarbonate ions. The mucus secretion is stimulated by excitation of parasympathetic nerves. Therefore, during extreme stimulation (e.g., as a result of emotions) large amounts of mucus are secreted, resulting in the passage of stringy mucus as often as every 30 minutes with little or no feces (Guyton 1986, p. 785). Mucus protects the wall of the large intestine from trauma by the acids formed in the feces, and it binds the fecal material together. Mucus also protects the intestinal wall from bacterial activity.

The colon transports the products of digestion, flatus and feces, which are eventually eliminated through the anal canal. **Flatus** is largely air and the by-products of the digestion of carbohydrates. The colon additionally serves to eliminate waste products, that is, **feces.** Three types of movements propel the chyme along the colon: haustral shuffling, contractions of the haustra, and peristalsis. See Figure 40–3. **Haustral shuffling** involves movement of the chyme back and forth within the haustra. In addition to mixing the contents, this action aids in the absorption of water and moves the contents forward to the next haustra.

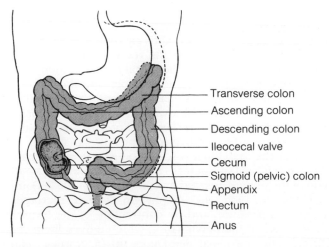

Figure 40–1 The large intestine and rectum

Transverse colon
Ascending colon
Descending colon
Ileocecal valve
Cecum
Sigmoid (pelvic) colon
Appendix
Rectum
Anus

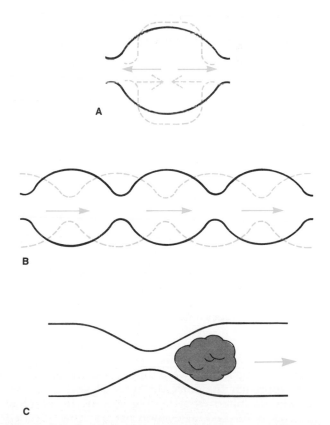

Figure 40–3 Three types of intestinal movements: **A,** haustral shuffling; **B,** contraction of the haustra; **C,** peristalsis

Contractions of the haustra, also called **segmentation,** help propel the liquid and semisolid contents along the colon. This kind of movement is less effective when it involves formed feces (Vick 1984, p. 738). These contraction movements normally occur intermittently, averaging one every 2 hours during fasting and about one every hour after a meal (Vick 1984, p. 739). **Peristalsis,** the third type of colonic movement, involves a wave of muscular contraction that advances the length of the colon, usually toward the anus. About 50% of people experience one or more peristaltic waves in the distal colon each day, commonly after breakfast.

There are three folds of tissue in the rectum that extend across the rectum and several folds that extend vertically. Each of the vertical folds contains a vein and an artery. It is believed that these folds help retain feces within the rectum. When the veins become distended, as they can with repeated pressure, a condition known as *hemorrhoids* occurs, which may be associated with constipation or pain, itching, or bleeding upon defecation.

The anal canal is bounded by an internal and an external sphincter muscle. See Figure 40–4. The **internal sphincter** is under involuntary control, innervated by the autonomic nervous system. The **external sphincter** normally is voluntarily controlled and its action is augmented by the levator ani muscles of the pelvic floor. The external sphincter is innervated by the somatic nervous system.

Normal feces are brown, due to the bilirubin derivatives stercobilin and urobilin and to the action of the normal bacteria within the intestine. **Bilirubin** is a yellow pigment in the bile. Feces may have other colors, especially when there are abnormal constituents (e.g., black, tarry feces may indicate the presence of blood from the stomach or small intestine; clay-colored feces usually indicate the absence of bile; and green or orange stools may indicate the presence of an intestinal infection). Food may also affect the color of feces; for example, beets can color stool red or sometimes green. Medications, too, can alter the color of feces; iron, for example, can make stool black. See Table 40–1. Feces are usually formed, but soft, and contain about 75% water if the person has an adequate fluid intake. The other 25% is solid materials. See Table 40–2.

The frequency of defecation is highly individual, varying from several times per day to two or three times per week. The amount defecated also varies from person to person. When peristaltic waves move the feces into the sigmoid colon and the rectum, the sensory nerves in the rectum are stimulated and the individual becomes aware of the need to defecate.

Defecation is normally initiated by two defecation reflexes. When feces enter the rectum, distention of the rectum initiates a signal that spreads through the mesenteric plexus to initiate peristaltic waves in the descending and sigmoid colons and in the rectum. These waves force the feces toward the anus. As the peristaltic waves approach the anus, the internal anal sphincter becomes inhibited from closing and, if the external sphincter is relaxed, defecation occurs. This is called the **intrinsic defecation reflex.**

The second reflex, called the **parasympathetic**

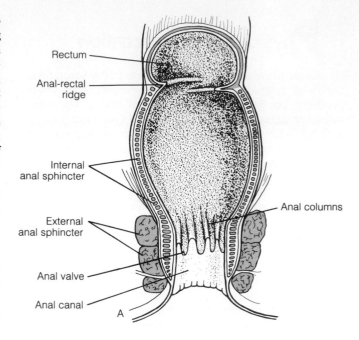

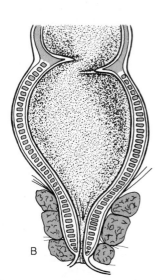

Figure 40–4 The rectum, anal canal, and anal sphincters: **A,** open; **B,** closed

defecation reflex, is also actively involved in defecation. When nerve fibers in the rectum are stimulated, signals are transmitted to the spinal cord and then back to the descending and sigmoid colons and the rectum. These parasympathetic signals intensify the peristaltic waves, relax the internal anal sphincter, and intensify the intrinsic defecation reflex. The internal anal sphincter relaxes, and feces move into the anal canal.

After the individual is seated on a toilet or bedpan, the external anal sphincter is relaxed voluntarily. Expulsion of the feces is assisted by contraction of the abdominal muscles and the diaphragm, which increases abdominal pressure, and by contraction of the levator ani muscles of the pelvic floor, which moves the feces through the anal canal. See Figure 40–5. Normal defecation is facilitated by thigh flexion, which increases

Table 40–1 Characteristics of Normal and Abnormal Feces

Characteristic	Normal	Abnormal	Possible Cause
Color	Adult: brown	Clay or white	Bile obstruction
	Infant: yellow	Black; tarry	Drug, e.g., iron; upper gastrointestinal bleeding
		Red	Lower gastrointestinal bleeding; some foods, e.g., beets
		Pale	Malabsorption of fat
Consistency	Formed; moist	Hard	Constipation
		Watery	Diarrhea, e.g., intestinal irritation
Odor	Aromatic: affected by ingested food	Pungent	Infection, blood
Frequency	Adult: varies from 1–3 movements per day to once every 3 days	More than 3 movements per day; fewer than 1 movement per week	
	Infant: 1–6 movements per day	More than 6 movements per day; fewer than 1 movement every 2 days	
Shape	Cylindrical (contour of rectum)	Narrow	Obstruction
Amount	100–400 g per day (varies with diet)		

the pressure within the abdomen, and a sitting position, which increases the downward pressure on the rectum.

If the defecation reflex is ignored, or if defecation is consciously inhibited by contracting the external sphincter muscle, the urge to defecate normally disappears for a few hours before occurring again. Repeated inhibition of the urge to defecate can result in expansion of the rectum to accommodate accumulated feces and eventual loss of sensitivity to the need to defecate. Constipation can be the ultimate result.

Factors Affecting Defecation

Age

Age affects not only the character of fecal elimination but also its control. The very young are unable to control elimination until the neuromuscular system is developed, usually between the ages of 2 and 3 years.

Table 40–2 Composition of Normal Feces

Constituent	Percentage of Feces	Percentage of Solid Constituents
Water	75	
Solid materials	25	
Dead bacteria		30
Fat		10 to 20
Inorganic matter		10 to 20
Protein		2 to 3
Undigested roughage and dried constituents of digestive juices (e.g., bile pigment and sloughed epithelial cells)		30

Adapted from A. C. Guyton, *Textbook of medical physiology,* 7th ed. (Philadelphia: W. B. Saunders Co., 1986), p. 796.

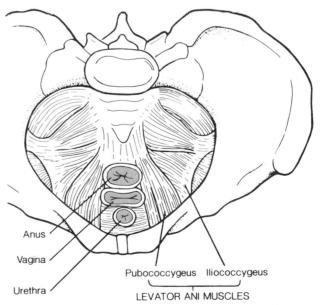

Figure 40–5 The levator ani muscles of the pelvic floor aid in expulsion of feces

lihood of intestinal spasm and premature ejection of the solution. Rolling up the container prevents subsequent suctioning of the solution.

10. After all the solution has been instilled or when the client cannot hold any more and wants to defecate, close the clamp and remove the rectal tube from the anus.
    Rationale: The urge to defecate usually indicates that sufficient fluid has been administered.

11. Apply firm pressure over the anus with tissue wipes or press the buttocks together to assist retention of the enema. Ask the client to remain lying down. Encourage the client to hold the enema.
    Rationale: Some enemas are more effective if they are retained from 5–10 minutes. The time depends on the type of enema. It is easier for a person to retain the enema when lying down than when sitting or standing because gravity promotes drainage and peristalsis.

12. Assist the client to a sitting position on the bedpan, commode, or toilet. If a specimen of feces is required, ask the client to use a bedpan or commode.
    Rationale: A sitting position is preferred because it promotes defecation.

13. Ask the client not to flush the toilet if he or she is using one.
    Rationale: The nurse needs to observe the feces.

14. Record administration of the enema; the amount, color, consistency of returns; the presence of unusual constituents, eg, worms; and the relief of flatus and abdominal distention.

Sample Recording

Date	Time	Notes
6/29/89	2100	1,000 ml saline enema given. Returned large amount of hard, white stool and large amount of flatus. Abdomen soft and less distended. —— —— Roxy-Ann B. Stanley, NS

15. Teach the client practices that develop regular and normal defecation, such as
    a. Eating a balanced diet containing adequate bulk (roughage and fiber content). Bulk is found primarily in unrefined breakfast cereals, whole wheat flour, raw fruits, and raw vegetables.
    b. Maintaining an adequate fluid intake, eg, 1500 ml daily.
    c. Eating regular meals.
    d. Establishing a regular time for defecation and allowing adequate time to defecate.
    e. Doing regular and sufficient amounts of exercise.

Administering an Enema to an Incontinent Client

Occasionally, a nurse needs to administer an enema to a person who is unable to control his or her external sphincter muscle and thus cannot retain the enema solution for even a few minutes. In that case the client assumes

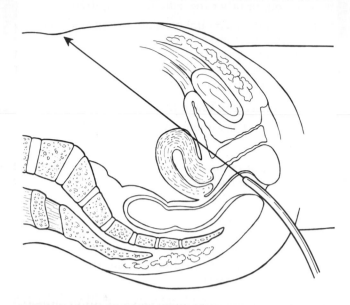

Figure 40–10

a supine position on a bedpan. The head of the bed can be elevated slightly, eg, to 30° if necessary, and the client's head and back are supported by pillows. The nurse wears a glove over the hand that holds the rectal tube, to prevent direct contact with the solution and feces that are expelled over the hand into the bedpan during administration of the enema.

Administering a Return Flow Enema

The return flow enema (Harris flush or colonic irrigation) is a repetitive instillation and drainage of fluid to and from the rectum. It is similar to administering and siphoning an enema. Initially, the solution (100–200 ml for an adult) is instilled into the client's rectum and sigmoid colon. Then the solution container is lowered so that the fluid flows back out through the rectal tube into the container. This alternating flow of fluid into and out of the large intestine stimulates peristalsis and the expulsion of flatus. The inflow-outflow process is repeated five or six times, and the solution is replaced several times during the procedure as it becomes thick with feces. A total of about 1000 ml of solution is usually used for an adult.

Siphoning an Enema

In some instances a client may be unable to expel the solution after administration of an enema. The solution must then be siphoned off. In siphoning, the nurse uses the force of gravity to draw the fluid out of the rectum and colon.

The equipment required is a bedpan, a funnel and rectal tube, lubricant, and a container of water at 40 C (105 F). During siphoning, the client assumes a right side–lying position so that the sigmoid colon is uppermost, thus facilitating drainage of the solution from the rectum and the colon. The client lies on the bed with hips close to the side of the bed. The nurse places a bedpan on a chair at the side of the bed near the client's hips. The chair must be lower than the bed. The rectal tube is lubricated and attached to the funnel. The tube and half of the funnel are filled with solution, then the tube is pinched and gently inserted into the rectum as for an enema. The nurse holds the funnel about 10 cm (4 in.) above the anus, releases the pinched rectal tube, and quickly lowers the funnel over the bedpan. This action should draw the fluid from the colon and rectum, permitting it to flow through the rectal tube and funnel into the bedpan. The nurse then notes the amount of fluid siphoned off as well as the color, odor, and presence of any feces or abnormal constituents, such as blood or mucus.

Digital Removal of a Fecal Impaction

Digital removal of a fecal impaction is sometimes necessary. The nurse breaks up the fecal mass digitally and then removes portions of it. This procedure is distressing and uncomfortable, and clients may desire the presence of another nurse or family member for support. Care must be taken to avoid injuring the bowel mucosa and thus to prevent bleeding. Also, rectal stimulation is contraindicated for some clients, since it may cause an excessive vagal response, resulting in cardiac arrhythmia. For these reasons, agency policies vary about who may remove impactions digitally. After disimpaction, follow-up measures to encourage normal defecation, such as administering enemas or suppositories, are implemented for a few days.

Encouraging Appropriate Diet and Exercise

Diets to promote normal elimination vary, depending on the current state of the client's feces, the frequency of defecation, and the client's past experience with foods that prompt defecation. In general, clients who are constipated can increase daily fluid intake and include bulk in the diet, e.g., foods such as prunes, raw fruit, and bran products.

The client with diarrhea should be encouraged to take fluids and food. Because ingestion of foods and fluids stimulates the gastrocolic and duodenocolic reflexes, thus inducing more stool, the client may be reluctant to eat or drink. Eating small amounts of bland foods can be helpful, since they are more easily absorbed. Potassium losses due to diarrhea may be great, and the nurse should encourage the client to take food or fluids containing potassium. See the discussion of hypokalemia in Chapter 43. Excessively hot or cold fluids should be avoided, because they stimulate peristalsis.

Regular exercise helps the constipated client develop a more normal defecation pattern. Walking and swimming, for example, help stimulate normal motility of the intestines. Regaining normal intestinal motility is one reason why postsurgical clients are encouraged to ambulate.

Decreasing Flatulence

There are several ways to reduce or prevent flatulence: not providing gas-producing foods, encouraging exercise, and repositioning clients are recommended. Encouraging ambulation is an effective means of reducing flatulence, since the motility stimulates reabsorption of gases in intestinal capillaries. A method of treating flatulence is to insert a rectal tube into the rectum and leave it there for varying lengths of time (generally no longer than 30 minutes, to prevent undue irritation to the rectal lining). The tube can then be reinserted, as needed, every 2 to 3 hours. Some nurses advocate connecting the open end of the rectal tube, via another tube, to a collecting receptacle. The passage of flatus is confirmed by noting bubbles in the water.

Caring for Clients with Bowel Diversion Ostomies

Bowel diversion ostomies are often classified according to their permanent or temporary nature, their anatomic location, and the construction of the **stoma** (artificial opening in the abdominal wall). An *ileostomy* is an opening into the ileum (small bowel). A *colostomy* is an opening into the colon (large bowel). Figure 40–11 shows a colostomy stoma with the surgical incision to the right and retention sutures supporting the incision.

Colostomies can be either temporary or permanent. Temporary colostomies are generally performed for traumatic injuries or inflammatory conditions of the bowel. They allow the distal diseased portion of the bowel to rest and heal. Permanent colostomies are performed to provide a means of elimination when the rectum or anus is nonfunctional as a result of disease or birth defect. They are commonly performed for diseases such as cancer of the bowel. The diseased portion may or may not be removed.

An ileostomy generally empties from the distal end of the small intestine. A cecostomy empties from the

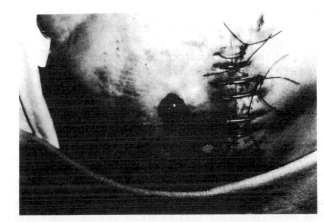

Figure 40–11 A colostomy stoma, with the surgical incision to the right. Note the retention sutures supporting the incision.

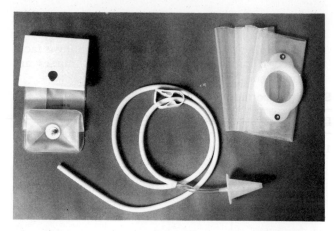

Figure 40–22 A commercially prepared colostomy irrigation set. The irrigation solution bag is on the left and the collecting bag (irrigation drainage sleeve) on the right; the stoma cone is fitted to the catheter.

Chapter Highlights

Patterns of fecal elimination vary greatly among people; regular fecal elimination is usually important.

The main functions of the colon are absorption, protection, and elimination.

A variety of factors affect defecation, including age, diet, fluid intake, muscle tone, and psychologic factors.

Anesthesia and surgical procedures often impair intestinal movements temporarily.

Sufficient fluid and fiber intake helps keep feces soft.

Lack of exercise, irregular defecation habits, stress, and bland diets are all thought to contribute to constipation.

Constipation can cause straining and use of the Valsalva maneuver during defecation, which can lead to hemorrhoids and increased intrathoracic pressure.

A client with a fecal impaction may excrete liquid or loose feces.

Caution is necessary during digital removal of an impaction because vagal nerve stimulation can depress cardiac rate.

Diarrhea can lead to serious fluid and electrolyte imbalances.

Flatulence is chiefly the result of gas formed in the intestines.

When assessing fecal elimination, the nurse considers the nursing history data, physical health examination data, pattern of defecation, nature of feces, and diagnostic test data.

The nurse can promote normal defecation by pro-

viding privacy and assisting the client to a normal squatting position.

An enema involves the instillation of fluid into the rectum and sigmoid colon.

The position of a bowel diversion ostomy greatly affects the character and management of the fecal drainage.

When assessing a bowel diversion ostomy, the nurse notes the color of the stoma, presence of stoma swelling, condition of peristomal skin, amount and type of feces, tape allergy, and presence of abdominal discomfort or distention.

Clients who have a bowel diversion ostomy require instruction to manage the ostomy.

Nurses caring for clients with ostomies must consider psychosocial factors.

Protecting the peristomal skin is important because fecal effluent irritates the skin.

A colostomy irrigation is similar to an enema except that the client cannot control the expulsion of fluid and feces.

Selected References

Alterescu, V. November 1985. The ostomy. What do you teach the patient? *American Journal of Nursing* 85:1250–53.

Behm, R. M. July/August 1985. A special recipe to banish constipation. *Geriatric Nursing* 6:216–17.

Broadwell, D. C., and Jackson, B. S. (eds.) 1982. *Principles of Ostomy Care.* St. Louis: C. V. Mosby.

Eliopoulos, C. 1984. *Health Assessment of the Older Adult.* Menlo Park, Calif.: Addison-Wesley.

Guyton, A. C. 1986. *Textbook of Medical Physiology,* 7th ed. Philadelphia: W. B. Saunders Co.

Hahn, A. B.; Barkin, R. L.; and Oestreich, S. J. K. 1982. *Pharmacology in Nursing,* 15th ed. St. Louis: C. V. Mosby.

Logio, T. February 1985. Suppository insertion—which end is first? *Nursing 85* 15:10.

Mager-O'Connor, E. May/June 1984. How to identify and remove fecal impactions. *Geriatric Nursing* 5:158–61.

Miller, J. February 1985. Helping the aged manage bowel function. *Journal of Gerontological Nursing* 11:37–41.

Northridge, J. A. S. April 1982. Helpful hints for assessing the ostomate. *Nursing 82* 12:72–77; Canadian edition 12:8–13.

Resnick, B. July/August 1985. Constipation: Common but preventable. *Geriatric Nursing* 6:213–15.

Ritter, M. January/February 1983. Karaya reconsidered . . . The original skin barrier for persons with an ostomy. *Journal of Enterostomal Therapy* 10:35–36.

Smith, D. B. January/February 1983. Colostomy irrigations—so simple . . . Irrigation takes on complex variables and requires individualization in each situation. *Journal of Enterostomal Therapy* 10:22–23.

Smith, D. B. November 1985. The ostomy, how is it managed? *American Journal of Nursing* 85:1246–49.

Vick, R. L. 1984. *Contemporary Medical Physiology.* Menlo Park, Calif.: Addison-Wesley.

Watt, R. C. November 1985. The ostomy, why is it created? *American Journal of Nursing* 85:1242–45.

CHAPTER 41

Urinary **E**limination

OBJECTIVES

Describe the process of micturition.

Identify developmental variations in urinary elimination.

Describe common alterations in urinary production and elimination.

Identify factors that influence urinary elimination.

Recognize normal and abnormal characteristics and constituents of urine.

Describe diagnostic measures to assess kidney function and urinary tract abnormalities.

Explain how to collect urine specimens and perform simple urine tests.

Identify nursing diagnoses related to urinary elimination.

Describe interventions to maintain normal urinary elimination and assist clients with urinary incontinence and retention.

List guidelines for preventing urinary infection.

Identify outcome criteria to evaluate client responses to nursing interventions for alterations in urinary elimination.

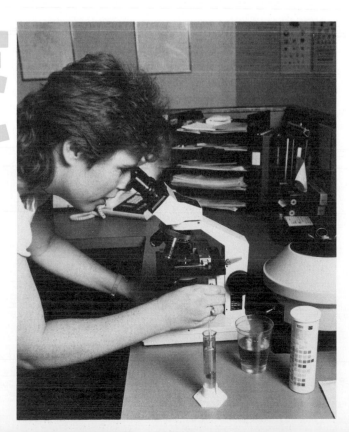

Urinary Elimination

Urinary elimination depends on effective functioning of four urinary tract organs: kidneys, ureters, bladder, and urethra. See Figure 41–1. The **kidneys** filter from the blood any products for which the body has no use. Each kidney has one renal artery that originates from the abdominal aorta and enters the kidney at the hilum. (See Figure 41–1.) The renal vein exits through the hilum and joins the inferior vena cava. It is estimated that, in the average adult, 1200 ml of blood passes through the kidneys every minute, representing about 21% of the cardiac output (5600 ml per minute). The body's total blood supply circulates through the kidneys approximately 12 times per hour (Richard 1986, p. 13).

The nephrons (the functional units of the kidney—see Figure 41–2) convert the blood that circulates through the kidneys into a fluid (consisting of water, electrolytes, creatinine, glucose, urea, amino acids, uric acid, bicarbonate, and other electrolytes) called **glomerular filtrate** (about 180 liters daily, or 25 ml per minute). This volume-time ratio is referred to as the **glomerular filtration rate** (GFR). The **glomerulus** is a tuft or cluster of blood vessels surrounded by Bow-

man's capsule. Because the glomerular membrane is relatively porous, water and all of the dissolved constituents of plasma proteins do not filter through to Bowman's capsule. Thus, the glomerular filtrate is chemically almost the same as plasma, except that it has only minute quantities of protein (0.03%) compared to plasma (7%). After the filtrate enters Bowman's capsule, it passes into the tubular system, where about 99% of it is reabsorbed into the bloodstream. The remaining 1% forms the urine to be excreted from the body (Guyton 1986, p. 398). The main function of the nephrons is to return the majority of glomerular filtrate to the circulation.

Once the urine is formed in the kidneys, it enters the **ureters** via collecting ducts and then passes to the bladder. See Figure 41–1. The upper end of each ureter is funnel-shaped as it enters the kidney, forming what is referred to as the **renal pelvis.** The lower ends of the ureters enter the bladder at the posterior corners of the floor of the bladder. At this junction between the ureter and the bladder there is a flaplike fold of mucous membrane that acts as a valve to prevent the backflow (**reflux**) of urine up the ureters to the kidneys.

The **urinary bladder** is a hollow, muscular organ that serves as a reservoir for urine and as the organ of excretion. When empty it lies behind the symphysis pubis. In the male, the bladder lies in front of the rectum

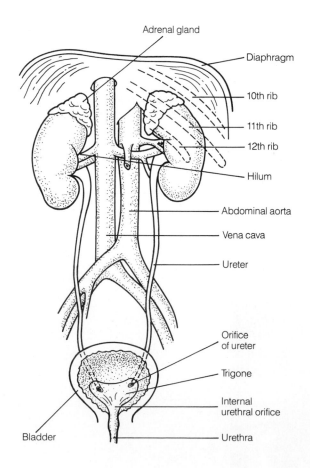

Figure ▪ 41–1 ▪ Anatomic structures of the urinary tract

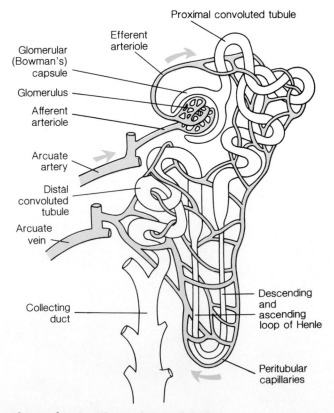

Figure 41–2 The nephrons of the kidney are composed of five parts: Bowman's capsule, proximal convoluted tubule, loop of Henle, distal convoluted tubule, and collecting duct

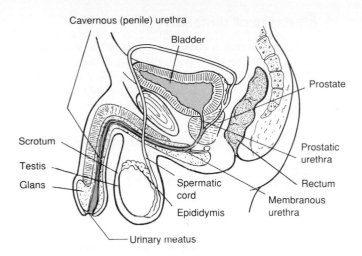

Figure 41-3 The male urogenital system

and above the prostate gland (see Figure 41-3). In the female, it lies in front of the uterus and vagina (see Figure 41-4).

The amount of urine normally stored in the bladder varies to some degree among individuals and with age. For an adult, the desire to void is normally experienced when the bladder contains between 250 and 450 ml of urine. Normal output of urine for an adult is about 1500 ml/day. The bladder is capable of considerable distention because of **rugae** (folds) in the mucous membrane lining and because of the elasticity of its walls. When full, the dome of the bladder may extend above the symphysis pubis; in extreme situations it may extend as high as the umbilicus. Urine exits from the bladder through the urethra.

The **urethra** extends from the bladder to the urinary **meatus** (opening, or passage) and is the exit passageway for the urine. It is lined with mucous membrane. In the adult male, the urethra functions as a passageway for semen as well as urine. In the adult female, the urethra lies directly behind the symphysis pubis,

anterior to the vagina. See Figure 41-4. It serves only as a passageway for the elimination of urine. The urinary meatus is located between the labia minora, in front of the vagina and below the clitoris (see Figure 41-5).

In both the male and the female, the urethra has two **sphincter** muscles. The internal sphincter muscle is situated at the base of the urinary bladder and is involuntary. The second sphincter muscle is under voluntary control. In the female it is situated at about the midpoint of the urethra; in the male it is distal to the prostatic portion of the urethra. The urethra has a mucous membrane lining that is continuous with the bladder and the ureters. Thus, an infection of the urethra can readily extend through the urinary tract to the kidneys. Women are particularly prone to urinary tract infections because of the shortness of their urethras.

▪ Micturition

Micturition (*voiding, urination*) refers to the voluntary process of emptying the urinary bladder. Urine collects in the bladder until pressure stimulates special sensory nerve endings in the bladder wall called *stretch receptors*. Once excited, the stretch receptors transmit impulses to the spinal cord, specifically to the voiding reflex center located at the level of the second to fourth sacral vertebrae. Some impulses continue up the spinal cord to the voiding control center in the cerebral cortex. If the time is appropriate to void, the brain then sends impulses through the spinal cord to the motor neurons in the sacral area, causing stimulation of the parasympathetic nerves.

As a result, urine can be released from the bladder, but it is still impeded by the external urinary sphincter. If the time and place are appropriate for urination, the conscious portion of the brain relaxes the external ure-

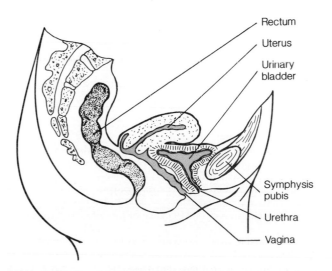

Figure 41-4 The female urogenital system

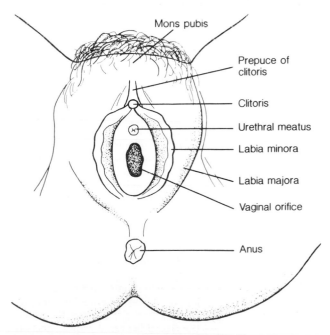

Figure 41-5 Location of the female urinary meatus in relation to surrounding structures

thral sphincter muscle, and urination takes place. If the time and place are inappropriate, the micturition reflex usually subsides until the bladder becomes more filled and the reflex is stimulated again. The sympathetic nervous system also innervates the bladder, causing it to relax.

Voluntary control of voiding is possible only if the nerves supplying the bladder and urethra, the projection tracts of the cord and brain, and the motor area of the cerebrum are all intact. Injury to any of these parts of the nervous system (e.g., by a cerebral hemorrhage or spinal cord injury above the level of the sacral region) results in intermittent involuntary emptying of the bladder, **incontinence.** When there is damage to the spinal cord above the sacral vertebrae, the micturition reflex may remain intact and urination may occur reflexively. This situation is referred to as an **automatic bladder.**

Occasionally, a person is unable to void even though the bladder contains an excessive amount of urine. This condition is known as **retention.** A more serious complication, which is also characterized by the inability to void, is called **suppression.** In this situation the person cannot void because the kidneys are not secreting any urine; the bladder is empty.

Developmental Variables

Urinary elimination functioning changes throughout the life cycle. Table 41–1 outlines these changes. Consideration of developmental variables in urination is important in all phases of the nursing process to ensure provision of appropriately individualized care.

Patterns of Urination

Although people's patterns of urination are highly individual, most people void about five or more times a day. People usually void when they first awaken in the morning, before they go to bed, and around meal times. Most people void about 70% of their daily urine during the waking hours and do not need to void during the night.

Alterations in Urine Production

Polyuria

Polyuria, or **diuresis,** refers to the production of abnormally large amounts of urine by the kidneys, such as 2500 ml/day, without any increase in fluid intake. This can happen as a result of:

1. The ingestion of substances containing caffeine and alcohol
2. Diabetes mellitus
3. Hormone imbalances (e.g., deficiency of antidiuretic hormone)
4. Chronic kidney disease

Alcohol inhibits the release of antidiuretic hormone (ADH) and thus promotes urine formation. Coffee, tea, and cola drinks, which usually contain caffeine, increase the frequency and volume of micturition. Other signs often associated with diuresis are **polydipsia** (intense thirst), dehydration, and weight loss.

Table 41–1 Changes in Urinary Elimination Through the Life Cycle

Stage	Variations
Fetus	The fetal kidney begins to excrete urine between the 11th and 12th week of development.
	Fetal urine is hypotonic to plasma.
	The placenta serves as a pseudo-kidney in regulating fetal fluid and electrolyte balance.
	The kidney does not function independently until after birth.
Infant	Ability to concentrate urine is minimal; therefore urine appears light yellow.
	Voluntary urinary control is absent.
Children	Kidney function reaches maturity between the first and second year of life; urine is concentrated effectively and appears a normal amber color.
	Voluntary control of urine begins at 18 to 24 months of age, when the child starts to recognize bladder fullness, holds urine beyond the urge to void, and warns parents of the urge to void.
	Full urinary control is not gained until age 4 or 5 years; daytime control is usually achieved by age 2 years.
	Boys are slower than girls in gaining control.
	The kidneys grow in proportion to overall body growth.
Adults	The kidneys reach maximum size between 35 and 40 years of age.
	After age 50 the kidneys begin to diminish in size and function. Most shrinkage occurs in the cortex of the kidney, due primarily to the loss of glomeruli.
Elderly adults	There is an estimated 30% loss of glomeruli by age 80 (Richard 1986, p. 38).
	Renal blood flow decreases because of vascular changes and a decrease in cardiac output.
	Urine concentratability declines.
	Excessive urination at night and increased frequency of urination occur because of loss of concentratability and diminished bladder muscle tone.
	Residual urine may increase due to diminished bladder muscle tone and contractibility, which increases the risk of bacterial growth and infection.
	Urinary incontinence may occur due to mobility problems or neurologic impairments.

Oliguria and Anuria

Oliguria refers to production of scant amounts of urine, such as 100 to 500 ml/day. **Anuria** refers to the production of less than 100 ml/day. The terms complete kidney shutdown, renal failure, and urinary suppression have the same meaning as anuria. Oliguria may result from an extremely low fluid intake but may also follow disease. Both anuria and oliguria can result from kidney disease, severe heart failure, burns, and shock. These clinical signs can be fatal if some other means (e.g., hemodialysis) is not used to remove body wastes.

Oliguria may also normally accompany fever and heavy perspiration. Because of excessive fluid losses via the skin, urine production is decreased. Urine that is produced during febrile conditions is usually concentrated. The elevated metabolism associated with fever increases the accumulation of body wastes.

Alterations in Urinary Elimination

Frequency

Frequency is generally considered voiding at shortened intervals, that is, more often than usual. Normally, with an increased intake of fluid, there is some increase in the frequency with which a person voids. Frequency without an increase in fluid intake may be the result of **cystitis** (inflammation of the bladder), stress, or pressure on the bladder (because of pregnancy, for example). With frequency, the total amount of urine voided may be normal, since the amounts voided each time are small, such as 50 to 100 ml. **Nocturia** is increased frequency at night that is not a result of an increase in fluid intake.

Urgency

Urgency is the feeling that the person *must* void. There may or may not be a great deal of urine in the bladder, but the person feels a need to void immediately. Often the person hurries to the toilet with the fear of being incontinent if he or she does not urinate. Urgency accompanies psychologic stress and irritation of the trigone and urethra. It is also common in young children who have poor external sphincter control.

Dysuria

Dysuria means voiding that is either painful or difficult. It can accompany a stricture of the urethra, urinary infections, and injury to the bladder and/or urethra. Often clients say they have to push to void or that burning accompanies or follows voiding. Burning during micturition is often due to an irritated urethra; burning following urination may be the result of a bladder infection. The burning may be described as severe, like a hot poker, or more subdued, like a sunburn. Often, **hesi-**

tancy (a delay and difficulty in initiating voiding) is associated with dysuria.

Enuresis

Enuresis is defined as repeated involuntary urination in children beyond the age when voluntary bladder control is normally acquired, usually 4 or 5 years of age (Whaley and Wong 1983, p. 662). There are many reasons for enuresis; several causes or contributing factors may exist in each individual situation. These factors include:

1. Heredity. High frequency of bed wetting among parents, siblings, and other near relatives of the affected child; possible inherited difficulty inhibiting the mechanisms that regulate bladder emptying.
2. Smaller-than-normal bladder capacity.
3. Sleeping soundly. Inattention to signals from the bladder indicating the need to urinate until it is too late to get out of bed and to the bathroom.
4. Irritable bladder. Inability to hold large quantities of urine.
5. Socioeconomic conditions. Higher frequency among children who live in homes where toilet facilities are not readily accessible, the temperature is cold at night, the child sleeps with a bed wetting sibling, and cleanliness practices are poor.
6. Too early and too vigorous bladder training. May be an expression of an unconscious desire to regress and to receive the attention and care the child had when younger or of resentment toward the parents.
7. Parental attitudes. Parents who believe the child will outgrow the habit and thus do not try to train the child.
8. Disease. Infections of the urinary tract, or physical or neurologic defects of the urinary system.
9. Diet. Foods such as pickles and relishes, which are irritating to the urinary system.
10. Fear of the dark. May prevent the child from walking down a dark corridor to the bathroom at night.

Incontinence

Incontinence is involuntary leakage or loss of urine from the bladder. In **total incontinence** there is nearly continuous, unpredicted urine leakage. Common causes are injury to the external urinary sphincter in the male, injury to the perineal musculature or a fistula between the bladder and vagina in the female, and congenital or acquired neurogenic disease. With **functional incontinence,** environmental barriers, disorientation, or physical barriers interfere with the person's ability to reach the toilet in time to control voiding. **Stress incontinence,** leakage of urine is a result of a sudden increase in intraabdominal pressure, may occur when the person coughs, sneezes, laughs, or otherwise exerts physical strain. This type of incontinence occurs most frequently in females who suffer pelvic relaxation due to childbirth trauma, loss of tissue tone, or aging.

Urge incontinence follows a sudden strong desire to urinate. The client is unable to stop urine flow when it starts and often fails to get to the bathroom on time. Urge incontinence is different from stress incontinence in that loss of urine occurs at any time, not just with straining. It often occurs with cystitis in women and with other bladder diseases, such as calculi and tumors, in both men and women. Psychologic factors may also stimulate voiding. There is a high incidence of urge incontinence in older adults, although the reasons are not completely understood. Inhibitory impulses that normally calm the bladder may be too weak, or some other imbalance of voiding reflexes may exist due to central nervous system disease, such as cerebral arteriosclerosis.

Overflow incontinence is a dribbling incontinence that results when the client's bladder is greatly distended with urine because of an obstruction at the bladder level or below, often secondary to a flaccid neurogenic bladder. **Neurogenic bladder** results from neurologic impairment or dysfunction. A flaccid type of neurogenic bladder occurs following spinal injury or other disease at the sacral level (below T12). The client is unaware of bladder-filling; the bladder walls become overstretched and atonic. Urine "overflows" or dribbles when the pressure increases in the bladder to a point where it surpasses the urethral sphincter's resistance to urine. This condition is also called **reflex incontinence.**

Urinary retention is the accumulation of urine in the bladder with associated inability of the bladder to empty itself. Because urine production continues, retention distends the bladder. An adult urinary bladder normally holds 250 to 450 ml of urine when the micturition reflex is triggered. With urinary retention, some adult bladders may distend to hold 3000 ml of urine. Distention of 1000 ml or more can mean weeks or months until full recovery of bladder tone; in some cases the result is permanent loss of bladder tone (McConnell and Zimmerman 1983, p. 40). Prolonged retention leads to **stasis** (a slowing of the flow of urine) and stagnation of urine, which increase the possibility of urinary tract infection. Clinical signs of retention are summarized in the accompanying box. Retention is distinguished from oliguria or anuria by the bladder distention. Bladder distention can be assessed by palpation and percussion above the symphysis pubis. Percussion of the suprapubic area produces a "kettle-drum" or dull sound when the bladder is full. The most common type of retention is postoperative retention.

Urinary Retention: Clinical Signs

▪ Discomfort in the pubic area
▪ Bladder distention
▪ Inability to void or frequent voiding of small volumes (25 to 50 ml)
▪ A disproportionately small amount of fluid output in relation to intake
▪ Increasing restlessness and need to void

Medications Causing Urinary Retention

Anticholinergic/antispasmodic medications, such as atropine, belladonna, Donnatal (containing atropine), and papaverine
Antidepressant/antipsychotic agents, such as phenothiazines and MAO inhibitors
Antiparkinsonism drugs, such as levodopa, trihexyphenidyl (Artane), and benztropine mesylate (Cogentin)
Antihistamine preparations, such as Actifed and Sudafed
Beta-adrenergic blockers, such as propanolol (Inderal)
Antihypertensives, such as hydralazine (Apresoline) and methyldopa (Aldomet)

Postpartum retention is commonly due to swelling of the urinary meatus that results from perineal trauma associated with vaginal delivery. It is also caused by conditions that contribute to spasm of the perineal musculature. Many medications interfere with the normal urination process and may cause retention. Examples are listed in the accompanying box.

Certain **psychosocial factors** may be associated with retention. Many people have developed a set of behaviors that help stimulate the micturition reflex. Examples are privacy, comfortable position, sufficient time, and, occasionally, running water. North Americans, in contrast to many Europeans, expect private toilet facilities. There are also sex differences in privacy needs. Women are used to enclosed cubicles in public facilities; men are used to sharing more open facilities. Circumstances that counter the client's usual set of behaviors may produce anxiety and muscle tension. In persons who are unable to relax abdominal and perineal muscles and the external urethral sphincter, voiding may be incomplete and result in urinary retention.

Assessing Urinary Elimination

When assessing urinary elimination, the nurse should consider the client's history, physical examination, and data obtained from diagnostic procedures performed. Guidelines for assessment are summarized in the accompanying box.

The nurse determines the client's usual **pattern** and **frequency** of urination by asking the client when voiding occurs each day and whether there have been any changes in usual elimination patterns. The nurse structures the nursing history to determine recent changes and/or problems in urinary elimination patterns. Table 41–2 summarizes altered urinary patterns and influencing factors the nurse should assess.

GUIDELINES

Assessing Urinary Elimination

Complete assessment includes:

Developmental variables (see section earlier in this chapter)

Usual patterns of urination

Identification of any alterations in urinary elimination and influencing or associated factors

Physical assessment (see the section to follow)

Volume and characteristics of the client's urine

Review of data obtained from diagnostic tests and examinations

Past illnesses or surgery

In addition to assessing conditions that affect urinary function directly, the nurse needs to consider problems the client may have with mobility. Diseases such as rheumatoid arthritis or other degenerative musculoskeletal or neurologic disorders that impair the client's mobility may result in functional incontinence. Clients who have impaired hand coordination may have difficulty manipulating clothing fasteners. Assessment of these related conditions permits the nurse to identify relevant nursing diagnoses.

The client's medical history of elimination problems and urinary tract disease or surgery and other diseases may affect urinary elimination problems. Some of these conditions are:

1. Urinary tract infections of the kidney, bladder, or urethra
2. Urinary calculi
3. Urinary tract surgery, such as kidney surgery, bladder surgery, prostate removal, or other surgical procedures that alter urinary routes, e.g., ureterostomy
4. Cardiovascular disease such as hypertension or heart disease
5. Chronic diseases that alter urinary characteristics or impair urinary function, such as diabetes mellitus, neurologic disease (e.g., multiple sclerosis), and cancer.

Table 41–2 Assessing Factors Associated with Altered Urinary Elimination Patterns

Altered Pattern	Selected Influencing and Associated Factors to be Determined
Polyuria	Increases in fluid intake and ingestion of fluids containing caffeine or alcohol
	Whether diuretics are prescribed (note type and dosage)
	Presence of thirst, dehydration, and weight loss
	Presence of, or familial history of, diabetes insipidus or kidney disease
Oliguria, anuria	Decreases in fluid intake and signs of dehydration (see Chapter 43)
	Presence of known kidney disease or familial history of kidney disease
	Signs of renal failure, such as the presence of uremic frost (urea crystals) on the skin, an elevated BUN, and an aromatic odor to the skin, and signs of fluid and electrolyte imbalances (see Chapter 43)
	Presence of febrile condition
Frequency or nocturia	Whether client is pregnant
	Increases in fluid intake
	Presence of known urinary tract inflammation or infection
	Any known contributing or initiating causes, such as stress
Urgency	Presence of psychologic stress
	Presence of known urinary tract inflammation or infection
Dysuria	Presence of known urinary tract inflammation, infection, or injury
	Presence of other signs that may accompany dysuria, such as hesitancy, hematuria, pyuria, and frequency.
Enuresis	Family history of enuresis
	Access to toilet facilities and home cleanliness habits
	Home stresses
	Bladder training methods used
Incontinence	Whether urine leakage is continuous, occurs as a result of increased intraabdominal pressure, follows a strong desire to urinate, or is dribbling associated with a distended bladder
	Medical history and surgery for associated causes
	Presence of known bladder inflammation or other disease
	The client's age and mobility
Retention	Amounts and frequency of voiding
	Presence of distended bladder by palpation and percussion
	Associated signs, such as pubic discomfort, restlessness
	Whether fluid intake is low
	Recent anesthesia and type
	Type of surgery
	Time period between administration of perspective medications and anesthesia
	Amount of activity after recovery from anesthesia
	Presence of perineal swelling
	Types of medications prescribed
	Whether sufficient privacy or other factors that initiate micturition are lacking

Physical Assessment

Complete physical assessment of the urinary tract is usually performed by a physician or nurse practitioner. It includes percussion of the kidneys to detect areas of tenderness and palpation for contour, size, tenderness, and lumps. Palpation and percussion of the bladder are performed also. These aspects of physical assessment are included in the ongoing assessment of the client as well and are routinely performed by the assigned nurse. The urethral meatus of both male and female clients is inspected during examination of the genitals (either during the physical examination or when bathing the client) for swelling, discharge, and inflammation.

Assessment of Urine

Normal urine consists of 96% water and 4% solutes. Organic solutes include urea, ammonia, creatinine, and uric acid. Urea is the chief organic solute. Inorganic solutes include sodium, chloride, potassium, sulfate, magnesium, and phosphorus. Sodium chloride is the most abundant inorganic salt. Assessment of urine involves measuring the volume of urine; comparing the output to the client's intake; inspecting the urine for color, clarity, and odor; testing urine for specific gravity, glucose, ketone bodies, blood, and pH; and reviewing of data obtained from diagnostic tests. Characteristics of normal and abnormal urine are summarized in Table 41–3.

Urine volume depends on the amount of solutes to be excreted, loss of fluid in perspiration and exhaled air, the cardiac status and renal status of the client, hormonal influences, and the amount of fluid ingested. Normally, the kidneys produce urine continuously at the rate of 30 to 60 ml per hour (720 to 1440 ml per day) in the adult, but the rate may be as high as 2000 ml per day if fluid intake is high. Fluid balance and measurement of all fluid intake and output are discussed in Chapter 43. Urine outputs below 30 ml per hour may indicate kidney malfunction and must be reported. Urine production of more than 2000 ml per day or 80 ml per hr constitutes polyuria. In children, normal values for urine volumes are 300 to 1500 ml per day.

Normal urine is straw-colored or amber-colored. The latter is most likely early in the morning, when urine is most concentrated. Increased fluid intake throughout the day normally makes the urine less concentrated, and so it becomes paler in color. Abnormal urine colors can occur a number of reasons. Table 41–4 summarizes some causes of urine discoloration.

Normal, freshly voided urine is clear or transparent. Urine may become cloudy due to the presence of mucus or pus, or because of a high protein concentration (e.g., with kidney disease). Urine that is left to stand for a while normally becomes cloudy. Similarly, normal, freshly

Table 41–3 Characteristics of Normal and Abnormal Urine

Characteristic	Normal	Abnormal	Possible Causes
Amount in 24 hours (adult)	1200–1500 ml	Under 1200 ml	Decreased fluid intake Kidney failure
		Over 1500 ml	Diabetes Diuretics Increased fluid intake
Color	Straw, amber	Dark amber	Insufficient fluid intake resulting in concentrated urine
	Transparent	Cloudy	Infectious process
		Dark orange	Drugs, e.g., pyridium
		Red or dark brown	Disease process causing blood in urine
Consistency	Clear liquid	Mucous plugs, viscid, thick	Infectious process
Odor	Faint aromatic	Offensive	Infectious process
Sterility	No microorganisms present	Microorganisms present	Infection of the urinary tract
pH	4.5 to 8	Under 4.5	Uncontrolled diabetes
		Over 8	Urinary tract infections Starvation Dehydration
Specific gravity	1.010 to 1.025	Under 1.010	Diabetes insipitus Kidney disease Overhydration
		Over 1.025	Diabetes mellitus Underhydration
Glucose	Not present	Present	Diabetes mellitus
Ketone bodies (acetone)	Not present	Present	Diabetic coma Starvation Prolonged vomiting
Blood	Not present	Occult	Kidney disease
		Bright red	Hemorrhage

Table 41–4 Selected Causes of Urine Discoloration

Color	Cause	Color	Cause
Almost colorless (very pale greenish yellow)	Alcohol ingestion		Porphyrin
	Chronic kidney disease		Rifampin (Rifadin)
	Diabetes insipidus	Green or blue-green (often blue mixed with yellow)	Amitriptyline (Elavil hydrochloride)
	Diabetes mellitus		Azuresin (Diagnex Blue)
	Diuretic therapy		Bilirubin-biliverdin
	Large fluid intake		Phenylsalicylate
	Nervousness		Vitamin B complex
	Severe iron deficiency		Yeast concentrate
Yellow	Acriflavine		
	Cascara		Pyrenium
	Nitrofurantoin (Furadantin)	Pale blue	
	Phenacetin	Brown or black	Bilirubin-biliverdin
	Quinacrine hydrochloride (Atabrine)		Cascara (in acid urine)
	Riboflavin (vitamin B_2)		Chloroquine phosphate (Aralen)
Orange	Azo Gantrisin		Furazolidone (Furoxone)
	Bilirubin		Iron compounds (injectable)
	Concentrated urine		Levodopa (L-dopa)
	Multivitamins		Melanin
	Nitrofurantoin		Nitrofurantoin
	Phenazopyridine hydrochloride (Pyridium)		Phenol
			Phenylhydrazine
	Restricted fluid intake		Porphyrin
	Rhubarb, senna, santonin, cascara (in acid urine)		Sinemet
	Sulfonamides	Cloudy	Bacteria
	Thiamine hydrochloride		Calculi "gravel"
	Urobilin in excess		Clumps, pus, tissue
Pink, red, or reddish orange	Azo Gantrisin		Fecal contamination
	Beets		Leukocytes
	Cascara (in alkaline urine)		Mucin, mucous threads
	Chlorpromazine hydrochloride (Thorazine)		Phosphates, carbonates
			Prostatic fluid
	Dorbantyl		Red blood cells (smoky)
	Doxidan		X-ray contrast media
	Ex-Lax		
	Hemoglobin	Milky	Fat (lipuria, opalescent; chyluria, milky)
	Phenothiazine		
	Phenytoin (Dilantin)		Pyuria

Source: Adapted from C. J. Byrne, D. F. Saxton, P. K. Pelikan, and P. M. Nugent, *Laboratory Tests Implications for Nursing Care* 2d ed. (Menlo Park, Calif.: Addison-Wesley, 1986), pp. 10–12. Used by permission.

voided urine has a characteristically faint aromatic odor but acquires a stronger odor the more concentrated it becomes. Bacterial decomposition may change the odor after urine stands for any length of time. Decomposition produces the characteristic pungent odor of ammonia. Additional odors may be due to a variety of causes (Byrne et al. 1986, p. 9), such as:

1. *A sweet or fruity smell.* Due to acetone and aceto-acetic acid, which is associated with starvation, diabetes mellitus, or dehydration.
2. *An offensive odor.* Due to bacterial action on pus in heavily infected urine (**pyuria**).
3. *Certain ingested foods.* E.g., garlic or asparagus produce characteristic odors.
4. *Certain medications.* E.g., menthol, antibiotics, paraldehyde, and vitamins give characteristic odors.

Several simple **urine tests** are often done by nurses on the nursing units or are taught to clients, who perform them independently. Tests commonly performed on urine include those for specific gravity, pH, and presence of occult blood. **Specific gravity** is the weight or degree of concentration of a substance compared with that of an equal volume of another, such as distilled water, taken as a standard. The specific gravity of distilled water is 1.00 g/ml (in other words, 1 ml of water weighs 1 g).

The specific gravity of urine can be measured by a urinometer (**hydrometer**), calibrated in units of 0.001. The instrument is placed in a glass cylinder containing the urine. See Figure 41–6. The scale on the urinometer progresses from 1.000 at the top to 1.060 at the bottom. The specific gravity of urine is normally about 1.010 to 1.025 g/ml. A low specific gravity is often the result of overhydration or a disease that affects the kidneys' ability to concentrate solutes in the urine. A high specific gravity may indicate dehydration or a disease that increases water reabsorption by the kidneys, causing concentrated urine. False positive results are caused by

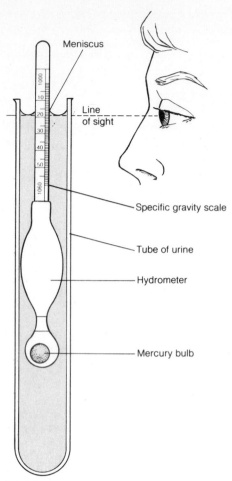

Figure 41–6 A urinometer measurement of specific gravity is taken at the base of the meniscus.

drugs such as dextran and radiopaque materials used in x-ray examination of the urinary tract. To measure specific gravity with a urinometer, the nurse can do the following:

1. Pour at least 20 ml of a fresh urine sample in a glass cylinder, or fill the cylinder three-quarters full.
2. Place the urinometer into the cylinder and give it a gentle spin to prevent it from adhering to the sides of the cylinder.
3. Hold the urinometer at eye level, and read the measurement at the base of the meniscus at the surface of the urine. See Figure 41–6.

The concentration of the urine affects the degree to which the urinometer will float. The depth to which it sinks indicates the specific gravity.

Specific gravity can also be measured with a *spectrometer* or *refractometer.* In this instance the nurse places one or two drops of urine on a slide, turns on the instrument light, and looks into the instrument. The specific gravity appears on a scope. Manufacturer's directions are usually available for specific models.

Urinary pH is a measurement of the concentration of hydrogen ions in the client's urine, which indicates its acidity or alkalinity. Discrete measurements of pH are made on a scale of 1 to 14, in which the value 7 is

neutral, below 7 is acid, and above 7 is alkaline (base). Such quantitative measurements, however, are conducted in the agency laboratory, where specific reactive agents are used.

Urine becomes increasingly acidic when increasing amounts of sodium and excess acid are retained in the body. Ingestion of various foods also affects urinary pH. A diet rich in animal protein and cranberry juice decreases the pH and produces an acid urine. A diet high in citrus fruits, most vegetables, milk, and other dairy products increases the pH and produces an alkaline urine. Urine left at room temperature for several hours gradually becomes alkaline because of bacterial action.

Control of the urine pH is an important factor in certain medical therapies. For example, the formation of renal stones is partially dependent on the urinary pH; therefore, clients being treated for stones are often given diets or medications to alter the pH and prevent stone formation. Certain medications, such as streptomycin, neomycin, and kanamycin, are more effective for treating urinary tract infections if the urine is alkaline.

Measurement of pH involves dipping a strip of either red or blue litmus paper into the urine specimen, observing the color of the litmus paper, and comparing it to a standardized color chart on the bottle. The blue litmus paper, more commonly used, remains blue if the urine is alkaline and turns red if it is acidic. The red litmus paper remains red in the presence of acid urine and turns blue if the urine is alkaline. Whichever litmus strip is used, red always indicated acid urine; blue, alkaline urine.

Normal urine is free of blood and has negligible amounts of glucose and acetone. When blood is present, it may be clearly visible or not visible (occult). Commercial reagent strips and tablets are used to test the urine for these substances. The nurse dips the reagent strip into a sample of urine or applies a drop of urine to the tablet and compares the color change with a color chart.

▪ Diagnostic Tests

Diagnostic tests and procedures to determine urinary tract disease or disorders of other body systems influencing the production of urine include laboratory analysis of urine (**urinalysis**), urine culture, radiographic examinations (KUB and IVP), cystoscopy, and blood tests. A **routine screening urinalysis** is usually performed on all clients when they are admitted to a health care agency. Routine urine examination is usually done on the first voided specimen in the morning, because it tends to have a higher, more uniform concentration and a more acid pH than specimens later in the day (Byrne et al. 1986, p. 5). In addition to the routine tests discussed previously (i.e., specific gravity, pH, presence of glucose, ketone bodies, and blood), the physical examination of the urine sample provides data about the presence of other abnormal constituents, such as protein, bilirubin, urobilinogen, and nitrite determinations. Microscopic examination provides information on urinary constituents such as red and white blood cells, epithelial cells, casts, crystals, bacteria, parasites, and yeast (Byrne et al. 1986, p. 37).

Urine culture and sensitivity tests are done to identify specific causative microorganisms of urinary tract infections and appropriate antimicrobial agents. The nurse's role in bacteriologic urine culture tests is to obtain a clean-catch specimen, also referred to as a clean voided midstream urine (CVMS). In the past, catheterization was the preferred method for acquiring uncontaminated culture specimens, particularly from females. Today, even though the clean-catch specimen may be somewhat contaminated by skin bacteria, it is considered better to have a contaminated specimen than to risk causing infection of the client's urinary tract by introducing a microorganism through catheterization. If a client has an indwelling catheter, the aspiration method is used.

Radiographic examinations involving the urinary tract include intravenous pyelography (IVP), x-ray films of the kidneys, ureters, and bladder (KUB), and renal scanning. These examinations provide data about the presence of tumors or other obstructions within the organs and distortions in the shapes or densities of the organs. Two **blood tests** commonly conducted to examine renal function are the **blood urea nitrogen** (BUN) clearance test and the **creatinine** clearance test. These measure how effectively the kidneys are excreting the respective substances.

The nurse is responsible for collecting urine specimens for a number of tests: *clean voided specimens* for routine urinalysis, *clean catch or midstream urine specimens* for urine culture, and *timed urine specimens* for a variety of tests that depend on the client's specific health problem. Clients need varying degrees of instruction and assistance to provide *clean voided* specimens. Many clients are able to provide the specimen independently. Male clients generally have little difficulty voiding directly into the specimen container, but female clients usually need to stand over a toilet bowl and hold the container between their legs during the process of voiding. About 120 ml (4 oz) of urine is generally required. Clients who are seriously ill, physically incapacitated, or disoriented may need to use a bedpan or urinal in bed; others may require supervision and/or assistance in the bathroom. Whatever the situation, explicit directions are required.

The nurse should explain that all specimens must be free of fecal contamination, so voiding needs to occur at a different time from defecation. Instruct female clients to discard the toilet tissue in the toilet or in a waste bag rather than in the bedpan, since tissue in the specimen makes laboratory analysis more difficult. When the specimen is obtained, put the lid tightly on the container to prevent spillage of the urine and contamination of other objects. If the outside of the container has been contaminated by urine, clean it with a disinfectant. Make sure that the specimen label and the laboratory requisition carry the correct information, and attach them securely to the specimen. Inappropriate identification of the specimen can lead to errors of diagnosis or therapy for the client.

Clean-catch or *mid-stream specimens* must be as free as possible from external contamination by microorganisms near the urethral opening. Sterile specimen containers and lids are used for these specimens. Procedure 41–1 describes the steps involved in obtaining these specimens.

PROCEDURE 41–1

Collecting a Clean-Catch Urine Specimen

Equipment

The equipment used varies from agency to agency. Some agencies use commercially prepared disposable clean-catch kits. See Figure 41–7. Others use agency-prepared sterile trays. Both prepared trays and kits generally contain the first four following items:

- Sterile cotton balls or 2 × 2 inch gauze pads to clean and dry the genitals and perineal area.
- An antiseptic, such as povidone iodine. The antiseptic may need to be added to an agency-prepared tray.
- A sterile specimen container for the urine specimen.
- A specimen identification label.
- A container of sterile water to rinse the perineal area after cleaning.
- Sterile gloves for the nurse to wear when assisting a client.

- A completed laboratory requisition form.
- A bath blanket, if the client is not ambulatory.

Intervention

1. Inform the client that a urine specimen is required; give the reason for it, and explain the method to be used to collect it.
2. Ask the client to wash and dry the genitals and perineum thoroughly with soap and water. A clean per-

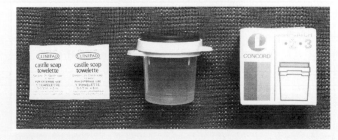

Figure 41–7 A commercially prepared disposable clean-catch kit

ineum is essential to reduce the number of skin bacteria and to minimize contamination of the specimen.

3. Assist the ambulatory client to the bathroom. The preferred method to collect the specimen from ambulatory people is to have them provide the specimen while standing over the toilet in the bathroom.

4. Assist nonambulatory clients to an upright sitting position on a urine receptacle. Provide appropriate covers for the client. Fold back the top bed linen to the bottom of the bed and drape the client in a bath blanket, exposing only the perineal area.

5. Assist females to spread their legs apart enough to ensure that the urine will not touch the legs.

6. Open the sterile kit or tray, using sterile technique. *Rationale:* Sterile technique is essential to maintain the sterility of the specimen container.

7. Put on the sterile gloves.

8. Pour the antiseptic solution over the cotton balls.

9. Clean the client's vulvar area or the tip of the penis with the antiseptic.
Rationale: The antiseptic reduces the number of bacteria near the urethral opening and minimizes contamination of the urine specimens.

10. For female clients:
a. Swab the labia minora from front to back, using one swab for each wipe.
Rationale: Swabbing from front to back cleans from the area of least contamination to the area of greatest contamination.
b. Spread the labia minora well apart, using the thumb and another finger, eg, the third finger, of one hand.
c. Swab between the labia minora over the urethra from front to back.
Rationale: The urethra is considered less contaminated than the vagina and anus.
d. Rinse the area with sterile water.
Rationale: Rinsing removes the antiseptic and other external contaminants.
e. Dry the area with sterile cotton balls.

11. For male clients:
a. Hold the penis with one hand and clean the urinary meatus by using a circular motion. Retract the foreskin of an uncircumcised male.

b. Wash outward from the meatus in a circular motion, using one swab for each wipe.
Rationale: This cleans from the area of least contamination to the area of greatest contamination.
c. Rinse the area with sterile water.
d. Dry the area with cotton balls, in the same manner used for cleaning.

12. Ask the client to start voiding.
Rationale: Initial voiding clears additional external contaminants at the urethral opening.

13. After the client has begun to void, place the specimen container under the stream of urine to collect 30–60 ml of midstream urine. Handle only the outside of the container.
Rationale: Handling only the outside protects the sterility of the inside.

14. Put the sterile cap tightly on the specimen container, touching only the outside of the cap.
Rationale: Capping the container prevents spillage of urine and contamination of other objects. Touching only the outside of the cap retains the sterility of the inside of the cap.

15. Inspect the urine for normal and abnormal characteristics. See Table 41–3.

16. Clean the outer surface of the container with soap and water.
Rationale: Cleaning the outer surface prevents the transfer of microorganisms to others.

17. Remove your gloves and wash hands.

18. Ensure that the specimen label and the laboratory requisition have the correct information on them. Attach them securely to the specimen container.
Rationale: Inaccurate identification and/or information on the specimen container can lead to errors of diagnosis or therapy.

19. Arrange for the specimen to be sent to the laboratory immediately.
Rationale: Bacterial cultures must be started immediately, before any contaminating organisms can grow and multiply.

20. Record collection of the specimen, any pertinent observations of the urine in terms of color, odor, or consistency, and any difficulty in voiding that the client experienced.

Several urine tests require *timed specimens.* Urine specimens are collected at timed intervals, for short periods (1 to 2 hours) or long periods (12 to 24 hours). All timed urine specimens should be refrigerated to prevent bacterial growth and decomposition of the urine components, unless a special preservative has been added. Each voiding of urine is collected in a small, clean container and then emptied immediately into the large refrigerated bottle or carton. Some of the tests performed on timed urine specimens include:

1. **Quantitative albumin** (24 hours): Determines the daily amount of albumin lost in the urine in such

conditions as kidney disease, hypertension, drug toxicity, or severe heart failure involving kidney damage.

2. **Amino acid** (24 hours): Determines acquired or congenital disease of the kidneys.

3. **Amylase** (2, 12, or 24 hours): Determine the amount of amylase, a pancreatic enzyme that may be excreted in the urine in certain diseases of the pancreas.

4. **Quantitative chlorides** (24 hours): Determines the total excretion of chloride; may be performed in the management of cardiac clients who are on low-salt diets.

5. **Concentration and dilution:** Determines disorders of the kidney tubules in concentrating and diluting urine. These specimens are collected over varying periods of time. Specimens are commonly collected at hourly intervals for 2 to 4 hours after the client has been given a specified amount of clear fluid to drink.

6. **Creatinine** or **creatinine clearance** (24 hours): Reflects the degree of kidney impairment. Creatinine is formed in the muscles from creatine in relatively constant daily amounts and is excreted in the urine. Elevated creatinine content indicates a disturbance in kidney function.

7. **Estriol determination** (24 hours): Measures the level of this hormone in the urine of high-risk pregnant women, e.g., those with toxemia or diabetes. Estriol is the major form in which estrogen is excreted in the urine. Low levels can indicate inadequate function of the placenta and possible fetal distress.

8. **Glucose tolerance** (24 hours): Determines disorders of glucose metabolism that may arise from malfunction of the liver or pancreas. Tests are performed on both the blood and the urine after the client is given a large amount of glucose orally or intravenously.

9. **17-hydroxycorticosteroid** (24 hours): Assesses the functioning of the adrenal cortex. Corticosteroids are hormones that are produced in the adrenal cortex, altered, and then excreted in the urine.

10. **Urobilinogen** (random times or 2 hours): Determines obstruction of the biliary tract, excessive destruction of red blood cells, or liver damage. These specimens need to be protected from light.

Appropriate specimen containers with or without preservative in accordance with the specific test are generally obtained from the laboratory and placed in the client's bathroom or in the utility room. Alert signs are placed in the client's unit to remind staff of the test in progress. Specimen identification labels need to indicate the date and time of each voiding in addition to the usual identification information. They may also be numbered sequentially, e.g., 1st specimen, 2nd specimen, 3rd specimen.

Clients need to be told explicitly why the test is being done and how they can assist. The nurse tells the client when the specimen collection will begin and end; e.g., a 24-hour urine test may begin at 0700 hours and ends at the same hour the next day. Instructions should include the following facts:

1. All urine must be saved and placed in the specimen containers once the test starts.
2. The urine must be free of fecal contamination and toilet tissue.
3. Each specimen must be given to the nursing staff immediately so that it can be placed in the appropriate specimen bottle.

The collection period is started by having the client void in the toilet or bedpan or urinal. This urine is usually discarded, but agency procedure needs to be checked.

All subsequent urine specimens are collected, including the one at the end of the period.

The nurse needs to make sure that the client ingests a required amount of liquid for certain tests and instructs the client to void all subsequent urine into the bedpan or urinal and to notify the nursing staff for assistance and after each voiding. Some tests require that the client void at specified times. Each specimen must be placed in the appropriately labeled container. The nurse asks the client to provide the last specimen 5 to 10 minutes before the end of the collection period and informs the client that the test is completed. The starting time of the test and completion of the specimen collection are recorded on the client's chart. In addition, if indicated for the specific test, the time each urine specimen was collected is noted, as are the volume of each specimen, the appearance of the urine, and other relevant data such as fluid intake or restrictions.

Nursing Diagnoses for Clients with Urinary Elimination Problems

Nursing diagnostic categories that relate specifically to urinary tract function and urinary patterns include alteration in urinary elimination pattern, stress incontinence, reflex incontinence, functional incontinence, total incontinence, urge incontinence, and urinary retention. Other relevant categories to consider are potential for infection, altered comfort, potential fluid volume deficit or excess, disturbance in self-concept, and potential impairment of skin integrity. Specific examples are provided in the accompanying box.

Clients who have urinary retention not only experience discomfort but are also at risk of urinary tract infection. Distention of the bladder reduces blood flow to the mucosal layers, and tissues become more susceptible to bacterial invasion. Stasis of urine in the bladder provides an ideal medium for bacterial growth and reproduction. Depending on the acidity and urea concentration of this urine in the bladder, infection may occur. Bacteria favor an alkaline medium and a certain concentration of urea.

The most common cause of urinary tract infection is an invasive procedure such as catheterization or cystoscopic examination. In catheterization, a urine drainage tube is inserted through the urethra into the bladder; during cystoscopic examination, a lighted instrument is inserted. These procedures provide a direct route for microorganisms to ascend through the urethra to the bladder and beyond into the ureters and kidneys. A catheter may also irritate urethral and bladder tissues, thus predisposing them to further risk of bacterial invasion.

Females in particular are prone to ascending urinary tract infections because of their short urethras. Microorganisms are normally present in the perineal area surrounding the urinary meatus, in the distal urethra, and in the vagina. Males, who have longer urethras and

NURSING DIAGNOSIS

Urinary Elimination Problems

- Stress incontinence related to weak pelvic muscles and structural supports associated with increased age
- Functional urinary incontinence related to mobility deficit
- Reflex incontinence related to spinal cord lesion
- Total incontinence related to dysfunction causing triggering of micturition at unpredictable times
- Total incontinence related to independent contraction of detrusor reflex associated with surgery
- Total incontinence related to fistula between bladder and vagina
- Total incontinence related to trauma affecting spinal cord nerves
- Urge incontinence related to decreased bladder capacity
- Urge incontinence related to irritation of bladder stretch receptors, causing spasm
- Urge incontinence related to overdistention of bladder
- Urinary retention related to urethral blockage associated with enlarged prostate gland
- Urinary retention related to inhibition of micturition reflex arc
- Potential for urinary tract infection related to indwelling urethral catheter
- Potential for urinary tract infection related to urinary retention and stasis of urine
- Potential for impaired skin integrity related to incontinence
- Disturbance in self-concept related to inability to control urine
- Disturbance in self-concept related to enuresis
- Potential for fluid imbalance related to urinary retention

prostatic secretions containing antibacterial substances, are less prone to infection. Factors contributing to urinary infections in females include poor perineal hygiene, failure to wipe from the front to the back after voiding or defecating, inadequate hand washing, and frequent sexual intercourse.

Clients with lower urinary tract infections often experience **dysuria** (burning during urination) due to passage of urine over inflamed tissues; frequency and urgency resulting from irritated tissues and disruption of normal micturition mechanisms; and, if the infection is acute, fever, chills, nausea, vomiting, and malaise. Urine appears cloudy due to the presence of pus (**pyuria**). Clients with upper urinary tract infections experience flank pain and tenderness, and chills.

Planning Care for Clients with Urinary Elimination Problems

The overall goals for clients with potential or actual urinary elimination problems are maintenance or restoration of the client's normal urinary elimination pattern and prevention of associated risks such as infection, skin breakdown, fluid and electrolyte imbalance, and lowered self-esteem. The client's need for education must also be considered. For example, a female may need education about perineal hygiene; a male, about self-care in regard to catheter care or insertion. Planning also involves the establishment of outcome criteria. For suggestions, see the section on evaluation, later in this chapter.

Implementing Nursing Strategies

Maintaining Normal Urinary Elimination

Most interventions to maintain normal urinary elimination are independent nursing functions. These include maintaining an adequate fluid intake and promoting normal voiding habits. Increasing fluid intake increases urine production, which in turn stimulates the micturition reflex. A normal, average daily intake of 1200 to 1500 ml of fluids is adequate for most clients. Additional amounts are required by clients with increased fluid demands, e.g., those who have abnormal fluid losses from other routes, such as excessive perspiration, vomiting, or diarrhea.

Immobilized clients, susceptible to calculi formation, should be provided daily intakes of 2000 to 3000 ml per day (unless medically contraindicated). Dilute urine prevents urinary tract stones and infection. Increased fluid intakes are contraindicated in clients who require fluid restrictions, e.g., those with renal impairment or congestive heart failure. Fluid intake can be increased by encouraging the client to eat plenty of raw fruits and vegetables, which have a high water content. Assisting clients to use bedpans is discussed in Chapter 40. Some female clients may prefer to use a female urinal. Figure 41–8, *B,* shows a female urinal; Figure 41–8, *A,* shows a male urinal.

Hospital routines and prescribed medical therapies can interfere with a client's normal voiding habits. Guidelines for helping clients maintain normal voiding habits are summarized in the accompanying box.

Nursing Interventions for Urinary Incontinence

Independent nursing interventions for clients with urinary incontinence include a bladder-training program, meticulous skin care, and for males, application

GUIDELINES

Maintaining Normal Voiding Habits

Positioning

- Assist the client to a normal position for voiding: standing for males; for females, squatting or sitting.

- Use bedside commodes as necessary for females and urinals for males standing at the bedside.

- Encourage the client to push over the pubic area with the hands or to lean forward to increase intraabdominal pressure and external pressure on the bladder.

Relaxation

- Provide privacy for the client.

- Allow the client sufficient time to void.

- Suggest the client read or listen to music.

- Provide sensory stimuli that may help the client relax. Pour warm water over the perineum of a female or have the client sit in a warm bath to promote muscle relaxation. Applying a hot-water bottle to the lower abdomen of both men and women may also foster muscle relaxation.

- Turn on running water within hearing distance of the client to mask the sound of voiding for persons who find this embarrassing.

- Relieve physical and emotional discomfort to decrease muscle tension and encourage the mental concentration that may be needed for micturition. Make sure to provide ordered analgesics and emotional support.

Timing

- Assist clients who have the urge to void immediately. Delays only increase the difficulty in starting to void, and the desire to void may pass.

- Offer toileting assistance to the client at his or her usual times of voiding, e.g., on awakening, before or after meals, and at bedtime.

For bed-confined clients

- Warm the bed pan. A cold bedpan may prompt contraction of the perineal muscles and inhibit voiding.

- Elevate the head of the client's bed to Fowler's position, place a small pillow or rolled towel at the small of the back to increase physical support and comfort, and have the client flex the hips and knees. This position simulates the normal voiding position as closely as possible.

of an external drainage device (**condom**). The physician may order urinary catheterization for clients unable to voluntarily control micturition. Nursing interventions for catheterized clients are discussed in the next section.

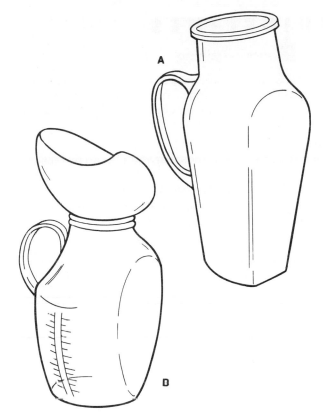

Figure 41–8 Two types of urinals: **A,** male urinal; **B,** female urinal

A **bladder-training program** requires involvement of the nurse, the client, and support persons. Guidelines for bladder-training are summarized in the accompanying box.

Skin that is continually moist becomes macerated. Over a period of time urine that accumulates on the skin is converted to ammonia, which is very irritating to the skin. Since both skin irritation and maceration predispose the client to skin breakdown and decubitus ulcers, the incontinent person requires meticulous skin care. To prevent alterations in skin integrity, the nurse washes the client's perineal area with soap and water after periods of incontinence, dries it thoroughly, and provides clean, dry clothing or bed linen. If the skin is irritated, the nurse applies barrier creams such as zinc oxide ointment to protect it from contact with urine. If it is necessary to pad the client's clothes for protection, the nurse should use products that absorb wetness and leave a dry surface in contact with the skin.

The application of a **condom**, also referred to as a **urinary sheath (urosheath)** or **external catheter,** and attachment of its base to a urinary drainage system are commonly prescribed for incontinent males. Use of a condom appliance is preferable to insertion of a retention catheter, because it avoids entrance into the urethra and bladder and minimizes the risk of urethral or bladder infection.

Methods of applying condoms vary with the duration the condom is to be worn. Condoms that are to be

pertinent observations, such as irritated areas on the penis.

14. Observe the penis for swelling and discoloration 30 minutes following the application of the condom and regularly thereafter. Also check urine flow. *Rationale:* Swelling and discoloration could indicate that the condom is too tight. Normally, some urine will be present in the tube if the flow is not obstructed.

Removing the Condom

15. Remove the tape, if it was applied, and roll off the condom. Remove the plasticized skin spray (it peels off readily) or the skin protector every 1–2 days to provide skin care to the penis. Wash the penis with soapy water, rinse, and dry it thoroughly.
16. Change the condom daily, and assess the foreskin for signs of irritation, swelling, and discoloration.

Nursing Interventions for Urinary Retention

Urinary catheterization may be ordered for the client with retention. It involves the introduction of a catheter (a rubber or plastic tube) through the urethra into the urinary bladder. Catheterization is usually performed only when absolutely necessary, since it poses certain risks. Because the urinary structures are normally sterile except at the end of the urethra, the danger exists of introducing microorganisms into the bladder. This hazard is greatest for clients who have lowered resistance due to disease processes. Once an infection is introduced into the bladder, it can ascend the ureters and eventually involve the kidneys. Even after the catheter has been inserted and left in place for a time, the hazard of infection remains, since pathogens can be introduced through the catheter lumen. Thus, strict surgical asepsis is used for catheterizations.

Another hazard of catheterization is trauma, particularly in the male client, whose urethra is longer and more tortuous. It is important to insert a catheter along the normal contour of the urethra. Damage to the urethra can occur if the catheter is forced through strictures or at an incorrect angle. For females, the urethra lies posteriorly, then takes a slightly anterior direction toward the bladder. See Figure 41–4. For males, the urethra is normally curved (see Figure 41–3), but it can be straightened by elevating the penis to a position perpendicular to the body.

Two categories of urinary catheters are straight catheters and retention catheters. The **straight (Robinson) catheter** is a single-lumen tube with a small eye or opening about 1¼ cm (½ in) from the insertion tip. See Figure 41–12, *A.* It is used for obtaining specimens and checking residual urine.

Residual urine is normally not present in the bladder or consists of only a few milliliters. However, whenever there is a bladder outlet obstruction (e.g., enlargement of the prostate gland) or loss of bladder muscle tone, there can be large amounts of residual urine. Incomplete emptying of the bladder may be suspected when the client experiences frequency and when only small amounts of urine are voided at a time (e.g., 100 ml in an adult). The purposes of measuring the residual urine are to determine the degree to which the bladder is emptying, and to assess the need to establish therapy that will empty the bladder (e.g., insertion of a retention catheter). To measure the residual urine, the nurse asks the client to void and then immediately catheterizes the client. Both the amount of urine voided and the amount of residual urine are measured and recorded. Generally, if the amount of residual urine exceeds 50 ml, an in-dwelling (retention) catheter is inserted.

The **retention (indwelling or Foley) catheter** contains a second, smaller tube throughout its length on the inside. This tube is connected to a balloon near the insertion tip. After catheter insertion, the balloon is inflated to hold the catheter in place within the bladder. The outside end of the retention catheter is bifurcated, that is, it has two openings, one to drain the urine, the other to inflate the balloon. See Figure 41–12, *B.*

There are several other types of retention catheters. One that is frequently used for a client requiring con-

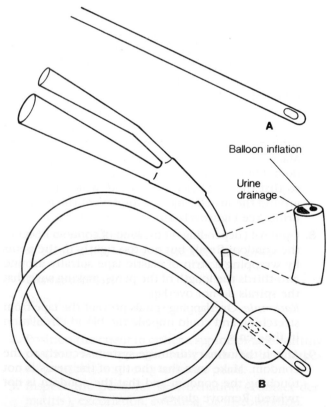

Balloon inflation

Urine drainage

Figure 41–12 Two types of commonly used catheters: **A,** a straight (Robinson) catheter; **B,** a retention (Foley) catheter with the balloon inflated

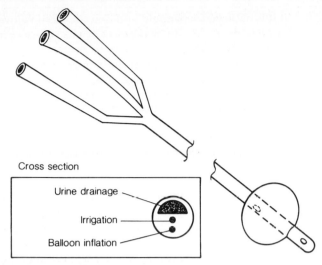

Cross section

Urine drainage

Irrigation

Balloon inflation

Figure 41–13 A three-way Foley catheter

tinual or periodic bladder irrigations is the **three-way Foley catheter.** It is similar to the two-way Foley catheter described above, except that it has a third channel through which sterile fluid can flow into the urinary bladder. See Figure 41–13.

All types of catheters are sized by the diameter of the lumen and are categorized according to the French scale of numbers: the larger the number, the larger the lumen. Small sizes, such as #8 or #10, are used for children; #14, #16, and #18 are commonly used for adults. Men frequently require a larger size than women. The balloons of retention catheters are sized by the volume of fluid or air used to inflate them. The two commonly used sizes are 5 ml and 30 ml balloons. The size of the balloon is indicated on the catheter along with the diameter, e.g., "#18 Fr.—5 ml." Catheterization of females and males, using straight catheters, is described in Procedures 41–3 and 41–4, respectively. Procedure 41–5 outlines how to insert retention catheter.

PROCEDURE 41–3

Female Urinary Catheterization Using a Straight Catheter

Equipment

A sterile catheterization kit containing

- Gloves.
- Drapes to protect the bed and to provide a sterile field.
- A fenestrated drape (optional) to place over the perineum.
- An antiseptic solution recommended by agency policy, eg, aqueous benzalkonium chloride (Zephiran) 1:750, to clean the labia and urinary meatus.
- Cotton balls or gauze squares to apply the antiseptic.
- Forceps to apply the antiseptic.
- A water-soluble lubricant to lubricate the insertion tip of the catheter to facilitate insertion and reduce the chance of trauma to the mucous membrane lining the urethra.
- A catheter of appropriate size (#14 or #16).
- A receptacle for the urine. Often, the base of the kit serves this purpose.
- A specimen container if a specimen is to be acquired.
- A bag or receptacle for disposal of the cotton balls.
- A flashlight or lamp to provide light on the genital area.
- A mask, clean gown, and cap, if required by agency policy.
- A bath blanket.

- Soap, a basin of warm water, a washcloth, and a towel.
- Disposable gloves.

Intervention

1. To assess for urinary retention, palpate or percuss the bladder just above the symphysis pubis. To palpate the bladder, indent the skin more than 1.3 cm (0.5 in.) by pressing the fingers of one hand upon the fingers of the other. See Figure 41–14. This increases the pressure for palpation. To percuss the bladder, place the middle finger of one hand against the skin, and strike it sharply with the middle finger of the other hand. The resulting sound when the bladder is full will be duller than normal.

2. Obtain assistance if the client requires help to maintain the required position.

3. Explain the catheterization to the client. Some people fear that the procedure will be painful. Normally, a catheterization is painless; there may only be a slight sensation of pressure.
   Rationale: Relieving the person's tension can facilitate insertion of the catheter, because the urinary sphincters are more likely to be relaxed.

4. Provide privacy. Exposure of the genitals is embarrassing to most people.

5. Assist the client to a supine position with knees flexed and thighs externally rotated. Pillows can be used to support the knees and elevate the buttocks.
   Rationale: Raising the pelvis gives the nurse a better view of the urinary meatus.

6. Drape the client. Use a bath blanket to cover the

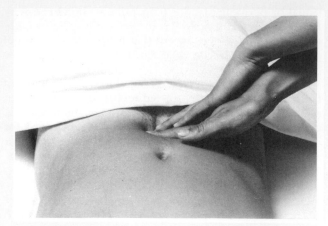

Figure 41-14

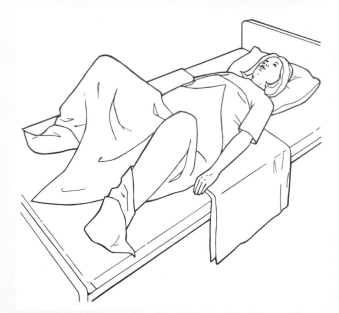

Figure 41-15

chest and abdomen. Pull the client's gown up over her hips. Cover her legs and feet with the bed sheet or another blanket. Place it diagonally on the client with a corner around each foot. See Figure 41-15.

7. Don disposable gloves and wash the perineal-genital area with warm water and soap; rinse and dry.
Rationale: Gloves protect the nurse's hands from contact with the client's body secretions. Cleanliness reduces the possibility of introducing microorganisms with the catheter. Appropriate rinsing removes soap that could inhibit the action of the antiseptic used later.

8. Adjust the light for vision of the urinary meatus. It may be necessary to use a flashlight or to place a gooseneck lamp at the foot of the bed, so that it focuses on the perineal area.

9. Put on a mask if required by agency policy. Some agencies also advocate the use of a clean gown and a surgical cap if the nurse's hair is long.

10. At the bedside, open the sterile kit and the catheter,

if it is packaged separately, and don the sterile gloves (see Procedure 23-3). The kit can be placed between the client's thighs.

11. Drape the client with the sterile drapes, being careful to protect the sterility of your gloves. Use the first drape as an underpad, and place it under the buttocks. Keep the underpad edges cuffed over your gloves to prevent contamination of the gloves against the client's buttocks. If the other drape is fenestrated, place it over the perineal area exposing only the labia. Place thigh drapes from the side farthest to the side nearest you. If an underpad is not available, place the two thigh drapes so that they overlap between the client's thighs.

12. Pour the antiseptic solution over the cotton balls, if they are not already prepared.

13. Lubricate the insertion tip of the catheter liberally. Place it aside in the sterile container ready for use.
Rationale: Water-soluble lubricant facilitates insertion of the catheter by reducing friction. It is important to lubricate at this point because the nurse will subsequently have only one sterile hand available.

14. Separate the labia majora with the thumb and index or other finger of one hand, and clean the labia minora on each side using forceps and cotton balls soaked in antiseptic. Use a new swab for each stroke, and move downward from the pubic area to the anus. See Figure 41-16. Then separate the labia minora with two other fingers, still using the same hand. See Figure 41-17.
Rationale: The hand that touches the client becomes contaminated. It remains in position exposing the urinary meatus, while the other hand remains sterile holding the sterile forceps. Cleaning from anterior to posterior cleans from the area of least contamination to the area of greatest contamination.

15. Expose the urinary meatus adequately by retracting the tissue of the labia minora in an upward (anterior) direction. See Figure 41-17. Clean first from the meatus downward and then on either side, using a new swab for each stroke. Once the meatus is cleaned, do not allow the labia to close over it.
Rationale: Keeping the labia apart prevents the risk of contaminating the urinary meatus.

16. Inspect the tissues for excoriation around the urinary meatus, swelling of the urinary meatus, or the presence of discharge around the urinary meatus.

17. Place the drainage end of the catheter in the urine receptacle. Then pick up the insertion end of the catheter with the uncontaminated, sterile, gloved hand, holding it 5-8 cm (2-3 in.) from the insertion tip for an adult and 2-3 cm (1 in.) for an infant or small child. If agency policy requires, use sterile forceps to pick up the catheter.
Rationale: The adult female urethra is approximately 4 cm (1.5 in.) long. The nurse holds the catheter far enough from the end to allow full insertion into the bladder and to maintain control of the tip of the catheter so it will not accidentally become contaminated.

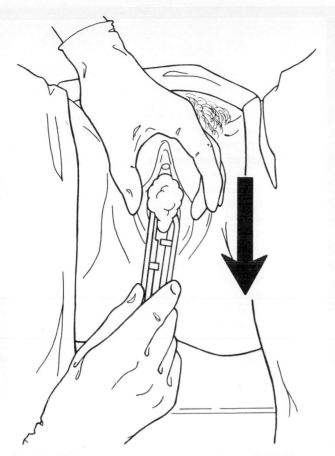

Figure 41—16

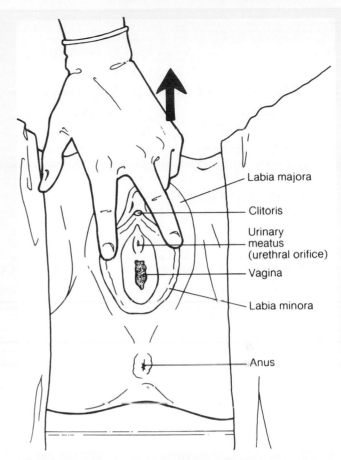

Labia majora

Clitoris

Urinary meatus (urethral orifice)

Vagina

Labia minora

Anus

Figure 41—17

18. Gently insert the catheter into the urinary meatus about 5 cm (2 in.) for an adult, 2.5 cm (1 in.) for a small child, or until urine flows. Insert the catheter in the direction of the urethra. If the catheter meets resistance during insertion, do not force it. Ask the client to take deep breaths. If this does not relieve the resistance, discontinue the procedure, and report the problem to the nurse in charge. Exercise caution to prevent the catheter tip from becoming contaminated. If it becomes contaminated, discard it.
Rationale: Forceful pressure exerted against the urethra can produce trauma. Deep breaths by the client may relax the external sphincter.

19. When the urine flows, transfer the hand from the labia to the catheter to hold it in place at the meatus.

20. Collect a urine specimen. Pinch the catheter, and transfer the drainage end of it into the sterile specimen bottle. Usually, 30 ml of urine is sufficient for a specimen.

21. Empty the bladder or drain the amount of urine specified in the order. For adults experiencing urinary retention, some agencies limit the amount of urine drained to 700–1000 ml. Whether or not to limit the amount of urine drained is currently controversial (Nurse's Reference Library 1983, p. 588). Remove the catheter slowly.
Rationale: Removing large amounts of urine too quickly is thought to induce engorgement of the

pelvic blood vessels and hypovolemic shock. Usually, the physician prescribes the amount to be removed and times at which the remaining urine is to be withdrawn.

22. Dry the perineum with a towel or drape.

23. Assess the urine for color, clarity, odor, and the presence of any abnormal constituents, such as blood. Measure the amount of urine.

24. Remove gloves.

25. Send the specimen to the laboratory.

26. Document the catheterization, the reason for it, nursing assessments, and whether a specimen was sent to the laboratory.

Sample Recording

Date	Time	Notes
1/26/89	1900	C/o pubic discomfort. Has not voided since surgery. Bladder palpable above symphysis pubis. Is restless. Catheterized for 650 ml clear amber urine. Discomfort relieved. Resting s̄ complaint. —————— Sylvia F. Tompkins, RN

PROCEDURE 41–4

Male Urinary Catheterization Using a Straight Catheter

Equipment

See Procedure 41–3. A #16 or #18 catheter is usually used for an adult male.

Intervention

1. Follow Procedure 41–3, steps 1–4.

2. Assist the client to a supine position with the knees slightly flexed and the thighs slightly apart.
   Rationale: This allows greater relaxation of the adbominal and perineal muscles and permits easier insertion of the catheter.

3. Drape the client by folding the top bedclothes down so that the penis is exposed and the thighs are covered. Use a bath blanket to cover the chest and abdomen.

4. Follow Procedure 41–3, steps 7–9.

5. Open the sterile tray, and don the sterile gloves (see Procedure 23–3). Place the tray directly on the client's thighs, if he is not restless.

6. Place a drape under the penis and a second drape above the penis over the pubic area. If a fenestrated drape is available, place it over the penis and pubic area, exposing only the penis.

7. Pour the antiseptic solution over the cotton balls if they are not already prepared.

8. Lubricate the insertion tip of the catheter liberally for about 5–7 cm (2–3 in.). Place it aside on the sterile tray ready for insertion.
   Rationale: Water-soluble lubricant facilitates insertion of the catheter by reducing friction. It is important to do this step before cleaning, since the nurse will subsequently have only one sterile hand available.

9. Clean the urinary meatus with antiseptic swabs. Grasp the penis firmly behind the glans, and spread the meatus between the thumb and forefinger. Retract the foreskin of an uncircumcised male. The hand holding the penis is now considered contaminated. With the other hand, use sterile forceps to pick up a swab. Clean the meatus first, and then wipe the tissue surrounding the meatus in a circular fashion. Discard each swab after only one wipe.
   Rationale: To avoid stimulating an erection, firm pressure rather than light pressure is used to grasp the penis. Using forceps maintains the sterility of the nurse's glove.

10. Place the drainage end of the catheter in the urine receptacle. Then pick up the insertion end of the catheter with the uncontaminated, sterile, gloved hand, holding it about 8–10 cm (3–4 in.) from the insertion tip for an adult or about 2.5 cm (1 in.) for a baby or small boy. In some agencies the catheter is picked up with forceps.
    Rationale: The male urethra is approximately 20 cm (8 in.) long. The nurse holds the catheter far enough from the end to maintain control of the tip of the catheter so it will not accidentally become contaminated.

11. To insert the catheter, lift the penis to a position perpendicular to the body and exert slight traction. Insert the catheter steadily about 20 cm (8 in.) or until urine begins to flow. To bypass slight resistance at the sphincters, twist the catheter or wait until the sphincter relaxes. Have the client take deep breaths or try to void. If difficult resistance is met, discontinue the procedure and report the problem to the nurse in charge.
    Rationale: Lifting the penis perpendicular to the body straightens the downward curvature of the urethra. Slight resistance is normally encountered at the external and internal urethral sphincters. Deep breaths by the client can help to relax the external sphincter. Forceful pressure exerted against a major resistance can traumatize the urethra.

12. While the urine flows, lower the penis and hold the catheter in place at the meatus with the hand that held the penis.

13. Collect a urine specimen (if required) after the urine has flowed for a few seconds. Pinch the catheter, and transfer the drainage end of the catheter into the sterile specimen bottle. Usually, 30 ml of urine is sufficient for a specimen.

14. Empty the bladder or drain the amount of urine specified in the order. For adult clients experiencing urinary retention, limit the amount of urine drained to 700–1000 ml if agency policy indicates. Remove the catheter slowly.
    Rationale: Removing large amounts of urine too quickly may induce engorgement of the pelvic blood vessels and hypovolemic shock. Usually, the physician prescribes the amount to be removed and times at which the remaining urine is to be withdrawn.

15. Replace the foreskin to normal position and dry the client's penis with a towel or drape.
    Rationale: Replacement of the foreskin prevents risk of restricted circulation.

16. Follow Procedure 41–3, steps 23–26.

PROCEDURE 41-5

Inserting a Retention Catheter

The procedure for inserting a urinary retention catheter is similar to the basic catheterization procedure, with differences occurring primarily after the catheter is inserted. Prior to insertion of the catheter, the nurse needs to test the balloon of the retention catheter to see that it is intact, and following the insertion, the nurse inflates the balloon and attaches a urinary drainage system.

A simple urinary drainage system consists of a reten-tion catheter, tubing, and a receptacle (collecting bag) for the urine. This is called a straight drainage system, and it depends on the force of gravity to move the urine from the urinary bladder to the collecting bag. When this system is not or cannot be opened anywhere along it from the catheter to the bag, it is referred to as a closed system. See Figure 41–18. Closed systems are being used increasingly because of the danger of microorganisms entering the urinary tract whenever the system is opened.

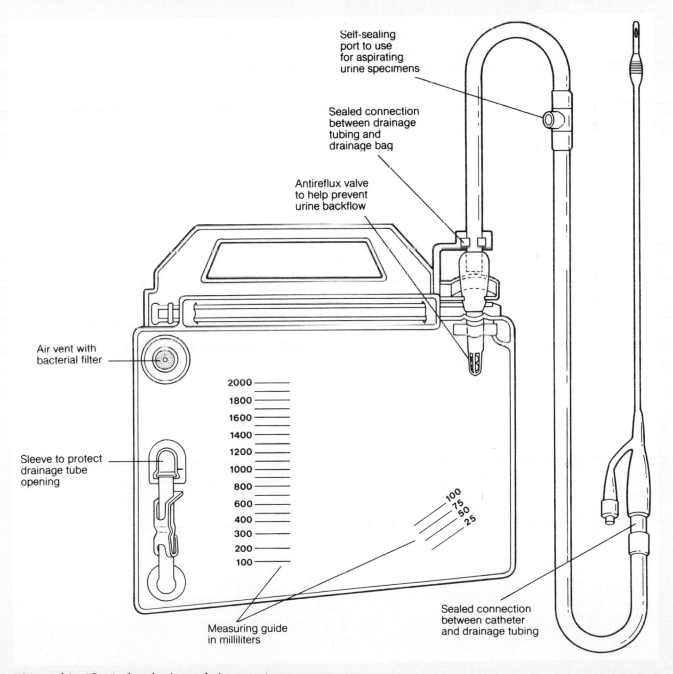

Self-sealing port to use for aspirating urine specimens

Sealed connection between drainage tubing and drainage bag

Antireflux valve to help prevent urine backflow

Air vent with bacterial filter

Sleeve to protect drainage tube opening

2000
1800
1600
1400
1200
1000
800
600
400
300
200
100

100
75
50
25

Measuring guide in milliliters

Sealed connection between catheter and drainage tubing

Figure 41–18 A closed urinary drainage system

The more traditional type of system is the open system, in which the tubing may be separated from the catheter to perform such techniques as a bladder irrigation.

Equipment

In addition to the equipment used for a straight catheterization, the following equipment is needed:

- A retention catheter #14 or #16 for adults, #8 or #10 for children. The catheter may be supplied separately from the sterile set in some agencies. The catheter may be attached to a closed drainage system. If these are not in the set, acquire a drainage bag and tubing.
- A prefilled syringe to inflate the balloon of the catheter. Sterile water is often used.
- Nonallergenic tape to secure the catheter to the client.
- A safety pin or clip to attach the catheter tubing to the bedding.

Intervention

1. Explain the reason for inserting the retention catheter, how long it will be in place, and the ways in which the urinary drainage equipment needs to be handled to maintain and facilitate the drainage of urine. Reassure the client that the procedure is painless. Some clients fear spillage of urine when they experience the urge to void during insertion of the catheter and for a short period of time after the catheter is in place. Reassure these clients that the catheter drains the urine and that the urge to void will disappear.

2. Follow the technique for a straight catheterization up to and including draping the client.

3. Test the catheter balloon by attaching the prefilled syringe to the balloon valve and injecting the fluid. The balloon should inflate appropriately and should not leak. Withdraw the fluid, and set aside the catheter with the syringe attached for later use. If the balloon leaks or does not inflate adequately, replace the catheter. In such a case, withdraw the fluid and detach the syringe for later use. Ask another nurse to obtain a second catheter and open the package for you, then test the new balloon.

   or

   Remove the equipment and obtain another catheter. Then start the intervention over again with the new sterile equipment.

4. Follow the steps for straight catheterization to
   a. Lubricate the injection tip of the catheter.
   b. Remove the sterile cap from the specimen container.
   c. Separate and clean the urinary meatus and surrounding tissues.
   d. Insert the catheter.
   e. Collect a urine specimen as required.

5. Insert the catheter an additional 2.5–5 cm (1–2 in.) beyond the point at which urine began to flow. *Rationale:* The balloon of the catheter is located

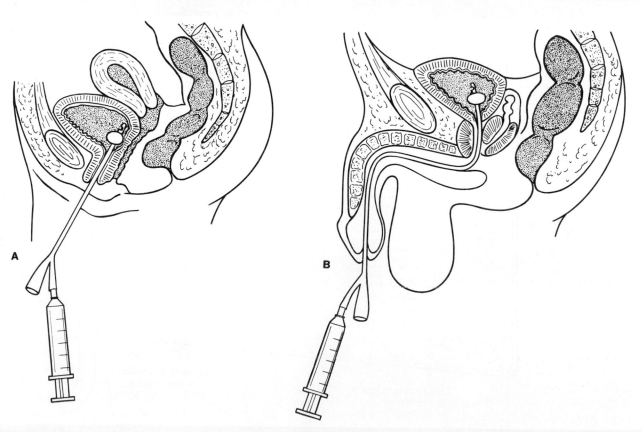

Figure 41–19

behind the opening at the insertion tip, and sufficient space needs to be provided to inflate the balloon. This ensures that the balloon is inflated inside the bladder and not in the urethra, where it could produce trauma.

6. Inflate the balloon by injecting the contents of the prefilled syringe into the valve of the catheter. See Figure 41–19, *A*. Placement of the catheter and balloon in a male client is shown in Figure 41–19, *B*. If the client complains of discomfort or pain during the balloon inflation, withdraw the fluid, insert the catheter a little farther, and inflate the balloon again. Insert no more fluid than the balloon size indicates (eg, 5 ml or 30 ml), and remove the syringe. A special valve prevents backflow of the fluid out of the catheter. When 30-ml balloons are used, some agency policies state that only 15 ml of fluid is injected for inflation.

7. When the balloon is safely inflated, apply slight tension on the catheter until you feel resistance. Then move the catheter slightly back into the bladder. *Rationale:* Resistance indicates that the catheter balloon is inflated appropriately and the catheter is well anchored in the bladder. Moving the catheter slightly back into the bladder keeps the balloon from exerting undue pressure on the neck of the bladder.

8. If the drainage bag and tubing are not already attached to the end of the catheter, remove the protective cap or plug from the tubing, and attach the catheter. Handle the ends of both the catheter and the drainage tube at least 2.5 cm (1 in.) away from their tips. To ensure closure, apply waterproof tape around the connection site of the catheter and tubing. *Rationale:* The sterility of the tips of both the catheter and the drainage tube must be maintained so that microorganisms do not enter the system and move to the bladder.

9. Ensure that the emptying base of the drainage bag is closed. Secure the drainage bag to the bed frame by using the hook or strap provided. Suspend the bag off the floor, but keep it below the level of the client's bladder. See Figure 41–20. *Rationale:* Urine flows by gravity from the bladder to the drainage bag. The bag should be off the floor so that the emptying portion does not become grossly contaminated.

10. Retract the foreskin to its normal position and anchor the catheter with nonallergenic tape to the inside of a female's thigh or to the thigh or abdomen of a male client. See figures 41–21 and 41–25. *Rationale:* Taping restricts the movement of the catheter, thus reducing friction and irritation in the urethra when the client moves. It also prevents skin excoriation at the penile-scrotal junction in the male.

11. Coil the drainage tubing beside the client so that the tubing runs in a straight line down to the drainage bag, and fasten it to the bedclothes with tape, a tubing clamp, or a safety pin. See figures 41–20 and 41–21.

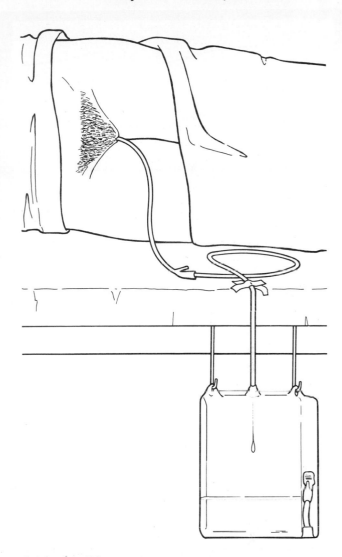

Figure 41–20

Rationale: The drainage tubing should not loop below its entry into the drainage bag, since this impedes the flow of urine by gravity.

12. Dry the client's perineum or penis with a towel or drape.

13. Record the time and date of the catheterization; the reason; pertinent observations, such as the color and amount of urine; whether a specimen was taken and sent to the laboratory; whether all urine was emptied from the bladder; and the nursing assessments.

Sample Recording

Date	Time	Notes
7/12/89	2000	#18 5-ml Foley catheter inserted and connected. 750 ml clear amber urine drained, and catheter clamped. Stated burning pain over pubic area relieved. Instructed about I & O. Dr. Bradley notified, and bladder decompression regimen established q.2h. ———————————— Ron J. Randall, SN

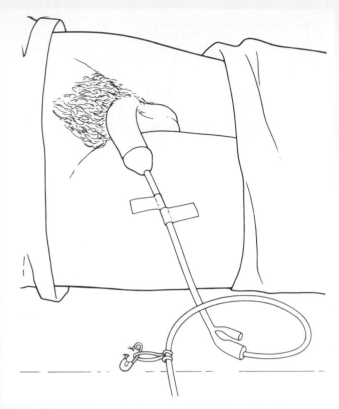

Figure 41–21

14. Observe the flow of urine every 2–3 hours, and note color, odor, and any abnormal constituents. If blood clots are present, check the catheter more frequently to ascertain whether it is plugged.
15. Empty the drainage bag regularly. Apply povidone-iodine (or other antiseptic used in the agency) to the end of the drainage tube before replacing it in the sleeve of the bag.
Rationale: Antiseptics applied to the drainage tube spout prevent microorganisms from entering the system and the client's bladder.

16. Ascertain the agency's policies about changing catheters and drainage systems. Some agencies advocate changes weekly or every other week. Others change the catheter only when sediment accumulates at the distal end. Sediment is present if you feel sandy particles when rolling the end of the catheter between your thumb and fingers. The drainage bag and tubing are generally changed along with the catheter but need to be changed more frequently if sediment accumulates, if leakage occurs, or if a strong odor is evident. Clean the catheter-tubing junction with an antiseptic solution prior to the change.

17. Inspect the patency of the urinary drainage system to ensure that:
    a. There are no obstructions in the drainage. Check that there are no kinks in the tubing, the client is not lying on the tubing, and the tubing is not clogged with mucus or blood.
    b. There is no tension on the catheter or tubing, that the catheter is securely taped to the client's thigh or abdomen, and that the tubing is fastened appropriately to the bedclothes.
    c. Gravity drainage is maintained. For example, check that there are no loops in the tubing below its entry to the drainage receptacle and that the drainage receptacle is below the level of the client's bladder.
    d. The drainage system is well sealed or closed. Check that there are no leaks at the connection sites in open systems.

Nursing care of the client with an indwelling catheter and continuous drainage is largely directed toward preventing infection of the urinary tract and encouraging urinary flow through the drainage system. Interventions include encouraging large amounts of fluid intake, accurately recording of the fluid intake and output, providing perineal-genital care, providing catheter care, changing the retention catheter and tubing, maintaining the patency of the drainage system, preventing contamination of the drainage system, and teaching these measures to the client.

Fluid balance is essential for the client with a retention catheter to minimize the risk of infection. The nurse encourages the client to drink up to 3000 ml per day if permitted. Large amounts of fluid ensure a large urine output, which keeps the bladder flushed out and decreases the likelihood of urinary stasis and subsequent infection. Large volumes of urine also minimize the risk of sediment or other particles obstructing the drainage tubing. Accurate recording of fluid intake and output is discussed in Chapter 43.

Many agencies implement prophylactic measures to acidify the client's urine to prevent urinary infection. By changing the composition of the *diet,* the urine can be made either acid or alkaline. Most vegetables and fruits yield an alkaline urine, whereas meat, fish, fowl, eggs, and cereals yield an acid urine. Alkalinization of the urine may be warranted to soothe an irritated bladder.

Perineal-genital care is recommended at least twice daily or as needed for the client with an indwelling catheter. It is considered one of the most significant measures for reducing the incidence of infection. Any secretions or encrustations that accumulate at the urethral orifice provide an excellent medium for pathogens, which can ascend the tract. Most agencies recommend specific cleaning methods. Some advocate routine perineal-genital care with warm water and soap. For the uncircumcised male client, the foreskin is retracted to clean well under it.

Clients with retention catheters require **special catheter care** once or twice a day in addition to perineal-genital care. This is because microorganisms on the catheter and at the urinary meatus can ascend into the urethra and bladder and cause an infection. Catheter care is usually given directly after perineal-genital care. Because catheter care varies considerably from agency to agency, the nurse should check agency practice. Agencies provide different types of equipment and solutions for cleaning clients who have catheters. See Procedure 41–6 for steps in providing catheter care.

PROCEDURE 41–6

Providing Catheter Care

Equipment

A sterile catheter care kit containing:

- A drape to cover the legs and perineal area around the catheter and the urinary meatus
- Gloves to wear during the procedure
- An antiseptic solution, such as a water-soluble iodine solution
- Cotton balls or applicator swabs
- An antibiotic ointment, such as neomycin
- Sterile forceps
- A small receptacle for the discarded balls or swabs
- A bath blanket (optional)

Intervention

1. Discuss the possibility that the client may provide the care. Because of exposure of the genital area, some people find this procedure embarrassing and often prefer to learn to do it themselves.
2. Arrange the bedclothes or bath blanket so that only the perineal area is exposed.
3. Open the sterile catheter care kit by using surgical aseptic technique.
4. Don the sterile gloves.
5. Drape the client.
6. Pour antiseptic on the cotton balls or swabs.
7. Put some sterile ointment on one cotton ball or swab.
8. Assess the area around the urinary meatus for inflammation, swelling, and discharge. Determine the color, amount, and consistency of any discharge. Note any odor from the area.
9. Clean the perineal-genital area, using forceps and cotton balls or swabs. Use each swab only once.
   a. For a female client, clean the labia majora, moving downward. Then separate the labia majora with your thumb and fourth finger, and clean the labia minora. Then separate them with the index and middle fingers of the same hand. Expose the urinary meatus adequately by retracting the tissue of the labia minora in an upward (anterior) direction. Clean first from the meatus and catheter downward and then on either side.
   b. For a male client, clean the meatus by grasping the penis behind the glans and spreading the urinary meatus between your thumb and forefinger. Retract the foreskin of an uncircumcised male. Clean the meatus around the catheter first, and then wipe the tissue surrounding the meatus in a circular fashion.
10. Assess the area around the urinary meatus for
    a. Discomfort experienced by the client.
    b. Inflammation or swelling.
    c. Discharge (note the color, amount, and consistency).
    d. Odor.
11. Using a new swab, clean along the catheter for about 10 cm (4 in.). Use a circular motion to ensure that all sides of the catheter are cleaned.
12. Apply antiseptic ointment around the base and along about 2.5 cm (1 in.) of the catheter.
    Rationale: This protects the urethra from infection.
13. Inspect the patency of the drainage system.
14. Record on the client's chart the technique, the time, and the assessment data. Report any problems to the nurse in charge.

Sample Recording

Date	Time	Notes
4/30/89	0900	Catheter care given. No apparent urethral redness or swelling. Small amount of thick white discharge around base of catheter. No complaints of discomfort.———————— Yvonne A. Able, NS

Agency policies may specify the frequency of **catheter** and **tubing changes.** Some agencies advocate that both be changed weekly or every other week; others change the catheter only when sediment accumulates at the distal end. Sediment is present if sandy particles are felt when the end of the catheter is rolled between the thumb and fingers. The drainage bag and tubing are generally changed along with the catheter but need to be changed more frequently if sediment accumulates, if leakage occurs, or if a strong odor is evident. Recommendations for changes are made on the basis of reducing the incidence of infection and preventing unpleas-

GUIDELINES

Ongoing Assessment of Clients with Retention Catheters

Ensure that there are no obstructions in the drainage. Check that there are no kinks in the tubing, the client is not lying on the tubing, and the tubing is not clogged with mucus or blood.

Check that there is no tension on the catheter or tubing, that the catheter is securely taped to the thigh or abdomen, and that the tubing is fastened appropriately to the bedclothes.

Ensure that gravity drainage is maintained. Make sure there are no loops in the tubing below its entry to the drainage receptacle and that the drainage receptacle is below the level of the client's bladder.

Ensure that the drainage system is well sealed or closed. Check that there are no leaks at the connection sites in open systems. Apply waterproof tape around the connection site of the catheter and tubing.

Observe the flow of urine every 2 or 3 hours, and note color, odor, and any abnormal constituents. If blood clots are present, check the catheter more frequently to ascertain whether it is plugged.

ant odors. Some authorities recommend that catheters be changed as infrequently as possible.

During tubing changes, strict surgical asepsis is essential to prevent contamination of the distal lumen of the catheter. The nurse acquires a new sterile drainage bag and tubing, a sterile towel or sterile gauzes, clamp, and antiseptic solution. After washing the hands well and setting up a sterile field, the nurse removes the protective cap from the drainage tube, and places the open end of the tubing on the sterile field. She or he then clamps the catheter above the tubing connector and cleans the catheter-tubing junction with an antiseptic solution. The nurse then disconnects the catheter from the old tubing, being careful not to contaminate the end of the catheter, and connects the catheter to the new tubing. She or he then unclamps the catheter, and establishes drainage by securing the tubing and drainage receptacle to the bed at an appropriate level. Applying waterproof tape around the connection site of the catheter and the tubing ensures a closed drainage system.

Ongoing assessment of clients with retention catheters is a high priority. The accompanying box provides guidelines.

When emptying the drainage bag, the nurse must maintain surgical aseptic technique. The bag is emptied usually at the end of each shift of duty, and the tube at the bottom of the bag is used to drain the bag. The amount of drainage is noted in accordance with calibrations on the bag, or a graduated pitcher is brought to the bedside to assess the output. It is important for the nurse not to contaminate the end of the tubing and to reattach it appropriately when the bag is emptied.

Some agencies recommend instillation of hydrogen peroxide in the drainage bag of open systems to prevent the growth of microorganisms in the bag and to reduce odor. Agency policies vary, however. Guidelines to prevent catheter-associated urinary tract infections are given in the accompanying box.

Usually nurses need to **teach** the client some principles about the gravity drainage system and the importance of maintaining a closed system. The client has to understand that the drainage tubing and drainage bag need to be kept lower than the bladder at all times. The client also needs to know how to prevent tension on the catheter tubing, to prevent loops or kinks in the drainage tubing, and to avoid lying on the tubing. Understanding how to manipulate the system when ambulating can give the client a sense of independence. Some clients also benefit from instruction about fluid intake measurement and perineal-genital care. Clients who wish to be involved in recording fluid intake measurements need information about how to compute these values and which foods are considered fluids.

Retention catheters are **removed** after their purpose has been achieved, usually on the order of the physician. A few days prior to removal the catheter may be clamped for specified periods of time (e.g., 2 to 4 hours) and then released. This causes some distention of the bladder and stimulation of the bladder musculature and may be ordered as "bladder training." See Procedure 41–7 for steps to remove a retention catheter.

GUIDELINES

Preventing Catheter-Associated Urinary Infections

Have an established infection control program.

Catheterize clients only when necessary, by using aseptic technique, sterile equipment, and trained personnel.

Maintain a sterile closed-drainage system.

Do not disconnect the catheter and drainage tubing unless absolutely necessary.

Remove the catheter as soon as possible.

Follow and reinforce good handwashing technique.

Changing indwelling catheters at arbitrary, fixed intervals and regular bacteriologic monitoring of catheterized clients are not cost-effective practices and should not be performed.

Avoid other measures until further data are available. New products that appear to be questionable or gimmicky probably should be avoided.

Although instillation of H_2O_2 into the outlet tube of the drainage set or into the drainage bags has been associated with a reduction in bag contamination, studies indicate no difference in the rate of bag-source infection in clients with the suggested instillation of H_2O_2 into the drainage bag when compared with clients who had conventional closed-drainage systems. (Epstein 1985)

PROCEDURE 41–7

Removing a Retention Catheter

Equipment

- A receptacle for the catheter after its removal, eg, a kidney basin.
- A syringe to deflate the balloon. A needle may also be required to deflate some types of balloons.
- Cotton balls to dry the genital area.
- Disposable gloves for the nurse.

Intervention

1. Don gloves.
2. Clamp the catheter.
   Rationale: This prevents spillage of urine that might remain in the catheter.
3. Insert the syringe into the balloon inflation tube of the catheter and draw out all the fluid.
   Rationale: The balloon needs to be completely deflated to prevent trauma to the urethra when the catheter is withdrawn.
4. Gently withdraw the catheter from the urethra.
5. Place the catheter in the kidney basin or other receptacle.
6. Dry the genital area with cotton balls.

7. Measure the urine in the drainage bag.
8. Record the time the catheter was removed and the amount, color, and consistency of the urine in the drainage bag.
9. Adjust the nursing care plan to
   a. Encourage the client to drink up to 3000 ml of fluid daily if not contraindicated.
   Rationale: If the urethra has been irritated by the catheter, the client may experience some burning when voiding. This problem is minimized by diluting the urine with an increased fluid intake.
   b. Monitor the client's fluid intake and output.
10. Assess the frequency of voiding, or any unusual symptoms related to voiding following the procedure. Prolonged, continuous drainage of urine through an indwelling catheter causes loss of bladder tone. The bladder remains relatively empty and thus is never stretched to its capacity. When a muscle fails to be stretched regularly, atrophy develops. When a catheter is removed, the client may have difficulty regaining urinary control.
11. Assess fluid intake and output following the removal of the catheter.

Sterile urine specimens can be obtained from closed drainage systems by inserting a sterile 1-in needle (#21 to #25 gauge), attached to a 3-ml syringe, into the end of the catheter or through a drainage port in the tubing. See Figure 41–22. Aspiration of urine from catheters can be done only with self-sealing rubber catheters, not plastic, silicone, or Silastic catheters.

First, the nurse dons gloves and cleans the entry point of the needle with a disinfectant swab. The needle is then inserted at an angle, to facilitate self-sealing, and at a place where it will not puncture the tube leading to the balloon. If the urine is not readily available, the drainage tubing is elevated slightly to return urine to the area or the catheter is pinched or clamped about 5 to 7 cm (3 in) from its tip for a short period until urine appears. After the urine is drawn into the syringe, the nurse transfers it to a sterile specimen container, caps the container, labels it, and sends it to the laboratory immediately for analysis or refrigeration.

Urinary Irrigations and Instillations

An **irrigation** is a flushing or washing out using a specified solution. A **bladder irrigation** is carried out on a physician's order, usually to wash out the bladder and/or apply an antiseptic solution to the bladder lining

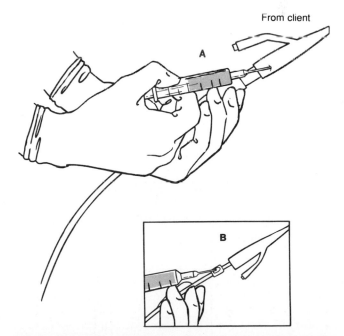

Figure 41–22 Obtaining a urine specimen from a retention catheter: **A,** from a specific area, sometimes designated by a patch, near the end of the catheter; **B,** from a drainage port in the tubing

to treat a bladder infection. Surgical aseptic technique is used. **Catheter irrigations** are usually carried out to maintain or restore the patency of a catheter, e.g., to remove pus or blood clots that have formed in the bladder and are blocking the catheter. A physician's order may or may not be required, depending on agency policy.

In a **bladder instillation,** a small amount of liquid is placed in the bladder and allowed to remain there for a specific period of time. For example, an antiseptic solution may be instilled through a catheter, which is then clamped for 30 minutes so that the antiseptic will remain in contact with the walls of the bladder. Bladder instillations and irrigations are not performed routinely because of the danger of transmitting microorganisms into the urinary bladder, but rather for specific therapeutic purposes.

For a bladder irrigation, the frequency and the type, amount, and strength of solution to be used are ordered by the physician. If the physician has not specified these on the client's chart, the nurse should check agency policies. Some agencies recommend the use of sterile normal saline at room temperature for both catheter and bladder irrigations. To irrigate an adult bladder, 1000 ml is commonly used; for a catheter irrigation, 200 ml is normally required. The strength, amount, and kind of medication for a bladder instillation are specified by the physician.

Intermittent bladder irrigations may be performed through the standard type of closed or open bladder drainage systems. A closed bladder or catheter irrigation is done to assess the patency of an indwelling catheter and to reestablish patency if the catheter is plugged by

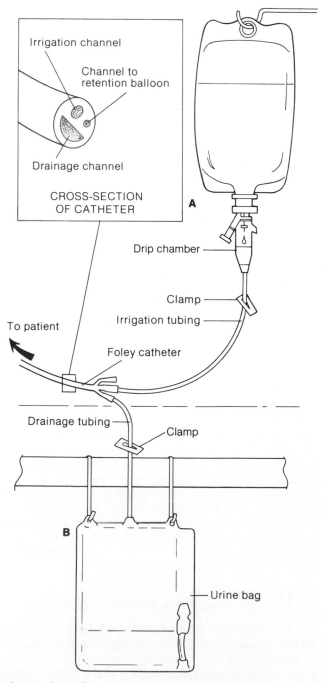

Figure 41–23

Figure 41–24 An intermittent bladder irrigation

mucus shreds or small calculi. Because the system is closed, the irrigating solution is instilled through an injection or irrigation port by using a syringe and needle. A medication can also be instilled into a closed system by this method. Medications are instilled to treat bladder infections.

Open bladder or catheter irrigations are performed by interrupting the drainage system temporarily, i.c., detaching the catheter at the tubing connection site. This procedure is also performed to assess patency of the catheter and to instill medications. In addition, it is also performed to remove clots and to relieve bladder spasms following surgery.

Intermittent bladder irrigations are often administered by attaching a Y-connector to a two-way Foley catheter. See Figure 41–23. When a Y-attachment is used, the stem of the Y is attached to the catheter; one arm of the Y is connected by tubing to a drip chamber and then to a container of sterile irrigation solution. The other arm is connected by tubing to a urine drainage bag. Continuous or intermittent bladder irrigations can also be administered via a triple lumen catheter. When a triple-lumen catheter is used, one lumen of the three-way catheter is connected by tubing to a drip chamber and then to a container of sterile solution. The second lumen is attached to tubing and then to a urine receptacle. See Figure 41–24. There are clamps on both tubes. For an intermittent irrigation, the clamp from the solution container (A) is released while the clamp to the urine bag (B) is closed. The fluid enters and remains in the bladder. The container tubing is then reclamped, and the urine receptacle tubing is unclamped, permitting the solution to flow out of the bladder. This process is carried out regularly. For continuous irrigations the flow of fluid leaving the solution container is carefully regulated and permitted to flow freely out of the bladder into the urine bag.

This type of irrigation system is used following bladder or prostate surgery to flush out blood clots. A mild hemostasis is also provided by the pressure from the irrigating fluid. Triple-lumen catheter irrigating systems are usually set up in the operating room. The nurse then monitors and maintains the system. Procedure 41–8 describes the steps involved in irrigating a catheter or bladder and instilling a medication into a bladder.

PROCEDURE 41–8

Irrigating a Catheter or a Bladder and Instilling Medication into a Bladder

Equipment

- Gloves for the nurse.

For using a syringe with a closed drainage system, a sterile irrigation or instillation set containing:

- A sterile container for the solution. Check that the container is large enough to hold the amount of fluid to be used.
- Absorbent cotton balls or gauze squares with a disinfectant.
- A drape to protect the bedding and to provide a sterile field.
- A standard syringe (30 or 50 ml) with a #18 or #19 gauge needle.
- The sterile irrigating solution or medication to be instilled into the bladder. Normal saline or antibiotic solutions are commonly used. The solution is generally room temperature, although warming it to body temperature makes it more comfortable for the client.
- A tubing clamp.
- A bath blanket.

For using a syringe with an open drainage system, the following additional equipment is required:

- A sterile drainage tube protector. The inside of a sterile foil package can be used if a protector is not available.
- A sterile Asepto or catheter syringe to instill the solution. The Asepto (or bulb) syringe is a plastic or glass syringe with a rubber bulb. See Figure 41–25, A. Bulb syringes come in different sizes, eg, 2 oz, 4 oz. The bulb pushes the solution into the catheter and can also be used to create suction for withdrawing the solution. A second type of syringe is the catheter syringe with an adapter tip. See Figure 41–25, B.
- A sterile drainage receptacle, if an irrigation is being performed.

For irrigations using a Y-connector and a two-way Foley catheter:

- A container of sterile irrigating solution.
- A sterile Y-connector, with sterile tubing to connect to the solution container, a drip chamber, and a clamp.
- An IV pole.
- Sterile drainage tubing, a clamp, and a drainage receptacle. The tubing connects the catheter to the drainage receptacle.
- A bath blanket.

For irrigations using a three-way Foley catheter:

- A container of sterile irrigating solution.
- Sterile irrigation tubing, a drip chamber, and a clamp.
- An IV pole.
- Sterile drainage tubing and a drainage bag. The tubing connects the catheter to the bag.
- A bath blanket.

of the three-way catheter is connected to the irrigation tubing and the other is connected to the drainage tubing. See Figure 41–24. In some closed systems, the tubings are already connected to the catheter.

45. Open the flow clamp on the drainage tubing.

46. Adjust the flow rate, using the clamp on the irrigation tubing, as specified by the physician. If the order does not specify, the rate should be 40–60 drops per minute.

47. Inspect the fluid returns for amount, color, and clarity. The amount of returning fluid should correspond to the amount of fluid entering the bladder.

48. Document all assessments and interventions.

Sample Recording

Date	Time	Notes
9/24/89	1900	Catheter irrigated with 200 ml normal saline at room temperature. Returns slightly blood-tinged with some small blood clots. Catheter running freely. No discomfort verbalized. ————— ————— Sandi R. Bailey, NS

Suprapubic Catheter Care

Suprapubic catheters, inserted through the abdominal wall above the **symphysis pubis** into the urinary bladder (see Figure 41–27), have the following advantages over urethral catheters:

1. They are associated with a lower rate of urinary tract infections.
2. They are more comfortable for the client.
3. They allow the opportunity to evaluate the client's ability to void normally; the client is asked to void normally when the suprapubic catheter is clamped. To assess the client's ability to void normally with a urethral catheter, you must first remove the catheter.
4. They facilitate evaluation of the client's residual urine.

The physician inserts the catheter using local anesthesia, in the client's bed unit, or using general anesthesia in conjunction with bladder or vaginal surgery, in the operating room. The catheter may be secured in place either with sutures or with a commercial retention body seal, or with both sutures and a body seal. It is then attached to a closed drainage system. When the catheter is removed, the muscle layers of the bladder contract over the insertion site to seal off the opening.

Two commonly used suprapubic catheters are the **Cystocath** and the **Bonanno** catheter. See Figure 41–28. These are narrow-lumen catheters with a curl at the distal end that prevents the catheter from being expelled by the bladder through the urethra. The Cystocath has a disc that holds the catheter in place on the abdominal wall; the Bonanno catheter has wings for that purpose. Attachments of the catheter to the drainage system tubing also vary: The Cystocath is joined with a stopcock; the Bonanno with a Luer-Lok adapter.

The most common problem with the suprapubic catheter is blockage of drainage due to sediment, clots, or the bladder wall itself obstructing the catheter or catheter tip. Dislodgement of the catheter and hematuria following the use of a large-bore catheter are less common problems. Care of clients with suprapubic catheters includes regular assessments of the client's urine, fluid intake, and comfort; maintenance of a patent drainage system; skin care around the insertion site; periodic clamping of the catheter preparatory to removing it; and measurement of residual urine. The physician's orders generally include leaving the catheter open to drainage for 48 to 72 hours then, clamping the catheter for 3- to 4-hour periods during the day until the client can void satisfactory amounts.

Satisfactory voiding is determined by measuring the client's residual urine after voiding. The client's urine needs to be assessed for color, consistency, clarity, and amount of urine drained, hourly for the first 24 hours and then at least three times daily. Fluid intake is carefully monitored to ensure it is adequate to maintain a satisfactory urine output. Bladder discomfort may occur because of bladder spasms, especially during the first 24 to 48 hours. Spasms are identified by the presence of intermittent pain that does not affect the amount of urinary output.

Patency of the drainage system is maintained in the same manner as an indwelling catheter urinary drainage system. Dressings around the suprapubic catheter are changed whenever they are soiled with drainage to pre-

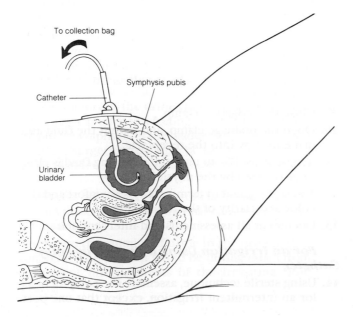

Figure 41–27 A suprapubic catheter in place

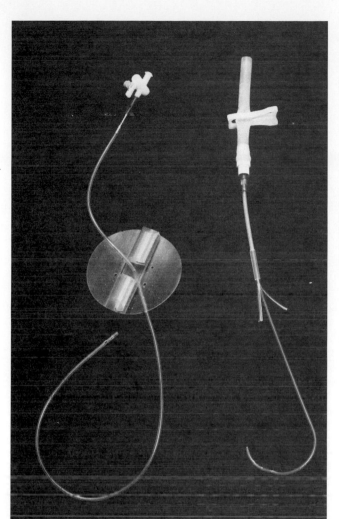

Figure 41–28 Two types of suprapubic catheters: a Cystocath (left) and a Bonanno (right)

vent bacterial growth around the insertion site and reduce the potential for infection. Procedures for cleaning wounds and changing dressings are discussed in Chapter 45. Any redness and discharge at the skin around the insertion site must be reported.

To ascertain the residual urine, the nurse first closes suprapubic catheter with a clamp for 2 to 4 hours. The client then voids by the normal route, emptying the bladder as completely as possible. After this the residual urine is obtained by releasing the suprapubic catheter and allowing any remaining urine to drain into the drainage bag. Both the amount of urine voided and the amount of residual urine are measured. If the client can void a satisfactory amount (e.g., 150 to 350 ml) and the residual urine is less than 50 to 100 ml (or a volume specified by the physician), the catheter is removed.

To remove a suprapubic catheter, the nurse first removes the dressing and any sutures holding the catheter in place. Suture removal is described in Chapter 45. The nurse then removes the catheter with a steady, continuous pull, applies pressure over the insertion site with gauze squares, cleans the site with antiseptic solution or swabs, and applies povidone-iodine ointment and an Elastoplast bandage.

OUTCOME CRITERIA

Urinary Problems

The client will have:

- Normal color, odor, and consistency of urine
- A residual urine of 30 ml
- A urinary output in balance with fluid intake
- Intact skin around the urinary meatus and perineum
- Intact skin under condom appliance
- A negative urine culture
- No dysuria or frequency
- Urinary pH of less than 5.5
- Absence of signs of fluid or electrolyte imbalance
- Urinary output of at least 1500 ml/day
- Fluid intake of at least 2500 ml/day

Evaluating Client Responses

Examples of outcome criteria to evaluate the client's goal achievement and the effectiveness of nursing interventions are shown in the accompanying box.

Chapter Highlights

- Urinary elimination depends on normal functioning of the urinary, cardiovascular, and nervous systems.
- The normal process of micturition includes sufficient accumulation of urine in the bladder to stimulate the sensory stretch nerves in the bladder wall. Impulses from these stretch receptors then travel to the spinal cord to the voiding reflex center and to the voiding control center in the cerebral cortex, where conscious control of micturition is regulated.
- In the adult, micturition generally occurs after 250 to 450 ml of urine has collected in the bladder.
- Many factors influence a person's urinary elimination, including fluid intake, stress, activity, diuretics, and various diseases.
- When assessing a person's urinary function, the nurse needs to systematically consider patterns of urination, problems with urinary elimination and influencing factors, physical assessment data, characteristics of the urine, past illnesses or surgery, and data obtained from diagnostic tests and examinations.
- Nursing diagnoses that relate to urinary tract function and urinary patterns include specific problems of urination and associated problems (e.g., potential for infection, impaired skin integrity).
- Incontinence can be physically and emotionally distressing to clients because it is considered socially unacceptable.
- Clients who have urinary retention not only experience discomfort but are also at risk of urinary tract infection.

■ The most common cause of urinary tract infection are invasive procedures such as catheterization and cystoscopic examination.

■ Females in particular are prone to ascending urinary tract infections because of their short urethras.

■ Nursing interventions related to urinary elimination are generally directed toward facilitating the normal functioning of the urinary system or toward assisting the client with particular problems.

■ Interventions include assisting the client to maintain an appropriate fluid intake and normal voiding patterns, monitoring the client's daily fluid intake and output, and maintaining cleanliness of the genital area.

■ Urinary catheterization (a sterile technique) is frequently required for clients with urinary retention but is performed only when all other measures to facilitate voiding fail.

■ Care of clients with indwelling catheters is directed toward preventing infection of the urinary tract and encouraging urinary flow through the drainage system.

Selected References

Birdsall, C. November 1985. How do you teach female self-catheterization? *American Journal of Nursing* 85:1226–27.

Byrne, C. J.; Saxton, D. F., Pelikan, P. K.; and Nugent, P. M. 1986. *Laboratory tests: Implications for nursing care.* 2d ed. Menlo Park, Calif. Addison-Wesley.

Carpenito, L. J. 1987. *Nursing Diagnosis,* 2d ed. Philadelphia: J. B. Lippincott.

Epstein, S. E. December 1985. Cost-effective application of the Centers for Disease Control Guideline for prevention of catheter-associated urinary tract infections. *American Journal of Infection Control* 13:272–75.

Frye, S., and Melman, A. January 15, 1985. Urinary tract infection: Aspects of asymptomatic UTI in elderly patients. *Consultant* 25:51–2, 62–3.

Greengold, B. A., and Ouslander, J. G. June 1986. Bladder retraining: Program for elderly patients with post-indwelling catheterization. *Journal of Gerontological Nursing* 12:31–35.

Gurevich, I. July 1985. Selection of closed urinary drainage systems—an update. *Infection Control* 6:289–90.

Guyton, A. C. 1986. *Textbook of Medical Physiology,* 7th ed. Philadelphia: W. B. Saunders Co.

Hart, J. A. 1985. The urethral catheter: A review of its implication in urinary tract infection. *International Journal of Nursing Studies* 22(1):57–59.

Hart, M., and Adamek, C. July/August 1984. Do increased fluids decrease urinary stone formation? *Geriatric Nursing* 5:245–48.

Kniep-Hardy, M. J.; Votava, K.; and Stubbings, M. J. September/October 1985. Managing indwelling catheters in the home. *Geriatric Nursing* 6:280–85.

Long, M. L. January 1985. Incontinence: Defining the nursing role. *Journal of Gerontological Nursing* 11:30–35, 41.

McConnell, J. November/December 1984. Preventing urinary tract infections. *Geriatric Nursing* 5:361–62.

McConnell, E. A., and Zimmerman, M. I. 1983. *Care of patients with urologic problems.* Philadelphia: J. B. Lippincott.

Richard, C. J. 1986. *Comprehensive nephrology nursing.* Boston: Little, Brown & Co.

Simons, J. June 1985. Does incontinence affect your client's self-concept? *Journal of Gerontological Nursing* 11:37–40, 42.

Voith, A. M., and Smith, D. A. December 1985. Validation of the nursing diagnosis of urinary retention. *Nursing Clinics of North America* 20:723–29.

Whaley, L. F., and Wong, D. L. 1987. *Nursing care of infants and children,* 3d ed. St. Louis: C. V. Mosby Co.

CHAPTER 42

Oxygenation

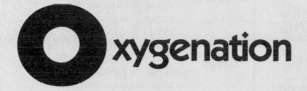

OBJECTIVES

Explain the three phases of respiration.

Describe the basic mechanics of breathing.

Identify the requirements of adequate ventilation.

Explain mechanisms regulating the respiratory process.

Describe factors that influence the rate of diffusion of gases through the respiratory membrane.

Explain how oxygen is transported to the tissues and how carbon dioxide is transported from the tissues.

Identify factors influencing respiratory and circulatory function.

Describe clinical signs of hypoxia.

Describe common altered breathing patterns.

List the signs of an obstructed airway.

Identify common responses to alterations in respiratory and circulatory status.

Describe positions that facilitate oxygenation.

Explain the importance of hydration in promoting adequate oxygenation.

Describe the use of selected inhalation therapy devices and practices.

Explain oropharyngeal and nasopharyngeal suctioning.

Describe various methods to administer oxygen.

Compare administering oxygen therapy by nasal cannula, nasal catheter, and face mask.

State outcome criteria for evaluating client responses to implemented measures to promote adequate oxygenation.

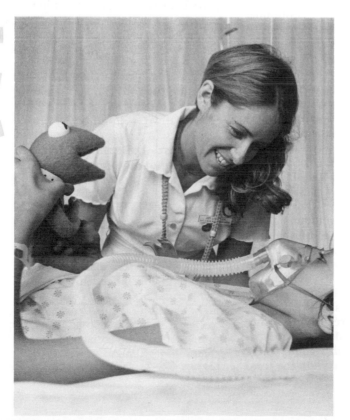

Terms Describing Oxygenation Status Breathing Patterns

Rate

- *Eupnea*—normal respiration that is quiet, rhythmic, and effortless
- *Tachypnea*—rapid respiration marked by quick, shallow breaths
- *Bradypnea*—abnormally slow breathing
- *Apnea*—cessation of breathing

Volume

- *Hyperventilation*—an increase in the amount of air in the lungs characterized by prolonged and deep breaths; may be associated with anxiety
- *Hypoventilation*—a reduction in the amount of air in the lungs; characterized by shallow respirations

Rhythm

- *Cheyne-Stokes breathing*—rhythmic waxing and waning of respirations, from very deep to very shallow breathing and temporary apnea; often associated with cardiac failure, increased intracranial pressure, or brain damage

Ease or Effort

- *Dyspnea*—difficult and labored breathing during which the individual has a persistent, unsatisfied need for air and feels distressed
- *Orthopnea*—ability to breathe only in upright sitting or standing positions

Breath Sounds

Audible without amplification

- *Stridor*—a shrill, harsh sound heard during inspiration with laryngeal obstruction
- *Stertor*—snoring or sonorous respiration, usually due to a partial obstruction of the upper airway
- *Wheeze*—a whistling respiratory sound on expiration that usually indicates a narrowing of the bronchial tree
- *Bubbling*—gurgling sounds heard as air passes through moist secretions in the respiratory tract

Audible by stethoscope

- *Rales*—rattling or bubbling sounds generally heard on inspiration as air moves through accumulated moist secretions
- *Rhonchi*—coarse, dry, wheezy, or whistling sound more audible during expiration as the air moves through tenacious mucus or narrowed bronchi
- *Creps* (crepitation)—a dry, crackling sound (like crumpled cellophane) produced by air in the subcutaneous tissue or by air moving through fluid in the alveoli
- *Pleural rub*—coarse, leathery, or grating sound produced by the rubbing together of the pleura; also called *friction rub*

Chest Movements

- *Intercostal retraction*—indrawing between the ribs
- *Substernal restraction*—indrawing beneath the breast bone
- *Suprasternal retraction*—indrawing above the breast bone
- *Supraclavicular retraction*—indrawing above the clavicles
- *Tracheal tug*—indrawing and downward pull of the trachea during inspiration
- *Flail chest*—the ballooning out of the chest wall through injured rib spaces; results in *paradoxical breathing,* during which the chest wall balloons on expiration but is depressed or sucked inward on inspiration

Secretions and Coughing

- *Hemoptysis*—the presence of blood in the sputum
- *Productive cough*—a cough accompanied by expectorated secretions
- *Nonproductive cough*—a dry, harsh cough without secretions

---

Which of the client's activities might cause these symptoms to occur?

2. *History of respiratory diseases.* Has the client had colds, asthma, croup, bronchitis, or pneumonia? How frequently have these occurred? How long did they last? How were they treated?
3. *The presence of a cough.* Is it productive (accompanied by expectorated secretions) or nonproductive? To **expectorate** is to cough and spit out secretions from the lungs, bronchi, and trachea. When a cough is productive, the nurse should question the client about the sputum: When is sputum produced? What is the amount, color, thickness, and odor?
4. *Life-style.* Does the client smoke? If so, how much? Does any member of the client's family smoke?
5. *Cardiovascular problems.* Does the client have a history of cardiac or blood circulation problems?
6. *Pain.* Does the client experience any pain associated with breathing or activity? Pain that is a result of activity may reflect a cardiovascular problem. Pain associated with breathing can indicate infections of the lungs or pleura, injured ribs, and trauma to the chest muscles.
7. *Risk factors.* Are any risk factors that can impair

oxygenation present? Some of these are family history of hypertension, obesity, sedentary life-style, and diet high in saturated fats.

8. *Medication history.* Has the client taken or does the client take any over-the-counter or prescription medications for heart, blood pressure, or breathing? Which ones? What are the dosages, times taken, and effects on the client, including side effects?

9. *Stressors.* What stressors exist in the client's life? For example, having an alcoholic partner, having to commute long distances to work each day, or working two jobs.

10. *Health status.* How does the client perceive his or her health status? Even though a client may present numerous problems, he or she may consider himself or herself to be well or even healthier than in previous years.

11. *Developmental status.* What activities does the client enjoy? Do alterations in respiratory function interfere with these activities? Can adaptations be made?

12. *Strengths.* What are the client's strengths at this time? For instance, does the client have any insight into his or her health problems? Does he or she comply with therapeutic regimens?

▪ Physical Assessment

In assessing a client's oxygenation status the nurse uses all four physical assessment techniques: inspection, palpation, percussion, and auscultation. She or he first observes the rate, depth, rhythm, and quality of respirations. The position the client assumes for breathing should be noted. Some clients with chronic respiratory problems prefer to bend forward at the waist to ease breathing or to sit leaning over a table because these positions permit greater lung expansion. Lying on the back or on either side restricts expansion of part of the thorax (the underlying portion). This relatively small increase in expansion may be important to a dyspneic client. Chapter 31 provides additional information on assessing respirations.

Variations in the **shape** of the thorax may indicate adaptation to chronic respiratory conditions. For example, clients with emphysema frequently develop a *barrel chest.* See Figure 32–31 on page 446 for an illustration of variations in the shape of the chest. The lungs and heart should be assessed very carefully. See Procedure 32–1 (pages 465–466) and Procedure 32–3 (pages 457–460) for guidelines.

▪ Diagnostic Procedures

The physician may order specific diagnostic tests to assess oxygenation. Among the more common are sputum specimens. Often it is a nurse who collects the specimens that are sent to the laboratory for analysis. **Sputum** is the mucus secretion from the lungs, bronchi, and trachea. It is important to differentiate it from *saliva,* the clear liquid secreted by the salivary glands in the mouth. Healthy individuals do not produce sputum. Clients need to cough to bring sputum up from the lungs, bronchi, and trachea into the mouth and then expectorate it into a collecting container. **Sputum specimens** are usually collected for one or more of the following reasons:

1. For *culture and sensitivity* to identify a specific microorganism and its drug sensitivities.

2. For *cytology* to identify the origin, structure, function, and pathology of cells. Specimens for cytology often require serial collection of three early morning specimens and are tested to identify cancer in the lung and its specific cell type.

3. For *acid-fast bacillus* (AFB), which also require serial collection, often for 3 consecutive days, to identify the presence of tuberculosis (TB). Some agencies use a special glass container when the presence of AFB is suspected.

4. To assess the *effectiveness of therapy.* Sputum specimens are often collected in the morning. Upon awakening, the client can cough up the secretions that have accumulated during the night. Sometimes specimens are collected during postural drainage, when the client can usually produce sputum. When a client cannot cough, the nurse must sometimes use pharyngeal suctioning to obtain a specimen.

To **collect a sputum specimen,** the nurse should have the client breathe deeply and cough up 1 to 2 tablespoons of sputum (15 to 30 ml, or 4 to 8 fluid drams). The client then expectorates into the specimen container, taking care that the sputum does not contact the outside of the container (see Figure 42–3). If the outside of the container becomes soiled, the nurse washes it with a disinfectant. The nurse's hands should be gloved to avoid direct contact with the client's sputum. The client might want to use a mouthwash after producing the specimen, to remove any unpleasant taste. When

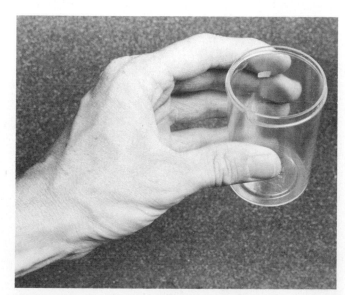

Figure 42–3 Sputum specimen container

recording the collection of the sputum specimen, the nurse should note the amount, color, odor, consistency (thick, tenacious, watery, etc.), and the presence of blood (hemoptysis). Normal sputum often contains the same kinds of microorganisms found in the upper respiratory passages. The normal flora found in sputum are listed in the accompanying box.

Measurement of **arterial blood gases** is another important diagnostic procedure. Specimens of arterial blood are normally taken by specialty nurses or medical technicians. Arterial blood is often tested for partial pressure of oxygen (PaO_2), partial pressure of carbon dioxide ($PaCO_2$), oxygen saturation (SO_2 or O_2Sat), hydrogen ion concentration (pH), and the amount of bicarbonate (HCO_3^-), and base excess (BE). Blood for these tests is taken from the radial, brachial, or femoral arteries. Because of the relatively great pressure of the blood in these arteries, it is important to prevent hemorrhaging by applying pressure to the puncture site for about 5 minutes after removing the needle.

Pulmonary function tests measure lung volume and capacity, discussed earlier in this chapter. Clients undergoing pulmonary function tests, which are usually carried out by a respiratory therapist, do not require an anesthetic. The client breathes into a machine. The tests are painless, but the client's cooperation is essential. Nurses need to explain the tests to people beforehand and help clients to get rest afterward, because the tests are often tiring.

Nursing Diagnoses for Clients with Respiratory Problems

Five main categories of nursing diagnoses relate to oxygenation: impaired gas exchange, ineffective airway clearance, ineffective breathing patterns, alterations in cardiac output, and impaired tissue perfusion. See the accompanying box for examples of nursing diagnoses

NURSING DIAGNOSIS

Oxygenation

- Alterations in respiratory function related to pain secondary to abdominal incision
- Alterations in respiratory function related to smoking 2 to 3 packs of cigarettes for 15 years
- Alterations in respiratory function related to allergy to unknown pollens
- Ineffective airway clearance related to ineffective coughing
- Ineffective airway clearance related to fear of pain
- Ineffective breathing pattern related to activity
- Alterations in cardiac output related to anemia
- Alterations in cardiac output related to medications

Normal Flora of Sputum

Bacteria

- *Bacteroides* species
- *Borrelia* species
- *Corynebacterium diphtheriae*
- *Fusobacterium* species
- *Haemophilus influenzae*
- *Neisseria catarrhalis*
- *Staphylococcus aureus*
- *Staphylococcus epidermidis*
- *Streptococcus* species (groups A, B, D)
- *Streptococcus pneumoniae*
- *Streptococcus viridans*

Fungi

- *Candida albicans* (Byrne et al. 1986, p. 513)

related to oxygenation. When clients are in acute distress (i.e., have life-threatening conditions that impair breathing or circulation of oxygenated blood), the nurse usually intervenes in collaboration with other health team members; thus, the client's health problems are termed collaborative or clinical problems, rather than nursing diagnoses in the strictest sense (i.e., problems that the nurse can address independently).

Planning Care to Modify Alterations in Respiratory Function

Planning for a client's actual or potential oxygenation problems involves facilitating pulmonary ventilation, the diffusion of gases, and the transport of oxygen and carbon dioxide. *Facilitating pulmonary ventilation* may include ensuring a patent airway, positioning, encouraging deep breathing and coughing, and ensuring adequate hydration. Other nursing interventions helpful to ventilation are suctioning, lung inflation techniques, postural drainage, and percussion and vibration. Nursing strategies to *facilitate the diffusion of gases* through the alveolar membrane include encouraging coughing, deep breathing, and suitable activity. To *promote the transport of oxygen and carbon dioxide,* the nurse can optimze cardiac output by reducing stress, planning appropriate activities, and positioning the client for improved vascular blood flow. A client's nursing care plan should also include appropriate dependent nursing interventions such as oxygen therapy, tracheostomy care, and maintenance of a chest tube.

Implementing Nursing Strategies

Positioning

Normally, adequate ventilation is maintained by frequent changes of position, ambulation, and exercise. In ill persons, however, respiratory functions may be inhibited for a variety of reasons. One common reason is immobility secondary to surgery or medical therapy. Lying too long in one position compresses the thorax, limits chest expansion, and thus inhibits the movement of air through the lungs. Sitting in a slumped position also inhibits chest expansion, since the abdominal contents are pushed up against the diaphragm. Another frequent cause of limited chest expansion is abdominal or chest pain. The client often voluntarily limits chest movements to relieve the pain.

Shallow respirations inhibit both diaphragmatic excursion and lung distensibility. The result of inadequate chest expansion is stasis and pooling of respiratory secretions, which ultimately harbor microorganisms and promote infection. This situation is often compounded in the hospitalized client who receives narcotics for pain, because narcotics further depress the rate and depth of respiration. Interventions by the nurse to **maintain the normal respirations** of clients include:

1. Positioning the client to allow for maximum chest expansion
2. Encouraging or providing frequent changes in position
3. Encouraging ambulation
4. Implementing measures that promote comfort, such as giving pain medications

The semi-Fowler's or high-Fowler's position allows maximum chest expansion in bedfast clients, particularly dyspneic clients. The nurse encourages clients who cannot assume this position to turn from side to side frequently, so that alternate sides of the chest are permitted maximum expansion. In the hospital, dyspneic clients often sit in bed and lean over their overbed tables (which are raised to a suitable height), usually with a pillow for support. This *orthopneic position* is an adaptation of the high-Fowler's position. It has a further advantage in that, unlike in high-Fowler's, the abdominal organs are not pressing on the diaphragm. Also, a client in the orthopneic position can press the lower part of the chest against the table to help in exhaling.

Deep Breathing and Coughing

In addition to positioning clients, the nurse can facilitate respiratory functioning by encouraging deep-breathing exercises and coughing to remove secretions. Breathing exercises are frequently indicated for clients with restricted chest expansion, e.g., people with chronic obstructive pulmonary disease (COPD) or clients recovering from thoracic surgery. Commonly employed breathing exercises are abdominal (diaphragmatic) and pursed-lip breathing, apical expansion, and basal expansion exercises.

Abdominal (diaphragmatic) breathing permits deep full breaths with little effort. After positioning the client for comfort in supine and semi-Fowler's positions with knees flexed (to help relax the abdominal muscles), the nurse should instruct the client to:

1. Breathe in deeply through the nose
2. Keep the mouth closed
3. Concentrate on feeling the abdomen rise as far as possible

The nurse may have to remind the client to stay relaxed and not to arch the back. When the diaphragm contracts, the chest cavity expands and the lungs fill with air. See Figure 42–1 on page 712. When properly performed, the client's abdomen should rise. If the client has difficulty raising the abdomen, the nurse should ask him or her to take a quick, forceful inhalation through the nose.

Next, the nurse should have the client purse the lips as if about to whistle and to breathe out slowly and gently, tightening the abdominal muscles to exhale more effectively. Pursing the lips creates a resistance to air flowing out of the lungs, increases pressure within the bronchi, and minimizes the collapse of smaller bronchioles, a common problem for clients with COPD. Regular practice of *pursed-lip breathing* enables the client to do this type of breathing without conscious effort and is an effective adaptive breathing technique for clients with COPD.

Apical expansion exercises are often required for clients who restrict their upper chest movement because of pain. The nurse instructs the client to concentrate on expanding the upper chest forward and upward while inhaling. This helps aerate the apical areas of the upper lung lobes. To promote aeration of the alveoli, the nurse encourages the client to hold the inhalation for a few seconds before slowly, quietly, and passively exhaling through the mouth or nose. Performing this exercise several times a day helps to re-expand lung tissue, move secretions to promote effective elimination, and minimize flattening of the upper chest wall from disuse.

When clients restrict lower chest movements because of pain due to disease or surgery, **basal expansion exercises** should be explained and encouraged. The nurse instructs the client to concentrate on moving the lower chest outward upon inhalation and then to slowly, quietly, and passively exhale. If the client appears to be having difficulty exhaling, or if there is an indrawing of the upper chest upon exhalation, the nurse should have the client do pursed-lip exhalation.

Hydration

Adequate hydration maintains the moisture of the respiratory mucous membranes. Normally, respiratory tract secretions are thin and therefore moved readily by ciliary action. However, when the client is dehydrated or when the environment has a low humidity,

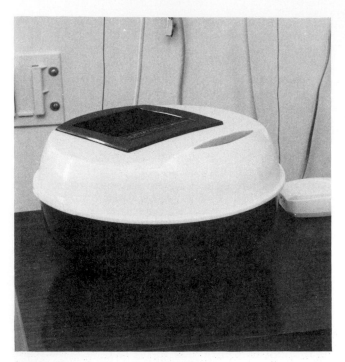

Figure 42–4 A room humidifier

the respiratory secretions can become thick and tenacious. The mucous membranes then become irritated and prone to infection. Nursing measures to increase and monitor fluid intake thus assume a high priority when providing care. Appropriate measures are discussed in Chapter 43.

Humidifiers are devices that add water vapor to inspired air. Their purposes are to prevent mucous membranes from drying and becoming irritated and to loosen secretions for easier expectoration. All humidifiers employ the simple method of passing the gas through distilled water so that water vapor is picked up before the gas reaches the client. The more bubbles created during this process, the more water vapor is produced. Some humidifiers heat the water vapor, which increases the humidity provided. Three main types are the room humidifier (ordinarily for home use), the cascade humidifier, and the cold bubble diffuser (humidifier).

A *room humidifier* (see Figure 42–4) can provide either cool mist or steam. Some types can be used with gas lines, e.g., oxygen, to provide moistened air directly to the client. A *cascade humidifier* can deliver 100% humidity at body temperature. The temperature of the vapor can be controlled, and the machine can be used to provide humidified oxygen to clients on ventilators.

A *cold bubble diffuser* or *humidifier* (see Figure 42–5) is used with all oxygen equipment to moisten the oxygen before it is inhaled. This device provides 20 to 40% humidity. The oxygen passes through sterile distilled water and then along a line to the device through which the moistened oxygen is inhaled (e.g., a cannula, nasal catheter, or oxygen mask). A *nebulizer* is used to deliver a fine spray of medication or moisture to a client. **Nebulization** is the production of a fog or mist.

There are two kinds of neubulization: atomization and aerosolization. In *atomization,* a device called an *atomizer* produces rather large droplets for inhalation. When the droplets are suspended in a gas, such as oxygen, the process is **inhalation** (aerosol) **therapy.** The smaller the droplets, the further they can be inhaled into the respiratory tract. When a medication is intended for the nasal mucosa, it is inhaled through the nose; when it is intended for the trachea, bronchi, and/or lungs, it is inhaled through the mouth.

A *large-volume nebulizer* can provide a heated or cool mist. It is used for long-term therapy, such as that following a tracheostomy. These nebulizers have a 250-ml capacity and deliver oxygen or room air. The *ultrasonic nebulizer* (see Figure 42–6) provides 100% humidity and can provide particles small enough to be inhaled deeply into the respiratory tract. There are two types of ultrasonic nebulizers: one has a cup that is filled with sterile distilled water; the other requires a continuous supply of sterile distilled water from a bag connected by tubing to the nebulizer bottle.

The *hand nebulizer* (see Figure 42–7) is a container of medication that can be compressed by hand to release the medication through a nosepiece or mouthpiece. The force with which the air moves through the nebulizer causes the large particles of medicated solution to break up into finer particles, forming a mist or fine spray. The *mini-nebulizer* is used with oxygen or a pressurized gas source, e.g., air. With this device, the

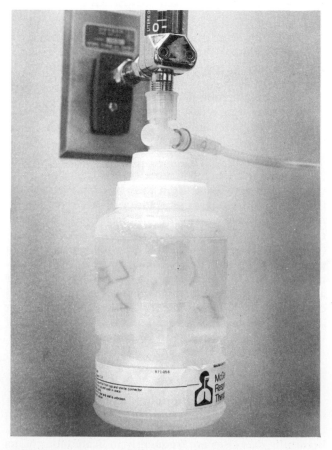

Figure 42–5 A cold bubble humidifier

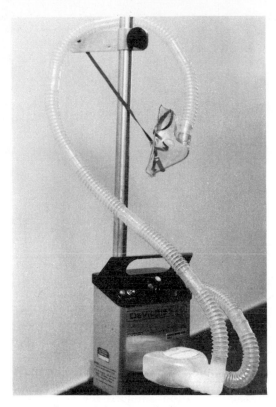

Figure 42—6   An ultrasonic nebulizer

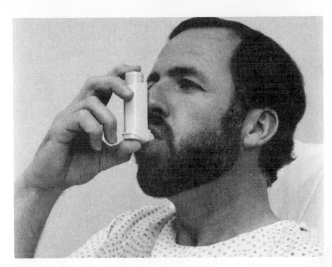

Figure 42—7   A hand nebulizer

client inhales and exhales independently. Medication is administered during inhalation. A *side-stream nebulizer* provides a medication to a client on a ventilator or receiving intermittent positive pressure breathing (IPPB) therapy. The gas, e.g., oxygen, passes through a device containing the medicated solution and then into the ventilator and to the client.

▪ Lung Inflation Devices

Lung inflation devices are used to:

1. Improve pulmonary ventilation
2. Counteract the effects of anesthesia and/or hypoventilation
3. Loosen respiratory secretions
4. Facilitate respiratory gaseous exchange
5. Expand collapsed alveoli

There are three types: blow bottles, sustained maximal inspiration (SMI) devices, and volume-oriented SMIs. *Blow bottles,* two bottles half-filled with water and connected by tubing, provide feedback about a client's respiratory *exhalation.* The client moves the water from one bottle to the other by blowing into a short tube connected to the first bottle. See Figure 42—8. Lung inflation is encouraged by the deep breath the client must take before blowing into the bottle. After the client transfers the fluid from the first bottle, the set is reversed, and the procedure is repeated.

Sustained maximal inspiration devices measure the flow of air inhaled through the mouthpiece. They there-

fore offer an incentive to improve inhalation and may also be referred to as **incentive inspirometers.** Two general types are the flow-oriented spirometer and the volume-oriented spirometer. The *flow-oriented SMI* consists of one or more clear plastic chambers that contain freely movable colored balls or discs. The balls or discs rise in the chamber as the client inhales. The client is asked to keep them elevated as long as possible with a maximal sustained inhalation. Figure 42—9 shows a

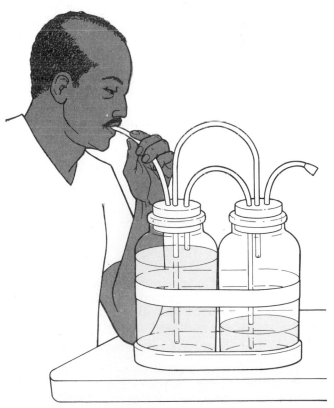

Figure 42—8   Blow bottles

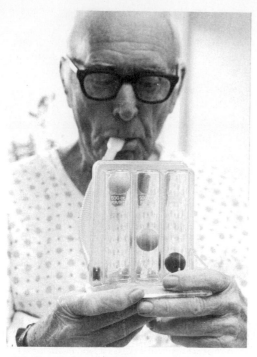

Figure 42–9 Sustained maximal inspiration device

Triflo II SMI. Flow-oriented SMIs are low-cost devices, are often disposable, and can be used independently by clients. They do not measure the specific volume of air inhaled, however.

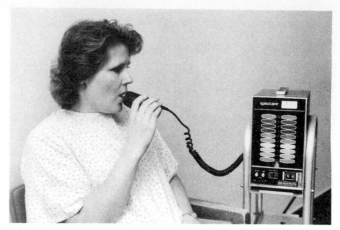

Figure 42–10 Volume-oriented SMI

The more expensive *volume-oriented SMIs* precisely measure the inhalation volume maintained by the client. These devices contain pistons or bellows that are raised by the client's inhalation to a predetermined volume. Some volume-oriented devices are designed with an achievement counter or light. The light will not turn on until the inspiration is held at the minimum predetermined volume for a specified time period. See Figure 42–10. Assisting clients to use these devices to promote lung inflation is explained in Procedure 42–1.

PROCEDURE 42–1

Teaching the Use of Lung Inflation Devices

Equipment
- Blow bottles
  or
- A flow-oriented SMI
  or
- A volume-oriented SMI
- A mouthpiece or breathing tube
- A nose clip (optional)

Intervention

1. Assist the client to an upright sitting position in bed or in a chair. If the person is unable to assume a sitting position for a flow spirometer, have the person assume any position.

   Rationale: A sitting position facilitates maximum ventilation.

For Blow Bottles

2. Instruct the client to
   a. Take in a slow, deep breath.

Rationale: A deep breath ensures maximum inflation of the alveoli, which facilitates gaseous exchange.

b. Seal the lips tightly around the mouthpiece, exhale slowly and steadily as long as possible into the bottle, and concentrate on moving the fluid from one bottle to the other.

Rationale: A tight lip seal prevents leakage of exhaled air outside the mouthpiece and ensures adequate movement and measurement of the fluid. As the client exhales, pressure in the bottle is increased and displaces the water with air. A prolonged exhalation against resistance creates an increase in alveolar pressure, reexpanding collapsed alveoli, preventing atelectasis (collapse of the lung), and strengthening the muscles of expiration.

c. Establish a goal of moving a certain portion of water into the second bottle with each exhalation (eg, one-quarter, one-third, one-half, or three-quarters). Provide practice periods about five times every hour, and set progressive increases in the volume of fluid to be moved.

Rationale: Initially, a client may be unable to move the entire contents of one bottle to the other with one breath. The nurse and the client need to establish realistic goals. Practice helps to increase the expiratory volume.

For a Flow-Oriented SMI

3. If the spirometer has an inspiratory volume-level pointer, set the pointer at the prescribed level. Check the physician's or respiratory therapist's order.
4. Instruct the client to
   a. Hold the spirometer in the upright position.
   Rationale: A tilted spirometer requires less effort to raise the balls or discs.

   b. Exhale normally.
   c. Seal the lips tightly around the mouthpiece; take in a slow deep breath to elevate the balls; and then hold the breath for 2 seconds initially, increasing to 6 seconds (optimum), to keep the balls elevated if possible. Instruct the client to avoid brisk low-volume breaths that snap the balls to the top of the chamber. The client may use a noseclip if the person has difficulty breathing only through the mouth.

   Rationale: A slow deep breath ensures maximal ventilation. Greater lung expansion is achieved with a very slow inspiration than with a brisk shallow breath, even though a slow inspiration may not elevate or keep the balls elevated while the client holds the breath (Luce, Tyler, and Pierson 1984). Sustained elevation of the balls ensures adequate alveolar ventilation.

   d. Remove the mouthpiece, and exhale normally.
   e. Cough productively, if possible, after using the spirometer.
   Rationale: Deep ventilation may loosen secretions, and coughing can facilitate their removal.

   f. Relax, and take several normal breaths before using the spirometer again.
   g. Repeat the procedure several times and then four or five times hourly.
   Rationale: Practice increases inspiratory volume, maintains alveolar ventilation, and prevents atelectasis.

For a Volume-Oriented SMI

5. Set the spirometer to the predetermined volume. Volume ranges vary from 0 to 5000 ml, depending on the type of spirometer. Check the physician's or respiratory therapist's order.
6. Since some SMIs are battery-operated, ensure that the spirometer is functioning. Place the device on the client's bedside table.
7. Instruct the client to
   a. Exhale normally.
   b. Seal the lips tightly around the mouthpiece, and take in a slow deep breath, until the piston is elevated to the present level. The piston level may be visible to the client or lights or the word "Hold" may be illuminated to identify the volume obtained.
   c. Hold the breath for 6 seconds to ensure maximal alveolar ventilation.
   d. Remove the mouthpiece, and exhale normally.
   e. Follow steps 4e–g.

For All Devices

8. Clean the mouthpiece with sterile water and shake it dry. Label the mouthpiece and a disposable SMI with the client's name, and store them in the bedside unit. Only the mouthpiece of a volume SMI is stored with the client, since volume SMIs are used by many clients. Disposable mouthpieces are changed every 24 hours.
9. Auscultate the client's lungs to compare with the baseline data.
10. Document the technique, including type of spirometer, number of breaths taken, volume or flow levels achieved, and results of auscultation. For a flow SMI, calculate the volume achieved by multiplying the setting by the length of time the client kept the balls elevated. For example, if the setting was 500 ml, and the balls were kept suspended for 2 seconds, the volume is 500 × 2, or 1000 ml. For a volume SMI, take the volume directly from the spirometer, eg, 1500 ml.

Sample Recording

Date	Time	Notes
7/6/89	1100	Instructed in use of Triflo II spirometer. 5 breaths taken at volume of 1,000 ml (500 ml × 2 sec). Bilateral breath sounds normal on auscultation before and after spirometry. ——————— — Nicholas Coscos, SN

Intermittent positive pressure breathing (IBBP) is a lung inflation technique for delivering air or oxygen into the lungs at positive (above atmospheric) pressure during inspiration and automatic releasing of the pressure when the predetermined positive pressure level is reached in the air passages. Thus, expiration occurs passively. Use of IPPB therapy has decreased since the advent of incentive spirometers. Advocates of IPPB therapy, however, believe that IPPB devices are more effective in expanding the lungs, moving secretions, promoting coughing, and delivering aerosol medications into the deeper, smaller air passages. Also, they require less effort by the client, and so they are prescribed for selected clients. Usually, IPPB treatments are given by respiratory

c. Don the sterile gloves or don a nonsterile glove on the nondominant hand and then a sterile glove on the dominant hand.

Rationale: The sterile gloved hand maintains the sterility of the suction catheter and the unsterile glove prevents the transmission of microorganisms to the nurse.

7. With your sterile gloved hand, pick up the catheter, and attach it to the suction unit. See Figure 42–13.

8. Make an approximate measure of the depth for the insertion. Mark the position on the tube with the fingers of the sterile gloved hand. An appropriate measure is the distance between the tip of the client's nose and the earlobe, or about 13 cm (5 in.) for an adult.

9. Moisten the catheter tip by dipping it in the container of sterile water or saline.

Rationale: Moistening reduces friction and eases insertion.

10. Test the suction and the patency of the catheter by applying your finger or thumb to the port or open branch of the Y-connector (the suction control) to create suction.

11. For a nasopharyngeal suction, insert the catheter gently through one nostril with your thumb away from the suction control (ie, not applying suction). Direct the catheter along the floor of the nasal cavity. If one nostril is obstructed, try the other. Never force the catheter against an obstruction.

or

For an oropharyngeal suction, insert the catheter through the mouth along one side into the oropharynx, without applying suction.

Rationale: Gentle insertion without applying suction during insertion prevents trauma to the mucous membrane. Directing the catheter along the floor of the nasal cavity avoids the nasal turbinates. Directing the catheter along one side of the mouth prevents gagging.

12. Apply your finger to the suction control port, and gently rotate the catheter. Apply suction for 5–10 seconds, then remove your finger from the control, and remove the catheter. It may be necessary during oropharyngeal suctioning to apply suction to secretions that collect in the vestibule of the mouth and beneath the tongue. A suction attempt should last only 15 seconds. During this time the catheter is inserted, the suction applied and discontinued, and the catheter removed.

Rationale: Placing the finger over the suction control port starts the suction. Gentle rotation of the catheter ensures that all surfaces are reached and prevents trauma to any one area of the respiratory mucosa due to prolonged suction.

13. Wipe off the catheter with sterile gauze if it is thickly coated with secretions, flush it with sterile water or saline, and repeat steps 9, 11–12, until the air passage is clear, but do not apply suction for more than 5 minutes in total.

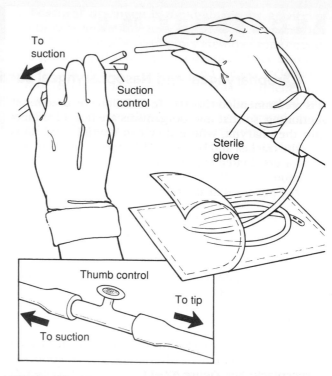

Figure 42–13

Rationale: Applying suction for too long can decrease the client's oxygen supply.

14. Encourage the client to breathe deeply and cough between suctions.

Rationale: Coughing and deep breathing help carry secretions from the trachea and bronchi into the pharynx, where they can be reached with the suction catheter.

15. If a specimen is required, use a sputum trap (see Figure 42–14):
    a. Attach the suction catheter to the rubber tubing of the sputum trap.
    b. Attach the suction tubing to the sputum trap air vent.
    c. Suction the client's nasopharynx or oropharynx. The sputum trap will collect the mucus during suctioning.
    d. Remove the catheter from the client. Disconnect the sputum trap rubber tubing from the suction catheter. Remove the suction tubing from the trap air vent.
    e. Connect the rubber tubing of the sputum trap to the air vent.

Rationale: This contains any microorganisms in the sputum trap.

16. Offer, or assist the client with, oral or nasal hygiene.

17. Dispose of the catheter, glove, water, and waste container. The catheter can be rolled inside the glove for disposal.

18. Ensure that equipment is available for the next suctioning. Change suction collection bottles and tubing daily or more frequently as necessary.

tinged mucus; or blood-flecked mucus. Also record nursing assessments and interventions.

Sample Recording

Date	Time	Notes
5/12/89	0200	Oropharyngeal suctioning for 5 min. 35 ml thick, greenish sputum. Respirations 20/min, wet. Cyanotic. No response to painful stimuli. Positioned in left Sims'.
		———————Rozelle L. Schwartz, RN

If the technique is carried out frequently eg, q1h, it may be appropriate to record only once, at the end of the shift however the frequency of the suctioning must be recorded.

Sample Recording

Date	Time	Notes
5/12/89	0700	Nasopharyngeal suctioning q.1h. for 3 min. × 6. Nares alternated. 175 ml thick, greenish sputum obtained with 6 suctionings. Respirations remain dyspneic, 30–32/min. No response to verbal stimuli. Position changed q.1h. × 6.
		———————Rozelle L. Schwartz, RN

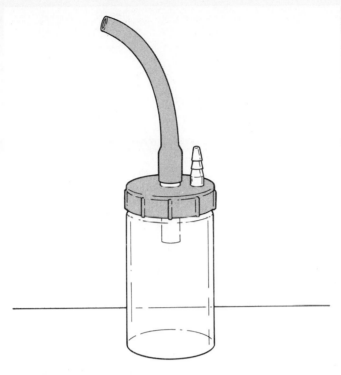

Figure 42–14

19. Assess the client's breathing. See the assessment guide for this chapter.
20. Document the amount, consistency, color, and odor of sputum, eg, foamy, white mucus; thick, green-

Deeper suctioning, called *endotracheal suctioning*, removes secretions from the trachea and the bronchi. Deep suctioning requires considerably more skill and is not usually performed by the inexperienced nurse. It is recommended that surgical aseptic technique be used for deep suctioning, so that microorganisms are not introduced. This is particularly important for debilitated clients, who are more susceptible to infection.

▣ Artificial Airways

Artificial airways are inserted to maintain a patent air passage for clients whose airway has become or may become obstructed. A patent airway is necessary so that air can flow to and from the lungs. Four of the more common types of intubation are oropharyngeal, nasopharyngeal, endotracheal, and tracheostomy.

Oropharyngeal intubation is done most frequently for clients who have had general anesthesia and for those who are semiconscious and are likely to obstruct their own airways with their tongues. An oropharyngeal tube is inserted in some instances for pharyngeal suctioning. It is not inserted in clients who are conscious, because it stimulates the gag reflex and thus can cause vomiting.

Oropharyngeal tubes are S-shaped and usually made of plastic. Adult, child, and infant sizes are available. The tube is inserted through the mouth and terminates in the posterior pharynx. See Figure 42–15. For insertion of the tube, the client should be in a supine position with the neck hyperextended so that the tongue cannot fall back to block the pharynx. This position may be contraindicated for clients with head, neck, or back injuries. Nursing interventions for clients with oropharyngeal airways in place include the following:

1. Remove the tube every 4 hours, or more often if necessary, and provide oral hygiene to maintain the health of oral mucosa.
2. Make sure a bite block is in place if the client is likely to bite the tube and thus obstruct the airway.
3. Maintain the client in a lateral or semiprone position so that blood, vomitus, and mucus will drain out of the mouth and not be aspirated.
4. Remove the airway once the client has regained consciousness and has the swallow, gag, and cough reflexes.

Nasopharyngeal intubation is carried out if the oropharyngeal route is contraindicated, e.g., following oral surgery. A nasopharyngeal tube may also be inserted to protect the nasal and pharyngeal mucosa during naso-

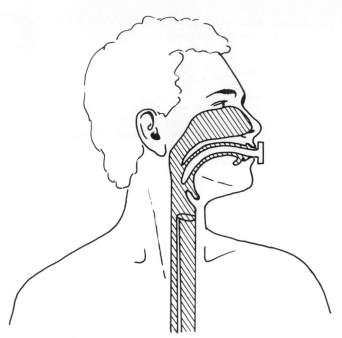

Figure 42–15   An oropharyngeal tube in place

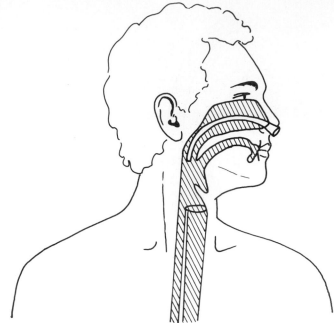

Figure 42–16   A nasopharyngeal tube in place

pharyngeal or nasotracheal suctioning. The tube is inserted through a nostril and terminates in the pharynx, below the upper edge of the epiglottis. See Figure 42–16. Tubes vary in size for adults, children, and infants. They are usually made of latex rubber. Nursing interventions for clients with nasopharyngeal tubes include the following:

1. Lubricate the tube with a water-soluble lubricant and/or a topical anesthetic agent prior to insertion, to prevent irritation of the nasopharyngeal mucosa and undue discomfort. The local anesthetic agent will be specified in the order.
2. Remove the tube, and insert it in the other nostril at least every 8 hours, or as ordered by the physician, or more often to prevent irritation of the mucosa.
3. Provide nasal hygiene every 4 hours, or more often if needed.
4. Monitor the client closely for stimulation of the vagus nerve if nasotracheal suctioning is carried out. Vagal stimulation can lead to cardiac arrest.

Endotracheal tubes are usually inserted by a physician for clients undergoing general anesthesia or when mechanical ventilation is required. An endotracheal tube is a curved polyvinylchloride tube that is inserted through either the mouth or the nose and into the trachea. See Figure 42–17. It terminates just above the bifurcation of the trachea into the bronchi. Nursing interventions for clients with endotracheal tubes in place include the following:

1. Maintain the client in a lateral or semiprone position so that blood, vomitus, or secretions can drain from the mouth and are not aspirated.
2. Provide oral or nasal hygiene every 3 hours or as needed.

3. For an oral insertion, provide a bite block so that the client cannot bite the tube and occlude the airway.
4. Assess the condition of the nasal or oral mucosa for irritation and notify the physician should the need to change a nasal endotracheal tube arise; reposition an oral endotracheal tube from one side of the mouth to the other every 8 hours or as required.
5. Closely monitor the air pressure in the endotra-

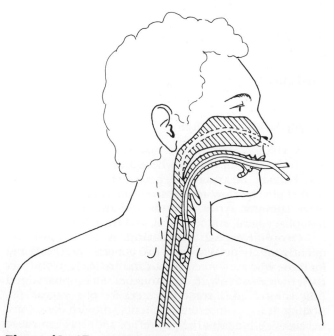

Figure 42–17   An endotracheal tube in place

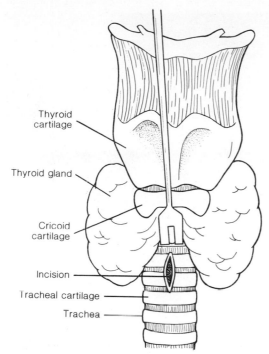

Figure 42–18 A site of a tracheostomy incision

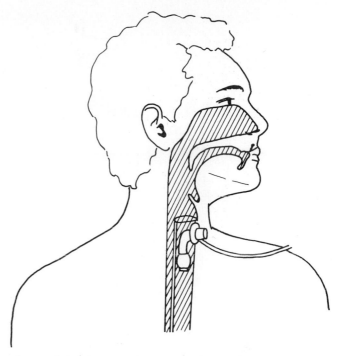

Figure 42–19 A tracheostomy tube in place

cheal cuff. If it is greater than 20 mm Hg, necrosis of the tracheal tissues can result.

6. Tape the airway in place to prevent accidental slippage or extubation.
7. Provide continuous humidification or aerosol therapy to prevent undue drying and irritation of the mucous membranes, if the tube is left in for more than a short time, e.g., for days or weeks.

Tracheostomy tubes are inserted to provide and maintain a patent airway, to remove tracheobronchial secretions from clients unable to cough, to replace endotracheal tubes, to permit the use of positive pressure ventilation, and to prevent unconscious clients from aspirating secretions. A tracheostomy tube is a curved tube that is inserted into a tracheostomy (a surgical incision in the trachea just below the first or second tracheal cartilage). See Figure 42–18. The tracheostomy tube extends through the tracheostomy stoma into the trachea. See Figure 42–19.

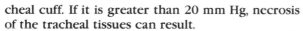 **Oxygen Therapy**

Additional oxygen is indicated for clients with *hypoxemia* (e.g., those with reduced lung diffusion of oxygen through the respiratory membrane, heart failure leading to inadequate transport of oxygen, or substantial loss of lung tissue due to tumors or surgery). Oxygen therapy is prescribed by the physician, who specifies the specific concentration, method, and liter flow per minute. When the administration of oxygen is an emergency measure, the nurse may initiate the therapy. The signs of hypoxemia generally include, in order of occurrence:

1. Increased rapid pulse
2. Rapid, shallow respirations and dyspnea
3. Increased restlessness or lightheadedness
4. Flaring of the nares
5. Substernal or intercostal retractions
6. Cyanosis

Oxygen is supplied in hospitals in two ways: by liquid portable systems (cylinders) and from wall outlets. Oxygen cylinders are made of steel. Large ones contain 244 cubic feet of oxygen stored at a pressure of 2200 pounds per square inch (psi). Smaller cylinders that are readily portable on stretchers are often used. Piped in oxygen is stored at much lower pressure, usually 50 to 60 psi. Oxygen administered from a cylinder or wall-outlet system is dry. Dry gases dehydrate the respiratory membranes. Humidifying devices are thus an essential adjunct of oxygen therapy. To use an oxygen wall outlet:

1. Attach the flowmeter to the wall outlet, exerting firm pressure. The flowmeter should be in the off position. See Figure 42–20.
2. Fill the humidifier bottle with distilled water. (This can be done before coming to the bedside.)
3. Attach the humidifier bottle to the base of the flow meter. See Figure 42–5 on page 722.
4. Attach the prescribed oxygen tubing and delivery device to the humidifier.
5. Regulate the flowmeter to the prescribed level.

Oxygen is administered by either low-flow or high-flow systems. The fraction of inspired oxygen (FiO_2) is variable, depending on the client's respiratory rate and volume and the oxygen liter flow. A low-flow system is contraindicated when a client requires a carefully monitored oxygen concentration. **Low-flow** administration devices include nasal cannula, simple face mask, nasal catheter, partial rebreathing mask, nonrebreathing mask,

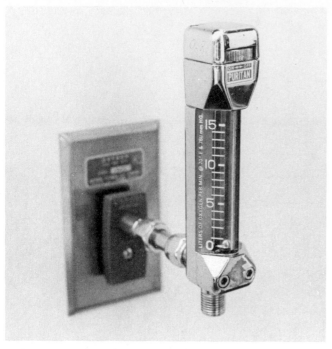

Figure 42–20 An oxygen flowmeter attached to a wall outlet

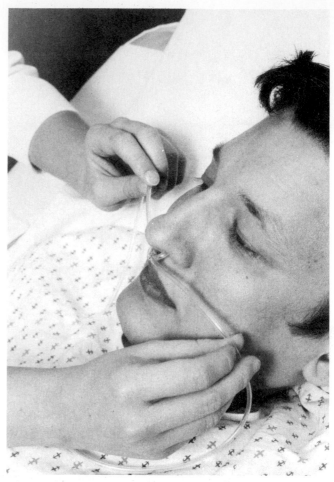

Figure 42–21 Client with nasal cannula

Croupette, and oxygen tent.

A high-flow oxygen system delivers all the gas required. It provides a precise amount of oxygen, regardless of the client's respirations. The ratio of room air to oxygen is regulated and does not vary with the client's respirations. The Venturi mask is an example of a **high-flow** administration device. Some devices can be used for both low- and high-flow administration, e.g., the face tent, oxygen hood, and incubator (Isolette).

The **nasal cannula** (nasal prongs) is the most commonly used device to administer oxygen. It consists of a rubber or plastic tube that extends around the face, with 0.6- to 1.3-cm (¼ to ½ in) curved prongs that fit into the nostrils. One side of the tube connects to the oxygen tubing and oxygen supply. The cannula is often held in place by an elastic band that fits around the client's head or under the chin. See Figure 42–21. For clients who are confused or particularly active, it may be helpful to secure the cannula in place with small pieces of tape on each side of the face.

The nasal cannula is easy to apply and does not interfere with the client's ability to eat or talk. It also is relatively comfortable and permits some freedom of movement. It delivers a relatively low concentration of oxygen (23 to 44%) at flow rates of 2 to 6 liters per minute. Higher concentrations and flow rates can be administered; however, above 6 liters per minute there is a tendency for the client to swallow air and for the nasal and pharyngeal mucosa to become irritated. Administering oxygen by cannula is explained in Procedure 42–3.

PROCEDURE 42-3

Administering Oxygen by Cannula

Equipment

- An oxygen supply with a flowmeter
- A humidifier with sterile distilled water
- A nasal cannula and tubing
- Tape, if needed, to secure the cannula in place
- Gauzes to pad the tubing over the cheekbones

Intervention

1. Assist the client to a semi-Fowler's position if possible.

   Rationale This position permits easier chest expansion and hence easier breathing.

2. Explain that oxygen is not dangerous when safety precautions are observed and that it will ease the discomfort of dyspnea. Inform the client and sup-

port persons about the safety precautions connected with oxygen use.

3. Set up the oxygen equipment and the humidifier as described earlier in this chapter.

4. Turn on the oxygen at the flow rate ordered.

5. Check that the oxygen is flowing freely through the tubing. The tubing should be free of kinks and the connections should be airtight. There should be bubbles in the humidifier as the oxygen flows through the water. Oxygen should be felt flowing at the outlets of the cannula.

6. Put the cannula over the client's face, with the outlet prongs fitting into the nares and the elastic band around the head. Some models have a strap to adjust under the chin. Make sure the prongs are turned upward so the oxygen is directed into the nasal passages and away from the tissues at the base of the nares.

7. If the cannula will not stay in place, tape it at the sides of the face. Slip gauze pads under the tubing over the cheekbones to prevent skin irritation.

8. Assess the client's color, ease of respirations, etc, and provide support for adjusting to the presence of cannula.

9. Assess the client in 15–30 minutes, depending on the client's health, and regularly thereafter. Assess

vital signs, color, breathing patterns, and chest movements.

10. Make sure that safety precautions are being followed.

11. Check the liter flow and the level of water in the humidifier in 30 minutes and whenever providing care.

12. Assess the client regularly for clinical signs of hypoxia.

13. Assess the client's nares for encrustations and irritation. Apply a water-soluble lubricant as required to soothe the mucous membranes.

14. Document initiation of the therapy and all nursing assessments.

Sample Recording

Date	Time	Notes
12/5/89	0730	P 96, R 24. Slightly cyanotic, dyspneic on exertion, and restless. O_2 by cannula at 3 l/min. applied. —————— ——————Susan de Camillis, NS
	0800	No cyanosis apparent. P 84, R 16. States "breathing is easier." Is less restless. —————— ——————Susan de Camillis, NS

The **nasal catheter** (low-flow device) is a rubber or plastic tube about 39 cm (16 in) long, with six or eight holes at the tip to disperse the oxygen. It is used to administer low to moderate concentrations of oxygen, but it can deliver higher concentrations than the nasal cannula. At flows of 1 to 5 liters per minute, the catheter can deliver concentrations of oxygen of 30 to 35%. It allows the client the same mobility as the cannula does.

Major problems associated with nasal catheters are laryngeal ulceration from the constant flow of oxygen into the larynx, and gastric distention caused by air and oxygen entering the stomach. Gastric distention can be relieved by inserting a nasogastric tube. Laryngeal ulceration may be prevented by moving the catheter from one nostril to the other every 8 hours (Fuchs 1980, p. 39). The details of administering oxygen by catheter are given in Procedure 42–4.

PROCEDURE 42–4

Administering Oxygen by Nasal Catheter

Equipment

▪ A nasal catheter of the appropriate size: #8 or 10 Fr. for children; #10 or 12 Fr. for women; #12 or 14 Fr. for men

▪ An oxygen supply with a flowmeter

▪ A humidifier with sterile distilled water

▪ Water-soluble lubricating jelly to facilitate catheter insertion and a gauze square to apply it

▪ Adhesive tape (nonallergenic is preferred) to secure catheter to the client's face

▪ A flashlight and a tongue blade for assessing correct placement of the catheter

▪ A container of sterile water to test the oxygen flow

Intervention

1. Follow Procedure 42–3, steps 1–4. Test the oxygen flow by turning on the flowmeter to 3 L/minute and inserting the tip of the catheter into a container of sterile water. Bubbling indicates that oxygen is flowing.

2. Determine how deeply to insert the catheter by placing the end of the catheter in a straight line between the tip of the client's nose and the earlobe. See Figure 42–22. This distance can be marked with tape.

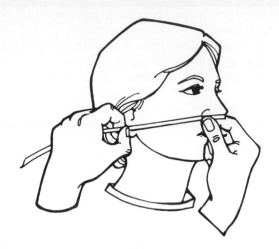

Figure 42—22

Rationale: This external distance approximates the distance from the nares to the oropharynx.

3. Lubricate the tip of the catheter with water-soluble jelly. Squeeze the lubricant onto a gauze square, and rotate the catheter tip through it. Do not use mineral oil or petroleum jelly.

Rationale: Lubrication facilitates insertion and prevents injury to the nasal mucosa. If aspirated, mineral oil or petroleum jelly can cause severe lung irritations or lipoid pneumonia.

4. Start the flow of oxygen at about 3 l/minute prior to inserting the tube.

Rationale: The flow of oxygen prevents the catheter from becoming plugged by secretions during insertion.

5. Introduce the catheter slowly through one nostril until the tip is at the entrance to the oropharynx (the marked distance). See Figure 42—23, *A*. Look into the client's mouth, using the flashlight and tongue blade, to check placement. The tip of the catheter will be visible through the mouth beside the uvula. See Figure 42—23, *B*.

6. Withdraw the tip slightly so that it can no longer be seen.

Rationale: When the catheter is in this position, the client is less likely to swallow oxygen.

7. Tape the catheter to the client's face at the side of the nose and the cheek (see Figure 42—24, *A*) or at the tip of the nose and the forehead. (see Figure 42—24, *B*). Pin the tubing to the client's pillow or gown, leaving slack in the tubing.

LATERAL VIEW

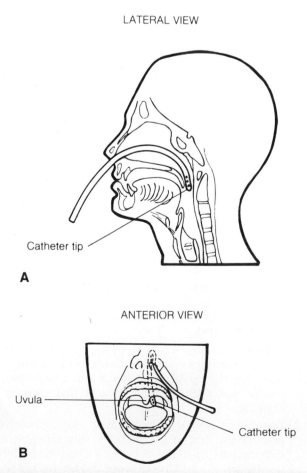

Catheter tip

A

ANTERIOR VIEW

Uvula

Catheter tip

B

Figure 42—23

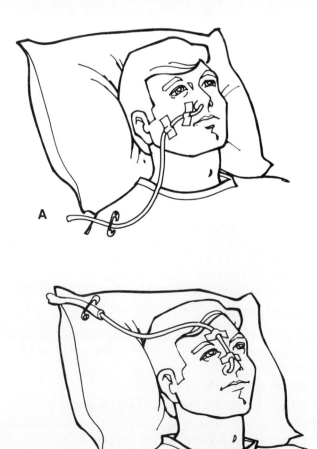

A

B

Figure 42—24

Rationale: If taped and pinned, the catheter will not be displaced when the client moves. Slack allows a person to move without pulling on the tubing.

8. Adjust the flow to the prescribed rate.
9. Assess the client's respirations, color, etc, and provide support for adjusting to the catheter.
10. Follow Procedure 42–3, steps 9–12.
11. Document the initiation of oxygen therapy, including the method, the flow rate, and the nursing assessments.

Face masks that cover the client's nose and mouth may be used for oxygen inhalation. Most masks are made of clear, pliable plastic that can be molded to fit the face. They are held to the client's head with elastic bands. Some have a metal clip that can be bent over the bridge of the nose for a snug fit. There are several holes in the sides of the mask (exhalation ports) to allow the escape of exhaled carbon dioxide.

Some masks have reservoir bags, which provide higher oxygen concentrations to the client. A portion of the client's expired air is directed into the bag. Because this air comes from the upper respiratory passages (e.g., the trachea and bronchi), where it does not take part in gaseous exchange, its oxygen concentration remains the same as that of inspired air. A variety of oxygen masks are available:

1. The *simple face mask* (low-flow system) delivers oxygen concentrations from 40 to 60% at liter flows of 5 to 8 liters per minute. See Figure 42–25.
2. The *partial rebreather mask* (low flow system) delivers oxygen concentrations of 35 to 60% at liter flows of 6 to 15 liters per minute. See Figure 42–26. The oxygen reservoir bag that is attached allows the client to rebreathe about the first third of the exhaled air. The partial rebreather bag must not totally deflate during inspiration. If this problem occurs, increase the liter flow of oxygen.
3. The *nonrebreather mask* (low-flow system) delivers the highest oxygen concentration possible by means other than intubation or mechanical venti-

lation, i.e., 60 to 90% at liter flows of 6 to 15 liters per minute. See Figure 42–27. Using a nonrebreather mask, the client breathes only the source gas from the bag. One-way valves on the mask and between the reservoir bag and the mask prevent the room air and the client's exhaled air from entering the bag. The nonrebreather bag must not totally deflate during inspiration. If it does, this problem can be corrected by increasing the liter flow of oxygen.

4. The *Venturi mask* (high-flow system) delivers oxygen concentrations precise to within 1% and is often used for clients with chronic respiratory disorders. See Figure 42–28. Oxygen concentrations vary from 24 to 40 or 50% at liter flows of 4 to 8 liters per minute. Optional humidification adapters are also available for clients who require them, e.g., those receiving oxygen concentrations in excess of 30%. When a Venturi mask is used, it is important to prevent occlusion of the air ports by bed linen, clothing, or other objects. Blood gas measurements are taken frequently to monitor the effectiveness of therapy

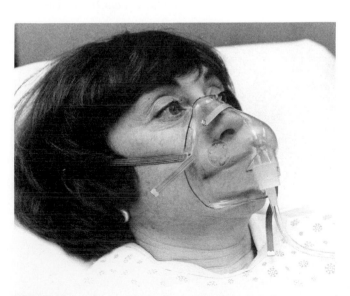

Figure 42–25 A simple face mask for a low-flow oxygen system

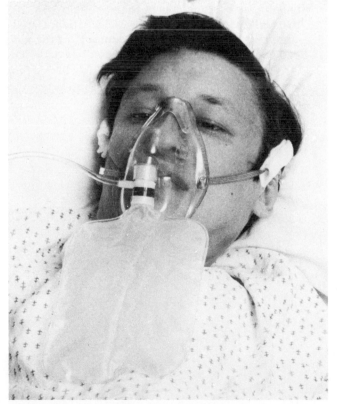

Figure 42–26 A partial rebreathing mask for a low-flow oxygen system

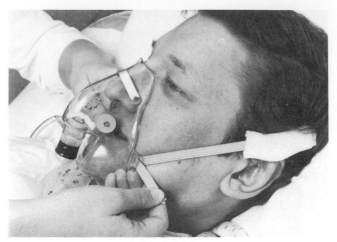

Figure 42—27 A nonrebreathing mask for a low-flow or a high-flow oxygen system

Initiating oxygen by mask is much the same as initiating oxygen by cannula or catheter, except that the nurse must find a mask of appropriate size. Smaller sizes are available for children. When fitting a client with a face mask, the nurse needs to:

1. Familiarize the client with the mask when possible. Allow the client to hold the mask, guide it toward the face, and get used to the sensation of the mask covering the nose and mouth. Instruct the client to put on the mask from the nose downward during expiration.
2. Turn on the oxygen to the prescribed rate of flow before placing the mask on the client. When the mask has a reservoir bag, the nurse should first flush the mask with oxygen until it is partially inflated.
3. Gradually fit the mask to the contours of the face, and encourage the client to breathe normally. The mask should be molded to prevent oxygen escaping

upward into the client's eyes or around the cheeks or chin. Pad the band behind the ears and over bony prominences to prevent skin irritation.

Face tents can replace oxygen masks when masks are poorly tolerated by clients (e.g., children). When a face tent alone is used to supply oxygen, the concentration of oxygen varies; therefore, it is often used in conjunction with a Venturi system. Face tents can provide 30 to 55% concentration of oxygen at 4 to 8 liters per minute. When a face tent is used, the nurse needs to inspect the client's facial skin frequently for dampness or chafing, and dry and treat as needed. See Figure 42—29.

▪ Chest Tubes

Chest tubes are made of pliable plastic or rubber. They are usually inserted through an intercostal space into the pleural cavity. See Figure 42—30. A **pneumothorax** is the collection of air in the pleural cavity. A **hemothorax** is an accumulation of blood in the pleural cavity. Chest tubes that are used to remove air are usually inserted superiorly, i.e., through the second intercostal space, and anteriorly, because air tends to rise in the pleural cavity. Tubes used to drain fluid are inserted more inferiorly, often in the eighth or ninth intercostal space, and more posteriorly. Sometimes a tube used to drain air is inserted inferiorly and threaded superiorly in the pleural space. When a client requires drainage of both fluid and air, two chest tubes may be inserted. These are sometimes joined externally by a Y-connector.

Chest tubes are inserted during surgery and in nonsurgical situations, e.g., in emergency treatment of injuries. Because the pleural cavity normally has negative pressure, any drainage system connected to it must be sealed so that air or liquid cannot enter. Such a drainage system is called a *water-sealed (underwater) drainage* or a *disposable pleural drainage system*. In water-sealed drainage, fluid in the bottom of the container prevents air from entering the chest tube and thus entering the pleural cavity. The system must be kept below the level

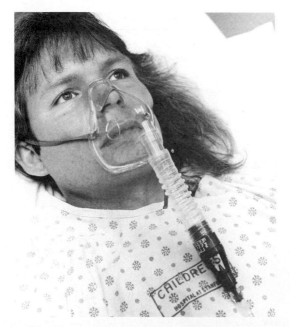

Figure 42—28 A Venturi mask for a high-flow oxygen system

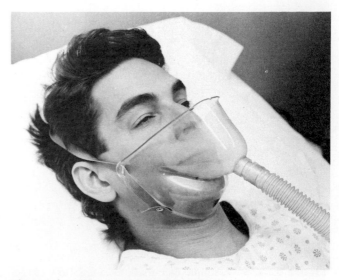

Figure 42—29 An oxygen face tent

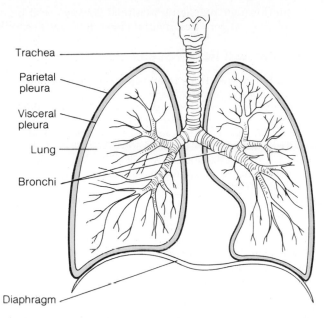

Figure 42–30 The pleural cavity is a potential space that lies between the visceral pleura and the parietal pleura. Chest tubes are inserted into this space.

Labels for the figure: Trachea, Parietal pleura, Visceral pleura, Lung, Bronchi, Diaphragm

of the client's chest so that the fluid in the container is not drawn into the pleural cavity by gravity. It is also very important to maintain the patency of the tubing.

Drainage systems use three mechanisms to drain fluid and air from the pleural cavity: positive expiratory pressure, gravity, and suction. When the pleural cavity contains some air or fluid, a positive pressure develops during expiration. This positive pressure is abnormal, but it does help expel the air and to some extent fluid from the space. Gravity acts as an evacuation force when the tubing is placed so that it descends from the insertion site to the drainage receptacle. Suction is used in conjunction with the other two forces in some drainage systems.

Evaluating Client Responses

Examples of outcome criteria used to evaluate clients' responses to nursing interventions related to oxygenation are listed in the accompanying box.

OUTCOME CRITERIA

Oxygenation

The client will:

- Have full lung expansion during deep breathing exercises
- Expectorate secretions when coughing
- Exhibit no adventitious breath sounds
- Have no chest retractions
- Have a blood pressure within normal range
- Have a normal Pao_2 and $Paco_2$

Chapter Highlights

- Respiration, the process of gaseous exchange between the individual and the atmosphere, involves pulmonary ventilation, diffusion of gases, and transport of oxygen and carbon dioxide to and from the body's cells.
- Pulmonary ventilation, the inflow and outflow of air between the atmosphere and the alveoli of the lungs, is accomplished through the mechanical act of breathing (inspiration and expiration).
- The volume to which the lungs expand during ventilation depends on the pattern of breathing, the size and position of the individual, medical or surgical conditions affecting the thorax, and developmental variations in the shape of the chest.
- Ventilation depends upon adequate atmospheric oxygen, clear air passages, adequate pulmonary compliance and recoil, and neurochemical regulation of respiration.
- Diffusion of oxygen and carbon dioxide is the movement of the gases from areas of greater pressure or concentration to areas of lower pressure or concentration.
- The rate of diffusion of gases through the respiratory membrane is influenced by the thickness of the membrane, surface area of the membrane, diffusion coefficient of the gases, and pressure difference on either side of the membrane.
- Factors affecting the rate of oxygen transport include: cardiac output, the number of erythrocytes present in the blood, exercise, and blood hematocrit.
- In healthy individuals, decreased concentration of carbon dioxide in the blood stimulates respiration. Clients with respiratory disorders such as COPD have what is called a *hypoxic drive,* i.e., decreased levels of blood oxygen stimulate respiration.
- Factors that influence oxygenation of the body's tissues include altitude, environment, emotions, exercise, health, and life-style.
- Respiratory function may be altered by any condition that affects the movement of air into or out of the lungs, changes the diffusion rate of oxygen and carbon dioxide between the alveoli and the pulmonary capillaries, or alters the transport of oxygen and carbon dioxide via the blood to and from the tissue cells.
- Hypoxia is insufficient oxygenation of body tissues.
- Clinical signs of hypoxia may be early (increased heart and respiratory rates and slight rise in systolic blood pressure) or late (decreased pulse and systolic blood pressure, dyspnea, cough, and hemoptysis). Cyanosis is not a reliable sign.
- Normal respiration (eupnea) is quiet, rhythmic, and effortless. Common altered breathing patterns include: tachypnea, bradypnea, dyspnea, orthopnea, hyperventilation, and hypoventilation.
- The signs of airway obstruction include: labored noisy respirations, extreme inspiratory effort without chest movement, sternal or intercostal retractions, altered arterial blood gas values, restlessness, dyspnea, and abnormal or absent breath sounds.

To assess respiratory function, the nurse conducts a nursing history, performs a complete physical assessment of the client, and reviews relevant diagnostic data.

The nursing history should be structured to obtain data about the client's present respiratory problem, history, presence of cough, smoking and other risk factors, medications, stressors, health and developmental status, and strengths.

Physical assessment should include general assessment and specific attention to cardiopulmonary status.

The nurse is responsible for obtaining specimens for diagnostic tests, preparing the client and family for diagnostic procedures, monitoring the client after selected procedures, and reviewing records and reports of diagnostic tests.

Nursing diagnoses for clients with respiratory problems include categories specific to respiration (impaired gas exchange, ineffective airway clearance, and ineffective breathing patterns) and related diagnostic categories, such as alterations in cardiac output and impaired tissue perfusion.

Planning care for clients with respiratory problems includes identifying strategies to facilitate pulmonary ventilation and diffusion and the transport of oxygen and carbon dioxide.

Interventions for clients with respiratory problems include positioning, deep breathing and coughing, hydration, assisting clients with lung inflation devices, implementing measures to clear secretions (e.g., percussion, vibration, postural drainage, and suctioning), managing artificial airways, and monitoring oxygen therapy and chest drainage systems.

Selected References

Acee, S. July/August 1984. Helping patients breathe more easily. *Geriatric Nursing* 5:230–33.

American Heart Association. 1986. Standards and guidelines for cardiopulmonary resuscitation (CPR) and emergency cardiac care (ECC). *Journal of the American Medical Association* 255:2841–3044.

Bellack, J. P., and Bamford, P. A. 1984. Nursing assessment: A multidimensional approach. Monterey, Calif.: Wadsworth Health Sciences Div.

Byrne, C. J.; Saxton, D. F.; Pelikan, P. K.; and Nugent, P. M. 1986. *Laboratory tests: Implications for nursing care.* 2d ed. Menlo Park, Calif.: Addison-Wesley Publishing Co.

Fuchs, P. L. December 1980. Getting the best out of oxygen delivery systems. *Nursing 80* 10:34–43.

Guyton, A. C. 1986. *Textbook of medical physiology.* 7th ed. Philadelphia: W. B. Saunders Co.

Luce, J. M.; Tyler, M. L.; and Pierson, D. J. 1984. *Intensive respiratory care.* Philadelphia: W. B. Saunders Co.

Teaching your patient to live with C.O.P.D. May/June 1985. *Nursing Life* 5:31–32.

Vick, R. L. 1984. *Contemporary medical physiology.* Menlo Park, Calif.: Addison-Wesley Publishing Co.

Weaver, T. May 1985. Chronic ineffective gas exchange when your patient goes from bad to worse. *Nursing 85* 15:7.

Wimsatt, R. November 1985. Unlocking the mysteries behind the chest wall. *Nursing 83* 15:58–63.

Winslow, E. H.; Lane, L. D.; and Gaffney, F. A. May/June 1985. Oxygen uptake and cardiovascular responses in control adults and acute myocardial infarction patients during bathing. *Nursing Research* 34:164–69.

43

Fluids and Electrolytes

OBJECTIVES

Describe factors affecting the proportion of body weight that is fluid.

Identify major constituents ('electrolytes') of intracellular and extracellular fluid compartments and body secretions.

Describe ways in which fluids and electrolytes move through the body.

Identify ways in which osmotic and hydrostatic pressures influence movement of fluid through membranes.

Describe how body mechanisms regulate fluid and electrolyte balance.

Describe the role of the kidneys and lungs in regulating acid-base balance.

Identify information to obtain in a health history to assess fluid and electrolyte balance.

List factors that influence fluid and electrolyte balance.

Describe techniques for monitoring fluid intake and output.

Identify diagnostic tests used to assess fluid and electrolyte balance and describe their significance.

Identify causes of extracellular fluid and electrolyte deficits and excesses.

Recognize clinical signs and laboratory findings of selected fluid and electrolyte imbalances.

Describe four primary acid-base disturbances.

Give examples of nursing diagnoses related to fluid,

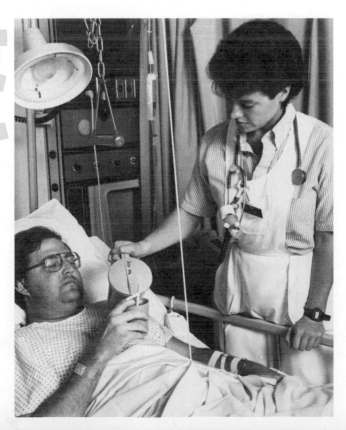

electrolyte, and acid-base imbalances.

Explain how to calculate infusion flow rates.

Identify factors influencing infusion flow rates.

Describe how to change intravenous containers and tubing.

Give guidelines for discontinuing an intravenous infusion.

State outcome criteria for evaluating the client's responses to strategies implemented to promote fluid and electrolyte balance.

Body Fluids and Electrolytes

Fluids and electrolytes are necessary to maintain good health, and their relative amounts in the body must be maintained within a narrow range. The balance of fluids and electrolytes in the body is maintained in health by the body's physiologic processes. Almost every illness, however, threatens the balance. Even in normal daily living, excessive temperatures or excessive activity can disturb the balance if adequate water or salt intake is not maintained. Some therapeutic measures for clients, such as the use of diuretics, can also disturb the balance unless water and electrolytes are replaced.

Distribution of Body Fluids

The body's fluid is divided into two major reservoirs, intracellular and extracellular. **Intracellular fluid (ICF)** is found within the cells of the body. It comprises two-thirds to three-quarters of the total body fluid. **Extracellular fluid (ECF)** is found outside the cells; it is subdivided into two compartments, *intravascular* (*plasma*, fluid found within the vascular system) and *interstitial* (fluid that surrounds the cells, including lymph). Extracellular fluids comprise one-third to one-fourth of total body fluids. Interstitial fluid comprises three-quarters of extracellular fluid. Extracellular fluid is in constant motion throughout the body. Although it is the smaller of the two compartments, it is the transport system that carries nutrients to and waste products from the cells.

Secretions and excretions are part of the extracellular fluid. A **secretion** (e.g., cerebrospinal fluid, synovial fluid, pericardial fluid, and alimentary secretions) is the product of a gland, for example, the salivary glands. An **excretion** is waste produced by the cells of the body. Just as balances exist between cellular and extracellular compartments, special balances exist between plasma and secretions and excretions.

The proportion of the human body composed of fluid is surprisingly large, considering that the external appearance suggests mostly solid tissue such as muscle and bone. Fluid comprises about 57% of the average healthy adult man's weight. In health, this volume (about 40 liters) of body fluid remains relatively constant. In fact, a healthy person's weight varies less than 0.2 kg (0.5 lb) in 24 hours, regardless of the amount of fluid ingested. The percentage of total body fluid varies according to the individual's age, body fat, and sex. See Table 43–1.

Since body fat is essentially free of fluid, the amount of fat a person has alters the proportion of body fluid to body weight. In other words, the less body fat present, the greater the proportion of body fluid. For example, a thin man's body may be 70% fluid, whereas an obese man's may be only 55%. This variable, body fat, also accounts for the difference in total body fluid between the sexes. After adolescence, women have proportionately more fat than men. Thus, they have a smaller percentage of fluid in relation to total body weight than do men.

Large volumes of fluid carry dissolved waste materials through the kidneys and through the gastrointestinal tract. However, in both instances, most of this fluid is reabsorbed into the vascular spaces and reused by the body. For example, of 6700 ml produced in the alimentary tract, only 100 ml is usually excreted in the feces, just enough to keep the feces lubricated. Of 180 liters of glomerular filtrate that filters through the kidneys per day, only 1.4 liters are excreted from the body under normal conditions. See Table 43–2.

Extracellular and intracellular fluids contain oxygen from the lungs; dissolved nutrients from the gastrointestinal tract; excretory products of metabolism; and dissolved particles called ions. Many salts dissociate in water, i.e., break up into electrically charged ions (e.g., the salt sodium chloride breaks up into one ion of sodium [Na^+] and one ion of chloride [Cl^-]). These charged particles are called **electrolytes** because they are capable of conducting electricity. Ions that carry a positive charge (e.g., sodium, potassium, calcium, and magnesium) are called **cations,** and ions carrying a negative charge (e.g., chloride, bicarbonate, monohydrogen phosphate, and sulfate) are called **anions.**

Table 43–1   Fluid Percentage of Body Weight, by Age

Developmental Stage	Percentage of Water (approximate)
Newborn	75
Adult male	57
Adult female	55
Elderly adult	45

Note: As age increases, proportion of body water decreases.

Table 43—2 Average Daily Fluid Output for an Adult

Route	Amount at Normal Temperature (ml)
Urine	1400
Insensible losses:	
Lungs	350
Skin	350
Sweat	100
Feces	100
Total	2300

Source: Adapted from A. C. Guyton, *Textbook of medical physiology,* 7th ed. (Philadelphia: W. B. Saunders Co., 1986), p. 383.

Electrolyte Composition of Body Fluids

The electrolyte composition of fluids varies from one compartment to another. The principal ions of extracellular fluid are sodium and chloride, while the principal ions of cellular fluid are potassium and phosphate. See Figure 43–1. The ion composition of the two extracellular fluid reservoirs (intravascular and interstitial) is similar; the main difference is that intravascular fluid (plasma) has a greater quantity of protein than interstitial fluid does. This is because large particles of protein have difficulty passing through the vascular (capillary) membranes into the interstitial fluid. All other electrolytes move readily between these two extracellular compartments.

The higher quantity of protein in plasma plays a significant role in maintaining the intravascular fluid volume and blood pressure. When quantities of plasma protein are low in the body, the blood volume diminishes noticeably and results in a state of **hypotension** (low blood pressure). This is particularly noticeable in people with diseases of the liver (the source of body plasma proteins), who are unable to produce sufficient quantities of plasma proteins.

Electrolyte balance is maintained in proportion to the quantities of fluid in the compartments. Although the specific numbers of cations and anions may differ in the fluid compartments, to be in balance, the total number of cations must equal the total number of anions within each compartment.

Body secretions and excretions also contain electrolytes. This is of particular concern when excretions are abnormally increased or decreased or when a secretion is lost from the body (for example, when gastric suction removes the gastric secretions). Fluid and electrolyte imbalance can result from prolonged loss through these routes. See Table 43–3 for the electrolyte composition of body secretions and excretions.

Measurement of Electrolytes

Electrolytes are measured in milliequivalents per liter of water (mEq/liter) or milligrams per 100 milliliters (mg/100 ml). The term **milliequivalent** means one thousandth of an equivalent; equivalent refers to the *chemical combining power* of a substance, or the power of cations to unite with anions to form molecules. It is important to realize that a laboratory analysis of serum electrolytes indicates the electrolyte status of only the extracellular fluid, since intracellular fluid is not easily accessible for examination. Examination of extracellular fluid indirectly indicates the electrolytes in the intracellular fluid, though not always precisely.

Movement of Body Fluids and Electrolytes

Movement of fluid and transport of substances occur in three areas.

1. Blood plasma moves around the body within the circulatory system.
2. Interstitial fluid and its components move between the blood capillaries and the cells.
3. Fluid and substances move between the interstitial fluid and the cells.

Methods of Movement

The methods by which body fluids and electrolytes move are: diffusion, osmosis, and active transport. **Diffusion** is the continual intermingling of molecules in liquids, gases, or solids brought about by the random movement of the molecules. For example, two gases

Table 43-3 Electrolyte Composition of Secretions and Excretions Compared to Plasma

Substance	Electrolyte (mEq/L)			
	Sodium (Na^+)	Potassium (K^+)	Chloride (Cl^-)	Bicarbonate (HCO_3^-)
Plasma	135–145	3.6–5.0	95–108	21–28
Gastric secretions	70	5+	140	5
Pancreatic juice	140+	5	35	115+
Hepatic duct bile	140+	5	100+	40
Jejunal secretions	140	5	135	30
Perspiration	80	5	85	—

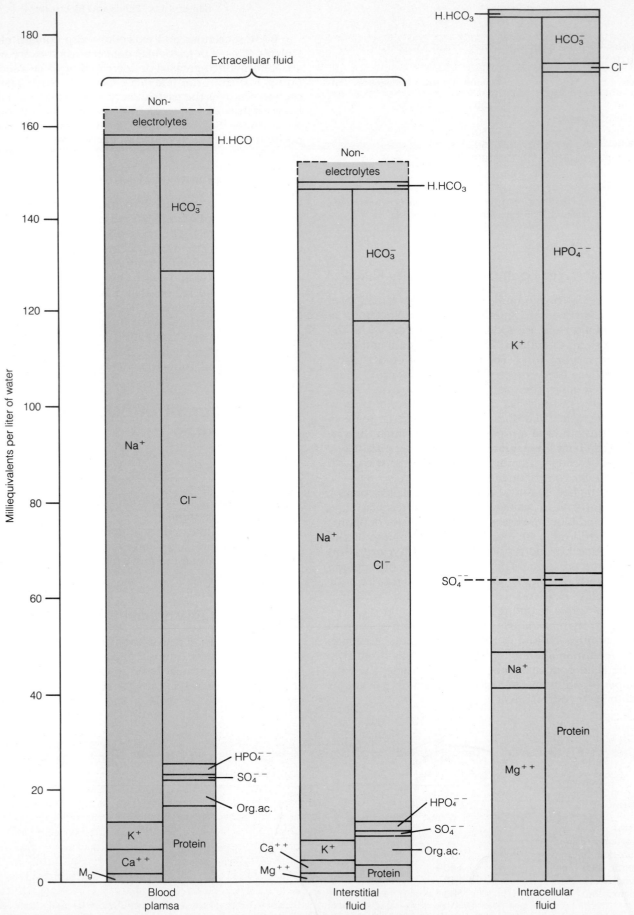

Figure 43–1 The composition of plasma, interstitial fluid, and intracellular fluid. *Source:* Adapted from A. C. Guyton, *Textbook of medical physiology,* 7th ed. (Philadelphia: W. B. Saunders Co., 1986), p. 386. Used by permission.

become mixed by the incessant motion of their molecules. The process of diffusion occurs even when two substances are separated by a thin membrane. In the body, diffusion of water, electrolytes, and other substances occurs through capillary membranes. The rate of diffusion of substances varies according to:

1. **Size of the molecules.** Larger molecules move less quickly than smaller ones, since they require more energy to move about.
2. **Concentration of the solution.** Molecules move more rapidly from a solution of higher concentration to a solution of lower concentration.
3. **Temperature of the solution.** Increases in temperature increase the rate of motion of molecules and therefore the rate of diffusion.

Osmosis is the movement of a solvent across cell membranes, from a less concentrated solution to a more concentrated solution. In other words, body water moves across a cell membrane toward the higher concentration of solute to dilute the concentration and make it equal to the solute concentration on the side of the cell membrane where the body water first was. A **solute** is a substance dissolved in a solution. A **solvent** is the component of a solution that can dissolve a solute. Osmosis is important in maintaining proper balance in the volumes of extracellular and intracellular fluid.

Substances can move across cell membranes from a less concentrated solution to a more concentrated one by **active transport.** This process differs from diffusion and osmosis in that metabolic energy is expended. In active transport, the substance combines with a carrier on the outside surface of the cell membrane. The combined carrier and substance then move to the inside surface. Once inside, they separate, and the substance is released to the inside of the cell. A specific carrier is required for each substance, and enzymes are required for active transport.

Active transport is of particular importance in maintaining the differences in sodium and potassium ion concentrations of extracellular and intracellular fluid. Under normal conditions, sodium concentrations are higher in the extracellular fluid, whereas potassium concentrations are higher inside the cells. To maintain this balance, the active transport mechanism (the **sodium-potassium pump**) moves sodium out of the cells and potassium into the cells.

Fluid Pressures

A number of pressures are exerted as part of the movement of fluid and electrolytes from one fluid compartment to another. Two of these are osmotic pressure and hydrostatic pressure, each of which can cause a flow of fluid through the capillary membranes. **Osmotic pressure** is the force exerted by solute particles drawing the solvent across membranes. The solute particles may be **crystalloids** (salts that dissolve readily into true solutions) or **colloids** (substances such as large protein molecules that do not readily dissolve into true solutions). Normally, the distribution of electrolytes on both sides of membranes is equal. If the concentration of sol-ute on one side of a membrane becomes greater, the osmotic pressure and attraction for the solvent increase on that side, and the fluid flows toward the solution of greater concentration until the concentration gradient disappears.

The principle of osmosis can be applied clinically in the administration of intravenous solutions. Usually, the solutions given are **isotonic,** having the same concentration (and thus, osmotic pressure) as blood plasma. This prevents sudden shifts of fluids and electrolytes. In some cases, however, hypertonic or hypotonic solutions are infused. **Hypertonic** solutions have a greater concentration (osmotic pressure) of solutes than plasma does; **hypotonic** solutions have a lesser concentration (osmotic pressure) of solutes.

Counterbalancing the osmotic pressure of plasma, which attracts fluid, is the hydrostatic pressure of the blood flowing through the capillaries, which pushes fluid out of the vascular space. **Hydrostatic pressure** is the pressure exerted by a fluid within a closed system. Thus, the hydrostatic pressure of blood is the force exerted by blood against the vascular walls, e.g., the artery walls. The principle involved in hydrostatic pressure is that fluids move from the area of greater pressure to the area of less pressure. For this reason, fluid moves out of blood vessels.

The net movement of water from plasma to tissue spaces thus depends on which force is greater: hydrostatic pressure, which forces fluid out of the blood vessels, or osmotic pressure, which draws fluid into the blood vessels. Normally, fluid moves out of capillaries at the arterial end, where the intravascular hydrostatic pressure exceeds the colloid osmotic pressure. At the venous end of the capillaries, where the colloid osmotic pressure is greater, fluid is drawn from the interstitial compartment into the intravascular compartment.

Selective Permeability of Membranes

Capillary and cellular membranes in the body are described as selectively permeable, because not all substances move with the same ease across the membranes. Compounds such as proteins and glycogen do not readily cross capillary and cellular membranes. Organic compounds such as glucose and amino acids move freely across capillary walls, although they often require active transport. Certain membranes, called **dialyzing membranes,** allow water molecules and particles in true solution (crystalloids), but not particles in colloid dispersion, to pass through. Most of the membranes that surround cells are dialyzing membranes.

Cellular (not capillary) membranes are particularly selective in regard to sodium and potassium ions. Movement of potassium across cell membranes depends on metabolic cellular activities. Administration of glucose or insulin accelerates the movement of potassium into the cells. Sodium enters in greater quantities when the cells lose potassium. Any factor that alters the properties of the cell membranes brings about changes in the distribution of sodium and potassium. Some of these factors are excitation of nerve and muscle cells, changes in pH, and anoxia.

Maintaining Balance

Factors Affecting Fluid and Electrolyte Balance

A number of factors influence the maintenance of fluid and electrolyte balance within individuals. Among these factors are age, environment, diet, stress, and illness. Fluid intake requirements vary with **age.** See Table 43–4 for approximate fluid requirements at different ages according to body weight. In elderly people, fluid and electrolyte imbalances are often associated with kidney or cardiac problems. Because the kidneys are less able to concentrate urine, the elderly person may need to take in additional fluid to meet his or her fluid needs.

Excessive heat in the **external environment** stimulates the sympathetic nervous system and causes the person to sweat. When the person is not acclimatized to the heat, the sweat glands are strongly stimulated, and he or she can lose as much as 700 ml to 2 liters per hour by sweating. The sodium chloride (NaCl) in the sweat is also lost. An unacclimatized person can lose as much as 15 to 30 g of salt each day (Guyton 1986, p. 853).

When an individual's **diet** is inadequate or nutritionally unbalanced, the body tries to preserve stored protein by breaking down glycogen and fat. Once these resources are gone, the body draws on protein stores, and the serum albumin level decreases. Serum albumin plays an important role in drawing fluid from the interstitial body compartment into the blood through osmosis. When fluid is not drawn normally into the bloodstream, it remains in the interstitial space, causing edema.

Stress increases cellular metabolism, blood glucose concentration, and muscle glycolysis. These mechanisms can lead to sodium and water retention. In addition, stress can increase production of the antidiuretic hormone, which in turn decreases urine production. The overall response of the body to stress is to increase the blood volume. See Chapter 16 for additional information.

Illness and extensive surgical procedures can change a person's fluid and electrolyte balance through a number of mechanisms. The stress response mentioned above is one of these. In addition, tissue trauma can cause the loss of fluid and electrolytes (principally potassium) from within the damaged cells. An example of such trauma is severe burns. The burned person loses plasma and interstitial fluid. Water vapor is lost from the burn site, blood leaks from damaged capillaries, and water and sodium move into the tissue cells (Metheny and Snively 1983, pp. 204–5). Impaired heart function can decrease blood flow to the kidneys and thus hinder the elimination of the waste products of metabolism. When urine output decreases, the body retains sodium, and circulatory overload (hypervolemia) can result. Fluid retention can also lead to pulmonary edema (fluid in the lungs).

Regulating Fluid Volume

In the healthy person, fluid intake is counterbalanced by fluid loss. Illness can upset this balance so that the body has too little or too much fluid. During periods of moderate activity at moderate temperature, the average adult drinks about 1500 ml per day, but actual fluid needs are 2500 ml per day. This added volume is acquired from foods (referred to as preformed water) and from the oxidation of these foods during metabolic processes.

The primary regulator of fluid intake is the body's *thirst mechanism.* The thirst center is situated in the supraoptic nuclei in the lateral preoptic area of the hypothalamus. A number of stimuli trigger this center:

1. Intracellular dehydration
2. Excess angiotensin II (a hormone released into the blood in response to very low blood pressure) in the body fluids
3. Hemorrhage
4. Low cardiac output resulting in lowered blood volume

Dryness of the mouth is often associated with thirst but can occur independently (for example, when a person's salivary glands do not secrete saliva). Thirst is normally relieved immediately after drinking a small amount of fluid, even before it is absorbed from the gastrointestinal tract. However, this relief is only temporary, and the thirst returns in about 15 minutes. The thirst is again temporarily relieved after the ingested fluid distends the upper gastrointestinal tract. These mechanisms protect the individual from drinking too much, because it takes from 30 minutes to 1 hour for the fluid to be absorbed and distributed throughout the body. If a person continued to drink during that time, the fluid ingested would overdilute the body fluids.

Fluid losses counterbalance the adult's daily intake of water. The main channel of excretion is the kidneys, which are responsible for an output of about 1500 ml per day in the adult. This approximates the amount of fluid an adult drinks per day. Oral intake and kidney

Table 43–4 Average Daily Water Requirements, by Age and Weight

Age	Water Requirement	
	ml	ml/kg Body Weight
3 days	250–300	80–100
1 year	1150–300	120–135
2 years	1350–1500	115–125
4 years	1600–1800	100–110
10 years	2000–2500	70–85
14 years	2200–2700	50–60
18 years	2200–2700	40–50
Adult	2400–2600	20–30

Sources: R. E. Behrman and V. C. Vaughan, *Nelson textbook of pediatrics,* 13th ed. (Philadelphia: W. B. Saunders Co., 1987), p. 115; and R. B. Howard and N. H. Herbold, *Nutrition in clinical care,* 2d ed. (New York: McGraw-Hill, 1982), p. 153.

output are frequently and easily measured in nursing practice. Three other routes of fluid output are:

1. Insensible loss through the skin as perspiration and through the lungs as water vapor in the expired air
2. Noticeable loss through the skin as sweat
3. Loss through the intestines in feces

Obligatory loss is the essential fluid loss required to maintain body functioning. Water lost as vapor in expired air and as vapor from the skin, a minimum volume of about 500 ml from the kidneys, and the fluid required to excrete the solid metabolic wastes produced daily are the obligatory losses, totaling about 1300 ml per day. Since the vaporized losses and the water in feces are not readily measured, the measured obligatory kidney loss becomes of prime importance in critical illness. An adult hourly urine volume of less than 30 ml or daily volume under 500 ml is cause for concern. Clients with inadequate output require immediate attention, and such a finding by the nurse must therefore be reported promptly.

Although losses from the skin, lungs, and intestines in health account for approximately half of the daily loss, they can account for a much larger percentage of loss from a client who has a fever or accelerated respiration. Increases in respiratory rate, fever, diaphoresis (sweating), and diarrhea can magnify fluid loss from the normal routes. Other routes of loss, such as from the stomach through emesis or suction or from abnormal body openings such as fistulas or surgically implanted drainage tubes, often account for significant losses, all of which require intake replacements.

The formation of urine by the kidneys and its subsequent excretion from the urinary bladder is the major avenue of fluid output. One of the major controls of urine formation is blood volume. When the volume of circulating blood becomes excessive, the stretch receptors in the walls of the left and right atria are triggered to transmit impulses to the brain. The brain reacts by inhibiting sympathetic nervous impulses to the kidneys, reducing the secretion of antidiuretic hormone (ADH), and dilating the body's peripheral capillaries. As a result of these mechanisms, the rate of urine output is increased and excess blood volume filters temporarily into the tissue spaces.

Another control mechanism is the osmoreceptor of sodium and antidiuretic hormone system. This feedback system adjusts the urine formation by controlling the concentration of sodium in the extracellular fluid. An increase in the sodium concentration of the extracellular fluid stimulates osmoreceptors, which are located in the supraoptic nuclei of the hypothalamus. These stimulate the production of *antidiuretic hormone (ADH)* by the hypothalamus and release of ADH by the posterior pituitary gland. ADH acts on the cells of the distal and collecting tubules of the glomeruli to make them more permeable to water. As a result, more fluid is reabsorbed into the bloodstream to dilute the sodium and other substances in the extracellular fluid, and less urine is formed. When the extracellular fluid becomes sufficiently diluted, the osmoreceptors respond to the decreased sodium concentration by reducing the production of ADH. Consequently, the antidiuretic effect ceases, and additional urine is produced.

Regulating Electrolytes

The major electrolytes of the body are the cations sodium, potassium, and calcium and the anion chloride. Other electrolytes (e.g., magnesium and phosphate) are also significant for normal body functioning. Normal **sodium** concentrations in the extracellular fluid are regulated by ADH and aldosterone. *Aldosterone,* a hormone produced by the adrenal cortex, acts to maintain sodium concentrations, although its action can be overridden by ADH and the thirst mechanism described earlier. ADH regulates the amount of water absorbed into the blood from the renal tubules. Aldosterone regulates the amount of sodium reabsorbed into the blood. When aldosterone is secreted and the reabsorption of sodium is increased, the sodium concentration of the extracellular fluid rises. In a feedback mechanism, the increased extracellular sodium causes the adrenal cortex to decrease the secretion of aldosterone. If the body must conserve sodium for any reason, it can excrete sodium-free urine.

Sodium not only moves into and out of the body but also moves in careful balance among the three fluid compartments. It is found in most body secretions, e.g., saliva, gastric and intestinal secretions, bile, and pancreatic fluid. Therefore, continuous excretion of any of these fluids, e.g., via intestinal suction, can result in a sodium deficit.

Sodium functions largely in the control and regulation of the body fluids. When sodium is reabsorbed into the blood from the tubules of the glomeruli, chloride is reabsorbed with it. The combined reabsorption increases the fluid held in the body, helping to maintain blood volume and interstitial fluid volume. With potassium, sodium helps maintain the electrolyte balance of intracellular and extracellular fluids by means of the active transport mechanism, the sodium-potassium pump.

Hyponatremia is a sodium deficit in the blood plasma. This condition occurs with overhydration (an excess of fluid in the body). Two situations commonly precede hyponatremia:

1. Sodium loss that exceeds corresponding water loss, e.g., due to prolonged, excessive sweating or to the prolonged use of strong diuretics
2. Intake of water that exceeds corresponding intake of sodium, e.g., due to drinking excessive quantities of water

Clients can lose abnormally large amounts of sodium through the gastrointestinal tract. The sodium content of pancreatic secretions and gastric mucus is especially high. Severe, prolonged diarrhea or a draining pancreatic fistula can result in abnormally high sodium loss. Gastric suction, which withdraws gastric mucus along with other gastric fluids, can be the cause as well. See Table 43–5 for a summary of data regarding hyponatre-

Table 43–5 Summary Data Regarding Fluid and Electrolytes

Clinical Factor	Body Normal	Predisposing Conditions	Deficit Symptoms	Excess Symptoms	Food Source
Extracellular fluid	Infant: 29% of body weight Adult: 15% of body weight	*Deficit:* Insufficient fluid intake, vomiting, diarrhea *Excess:* Excess administration or intake of fluid with NaCl	Weight loss, dry skin and mucous membrane, thirst, oliguria, low blood pressure, plasma pH above 7.45, urine pH above 7.0	Weight gain, edema, puffy eyelids, high blood pressure	Meats, fruits, vegetables, liquids
Sodium (Na^+)	135–145 mEg/L (plasma)	*Deficit:* Excessive perspiration, gastrointestinal suction, diarrhea *Excess:* Inadequate water intake	Apprehension, abdominal cramps, rapid and weak pulse, oliguria, plasma sodium below 135 mEq/L	Dry and sticky mucous membranes, fever, thirst, firm rubbery tissue turgor, plasma sodium above 145 mEq/L	Table salt (NaCl), cheese, butter and margarine, processed meat (ham, bacon, pork), canned vegetables, vegetable juice
Chloride (Cl^-)	98–108 mEq/L (plasma)	*Deficit:* Increased HCO_3^-, loss through vomiting, excessive ECF loss through intestinal fistula *Excess:* Increased Na^+, excessive fluid loss through kidneys, severe dehydration	*See* sodium	*See* sodium	Table salt, dairy products, meat
Potassium (K^+)	3.6–5.0 mEq/L (plasma)	*Deficit:* Diarrhea, vomiting, some kidney disease, diuretic therapy, increased stress *Excess:* Renal failure, burns, excessive administration	Muscle weakness, abnormal heart rhythm, anorexia, abdominal distention	Oliguria, intestinal colic, irritability, irregular pulse, diarrhea	Nuts, fruits, vegetables, poultry, fish
Calcium (Ca^{++})	4.3–5.3 mEq/L (plasma)	*Deficit:* Removal of parathyroid glands, excessive loss of intestinal fluids, massive infections *Excess:* Overactive parathyroid gland, excessive ingestion of milk	Muscle cramp, tingling in the fingers, tetany, convulsions	Relaxed muscles, flank pain, kidney stones, deep bone pain	Dairy products, meat, fish, poultry, whole grain cereals, greens, beans
Phosphate (PO_4)	1.2–3.0 mEq/L (plasma)	*Deficit:* Excessive use of phosphate-binding antacids, malabsorption syndrome *Excess:* Renal insufficiency, hypoparathyroidism, Vitamin D intoxication, myelogenous leukemia, lymphoma	Same as for calcium excess	Same as for calcium deficit	Milk, cheese, meat, poultry, whole grains
Magnesium (Mg^{++})	1.5–2.5 mEq/L (plasma)	*Deficit:* Chronic alcoholism, acute pancreatitis, prolonged gastric suction, diarrhea, intestinal malabsorption syndrome *Excess:* Excessive use of magnesium-containing antacids, renal failure, Addison's disease	Confusion, dizziness, convulsions, hyperactive reflexes	Flushed skin, warmth, lethargy, coma, depressed respations and pulse	Whole grains, green, leafy vegetables

mia and other electrolyte imbalances discussed in this section.

Hypernatremia is sodium excess in the blood plasma that occurs with dehydration (insufficient fluid in the body). Hypernatremia can occur when:

1. Sodium intake greatly exceeds water intake
2. Water loss exceeds sodium loss

For example, a client may lose more water than sodium through a draining intestinal wound and as a result become hypernatremic. A client who is not treated for watery diarrhea may experience hypernatremia on about the fifth or sixth day after onset.

Chloride is the major anion of extracellular fluid (see Figure 43–1, earlier). Chloride is found in blood, interstitial fluid, and lymph. A very small amount is found in intracellular fluid. It functions as sodium does to maintain the osmotic pressure of the blood. Its reabsorption in the kidney is secondary to that of sodium; i.e., each sodium ion reabsorbed is accompanied by the chloride or bicarbonate ion. Because aldosterone controls the reabsorption of sodium, it controls the reabsorption of chloride indirectly. **Hypochloremia** (a deficit in serum chloride) and **hyperchloremia** (an excess serum chloride) usually develop along with sodium disturbances.

Potassium is the major cation of intracellular fluid (see Figure 43–1, earlier). Potassium balance is regulated in the kidneys by two mechanisms: exchange with sodium ions in the kidney tubules and secretion of *aldosterone.* Aldosterone is extremely important in controlling potassium concentrations in extracellular fluids. The aldosterone-potassium feedback system works in three steps:

1. Increased potassium concentration in extracellular fluid causes an increase in the production of aldosterone.
2. The elevated aldosterone level increases the amount of potassium excreted by the kidneys.
3. As potassium excretion increases, the concentration of potassium in the extracellular fluid decreases, and, in turn, aldosterone production decreases.

Potassium affects the functions of most body systems, including the cardiovascular system, the gastrointestinal system, the neuromuscular system, and the respiratory system. Of particular importance is potassium's role in transmitting electrical impulses to the heart and other muscles, to lung tissues, and to intestinal tissues. Most of the body's potassium is found inside the cells. A small amount is found in the plasma and interstitial fluids.

Potassium is usually excreted by the kidneys. However, the kidneys do not regulate potassium excretion as effectively as sodium excretion. Therefore, an acute potassium deficiency can develop rapidly. Of the body's secretions, the gastrointestinal secretions are high in potassium. Like other electrolytes, potassium moves continually in and out of the cells. This movement from the interstitial fluid, which has less potassium, to the intracellular fluid, which has a greater concentration, is influenced by the adrenal steroids, testosterone, pH

changes, glycogen formation, and hyponatremia. Because potassium is the major intracellular ion, the body can lose potassium quickly if tissues are damaged.

Hypokalemia is a potassium deficit in the blood plasma. The combined effects of inadequate potassium intake and potassium loss because of prolonged diarrhea can deplete potassium stores acutely. The leading cause of potassium deficit is thought to be the use of powerful diuretics (Metheny and Snively 1983, p. 48). Surgical procedures, particularly those involving the digestive tract, often result in a potassium deficit unless supplemental potassium is supplied.

Hyperkalemia is a potassium excess in the blood plasma. Hyperkalemia is most often caused by a leakage of potassium from the body's cells, e.g., after severe burns. It can also occur as a result of excessive ingestion of potassium or the intravenous administration of excessive amounts of potassium when kidney function is impaired.

Calcium functions in bone formation and in the transmission of nerve impulses, muscle contraction, blood coagulation, and activation of certain enzymes, e.g., pancreatic lipase and phospholipase. Calcium is excreted in urine, feces, bile, digestive secretions, and sweat. The concentration of body calcium is controlled indirectly by the effect of *parathyroid hormone* on bone reabsorption. When calcium levels in extracellular fluid fall too low, the parathyroid glands are stimulated to increase parathyroid hormone (parathormone) secretion. This hormone acts directly on the bones to increase the release of calcium into the blood. When the bones run out of calcium, parathyroid hormone acts on both the kidney tubules and the intestinal mucosa to increase the reabsorption of calcium from the kidneys and the intestine.

Another hormone, *calcitonin,* has an effect nearly opposite that of the parathyroid hormone. Calcitonin reduces the concentration of calcium ions in the blood. Calcitonin, which is secreted by the thyroid gland, stimulates the deposition of calcium in bone and depresses the formation of osteoclasts in the bone. However, the effect of calcitonin on plasma concentration levels of adults is minimal (Guyton 1986, p. 947) because the parathyroid hormone counteracts the effect of calcitonin within hours.

Hypocalcemia is a calcium deficit in the blood plasma. Two common causes of hypocalcemia are removal of the parathyroid glands and excessive loss of intestinal secretions, which contain a great deal of calcium. Mild hypocalcemia may be reflected as a tingling sensation in the fingers and around the mouth, and as abdominal and skeletal muscle cramps. Severe depletion can cause **tetany** (muscle spasms, sharp flexion of the wrists and ankles, cramps), which can lead to convulsions. **Hypercalcemia** is an excess of calcium in the blood plasma.

The **phosphate anion** is found both in intracellular and extracellular fluid. See Figure 43–1, earlier. Together with calcium, phosphate is involved in bone and tooth formation. It is also involved in chemical actions within the body's cells. Many of the B vitamins are effective only when combined with phosphate (Metheny and Snively 1983, p. 58). Phosphate is absorbed exceedingly well from the intestine, and it is excreted in the urine.

Phosphate is a threshold substance because none is lost in urine when blood plasma concentrations fall below a critical level. When the concentration is above the critical level, however, it is excreted in proportion to the increase. Therefore, the kidneys regulate the concentration of phosphate in the extracellular fluid. In addition, phosphate excretion is regulated by the parathyroid hormone.

Magnesium is important for maintaining neuromuscular activity within the body. Like calcium, magnesium is regulated by the parathyroid glands. It is absorbed from the intestinal tract. The magnesium content of the body is affected by the potassium concentration. If magnesium is deficient, the kidneys tend to excrete more potassium. Increased extracellular magnesium levels (**hypermagnesemia**) depress nervous system activity and skeletal muscle contractions. Low magnesium concentrations (**hypomagnesemia**), by contrast, cause increased irritability of the nervous system, peripheral vasodilation, and cardiac arrhythmias (Guyton 1986, p. 872).

Fluid Volume Imbalances

Extracellular Fluid Deficit

An extracellular fluid (ECF) deficit is also called a fluid deficit, hypovolemia, or dehydration. **ECF deficit** can occur because of an abrupt decrease in fluid intake or a marked increase in fluid output, i.e., an acute loss of secretions or excretions. The body's initial response to a fluid deficit is depletion of the intravascular compartment. Then fluid is drawn into the intravascular compartment, depleting the interstitial compartment. To compensate for the decreased interstitial volume, the body then draws intracellular fluid (ICF) out of the cells. This depletion of fluid volume can occur with diarrhea and vomiting. **Isotonic** deficits occur when proportionate amounts of fluid and electrolytes are lost. **Hypertonic** deficits exist when there is a greater loss of water

than of electrolytes. **Hypotonic** deficits, the least common type, occur when there is a greater loss of electrolytes than of water. Most ECF volume deficits are isotonic. The clinical signs of a ECF deficit in an adult are listed in the accompanying box.

Isolated water deficits (hypertonic deficits) may occur because of insufficient water intake, excessive solute intake, profuse and prolonged sweating, and certain disorders creating large renal fluid losses (Harvey et al. 1980, pp. 53–54). Dehydration due to insufficient intake of water is usually confined to the very young, the very old, and persons too debilitated to satisfy their own water needs. Insufficient intake is especially likely during hot weather, when there is increased loss through the skin. When the greatest fluid loss is through perspiration, the sweating person may also lose significant amounts of sodium, resulting in a coexisting sodium deficit (in which case, the ECF deficit would be isotonic).

Excess solute intake is most commonly seen in ill, elderly clients who receive nasogastric tube feedings, which have high protein and sodium chloride contents (e.g., 120 g of protein and 10 g of salt). Such solute intakes result in obligatory excretion of urine in volumes between 1200 and 1500 ml per day (Harvey et al. 1980, p. 54). Urine volumes may exceed 2000 to 2500 ml per day in elderly people, who often have significant impairments in renal concentrating ability. Thus, a greatly increased water intake (e.g., up to 3 or 4 liters per day) may be required to meet the demand created by a high solute intake.

Normally, water deficits by renal loss are rare, since antidiuretic hormone (ADH) acts promptly to decrease the rate of loss when any significant water deficit elevates the osmolarity of plasma. However, certain disorders of the hypothalamus, posterior pituitary gland, and kidney can lead to excessive fluid loss through the kidneys. These include *diabetes insipidus* and impairments in the ability of the kidneys to concentrate urine.

Many illnesses are characterized by excessive losses of gastrointestinal fluids. Fluid loss accompanies vomiting, diarrhea, fistulas, tube drainages, and bowel obstructions (in which fluids are not reabsorbed). With such losses, varying amounts of solutes (electrolytes) are also lost. Urine and sweat losses also create deficits in electrolytes. For practical purposes, it is wise to assume that in other than mild dehydration, the body also loses sodium, chloride, and potassium.

The severity of ECF deficits depends on the rate and volume of loss. See Table 43–6. When the body is deprived of water, the ECF compartment, including interstitial fluid, is reduced. However, water passes into plasma immediately. The water gained passes by osmosis from the intracellular compartments through interstitial fluid to the plasma. This transfer of water tends to preserve the circulating blood plasma volume. If the kidneys are functioning normally, they will attempt to retain water and salt by reducing the excretion of sodium chloride and water to minimal amounts. As dehydration progresses, the concentrations of the sodium ion and the chloride ion in plasma rise, thus increasing blood concentration.

Clinical Signs of ECF Deficit

Observations

▪ Postural hypotension

▪ Weight loss

▪ Decreased tearing and salivation

▪ Dryness in the axillae and groin

▪ Inelastic skin

▪ Oliguria

▪ Increased pulse and respiratory rates

Laboratory data

▪ Increased specific gravity of urine

▪ Elevated hematocrit

Table 43—6 Severity of Fluid Deficit and Excess

Severity	Magnitude of Deficit or Excess (liters)	% of Body Water Deficit or Excess	Serum Na* (mEq/L)	Serum Osmolality* (mOsm/kg)
Fluid deficit				
Mild	1.5–2	3–4.5	149–151	294–298
Moderate	2–4	4.5–10	152–158	299–313
Severe	4–6	10–15	159–166	314–329
Very severe	>6	>15	>166	>330
Fluid excess				
Mild	1.5–4	3–8	139–132	275–261
Moderate	4–6	8–13	131–127	262–251
Severe	6–10	13–22	126–118	250–233
Very severe	>10	>22	<118	<233

*Normal serum Na is 144 mEq/liter and normal serum osmolality is 285 mOsm/kg.
Source: From A. M. Harvey, R. J. Johns, V. A. McKusick, A. H. Owens, and R. S. Ross, *The principles and practice of medicine,* 20th ed. (New York: Appleton-Lange, 1980), pp. 53, 57.

Clients go into shock when intravascular fluid compartments become greatly depleted. Shock indicates that the deficits are so great that the compensatory regulatory mechanisms of the body can no longer maintain the plasma volume. This blood volume reduction, called **hypovolemia,** is responsible for such manifestations as a rapid weak pulse, a fall in blood pressure, and increased concentration of blood solutes. Since the kidneys rely on sufficient arterial blood pressure to produce urine, hypovolemia results in **oliguria** (decreased urine production), which may progress to **anuria** (absence of urine) as the deficit increases in severity. As a consequence, metabolic wastes accumulate, the client quickly becomes disoriented and comatose, and death may occur because of the effects of the acid waste products on the cells.

Extracellular Fluid Excess

A fluid volume excess, also called overhydration, is characterized by an excessive amount of ECF. Excesses of ECF lead to **hypervolemia** (increased blood volume) and **edema** (excess fluid in the interstitial compartment). Normally, the interstitial fluid compartment is not bogged with water but compact, elastic, and expandable, with just enough fluid to fill the crevices between tissues. This compact state facilitates diffusion of nutrients from the plasma to the ICF and diffusion of the metabolic wastes from the cells to the plasma.

Edema increases the distance between the blood capillaries and the cells and thus hinders cell nutrition. **Pitting edema** is edema that leaves a small depression or pit after finger pressure is applied to the swollen area. The pit is caused by movement of fluid to adjacent tissue, away from the point of pressure. Within 10 to 30 seconds, the pit normally disappears. Pitting edema is not seen in clients with a pure water excess (Harvey et al. 1980, p. 56); therefore, it is considered a classic sign of ECF excess. (In nonpitting edema, the fluid in edematous tissues cannot be moved to adjacent spaces by finger pressure. Nonpitting edema often accompanies infections and traumas that cause fluid to collect and coagulate in tissue spaces. The coagulation prevents displacement of fluid to other areas by pressure.)

Overloading of the vascular fluid compartment increases blood hydrostatic pressure, which forces fluid into the interstitial spaces. Elderly people have inelastic blood vessels and tolerate only small increases in blood volume before the hydrostatic pressure is substantially increased. Greatly increased hydrostatic pressure may force large amounts of fluid through the alveolar-capillary membrane into the alveoli of the lungs, causing pulmonary edema, a serious problem that can result in death by suffocation. Manifestations of pulmonary edema are frothy sputum, dyspnea, cough, and gurgling sounds on respiration.

When fluid moves from the vascular compartment into the interstitial spaces, the blood volume drops. In response, the body releases antidiuretic hormone (ADH) and aldosterone, which stimulate the kidneys to retain fluid and sodium. This response adds to the existing problem because the retained fluid can also move into the interstitial spaces, thus augmenting the edema. Therefore, generalized edema (**anasarca**) is a self-perpetuating condition. See the accompanying box for the clinical signs of ECF excess.

Clinical Signs of ECF Excess

Observations

- Peripheral edema (pitting)
- Puffy eyelids
- Ascites
- Moist rales in the lungs
- Full, bounding pulse
- Sudden weight gain

Laboratory data

- Not significant

Acid-Base Balance

The body's cellular activity requires an alkaline medium. Alkalinity and its opposite, acidity, are measured in terms of hydrogen ion concentration, expressed on a scale called **pH.** Body fluids are normally maintained at a pH of about 7.4. Alterations of pH of even a few tenths can be incompatible with cellular activity.

Opposing the body's alkalinity are cellular chemical processes that are constantly producing large amounts of acid as by-products of metabolism. Fortunately, precise control mechanisms maintain the pH of body fluids within a very narrow range. The pH is controlled by dilution of hydrogen ions in the ECF, by buffer systems in all body fluids, and by respiratory and kidney regulatory systems. Three major buffer systems of the body fluids are the bicarbonate buffer, the phosphate buffer, and the protein buffer.

Bicarbonate Buffer System

The bicarbonate buffer system consists of sodium bicarbonate ($NaHCO_3$) or potassium bicarbonate ($KHCO_3$) and carbonic acid (H_2CO_3) in the same solution. Buffers do not neutralize; rather, acid-base buffers decrease the effect of strong acids and strong bases, so that the pH of a body fluid falls or rises only slightly. For example, if a strong acid such as hydrochloric acid (HCl) is introduced into a glass of water, the pH of the fluid drops significantly to 1 or 2. However, if a bicarbonate buffer system is already present in the water, the HCl quickly combines with the buffer, producing a weaker acid (carbonic acid), and the pH drops only slightly. A strong acid is a compound that completely dissociates its hydrogen ions; for example, HCl yields H^+ and Cl^-. A weak acid frees only some of its hydrogen ions; for example, H_2CO_3 yields H^+ and HCO_3^-. One hydrogen ion is free, the other is not.

Alkalis (bases) undergo a similar change. When a strong base such as sodium hydroxide is added to body fluids, it combines with carbonic acid to form a weaker base, sodium bicarbonate. Although the bicarbonate buffer system is not the strongest buffer system in the body (the most powerful and plentiful one consists of the proteins of plasma and cells), it is important, because the concentration of carbonic acid by the lungs and the concentration of sodium bicarbonate is regulated by the kidneys. Table 43–7 summarizes acid-base balance.

Respiratory Regulation

The carbon dioxide that a person exhales comes from carbonic acid. The more carbon dioxide exhaled, the more carbonic acid is removed from the blood, thus changing the blood pH to a more alkaline level. Hyperventilation is an example of a mechanism by which respiratory regulation of acid-base balance is achieved. Increasing the ventilation rate raises the pH. By contrast, holding one's breath, or hypoventilating, causes the body to retain carbon dioxide, which is then available to form

Table 43-7 Acid-Base Balance

Clinical Factor	Body Normal	Primary Regulator	Predisposing Conditions	Deficit Symptoms	Excess Symptoms
Carbonic acid (H_2CO_3)	$Paco_2$ 35–45 mm Hg, plasma pH 7.35–7.45 (arterial blood)	Lungs	*Deficit:* Oxygen lack, fever, anxiety, pulmonary infections, hyperventilations *Excess:* Hypoventilation, chronic asthma, emphysema, barbiturate poisoning	Respiratory alkalosis, deep and rapid breathing, unconsciousness, plasma pH above 7.45, low $Paco_2$	Respiratory acidosis, disorientation, shallow respirations, plasma pH below 7.35, high $Paco_2$
Bicarbonate (HCO_3^-)	Plasma bicarbonates 21–28 mEq/L, urine pH 4.6–8.0, plasma pH 7.35–7.45 (arterial blood)	Kidneys	*Deficit:* Uncontrolled diabetes mellitus, starvation, severe infectious disease, renal insufficiency *Excess:* Loss of Cl^- and H^+ through vomiting, gastric suction, hyperadrenalism, prolonged insertion of alkali	Metabolic acidosis, disorientation, weakness, shortness of breath, sweet fruity odor to breath, plasma pH below 7.35, HCO_3^- below 25 mEq/L	Metabolic alkalosis, slow and shallow respirations, tetany, hypertonic muscles, plasma pH above 7.45, HCO_3^- above 30 mEq/L

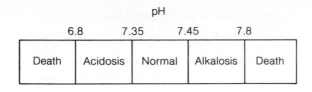

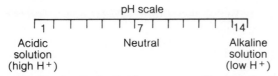

Figure 43–2 Body fluids are normally slightly alkaline, between a pH of 7.35 and 7.45.

carbonic acid, reducing the pH and acidifying body fluids. Respiratory alterations, therefore, change the pH of body fluids significantly and rapidly.

▮ Renal Regulation

The kidney's role in maintaining acid-base balance is complex. A simplified account of the process follows. The kidneys excrete hydrogen ions and form bicarbonate ions in specific amounts as indicated by the pH of the blood. When the plasma pH drops (becomes more acidic), hydrogen ions (acid) are excreted, and bicarbonate ions (base) are formed and retained. Conversely, when the plasma pH rises (becomes more alkaline), hydrogen ions are retained in the body, and bicarbonate ions are excreted.

▮ Primary Imbalances

The normal pH range of extracellular fluid is 7.35 to 7.45. See Figure 43–2. This precise balance is maintained as long as the ratio of 1 carbonic acid molecule to 20 bicarbonate ions is maintained in the extracellular fluid. The ratio, rather than the specific amount of each, is important. Imbalances in pH can result in either acidosis or alkalosis.

Clinical Signs of Respiratory Acidosis

Observations

▪ Hypoventilation evidenced by shallow respirations, poor exhalation, or respiratory embarrassment

▪ Loss of mental alertness and disorientation progressing to stupor, indicating central nervous system depression

Laboratory findings

▪ Low plasma pH (below 7.35) or a normal pH (if compensated)

▪ Low urine pH (below 6)

▪ High $Paco_2$ (above 45 mm Hg)

▪ Normal or high plasma bicarbonate (HCO_3^-) (if compensated):
  — Above 28 mEq/L in adults
  — Above 25 mEq/L in children

▪ Base excess (BE) is 0 or positive with chronic conditions that are compensated

Acidosis (blood pH below 7.35) occurs with increases in blood carbonic acid or with decreases in blood bicarbonate. **Alkalosis** (blood pH above 7.45) occurs with increases in blood bicarbonate or decreases in blood carbonic acid. A client will not become acidotic or alkalotic, however, unless the normal ratio of 1 carbonic acid molecule to 20 bicarbonate ions is altered.

The primary general cause or origin of a pH imbalance is indicated by the terms **metabolic** or **respiratory**. Metabolic acidosis and metabolic alkalosis are imbalances brought about by changes in bicarbonate levels as a result of metabolic alterations. Respiratory acidosis and respiratory alkalosis are imbalances brought about by changes in carbonic acid levels as a result of respiratory alterations. See Table 43–8 for laboratory indications of acid-base imbalances.

Table 43—8 Laboratory Indications of Acid-Base Imbalance

Sign	Normal	Interpretation
Plasma pH	7.35–7.45	Less than 7.35 → acidosis More than 7.45 → alkalosis
Urine pH	4.6–8.0	Below 6 → acidosis Above 7 → alkalosis
$Paco_2$	35–45mm Hg	Less than 35 → respiratory alkalosis More than 45 → respiratory acidosis
Bicarbonate (HCO_3^-)	21–28 mEq/L (about 25 mEq/L)	Less than 21 → metabolic acidosis More than 28 → metabolic alkalosis
Base excess (BE)	Male: −3.3 to +1.2 Female: −2.4 to +2.3	Positive results → alkaline excess Negative results → alkaline deficit These values do not always indicate a state of acidosis or alkalosis but show deficits or excesses of base.
Pao_2	80 to 100 mm Hg	May be greater than 100 mm Hg if client is on oxygen and less than 75 if there is a pulmonary problem.

In all acid-base imbalances, there is a corrective body response by both the kidneys and the lungs called **compensation.** Any given acid-base imbalance can be described as compensated until body reserves are used up. Then the condition is described as uncompensated. In compensated acidosis or alkalosis, the kidneys and lungs are able to restore the altered ratio of 1 carbonic acid molecule to 20 bicarbonate ions, thereby maintaining a normal pH. For example in (compensated) respiratory acidosis, the plasma pH is maintained at normal even though there is an increase in the carbonic acid because the kidneys retain bicarbonate.

Respiratory acidosis (carbonic acid excess) occurs when exhalation of carbonic dioxide is inhibited. Hypoventilation is its general cause. Two major conditions that cause hypoventilation are central nervous system depression and obstructive lung disease. Morphine poisoning and anesthesia are examples of central nervous system depression, whereas asthma and emphysema are obstructive lung diseases. See the accompanying box for the clinical signs of respiratory acidosis.

Metabolic acidosis (base bicarbonate deficit) occurs when levels of base bicarbonate are low in relation to carbonic acid blood levels. The kidneys normally retain bicarbonate (HCO_3^-) or excrete hydrogen ions (H^+) in response to altered blood pH. Starvation, renal impairment, and diabetes mellitus are among the conditions that deluge the plasma with acid metabolites. With renal impairment, related electrolyte imbalances may develop. Prolonged diarrhea can decrease bicarbonate. See the accompanying box for the clinical signs of metabolic acidosis.

Respiratory alkalosis (carbonic acid deficit) occurs when exhalation of carbonic dioxide is excessive, resulting in a carbonic acid deficit. Its root cause is hyper-

ventilation, which can be due to fever, anxiety, or pulmonary infections. A hyperventilating client blows off abundant carbon dioxide, resulting in lowered carbonic acid blood levels. The clinical signs of respiratory alkalosis are listed in the accompanying box. These signs reflect the primary imbalance, renal compensation, and associated electrolyte imbalances.

Metabolic alkalosis (bicarbonate excess) occurs when the level of base bicarbonate is high. Metabolic alkalosis may be due to excess intake of baking soda and other alkalis, prolonged vomiting, and other conditions that flood plasma with the bicarbonate anion. Prolonged vomiting causes the body to lose chloride and hydrogen ions. Loss of chloride ions causes a proportionate increase

---

Clinical Signs of Respiratory Alkalosis

Observations

- Hyperventilation (deep and/or rapid breathing)
- Paresthesias
- Mental restlessness and agitation progressing to hysteria and finally unconsciousness

Laboratory findings

- High plasma pH (above 7.45)
- High urine pH (above 7)
- Low plasma bicarbonate as a compensatory measure:
  — Below 21 mEq/l in adults
  — Below 20 mEq/l in children
- Low $Paco_2$ (below 35 mm Hg)
- Base excess: 0

Clinical Signs of Metabolic Acidosis

Observations

- Kussmaul breathing (deep rapid respirations), a compensatory mechanism, though absent in infants
- Weakness
- Disorientation
- Coma

Laboratory findings

- Low plasma pH (below 7.35) or a normal pH (if compensated)
- Low urine pH (below 6)
- Normal $Paco_2$ or low (if compensated in an attempt by the lungs to blow off more acid)
- Low plasma bicarbonate:
  — Below 21 mEq/l in adults
  — Below 20 mEq/l in children
- Base excess with negative results
- Hyperkalemia

Clinical Signs of Metabolic Alkalosis

Observations

- Depressed respiration (compensatory)
- Hypertonic muscles
- Tetany
- Mental dullness

Laboratory findings

- High plasma pH (above 7.45)
- High urine pH (above 7)
- High plasma bicarbonate:
  — Above 28 mEq/l in adults
  — Above 25 mEq/l in children
- Normal or high $Paco_2$ (above 45 mm Hg) as a compensatory elevation
- Base excess: positive results indicating an excess
- Hypokalemia

of bicarbonate in the blood. Related electrolyte imbalances acccount for some of the clinical signs. The clinical signs of metabolic alkalosis are summarized in the accompanying box.

Assessing Clients for Fluid and Electrolyte Balance

To assess a client's fluid and electrolyte balance, the nurse takes a nursing history, physically assesses the client, and refers to data in laboratory reports. The accompanying box summarizes the clinical status of a well-hydrated person.

Nursing History

A client's nursing history should include data about elimination patterns (see Chapters 40 and 41), oxygenation (see Chapter 42), and food and fluid intake (see Chapter 39). Specific data related to fluid and electrolyte balance should be included. See the accompanying box.

NURSING HISTORY

Fluid and Electrolyte Balance

Determine:

- Amount, type, and frequency of fluid intake
- Recent changes in health, e.g., draining wound
- Medications
- Dietary restrictions
- Health problems that affect fluid or electrolyte balance, e.g., vomiting

Physical Assessment

The client is examined for clinical signs of fluid, electrolyte, and acid-base imbalances. The nurse needs a knowledge of significant signs as well as the normal clinical picture presented by the client. Specific assessments should include body weight and assessment of each body system where potential or actual problems exist. Tables 43–5, 43–6, and 43–7, earlier, describe some common clinical signs of fluid, electrolyte, and acid-base imbalances.

Laboratory Reports

Diagnostic laboratory studies used to assess the client's fluid and electrolyte balance include analysis of serum electrolytes and arterial blood gas determinations. **Serum electrolyte levels** are frequently tested to determine the acid-base and electrolyte balance of the body fluids. The most commonly ordered serum tests are for sodium, potassium, carbon dioxide (bicarbonate), and chloride.

Serum sodium and potassium tests are done to determine changes in fluid and sodium balances in clients who have fluid imbalances, have cardiac, renal, or endocrine disorders, or are receiving intravenous infusions with electrolytes. Variations in the serum chloride level usually occur with changes in sodium level. Elevated serum chloride is found in such disorders as prostatic obstruction and renal failure. Decreased chloride levels may be found in clients with congestive heart failure or burns.

Tests normally carried out to determine acid-base balance are called **blood-gas determinations** and routinely include: blood pH, $Paco_2$ (carbonic acid concentration), total CO_2 (bicarbonate ion plus carbonic acid), Pao_2, and O_2 saturation. Specimens of arterial blood are taken for these tests. The *pH*, a measure of the concentration of hydrogen ions, indicates the blood's acidity or alkalinity. Normal blood pH is 7.35–7.45. The $Paco_2$ is a measure of the pressure exerted by carbon dioxide gas dissolved in the blood. The *Pa* stands for **partial arterial pressure** (the pressure exerted by CO_2 in the arterial blood). This pressure is regulated by the lungs and reflects the amount of carbonic acid available to the bicarbonate and carbonic acid buffer system. A normal $Paco_2$ is 35 to 45 mm Hg.

Total CO_2 content is the measure of both the bicarbonate ion and carbonic acid in the blood. The total CO_2 measure provides an accurate guide to the functioning of the bicarbonate and carbonic acid buffer system. The combined measurement in arterial blood is normally 21 to 30 mEq/liter. Partial pressure of oxygen (Pao_2) is the pressure exerted by the small amount of oxygen that is dissolved in the plasma. This oxygen is separate from the oxygen carried by the hemoglobin of the erythrocytes. Normal values of Pao_2 are 80 to 100 mm Hg in arterial blood. Oxygen saturation (O_2 *Sat*) is the ratio of the oxygen in the blood to the maximum amount of oxygen the blood can carry. Normal values are 95 to 98% in arterial blood and 60 and 85% in venous blood. Oxygen saturation provides some indication of the functioning of the client's lung ventilation.

Nursing Diagnoses for Clients with Fluid and Electrolyte Imbalances

After analyzing the assessment data collected, the nurse identifies specific nursing diagnoses for individual clients. Client problems may reflect not only the primary imbalance (e.g., fluid, electrolyte, or acid-base), but also secondary imbalances, which may be related. Additionally, problems of mobility, impaired skin integrity, altered tissue perfusion, and potential for injury may be identified. Examples of nursing diagnoses for clients with fluid and electrolyte imbalances are given in the accompanying box.

Planning Care to Promote Fluid and Electrolyte Balance

When planning interventions for a client who has fluid and electrolyte imbalances, nurses should consider the following:

1. Monitoring fluid intake and output
2. Identifying signs and symptoms of imbalances
3. Correcting fluid and/or electrolyte imbalances
4. Maintaining fluid and/or electrolyte balances
5. Preventing/treating problems secondary to imbalances or therapy

Planning also includes establishing outcome criteria by which to gauge whether or not a client's problem is

Fluid and Electrolyte Imbalances: Clients at Risk

- Postoperative clients
- NPO clients
- Clients with intravenous infusions
- Clients with retention catheters and urinary drainage systems
- Clients with special drainages or suctions, such as a nasogastric suction
- Clients receiving diuretics
- Clients with excessive fluid losses, requiring increased intake
- Clients who retain fluids
- Clients with fluid restrictions
- Elderly clients who may not be taking in adequate fluids

resolved. For outcome criteria, see the section on evaluation later in this chapter.

Implementing Strategies to Maintain Balance and Correct Imbalances

Monitoring Fluid Intake and Output

Clients who have actual or potential fluid and/or electrolyte imbalances need to have their fluid intake and output monitored. The accompanying box lists

NURSING DIAGNOSIS

Fluid and Electrolyte Imbalances

- Fluid volume deficit related to inability to swallow
- Fluid volume deficit related to diarrhea
- Fluid volume excess related to inability to excrete fluids/sodium
- Fluid volume excess related to excessive intake of salty foods
- Impaired tissue integrity related to peripheral edema
- Potential for injury related to seizures secondary to hypomagnesemia
- Potential decreased cardiac output related to cardiac dysrythmias secondary to hyperkalemia
- Decreased periheral tissue perfusion related to hypovolemia
- Ineffective breathing pattern (hyperventilation) related to anxiety about anticipated surgery

Commonly Used Fluid Containers and Their Volumes

Water glass	200 ml
Juice glass	120 ml
Cup	180 ml
Soup bowl	
Adult	180 ml
Child	100 ml
Teapot	240 ml
Creamer	
Large	90 ml
Small	30 ml
Water pitcher	1000 ml
Jello, custard dish	100 ml
Ice cream dish	120 ml
Paper cup	
Large	200 ml
Small	120 ml

groups of clients who are commonly monitored in this way.

The unit used to measure intake and output (I & O) is the milliliter (ml) or cubic centimeter (cc); these are equivalent metric units of measurement. In household measures, 30 ml is roughly equivalent to 1 fluid ounce, 500 ml is about 1 pint, and 1000 ml is about 1 quart. To measure fluid intake, nurses must convert household measures such as a glass, cup, or soup bowl to metric units. Most agencies provide conversion tables, since the sizes of dishes vary from agency to agency. A table is often provided on or with the bedside I & O record. See the accompanying box for examples of equivalents.

Most agencies have a form for recording I & O, usually a bedside record on which the nurse lists all items measured and their quantities per shift. Some agencies have another form for recording the specifics of intravenous fluids, such as the type of solution, additives, time started, amounts absorbed, and amounts remaining per shift. Procedure 43–1 gives guidelines for measuring intake and output.

PROCEDURE 43–1

Monitoring Fluid Intake and Output

Equipment

■ A bedside I & O form and a pencil or pen

■ A bedside bedpan, commode, or urinal for the client

■ A calibrated container in which to measure the urine

Intervention

1. Explain to the client that an accurate measurement of fluid intake and output is required, the reason for it, and the need to use a bedpan or urinal (unless a urinary drainage system is in place). Many people wish to be involved in recording these measurements and need to be given further information about how to compute the values and what foods are considered fluids.

2. Establish with the client a plan for ingesting the required amount of fluid. Generally, one-half the total volume is ingested on the day shift, and the other half is divided between the evening and night shifts, with the majority on the evening shift.

To Measure Fluid Intake

3. Following meals, record on the I & O form the amount of each fluid item taken, if the client has not already done so. Specify the kind of fluid and the time. Measure all obvious fluids, such as water, milk, juice, soft drinks, coffee, tea, cream, soup, sherry, and wine. Also include such foods as ice cream, sherbet, custard, and gelatin (Jello), ie, any food that turns to liquid at room temperature. Do not measure foods that are pureed.
   Rationale: Pureed foods are simply solid foods prepared in a different form.

4. Determine whether the client had taken any other fluids ingested between meals, and add the amounts to the form. Include water that is taken with medications. To assess the amount of water used from a water pitcher, measure what remains, and subtract this amount from the full amount of the pitcher. Then refill the pitcher.

5. Total the measurements at the end of the shift (every 8 or 12 hours), and transfer these totals onto the client's record. Include the total volumes of intravenous fluids, including blood transfusions. In some critical care settings, you may need to record intake hourly.

To Measure Fluid Output

6. Following each voiding, pour the urine into the measuring container, observe the amount, and record it and the time of voiding on the bedside I & O form. Clean the bedpan and measuring container, and return the bedpan to the client.

7. For clients with retention catheters, note and record the amount of urine at the end of the shift, and then empty the drainage bag. The drainage bag usually has markings that indicate the amount of urine. If there is any doubt about the amount in the drainage bag, empty it first into an accurate measuring container.

8. Record any other output, such as emesis, liquid feces, and other drainage. Specify the type of fluid and the time.

9. If the client is incontinent of urine or is extremely diaphoretic, estimate and record these "outputs." For example, of an incontinent client you might record "Incontinent × 3," or "Drawsheet soaked in 12-in. diameter." Of a diaphoretic client you might record: "Perspiring profusely [or + + +]. Gown and drawsheet changed × 2." Follow agency practices in this regard.

10. At the end of the shift (every 8 or 12 hours), total the measurements, and transfer the totals to the correct column on the record. In some critical care units, you may need to total the fluid measurements hourly.

11. Compare the total fluid output measurement with the total fluid intake measurement and compare both measurements to previous measurements.
    Rationale: Determines whether the fluid output

reflects the fluid intake and any changes in fluid balance.

12. Observe the client for signs of dehydration or over-hydration. Weigh the client daily, if indicated. Weigh the client at the same time and with the same clothing, to assess weight gain or loss accurately (eg, before breakfast, dressed in a hospital gown, dressing gown, and slippers). Assess ankle edema daily by measuring the ankle circumference with a measuring tape.

13. Report to the nurse in charge inadequate intakes and outputs. An adult urine output of less than 500 ml in 24 hours or less than 30 cc/hour is considered inadequate.

14. Document pertinent assessment data.

15. Adjust the nursing care plan as needed to ensure appropriate fluid intake for the client and appropriate measurement of I & O.

Considerations for the Elderly

The sensation of thirst generally induces sufficient intake of fluid in elderly individuals; however, some people with chronic illness may lose this regulatory capacity.

Worthington (1979) points out that in institutions the fluid needs of some elderly people may not be met if a prolonged period of time elapses between dinner and breakfast. Dehydration can easily develop if dinner has been served early and breakfast served late. It is recommended that elderly people be served an evening fluid snack to prevent this potential fluid deficit.

Providing Fluids and Electrolytes Orally

When the client's health permits, fluid and electrolytes may be replaced orally. Some clients may need to drink a large volume of fluid, e.g., over 3000 ml daily. For others, oral intake may be restricted. Fluid restrictions vary from "nothing by mouth" (NPO) to a precise amount ordered by a physician. In addition, a client may be limited to only fluids or only clear fluids. See Chapter 39. It is important that the client and support persons understand the fluid requirements and the reasons for them so that the client does not mistakenly take fluids that are not permitted. Electrolytes can often be provided orally through food and fluids. Potassium commonly needs to be supplemented. See Table 43–9 for foods high in specific electrolytes. Nurses can often help clients by giving them a list of foods and fluids high in the electrolyte they require.

Maintaining Intravenous Therapy

Intravenous (I.V.) fluid therapy is a common practice today. It is an efficient and effective method of supplying fluids directly into the extracellular fluid compartment, specifically the venous system. Intravenous fluid therapy is ordered by the physician. The nurse is responsible for administering and maintaining the therapy.

Intravenous therapy can be prescribed:

1. To supply fluid when clients are unable to take in an adequate volume of fluids by mouth
2. To provide salts needed to maintain electrolyte balance
3. To provide glucose (dextrose), the main fuel for metabolism
4. To provide water-soluble vitamins and medications
5. To establish a lifeline for rapidly needed medications

Common I.V. solutions include nutrient solutions, electrolyte solutions, alkalizing and acidifying solutions, and blood volume expanders. **Nutrient solutions** contain some form of carbohydrate (e.g., dextrose, glucose, or levulose) and water. Water is supplied for fluid requirements and carbohydrate for calories and energy. For example, 1 liter of 5% dextrose provides 170 calories. Nutrient solutions are useful in preventing dehydration and ketosis but do not provide sufficient calories to promote wound healing, weight gain, or normal growth in children. Common nutrient solutions are 5% dextrose in water (D5W) and 5% dextrose in 0.45% sodium chloride (dextrose in half-strength saline).

Electrolyte solutions contain varying amounts of cations and anions. Commonly used solutions are normal saline (0.9% sodium chloride solution), Ringer's solution (which contains sodium, chloride, potassium, and calcium), and lactated Ringer's solution (which contains sodium, chloride, potassium, calcium, and lactate). Lactate is a salt of lactic acid that is metabolized in the liver to form bicarbonate (HCO_3^-). Saline solutions are frequently used as initial hydrating solutions. Multiple electrolyte solutions approximate the ionic profile of plasma and are used to prevent dehydration or to restore or correct fluid and electrolyte imbalances.

Alkalizing solutions are administered to counteract metabolic acidosis. One commonly used solution is lactated Ringer's solution. **Acidifying solutions,** in contrast, are administered to counteract metabolic alkalosis. Examples of acidifying solutions are 5% dextrose in 0.45% sodium chloride and 0.9% sodium chloride solution.

Table 43–9 Major Food Sources of Selected Electrolytes

Electrolyte	Sources
Sodium (Na)	Table salt, cheese, ham, processed meats, canned foods, fish
Potassium (K)	Dark leafy greens, bananas, oranges, nuts, meat, fish, liver
Calcium (Ca)	Milk, cheese, yogurt
Magnesium (Mg)	Nuts, peanut butter, whole grains
Phosphorus (P)	Milk, poultry, fish, cereals

Blood volume expanders are used to increase the volume of blood following severe loss of blood (e.g., from hemorrhage) or plasma (e.g., from severe burns, which draw large amounts of plasma from the bloodstream to the burn site). Common blood volume expanders are dextran, plasma, and human serum albumin.

Agency practices vary about which nurses perform venipunctures and start intravenous infusions. In many settings, nurses must be supervised and certified before they are permitted to start infusions on their own. Some agencies have teams of specially prepared nurses who initiate all intravenous infusions.

An important nursing function is to **regulate the flow rate of an intravenous infusion.** The physician usually specifies in the I.V. order how long an infusion should last, e.g., 3000 ml over 24 hours. It is then a nursing responsibility to calculate the correct flow rate and regulate the infusion. There are a number of commercially prepared infusion sets (see Figure 43–3 for an example), and each has its own type of drip chamber, so it is important to know the number of drops per milliliter of solution for a particular drip chamber before calculating a drip rate. This rate is called the **drop** or **drip factor** and is printed on most commercially prepared packages. Common drop factors are 10, 15, and 20 for macrodrips (regular infusion sets) and 60 for microdrips (minidrip infusion sets).

Flow rates must contain a volume to be infused in a specified time segment. Two commonly used methods of indicating flow rates are designating the number of drops of solution to be given in 1 minute (gtts/min) or the number of milliliters to be administered in 1 hour (ml/hr). Since 1 milliliter of fluid displaces 1 cubic centimeter of space, the volume to be infused may also be designated as cubic centimeters per hour (cc/hr).

Hourly rates of infusion can be calculated by dividing the total infusion volume by the total infusion time in hours. For example, if 3000 ml is infused in 24 hours, the number of milliliters per hour is 125. Nurses should check infusions at least every hour to ensure that the indicated milliliters per hour have been infused. A strip of adhesive marking the exact time and/or amount to be infused may be taped to the solution bottle. Some agencies make premarked labels available. See Figure 43–4.

Unless a regulating device (i.e., a controller, infusion pump, or in-line manual adjuster) is being used, the nurse administering the intravenous solution must regulate the drops per minute manually by using the roller clamp (see Figure 43–3) to ensure that the prescribed

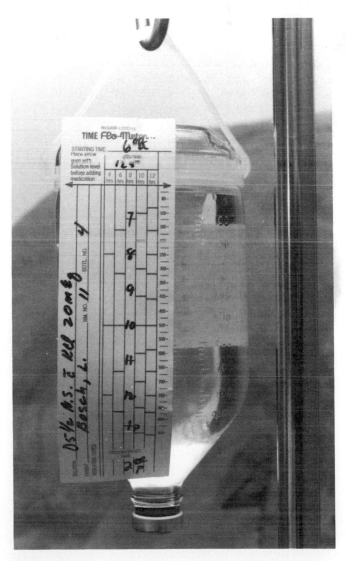

Figure 43–3

Figure 43–4 Timing label on an intravenous container

amount of solution will be infused in the desired time span. Drops per minute are calculated by multiplying the total volume to be infused by the drip factor and then dividing that figure by the total time of the infusion in minutes. For example, if the requirements are 1000 ml in 8 hours (480 minutes) and the drip factor is 20 gtts/ml, the drops per minute should be 41 gtts/min. The nurse must then regulate the drops per minute by tightening or releasing the intravenous tubing clamp and counting the drops in the drip chamber.

No matter how often flow rates are regulated, several **factors may alter the rate** of flow of an I.V. infusion. If an infusion is too fast or too slow, the nurse needs to consider several factors:

1. *The position of the forearm.* Sometimes a change in the position of the client's arm increases flow. Slight pronation, supination, extension, or elevation of the forearm on a pillow can increase flow.
2. *The position and patency of the tubing.* Not infrequently, the tubing is obstructed by the client's weight, a kink, or a clamp closed too tightly. The flow rate also diminishes when part of the tubing dangles below the puncture site.
3. *The height of the infusion bottle.* Elevating the infusion bottle a few inches can speed the flow by creating more pressure.
4. *Possible infiltration or fluid leakage.* Swelling, a feeling of coldness, and tenderness at the venipuncture site may indicate infiltration.

As part of the ongoing assessment of each client receiving intravenous therapy, the nurse should inspect the infusion site for fluid **infiltration** (the escape of intravenous fluid into the interstitial tissues). Infiltration occurs when the catheter has become dislodged from the client's vein, allowing the intravenous fluid to flow into the subcutaneous tissue. The clinical signs are swelling, coolness, pain, pallor at the site, and discomfort. To ascertain the presence of infiltration, the nurse:

1. Palpates the surrounding tissue for edema
2. Feels the surrounding skin for changes in temperature

If infiltration is not evident, the following measures can also be used to determine whether the needle is dislodged from the vein:

1. If the tubing does not have a backcheck valve, lower the infusion bottle below the level of the venipuncture site to see if blood returns. Blood may indicate that the intravenous needle is still in the vein. This method is not foolproof, however, because the needle may be only partially penetrating the vein wall.
2. Use a sterile syringe of saline to withdraw fluid from the rubber at the end of the tubing near the venipuncture site. If blood does not return, discontinue the intravenous infusion.
3. Try to stop the flow by applying a tourniquet 10 to 15 cm (4 to 6 in) above the insertion site and opening the roller clamp wide. If the infusion continues to flow slowly, the needle is in subcutaneous tissue (it has infiltrated).

When the nurse determines that the infusion has infiltrated, she or he should immediately discontinue the infusion. Discontinuing an infusion is not an uncomfortable procedure; in fact, it is usually a relief for the client and takes only a couple of minutes. The nurse first clamps the tubing to prevent fluid from flowing out when the catheter is removed. Next, the nurse loosens the tape at the venipuncture site, holds a swab above the site, and withdraws the catheter by pulling it out along the line of the vein. Gentle pressure is applied over the site for 2-3 minutes before the nurse applies a sterile dressing. If bleeding persists at the site, the nurse elevates the limb to decrease blood flow to the area. After removing the catheter, the nurse should inspect it to ensure that it is intact. The nurse should report a broken catheter to the physician so that it can be removed. Particles of the catheter remaining in the vein could become dislodged and travel toward the heart and lungs, potentially causing a serious problem.

The nurse should also include inspection for the presence of **phlebitis** (inflammation of a vein) as part of the initial and ongoing assessment of each client receiving intravenous therapy. Phlebitis can occur as a result of injury to a vein, e.g., because of mechanical trauma or chemical irritation. Chemical injury to a vein can occur from intravenous electrolytes (especially potassium and magnesium) and medications. The clinical signs are redness, warmth, and swelling at the intravenous site and burning pain along the course of a vein. Should phlebitis be detected, the infusion should be discontinued, warm compresses applied to the venipuncture site, and the injured vein should not be used for further infusions.

Being alert to signs of circulatory overload is another significant part of the nurse's ongoing assessment of the client. **Circulatory overload** means that the circulatory system contains more fluid than normal. An adult normally has about 6 liters of blood in circulation. A significant increase in this volume, e.g., when an I.V. is administered too quickly, can cause circulatory overload, which may result in pulmonary edema and cardiac failure. The clinical signs of cardiac failure are dyspnea, reduced urine output, edema, weak and rapid pulse, and shallow, rapid respirations. The clinical signs of pulmonary edema are dyspnea, coughing, frothy sputum, and rales on auscultation.

Ongoing assessment should also include inspection for **bleeding** at the intravenous site. Oozing or bleeding into the surrounding tissues can occur while an I.V. is patent (freely flowing) but is more likely to occur after the needle has been removed from the vein. The site of insertion should always be inspected for evidence of blood, particularly in clients who bleed readily, e.g., clients receiving anticoagulants.

Another nursing responsibility is to ensure that the **correct solution** is being infused. If the solution is incorrect, the nurse slows the rate of flow to a minimum to maintain the patency of the catheter. If the I.V. is terminated, the client will have to have another venipuncture before the new solution is administered. The error is reported to the nurse in charge and the solution is changed to the correct one. Agencies have different policies about how and to whom to report an incident.

In addition to assessing the client, the nurse should also **inspect the system** to make sure that it is intact. If there is leakage, the nurse locates the source. If the leak is at the catheter connection, the tubing into the catheter is tightened. If the leak cannot be stopped, the nurse slows the I.V. as much as possible without stopping it and replaces the tubing with a new sterile set. The system should be inspected for blockages. The flow of solution can be blocked or impeded for several reasons, and systematic assessment helps the nurse identify and correct problems rapidly. If blockage is suspected:

1. Check the tubing for any kinks. Arrange the tubing so that it is lightly coiled and under no pressure. Sometimes the tubing becomes caught under the client's arm, and the weight of the arm blocks the flow.
2. Determine whether the bevel of the catheter is blocked against the wall of the vein. If it is blocked, pull back gently, turn it slightly, or carefully raise or lower the angle of insertion slightly, using a sterile gauze pad underneath to protect the skin and change the position of the catheter bevel.
3. Examine the tubing clamp. If it is closed, adjust it to the open position.
4. Observe the position of the solution container. If it is less than 1 m (3 ft) above the I.V. site, readjust it to the correct height on the pole. If the container is too low, the solution may not flow into the vein because there is insufficient gravitational pressure to overcome the pressure of the blood within the vein.

5. Observe the position of the tubing. If it is dangling below the venipuncture, coil it carefully on the surface of the bed. The solution cannot flow upward into the vein against the force of gravity.
6. If the drip chamber is less than half full, the nurse should squeeze the chamber (see Figure 43–5) to allow the correct amount of fluid to flow in.

The nurse needs to teach clients when to call for assistance. To help the client maintain an intravenous infusion, the nurse should caution him or her to:

1. Avoid sudden twisting or turning movements of the arm with the needle or catheter.
2. Avoid stretching or placing tension on the tubing.
3. Try to keep the tubing from dangling below the level of the needle.
4. Notify a nurse if:
   a. There is a sudden change in the flow rate.
   b. The solution container is nearly empty.
   c. There is blood in the I.V. tubing.
   d. He or she feels discomfort at the I.V. site.

Most clients receiving intravenous therapy have a peripheral line in place, but in some instances a central venous line is inserted. A **central venous line** is a catheter inserted into a large vein located centrally in the body. The tip of the catheter may terminate in the vein, e.g., the superior vena cava, or in the right atrium of the heart. See Figure 43–6. Central venous lines are inserted primarily for the following reasons:

1. To administer nutritional solutions that are highly irritating to smaller veins
2. To administer irritating medications
3. To monitor central venous pressure (CVP)
4. To withdraw central venous blood samples

To aid the nurse in monitoring intravenous therapy several kinds of pumps and controllers are used with I.V. infusions. Each should be set up according to the manufacturer's directions.

A number of kinds of electronic pumps and controllers are available to control I.V. flow rates more precisely than the standard I.V. system. A pump (see Figure 43–7) delivers I.V. fluids by exerting positive pressure on the I.V. tubing or on the I.V. fluid. In situations where the I.V. fluid flow is unrestricted, the pump pressure is comparable to that of gravity flow. However, if restrictions develop (e.g., increased venous resistance) the pump can maintain the fluid flow by increasing the pressure applied to the fluid. A controller, on the other hand, operates solely by gravitational force (see Figure 43–8). The delivery pressure depends on the height of the I.V. container in relation to the venipuncture site. The I.V. container must be at least 76 cm (30 in) above the venipuncture site for a controller to work. A controller does not have the ability to add pressure to the line to overcome resistances to fluid flow.

Two types of delivery systems are provided: drops per minute and milliliters per hour. The drops-per-minute models, also referred to as rate-consistent devices, are useful when fluid needs to be delivered at a constant

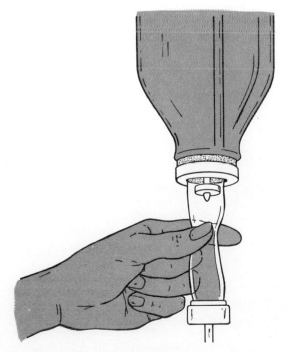

Figure 43–5

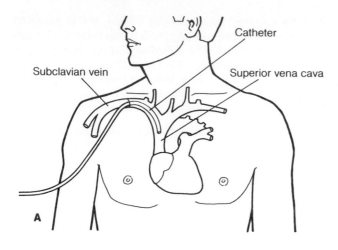

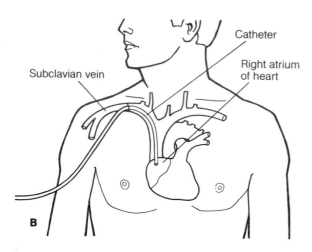

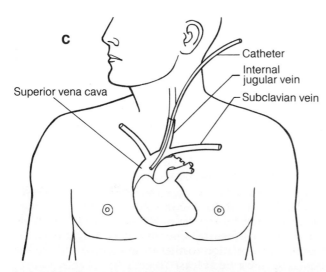

Figure 43–6 Central venous lines with: **A,** the catheter tip in the superior vena cava; **B,** the catheter tip in the right atrium of the heart; and **C,** left jugular insertion and catheter tip placement in the superior vena cava.

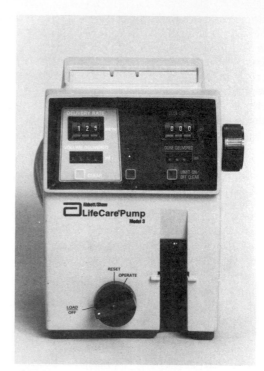

Figure 43–7 An intravenous infusion pump

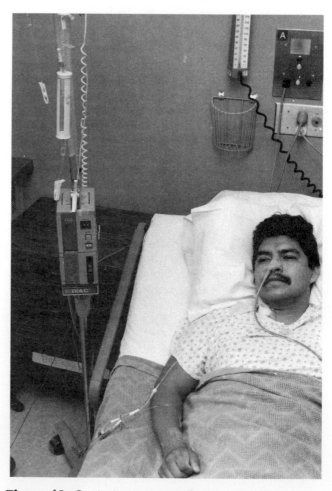

Figure 43–8 An intravenous infusion controller

and consistent rate to maintain a specific drug level in the client's blood or to achieve a desired client response. The milliliters-per-hour system, or volumetric device, is useful when a specific volume of fluid is to be delivered over a unit of time, e.g., 500 ml in 2 hours. Newborns, burn victims, and clients with renal or congestive heart failure usually require volumetric accuracy.

Some or all of the following special features may be included on pumps and controller.

■ **Alarms.** Both visible and audible alarms are usually available. In controllers the alarm is triggered when the infusion flow cannot be maintained by gravity to the selected rate. In pumps an occlusion alarm sounds when a restriction to flow cannot be overcome as the pump increases its pressure. When an alarm is activated some devices automatically stop; others maintain a low flow rate (e.g., 1–4 ml/hour) to keep the vein open. Some devices may also be equipped to trigger a remote alarm at the nurse-call system. The nurse needs to explain and demonstrate the alarm to clients so that they will know what to expect if it comes on later.

■ **Meters.** Some meters indicate the amount of I.V. fluid that has been delivered; others indicate the amount of fluid to be delivered.

■ **Flow Rate Settings.** On most models the flow-rate setting is simply set to the desired rate, i.e., in either drops/min or ml/hour.

■ **Drop Sensor.** The drop sensor is a photoelectric device that is placed on the drip chamber. It detects drops as they form and activates the alarm when no drops are formed (e.g., when the solution container is empty or when the I.V. tubing is occluded).

■ **Air Detector.** Some models activate an alarm when air is in the I.V. tubing.

■ **Occlusion Detector.** The pump sensor activates an alarm when back pressure becomes greater than the pump's preset limit (e.g., 10 or 15 psi). Most pumps have a psi rating that describes the maximum pressure at which the pump will trigger an occlusion alarm. This pressure rating differs from the actual pressure of fluid delivery. Excessive back pressure may be caused by infiltration, kinked or pinched I.V. tubing, an unopened tubing clamp, or an obstructed in-line filter or bottle airway. Accurate functioning of the occlusion alarm can be ascertained by pinching or clamping the I.V. tubing once or twice each shift.

■ **Battery.** To allow client mobility, most models are equipped with a rechargeable battery that operates the device from 1–4 hours.

If the equipment has an alarm system, explain the alarm to the client, and let the client hear it so that he or she will know what to expect if the alarm comes on later. Procedure 43–2 provides guidelines for using pumps and controllers.

PROCEDURE 43–2

Using an Infusion Pump or Controller

Equipment

- The controller or pump
- The I.V. solution or medication
- An I.V. pole
- An I.V. administration set with compatible I.V. tubing
- Sterile peristaltic tubing or a cassette if required
- Alcohol swabs and tape

Intervention

Setting Up an Infusion Controller

1. Plug the machine into the electric outlet, unless battery power is used.
2. Attach the controller to the I.V. pole so that it will be below and in line with the I.V. container.
3. Open the I.V. container, maintaining the sterility of the port, and spike the container with the administration set.

4. Place the I.V. container on the I.V. pole, and position the drip chamber 76 cm (30 in.) above the venipuncture site.
   Rationale: This provides sufficient gravitational pressure for the fluid to flow into the client.
5. Fill the drip chamber of the I.V. tubing one-third full.
   Rationale: If the drip chamber is filled more than halfway, the drops may be miscounted.
6. Rotate the drip chamber.
   Rationale: This removes vapor that could make the drop count inaccurate.
7. Prime the tubing, and close the clamp. Nonvolumetric controllers (regulators that measure the infusion in drops/minute) use standard tubing that is gravity-primed.
   Rationale: Priming expels all the air from the tubing.
8. Attach the I.V. drop sensor to the drip chamber so that the top edge of the sensor is in line with the drip orifice. Make sure the sensor is plugged into the controller.

Rationale: This placement ensures an accurate drop count. If the sensor is placed too high it can miss drops; if placed too low it may mistake splashes for drops.

9. Insert the tubing into the controller according to the manufacturer's instructions.

10. Perform a venipuncture or connect the tubing to the primary I.V. tubing or catheter. Don gloves before performing a venipuncture.

11. Open the I.V. control clamp completely.

12. Set the dials on the front of the controller to the appropriate infusion rate and volume. Set the volume at 50 ml less than the required amount, if the controller counts the volume infused.
Rationale: This will give the nurse time to attach a new container before the present one runs out completely.

13. Press the power button and the start button. Turn on the alarm switch.

14. Count the drops for a full minute.
Rationale: The nurse verifies that the rate has been correctly set and the controller is operating accurately.

15. Some nurses recommend that all connections be taped. Count the drop rate again after the taping.
Rationale: Taping could change the drop rate.

16. Record starting the I.V. with the controller, giving the data required for an intravenous infusion.

Setting Up an Infusion Pump

17. Check the manufacturer's directions before using an I.V. filter or before infusing blood.
Rationale: Infusion pump pressures may damage filters or cause rate inaccuracies. Certain models may also cause hemolysis of red blood cells.

18. Plug the machine into the electric outlet, unless battery power is used.

19. Attach the pump to the I.V. pole, usually at eye level.

Rationale: Because the pump does not depend on gravity pressure, it can be placed at any level. Eye level is convenient for checking its functioning.

20. Open the I.V. container, maintaining the sterility of the port, and spike the container with the administration set.

21. Place the I.V. container on the I.V. pole above the pump.

22. Follow steps 5 and 6.

23. Prime the tubing, and close the clamp. Most volumetric chamber pumps, ie, pumps calibrated to infuse a specific volume of fluid at a specific rate (ml/ hour), have a cassette that must also be primed. Manufacturers give instructions for doing this. Often the cassette must be inverted or tilted to be filled with fluid. Some volumetric pumps use special tubing, which is gravity-primed.

24. Position the drop sensor, if required, on the drip chamber. See step 8.

25. Load the machine according to the manufacturer's instructions.

26. Follow steps 10–16.

Monitoring an Infusion Pump or Controller

27. Monitor the drop rate and assess the client at least every hour. Observe the infusion, eg, for infiltration at the venipuncture site or leakage. A pump can increase the risk of extensive infiltration.

28. If the alarm sounds, check that
   a. The drip chamber is correctly filled.
   b. The I.V. tubing clamp is fully open.
   c. The container still has solution.
   d. The drop sensor is correctly placed.
   e. The I.V. container is correctly placed.
   f. The tubing is not pinched or kinked.

29. Discontinue the same way an intravenous infusion is terminated.

Intravenous solution containers are changed when only a small amount of fluid remains in the neck of the container and fluid still remains in the drip chamber. The Centers for Disease Control (CDC) recommend that tubing be changed every 48 hours to decrease the incidence of phlebitis and infection. Usually the tubing is changed at a time when the container is being changed. It is important to know agency practices regarding the frequency of changing infusion tubing and cleaning venipuncture sites. Procedure 43–3 provides guidelines for changing tubing.

PROCEDURE 43–3

Changing an Intravenous Container and Tubing

Equipment

To change the container:

▪ A container with the correct kind and amount of sterile solution.

To change the tubing:

▪ An administration set with sterile tubing, drip chamber, etc.

▪ Tape for taping the catheter and new tubing.

■ A sterile gauze square for positioning the needle.

■ Antiseptic solution and/or ointment for cleaning the site. Check agency practice.

■ Sterile swabs.

■ A receptacle (eg, a kidney basin) for discarded fluid.

■ Gloves to protect the nurse from contamination by the client's body secretions.

Intervention

1. Before starting, compare the number of the new container against the number on the used container. Read the label of the new container.

2. Assess the client for signs of infiltration, circulatory overload, and phlebitis. Also inspect the I.V. system for blockages.

3. Open the administration set and attach it to the container, using sterile technique.

4. Tighten the clamp and hang the container on the pole if it is not already hung.

5. Remove the protective cap from the end of the tubing, and prime the tubing. Clamp the tubing, and replace the protective cap.
   Rationale: Replacing the cap maintains the sterility of the end of the tubing.

6. Remove the tape and the dressing carefully from around the catheter. Take care not to dislodge the needle from the vein.

7. Place a sterile swab under the hub of the catheter to absorb any leakage that might occur when the tubing is disconnected. Clamp the old tubing.

8. Don gloves. While holding the hub of the catheter with the fingers of one hand, remove the tubing with the other hand, using a twisting, pulling motion. Place the end of the tubing in the kidney basin or other receptacle.
   Rationale: Holding the catheter firmly but gently maintains its position in the vein.

9. Continue to hold the catheter, and grasp the new tubing with the other hand. Remove the protective cap, and, maintaining sterility, insert the tubing end tightly into the catheter hub.

10. Open the clamp to start the solution flowing.

11. Clean the venipuncture site, working from the insertion point outward in a circular manner. Iodine or ethyl alcohol is frequently used. Some agencies

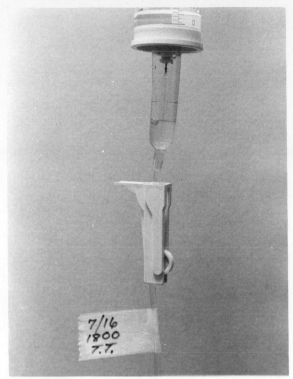

Figure 43–9

also place water-soluble iodine ointment, eg, Betadine, at the site.

12. Apply a sterile dressing over the site and tape the catheter in place. Apply a labeled tape over the dressing. The label should include the date and time the dressing is applied; the original date and time of the venipuncture; the size of the catheter; and your initials, as the nurse who changed the dressing.

13. Tape a label on the new tubing with the date and time of the change and your initials. See Figure 43–9.

14. Regulate the rate of flow of the solution according to the order on the chart.

15. Record the change of the solution container and/or tubing in the appropriate place on the client's chart. Also record the fluid intake according to agency practice. Some agencies have special flow sheets or intake and output records for recording I.V.s. Record the number of the container if the containers are numbered at the agency. Also record your assessments.

Evaluating Client Responses

Specific outcome criteria appropriate for the client's individual nursing diagnoses and goals should be selected. See the accompanying box for examples of outcome criteria related to fluid and electrolyte balances.

Chapter Highlights

■ A balance of both fluids and electrolytes in the body is necessary for health and life.

■ Extracellular fluid (ECF), subdivided into two compartments: intravascular (plasma) and interstitial,

OUTCOME CRITERIA

Fluid and Electrolyte Imbalances

The client will:

- Drink 3000 ml of fluid daily
- Have good tissue turgor
- Have a normal serum potassium
- Lose 3 pounds in 2 days
- Have a normal urine specific gravity
- Have a normal $Paco_2$

comprises about one-quarter to one-third of total body fluid.

Intracellular fluid (ICF) is the fluid inside the cells.

There are two types of body electrolytes (ions): positively charged ions (cations) and negatively charged ions (anions). The principal ions of ECF are sodium and chloride. The principal ions of ICF are potassium and phosphate.

Fluids move among the body compartments by diffusion, osmosis, and active transport. The major fluid pressures are osmotic pressure and hydrostatic pressure.

The three sources of body fluid are fluids taken orally, food ingested, and the oxidation of food. Fluid intake is regulated by the thirst mechanism.

Fluid output is chiefly through the excretion of urine, although body fluid is also lost through sweat, feces, and insensible vapor loss.

The most common electrolyte imbalances are deficits or excesses in sodium, potassium, and calcium.

The acid-base balance of the body is controlled by three buffer systems: bicarbonate, phosphate, and protein.

Acid-base imbalance occurs when the body fluids are higher or lower than the normal pH range: 7.35 to 7.45.

There are two types of acid-base disturbance, respiratory and metabolic, which can result in acidosis or alkalosis.

Parenteral therapy includes the administration of fluids and electrolytes intravenously (I.V.).

Assessment of a client's hydration and electrolyte status is an important nursing responsibility.

Selected References

Bellack, J. P., and Bamford, P. A. 1984. *Nursing assessment: A multidimensional approach.* Monterey, Calif.: Wadsworth Health Sciences Division.

Byrne, C. J.; Saxton, D. F.; Pelikan, P. K.; and Nugent, P. M. 1986. *Laboratory tests: Implications for nursing care.* 2d ed. Menlo Park, Calif.: Addison-Wesley Publishing Co.

Centers for Disease Control. 1982. Guidelines for prevention of intravascular infections. *Infection Control* 3:61–72.

Christian, J. L., and Greger, J. L. 1985. *Nutrition for living.* Menlo Park, Calif.: Benjamin/Cummings Publishing Co.

Feldstein, A. G. March 1985. Action stat catheter embolus. *Nursing 85* 15:59.

Feldstein, A. January 1986. Detect phlebitis and infiltration before they harm your patient. *Nursing 86* 16:44–47.

Folk-Lighty, M. February 1984. Solving the puzzles of patients' fluid imbalances. *Nursing 84* 14:34–41.

Frawley, L. W. December 1985. Cost-effective application of the Centers for Disease Control guideline for prevention of intravascular infections. *American Journal of Infection Control* 13:275–77.

Guyton, A. C. 1986. *Textbook of medical physiology.* 7th ed. Philadelphia: W. B. Saunders Co.

Harvey, A. M.; Johns, R. J.; McKusick, V. A.; Owens, A. H.; and Ross, R. S. 1980. *The principles and practice of medicine.* 20th ed. New York: Appleton-Century-Crofts.

Howard, M.; Puri, V.; and Paidipaty, B. November 1984. The effects of fluid resuscitation in the critically ill patient. *Heart and Lung* 13:649–54.

Huey, F. L. 1983. Setting up and troubleshooting. *American Journal of Nursing* 83:1026–28.

Keithley, J. K., and Fraulini, K. E. March 1982. What's behind that IV line? *Nursing 82* 12:32–42.

Metheny, N. M., and Snively, W. D. 1983. *Nurses' handbook of fluid balance.* 4th ed. Philadelphia: J. B. Lippincott Co.

Nelson, R., and Miller, H. March 1986. Keeping air out of IV lines. *Nursing 86* 16:57–59.

Vick, R. E. 1984. *Contemporary medical physiology.* Menlo Park, Calif.: Addison-Wesley Publishing Co.

Wiseman, M. April 1985. Setting standards for home IV therapy. *American Journal of Nursing* 85:421–23.

Wittig, P., and Semmler-Bertanzi, D. J. July 1983. Pumps and controllers: A nurse's assessment guide. *American Journal of Nursing* 83:1022–25.

Implementing Special Nursing Measures

9

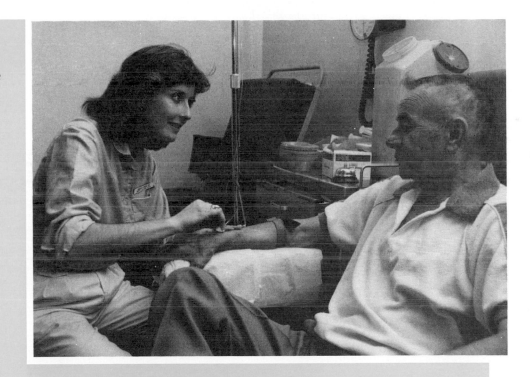

44

Medications

O B J E C T I V E S

Define selected terms related to administration of medications.

Describe legal aspects of administering drugs.

Identify physiologic factors and individual variables affecting drug action.

Describe various routes of drug administration.

Identify essential parts of a drug order.

Give examples of various types of medication orders.

Recognize abbreviations commonly used in medication orders.

List five essential steps to follow when administering drugs.

Describe physiologic changes in elderly persons that alter drug administration and effectiveness.

Outline steps required to administer oral medications safely.

Identify equipment required for parenteral medications.

Describe how to mix selected drugs from vials and ampules.

Identify sites used for subcutaneous, intramuscular, and intradermal injections.

Describe essential steps for safely administering parenteral medications by intradermal, subcutaneous, intramuscular, and intravenous routes.

Describe essential steps in safely administering topical medications: dermatologic, ophthalmic, otic, nasal, vaginal, and rectal preparations.

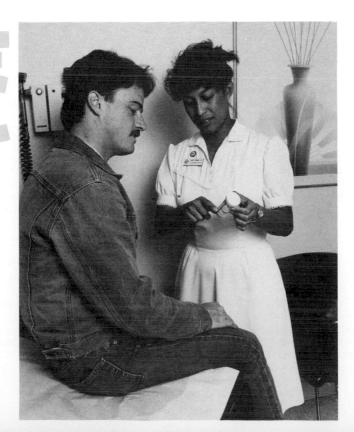

Names and Types of Medications

Medications have been known and used since antiquity. Crude drugs such as opium, castor oil, and vinegar were used in ancient times. Over the centuries the number of drugs available has increased greatly, and knowledge about these drugs has become correspondingly more accurate and detailed. A **medication** is a substance administered for the diagnosis, cure, treatment, mitigation (relief), or prevention of disease. In the health care context, the words **medication** and **drug** are generally used interchangeably. The term **drug** also has the connotation of an illicitly obtained substance such as heroin, cocaine, or amphetamines.

In the United States and Canada, medications are usually dispensed on the order of physicians and dentists. In some states in the United States, specially qualified nurse practitioners may also prescribe drugs. The written direction for the preparation and administration of a drug is called a **prescription.** One drug can have as many as four kinds of names: its generic name, official name, chemical name, and trademark or brand name. The **generic** name is given before a drug becomes official. The **official** name is the name under which it is listed in one of the official publications (e.g., the *United States Pharmacopeia*). The **chemical** name is the name by which a chemist knows it; this name describes the constituents of the drug precisely. The **trademark,** or **brand** name, is the name given by the drug manufacturer. Because one drug may be manufactured by several companies, it can have several trade names; for example, the drug hydrochlorothiazide (official name) is known by the trade names Esidrix and Hydro–Diuril. Medications are often available in a variety of forms. Common types of drug preparations are described in Table 44 –1.

Drug Standards

Drugs may have natural (e.g., plant, mineral, and animal) sources or they may be synthesized in the laboratory. For example, digitalis and opium are plant derived, iron and sodium chloride are minerals, insulin and vaccines have animal or human sources, and the sulfonamides and propoxyphene hydrochloride (the analgesic Darvon) are the products of laboratory synthesis. Early drugs were derived from the three natural sources only. During the past 45 years, however, more and more drugs have been produced synthetically.

Drugs vary in strength and activity. Drugs derived from plants, for example, vary in strength according to the age of the plant, the variety, the place in which it is grown, and the method by which it is preserved. Drugs must be pure and of uniform strength if drug dosages are to be predictable in their effect. Drug standards have therefore been developed to ensure uniform quality. In the United States, official drugs are those so designated by the Federal Food, Drug, and Cosmetic Act. These

Table 44–1 Types of Drug Preparations

Type	Description
Aqueous solution	One or more drugs dissolved in water.
Aerosol spray or foam	A liquid, powder, or foam deposited in a thin layer on the skin by air pressure
Aqueous suspension	One or more drugs finely divided in a liquid such as water
Capsule	A gelatinous container to hold a drug in powder, liquid, or oil form
Cream	A nongreasy, semisolid preparation used on the skin
Elixir	A sweetened and aromatic solution of alcohol used as a vehicle for medicinal agents
Extract	A concentrated form of a drug made from vegetables or animals
Fluid extract	An alcoholic solution of a drug from a vegetable source; the most concentrated of all fluid preparations
Gel or jelly	A clear or translucent semisolid that liquefies when applied to the skin
Liniment	An oily liquid used on the skin
Lotion	An emollient liquid that may be a clear solution, suspension, or emulsion used on the skin
Lozenge (troche)	A flat, round, or oval preparation that dissolves and releases a drug when held in the mouth
Ointment	A semisolid preparation of one or more drugs used for application to the skin and mucous membrane
Paste	A preparation like an ointment, but thicker and stiffer, that penetrates the skin less than an ointment
Pill	One or more drugs mixed with a cohesive material, in oval, round, or flattened shapes
Powder	A finely ground drug or drugs; some are used internally, others externally
Spirit	A concentrated alcoholic solution of a volatile substance
Suppository	One or several drugs mixed with a firm base such as gelatin and shaped for insertion into the body; the base dissolves gradually at body temperature, releasing the drug
Syrup	An aqueous solution of sugar often used to disguise unpleasant-tasting drugs
Tablet	A powdered drug compressed into a hard small disc; some are readily broken along a scored line; others are enteric-coated to prevent them from dissolving in the stomach
Tincture	An alcoholic or water-and-alcohol solution prepared from drugs derived from plants

drugs are officially listed in the *United States Pharmacopeia (USP)* and described according to their source, physical and chemical properties, tests for purity and identity, method of storage, assay, category, and normal dosages. In Canada, the *British Pharmacopoeia* is used for the same purpose, although some drugs used in Canada conform to the *USP* because they are obtained from the United States.

A **pharmacopoeia** is a book containing a list of products used in medicine, with descriptions of the product, chemical tests for determining identity and purity, and formulas for certain mixtures. A **formulary** is a collection of formulas and prescriptions. The United States' *National Formulary* lists drugs and their therapeutic value and can include drugs that may still be used but not listed in the *USP*. The *Canadian Formulary* lists drugs used extensively in Canada but not necessarily listed in the *British Pharmacopoeia*.

Pharmacopoeias and formularies are invaluable reference sources for nurses and nursing students. Nurses not only administer thousands of medications but also are responsible for assessing their effectiveness and recognizing unfavorable reactions to drugs. Since it is impossible to commit to memory all pertinent information about a very large number of drugs, nurses must have a reliable reference readily available.

Legal Aspects of Drug Administration

The administration of drugs in both the United States and Canada is controlled by law. In the United States the major federal acts controlling drugs are the Food, Drug, and Cosmetic Act (1938), its amendments, and the Comprehensive Drug Abuse Prevention and Control Act (1970) (Controlled Substances Act). In Canada, three federal acts control drugs: the Food and Drugs Act (1953), the Proprietary or Patent Medicine Act (1908), and the Narcotics Control Act (1961). See Table 44–2 for a summary of U.S. drug legislation. Table 44–3 provides a summary of Canadian drug legislation.

It is important for nurses to know how nursing practice acts in their areas define and limit their functions; it is equally important to recognize the limits of their own knowledge and skill. To function beyond the limits of nursing practice acts or one's ability is to endanger clients' lives and leave oneself open to malpractice suits. Under the law, nurses are responsible for their own actions regardless of whether there is a written order. If a physician writes an incorrect order (e.g., Demerol 500 mg instead of Demerol 50 mg), a nurse who administers the written incorrect dosage is responsible for the error. Therefore, nurses should question any order that appears unreasonable and refuse to give the medication until the order is clarified.

Another aspect of nursing practice governed by law is the use of narcotics and barbiturates. In hospitals, narcotics are kept under double lock in a drawer or

cupboard. Other medications, including barbiturates, are kept under single lock, although in some places barbiturates are kept with narcotics. Agencies have special forms for recording narcotics. The information required usually includes the name of the client, date and time of administration, name of the drug, dosage, and signature of the person who prepared and gave the narcotic. The name of the physician who ordered the narcotic may also be part of the record.

Included on the record are narcotics wasted during preparation. In most agencies, narcotic and barbiturate counts are taken at the end of each shift. The count total should tally with the total at the end of the last shift minus the number used. If the totals do not tally, the discrepancy must be reported immediately.

Table 44-2 United States Drug Legislation

Legislation	Content
Food, Drug, and Cosmetic Act (1938)	Implemented by Food and Drug Administration (FDA); requires that labels be accurate and that all drugs be tested for harmful effects
Durkham-Humphrey Amendment (1952)	Differentiates clearly between drugs that can be sold with and without a prescription
Kefauver-Harris Amendment (1962)	Requires proof of safety and efficacy of a drug for approval
Comprehensive Drug Abuse Prevention and Control Act (1970) (Controlled Substances Act)	Categorizes controlled substances (e.g., narcotics, amphetamines, barbiturates, and tranquilizers) and limits how often a prescription can be filled

Table 44-2 Canadian Drug Legislation

Legislation	Content
Proprietary or Patent Medicine Act (1908)	Protects the public against unsafe and ineffective over-the-counter drugs
Canada Food and Drugs Act (1953)	Prohibits advertising any food, drug, cosmetic, or device as a cure for certain specified diseases. Prohibits the sale of certain drugs unless approved by the federal government
Canadian Narcotic Control Act (1961)	Allows only authorized people to possess narcotics. Specifies records about narcotics that must be kept

The Actions of Drugs upon the Body

The action of a drug in the body can be described in terms of its **half-life,** the time interval required for the body's elimination processes to reduce the concentration of the drug in the body by one-half. For example, if a drug's half-life is 8 hours, then the amount of drug in the body is:

Initially	100%
After 8 hours	50%
After 16 hours	25%
After 24 hours	12.5%
After 32 hours	6.25%

Since the purpose of most drug therapy is to maintain a constant drug level in the body, repeated doses are required to maintain that level. When an orally administered drug is absorbed from the gastrointestinal tract into the blood plasma, its concentration in the plasma increases until the elimination rate equals the rate of absorption. This point is known as the **peak plasma level.** See Figure 44–1. Unless the client receives another dose of the drug, the concentration steadily decreases. Key terms related to drug actions are listed and described in the accompanying box. The actions of drugs on the body can be described in terms of four general principles (Reiss and Melick 1984, pp. 14–15). These principles are summarized in the accompanying box.

A drug that interacts with a receptor to produce a response is known as an **agonist.** Drugs that have no special pharmacologic action of their own but that inhibit or prevent the action of an agonist are called **specific antagonists.** There are also **partial agonists,** that is, drugs that interact with a receptor to elicit some response but at the same time have an antagonistic action. For

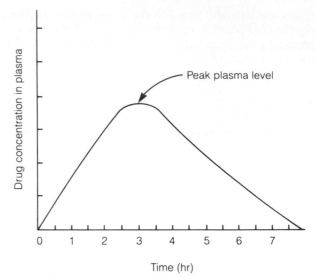

Figure 44–1 A graphic plot of the concentration of a drug in the blood plasma following a single dose

example, morphine, an agonist in depressing the central nervous system, will have its action blocked if a client is also given an antagonist, such as naloxone.

Variables Influencing Drug Action

A number of factors influence the actions of drugs upon the body. Among them are age, weight, sex, genetic and psychologic factors, illness and disease, time of administration, and environment. **Age** is a factor in that very young people and elderly people often are highly responsive to drugs and thus require lower doses. Immature liver and kidney function as well as diminished renal functioning due to aging can affect the action of a drug. **Body weight** also directly affects drug action; the greater the body weight, the greater the dosage required.

Sex-linked differences in the way men and women respond to drugs are chiefly due to two factors: differences in distribution of fat and water and hormonal differences. Because women usually weigh less than men, equal drug dosages are likely to affect women more than men. Women usually have more fatty pads than men, and men have more body fluid than women. Some drugs may be more soluble in fat, whereas others are more soluble in water. Thus, men absorb some drugs more readily than women, and vice versa.

Individuals may react differently to drugs as a result of **genetic factors.** A client may be abnormally sensitive to a drug or may metabolize a drug differently than most people because of genetic influences. Sometimes these reactions are mistaken for allergic reactions. **Psy-**

Key Terms Related to Drug Action

▪ Onset of action	The time after administration when the body initially responds to the drug
▪ Peak plasma level	The highest plasma level achieved by a single dose when the elimination rate of a drug equals the absorption rate
▪ Drug half-life (elimination half-life)	The time required for the elimination process to reduce the concentration of the drug to one half what it was at initial administration
▪ Plateau	When a drug's concentration in the plasma is maintained during a series of scheduled doses

General Principles Related to Drug Actions

Drugs act on existing cellular functions; they do not create new cellular function. For example, an antibiotic can slow microbial growth; laxatives can increase peristalsis.

Drugs act on the body in a number of ways. Some drugs alter the chemical composition of a body fluid; e.g., an antacid decreases the acidity of the gastric contents. Other drugs accumulate in certain body tissues because of their attraction to that tissue; e.g., propylthiouracil (PTU) is an antithyroid drug with an affinity for the thyroid gland, which thereby prevents the formation of thyroid hormones in the gland. Still other drugs act by forming a chemical bond with a receptor in the body. This binding occurs only when the drug and the receptor are compatible.

Drugs that reach the same receptor can be expected to produce a similar drug response in a client. For example, most penicillins, such as amoxicillin and cyclacillin, have a similar action.

chologic factors influence how one feels about a drug and what one believes it can do. A traditional example is the reaction of some people to a placebo, a substance (such as normal saline) often given to relieve pain. For some clients, the placebo has the same effect as an analgesic. See Chapter 38 for further information.

Illness and **disease** can also affect the action of drugs. For example, aspirin can reduce the body temperature of a feverish client but has no effect on the body temperature of a client without fever. Drug action is altered in clients with circulatory, liver, or kidney dysfunction. Diabetics need larger doses of insulin with fever or infection.

The **time of administration** of oral medications affects the relative speed with which they act. Orally administered medications are absorbed more quickly if the stomach is empty. Thus, oral medications taken 2 hours before meals act faster than those taken after meals. However, some medications irritate the gastrointestinal tract and need to be given after a meal, when they will be better tolerated, for example, iron preparations. A client's sleep-wake rhythm may affect the action of a drug. Circadian variations in urine output and blood circulation, for example, may affect a client's response to a drug.

The client's **environment** can affect the action of drugs, particularly those used to alter behavior and mood. Therefore, nurses assessing the effects of a drug need to consider the drug itself as well as the client's personality and milieu. Environmental temperature may also affect drug activity. When environmental temperature is high, the peripheral blood vessels dilate, thus intensifying the action of vasodilators. In contrast, a cold environment and the consequent vasoconstriction inhibit the action of vasodilators but enhance the action of vasoconstrictors.

Pharmacokinetics

Pharmacokinetics is the study of the absorption, distribution, biotransformation, and excretion of drugs. **Absorption** is the process by which a drug passes into the bloodstream. Unless the drug is administered directly into the bloodstream, absorption is the first step in the movement of the drug through the body. For absorption to occur, the correct form of the drug must be given by the route intended.

The rate of absorption of a drug in the stomach is variable. Food, for example, can delay the dissolution and absorption of some drugs as well as their passage into the small intestine, where most drug absorption occurs. Food can also combine with molecules of certain drugs, thereby changing their molecular structure and subsequently inhibiting or preventing their absorption. Another factor that affects the absorption of some drugs is the acid medium in the stomach. Acidity can vary according to the time of day, foods ingested, and the age of the client. Some drugs do not dissolve or have limited ability to dissolve in the gastrointestinal fluids, decreasing their absorption into the bloodstream. Some drugs are absorbed by tissues before they reach the stomach. For example, nitroglycerin is administered sublingually (under the tongue), where it is absorbed into the blood vessels that carry it directly to the heart, the intended site of action. If swallowed, this drug will be absorbed into the bloodstream and carried to the liver, where it will be destroyed.

A drug administered directly into the bloodstream, i.e., intravenously, is immediately in the vascular system without having to be absorbed. This then is the route of choice for rapid action. Because subcutaneous tissue has a poorer blood supply than muscle tissue, absorption from subcutaneous tissue is slower. The rate of absorption of a drug can be accelerated by the application of heat, which increases blood flow to the area; conversely, absorption can be slowed by the application of cold. In addition, the injection of a vasoconstrictor drug such as epinephrine into the tissue can slow absorption of other drugs. Some drugs intended to be absorbed slowly are suspended in a low-solubility medium such as oil. The absorption of drugs from the rectum into the bloodstream tends to be unpredictable. Therefore, this route is used when other routes are unavailable or when the intended action is localized to the rectum or sigmoid colon (Reiss and Melick 1984, p. 16).

Distribution is the transportation of a drug from its site of absorption to its site of action. When a drug enters the bloodstream it is carried to the most vascular organs, i.e., liver, kidneys, and brain. Body areas with lower blood supply, i.e., skin and muscles, receive the drug later. The chemical and physical properties of a drug largely determine the area of the body to which the drug will be attracted. For example, drugs that are fat soluble will accumulate in fatty tissue, whereas other drugs may bind with plasma proteins.

Biotransformation, also called **detoxification,** is a process by which a drug is converted to a less active form. Most biotransformation takes place in the liver.

There are many drug-metabolizing enzymes in the liver cells that detoxify the drugs. The products of this process are called *metabolites*. There are two types of metabolites: active and inactive. An *active metabolite* has a pharmacologic action itself, whereas an *inactive metabolite* does not.

The biotransformation capability of a client's liver may be impaired. For example, an elderly client, just like a client with hepatic damage, may have a decreased ability to metabolize drugs. In these situations, nurses must be alert to the accumulation of the active drug in the client and to subsequent toxicity.

Excretion is the process by which metabolites and drugs are eliminated from the body. Most metabolites are eliminated by the kidneys in the urine; however, some are excreted in the feces, the breath, perspiration, saliva, and breast milk. Certain drugs, e.g., general anesthetic agents, are excreted in an unchanged form via the respiratory tract. In addition to metabolites, alcohol is eliminated, unchanged, through the lungs. The efficiency with which the kidneys excrete drugs and metabolites diminishes with age. Elderly people may require smaller doses of a drug because the drug and its metabolites may accumulate in the body. Also, kidney disease can impair excretion of drugs and metabolites.

Routes of Administration

Pharmaceutical preparations are generally designed for one or two specific routes of administration. See Table 44–4. The route of administration should be indicated when the drug is ordered. When administering a drug, the nurse should ensure that the pharmaceutical preparation is appropriate for the route specified.

Table 44–4 Routes of Administration

Route	Advantages	Disadvantages
Oral	Most convenient Usually least expensive Safe, does not break skin barrier Administration usually does not cause stress	Inappropriate for clients nauseated or vomiting Drug may have unpleasant taste or odor Inappropriate when gastrointestinal tract has reduced mobility Inappropriate when client cannot swallow or is unconscious Cannot be used before certain diagnostic tests or surgical procedures Drug may discolor teeth, harm tooth enamel Drug may irritate gastric mucosa Drug can be aspirated by seriously ill clients
Sublinqual	Same as for oral, *plus;* Drug can be administered for local effect Drug is rapidly absorbed into the bloodstream Ensures greater potency because drug directly enters the blood and bypasses the liver	If swallowed, drug may be inactivated by gastric juice Drug must remain under tongue until dissolved and absorbed
Buccal	Same as for sublingual	Same as for sublingual
Rectal	Can be used when drug has objectionable taste or odor Drug released at slow, steady rate	Dose absorbed is unpredictable
Skin	Provides a local effect Few side-effects	May be messy and may soil clothes Drug can rapidly enter body through abrasions and cause systemic effects
Subcutaneous	Onset of drug action faster than oral	Must involve sterile technique because breaks skin barrier More expensive than oral Can administer only small volume Slower than intramuscular administration Some drugs can irritate tissues and cause pain Can be anxiety-producing
Intramuscular	Pain from irritating drugs is minimized Can administer larger volume than subcutaneous Drug is rapidly absorbed	Breaks skin barrier Can be anxiety-producing
Intradermal	Absorption is slow (this is an advantage when testing for allergies)	Amount of drug administered must be small Breaks skin barrier
Intravenous	Rapid effect	Limited to highly soluble drugs Drug distribution may be inhibited by poor circulation
Inhalation	Introduces drug throughout the respiratory tract Rapid localized relief Drug can be administered when client is unconscious	Drug intended for localized effect can have systemic effect Only of use for the respiratory system

Oral

Oral administration is the most common, least expensive, and most convenient route for most clients. It is also a safe method of administration in that the skin is not broken as it is for an injection.

Sublingual

A drug may be placed under the tongue (**sublingually**), where it dissolves. See Figure 44–2. In a relatively short time the drug is largely absorbed into the blood vessels on the underside of the tongue. The medication should not be swallowed. Drugs such as nitroglycerin are commonly given in this manner.

Buccal

Buccal means "pertaining to the cheek." In buccal administration, a medication (e.g., a tablet) is held in the mouth against the mucous membranes of the cheek until the drug dissolves. See Figure 44–3. The drug may act locally on the mucous membranes of the mouth or systemically when it is swallowed in the saliva.

Parenteral

Parenteral administration is administration other than through the alimentary tract, i.e., by needle. Some of the more common routes for parenteral administration are:

1. **Subcutaneous** (hypodermic). Into the subcutaneous tissue, just below the skin
2. **Intramuscular.** Into a muscle
3. **Intradermal.** Under the epidermis (into the dermis)
4. **Intravenous.** Into a vein

Some of the less commonly used routes for parenteral administration are **intraarterial** (into an artery), **intracardiac** (into the heart muscle), **intraosseous**

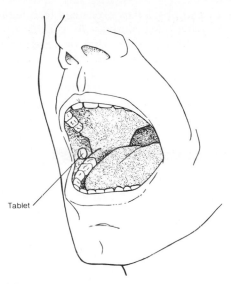

Figure 44–3   Buccal administration of a tablet

(into a bone), and **intrathecal** or **intraspinal** (into the spinal canal). These less common injections are normally administered by physicians. Sterile equipment and sterile drug solutions are essential for all parenteral therapy.

Topical

Topical applications are those applied to a circumscribed surface area of the body. They affect only the area to which they are applied. Topical applications include:

1. **Dermatologic preparations.** Applied to the skin.
2. **Instillations and irrigations.** Applied into body cavities or orifices such as the urinary bladder, eyes, ears, nose, rectum, or vagina.
3. **Inhalations.** Administered into the respiratory tract by nebulizers or positive pressure breathing apparatuses. Air, oxygen, and vapor are generally used to carry the drug into the lungs. See Chapter 42.

Medication Orders

A physician is the person who usually determines the clients' medications needs and orders medications, although in some settings nurse practitioners now order some drugs. Usually, the order is written, although telephone and verbal orders are acceptable in a number of agencies. Nursing students need to know the agency policies about medication orders. In some hospitals, for example, only licensed nurses are permitted to accept telephone and verbal orders.

Policies about physicians' orders vary considerably from agency to agency. For example, a client's orders are frequently automatically canceled after surgery or an examination involving an anesthetic agent. New orders must then be written. Most agencies also have lists of abbreviations officially accepted for use in the agency.

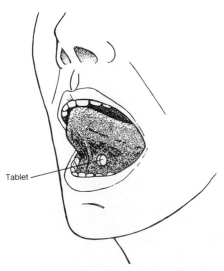

Figure 44–2   Sublingual administration of a tablet

Both nurses and physicians may need to refer to these lists if they have been working in a different agency. These abbreviations can be used on legal documents, such as clients' charts. See Table 44–5. The drug order has six essential parts, as listed in the accompanying box. In addition, unless it is a standing order, it should state the number of doses or the number of days the drug is to be administered.

> ## Drug Order: Essential Parts
>
> **Full name** of the client
> **Date** the order is written
> **Name of the drug** to be administered
> **Dosage** of the drug
> **Method** of administration
> **Signature** of the physician or nurse practitioner

Types of Medication Orders

Four common medication orders are the stat order, the single order, the standing order, and the p.r.n. order:

1. A **stat** order indicates that the medication is to be given immediately and only once, e.g., Demerol 100 mg IM stat.
2. The **single** order is for a medication to be given once at a specified time, e.g., Seconal 100 mg h.s. before surgery.
3. The **standing** order may or may not have a termination date. A standing order may be carried out indefinitely (e.g., multiple vitamins daily) until an order is written to cancel it, or it may be carried out for a specified number of days (e.g., Demerol 100 mg IM q.4h. × 5 days). In some agencies, standing orders are automatically canceled after a specified number of days and must be reordered.

4. A **p.r.n.** order permits the nurse to give a medication when in her or his judgment the client requires it, e.g., Amphojel 15 ml p.r.n. The nurse must use good judgment as to when the medication is needed and when it can be safely administered.

Communicating a Medication Order

A drug order is written on the client's chart by a physician or by a nurse receiving a telephone or verbal order from a physician. Most agencies have a specified time frame (e.g., 24 or 48 hours) in which the physician issuing the telephone or verbal order must co-sign the order written by the nurse. The medication order is then copied by a nurse or clerk to a Kardex and to a medication card. Increasingly nurses are being provided with

Table 44–5 Common Abbreviations Used in Medication Orders

Abbreviation	Explanation	Example of Administration Time	Abbreviation	Explanantion	Example of Administration Time
a.c.	before meals	0700, 1100, and 1700 hours	q.2h.	every 2 hours	0800, 1000, 1200 hours, etc.
ad lib	freely, as desired		q.3h.	every 3 hours	0900, 1200, 1500 hours, etc.
agit	shake, stir				
aq	water		q.4h.	every 4 hours	1000, 1400, 1800 hours, etc
aq dest	distilled water				
b.i.d.	twice a day	0900 and 2100 hours	q.6h.	every 6 hours	0600, 1200, 1800, 2400 hours
c̄	with				
cap	capsule		q.h.s.	every night at bedtime	
comp	compound				
dil	dissolve, dilute		q.i.d.	four times a day	1000, 1400, 1800, 2200 hours
elix	elixir				
h.	an hour		q.o.d.	every other day	0900 hours on odd dates
h.s.	at bedtime				
I.M.	intramuscular		q.s.	sufficient quantity	
I.V.	intravenous		rept	may be repeated	
M. or m.	mix		Rx	take	
no.	number		s̄	without	
non rep	do not repeat		s.c.	subcutaneous	
OD	right eye		Sig. or S.	label	
OS or o.l.	left eye		s.o.s.	if it is needed	
OU	both eyes		ss or s̄s̄	one half	
p.c.	after meals	0900, 1300, and 1900 hours	stat	at once	
			sup or supp	suppository	
p.o.	by mouth		susp	suspension	
p.r.n.	when needed		t.i.d.	three times a day	1000, 1400, and 1800 hours
q.	every				
q.d.	every day		Tr. or tinct	tincture	
q.ᴀᴍ (o.m.)	every morning	1000 hours			
q.h. (q.1h.)	every hour				

computer printouts of a client's medications instead of copying the physician's order. This method avoids errors of copying and saves nursing time.

Administering Medications Safely

The nurse should always assess a client's physical status prior to giving any medication. The extent of the assessment depends on the client's illness or current condition and the intended drug and route of administration. For example, the nurse assesses a dyspneic client's respirations carefully before administering any medication that might affect breathing. In general, the nurse assesses the client *prior* to administering any medication to obtain baseline data by which to evaluate the effectiveness of the medication.

▪ Process of Administering Medications

When administering any drug, regardless of the route of administration, the nurse must do the following.

▪ Identify the Client. Errors can and do occur, usually because one client gets a drug intended for another. In hospitals, most clients wear some sort of identification, such as a wristband with name and hospital identification number. Before giving the client any drug, the nurse should check the identification band with the medication card or medication administration record (MAR). As a double check, nurses also ask the client's name or ask another nurse to identify the client before administering any medication.

▪ Administer the Drug. Medication orders and cards or lists need to be read carefully and checked against the name on the medication envelope or on the drawer in which the client's medications are kept if a medication cart is used. The medication is then administered in the prescribed dosage, by the route ordered, at the correct time.

▪ Provide Adjunctive Interventions as Indicated. Clients may need help when receiving medications. They may require physical assistance, for instance, in assuming positions for intramuscular injections, or they may need explanations about the medications and guidance about measures to enhance drug effectiveness and prevent complications, e.g., drinking fluids. Some clients convey fear about their medications. The nurse can allay fears by listening carefully to clients' concerns and giving correct information.

▪ Record. The facts recorded in the chart, in ink or by computer printout, are name of the drug, dosage, method of administration, specific relevant data such as pulse rate (taken in most settings prior to the adminis-

tration of digitalis), and any other pertinent information. The record should also include the exact time of administration and the signature of the nurse providing the medication. Many medication records are designed so that the nurse signs her or his name once on the page and initials each medication administered. Often medications that are given regularly are recorded on a special flow record, and p.r.n. or stat medications are recorded separately.

▪ Evaluate the Client's Response to the Drug. The kinds of behavior that reflect the action or lack of action of a drug, and its untoward effects (both minor and major), are as variable as the purposes of the drugs themselves. The anxious client may show the desired effects of a tranquilizer by behavior that reflects a lowered stress level (e.g., slower speech or fewer random movements). The effectiveness of a sedative can often be measured by how well a client slept; the effectiveness of an antispasmodic, by how much pain the client feels. In all nursing activities, nurses need to be aware of the medications that a client is taking and record their effectiveness as assessed by the client and the nurse on the client's chart. The nurse may also report the client's response directly to the senior nurse and physician.

See the accompanying box for the five "rights" to accurate drug administration. In addition to adhering to these five "rights," the nurse should also be aware of clients' rights regarding medications. These are listed in the accompanying box.

Drug Administration: Five "Rights"

- Right **drug**
- Right **dose**
- Right **time**
- Right **route**
- Right **client**

Client's Rights According to the Patient's Bill of Rights

- To be informed of the drug's name, purpose, action and any possible adverse side effects.

- To refuse any medication.

- To have a qualified person, i.e., nurse or physician, assess your medication history including allergies.

- To have complete information about the experimental use of any drug and to refuse or consent to its use.

- To receive labelled medications safely.

- To receive appropriate therapy adjunctive to the drug therapy.

- Not to be given unnecessary medications.

Developmental Considerations

Knowledge of growth and development is essential for the nurse administering medications to children. Oral medications for children are usually prepared in sweetened liquid form to make them more palatable. The parents may provide suggestions about what method is best for their child. Necessary foods such as milk or orange juice should not be used to mask the taste of medications because the child may develop unpleasant associations and refuse that food in the future.

Children tend to fear any procedure in which a needle is used because they anticipate pain or because the procedure is unfamiliar and threatening. The nurse needs to acknowledge that the child will feel some pain. Denying this fact only deepens the child's distrust. After the injection, it is important for the nurse (or the parent) to cuddle and speak softly to the infant and give the child a toy to dispel the child's association of the nurse only with pain.

Older people can present special problems in relation to medications. Most of their problems are related to physiologic changes, to past experiences, and to established attitudes toward medications. The physiologic changes in elderly persons that may affect the administration and effectiveness of medications are included in the accompanying box.

Many of these changes enhance the possibility of cumulative effects and toxicity. For example, impaired circulation delays the action of medications given intramuscularly or subcutaneously. Digitalis, which is frequently taken by elderly people, can accumulate to toxic levels and be lethal. It is not uncommon for elderly clients to take several different medications daily. The possibility of error increases with the number of medications

taken, whether self-administered at home or administered by nurses in a hospital. The greater number of medications also compounds the problem of drug interactions, because much is yet to be learned about the effects of drugs given in combinations. A general rule to follow is that elderly clients should take as few medications as possible.

Elderly persons usually require smaller dosages of drugs, especially sedatives and other central nervous system depressants. Reactions of the elderly to medications, particularly sedatives, are unpredictable and often bizarre. It is not uncommon to see irritability, confusion, disorientation, restlessness, and incontinence as a result of sedatives. Nurses therefore need to observe clients carefully for untoward reactions. The use of alcohol (e.g., brandy) as a bedtime relaxant and as an appetizer before meals is becoming more common. The moderate use of alcohol by people who are accustomed to it can contribute to a sense of well-being.

Attitudes of elderly people toward medical care and medications vary. Elderly people tend to believe in the wisdom of the physician more readily than younger people. Some older people are bewildered by the prescription of several medications and may passively accept their medications from nurses but not swallow them, spitting out tablets or capsules after the nurse leaves the room. For this reason, the nurse is advised to stay with clients until they have taken the medications. Others may be suspicious of medications and actively refuse them.

Elderly people are mature adults capable of reasoning. Therefore, the nurse needs to explain the reasons for and effects of medications, particularly to ambulatory geriatric clients. This education can prevent the common occurrence of clients taking medications long after there is a need for them, or it can prevent clients from discontinuing a drug too quickly. For example, clients should know that diuretics will cause them to urinate more frequently and may reduce ankle edema. Instructions about medications need to be given to all clients prior to discharge from a hospital. These instructions should include when to take the drugs, what effects to expect, and when to consult a physician.

Because some clients are required to take several medications daily and because visual acuity and memory may be impaired, it is important for the nurse to develop simple, realistic plans for clients to follow at home. For example, most people, including elderly people, can have difficulties remembering to take drugs. If they are scheduled to be taken with meals or at bedtime, clients are not as likely to forget. Some clients may take their medications and then an hour later not remember whether they took them. One solution to forgetfulness is to use a special container or glass strictly for medications. If the container or glass is empty, the person knows that he or she took the pills. Loss of visual acuity presents problems that can be overcome by writing out the plan in block letters large enough to be read. In some situations the help of a spouse, son, or daughter can be enlisted.

Physiologic Changes Associated with Aging that Influence Medications

Altered **memory**

Less acute **vision**

Decrease in **renal function** resulting in slower elimination of drugs and higher drug concentrations in the bloodstream for longer periods

Less complete and slower **absorption** from the gastrointestinal tract

Increased proportion of **fat** to lean body mass, which facilitates retention of fat-soluble drugs and increases potential for toxicity

Decreased **liver function,** which hinders biotransformation of drugs

Decreased **organ sensitivity,** which means that the response to the same drug concentration in the vicinity of the target organ is less in older people than in the young

Altered quality of **organ responsiveness,** resulting in adverse effects becoming pronounced before therapeutic effects are achieved

▪ Oral Medications

The oral route is the most common route by which medications are given. As long as a client can swallow and retain the drug in his or her stomach, this is the route of choice. See Procedure 44–1. Oral medications are contraindicated when a client is vomiting, has gastric or intestinal suction, or is unconscious and unable to swallow. Such clients in a hospital usually are on orders "nothing by mouth" (NPO). Critical elements of administering oral medications are listed in the accompanying box.

PROCEDURE 44–1

Administering Oral Medications

Oral medications are generally the most easily taken of all drugs. Adjustments may be necessary for the very young, the very old, or for those who have difficulty swallowing solids. For easier ingestion, tablets can be crushed and mixed with a small amount of liquid or soft food, such as jelly or applesauce. It is preferable, however, to obtain a more suitable dosage form, eg, a liquid medication. Enteric-coated tablets and capsules should not be broken, because the coating is intended to prevent the medicine from being activated and absorbed in the stomach.

Arrange a time when the preparation of medications will not be interrupted. Concentration is necessary to prevent drug errors. Once prepared, medications should always remain within the nurse's sight unless they are stored with appropriate precautions.

Equipment

■ A medication tray or cart.

■ Medication cards or medication administration record (MAR). To save time and avoid retracing steps, arrange in the order in which the medications will be given. Plan to give medications first to clients who do not require assistance and last to those who do.

■ Disposable medication cups. Small paper cups are needed for tablets and capsules; for liquids, waxed or plastic calibrated medication cups are needed.

Intervention

1. Check the date on the medication order, and verify the order for accuracy. Records of medication orders include the physician's order, which is usually on the client's chart, the Kardex record, and the medication card or MAR. The surest check is to compare the medication card or MAR against the physician's order. In some settings a medication Kardex or computer printout is used instead of medication cards. This Kardex or printout is usually kept in the medication room or in the medication cart. Any discrepancies in the order should be brought to the notice of the nurse in charge or the physician, whichever is appropriate in the agency.

2. Read the medication card or MAR, and take the appropriate medication from the shelf, drawer, or refrigerator. The medication may be dispensed in a bottle, box, or envelope.

3. Compare the label of the medication container against the order on the medication card or MAR. If these are not identical, recheck the chart. If there is still a discrepancy, check with the nurse in charge.

4. Prepare the correct amount of medication for the required dose, without touching the medication.
   a. If administering tablets or capsules from a bottle, pour the required number into the bottle cap (see Figure 44–4), and then transfer the medication to the paper cup. Usually, all tablets or capsules to be given to the client are placed in the same paper cup. However, keep medications that require specific assessments—eg, pulse measurements, respiratory rate or depth, or blood pressure—separate from the others.
   b. If administering a liquid medication, remove the cap, and place it upside down on the countertop to avoid contaminating it. Hold the bottle with the label next to your palm so that if any spills, the label will not become soiled and illegible. See Figure 44–5. Hold the medication cup at eye level and fill it to the desired level, using the bottom of the meniscus (crescent-shaped upper surface of a column of liquid) as the measurement guide. See Figure 44–6.
   c. If administering an oral narcotic from a narcotic dispenser, expose the tablet by turning the dial or

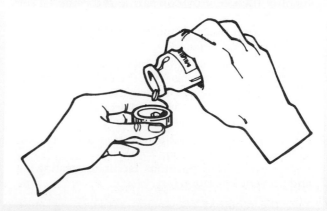

Figure 44–4

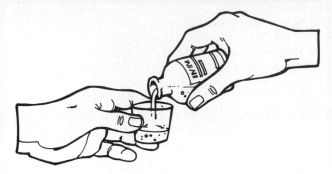

Figure 44–5

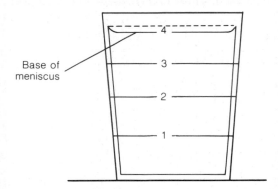

Base of meniscus

Figure 44–6

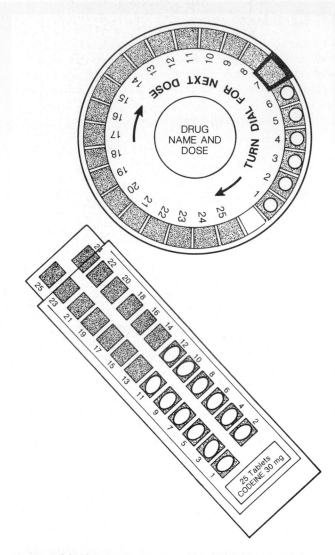

Figure 44–7

sliding out the numbered dose, and drop it into the cup. These containers are sectioned and numbered. See Figure 44–7. After removing a tablet, record the fact on the appropriate narcotic control record and sign it.

d. Open unit-dose medications at the client's bedside.

5. Place the prepared medication and medication card together on the tray or cart.

6. Check the label on the container again, and return the bottle, box, or envelope to its storage place.

7. Identify the client by comparing the name on the medication card or MAR with the name on the client's identification bracelet and by asking the client to state his or her name.

8. Explain the purpose of the medication and how it will help, using language that the client can understand. Include relevant information about effects, eg, tell the client receiving a diuretic to expect an increase in urine.

9. Assist the client to a sitting position or, if not possible, to a lateral position.
Rationale: These positions facilitate swallowing and prevent aspiration.

10. Take the required assessment measures, eg, pulse and respiratory rates or blood pressure. The pulse rate is taken before administering digitalis prepa-

rations. Blood pressure is taken before giving hypotensive drugs. The respiratory rate is taken prior to administering narcotics, since narcotics depress the respiratory center. If the rate is below 12, the nurse in charge should be consulted.

11. If appropriate, give the client sufficient water or juice to swallow the medication.
Rationale: Fluids ease swallowing and facilitate absorption from the gastrointestinal tract. Liquid medications are generally diluted with 15 ml (½ oz) of water to facilitate absorption.

12. If the client is unable to hold the pill cup, use the pill cup to introduce the medication into the mouth.
Rationale: Putting the cup to the mouth avoids contamination of the nurse's hands.

13. If the client has difficulty swallowing, direct the client to place the medication on the back of the tongue before taking the water.
Rationale: Stimulation of the back of the tongue produces the swallowing reflex.

14. If the medication is harmful to tooth enamel or irritating to the oral mucous membrane (eg, liquid iron preparations), have the client use a glass straw to ingest the medication and drink water following the medication.
15. If the client says that the medication you are about to give is different from what the person has been receiving, do not give the medication without checking the original order.
16. If the medication has an objectionable taste, have the client suck a few ice chips before administering it, or give the medication with juice, applesauce, or bread.

Rationale: The cold will desensitize the taste buds, and juices, bread etc, can mask the taste of the medication.

17. Stay with the client until all medications have been swallowed.
18. Record the medication given, dosage, time, nursing assessments and interventions, and your signature.
19. Return the medication card to the slot of the next time it is due.
20. Return to the client when the medication is expected to take effect to evaluate the effects of the medication, eg, relief of pain.

Parenteral Medications

Parenteral medications are medications administered by a route other than the alimentary canal. They are given by nurses subcutaneously, intramuscularly, intradermally, or intravenously. Because parenteral medications are absorbed more quickly than oral medications and are irretrievable once injected, it is essential that the nurse prepare and administer them carefully and accurately. Administering parenteral drugs requires the same nursing knowledge as administering oral and topical drugs, plus considerable manual dexterity and the use of sterile technique.

To administer parenteral medications, injectable equipment (i.e., syringes, needles, vials, and ampules) are used. **Syringes** have three parts: the tip, which connects with the needle; the barrel, or outside part, on which the scales are printed; and the plunger, which fits inside the barrel. See Figure 44–8. Most syringes used today are made of plastic and are individually packaged for sterility in a paper wrapper or a rigid plastic container.

There are several kinds of syringes, differing in size, shape, and material. The three most commonly used types are the standard hypodermic syringe, the insulin syringe, and the tuberculin syringe. See Figure 44–9. **Hypodermic syringes** come in 2, 2.5, and 3 ml sizes. They usually have two scales marked on them: the minim and the milliliter. The milliliter scale is the one normally used; the minim scale is used for very small dosages.

Insulin syringes are similar to hypodermic syringes, except that they have a scale specially designed for insulin: a 100-unit calibrated scale intended for use with U-100 insulin. Low-dose insulin syringes can hold a maximum of 50 units (½ ml) and frequently have a nonremovable needle. The **tuberculin syringe** was designed to administer tuberculin. It is a narrow syringe, calibrated in tenths and hundredths of a milliliter (up to 1 ml) on one scale and in sixteenths of a minim (up to 1 min) on the other scale. This type of syringe can also be useful in administering other drugs, particularly when small or precise measurement is indicated (e.g., pediatric dosages). Syringes are made in other sizes as well, for example, 5, 10, 20, and 50 milliliters. These are not generally used to administer drugs directly but can be useful for adding medications to intravenous solutions or for irrigating wounds.

The **disposable plastic syringe** is most frequently used today. The syringe is supplied with a needle, which

Administering Oral Medications: Critical Elements

Know the expected action of the medication, undesirable side effects, and signs of toxicity.
Check the physician's order against other sources, e.g., the Kardex, medication card or MAR, and medication label.
Confirm the correct route of administration.
Maintain medical asepsis.
Prepare and administer the correct drug and dosage to the correct client by the right route and at the right time.
Take required assessment measures, e.g., pulse and respiratory rates or blood pressure.
Document the administered medication according to agency protocol.

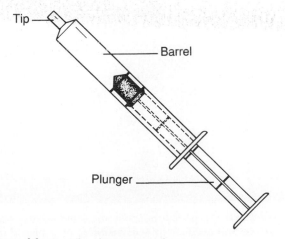

Figure 44–8 The three parts of a syringe

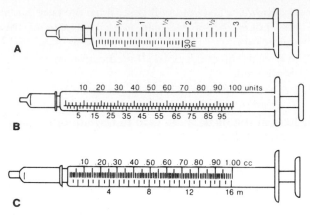

Figure 44–9 Three kinds of syringes: **A,** hypodermic; **B,** insulin; **C,** tuberculin.

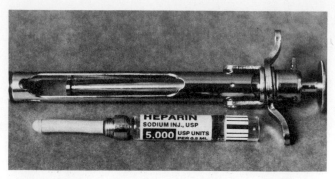

Figure 44–11 Metal cartridge holder and prefilled cartridge of heparin

may have a plastic cap over it. The syringe and needle may be packaged together or separately in a paper wrapper or in a rigid plastic container. See Figure 44–10.

Injectable medications are frequently supplied in **prefilled unit-dose syringes** with needles or cartridge-needle units. These prefilled syringes and cartridge-needle units are disposable. The cartridge-needle units, however, require special metal or plastic cartridge holders or syringes for administration. These syringes and cartridges come with manufacturer's directions for use. See Figure 44–11.

Needles are made of stainless steel and most are disposable. Reusable needles (e.g., for special procedures) need to be sharpened periodically before resterilization, because the points become dull with use and are occasionally damaged or acquire burrs on the tips. A dull or damaged needle should **never** be used.

A needle has three discernible parts: the hub, which fits onto the syringe; the cannula, or shaft, which is attached to the hub; and the bevel, which is the slanted part at the tip of the needle. See Figure 44–12. A dis-

posable needle has a plastic hub. Needles used for injections have three variables:

1. **Slant or length of the bevel.** The bevel of the needle may be short or long. Longer bevels provide the sharpest needles and cause less discomfort and are commonly used for subcutaneous and intramuscular injections. Short bevels are used for intradermal and intravenous injections, because a long bevel can become occluded if it rests against the side of a blood vessel.
2. **Length of the shaft.** The shaft length of commonly used needles varies from ¼ to 5 in.
3. **Gauge (or diameter) of the shaft.** The gauge varies from #14 to #27. The larger the gauge number, the smaller the diameter of the shaft. Smaller gauges

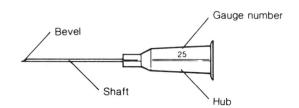

Figure 44–12 The parts of a needle

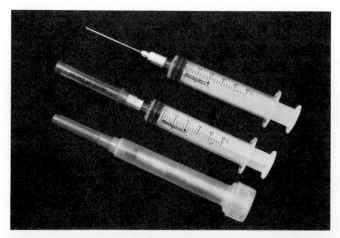

Figure 44–10 Disposable plastic syringes and needles: **top,** with syringe and needle exposed; **middle,** with plastic cap over the needle; **bottom,** with plastic case over the needle and syringe

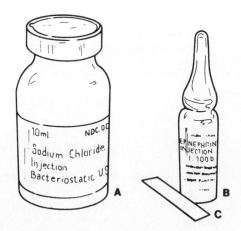

Figure 44–13 **A,** vial; **B,** ampule; **C,** ampule file

produce less tissue trauma, but larger gauges are necessary for viscous medications, such as penicillin.

For subcutaneous injections, it is usual to use a needle of #24 to #26 gauge and ⅜ to ⅝ in long. Obese clients may require a 1-in needle. For intramuscular injections, a longer needle, e.g., 1 to 1½ in, with a larger gauge, e.g., gauge #20 to #22, is used.

Ampules and **vials** are frequently used to package sterile parenteral medications. See Figure 44–13. An **ampule** is a glass container usually designed to hold a single dose of a drug. It is made of clear glass and has a distinctive shape with a constricted neck. Some ampule necks have colored marks around them, indicating where they are prescored for easy opening. If the neck is not scored, it should be filed with a small file, then broken off at the neck. A **vial** is a small glass bottle with a sealed rubber cap. Vials come in different sizes, from single to multidose vials. They usually have a metal or plastic cap that protects the rubber seal. Procedure 44–2 describes how to prepare medications from ampules and vials.

PROCEDURE 44–2

Preparing Medications from Ampules and Vials

Equipment

- The vial or ampule of sterile medication.
- Sterile gauze.
- A needle and syringe.
- Special filter needle (optional) for withdrawing pre-mixed liquid medications from multidose vials or from ampules to filter out glass slivers.
- Antiseptic solution.
- Sterile water, if necessary. Some vials contain only a powder, and it is necessary to instill a liquid such as sterile water to prepare the medication. The manufacturer specifies preparation directions.
- File if required to open the ampule.
- Medication card or computer printout.

Intervention

1. Check the label on the ampule or vial carefully against the medication card, computer printout, or client's chart to make sure that the correct medication is being prepared.
2. Follow the three checks for administering medications. Read the label on the medication before it is taken off the shelf, before withdrawing the medication, and after placing it back on the shelf.

Ampules

3. Flick the upper stem of the ampule several times with a fingernail or, holding the upper stem of the ampule, make a large circle with the arm extended.
   Rationale: This will bring all the medication down to the main portion of the ampule.
4. Partially file the neck of the ampule if necessary to start a clean break.
5. Place a piece of sterile gauze between nurse's thumb and the ampule neck or around the ampule neck, and break off the top by bending it toward the gauze,

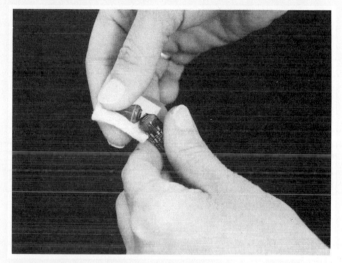

Figure 44–14

ie, away from the nurse. See Figure 44–14.
   Rationale: The sterile gauze protects the nurse's fingers from the broken glass.
6. Assemble the syringe and needle, if not preassembled. Hold the barrel of the syringe in the middle, and insert the plunger, maintaining the sterility of the plunger except at its uppermost end (which you are holding). Attach the needle to the barrel by holding the hub of the needle and maintaining the sterility of the remainder of the needle and the tip of the syringe. Needles have protective caps to help maintain their sterility.
7. Remove the cap from the needle, insert the needle in the ampule, and withdraw the amount of drug required for the dosage. See Figure 44–15. With a single-dose ampule, hold the ampule slightly on its side, if necessary, to obtain all the medication. Some nurses recommend using a needle with a filter to withdraw the medication in case there is any broken glass from the ampule in the medication.

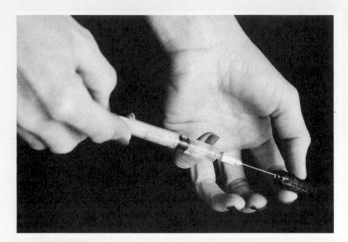

Figure 44–15

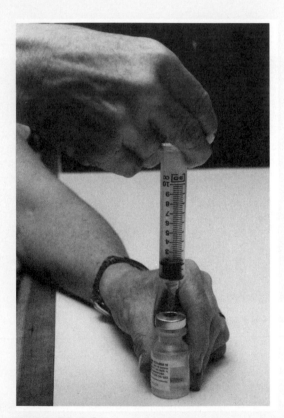

Figure 44–16

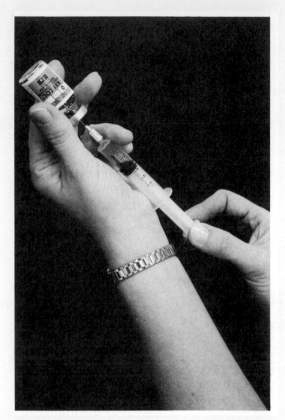

Figure 44–17

Rationale: The antiseptic cleans the cap so that the needle will remain sterile when it is inserted.

10. Remove the cap from the needle; then draw up into the syringe the amount of air equal to the volume of the medication to be withdrawn. In some agencies, a special filter needle is used to draw up premixed liquid medications from multidose vials. The filter needle is then replaced by a regular needle to inject the medication into the client. The filter prevents any solid material from being drawn up through the needle.

11. Carefully insert the needle into the vial through the center of the rubber cap, maintaining the sterility of the needle.

12. Inject the air into the vial, keeping the bevel of the needle above the surface of the medication. See Figure 44–16.
    Rationale: The air will allow the medication to be drawn out easily, since negative pressure is not created inside the vial. The bevel is kept above the medication to avoid creating bubbles in the medication.

13. Invert the vial and hold it at eye level while withdrawing the correct dosage of the drug into the syringe. See Figure 44–17.

14. Withdraw the needle from the vial, and replace the cap over the needle, thus maintaining its sterility. To recap an unused needle safely, hold the cap between two fingers and brace the barrel against

Vials

8. Mix the solution, if necessary, by rotating the vial between the palms of the hands, not by shaking.
   Rationale: Some vials contain aqueous suspensions, which settle when they stand. In some instances shaking is contraindicated because it may cause the mixture to foam.

9. Remove the protective metal cap, and clean the rubber cap with an antiseptic, such as 70% alcohol on a sterile gauze, by rubbing in a rotary motion.

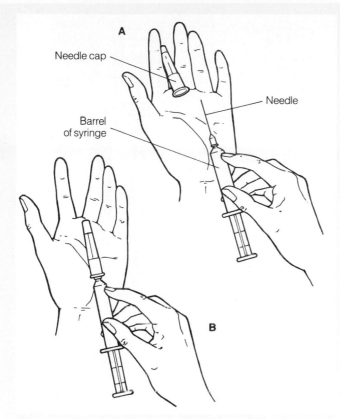

A

Needle cap

Needle

Barrel
of syringe

B

Figure 44–18 Recapping an unused needle

the palm. See Figure 44–18A. Gently guide the tip of the needle into the opening of the cap and release the fingers, allowing the cap to slide over the needle. See Figure 44–18B. Tighten the cap. If a filter needle was used to withdraw the medication, replace it with a regular needle before injecting the client.

Preparing Powdered Drugs

Several drugs (eg, penicillin) are dispensed as powders in vials. A liquid (solvent or diluent) must be added to a powdered medication before it can be injected. The technique of adding a solvent to a powdered drug to prepare it for administration is called reconstitution. Powdered drugs usually have printed instructions (enclosed with each packaged vial) that describe the amount and kind of solvent to be added. Commonly used solvents are sterile water or sterile normal saline. Some preparations are supplied in individual-dose vials; others come in multidose vials.

15. Read the manufacturer's directions. The following are two examples of the preparation of powdered drugs:

    a. *Single-dose vial:* Instructions for preparing a single-dose vial direct that 1.5 ml of sterile water be added to the sterile dry powder, thus providing a single dose of 2 ml. The volume of the drug powder was 0.5 ml. Therefore the 1.5 ml of water plus the 0.5 ml of powder results in 2 ml of solution. In other instances the addition of a solution does *not* increase the volume. Therefore it is important to follow the manufacturers' directions.

    b. *Multidose vial:* A dose of 750 mg of a certain drug is ordered for a client. On hand is a 10-g multidose vial. The directions for preparation read: "Add 8.5 ml of sterile water, and each milliliter will contain 1.0 g or 1000 mg." Thus, after adding the solvent, the nurse will give $\frac{750}{1000}$ or $\frac{3}{4}$ ml (0.75 ml) of the medication.

16. Withdraw an equivalent amount of air from the vial before adding the solvent, unless otherwise indicated by the directions.

17. Add the amount of sterile water or saline indicated in the directions.

18. If a multidose vial is reconstituted, label the vial with the date, time it was prepared, the amount of drug contained in each milliliter of solution, and your initials. Time is an important factor to consider in the expiration of these medications.

19. Once reconstituted, store the medication in the vial in a refrigerator or as recommended by the manufacturer.

Frequently clients need more than one drug injected at the same time. To spare the client the experience of being injected twice, two drugs (if compatible) are often mixed together in one syringe and given as one injection. It is common, for instance, to combine two types of insulin in this manner or to combine injectable preoperative medications such as morphine or meperidine (Demerol) with atropine or scopolamine. Drugs can also be mixed in intravenous solutions. When uncertain about drug compatibilities, the nurse should consult a pharmacist before mixing the drugs.

When withdrawing and **mixing medications** from two different vials, the nurse takes care not to contaminate the medication remaining in one vial with the other medication. To do this safely, the nurse inserts into vial A a needle attached to a syringe containing the needed volume of air and injects a volume of air equal to the volume of medication to be withdrawn. The tip of the needle must not touch the solution. The nurse withdraws the needle and repeats the procedure with vial B; the nurse again injects a volume of air equal to the volume of medication to be withdrawn. The nurse then withdraws the required amount of medication from vial B. In this way vial B is not contaminated by medication from vial A. When possible, the nurse then attaches a new, sterile needle to the syringe, inserts it into vial A, and withdraws the required amount of medication into the syringe. The syringe now contains a mixture of medications from vials A and B, and neither vial is contaminated by microorganisms or by medication from the other vial.

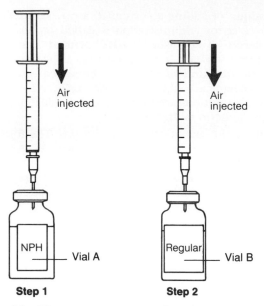

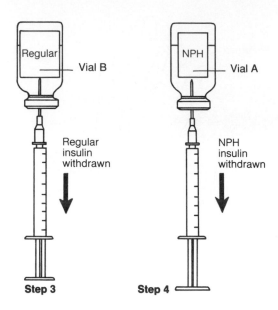

Figure 44–19 Mixing two types of insulin

Often clients are given two types of insulin, short- and long-acting; these two types vary in content. Chemically, insulin is a protein that, when hydrolyzed in the body, yields a number of amino acids. Some insulin preparations contain an additional modifying protein, such as globulin or protamine, that slows absorption. This fact is particularly relevant when mixing two insulin preparations for injection, as many insulin syringes have needles that cannot be changed. A vial of insulin that does **not** have the added protein should never be contaminated with insulin that does have the added protein. For example, a vial of regular insulin should never be entered with a needle that had been previously used to withdraw protamine zinc, globin zinc, or isophane (NPH) insulins, all of which have added protein. See Figure 44–19.

Because ampules do not require the addition of air prior to withdrawal of the drug, it is recommended that the nurse prepare the medication from the vial first, and then withdraw the medication from the ampule. To mix two medications from a cartridge and a vial or ampule, the nurse first ensures that the correct dose of the medication is in the cartridge. Any excess medication should be discarded. Then the nurse should draw up the required medication from a vial or ampule into the cartridge. If the total volume to be injected exceeds the capacity of the cartridge, a syringe with sufficient capacity should be used to withdraw the desired amount of medication from the vial/ampule, and the required amount from the cartridge should be transferred to the syringe.

■ **Intradermal Injections.** An intradermal injection is the administration of a drug into the dermal layer of the skin just beneath the epidermis. Usually only a small amount of liquid is used, for example, 0.1 ml. This method of administration is frequently indicated for allergy and tuberculin tests and for vaccinations. Common sites for intradermal injections are the inner lower arm, the upper chest, and the back beneath the scapulae. See Figure 44–20.

The equipment normally used is a 1-ml syringe calibrated into hundredths of a milliliter. The needle is short and fine, frequently a #25, #26, or #27 gauge, ¼ inch to ⅝ inch long. After the site is cleaned, the skin is held tautly, and the syringe is held at about a 15° angle to the skin, with the bevel of the needle upward. The needle is then inserted through the epidermis into the dermis, and the fluid is injected. The drug produces a small bleb just under the skin. See Figure 44–21. The needle is then withdrawn quickly, and the site is very lightly wiped with an antiseptic swab. The area is not massaged because the medication may disperse into the tissue or out through the needle insertion site. Intradermal injections are absorbed slowly through blood capillaries in the area.

■ **Subcutaneous Injections.** A subcutaneous injection is the introduction of a medication into the subcutaneous tissues. It may also be referred to as a

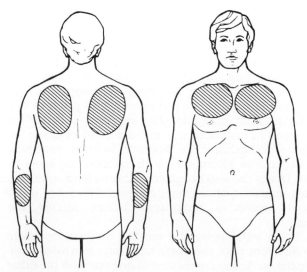

Figure 44–20 Body sites commonly used for intradermal injections

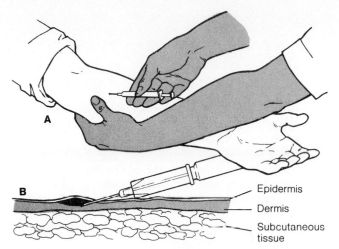

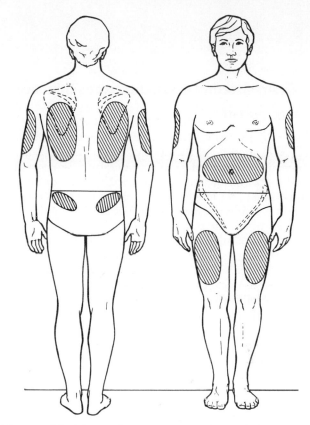

Epidermis

Dermis

Subcutaneous
tissue

Figure 44–21   For an intradermal injection: **A,** the needle enters the skin at a 15° angle; and **B,** the medication forms a bleb under the epidermis

hypodermic injection. Among the many kinds of drugs administered subcutaneously are vaccines, preoperative medications, narcotics, insulin, and heparin. Common sites for subcutaneous injections are the outer aspect of the upper arms and the anterior aspect of the thighs. These areas are convenient and normally have good blood circulation. Other areas that can be used are the abdomen, the scapular areas of the upper back, and the upper ventro/dorso gluteal areas. See Figure 44–22. Clients who administer their own injections, such as diabetics requiring insulin, usually use the abdomen and anterior thigh sites.

Subcutaneous injection sites need to be rotated in an orderly fashion to minimize tissue damage, aid absorption, and avoid discomfort. This is especially important for clients who must receive repeated injec-

Figure 44–22   Body sites commonly used for subcutaneous injections

tions, e.g., diabetics. To accomplish this, the nurse or client can prepare a diagram indicating the sites to be used and after each injection mark its location on the diagram. See Figure 44–23. The steps for administering a subcutaneous injection are described in Procedure 44–3.

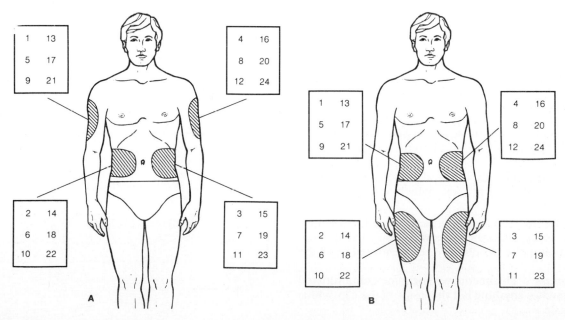

Figure 44–23   A commonly used system of rotating body injection sites for insulin administration; **A,** sites used by the nurse; **B,** sites used by the client.

PROCEDURE 44–3

Administering a Subcutaneous Injection

Equipment

- The client's medication card or computer printout.
- A vial or ampule of the correct sterile medication.
- A sterile syringe and needle. Generally, a 2-ml syringe and a #25 gauge needle are used for subcutaneous injections. The length of the needle depends on the amount of adipose tissue at the site and the angle used to administer the injection. Generally, a ⅝-in. needle is used for adults when the injection is administered at a 45° angle; a ½-in. needle is used at a 90° angle. Shorter needles, eg, ⅜ in., may be used for children, and longer ones, eg, 1 in., may be necessary for very obese adults. To determine the appropriate length of the needle for a 90° angle injection, pinch a fold of skin between your thumb and forefinger at the injection site, then measure the width of the skin fold by placing a needle that will not be used for the injection against the skin surface. The appropriate needle length is one-half the width of the skin fold (Pitel 1971, p. 78). When this method of measuring is used, the needle is inserted without pinching the skin.
- Sterile antiseptic-soaked swabs to clean the top of a medication vial and the injection site.
- Dry sterile gauze for opening an ampule.

Intervention

1. Check the medication order. See Procedure 44–2, steps 1 and 2.
2. Prepare the drug dosage from a vial or ampule. See Procedure 44–2.
3. Select a site free of tenderness, hardness, swelling, scarring, itching, burning, or localized inflammation. Select a site that has not been used frequently.
   Rationale: These conditions could hinder the absorption of the medication and also increase the likelihood of an infection at the injection site.
4. As agency policy indicates, clean the site with an antiseptic swab. Start at the center of the site and clean in a widening circle. Allow the area to dry thoroughly. Place the swab between the third and fourth fingers of the nondominant hand for later use.
   Rationale: The mechanical action of swabbing removes skin secretions, which contain microorganisms.
5. Remove the needle cap while waiting for the antiseptic to dry. Pull the cap straight off to avoid contaminating the needle by the outside edge of the cap.
   Rationale: The needle will become contaminated if it touches anything but the inside of the cap, which is sterile.
6. Expel any air bubbles from the syringe by inverting the syringe and gently pushing on the plunger until a drop of solution can be seen in the needle bevel. If air bubbles still remain, flick the side of the syringe barrel.
   or
7. When it is important that the entire amount of medication be administered, Wong (1982, p. 1237) recommends leaving 0.2 ml of air in the syringe. This is referred to as the air-bubble technique. Others (Chaplin, Shull, and Welk 1985, p. 59) do not recommend this technique.
   Rationale: Users of the air-bubble technique believe that this small amount of air ensures that only air remains in the needle bore and that all the medication is injected into the client. Nonusers believe that the risk of medication error is increased when the "dead-space volume" (residual amount of drug in the syringe hub and needle) is expelled during injection, since it is *not* part of the syringe barrel calibration.
8. Grasp the syringe in your dominant hand by holding it between your thumb and fingers with palm facing to the side or upward for a 45° angle insertion or with the palm downward for a 90° angle insertion. See Figure 44–24.
9. Using the nondominant hand, pinch or spread the skin at the site, and insert the needle, using the dominant hand and a firm steady push. See Figure 44–25.
   Rationale: Recommendations vary about whether to pinch or spread the skin. Pinching the skin is thought to desensitize the area somewhat and thus lessen the sensation of needle insertion. Spreading the skin can make it firmer and facilitate needle insertion. Some recommend neither pinching nor spreading the skin (Pitel 1971, p. 79). The nurse needs to judge which method to use depending on the client's tissue firmness.

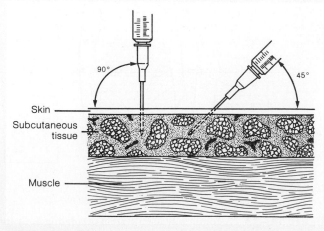

Figure 44–24

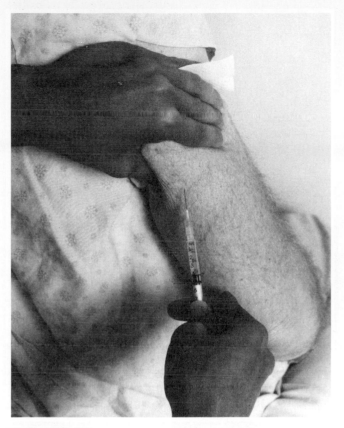

Figure 44-25

10. When the needle is inserted, move your nondominant hand to the end of the plunger. Some nurses find it easier to move the nondominant hand to the barrel of the syringe and the dominant hand to the end of the plunger.

11. Aspirate by pulling back on the plunger. If blood appears in the syringe, withdraw the needle, discard the syringe, and prepare a new injection. If blood does not appear, continue to administer the medication.
    Rationale: This step determines whether the needle has entered a blood vessel. Subcutaneous medications may be dangerous if placed directly into the bloodstream; they are intended for the subcutaneous tissues, where the absorption time is greater.

12. Inject the medication by holding the syringe steady and depressing the plunger with a slow, even pressure.
    Rationale: Holding the syringe steady and injecting the medication at an even pressure minimizes discomfort for the client.

13. Remove the needle quickly, pulling along the line of insertion while depressing the skin with your nondominant hand.

■ **Intramuscular Injections.** The intramuscular (IM) injection route is ordered for the following reasons:

1. The speed of absorption is faster than by the sub-

Rationale: Depressing the skin places countertraction on it and minimizes the client's discomfort when the needle is withdrawn.

14. Massage the site lightly with a sterile antiseptic-soaked swab, or apply slight pressure.
    Rationale: Massage is thought to disperse the medication in the tissues and facilitate its absorption. Massaging is omitted with heparin and insulin injections.

15. If bleeding occurs, apply pressure to the site with a dry sterile gauze until it stops. Bleeding rarely occurs after subcutaneous injection.

16. Dispose of supplies according to agency procedure.
    Rationale: Proper disposal protects the nurse and others from injury and contamination.

17. Document the medication given, dosage, time, route, assessments, and your signature. Many agencies prefer that medication administration is recorded on the medication record. The nurse's notes are used when p.r.n. medications are given or when there is a special problem.

18. Assess the effectiveness of the medication when it is expected to act.

Variations for a Heparin Injection

The subcutaneous administration of heparin requires special precautions because of the drug's anticoagulant properties.

19. Select a site on the abdomen above the level of the iliac crests.
    Rationale: These areas are away from major muscles and are not involved in muscular activity, as the arms and legs are; thus, the possibility of hematoma is reduced.

20. Use a ½-in., #25 or #26 gauge needle, and insert it at a 90° angle. Draw 0.1 ml of air into the syringe when preparing the heparin, and inject it after the heparin.
    Rationale: This step fills the needle with air and prevents any leakage of heparin into the intradermal layers when the needle is inserted and when the needle is withdrawn, thus minimizing the possibility of a hematoma.

21. Check agency practices regarding aspiration.
    Rationale: Some nurses recommend not to aspirate to determine needle placement because this can cause the needle to move, possibly damaging tissue and rupturing small blood vessels, causing bleeding and severe bruising.

22. Do not massage the site after the injection.
    Rationale: Massaging could cause bleeding and ecchymoses.

23. Alternate sites of subsequent injections.

cutaneous route because of the greater blood supply to the body muscles.

2. Muscles can usually take a larger volume of fluid without discomfort than subcutaneous tissues,

although the amount varies among people, chiefly with muscle size and condition.

3. Medications that irritate subcutaneous tissue may safely be given by intramuscular injection.

A number of body **sites** are used for intramuscular injections. Frequently used sites are the dorsogluteal, ventrogluteal, vastus lateralis, rectus femoris, deltoid, and triceps muscles. Only healthy muscles should be used for injections. The **dorsogluteal** site is composed of the thick gluteal muscles of the buttocks. See Figure 44–26. The dorsogluteal site can be used for adults and for children with well-developed gluteal muscles. Because these muscles are developed by walking, it should not be used for infants under 3 years. The injection site must be chosen carefully to avoid striking the sciatic nerve, major blood vessels, or bone. The nurse should palpate the posterior superior iliac spine, then draw an imaginary line to the greater trochanter of the femur. This line is lateral to and parallel to the sciatic nerve. The injection site is then lateral and superior to this line. See Figure 44–27. It is important to palpate the ilium and the trochanter. Visual calculations alone can result in an injection that is placed too low and injures other structures.

To administer an injection into the dorsogluteal site, the nurse has the client assume a prone position with the toes pointing medially. A side-lying position can also be used, with the upper leg flexed at the thigh and the knee and placed in front of the lower leg. Both positions promote relaxation of the gluteal muscles. In the past, the dorsogluteal site was most commonly used for intramuscular injections. However, because of the problems caused by inaccurately locating the site, it is losing favor as the best intramuscular site.

The **ventrogluteal** site is the preferred site for intramuscular injections because there are no large nerves or blood vessels in the area and less fat than in the buttock area. It is also farther from the rectal area and tends to be less contaminated, which is a consideration when giving injections to infants and incontinent adults. The ventrogluteal site, also known as von Hochstetter's

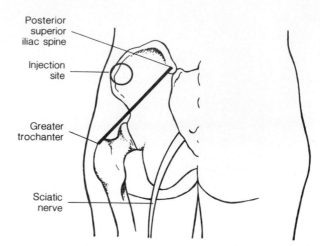

Figure 44–27 One method for establishing the dorsogluteal site for an intramuscular injection

site, is in the gluteus medius muscle, which lies over the gluteus minimus. See Figure 44–26. To establish the exact site, the nurse places the heel of the hand on the client's greater trochanter, with the fingers pointing toward the client's head. The right hand is used for the left hip, and the left hand for the right hip. With the index finger on the client's anterior superior iliac spine, the nurse stretches the middle finger dorsally, palpating

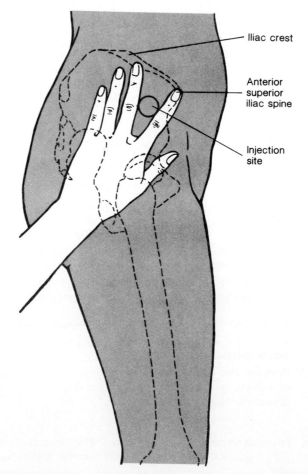

Figure 44–28 The ventrogluteal site for an intramuscular injection

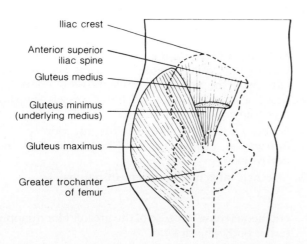

Figure 44–26 Lateral view of the right buttock showing the three gluteal muscles used for intramuscular injections

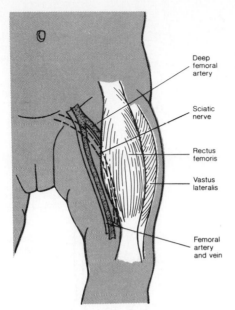

Figure 44–29 The vastus lateralis muscle of the upper thigh, used for intramuscular injections

the crest of the ilium and then pressing below it. The triangle formed by the index finger, the third finger, and the crest of the ilium is the injection site. See Figure 44–28. This site is suitable for infants, children, and adults. It is particularly suitable for immobilized clients whose dorsogluteal muscles may be atrophying. The client position for the injection can be a back- or side-lying position with the knee and hip flexed to relax the gluteal muscles.

The **vastus lateralis muscle** is usually thick and well developed in both adults and children. It is increasingly recommended as the site of choice for intramuscular injections for infants because there are no major

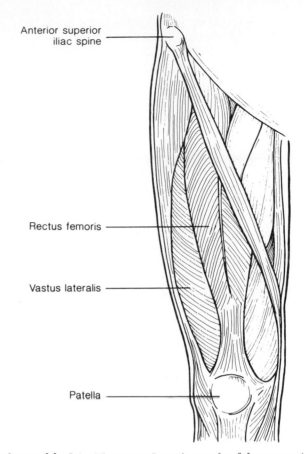

Figure 44–31 The rectus femoris muscle of the upper right thigh, used for intramuscular intejections

blood vessels or nerves in the area. It is situated on the anterior lateral aspect of the thigh. See Figure 44–29. The middle third of the muscle is suggested as the site. It is established by dividing the area between the greater

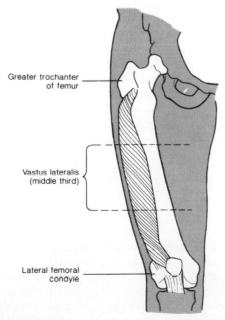

Figure 44–30 The vastus lateralis site for an intramuscular injection

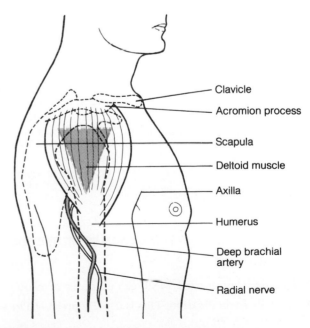

Figure 44–32 The deltoid muscle of the upper arm, used for intramuscular injections

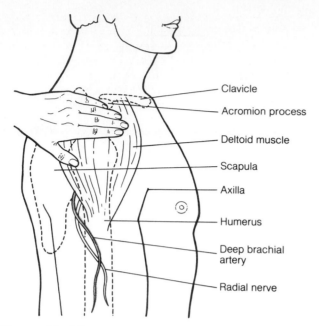

Figure 44–33 A method for establishing the deltoid muscle site for an intramuscular injection

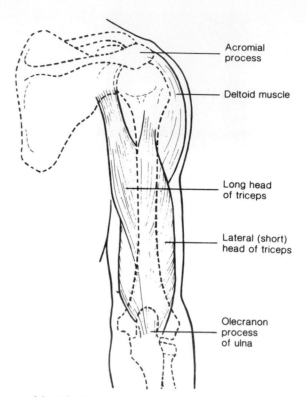

Figure 44–34 Posterior view of the upper right arm showing the triceps muscle, used for intramuscular injections

trochanter of the femur and the lateral femoral condyle into thirds and selecting the middle third. See Figure 44–30. The client can assume a back-lying or a sitting position for an injection into this site.

The **rectus femoris muscle**, which belongs to the quadriceps muscle group, can also be used for intramuscular injections. It is situated on the anterior aspect of the thigh. See Figure 44–31. This site can be used for occasional infections for infants and children and for adults when other sites are contraindicated. Its chief advantage is that the client who administers his or her own injections can reach this site easily. Its main disadvantage is that an injection here may cause considerable discomfort for some people. The client assumes a sitting or back-lying position for an injection at this site.

The **deltoid muscle** is found on the lateral aspect of the upper arm. It is not used often for intramuscular injections because it is a relatively small muscle and is very close to the radial nerve and radial artery. To locate the densest part of the muscle, the nurse palpates the lower edge of the acromion and the midpoint on the lateral aspect of the arm that is in line with the axilla. A triangle within these boundaries indicates the deltoid muscle about 5 cm (2 in) below the acromion. See Figure 44–32. Another method of establishing the deltoid site is to place four fingers across the deltoid muscle, with the first finger on the acromion; i.e., the site is three finger breadths below the acromion. See Figure 44–33.

The lateral head of the **triceps muscle** on the posterior aspect of the upper arm can also be used as an injection site. The site of choice is about midway between the acromion and the olecranon of the ulna (the elbow). See Figure 44–34. This site is not often used unless other sites are contraindicated. Sitting or lying positions can be assumed for injections in the deltoid and triceps sites. Procedure 44–4 describes how to administer an intramuscular injection.

PROCEDURE 44–4

Administering an Intramuscular Injection

Equipment

- The medication card, MAR, or computer printout.
- The sterile medication. This is usually provided in an ampule or vial.
- A sterile syringe and needle. Choose the size of syringe appropriate for the amount of solution to be admin-

istered. Usually, a 2–5 mL syringe is needed. Some medications, such as paraldehyde, require a glass syringe because the medication interacts with plastic. The size and length of the needle are determined by the muscle to be used, the type of solution, the amount of adipose tissue covering the muscle, and the age of the client. A large muscle, such as the gluteus medius, usually requires a #20–23 gauge needle, 1½ to 3 in.

long, whereas the deltoid muscle requires a smaller, #23–25 gauge needle, ⅝–1 in. long. Oily solutions such as paraldehyde require a thicker needle, eg, #21 gauge instead of #23 gauge. Also, the greater the amount of adipose tissue over the muscle, the longer the needle must be to reach the muscle. Therefore, 3-in. needles may be needed for obese clients, whereas ½-in. needles are used for thinner people. Infants and young children usually require smaller, shorter needles (#22–25 gauge, ⅝–1 in. long).

- A swab saturated in an antiseptic solution for cleaning the site.

- Dry sterile gauze or an unopened alcohol swab, if an ampule must be opened.

Intervention

1. Check the medication order. See Procedure 44–2, steps 1 and 2.

2. Prepare the correct dosage of the drug from a vial or ampule. See Procedure 44–2, steps 2–19.

3. If the medication is particularly irritating to subcutaneous tissue, change the needle on the syringe before the injection.
   Rationale: Because the outside of the new needle is free of medication, it does not irritate subcutaneous tissues as it passes into the muscle.

4. Select the intramuscular site for adequate muscle mass. The skin surface over the site should be free of bruises, abrasions, and infection. Determine if the size of the muscle is appropriate to the amount of medication to be injected. An average adult's deltoid muscle can usually absorb 0.5 ml of medication, although some authorities believe 2 ml can be absorbed by a well-developed deltoid muscle, and the gluteus medius muscle can absorb 1–5 ml (Newton and Newton 1979, p. 19), although 5 ml may be very painful. The site should not have been used frequently. If injections are to be frequent, sites should be alternated. If necessary, discuss an alternate method of providing the medication with the physician prescribing it.

5. Establish the exact site for the injection and assist the client to an appropriate position. See the discussion of sites earlier in this procedure.

6. Clean the site with an antiseptic swab. Using a circular motion, start at the center and move outward about 5 cm (2 in.).

7. Remove the needle cover without contaminating the needle.

8. Invert the syringe and expel any excess air that may have accidentally entered the syringe, leaving only 0.2 ml of air if the air-bubble technique is being used. It may be necessary to flick the syringe to move the bubbles out. The remaining air will rise to the plunger end when the needle is pointed downward. See Figure 44–35.
   Rationale: Users of the air-bubble technique for IM injections believe that, in addition to clearing the medication from the bore of the needle, this technique prevents medication from leaking into

subcutaneous tissue and onto the skin surface, where it can cause pain and tissue damage (Wong 1982, p. 1237). Others believe that the best way to prevent leakage is to use the Z-track method described below. However, if the nurse is administering (a) Wyeth's vaccines of diphtheria and tetanus toxoids prepared with aluminum adjuvant, or (b) diphtheria and tetanus toxoids and pertussis vaccine, or (c) tetanus toxoid, it is recommended that the air-bubble technique be used to prevent abscess formation (Chaplin, Shull, and Welk 1985, p. 59).

9. Use the nondominant hand to spread the skin at the site.
   Rationale: Spreading the skin makes it firmer and facilitates needle insertion. Under some circumstances, eg, when the client is emaciated or an infant, the muscle may be pinched.

10. Holding the syringe between the thumb and forefinger, pierce the skin quickly at a 90° angle (see Figure 44–36), and insert the needle into the muscle (see Figure 44–37).
    Rationale: Using a quick motion lessens the client's discomfort.

11. Aspirate by holding the barrel of the syringe steady with your nondominant hand and by pulling back on the plunger with your dominant hand. If blood appears in the syringe, withdraw the needle, discard the syringe, and prepare a new injection.
    Rationale: This step determines whether the needle is in a blood vessel.

12. If blood does not appear, inject the medication steadily and slowly, holding the syringe steady.
    Rationale: Injecting medication slowly permits it to disperse into the muscle tissue, thus decreasing

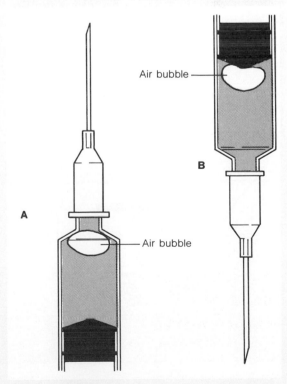

Figure 44–35

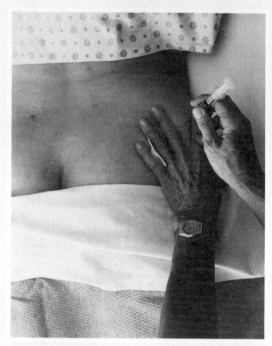

Figure 44-36

the client's discomfort. Holding the syringe steady minimizes discomfort.

13. See Procedure 44-3, steps 13-18, for withdrawing the needle, massaging the site, disposing of supplies, recording, and conducting follow-up assessment.

Sample Recording

Date	Time	Notes
12/5/89	0800	Penicillin G 500 mg IM into left vastus lateralis. No discomfort, walking without complaint. ——————— ——————— Rebecca I. Feinstein, NS

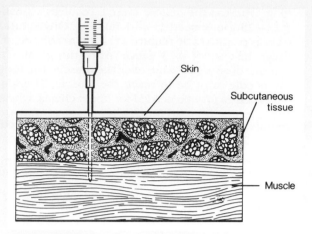

Figure 44-37

Variation for a Z-Tract Injection

This is a variation of the standard intramuscular technique. This variation is used to administer intramuscular medications that are highly irritating to subcutaneous and skin tissues.

14. Follow steps 1-8.

15. Attach a clean sterile needle to the syringe.
    Rationale: A new needle will not have any medication adhering to the outside that could be irritating to tissues.

16. With the nondominant hand, pull the skin and subcutaneous tissue about 2.5-3.5 cm (1-1¼ in.) to one side at the injection site (see Figure 44-38, *A*).

17. Insert the syringe and medication as in steps 10-12. Withdraw the plunger with the dominant hand while holding the syringe to ascertain placement of the needle.

18. Maintain the traction while removing the needle, and then permit the skin to return to its normal position.

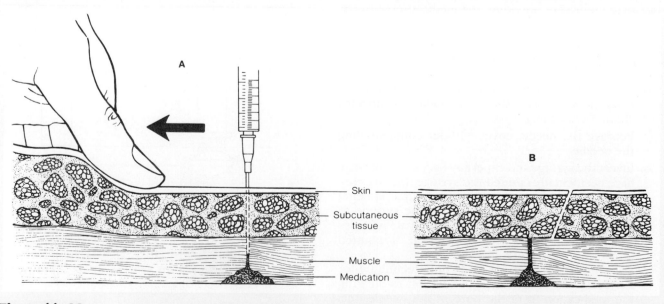

Figure 44-38

Rationale: During this time, muscle tissues relax and begin to absorb the medication. When the skin returns to its normal position, the needle track is interrupted, and the medication does not seep into the needle track or subcutaneous tissue. See Figure 44–38, *B.*

19. Do not massage.
    Rationale: Massage might cause seepage into delicate tissue.

Intramuscular Injections: Critical Events

Select needle size appropriate for the client

Select an appropriate muscle, one that has not been used frequently, has healthy intact skin, and adequate muscle mass

Locate the correct site for the injection

Position the client appropriately

Expel air from the syringe before the administration unless the air bubble technique is used

Aspirate for blood before injecting the medication

Minimize discomfort:

■ Spread the skin at the site before inserting the needle

■ Insert the needle quickly

■ Hold the syringe steady

■ Inject the medication slowly and steadily

■ Remove the needle quickly while depressing the skin

Use the Z-track technique for medications that irritate subcutaneous tissues:

■ Attach a clean needle before injection

■ Pull the skin to one side before the needle is inserted

■ Maintain the skin traction for 10 seconds before withdrawing the needle

■ Do not massage the site after the injection

■ **Intravenous Medications.** Because **intravenous (I.V.) medications** enter the client's bloodstream directly, they are appropriate when a rapid effect is required (e.g., in a life-threatening situation such as cardiac arrest). The I.V. route is also appropriate when medications are too irritating to tissues to be given by other routes. When an I.V. line is already established, this route is desirable because it avoids the discomfort of other parenteral routes. Medications are administered intravenously via:

1. Intravenous bottle or bag (continuous infusion)
2. Additional intravenous container (intermittent infusion by piggy-back [I.V.P.B.] or partial-fill [I.V.P.F.])
3. Volume-control administration set (often used for children)
4. Intravenous push (I.V.P. or bolus)

There are, however, potential hazards in giving I.V. medications: infection and rapid, severe reactions to the medication. To prevent infection, sterile technique is used during all aspects of I.V. medication techniques. To safeguard the client against severe reactions, the nurse must administer the drug slowly, following the manufacturer's recommendations. The client is assessed closely during the administration, and the medication is discontinued immediately if an untoward reaction occurs.

For **continuous infusions,** I.V. medications can be added to a new fluid container prior to hanging it or to a fluid container that is already attached and running. Electrolytes (e.g., potassium chloride) and vitamins (e.g., Solu-B) are commonly administered by this method. Before administering any intravenous medication, the nurse inspects and palpates the intravenous insertion site for signs of infection, infiltration, or a dislocated catheter. Also, the surrounding skin is inspected for redness, pallor, or swelling, and the surrounding tissues are palpated for coldness and presence of edema, which could indicate leakage of the I.V. fluid into the tissues. The nurse than takes the vital signs for baseline data. It is also important to make sure that the drug and solutions are compatible. A nurse may need to consult a pharmacist for this information. An **incompatibility** is an undesired chemical or physical reaction between a drug and an infusion solution, between two or more drugs, or between a drug and the container or tubing. See Procedure 44–5.

PROCEDURE 44–5

Adding an I.V. Medication to an I.V. Bottle or Bag

Equipment

■ The correct solution container, if a new one is to be attached. Confirm its sterility by ensuring that there are no container cracks or leaks, fluid discoloration, or seal damage.

■ The medication card or computer printout.

■ The correct sterile medication. If the medication is in a powdered form, a diluent (eg, sterile saline solution or water) will also be necessary.

■ Antiseptic swabs.

■ A sterile syringe of appropriate size (eg, 5 or 10 ml) and a 1- to 1½-in., #20 or #21 gauge sterile needle.

■ A medication label to attach to the I.V. solution container.

Intervention

1. Check the physician's orders carefully for the medication, dosage, and route. Verify which infusions are to be used with the medication. For example, the order may say to infuse the medication with 1000 ml of 5% dextrose and water rather than with normal saline.

2. Confirm the compatibility of the drugs and solutions being mixed. The nurse may need to consult a pharmacist for this information. An incompatibility, in terms of I.V. therapy, is an undesired chemical or physical reaction between a drug and an infusion solution, between two or more drugs, or between a drug and the container or tubing.

3. Prepare the medication from a vial or ampule as described in Procedure 44–2. Check the agency's practice about whether a special filter needle is to be used when withdrawing the medication. A filter needle may be used to draw up premixed liquid medications from multidose vials.

4. For a glass I.V. container, remove the metal cap and the rubber disc, if the bottle is vented. Locate the injection port.

    or

    For a plastic container, locate the separate, self-sealing, soft rubber injection port. An injection port may be designated in several ways, eg, by a triangular indentation or by the word *add.* It is important not to inject medication through the port for the administration spike or through an air vent port if there is an injection port.

5. Clean the injection port with an antiseptic swab.

6. Remove the needle cover from the medication syringe, and inject the medication into the port. See Figure 44–39.

7. Remove the needle. For a glass container, cover the top immediately either with

    a. An antiseptic swab with the metal I.V. cap taped over it.

    or

    b. The special sterile cap provided by the manufacturer.

8. Attach the medication label upside down to the fluid container. See Figure 44–40 for the information to be included on the medication label.
    Rationale: This makes the label easy to read when the container is hanging.

9. Gently rotate the solution container to mix the drug with the solution.

10. Spike and hang the container, and regulate the flow rate according to the dosage required when the medication is to be administered.

11. Record the I.V. infusion and medication.

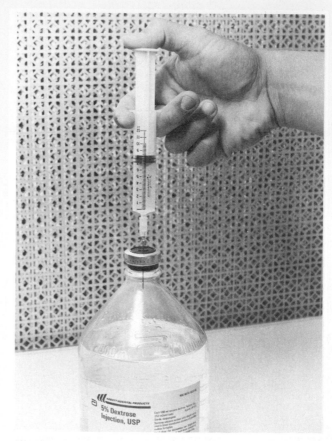

Figure 44–39

MEDICATION ADDED

PATIENT *Mendoza*   RM. *207-A*

DRUG *K-Cl*

AMOUNT *40 mEq*

ADDED BY *N.W. Armstrong, RN*

DATE *12/5/89*   TIME *0900*

START TIME *0900*   DATE *12/5/89* FLOW RATE *40*

EXP. DATE ———

THIS LABEL MUST BE AFFIXED TO ALL INFUSION
FLUIDS CONTAINING ADDITIONAL MEDICATION

Figure 44–40

12. Carefully monitor the I.V. infusion to maintain delivery of the medication and I.V. fluid at the specified rate.

13. During the administration, observe the client for signs of an adverse reaction, such as noisy respirations, changes in pulse rate, chills, nausea, or headache. If any adverse sign occurs, follow agency policy (ie, slow I.V. rate or stop flow), and notify the physician or nurse in charge. Also monitor the client for signs of the intended action of the medication.

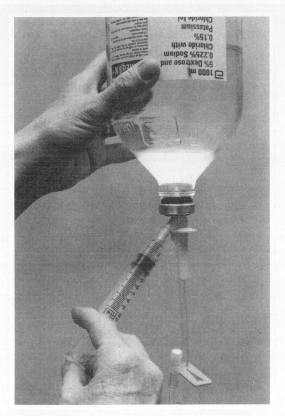

Figure 44–41

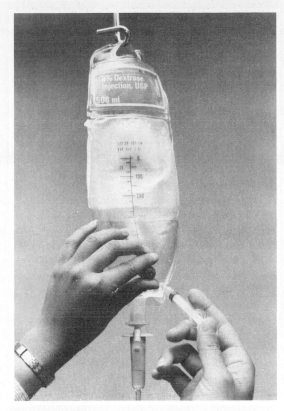

Figure 44–42

Variations for Adding Medications
to an Infusing Container

14. For an I.V. container with a vented administration set (ie, a nonvented container):
    a. Make sure there is sufficient solution in the bottle to ensure proper dilution of the drug.
    b. Close the I.V. flow clamp.
    Rationale: Closing the clamp is essential to prevent the medication from infusing to the client before it is properly diluted with the solution. Undiluted medication can produce a severe reaction.
    c. Detach the air vent cap, taking care not to contaminate the end.
    d. Insert the tip of the medication syringe, *without the needle,* into the air vent port. See Figure 44–41.
    e. Instill the medication.
    f. Reattach the air vent.
    or

15. For a vented I.V. bottle:
    a. After ensuring that there is sufficient solution in the bottle, close the I.V. flow clamp.
    b. Clean the medication port with an antiseptic swab.
    c. Insert the syringe needle through the port and instill the medication. The medication port is usually marked by a triangular imprint.
    or

16. For a plastic I.V. bag:
    a. After ensuring that there is sufficient solution in the bag, close the I.V. flow clamp.

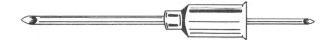

Figure 44–43

    b. Clean the medication port with an antiseptic swab.
    c. While supporting and stabilizing the bag with your thumb and forefinger, carefully insert the syringe needle through the port and inject the medication. See Figure 44–42.
    Rationale: The bag is supported while injecting the medication to avoid puncturing it.

17. For all infusing methods:
    a. Attach a medication label to the I.V. container.
    b. Gently lift and rotate the container.
    Rationale: This mixes the solution and medication.
    c. Open the I.V. flow clamp and regulate the rate as ordered.
    d. Follow steps 11–13.

Variation: Using a Transfer Needle

A special transfer needle (see Figure 44–43) can be used to put medications in vials into a plastic I.V. container, provided the entire amount of medication is to be transferred to the I.V. container. After cleaning the top of the medication vial and the medication port on the I.V. bag with an antiseptic sponge, the small end of the transfer needle is inserted into the medication vial and the large end into the port of the I.V. container. To mix the medication and solution:

▪ Invert the I.V. bag so that the medication bottle is on top.

▪ Gently squeeze the I.V. bag to transmit some air from the I.V. bag into the medication vial.

▪ Release the pressure on the I.V. bag to allow medication to drain into the I.V. bag.

▪ Repeat squeezing and releasing pressure until all the medication is transferred into the I.V. solution. The transfer needle may need to be pulled down so that all the medication is obtained from the vial.

▪ Remove the needle and gently rotate the bag to disperse the medication.

For **intermittent infusions,** additional fluid containers and secondary tubing sets are sometimes attached to a primary infusion to administer I.V. medications. These intermittent medications may be given simultaneously with the primary infusion (providing the medications are compatible and the client is able to tolerate the additional fluid), or the primary line may be clamped while the intermittent medication is infusing. The medication is commonly injected into a small container of intravenous solution (usually 50–100 ml of D5W or NS). At some facilities, these containers are called intravenous partial fills (I.V.P.F.) or additives (addits). When infusion pumps and controllers are used to administer intermittent medications via secondary lines, the nurse should follow the manufacturer's instructions for setting up the intermittent infusion.

Depending upon how the secondary infusion is set up, the intermittent infusion may be called an intravenous piggyback (I.V.P.B.) or a tandem intravenous alignment (see Figure 44–44). The term *piggyback* refers to the positioning of the additive container higher than the primary infusion container. Manufacturers provide an extension hook to lower the primary container. When the I.V.P.B. is connected to a port that has a backcheck valve, the valve automatically stops the flow of the primary infusion so that only the secondary infusion flows. See Figure 44–45. After the I.V.P.B. has infused and the

level of solution in the tubing is below the level of the primary infusion drip chamber, the backcheck valve is released and the primary infusion automatically starts running again. Thus, it is important that nurses leave the primary line unclamped when using this type of intermittent infusion setup.

When any intermittent medication is infusing, the nurse should calculate the desired flow rate and estimated time of infusion. The nurse then adjusts the flow rate by counting the drops per minute in the secondary set drip chamber, manually setting a flow adjustment device attached to the secondary set, or setting the rate on an infusion pump or controller. The nurse should assess the client at least every 15 minutes (or more frequently, e.g., when the client is receiving vasoactive drugs), to ensure that the medication is infusing satisfactorily. With some medications (e.g., potassium chloride), it may be necessary to dilute the medication in larger amounts of fluid (e.g., 250 ml) or infuse the medication at a slow rate with the primary line running at the usual rate to decrease irritation of the vein.

A *tandem intravenous alignment* may be set up by connecting the additive infusion to the primary line via a secondary port without a backcheck valve, more proximal to the client than the piggyback port. This type of setup requires a longer secondary tubing set than for a piggyback setup. Both the primary and the secondary infusions are positioned at the same height. Frequently, the primary infusion is temporarily clamped while the additive infuses, but this is only required when the two solutions are incompatible or when a more rapid infusion of the additive is desired. When the solutions are incompatible, the nurse must first clamp the primary line and flush the tubing between the secondary port and the client with a sterile solution (usually normal saline) before connecting and initiating the secondary infusion. The saline flush serves as a buffer between the two incompatible solutions. When the secondary infusion is complete, the nurse should again flush the line before restarting the primary infusion. Whenever the primary line is clamped, the nurse should carefully assess the client every 15 minutes (and more frequently when the secondary infusion is nearly complete), to maintain continuous patency.

Intermittent medications may also be administered by volume-control sets (e.g., Buretrol, Soluset, Volutrol, Pediatrol). They are small fluid containers (100 to 150

Administering Intravenous Medications: Critical Elements

Verify which infusions are to receive medications
Confirm compatibility of the medication and I.V. solution and equipment
Maintain sterility of the I.V. and medication equipment
Attach appropriate medication labels to the I.V. container
When adding medications to infusing containers:

▪ Make sure there is sufficient solution to dilute the drug
▪ Clamp the I.V. tubing before adding medications
▪ Insert medications only through designated medication ports
▪ If using an air-vent port insert the medication syringe *without the needle*

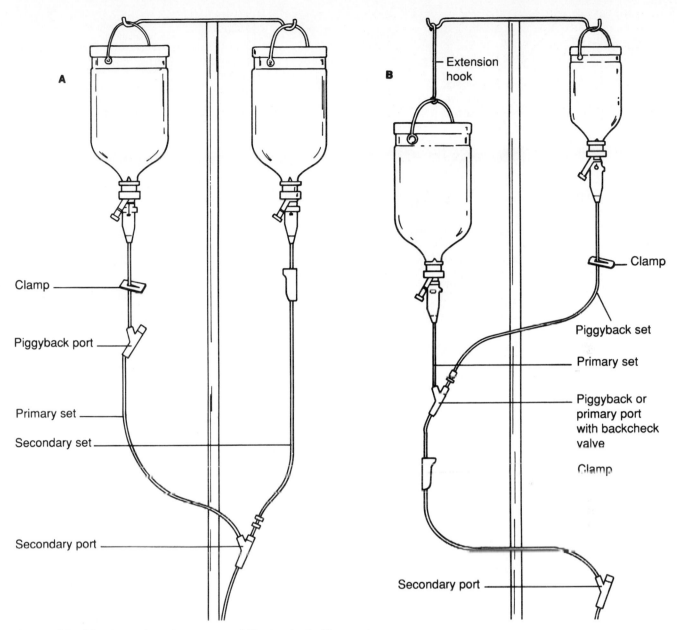

Figure 44–44 **A,** tandem alignment, and **B,** piggyback alignment

ml in size) attached below the primary infusion container. Volume-control sets are equipped with either a stationary membrane filter or a floating valve filter at the base of the container and are designed to finely control the amount of infusing fluid. See Figure 44–46. Volume-control administration sets serve the following purposes:

1. To administer I.V. medications (such as some antibiotics) that do not remain stable for the length of time it takes an entire solution container to infuse
2. To administer medications intermittently
3. To avoid mixing medications that are incompatible
4. To dilute a drug so that it is less irritating to the veins than if given by direct intravenous push
5. To deliver medications diluted in precise amounts of fluid

An **I.V. push** (I.V.P. or bolus) is the intravenous administration of a medication that cannot be diluted or that is needed in an emergency. Also, certain drugs are administered this way to achieve maximum effect. It is important to remember that the rapid administration of an I.V. push could be dangerous for the client. An I.V. push can be administered directly into a vein through venipuncture, into an existing intravenous apparatus through an injection port (see Figure 44–47), or through an intermittent infusion set (heparin lock) when the client does not have an I.V. running but does have a heparin lock in place. The heparin lock (Figure 44–48), also called a male adapter plug (MAP), is used primarily for clients who require regular intermittent I.V. medications but not the fluid volume of an intravenous infusion. The set usually consists of an indwelling catheter attached to a plastic tube with a sealed

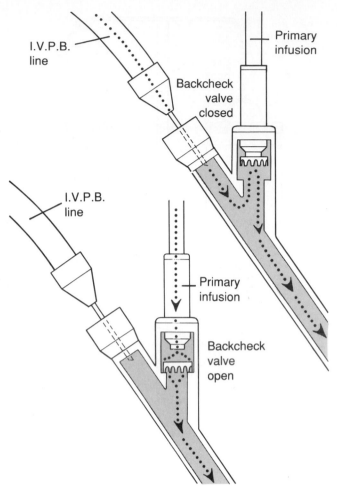

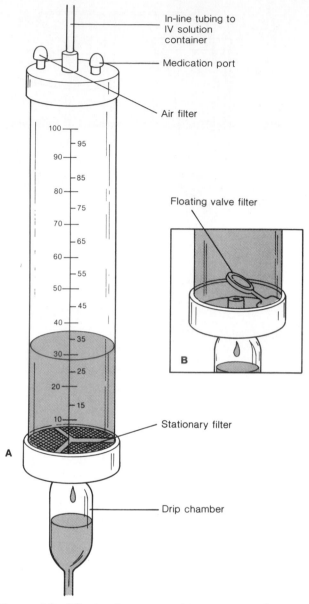

Figure 44–45

Figure 44–46 A volume-control intravenous infusion set: **A,** with a stationary filter; **B,** with a floating valve filter

injection tip. It is called a **heparin lock** because small amounts of heparin are injected into the catheter to maintain its patency. After administering an I.V. push, the nurse discards the used syringe and needle in a designated container without recapping the needle, as for any other type of injection.

Topical Medications

Dermatologic Medications.
Dermatologic medications are commonly applied for one of the following reasons:

1. To decrease itching (pruritus)
2. To lubricate and soften the skin
3. To cause local vasoconstriction or vasodilation
4. To increase or decrease secretions from the skin
5. To provide a protective coating to the skin
6. To apply an antibiotic or antiseptic to treat or prevent infection

In addition, some medications that are routinely administered by other routes may also be available for use transdermally by applying a "patch" to provide sustained action. Examples of these are nitroglycerin patches and anti–motion sickness preparations. Absorption is facil-

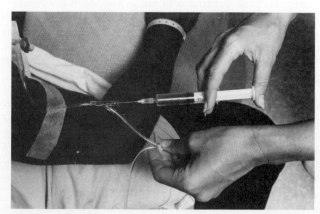

Figure 44–47

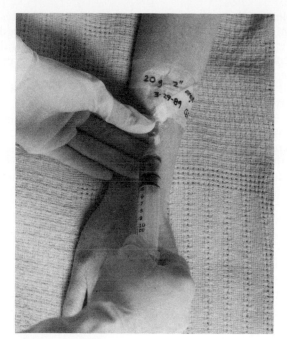

Figure 44–48

Table 44-6 Topical Applications

Medication	Application
Lotion	Shake before use to distribute suspended particles.
	Pour onto sterile gauze and pat onto affected area.
	Do not rub, to avoid aggravating affected area.
Liniment	Pour onto hands and rub into client's skin with long, smooth strokes.
Ointment and paste	Usually applied with a tongue blade or with gloves. Some must be applied thinly over the area, e.g., cortisone. Sterile dressing may be applied over ointment.
Powder	Sprinkle over the surface and cover with a dressing.

itated by washing the area well before the application. Dermatologic preparations include lotions, emollients, liniments, ointments, pastes, and powders. See Table 44–1, earlier in the chapter.

Unless contraindicated by a specific order, the nurse should wash and carefully dry the area, using a patting motion, before applying a dermatologic preparation. Skin encrustations and discharges harbor microorganisms and cause local infections. They can also prevent the medication from coming in contact with the area to be treated. Nurses should always use surgical asepsis when an open wound is present. If a client has lesions, the nurse must wear gloves or use tongue depressors. In this way the nurse's hand will not come in direct contact with microorganisms in and around the lesions. See Table 44–6 for general guidelines for applying topical medications.

■ **Irrigations and Instillations.** **Irrigation** (lavage) is the washing out of a body cavity by a stream of water or other fluid. **Instillation** is the insertion of a medication into a body cavity. Irrigation is performed for one or more of the following reasons:

1. To clean the area; i.e., to remove a foreign object or discharge
2. To apply heat or cold
3. To apply a medication, such as an antiseptic
4. To prepare an area for surgery, e.g., the eye

Surgical asepsis is required when there is a break in the skin (e.g., in a wound irrigation), or whenever a sterile body cavity (e.g., the bladder) is entered. Some irrigations (e.g., an eye irrigation to remove foreign material; or a vaginal, rectal, or gastric irrigation) are safely conducted using medical asepsis.

A number of different kinds of syringes are used for irrigations. The most common are the Asepto, the rub-

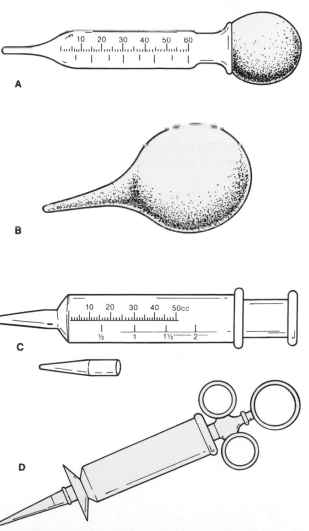

Figure 44–49 Four types of syringes commonly used for irrigations: **A,** Asepto; **B,** rubber bulb; **C,** Toomey with adaptor tip to fit into tubing; and **D,** Pomeroy.

ber bulb, the Toomey, and the Pomeroy. The syringes are often calibrated, permitting the nurse to determine the amount of irrigant being delivered at any given time. The **Asepto syringe** is a plastic (or glass) syringe with a rubber bulb. See Figure 44–49, *A*. Squeezing the air out of the bulb produces negative pressure, and fluid can be sucked into the syringe. When the bulb is squeezed again, the fluid is ejected from the syringe. Asepto syringes come in several sizes, e.g., 30 ml (1 oz), 60 ml (2 oz), and 120 ml (4 oz).

The **rubber bulb syringe** is often used for irrigating the ears. See Figure 44–49, *B*. Like the Asepto syringe, it comes in a range of sizes. The **Toomey syringe,** which is made of plastic or glass, is also calibrated. See Figure 44–49, *C*. This syringe has a remov-

able tip of metal or plastic that can fit into the end of tubing such as a catheter. Toomey syringes are used for deep-wound irrigations that require a catheter and for some types of bladder irrigations. The **Pomeroy syringe** is a metal syringe commonly used for ear irrigations. A shield near the tip prevents the solution from spraying outward (see Figure 44–49, *D*).

An **eye irrigation** is administered to wash out the conjunctival sac of the eye. In a hospital, sterile equipment is usually used. Medications for the eyes are instilled in the form of liquids or ointments. Usually, sterile preparations are used, but sterile technique is not always indicated. Prescribed liquids are usually dilute, e.g., less than 1% strength. Procedure 44–6 illustrates how to administer irrigations and instillations.

PROCEDURE 44–6

Administering Ophthalmic Irrigations and Instillations

Equipment

For an irrigation:

- A sterile container for the irrigating solution.
- Irrigating solution. Usually 60–235 ml (2–8 oz) of solution at 37 C (98.6 F) is appropriate.
- A sterile eye syringe or eye irrigator. An eyedropper can be used if only small amounts of solution are required.
- A sterile kidney basin.
- Sterile cotton balls.
- Sterile normal saline (optional).
- A moisture proof drape.
- Sterile gloves (optional).

For an instillation:

- The medication. Some eye medications are packaged in plastic containers that are also used to administer the preparation. Ointments are usually supplied in small tubes.
- A sterile eyedropper, if needed.
- Sterile absorbent sponges. Soak some sponges in sterile normal saline for cleaning the eyelid and eyelashes.
- A sterile eye dressing (pad) as needed and paper eye tape to secure it.
- Sterile gloves (optional).

Intervention

1. Verify the physician's order for the preparation, strength, and number of drops if it is a liquid instillation. Also verify the prescribed frequency of the instillation and which eye is to be treated. Abbreviations are frequently used to identify the eye: OD (right eye), OS (left eye), OU (both eyes).
   or
   For an irrigation, check the type, amount, temperature, and strength of the solution and the frequency of the irrigation.

2. Explain the technique to the client. The administration of an ophthalmic irrigating solution or medication is not usually painful. Ointments are often soothing to the eye, but some liquid preparations may sting initially.

3. Assist the client to a comfortable position either sitting or lying. Tilt the client's head toward the affected eye, and ensure that the light source does not shine into the person's eyes.
   Rationale: The head is tilted so that the solution will run from the eye to the basin at the side, not to the other eye. The light source is directed slightly away from the eye, particularly if the person is photophobic.

4. Place the drape to protect the client and the bedclothes, and position the basin against the cheek below the eye on the affected side.

5. Don gloves, if the eye is infected.

6. Assess:
   a. The eye for redness, the location and nature of any discharge, lacrimation, and swelling of the eyelids or of the lacrimal gland.
   b. Any complaints, eg, itching, burning, pain, blurring of vision, and photophobia.
   c. The client's behavior, eg, squinting, blinking excessively, frowning, or rubbing the eyes.

7. Clean the eyelid and lashes with sterile cotton balls, moistened with sterile irrigating solution or sterile

normal saline. Wipe from the inner canthus to the outer canthus.

Rationale: If not removed, material on the eyelid and lashes can be washed into the eye. Cleaning toward the outer canthus prevents contamination of the other eye and the lacrimal duct.

For an Irrigation

8. Expose the lower conjunctival sac by separating the lids with the thumb and forefinger (see Figure 44–50). Or, to irrigate in stages, first hold the lower lid down, then hold the upper lid up. Exert pressure on the bony prominences of the cheekbone and beneath the eyebrow when holding the eyelids.
   Rationale: Separating the lids prevents reflex blinking. Exerting pressure on the bony prominences minimizes the possibility of pressing the eyeball and causing discomfort.

9. Fill and hold the eye irrigator about 2.5 cm (1 in.) above the eye.
   Rationale: At this height the pressure of the solution will not damage the eye tissue, and the irrigator will not touch the eye.

10. Irrigate the eye, directing the solution onto the lower conjunctival sac and from the inner canthus to the outer canthus.
    Rationale: Directing the solution in this way prevents possible injury to the cornea and prevents fluid and contaminants from flowing down the nasolacrimal duct.

11. Irrigate until the solution leaving the eye is clear (no discharge is present) or until all the solution has been used.

12. Instruct the client to close and move the eye periodically.

Rationale: Eye closure and movement help to move secretions from the upper to the lower conjunctival sac.

13. Dry around the eye with cotton balls.

For an Instillation

14. Check the ophthalmic preparation as to name, strength, and number of drops if a liquid is used. Draw the correct number of drops into the shaft of the dropper if a dropper is used. If ointment is used, discard the first bead.
    Rationale: Checking medication data is essential to prevent a medication error. The first bead of ointment from a tube is considered to be contaminated.

15. Don gloves, if indicated.

16. Instruct the client to look up to the ceiling and give the client a piece of tissue.
    Rationale: The person is less likely to blink if looking up. While the client looks up, the cornea is partially protected by the top eyelid. A tissue is needed to press on the nasolacrimal duct after a liquid instillation (see step 21) or to wipe excess ointment from the eyelashes after an ointment is instilled.

17. Expose the lower conjunctival sac by placing the thumb or fingers of your nondominant hand on the client's cheekbone just below the eye and gently drawing down the skin on the cheek. If the tissues are edematous, handle the tissues carefully to avoid damaging them. See Figure 44–50.
    Rationale: Placing the fingers on the cheekbone minimizes the possibility of touching the cornea, avoids putting any pressure on the eyeball, and prevents the person from blinking or squinting.

18. Using a side approach, instill the correct number of drops onto the outer third of the lower conjunctival

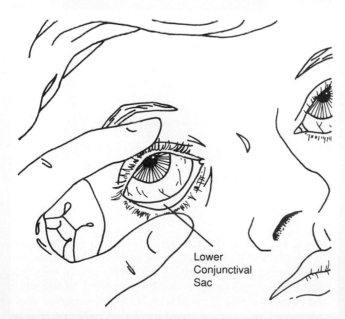

Lower Conjunctival Sac

Figure 44–50

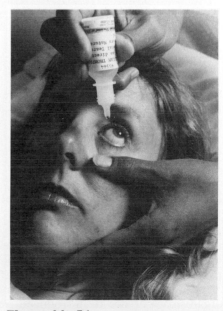

Figure 44–51

sac. Hold the dropper 1–2 cm (0.4–0.8 in.) above the sac. See Figure 44–51.

Rationale: The client is less likely to blink if a side approach is used. When instilled into the conjunctival sac, drops will not harm the cornea as they might if dropped directly on it. The dropper must not touch the sac or the cornea.

or

19. Holding the tube above the lower conjunctival sac, squeeze 3 cm (0.8 in.) of ointment from the tube into the lower conjunctival sac from the inner canthus outward. See Figure 44–52.

20. Instruct the client to close the eyelids but not to squeeze them shut.

Rationale: Closing the eye spreads the medication over the eyeball. Squeezing can injure the eye and push out the medication.

21. For liquid medications, press firmly or have the client press firmly on the nasolacrimal duct for at least 30 seconds. See Figure 44–53. Check agency practice.

Rationale: Pressing on the nasolacrimal duct prevents the medication from running out of the eye and down the duct.

22. Wipe the eyelids gently from the inner to the outer canthus, to collect excess medication.

23. Apply an eye pad if needed, and secure it with paper eye tape.

For an Irrigation and Instillation

24. Remove gloves if worn.

25. Assess the client's response in terms of the character and amount of any discharge; the appearance of the eye; and any discomfort, burning, etc. Assess any changes immediately after the instillation or irrigation and again after the medication should have acted.

26. Document nursing assessments and interventions relative to the instillation or irrigation. Include the name of the drug, the strength, the number of drops if a liquid, the time, and the response of the client.

Sample Recording

Date	Time	Notes
12/5/89	0900	C/o burning sensation OD. Moderate amount yellow purulent discharge at inner canthus and on eyelashes. Conjunctiva red. OD irrigated with 90 ml normal saline at 38C. Returns cloudy. Stated "eye feels better" following irrigation. —— Deborah M. Mondeau, NS

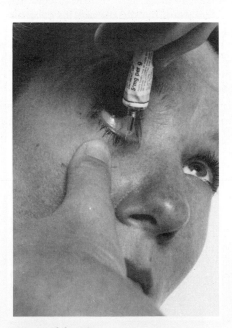

Figure 44–52

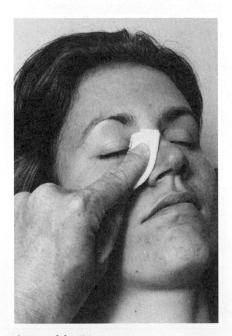

Figure 44–53

Irrigations of the external auditory canal are generally carried out for cleaning purposes, although applications of heat and of antiseptic solutions are sometimes prescribed. Irrigations are usually performed in a hospital, using sterile supplies and equipment so that microorganisms will not be introduced into the ear. Medical aseptic technique is used to instill medications to the ear unless the tympanic membrane is damaged, in which case sterile technique is used. The position of the external auditory canal varies with age. In the child under 3 years of age, it is directed upward. In the adult, the external auditory canal is an S-shaped structure about 2.5 cm (1 in) long. Procedure 44–7 explains how to administer otic irrigations and instillations.

PROCEDURE 44–7

Administering Otic Irrigations and Instillations

Equipment

For an irrigation:

- A container for the irrigating solution.

- Irrigating solution. About 500 ml (16 oz) of solution or as ordered. Normal saline is frequently used at body temperature: 37.0 C (98.6 F). Use a thermometer to make sure the temperature of the solution is appropriate.

- A syringe. A rubber bulb or Asepto syringe is frequently used.

- A basin (eg, kidney basin) to receive the irrigating solution.

- A moisture-resistant towel.

- Applicator swabs for cleaning the external ear.

- Absorbent cotton balls to dry the pinna of the ear after the irrigation.

- Gloves (optional).

For an instillation:

- The correct medication bottle with a dropper. To make the instillation more comfortable for the client, warm the container in your hand or place it in warm water for a short time.

- A cotton-tipped applicator to wipe the auditory meatus.

- A flexible rubber tip (optional) for the end of the dropper, which prevents injury from sudden motion, eg, by a child or disoriented client.

- A cotton fluff to cover the auditory meatus following the instillation.

Intervention

For an Irrigation

1. Verify the physician's order for the kind of medication or irrigation; the time, amount, and dosage (if it is an instillation) or strength (if it is an irrigation); the temperature (if it is an irrigation); and which ear is to be treated.

2. Explain to the client what you plan to do. The client may experience a feeling of fullness, warmth, and—occasionally—discomfort when the fluid comes in contact with the tympanic membrane.

3. Assist the client to a sitting or lying position with head turned toward the affected ear.
   Rationale: The solution can then flow from the ear canal to a basin.

4. Place the moisture-resistant towel around the client's shoulder under the ear to be irrigated and place the basin under the ear to be irrigated.

5. Assess the pinna of the ear and the meatus of the external auditory canal for signs of redness and abrasions, the type and amount of any discharge, and ask the client about complaints of discomfort. If indicated, use an otoscope to assess
   a. The external canal for any foreign bodies.
   b. The external canal for swelling, redness, and discharge. The lining should be intact, pink, and without lesions.
   c. The intactness and appearance of the tympanic membrane. If the tympanic membrane is not intact or if foreign bodies are present in the external canal, do not proceed with the irrigation; report your findings to the nurse in charge.

6. Don gloves, if indicated, and clean the pinna of the ear and the meatus of the ear canal with applicator swabs and solution.
   Rationale: Any discharge is removed so that it will not be washed into the ear canal.

7. Fill the syringe with solution.
   or

8. Hang up the irrigating container, and run solution through the tubing and the nozzle.
   Rationale: Solution is run through to remove air from the tubing and nozzle.

9. Straighten the auditory canal. For an infant, gently pull the pinna downward. See Figure 44–54. For an adult, pull the pinna upward and backward. See Figure 44–55.
   Rationale: The auditory canal is straightened so that the solution can flow the entire length of the canal.

10. Insert the tip of the syringe into the auditory meatus, and direct the solution gently upward against the top of the canal.
    Rationale: The solution will flow around the entire canal and out at the bottom. The solution is instilled

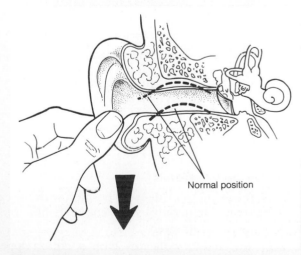

Normal position

Figure 44–54

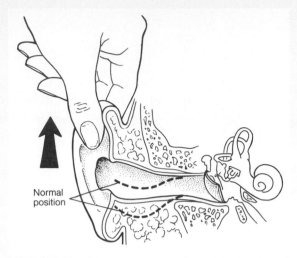

Normal position

Figure 44–55

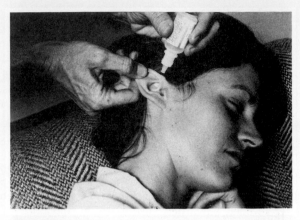

Figure 44–56

gently because strong pressure from the fluid can cause discomfort and damage the tympanic membrane.

11. Continue instilling the fluid until all the solution is used or until the canal is cleaned, depending on the purpose of the irrigation. Take care not to block the outward flow of the solution with the syringe.

12. Dry the outside of the ear with absorbent cotton balls. Place a cotton fluff in the auditory meatus, to absorb the excess fluid.

13. Assist the client to a side-lying position on the affected side.
    Rationale: Lying with the affected side down helps drain the excess fluid by gravity.

14. Assess the client for any discomfort, and the appearance and odor of the fluid returns.

15. Remove gloves, if worn.

16. Document assessments and interventions relative to the irrigation. Include the type, concentration, amount, and temperature of the solution used; the appearance of the returns; and the presence of any discomfort.

Sample Recording

Date	Time	Notes
12/5/89	1100	Irrigated left ear with 60 ml normal saline at 40 C. Returns clear with several dark brown flecks. No complaints of discomfort.———————————Josephine A. deSanto, NS

For an Instillation

17. Assist the client to a side-lying position with the ear being treated uppermost. See Figure 44–56.

18. Don gloves, if indicated.

19. Wipe the auditory meatus with a cotton-tipped applicator.

Rationale: The auditory meatus is cleaned to remove any drainage.

20. Partially fill the ear dropper with medication.

21. Straighten the ear canal. See step 9 and Figure 44–54 or Figure 44–55.

22. Instill the correct number of drops along the side of the ear canal.

23. Press gently but firmly a few times on the tragus of the ear.
    Rationale: Pressing on the tragus assists the flow of medication into the ear canal.

24. Have the client remain in the side-lying position for about 5 minutes.
    Rationale: This prevents the drops from escaping and allows the medication to reach all sides of the canal cavity.

25. Insert a small piece of cotton fluff loosely at the meatus of the auditory canal for 15–20 minutes. Do not press it into the canal.
    Rationale: The cotton helps retain the medication when the client is up. If pressed tightly into the canal, the cotton would interfere with the action of the drug and the outward movement of normal secretions.

26. Assess the character and amount of discharge, appearance of the canal, discomfort, etc after the instillation and again when the medication is expected to act. Inspect the cotton ball for any drainage.

27. Document nursing assessments and interventions relative to the instillation. Include the time, the dose, and any complaints of pain. Many agencies use flowsheets, others may require that a notation be made on the nurse's notes.

Sample Recording

Date	Time	Notes
12/5/89	0900	Auralgan instilled into left ear. States ear less painful. No discharge present.———————————Margaret N. Kerr, NS

Nasal instillations (nose drops) usually are instilled for their astringent effect (to shrink swollen mucous membranes) or to treat infections of the nasal cavity or sinuses. Prior to the instillation, the nurse should instruct the client to blow his or her nose to clear the nasal passages. Instilling nose drops requires that the client assume a back-lying position. For treating the opening of the eustachian (auditory) tube, the client can assume a dorsal recumbent position. The drops flow into the pharynx, where the eustachian tube opens. To treat the ethmoid and sphenoid sinuses, the client assumes a back-lying position, with the head over the edge of the bed or a pillow under the shoulders so the head is tipped backward. To treat the maxillary and frontal sinuses, the client assumes the same back-lying position, with the head turned toward the side to be treated. This is the Parkinson position. The nurse makes sure the client is positioned so that the correct side is accessible if only one side is to be treated. If the client's head is extended over the edge of the bed to facilitate instillation, it must be supported by the nurse's hands to prevent neck strain.

Once the client is supported in one of the above positions, the nurse administers the drops. The dropper is held just above the nostril, and the drops are directed toward the midline of the superior concha of the ethmoid bone as the client breathes through his or her mouth. If the drops are directed toward the base of the nasal cavity, they will run down the eustachian tube. The mucous membranes of the nostrils should not be touched, to avoid injury to tissue and contamination of the dropper. The nurse has the client remain in this position for 5 to 10 minutes so the solution will flow into the desired area. The nurse discards any medication remaining in the dropper before returning the dropper to the bottle.

Vaginal instillations are medications inserted as creams, jellies, foams, suppositories. **Vaginal irrigations** are also called *douches*. Vaginal creams, jellies, and foams are applied with a tubular applicator and plunger. Suppositories are inserted with the index finger of a gloved hand. Vaginal medications are inserted to treat a vaginal infection topically or to relieve vaginal discomfort, e.g., itching or pain.

Prior to the instillation, the nurse asks the client to urinate, since a full bladder can make treatment uncomfortable. Privacy is essential for this procedure. The nurse assists the client to a back-lying position, with the knees flexed and the hips rotated laterally. The client is draped as for catheterization. Adequate lighting on the vaginal orifice is necessary.

Suppositories are designed to melt at body temperature, so they are generally stored in the refrigerator to keep them firm for insertion. To prepare the vaginal suppository for instillation, the nurse should unwrap the suppository, place it on the opened wrapper, and don gloves to prevent contamination. Next, the nurse lubricates the smooth or rounded end of the suppository to facilitate its insertion. The rounded end is inserted first.

To insert the suppository, the nurse lubricates the gloved index finger of the dominant hand and exposes the vaginal orifice by separating the labia with the non-dominant hand. The suppository is placed about 8 to 10

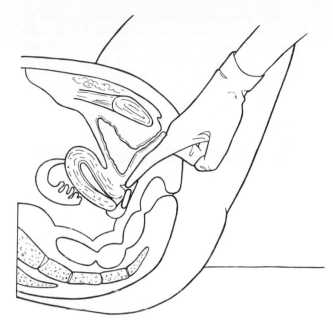

Figure 44—57 Instilling a vaginal suppository

cm (3 to 4 in) along the posterior wall of the vagina, or as far as it will go. See Figure 44—57. The nurse withdraws the finger, removes the gloves by turning them inside out, and discards them. Turning the gloves inside out prevents the spread of microorganisms. The client should be instructed to remain in the supine position for 5 to 10 minutes after the insertion to facilitate absorption and allow the melted medication to flow into the posterior fornix.

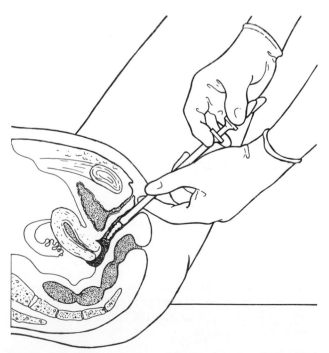

Figure 44—58 Instilling a vaginal cream using an applicator

To instill a vaginal cream, the nurse first fills the applicator with the prescribed cream, jelly, or foam. Directions are provided with the manufacturer's applicator. With the gloved nondominant hand, the nurse exposes the vaginal orifice. The nurse gently inserts the applicator about 5 cm (2 in) and pushes the plunger until the applicator is empty. See Figure 44–58. The applicator is removed and placed on a paper towel to contain microorganisms and prevent their spread. The client needs to remain supine for 5 to 10 minutes following the instillation. Finally, the nurse applies a clean perineal pad and a T-binder if there is excessive drainage.

A **vaginal irrigation** (douche) is the washing of the vagina by a liquid at a low pressure. It is similar to the irrigation of the external auditory canal in that the fluid returns immediately after being inserted. Vaginal irrigations are not necessary for ordinary female hygiene but are used to prevent infection by applying an antimicrobial solution that discourages the growth of microorganisms, to remove an offensive or irritating discharge, and to reduce inflammation or prevent hemorrhage by the application of heat or cold. Procedure 44–8 describes how to perform a vaginal irrigation.

PROCEDURE 44–8

Administering Vaginal Irrigations and Instillations

Equipment

For a vaginal irrigation:

- In hospitals, sterile supplies and equipment are used; in a home, sterility is not usually necessary because people are accustomed to the microorganisms in their environments. Sterile technique is indicated if there is an open wound.
- A vaginal irrigation set (these are often disposable), containing
- A nozzle
- Tubing and a clamp
- A container for the solution
- A moisture-resistant drape
- Irrigating solution. Usually, 1000–2000 ml at 40.5 C (105 F) is required. Check agency practice. Normal saline, tap water, sodium bicarbonate solution (8 ml of sodium bicarbonate to 1000 ml of water), and vinegar solution (8 ml of vinegar to 1000 ml of water) are commonly used.
- A thermometer to check the temperature of the solution. This is usually measured before the equipment is taken to the client.
- A moistureproof pad to protect the bedding.
- A bedpan to receive the irrigation returns.
- Tissues to dry the perineum.
- Gloves to protect the nurse from infection.
- An I.V. pole on which to hang the solution container.

For a vaginal instillation:

- The correct vaginal suppository or cream. Suppositories are designed to melt at body temperature, so they are generally stored in the refrigerator to keep them firm for insertion.
- Disposable gloves.
- Lubricant for a suppository.

- An applicator for vaginal cream.
- A paper towel.
- A clean perineal pad and T-binder or sanitary belt.

Intervention

1. Carefully check the physician's order for the specific medication or solution ordered, its dosage, and the time of administration.

2. Explain the technique to the client. A vaginal irrigation is normally a painless procedure and, in fact, may bring relief from itching and burning if an infection is present. It usually takes about 10 minutes. Many people feel embarrassed about these procedures, and some may prefer to perform the procedure themselves if instruction is provided.

3. Provide privacy, and ask the client to void.
   Rationale: If the bladder is empty, the client will have less discomfort during the treatment and the possibility of injuring the vaginal lining is decreased.

4. Don gloves.

5. Assess
   a. The vaginal orifice for inflammation.
   b. Any odor or discharge from the vagina.
   c. Complaints of vaginal discomfort.
   d. Clinical signs of generalized infection, eg, elevated body temperature, rapid pulse.

6. Assist the client to a back-lying position with the hips higher than the shoulders so that the solution will flow into the posterior fornix of the vagina. Position the client on a bedpan, and provide comfortable support for the lumbar region of the back with a roll or pillow. Place the waterproof drape under the bedpan to protect the bedding. Provide a drape for the legs so that only the perineal area is exposed.

7. Provide perineal care to remove microorganisms.
   Rationale: This decreases the chance of flushing microorganisms into the vagina.

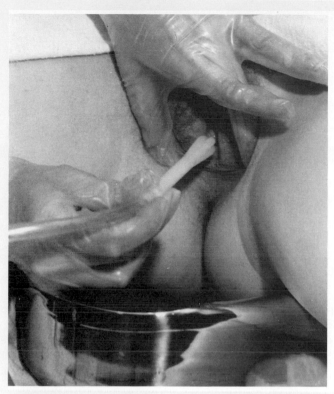

Figure 44–59

8. Clamp the tubing. Hang the irrigating container on the I.V. pole so that the base is about 30 cm (12 in.) above the vagina.
   Rationale: At this height the pressure of the solution should not be great enough to injure the vaginal lining.

9. Run fluid through the tubing and nozzle into the bedpan.
   Rationale: Fluid is run through the tubing to remove air and to moisten the nozzle.

10. Run some fluid over the perineal area, then insert the nozzle carefully into the vagina. Direct the nozzle toward the sacrum, following the direction of the vagina. See Figure 44–59.

11. Insert the nozzle about 7–10 cm (3–4 in.), start the flow, and rotate the nozzle several times.
    Rationale: Rotating the nozzle irrigates all parts of the vagina.

12. Use all the irrigating solution, permitting it to flow out freely into the bedpan.
    Rationale: Obstructing the flow of the returns could result in injury to the tissues from pressure.

13. Remove the nozzle from the vagina.

14. Assist the client to a sitting position on the bedpan.
    Rationale: Sitting on the bedpan will help drain the remaining fluid by gravity.

15. Dry the perineum with tissues.

16. Remove the bedpan.

17. Assess the color and consistency of the fluid returns.

18. Remove the moisture resistant pad and the drape.

19. Apply a dressing if indicated.

20. Remove gloves.

21. Record the administration of the irrigation. Note when it was administered; the amount, type, strength, and temperature of the irrigating solution; and all nursing assessments.

Rectal instillations (suppositories) are a convenient and safe method of giving certain medications. Rectal medications may have a local effect (e.g., a laxative suppository will soften feces and stimulate defecation) or a systemic effect (e.g., an aminophylline suppository will dilate the client's bronchi and ease breathing). The advantages of rectal instillation include:

1. It avoids irritation of the upper gastrointestinal tract.
2. Some medications are well-absorbed across the mucosal surface of the rectum.
3. Rectal suppositories are thought to provide higher bloodstream levels (titers) of medication, since the venous blood from the rectum is not transported through the liver (Hahn et al. 1982, p. 99).

Prior to the insertion, the nurse helps the client to a lateral position, with the upper leg acutely flexed. Next, the nurse unwraps the suppository, puts it on the opened wrapper, and dons a glove or fingercot on the hand that will insert the suppository. The glove or fingercot prevents contamination of the nurse's hand by rectal microorganisms and feces. The nurse lubricates the smooth, rounded end of the suppository to prevent anal friction and tissue damage during insertion and lubricates the gloved index finger as well. To relax the client's anal sphincter, the nurse asks the client to breathe through the mouth. The suppository is inserted gently into the anus and along the wall of the rectum with the gloved index finger. In adults, suppositories are inserted to a depth of 10 cm (4 in); in children or infants, 5 cm (2 in) or less. See Figure 44–60. To be effective, the suppository needs to be placed along the wall of the rectum rather than embedded in feces. The nurse withdraws the finger, removes the fingercot or glove by turning it inside out, and places it on a paper towel. Turning it inside out contains the rectal microorganisms and prevents their spread. To dispel the client's urge to expel the suppository, the nurse presses the client's buttocks together for a few seconds. If a laxative suppository has been given, the nurse asks the client to retain it for as long as possible (e.g., 15 to 20 minutes). The call signal should be within easy reach so that the client can summon assistance to use the bedpan or toilet.

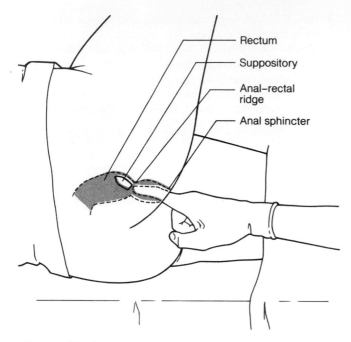

Rectum

Suppository

Anal–rectal ridge

Anal sphincter

Figure 44—60 A rectal suppository is inserted along the rectal wall beyond the internal anal sphincter.

Chapter Highlights

Nurse-practice acts define limits on the nurse's responsibilities regarding medications.

Federal drug legislation in the United States and Canada regulates the production, prescription, distribution, and administration of drugs.

Drugs are classified according to their overall action in the body.

Primary actions of drugs in the body are stimulation and inhibition of tissue or organ functions.

A drug may be incompatible with another drug or a particular food or an intravenous solution.

Repeated doses of a drug will achieve a sustained level in the bloodstream.

Obese clients require a larger dose of a drug than thin clients.

Drugs given parenterally act more quickly than drugs given orally or topically.

The five "rights" help ensure accurate administration of a drug.

Parenteral administration of medications employs sterile technique.

Clients receiving a series of injections should have the injection sites rotated.

Selected References

Chaplin, G.; Shull, H.; and Welk, P. C. September 1985. How safe is the air-bubble technique for I.M. injections? *Nursing 85* 15:59.

Gilman, A. G.; Goodman, L. S.; and Gilman, A. 1984. *The pharmacological basis of therapeutics,* 7th ed. New York: Macmillan.

Hahn, A. B.; Barkin, R. L.; and Oestreich, S. J. K. 1986. *Pharmacology in nursing.* 16th ed. St. Louis: C. V. Mosby Co.

Keen, M. F. July/August 1986. Comparison of intramuscular injection techniques to reduce site discomfort and lesions. *Nursing Research* 35:207–10.

Monahan, F. D. March/April 1984. When swallowing pills is difficult. *Geriatric Nursing* 5:88–89.

Motz-Harding, E., and Good, F. February 1985. The right solution: Mixing I.V. drugs thoroughly. *Nursing 85* 15:62–64.

Pitel, M. January 1971. The subcutaneous injection. *American Journal of Nursing* 71:76–79.

Reiss, B. S., and Melick, M. E. 1984. *Pharmacological aspects of nursing care.* Albany, New York: Delmar.

Todd, B. January/February 1983. Drugs and the elderly: Using eye drops and ointments safely. *Geriatric Nursing* 4(1):53–56.

———. May/June 1983. Drugs and the elderly: Topical analgesics. *Geriatric Nursing* 4(3):152, 192, 196.

———. July/August 1985. Drugs and the elderly: Identifying drug toxicity. *Geriatric Nursing* 6:231, 234.

Winfrey, A. July 1985. Single-dose I. M. injections: How much is too much? *Nursing 85* 15:38–39.

Wong, D. L. August 1982. Significance of dead space in syringes. *American Journal of Nursing* 82:1237.

CHAPTER 45

Wound Care

OBJECTIVES

Define terms commonly used to describe wounds.

State two basic ways in which wounds heal.

Describe factors that affect wound healing.

Identify the main complications of wound healing.

Describe assessment criteria of a clean, healing wound.

Identify nursing diagnoses for clients with various types of wounds.

List suggested nursing strategies to promote wound healing and prevent complications of wound healing.

Describe open and closed methods of wound care.

Identify commonly used dressing materials and binders.

Give reasons for selected steps of wound care procedures outlined in this chapter.

Identify physiologic responses to heat and cold and purposes of heat and cold.

Describe methods of applying dry and moist heat and cold.

List outcome criteria by which to gauge whether wound healing has been achieved.

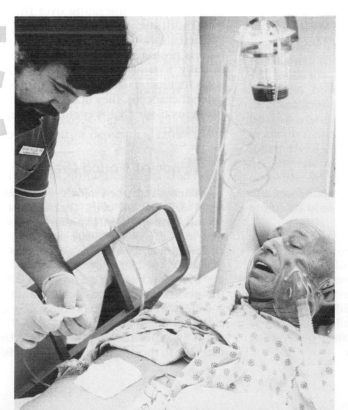

2. **Infection.** Infection of a surgical wound may become obvious 2 to 11 days postoperatively (Wright 1983, p. 143). Drainage from a suspected infected wound should be cultured. (Garner 1986, p. 79).

3. **Dehiscence with possible evisceration. Dehiscence** is the partial or total rupturing of a wound. Dehiscence often refers specifically to the opening of an abdominal wound in which the layers below the skin also separate. **Evisceration** is the protrusion of the internal viscera through an incision. A number of factors, including obesity, poor nutrition, multiple trauma, failure of suturing, excessive coughing, vomiting, and dehydration, heighten a client's risk of wound dehiscence. Wound dehiscence is more likely to occur when no healing ridge has appeared within 4 to 5 days postoperatively. This ridge normally develops along the entire length of an incision and is a sign that fibroplasia has occurred (LeMaitre and Finnegan 1980, p. 76).

Table 45–1 summarizes the clinical signs that indicate the presence of the complications of wound healing. The nurse should notify the physician if the signs of hemorrhage or infection are present. If dehiscence occurs, the area should be covered with sterile towels soaked in sterile saline to maintain tissue moistness, and the physician should be notified immediately. Wound dehiscence is an emergency situation requiring surgical resuturing. A nurse should remain with the client and support the wound, with gloved hands if necessary, to prevent evisceration.

Assessing Wounds

Nurses commonly assess both untreated and treated wounds. *Untreated wounds* usually are seen shortly after an injury (e.g., at the scene of an accident or in an emergency center). All untreated wounds should be assessed for bleeding and the presence of foreign material such as glass. *Treated wounds,* i.e., sutured wounds, are usually assessed during a dressing change. If a physician has not ordered dressing changes, the wound itself is not directly inspected; however, the dressing is inspected and other data regarding the wound, e.g., the presence of pain, are determined. Some surgical wounds are covered with a transparent occlusive dressing that permits observation of the wound without exposing it to the air.

Clinical Assessment

Wounds are assessed by visual inspection, palpation, and the sense of smell. They are assessed as to appearance, drainage, swelling, odor, dehiscence, and pain. The client is also assessed for any of the clinical signs of complications in Table 45–1.

As part of the ongoing assessment of each client with a wound, the nurse should first check the appearance of the wound itself for signs of healing and approximation (closing) of the wound edges. Taylor (1983, p. 44) and Bruno (1979, p. 670) outline the following *sequential* signs of **primary wound healing:**

1. *Absence of bleeding and a clot binding the wound edges.* After tissue is damaged, blood fills the area. A clot is formed from blood platelets, and the wound edges are well approximated and bound by fibrin in the clot within the first few hours after surgical closure.

2. *Inflammation (redness and swelling) at the wound edges* for 1 to 3 days. An inflammatory reaction begins after the clot sets, bringing white blood cells to ingest bacteria and cellular debris, and to demolish the clot.

3. *Reduction in inflammation when the clot diminishes,* as granulation tissue starts to bridge the area. Healthy tissue at the wound edges secretes nutrients, fibroblasts, and other building materials, e.g., epithelial cells, to bridge and close the wound within 7 to 10 days. Increased inflammation associated with fever and drainage is indicative of wound infection; the wound edges then appear brightly inflamed and swollen.

4. *Scar formation.* Fibroblasts in the granulation tissue secrete collagen, which forms scar tissue. Collagen synthesis starts 4 days after injury and continues for 6 months or longer.

5. *Diminished scar size* over a period of months or years. Collagen fibers shorten, and wound strength increases. An increase in scar size indicates keloid formation.

Additional assessment guidelines are presented in the accompanying box.

Laboratory Data

Laboratory data can often support the nurse's clinical assessment as to whether or not healing is taking

Table 45–1 Complications of Wound Healing		
Clinical Signs of Hemorrhage	**Clinical Signs of Infection**	**Clinical Signs of Dehiscence**
Increased pulse rate	Redness	Unexplained fever
Increased respiratory rate	Swelling	Unexplained tachycardia
Lowered blood pressure	Pain	Unusual wound pain
Restlessness	Induration (hardening of the tissues)	Prolonged paralytic ileus
Thirst	Fever	
Cold, clammy skin	Increased leukocyte count	

ASSESSMENT

Healing Wounds

Drainage: Inspect and record/report location, color, consistency, odor, and degree of saturation of dressings.

Swelling: Wearing sterile gloves, palpate wound edges for tension and tautness of tissues; minimal to moderate swelling is normal in early stages of wound healing.

Dehiscence: Observe for signs listed in Table 45–1. In addition, ask about pain/discomfort; severe to moderate postoperative pain may be present for 3–5 days; persistent severe pain or sudden onset of severe pain may indicate internal hemorrhaging or infection.

place. A **decreased leukocyte count** can delay healing and increase the possibility of infection. **Blood coagulation studies** are also significant to review. Prolonged coagulation times can result in excessive blood loss and prolonged clot absorption. Hypercoagulability can lead to intravascular clotting. Intraarterial clotting can result in ischemia to the wound area. **Serum protein analysis** provides an indication as to the body's nutritional reserves for rebuilding cells. **Wound cultures** can either confirm or rule out the presence of infection, and sensitivity studies are helpful in the selection of appropriate antibiotic therapy. Other laboratory tests may be ordered as needed for individual clients.

Nursing Diagnoses Relating to Wounds

Nursing diagnoses for clients with wounds largely reflect the need to prevent complications. See the accompanying box for examples of nursing diagnoses.

Planning Nursing Strategies to Augment Healing

Just as there are many types of wounds, there are many ways of caring for wounds. In general, the care varies with the type of wound, its size, the amount of exudate present, its state (open or closed), the location, the personal preference of the physician, and the presence of complicating factors. Planning includes both independent and dependent nursing strategies. Dependent strategies are those that stem largely from the wound care orders written by the physician. Both independent and dependent strategies are intended chiefly to promote healing and prevent infection.

Promoting wound healing is a goal for both the medical and nursing staff caring for a client with a wound. The physician approximates the wound edges with sutures to ensure a good blood supply to provide essential nutrients. The nurse provides ongoing assessment of the healing wound and keeps the area free from body excretions. In addition, the nurse protects the surrounding tissues from skin excoriation when a wound is draining. This is accomplished by changing saturated dressings as required and by cleaning and drying wounds and surrounding skin areas. When drainage is excessive, as in some bowel (colostomy) or urinary surgery, protective ointments or pastes may be applied to surrounding skin to prevent irritation and excoriation. The frequent removal of tape can also be irritating to the skin; thus, Montgomery straps (tie tapes) or newer tape products, which have minimal adhesive and are porous, are frequently used. These cause the least skin disruption.

The nurse can prevent infection from microorganisms entering a wound through the broken skin and mucous membranes by using surgical aseptic technique when caring for the wound, using antiseptic on the skin, and administering antibiotics as prescribed by the physician. Rubber or plastic tubes or drains are frequently put into wounds or ducts by surgeons to promote drainage. Some of these drains, commonly called **Penrose drains,** are shortened progressively throughout the healing process. They ensure removal of inflammatory exudates and blood prior to closure of the overlying skin. Just as the drain serves as an outlet for waste from the wound, it is also an inlet for infectious organisms. Therefore, the nurse keeps the area around the drain outlet clean to decrease the risk of wound infection. Planning wound care also involves establishing outcome criteria by which to evaluate the client's progress. For examples of outcome criteria, see the section on evaluation, later in this chapter.

Implementing Planned Care

Caring for Open and Closed Wounds

In the *open method* of wound care, no dressings are used. The *closed method* involves applying a dressing. Dressings have the following advantages:

1. Absorbing drainage and debriding the wound when removed

NURSING DIAGNOSIS

Wound Care

- Potential impaired skin integrity related to wound drainage
- Potential for infection related to an open wound
- Potential for infection related to the presence of a Penrose drain
- Altered comfort: pain related to incision
- Impaired physical mobility related to traction required to maintain proper alignment of left leg

2. Protecting the wound from external microbial contamination
3. Aiding in hemostasis when applied with elastic bandages
4. Approximating wound edges
5. Supporting and splinting the wound site, thus reducing mobility and trauma to the wound itself
6. Covering unpleasant disfigurements

In some situations, the physician applies a protective covering such as collodion spray instead of a gauze dressing. This spray hardens like nail polish and can be either peeled from the skin when the wound is healed or removed with a special solution. A spray covering is often preferred to a dressing, because friction is eliminated and the wound is always observable through the translucent covering. The wound is protected from external contamination because the spray is moisture-proof. For children, who are active and who heal quickly, spray is frequently used. It is not advised for wounds that have drainage.

The *open method* avoids certain disadvantages of dressings. For example, dressings produce dark, warm, moist environments in which resident and nonresident microorganisms can multiply, and dressings can irritate wounds by friction. Exposing wounds to the air produces drying. This discourages the growth of microorganisms, which need moisture. The open method is frequently employed for burns.

Caring for wounds involves cleaning (both open and closed wounds) and covering the wound. Some nurses prefer cotton balls to clean wounds because of their absorbent qualities; others prefer gauze squares, claiming that threads of cotton balls can stick to sutures.

Several sizes of gauze are available to cover wounds. See Figure 45–1. The standard sizes are 10 × 10 cm (4 × 4 in) and 10 × 20 cm (4 × 8 in). The size and the number of pads used depend on the nature of the wound, the amount of exudate, and the location of the wound. These decisions are left to the nurse's judgment. Sometimes the gauze is precut halfway through one side to make it fit around a drain, or it is folded in a special way.

Telfa gauze is a special type. It has a shiny, nonadherent surface on one or both sides and is applied with the shiny surface on the wound. Exudate seeps through this surface and collects on absorbent material on the other side or sandwiched between the two nonadherent surfaces. Since the dressing does not adhere, it does not cause injury to the wound when removed. **Petrolatum** gauze, another nonadherent type, is impregnated with petroleum jelly. It is placed against the wound and usually covered with 4 × 4 gauze. Nonadherent dressings should not be used when wound debridement is desired.

Larger and thicker gauze dressings, called **surgipads** or **abdominal pads,** are used to cover small gauzes. They not only hold the other gauzes in place but also absorb and collect excess drainage. Surgipads are more absorbent on one side, and this side is placed toward the wound; the less absorbent, more protective side is placed outward to protect the wound from external contamination. The outer side is often indicated with a blue stripe.

It is important to tape a dressing over a wound so that the dressing covers entire wound and the tape does not become dislodged. The correct type of tape must be selected for the purpose. Elastic tape can provide pressure; nonallergenic tape is used when a client is allergic to other tape. The nurse follows these steps:

1. Place the tape so that the dressing cannot be folded back to expose the wound. Place strips at the ends of the dressing, and space tapes evenly in the middle. See Figure 45–2.
2. Ensure that the tape is long and wide enough to

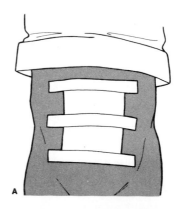

A

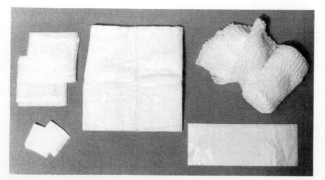

Figure 45–1 Some frequently used dressing materials (clockwise from bottom left): 2 × 2 gauze, 4 × 4 gauze, surgipad or abdominal pad, roller gauze, and nonadherent absorbent dressing

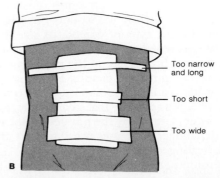

Too narrow and long

Too short

Too wide

B

Figure 45–2 The strips of tape should be placed at the ends of the dressing and must be sufficiently long and wide to secure the dressing. **A,** Correct taping; **B,** incorrect taping

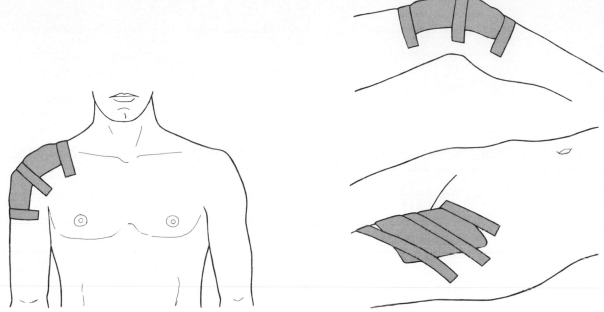

Figure 45–3 Dressings over moving parts must remain secure in spite of the movement.

adhere to the skin but not so long or wide that it loosens with activity. See Figure 45–2.

3. Place the tape in the opposite direction from the body action, e.g., across a body joint or crease, not lengthwise. See Figure 45–3.

After surgery, an elastic adhesive tape may be applied over wounds because of its ability to compress, thereby controlling hemorrhage. The original tape is removed during the initial dressing change, and a lighter dressing is applied. It is important to secure the dressing at both ends and across the middle and to use tape of a sufficient width for the dressing and the wound.

Montgomery straps (tie tapes) are commonly used for wounds requiring frequent dressing changes. See Figure 45–4. These straps prevent skin irritation and discomfort caused by removing the adhesive each time the dressing is changed. Nonallergenic tie tapes are available for people with sensitive skin. If these are not available, the nurse can protect the skin by applying tincture of benzoin applied to the site where the adhesive is to be placed.

▪ **S**upporting and Immobilizing Wounds

A **bandage** is a strip of cloth used to wrap some part of the body. Bandages are available in various widths, most commonly 1.5 to 7.5 cm (0.5 to 3 in). They are usually supplied in rolls for easy application to a body part. A **binder** bandage is designed for a specific body part; for example, the triangular binder (sling) fits the arm. Binders are used to support large areas of the body, such as the abdomen, arm, or chest. The purposes of bandages and binders are summarized in the accompanying box.

Before applying a bandage, the nurse needs to know its purpose and the area of the body to which it should be applied. Applying bandages to various parts of the body involves one or more of five basic bandaging turns: circular, spiral, spiral reverse, recurrent, and figure-eight. **Circular** turns are used to anchor bandages and to terminate them. They are also used to bandage certain areas, such as the proximal aspect of a finger or a wrist. Circular turns usually are not applied directly over a wound because of the discomfort the bandage would cause.

Spiral turns are used to bandage parts of the body that are fairly uniform in circumference, e.g., the upper arm or upper leg. **Spiral reverse** turns are used to bandage cylindrical parts of the body that are not uniform in circumference, e.g., the lower leg or forearm. **Recurrent** turns are used to cover distal parts of the body, e.g., the end of a finger, the skull, or the stump of an amputation. **Figure-eight** turns are used to bandage an elbow, knee, or ankle, because they permit some movement after application. Some basic guidelines for bandaging are listed in the accompanying box. Procedure 45–1 illustrates how to apply basic bandages using the turns described above.

▪ **P**urposes of Bandages and Binders

Supporting a wound, e.g., a fractured bone
Immobilizing a wound, e.g., a strained shoulder
Applying pressure, e.g., elastic bandages apply pressure to the lower extremities to improve venous blood flow
Securing a dressing, e.g., for an extensive abdominal surgical wound
Retaining splints (this applies chiefly to bandages)
Retaining warmth, e.g., a flannel bandage on a rheumatoid joint

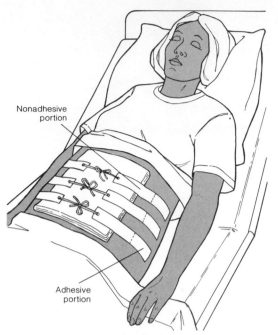

Nonadhesive portion

Adhesive portion

Figure 45—4 ▪ Montgomery straps, or tie tapes, are used to secure large dressings that require frequent changing.

GUIDELINES

Bandaging

Always bandage body parts by working from the distal end to the proximal end, to aid the return flow of the venous blood.

Whenever possible, bandage the part in its normal position, with the joint slightly flexed, to avoid putting strain on the ligaments and the muscles of the joint.

Pad between skin surfaces and over bony prominences to prevent friction from the bandage and consequent abrasion of the skin.

Bandage with even pressure so as not to impede blood circulation.

Whenever possible, leave the end of the body part (e.g., the finger) exposed so that the adequacy of blood circulation to the extremity can be assessed.

Cover dressings with bandages at least 5 cm (2 in) beyond the edges of the dressing to prevent the dressing and wound from becoming contaminated.

Face the client when applying a bandage, to maintain uniform tension and the appropriate direction of the bandage.

PROCEDURE 45–1

Basic Bandaging

Equipment

- A clean bandage of the appropriate material and width. The width of the bandage depends on the size of the body part to be bandaged. For example, a 2.5-cm (1-in.) bandage is used for a finger, a 5-cm (2-in.) bandage for an arm, and a 7.5-cm or 10-cm (3-in. or 4-in.) bandage for a leg. The larger the circumference of the part, the wider the bandage.

- Padding for bony prominences and for between skin surfaces. ABD pads and gauze squares are frequently used to cover bony prominences, such as the elbow, or to separate skin surfaces, such as the fingers.

- Tape, special metal clips, or a safety pin to secure the end of the bandage.

Intervention

1. Provide the client with a chair or bed, and arrange support for the area to be bandaged. For example, if a hand needs to be bandaged, ask the client to place the elbow on a table, so that the hand does not have to be held up unsupported.
   Rationale: Because bandaging takes a little time, holding up a body part without support can be very tiring.

2. Make sure that the area to be bandaged is clean and dry. Wash and dry the area if necessary.
   Rationale: Washing and drying remove microorganisms, which flourish in warm, moist areas.

3. Align the part to be bandaged with slight flexion of the joints, unless this is contraindicated.
   Rationale: Slight flexion places less strain on the ligaments and muscles of the joint.

Circular Turns

4. Hold the bandage in your dominant hand, with the roll uppermost and unroll the bandage about 8 cm (3 in.).
   Rationale: This length of unrolled bandage allows good control for placement and tension.

5. Apply the end of the bandage to the part of the body to be bandaged. Hold the end down with the thumb of the other hand. See Figure 45–5.

6. Encircle the body part a few times or as often as needed, each turn directly covering the previous turn.
   Rationale: This provides even support to the area.

7. Secure the end of the bandage with tape, metal clips, or a safety pin over an uninjured area.
   Rationale: Clips and pins can be uncomfortable when situated over an injured area.

Spiral Turns

8. See steps 1–5.

9. Make two circular turns.
Rationale: Two circular turns anchor the bandage.

10. Continue spiral turns at about a 30° angle, each turn overlapping the preceding one by two-thirds the width of the bandage. See Figure 45–6.

11. Terminate the bandage with two circular turns, and secure the end as in step 7.

Spiral Reverse Turns

12. See steps 1–5.

13. Anchor the bandage with two circular turns and bring the bandage upward at about a 30° angle.

14. Place the thumb of your free hand on the upper edge of the bandage. See Figure 45–7, *A.*
Rationale: The thumb will hold the bandage while it is folded upon itself.

15. Unroll the bandage about 15 cm (6 in.), then turn your hand so that the bandage falls over itself. See Figure 45–7, *B.*

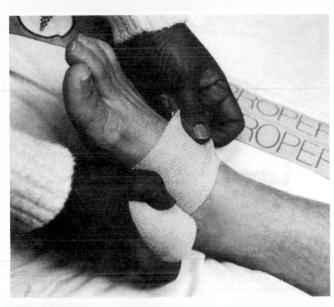

Figure 45–5

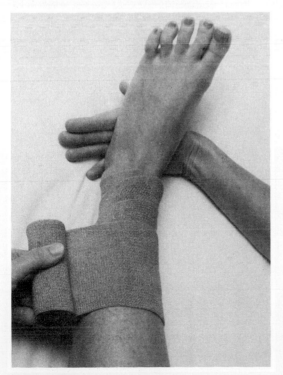

Figure 45–6

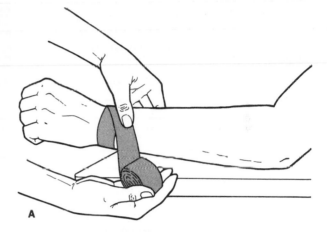

A

B

Circular turns

Bandage folded over to make spiral reverse turn

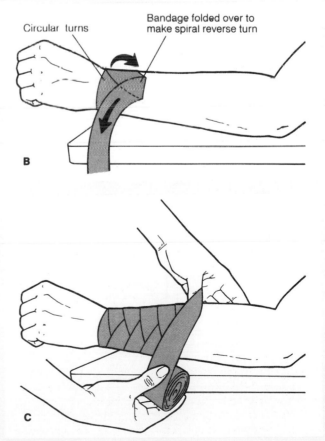

C

Figure 45–7

16. Continue the bandage around the limb, overlapping each previous turn by two-thirds the width of the bandage. Make each bandage turn at the same position on the limb so that the turns of the bandage will be aligned. See Figure 45–7, C.

17. Terminate the bandage with two circular turns, and secure the end as in step 7.

Recurrent Turns

18. See steps 1–5.

19. Anchor the bandage with two circular turns.

20. Fold it back on itself and bring it centrally over the distal end to be bandaged. See Figure 45–8.

21. Holding it with the other hand, bring it back over the end to the right of the center bandage but overlapping it by two-thirds the width of the bandage.

22. Bring the bandage back on the left side, also overlapping the first turn by two-thirds the width of the bandage.

23. Continue this pattern of alternating right and left until the area is covered. Overlap the preceding turn by two-thirds the bandage width each time.

24. Terminate the bandage with two circular turns. See Figure 45–9. Secure the end as in step 7.

Figure-Eight Turns

25. See steps 1–5 and then anchor the bandage with two circular turns.

26. Carry the bandage above the joint, around it, and then below it, making a figure eight. See Figure 45–10.

27. Continue above and below the joint, overlapping the previous turn by two-thirds the width of the bandage.

28. Terminate the bandage above the joint with two circular turns, and secure the end as in step 7.

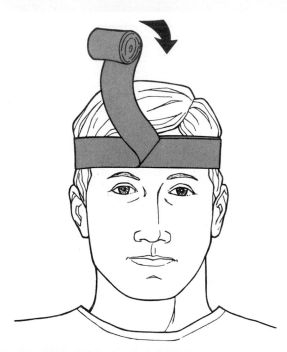

Figure 45–8

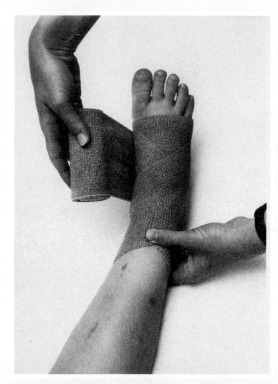

Figure 45–10

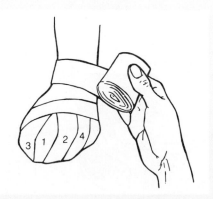

Figure 45–9

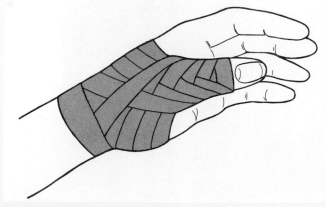

Figure 45–11

Spica Bandage

A spica bandage is a variation of the figure-eight bandage. It is commonly used to bandage the hip, groin, shoulder, breast, or thumb. This technique focuses on the thumb spica; other spica bandages are done in a similar way. A 2.5-cm (1-in.) bandage is frequently used for a thumb spica, and a 7.5-cm (3-in.) bandage is used for a hip or shoulder spica.

Thumb Spica

29. See steps 1–5.

30. Anchor the bandage with two circular turns around the wrist.

31. Bring the bandage down to the distal aspect of the thumb and encircle the thumb. Leave the tip of the thumb exposed if possible.
    Rationale: This enables the nurse to check blood circulation to the thumb.

32. Bring the bandage back up and around the wrist, then back down and around the thumb, overlapping the previous turn by two-thirds the width of the bandage.

33. Repeat steps 31 and 32, working up the thumb and hand until the thumb is covered. See Figure 45–11.

34. Anchor the bandage with two circular turns around the wrist, and secure the end as in step 7.

35. Document the type of bandage applied, the area to which it is applied, and nursing assessments, including skin problems or neurovascular problems.

Sample Recording

Date	Time	Notes
4/7/89	0700	Elastic spiral bandage applied to right leg. Toes warm and pink. No numbness.————————————————Laura R. Stenhouse, NS

Commonly used binders include the triangular arm binder or sling (Figure 45–12), and the single or double T-binder (Figure 45–13), used to retain pads, dressings, or packs in the perineal area. Single T-binders are often used for females, and double T-binders for males to prevent undue pressure on the penis. The double T-binder can also provide greater support for large dressings on both males and females. Another type of binder is the scultetus (many tailed) binder (Figure 45–14), which is used to provide support to the abdomen and, in some instances, to retain dressings.

▪ Preventing Infection

The Centers for Disease Control recommend the practices in the accompanying box to prevent wound infections.

▪ Changing Dressings

Sterile dry dressings are used for wounds such as surgical incisions that have minimal drainage, no tissue loss, and heal by *primary intention*. Most dressings have three layers:

1. A contact dressing that covers the incision and part of the surrounding skin and that collects fibrin, blood products, and debris from the wound

2. An absorbent gauze dressing that acts as a reservoir for excess secretions

3. A thicker outer dressing that protects the wound from external contamination

Not all surgical dressings require changing. Sometimes surgeons apply a dressing in the operating room that remains in place until the sutures are removed, and no further dressings are required. In most situations, how-

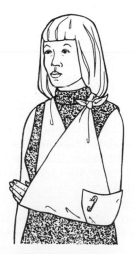

Figure 45–12 A large arm sling

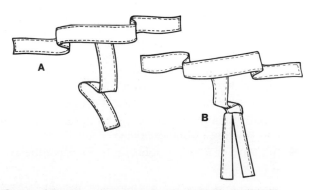

Figure 45–13 T-binders: **A**, single T; **B**, double T

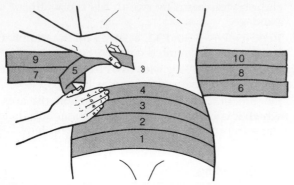

Figure 45–14 A scultetus (many-tailed) binder

Preventing Wound Infections

Wash hands before and after caring for surgical wounds.

Touch an open or fresh surgical wound only when wearing **sterile gloves** or using sterile forceps. After the wound is sealed, sterile gloves are no longer required.

Dressings over closed wounds should be removed or changed when they become wet or show signs of infection.

A **specimen** should be taken of any drainage from a wound that is suspected of being infected. The specimen should be sent to the laboratory for culture.

ever, surgical dressings are changed regularly to prevent the growth of microorganisms.

In some instances, a client may have a Penrose drain inserted. The main surgical incision is considered cleaner than the surgical stab wound made for the drain insertion, because there usually is considerable drainage. The main incision is therefore cleaned first, and under no circumstances are materials used to clean the stab wound used subsequently to clear the main incision. In this way, the main incision is kept free of the microorganisms around the stab wound. Changing a dry sterile dressing is detailed in Procedure 45–2.

PROCEDURE 45–2

Changing a Dry Sterile Dressing

Equipment

A sterile dressing set that includes

- A drape or towel.
- Cotton balls or gauze squares to clean the wound.
- A container for the cleaning solution.
- An antimicrobial solution.
- Two pairs of forceps (thumb or artery).
- Gauze dressings and surgipads.
- Applicators or tongue blades to apply ointments. If a set is not available, gather these items from a central supply cart.
- Additional supplies required for the particular dressing, eg, extra gauze dressings and ointment or powder, if ordered.
- Disposable gloves.
- Sterile gloves (optional).
- A mask.
- A moistureproof bag for disposal of the old dressings and the used cleaning gauzes.
- Tape or tie tapes to secure the dressing.
- A bath blanket, if necessary, to cover the client and prevent undue exposure.
- Acetone or another solution to loosen adhesive, if necessary.

Intervention

Preparing the Client

1. Acquire assistance for changing a dressing on a restless or confused adult.
   Rationale: The person might move and contaminate the sterile field or the wound.

2. Assist the client to a comfortable position, in which the wound can be readily exposed. Expose only the wound area, using a bath blanket to cover the client, if necessary.
   Rationale: Undue exposure is physically and psychologically distressing to most people.

3. Make a cuff on the moistureproof bag for disposal of the soiled dressings, and place the bag within reach. It can be taped to the bedclothes or bedside table.
   Rationale: Making a cuff keeps the outside of the bag free from contamination by the soiled dressings and prevents subsequent contamination of the nurse's hands or of sterile instrument tips when discarding dressings or sponges. Placement of the bag within reach prevents the nurse from reaching across the sterile field and the wound and potentially contaminating these areas.

4. Don a face mask.
   Rationale: Many agencies require that a mask be worn for surgical dressing changes to prevent con-

tamination of the wound by droplet spray from the nurse's respiratory tract.

Removing the Soiled Dressing

5. Remove binders, if used, and place them aside. Untie tie tapes, if used.

6. If adhesive tape was used, remove it by holding down the skin and pulling the tape gently but firmly toward the wound. Use a solvent to loosen the tape, if required.
Rationale: Pressing down on the skin provides countertraction against the pulling motion. Tape is pulled toward the incision to prevent strain on the sutures or wound. Moistening the tape with acetone or a similar solvent lessens the discomfort of removal, particularly from hairy surfaces.

7. Don gloves and remove the outer abdominal dressing or surgipad by hand if the dressing is dry, or using a disposable glove if the dressing is moist. Lift the dressing so that the underside is away from the client's face.
Rationale: The outer surgipad is considered contaminated by the client's clothing and linen. The appearance and odor of the drainage may be upsetting to the client.

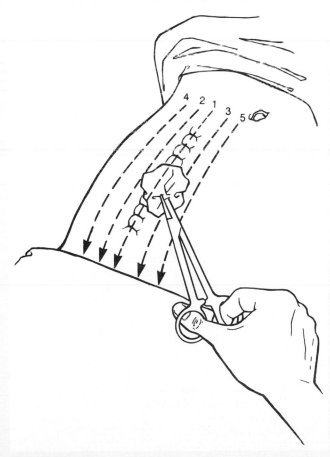

Figure 45–15

8. Place the soiled dressing in the waterproof bag without touching the outside of the bag.
Rationale: Contamination of the outside of the bag is avoided to prevent the spread of microorganisms to the nurse and subsequently to others.

9. Remove glove(s), dispose of them in the waterproof bag, and wash your hands.

10. Open the sterile dressing set.

11. Place the sterile drape beside the wound and don sterile gloves (optional). See Procedures 23–2 and 23–3.

12. Remove the under dressings with tissue forceps or sterile gloves, taking care not to dislodge any drains. If the gauze sticks to the drain, use two pairs of forceps, one to remove the gauze and one to hold the drain, or secure the drain with one hand.
Rationale: Forceps or gloves are used to prevent contamination of the wound by the nurse's hands and contamination of the nurse's hands by wound drainage.

13. Assess the location, type (color, consistency), and odor of wound drainage, and the number of gauzes saturated or the diameter of drainage collected on the dressings.

14. Discard the soiled dressings in the bag. To avoid contaminating the forceps tips on the edge of the paper bag, hold the dressings 10–15 cm (4–6 in.) above the bag, and drop the dressings into it. After the dressings are removed, discard the forceps, or set them aside from the sterile field.
Rationale: These forceps are now contaminated by the wound drainage.

Cleaning and Dressing the Wound

15. Clean the wound, using the second pair of artery or tissue forceps and gauze swabs moistened with antiseptic solution. Keep the forceps tips lower than the handles at all times. Use a separate swab for each stroke, cleaning from the top of the incision downward. Discard each swab after use.
Rationale: The wound is cleaned from the least to the most contaminated area, ie, from the top of the incision, which is drier, to the bottom of the incision, where any drainage will collect and which is considered more contaminated. Forceps tips are always held lower than the handle to prevent their contamination by fluid traveling up to the handle and back to the tips. The handle is contaminated by the nurse's bare hand.
    a. Clean with strokes from the top to the bottom, starting at the center and continuing to the outside. See Figure 45–15.
    or
    Clean with strokes outward from the incision on one side and then outward on the other side. See Figure 45–16.
    b. If a drain is present, clean it after the incision.
    c. For irregular wounds, such as a decubitus ulcer,

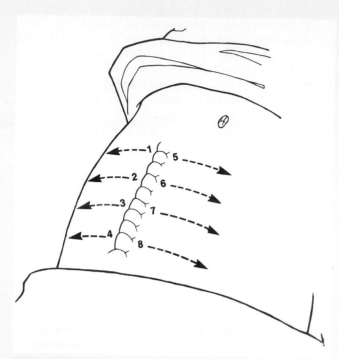

Figure 45-16

clean from the center of the wound outward, using circular strokes.

16. Repeat the cleaning process until all drainage is removed.

17. Dry the wound with dry gauze swabs, using the strokes described in step 15.

18. Assess the overall appearance of the wound.

19. Apply powder or ointment if required. Shake powder directly onto the wound; use sterile applicators or tongue blades to apply ointment.
    Rationale: If drainage is profuse, ointment can protect the skin from irritation. Antibiotic powders or other substances may be ordered by the physician.

20. Apply sterile dressings one at a time over the wound, using sterile forceps. Start at the center of the wound and move progressively outward. The final surgipad can be picked up by hand, touching only the outside, which is often marked by a blue line down the center.

21. Remove gloves if worn and discard.

22. Secure the dressing with tape, tie tapes, or a binder.

23. Document the dressing change and all nursing assessments.

Sample Recording

Date	Time	Notes
12/5/89	1500	Abdominal dressing changed. Incision cleaned with Alcohol 70%. Two 4 × 4 gauzes saturated with serous drainage at base of incision. Wound clean, edges closely approximated. No redness on incision line or surrounding tissue. 4 × 4 gauze and surgipads secured with tie tapes. No discomfort voiced.———————— ————————Evangeline R. Puritos, RN

Sterile wet-to-dry dressings may be prescribed for debridement of wounds with **extensive tissue loss** that heal by *secondary intention*. Examples of such wounds are burns, varicose ulcers, or decubitus ulcers. These wounds are not amenable to suturing. Although the basic processes of wound healing are essentially the same in primary intention and secondary intention healing, secondary intention healing is prolonged, produces extensive granulation tissue, and results in extensive scarring. In addition, the wound is more susceptible to infection

Table 45-2 Dressings for Chronic Wounds

Dressing	Description	Purpose
Dry-to-dry	A layer of wide-mesh cotton gauze lies next to the wound surface. A second layer of dry absorbent cotton or Dacron is on top.	Necrotic debris and exudate are trapped in the interstices of the contact (gauze) layer. These are removed when the dressing is removed.
Wet-to-dry	Next to the wound surface is a layer of wide-mesh cotton gauze saturated with saline or an antimicrobial solution. This layer is covered by a moist absorbent material, i.e., moistened with the same solution.	Necrotic debris is softened by the solution and then adheres to the mesh gauze as it dries. It is removed when the dressing is removed. Also, moisture helps dilute viscous exudate.
Wet-to-damp	A variation of the wet-to-dry dressing, this dressing is removed before it has completely dried.	The wound is debrided when the gauze is removed.
Wet-to-wet	A layer of wide-mesh gauze saturated with antibacterial or physiologic solution lies next to the wound surface. Above is a second layer of absorbent material saturated with the same solution. The entire dressing is kept moist with wetting agent.	The wound surface is continually bathed. Moisture dilutes viscous exudate.

Source: J. Z. Cuzzell, Wound care forum: Artful solutions to chronic problems, *American Journal of Nursing,* February 1985, 85:162—66. Copyright 1985 American Journal of Nursing Company. Reprinted with permission.

because the normal skin barrier to bacterial invasion has been lost.

Wet-to-dry dressings consist of a moistened contact dressing layer that touches the wound surface. This layer is allowed to dry between dressing changes every 4–6 hours. Wet-to-dry dressings are the treatment of choice for wounds requiring debridement, i.e., cleaning of infected and necrotic material from the wound. The wet gauze traps necrotic material in its spaces as it dries. Dry dressings do not trap the debris as effectively. Wet dressings that do not dry out enough to trap debris promote bacterial growth in the damp environment and can cause tissue breakdown. See Table 45–2 for dressings used for chronic wounds. Procedure 45–3 describes how to apply wet-to-dry dressings.

PROCEDURE 45–3

Applying Wet-to-Dry Dressings

Equipment

- A sterile dressing set. See Procedure 45–2.
- Sterile thin, fine-mesh gauze. Generally, 4 × 4 non-cotton-filled gauze dressings are used. Cotton fibers are contraindicated because they can pull loose and remain in the wound, encouraging bacterial growth and contamination.
- A sterile round or kidney-shaped container for the solution.
- The ordered solution. The type used depends on the condition of the wound and the purpose of the dressings. Normal saline is often used to moisten necrotic tissue to help loosen and remove it. Betadine (10% solution) is often used for draining wounds infected with *Staphylococcus* or aerobic bacteria; it can cause burning and stinging, and some clients may be allergic to it. Acetic acid (0.25% solution) is often used for wounds infected with *Pseudomonas* or gram-positive and gram-negative organisms; it can be irritating to the skin surrounding the wound. Hydrogen peroxide (3% solution), not used as frequently today as in the past, is a debriding agent that facilitates removal of necrotic tissue. Sodium hypochlorite (Dakin's solution) is an antiseptic that dissolves necrotic tissue and retards *Pseudomonas* growth. Dakin's solution can cause skin breakdown, so it is used only on necrotic tissue.
- Clean disposable gloves to remove soiled dressings.
- Sterile gloves for cleaning the wound and applying dressings.
- A mask.
- A moistureproof bag for soiled dressings.
- Tape or tie tapes.

Intervention

Clients are usually medicated before this procedure, so ensure that the ordered medication has been given.

1. Assemble all equipment, prepare the client, and remove the soiled dressings as in Procedure 45–2, steps 1–8.

2. Gradually free the dressing as quickly as possible. Do not moisten the dressing.
   Rationale: Wet-to-dry dressings are intended to clean wounds by debridement of the exudate or necrotic tissue.

3. Assess the character and amount of drainage on the dressings and the appearance of the wound, ie, the progress of healing by secondary intention. Observe the development and amount of granulation tissue.

4. Remove the disposable gloves and discard them in the bag.

5. Wash your hands.

6. Open the packages of the sterile dressing set, fine mesh gauze, and sterile solution container.

7. Pour the ordered solution into the solution container.

8. Don the sterile gloves.

9. Place the fine mesh gauze dressings into the solution container and thoroughly saturate them with solution.
   Rationale: The entire gauze must be moistened to enhance its absorptive abilities.

10. If agency policy indicates, clean the wound gently, using a circular motion. Work outward from the center of the wound to its edge and beyond. Use a separate gauze swab for each cleaning stroke.

11. Wring out excess moisture from the saturated fine mesh gauze dressings.
    Rationale: Dressings that are too wet will not dry out in 4–6 hours.

12. Pack the moistened dressings into all depressions and grooves of the wound, ensuring that all exposed surfaces are covered. If necessary, use forceps to feed the gauze gradually into deep depressed areas.
    Rationale: Necrotic tissue is usually more prevalent in depressed wound areas and needs to be covered with the wet-to-dry gauze.

13. Apply a dry 4 × 4 gauze over the wet dressings.
    Rationale: The dry gauze absorbs excess drainage.

14. Cover the dressings with a surgipad or abdominal pad.
    Rationale: The pad protects the wound from external contaminants.

15. Remove your gloves and discard them.

16. Secure the dressing at the edges only, with tape, tie tapes, bandage, or binder. Do not apply an airtight occlusive covering.

Rationale: Occlusive dressings prevent air circulation and hinder drying of the fine mesh gauze.

17. Document the dressing change and nursing assessments.

▪ Promoting Healing and Preventing Complications

Adequate nutrition is essential for wound healing. Proteins, vitamins, and trace metals play a major role in the healing process. During the healing process, it is important to prevent stress on a wound, e.g., vomiting, abdominal distention, or strenuous coughing. Vomiting is often prevented by withholding food and oral fluids until there is no nausea. For clients unable to eat a diet that provides sufficient calories and nutrients for wound healing, a central line for total parenteral nutrition or an enteral feeding tube may be inserted.

Abdominal distention often can be prevented by frequent position changes and early ambulation. Electrolyte imbalance also can contribute to abdominal distention and delayed wound healing (Cooper and Schumann 1979, p. 716). Specifically, imbalances due to hydrogen ion loss through gastric suctioning and excessive loss of potassium through the kidneys contribute to smooth muscle inactivity and abdominal distention. Ambulation improves respiration and blood circulation, aiding the delivery of nutrients and oxygen to the wound area. A distended urinary bladder can impair wound healing by displacing affected tissue and stretching an incision. Therefore, careful monitoring of fluid intake and output is important, as is prompt initiation of measures to promote urinary elimination when appropriate.

▪ Applying Heat and Cold

Heat and cold are applied to the body to promote the repair and healing of tissues. The form of thermal applications generally depends on their purpose. Cold applied to a body part draws heat from the area, whereas heat, of course, warms the area. The application of heat or cold produces physiologic changes in the temperature of the tissues, size of the blood vessels, capillary blood pressure, capillary surface area for exchange of fluids and electrolytes, and tissue metabolism. The duration of the application also affects the response. See Table 45–3 for a summary of the physiologic effects of heat and cold.

Heat can be applied to the body in both dry and moist forms. Dry heat is applied to the body in both dry and moist forms. Dry heat is applied locally, for heat conduction, by means of a hot water bottle, electric pad, aquathermia pad, or disposable heat pack. The heat lamp and bed cradle provide dry heat by radiation. Moist heat can be provided, through conduction, by compress, hot pack, soak, or sitz bath. Recommended temperatures for hot and cold applications are shown in Table 45–4.

Cold applications may also be dry or moist. Dry cold is applied with ice bags, ice collars, ice gloves, or disposable cold packs and creates a localized effect. Moist cold is applied for either localized or systemic effects. Cold moist compresses are administered to body parts for a localized effect; a tepid sponge bath is given for a systemic cooling effect.

▪ Heat. Heat is an old remedy for aches and pains; people often equate heat with comfort and relief. Heat causes **vasodilation** (an increase in the inner diameter of blood vessels) and increases blood flow to the affected area, bringing oxygen, nutrients, antibodies, and leukocytes. Heat accelerates the inflammatory process by increasing both the action of phagocytic cells that ingest microorganisms and other foreign material and the removal of the waste products of infection and metabolic processes. Vasodilation produces skin redness and warmth that can be assessed by touch.

Application of heat promotes soft tissue healing and increases **suppuration** (the formation of pus). The increase in blood flow also dissipates the heat, or draws it away from the affected area. Impaired circulation reduces heat dissipation, placing persons with this condition (e.g., clients with peripheral vascular disease) at

Table 45–3 Physiologic Effects of Heat and Cold

Body Part or Process	Effect of Heat	Effect of Cold
Local circulatory response	Vasodilation (reddened skin)	Vasoconstriction (pale, bluish skin)
Capillary permeability	Increased	Decreased
Cellular metabolism	Increased	Decreased
Inflammatory process	Increased	Decreased
Muscles	Relaxation	Decreased contractility
Nerves	Increased conduction rate	Decreased conduction rate
Connective tissue	Increased flexibility	Decreased distention
Synovial fluid	Decreased viscosity	Increased viscosity
Pain	Promotes comfort	Initial discomfort; later, numbness and paresthesia

Table 45—4   Recommended Temperatures for Hot and Cold Applications

Description	Centigrade	Fahrenheit	Application
Very cold	Below 15	Below 59	Ice bags
Cold	15–18	59–65	Cold pack
Cool	18–27	65–80	Cold compress
Tepid	27–37	80–98	Alcohol and tepid sponges
Warm	37–40	98–105	Warm bath
Hot	40–46	105–115	Aquathermia, soaks, sitz baths, irrigations, moist sterile compresses, hot water bags for debilitated or young clients
Very hot	Above 46	Above 115	Hot water bags for adults, heat cradles

risk for burns by applications that are normally considered safe. A possible disadvantage of heat is that it increases capillary permeability, which allows extracellular fluid and substances such as plasma proteins to pass through the capillary walls and may result in edema (excessive amounts of fluid in the tissues) or an increase in preexisting edema. Heat is often used for clients with musculoskeletal problems such as joint stiffness from arthritis, contractures, and low back pain; and for those with open wounds needing debridement. See Table 45–5.

Heat applied to a localized body area, particularly a large body area, may cause systemic effects, such as increased cardiac output and pulmonary ventilation. These increases are a result of excessive peripheral vasodilation, which diverts large supplies of blood from the internal organs and produces a drop in blood pressure. A significant drop in blood pressure can cause fainting. Clients who have heart or pulmonary disease and who have circulatory disturbances such as arteriosclerosis are more prone to this effect than healthy persons.

▪ **Cold.**   Cold therapy is more recent than heat therapy. Generally, its physiologic effects are opposite to the effects of heat. Cold lowers the temperature of the skin and underlying tissues and causes **vasoconstriction** (a decrease in the inner diameter of blood vessels). Vasoconstriction reduces blood flow to the affected area and thus reduces the supply of oxygen and metabolites, decreases the removal of wastes, and produces skin pallor, or a bluish discoloration, and coolness. Vasoconstriction and its consequent lowered blood flow to an area help control bleeding after injury. Prolonged exposure to cold results in impaired circulation, cell deprivation,

and subsequent damage to the tissues from lack of oxygen and nourishment. The signs of tissue damage due to cold are a bluish-purple mottled appearance of the skin, numbness, stiffness, pallor, and sometimes blisters and pain. Cold is most often used for active young people with sports injuries (e.g., sprains, strains, fractures) to limit postinjury swelling and bleeding. It is increasingly being used for clients with rheumatoid arthritis, since it is thought to inhibit the activity of certain destructive enzymes that exacerbate joint problems (Lehmann and DeLateur 1982b). See Table 45–6.

With extensive cold applications and subsequent vasoconstriction, a client's blood pressure can increase, because blood is shunted from the cutaneous circulation to the internal blood vessels. This shunting of blood, a normal protective response to prolonged cold, is the body's attempt to maintain its core temperature. Shivering, another generalized effect of prolonged cold, is a normal response as the body attempts to warm itself.

▪ **Applying Heat.**   The **aquathermia** or **aquamatic pad** (also referred to as a **K-pad**) is a device commonly used in hospitals to provide heat to a body part. The pad is attached by tubing to an electrically powered control unit that has an opening for water and a temperature gauge. See Figure 45–17. Some aquathermia pads have an absorbent surface through which moist heat can be applied. The other surface of the pad is waterproof. These pads are disposable.

The reservoir of an aquathermia unit should be filled two-thirds full. The desired temperature is set, the pad is covered, placed on the body part, and maintained in place with roller gauze if needed. The nurse should check

Table 45—5   Selected Indications for Heat

Indication	Effect of Heat
Muscle spasm	Relaxes muscles and increases their contractility
Inflammation	Increases blood flow, bringing more phagocytes (to facilitate exudate formation) and essential nutrients for healing; also enhances removal of wastes and debris formed in the inflammatory process. Moist heat softens exudates
Contracture	Reduces contractures and increases joint range of motion by allowing greater distention of muscles and connective tissue
Joint stiffness	Reduces joint stiffness by decreasing the viscosity of synovial fluid and increasing tissue distensibility
Pain	Relieves pain, possibly by promoting muscle relaxation, increasing circulation to ischemic areas, promoting psychologic relaxation and a feeling of comfort, and acting as a counterirritant

Source: P. S. Tepperman and M. Devlin, Therapeutic heat and cold. A practitioner's guide. *Postgraduate Medicine,* January 1983, 73:69.

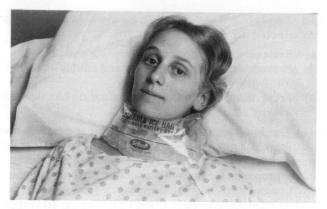

Figure 45—22 A disposable ice collar provides dry cold to the neck area (e.g., to control bleeding after a tonsillectomy).

squeezing, or kneading the package, the nurse activates chemical reactions that release the cold. The manufacturer's instructions must be followed. Most commercially prepared cold packs have soft outer coverings so that they can be applied directly to the body part. See Figure 45—22.

▪ Applying Compresses and Moist Packs.
Compresses and moist packs can be either hot or cold.

A **compress** is a moist gauze dressing applied frequently to an open wound. When hot compresses are ordered, the solution is heated to the temperature indicated by the physician, e.g., 40.5 (105 F). When there is a break in the skin or when the body part (e.g., an eye) is vulnerable to microbrial invasion, sterile technique is necessary; therefore sterile gloves or sterile forceps are needed to apply the compress. A hot or cold pack is a hot or cold moist cloth applied to an area of the body. Packs are usually unsterile; after application, they are covered with a water-resistant material (e.g., plastic wrap) to contain the moisture and prevent the transfer of airborne microorganisms to the area.

Hot compresses usually are applied to hasten the suppurative process and healing. Cold compresses are applied either to decrease or prevent bleeding or to reduce inflammation. Hot packs are applied to relieve muscle spasm or pain, to reduce the pressure of accumulated fluid in a tissue or joint, and to reduce congestion in an underlying organ. Cold packs are used to prevent swelling due to tissue trauma and inflammation, and to anesthetize tissues and temporarily reduce pain.

After a compress or a pack has been applied, it is advisable to apply external heat or cold, such as a hot water bottle, heating pad, or ice bag, to help maintain the temperature of the application. Application of compresses and moist packs is described in Procedure 45—4.

PROCEDURE 45—4

Applying Compresses and Moist Packs

Equipment

Compress:

- A container for the solution
- The solution at the strength and temperature specified by the physician or the agency
- A thermometer to test the temperature of the solution
- Petroleum jelly for surrounding skin areas
- Gauze squares to soak with the solution
- An insulating towel to help maintain the temperature of the compress
- Plastic to insulate the compresses and to retain the temperature and moisture
- A hot water bottle or aquathermia pad (optional) to provide additional heat and maintain the heat of a hot compress

  or
- An ice bag (optional) to maintain the cold of a cold compress
- Ties, eg, roller gauze, or masking tape to fasten the compress, towels, and plastic in place
- Disposable and/or sterile gloves

For a sterile compress, the solution, container, thermometer, towels, gauze squares, and petroleum jelly must be sterile. The jelly can be applied by using sterile cotton application sticks. In addition, sterile forceps or sterile gloves are required to maintain the sterility of the gauze when it is wrung out and applied. If a sterile thermometer is not available, pour a small amount of the solution into a clean basin, measure the temperature with a bath thermometer, and then discard the solution, since it is no longer sterile. Adjust the temperature of the solution according to your findings.

Moist pack:

- Flannel pieces or towel packs
- A hot-pack machine for heating the packs

  or
- A basin of water with some ice chips to cool the water
- Insulating material, eg, flannel or towels
- Plastic for insulation
- A hot water bottle (optional) to provide additional heat and maintain the heat of the pack

  or

- An ice bag (optional) to maintain the cold of the pack
- A thermometer if a specific temperature is ordered for the pack (eg, a cold pack of 24 C (75 F) may be ordered)
- Petroleum jelly to apply to surrounding skin areas if the pack tends to irritate them
- Ties, eg, roller gauze, to fasten the pack

For a sterile moist pack, the container, solution, thermometer, and all materials must be sterile. In addition, sterile gloves or forceps are required to maintain the sterility of the pack when it is wrung out and applied.

Intervention

1. Assist the client to a comfortable position, expose the area for the compress or pack, and provide support for the body part requiring the compress or pack.

Compress

2. Place the gauze in the solution.
3. Don disposable gloves and remove the wound dressing, if present. A dry, sterile dressing is often placed over open wounds between applications of moist heat or cold. To remove a sterile dressing, see Procedure 45–2.
4. With a cotton swab or an applicator stick, apply petroleum jelly to the skin surrounding the wound, not on the wound or open areas of the skin.
   Rationale: Jelly protects the skin from possible burns, maceration, and irritating effects of some solutions.
5. Wring out the gauze so that the solution does not drip from it. For a sterile compress, use sterile forceps or sterile gloves to wring out the gauze.
6. Apply the gauze lightly and gradually to the designated area and, if tolerated by the client, mold the compress close to the body. Pack the gauze snugly against all wound surfaces.
   Rationale: Air is a poor conductor of cold or heat, and molding excludes air.
7. Cover the gauze quickly with a dry towel and a piece of plastic.
   Rationale: The compress is insulated quickly to maintain its temperature.
8. Secure the compress in place with gauze ties or tape.
9. Optional: Apply a hot water bottle or aquathermia pad or ice bag over the plastic to maintain the heat or cold.
10. Document the technique, the time, and the type and strength of the solution. Note assessments,

including the appearance of the wound and surrounding skin area.

11. Assess the client frequently in terms of discomfort. If the client feels any discomfort, assess the area for erythema, numbness, maceration, or blistering. For applications to large areas of the body, note any change in the pulse, respirations, and blood pressure. In the event of unexpected reactions, terminate the treatment and report to the nurse in charge.
12. Remove the compress or pack at the specified time. Compresses and packs with external heat or cold usually retain their temperature anywhere from 15–30 minutes. Without external heat or cold, they need to be changed every 5 minutes.
13. Apply a sterile dressing if one is required.
14. When the compress or pack is removed, record the appearance of the area and any other assessments.

Moist Pack

15. Heat the flannel or towel.
16. Apply petroleum jelly to the surrounding skin if it appears reddened.
17. Wring out the flannel. For a sterile pack, use sterile gloves.
18. Apply the flannel to the body area, molding it closely to the body part.
19. Cover the flannel quickly with the insulating material, eg, a towel and the plastic.
20. Secure the pack in place with ties.
21. Optional: Apply a hot water bottle or ice bag over the pack.
22. Follow steps 10–14.

Sample Recording

Date	Time	Notes
5/12/89	0910	Sterile normal saline compress with K-Matic 37.7 °C applied to 2.5 cm sacral ulcer. Pink tissue surrounding ulcer. 1 cm diameter serosanguineous discharge on dressing. No discomfort voiced. ——— Olga R. Resnicoff, NS
	0940	Compress removed. No further discharge. Ulcer packed with petrolatum gauze and sterile dry dressing applied.——————————— Olga R. Resnicoff, NS

▪ Monitoring Wound Drains and Suction

Surgical drains are inserted to permit the drainage of excessive serosanguineous fluid and purulent material and to promote healing of underlying tissues. These

drains may be inserted and sutured through the incision line, but they are most commonly inserted through stab wounds a few centimeters away from the incision line so that the incision itself may be kept dry. Without a drain, some wounds would heal on the surface and trap the discharge inside. Then the tissues under the skin could not heal because of the discharge, and an abscess might form.

Drains vary in length and width. The length can be 25 to 35 cm (10 to 14 in), and the width 2.5 to 4 cm (0.5 to 1.5 in). To facilitate drainage and healing of tissues from the inside to the outside, or from the bottom to the top, the physician may order that the drain be pulled out or shortened 2 to 5 cm (1 to 2 in) each day. When a drain is completely removed, the remaining stab wound usually heals within a day or two. In some agencies this shortening procedure is performed only by physicians; in others, it is ordered by the physician and performed by nurses. When changing a dressing or a draining wound, the nurse should be careful not to dislodge the drain.

The plastic **bellows wound suction (Hemovac)** is frequently used to suction excessive drainage from surgical wounds. Suction is created by manually compressing and releasing the sides of the apparatus. This apparatus is advantageous in that it exerts a gentle, even pressure on tissues, is quiet and lightweight, and moves easily with the client. The unit consists of an evacuator bag, evacuator tubing with a Y-connector, and wound tubing with a needle. See Figure 45–23.

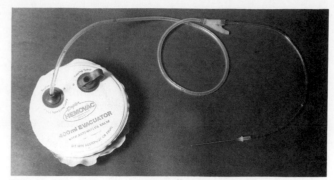

Figure 45–23   A wound suction (Hemovac)

The surgeon inserts the wound drainage tube during surgery. Generally the suction is discontinued from 3 to 7 days postoperatively or when the wound is free from drainage. Nurses are responsible for maintaining the patency of the tube used for wound suction, which hastens the healing process by draining excess exudate that might otherwise interfere with the formation of granulation tissue. See Procedure 45–5.

PROCEDURE 45–5

Establishing and Maintaining a Plastic Bellows Wound Suction

Equipment

To empty the evacuator bag:

- Disposable gloves to protect the nurse.
- A drainage receptacle, eg, a solution basin.
- A calibrated pitcher to measure the drainage.

To irrigate the tubing:

- Disposable gloves for the nurse.
- A sterile 50-ml syringe.
- A sterile #18 or #20 needle with a blunt bevel. The needle needs to fit snugly into the drainage tubing.
- Sterile irrigating solution as ordered, eg, normal saline.
- A sterile set with a sterile receptacle, eg, a kidney basin or solution basin and a sterile towel.

Intervention

Establishing Suction

Establish suction if it was not already initiated.

1. Place the evacuator bag on a solid, flat surface.
2. Open the drainage plug marked "B" on top of the bag, without contaminating it.
3. Compress the bag; while it is compressed, close the drainage plug to retain the vacuum. See Figure 45–24.

Emptying the Evacuator Bag

4. When the drainage fluid reaches the line marked "Full," don disposable gloves and open drainage plug B.
5. Invert the bag, and empty it into the collecting receptacle.
6. Reestablish suction as in steps 1–3.
7. Measure the amount of drainage, and note its characteristics.

Irrigating the Evacuator and Wound Tubing

Because the wound tubing of a portable wound suction is siliconized and perforated with many holes, occlusions of the tubing are rare. However, when the evacuator bag is compressed and no drainage appears, either the wound is free of exudate or the tubing is clogged. In the latter instance, notify the nurse in charge and/or the physician; an irrigation *may* be ordered.

8. Open the sterile set, prepare a sterile field, and don disposable gloves.
9. Fill the irrigating syringe with irrigating fluid, keeping the needle and plunger sterile.
10. Disconnect the wound tubing from the tubing connector, keeping the ends sterile to prevent contamination of the wound.

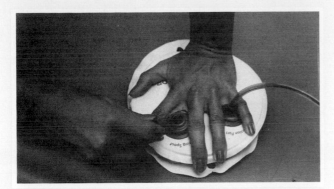

Figure 45-24

11. Insert the needle into the wound tubing, taking care not to perforate the tubing with the needle.
12. Instill the prescribed amount of irrigating fluid slowly and gently.
    Rationale: Too much force could injure the tissues.
13. Detach the syringe from the tubing and place the end of the wound tubing in a sterile container.
14. Refill the syringe, if necessary, and insert the needle into the Y-connector opening. Monitor the amount of fluid used. See Figure 45-25.
15. Irrigate the evacuator tubing until the fluid that runs into the evacuator bag is clear.
16. Reconnect the tubes securely, and empty the bag.

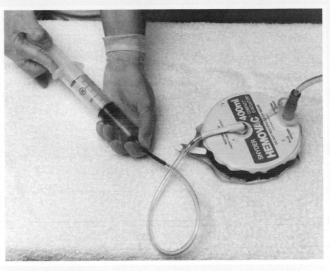

Figure 45-25

Calculate the amount of drainage by subtracting the amount of irrigating fluid used.
17. Reestablish the suction as in steps 1-3.
18. Assess the client's discomfort, relief from discomfort, etc.
19. Document the emptying of the evacuator bag, irrigation of the tubing, and nursing assessments.
20. The amount and type of drainage should be included on the intake and output record.

▌rrigating a Wound

An **irrigation (lavage)** is the washing or flushing out of an area. Sterile technique is required for a wound irrigation, because there is a break in the skin integrity. Wounds are usually irrigated to:

1. Clean the area
2. Apply heat and hasten the healing process
3. Apply a medication, such as an antimicrobial solution

Procedure 45-6 explains how to irrigate a wound.

PROCEDURE 45-6

▌rrigating a Wound

Equipment

- A sterile dressing set and dressing materials. See Procedure 45-2. Arrange the set as you would for a dressing change.
- A sterile irrigating syringe. A 50-ml piston syringe is frequently used. Piston syringes reduce the risk of aspirating drainage. For deep wounds with small openings, a sterile straight catheter may also be necessary.
- A sterile basin for the irrigating solution.

- A sterile basin to receive the irrigation returns.
- Irrigating solution, usually 200 ml (6.5 oz) of solution at 32-33 C (90-95 F), according to the agency's or physician's choice. Sterile normal saline, Dakin's solution, hydrogen peroxide, or antibiotic solutions are frequently used.
- Sterile gloves to wear during the irrigation.
- A moistureproof sterile drape to protect the client and the bed.
- Sterile petroleum jelly to protect the surround-

ing skin from irritation by certain solutions (eg, Dakin's solution).

- A sterile tongue blade to apply the petroleum jelly.

Intervention

1. Assist the client to a position in which the irrigating solution will flow by gravity from the upper end of the wound to the lower end and then into the basin.

2. Place the waterproof drape over the client and the bed, and position the sterile basin on it below the wound, to catch the irrigating solution.

3. Remove the old dressing, and clean the wound. See Procedure 45–2.

4. If an irrigating solution, such as Dakin's solution, is being used, apply sterile petroleum jelly to the skin around the wound, using the sterile tongue blade.

5. Using the syringe, gently instill a steady stream of irrigating solution into the wound. Make sure all areas of the wound are irrigated. If you are using a catheter, insert the catheter into the wound until

resistance is met. Do not force the catheter, since this can cause tissue damage.

6. Continue irrigating until the solution becomes clear (no exudate is present) or until all the solution has been used.
   Rationale: The irrigation washes away tissue debris and drainage so that later returns are clearer.

7. Using dressing forceps and sterile gauze, dry the area around the wound.
   Rationale: Moisture left on the skin promotes the growth of microorganisms and can cause skin irritation.

8. Assess the appearance of the wound, noting in particular the type and amount of exudate, and the presence and extent of granulation tissue.

9. Apply a sterile dressing to the wound. See Procedure 45–2.

10. Document the irrigation, the solution used, the appearance of the irrigation returns, and nursing assessments. Note the presence of any exudate and sloughing tissue.

▪ Assessing and Removing Sutures

Sutures are stitches used to sew body tissues together. *Suture* can also refer to the material used to sew the stitch. Policies vary about the personnel who may remove skin sutures. In some agencies, only physicians remove sutures; in others, registered nurses, licensed vocational nurses, and nursing students with appropriate supervision may do so. Various suture materials, e.g., silk, cotton, linen, wire, nylon, and Dacron (polyester fiber) threads are used. Silver wire clips are also available. The physician orders the removal of sutures. Usually, skin sutures are removed 7 to 10 days after surgery. Sterile technique and special suture scissors are used. The scissors have a short, curved cutting tip that readily slides under the suture. See Figure 45–26. Wire clips or staples are removed with a special instrument

that squeezes the center of the clip to remove it from the skin. See Figure 45–27.

Retention sutures (*stay sutures*) are very large sutures used in addition to skin sutures for some incisions. See Figure 45–28. They attach underlying tissues of fat and muscle as well as skin and are used to support incisions in obese individuals or when healing may be prolonged. They are frequently left in place longer than skin sutures (14 to 21 days) but in some instances are removed at the same time as the skin sutures. To prevent these large sutures from irritating the incision, the surgeon may place rubber tubing over them or a roll of gauze under them extending down the incision line. Several forms of retention sutures are used, and agency policies about them may vary. The nurse should verify whether they are to be removed and who may remove them.

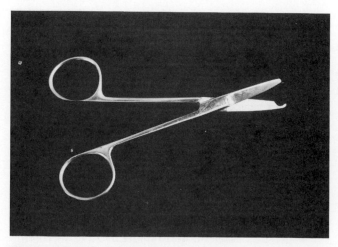

Figure 45–26 ▪ Suture scissors

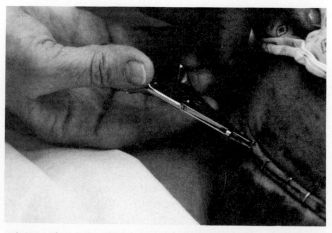

Figure 45–27 Removing metal clips (staples) with a clip remover

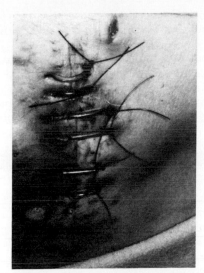

Figure 45—28 A surgical incision with retention sutures

There are various methods of suturing. Skin sutures can be broadly categorized as either **interrupted** (each stitch is tied and knotted separately) or **continuous** (one thread runs in a series of stitches and is tied only at the beginning and at the end of the run). Common sutures are illustrated in Figure 45—29. The technique for removing skin sutures is described in Procedure 45—7.

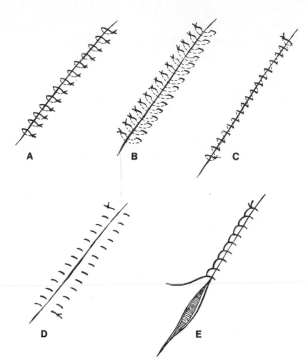

Figure 45—29 Common methods of suturing: **A,** plain interrupted; **B,** mattress interrupted; **C,** plain continuous; **D,** mattress continuous; **E,** blanket continuous

PROCEDURE 45—7

Removing Skin Sutures

Equipment

- A sterile dressing set. See Procedure 45—2.
- Sterile suture scissors.
- Sterile butterfly tape (optional) to hold the wound edges together if wound dehiscence occurs.
- A moistureproof bag to receive used dressings and supplies.
- A light sterile gauze pad and tape if a dressing is to be applied.

Intervention

1. Verify the physician's orders for suture removal. Many times only *alternate* interrupted sutures are removed one day, and the remaining sutures are removed a day or two later.
2. Inform the client that suture removal may produce slight discomfort, such as a pulling or stinging sensation, but it is not painful. Ask the client not to touch the wound during the suture removal, so as not to contaminate the wound.
3. Clean the incision as described in Procedure 45—2. The suture line is usually cleaned with an antimicrobial solution before and after suture removal as a prophylactic measure to prevent infection.

Plain Interrupted Sutures

4. Grasp the suture at the knot with a pair of forceps.
5. Place the curved tip of the suture scissors under the suture as close to the skin as possible, either on the side opposite the knot (see Figure 45—30) or directly under the knot. Cut the suture.
   Rationale: Sutures are cut as close to the skin as possible on one side of the visible part because the suture material that is visible to the eye is in contact with resident bacteria of the skin and must not be pulled beneath the skin during removal. Suture material that is beneath the skin is considered free from bacteria.
6. With the forceps, pull the suture out in one piece. Inspect the suture carefully to make sure that all suture material is removed.
   Rationale: Suture material left beneath the skin acts as a foreign body and causes inflammation.
7. Discard the suture onto a piece of sterile gauze or into the moistureproof bag, being careful not to contaminate the forceps tips. Sometimes the suture sticks to the forceps and needs to be removed by wiping the tips on a sterile gauze.
8. Continue to remove *alternate* sutures, ie, the third, fifth, seventh, etc.

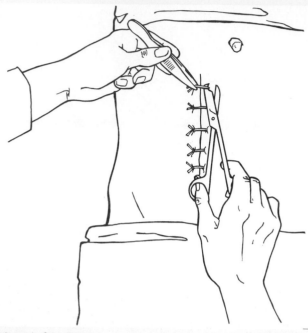

Figure 45–30

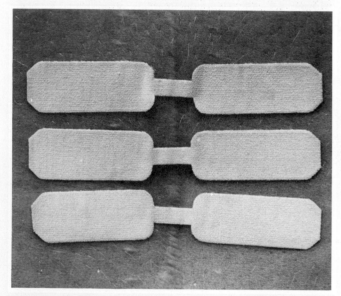

Figure 45–31

Rationale: Alternate sutures are removed first so that remaining sutures keep the skin edges in close approximation and prevent any dehiscence from becoming large.

9. If no dehiscence occurs, remove the remaining sutures. If dehiscence does occur, do not remove the remaining sutures, and report the dehiscence to the nurse in charge.

10. **a.** If a little wound dehiscence occurs, apply a sterile butterfly tape over the gap:

   ▪ Attach the tape to one side of the incision.

▪ Press the wound edges together.

▪ Attach the tape to the other side of the incision. See Figure 45–31.

Rationale: The butterfly tape holds the wound edges as close together as possible and promotes healing.

   b. If a large dehiscence occurs, cover the wound with sterile gauze and report the problem immediately to the nurse in charge or physician.

11. Clean the incision again with antimicrobial solution.

12. Apply a small, light, sterile gauze dressing, if any small dehiscence has occurred or if this is agency practice.

13. Instruct the client about follow-up wound care. Generally, if a wound is dry and healing well, the person can take showers in a day or two. Instruct the client to contact the physician if wound discharge appears.

14. Document the suture removal and assessment data on the appropriate records.

Sample Recording

Date	Time	Notes
12/5/89	1105	Abdominal sutures removed. Wound dry, edges approximated closely. No signs of inflammation. Gauze dressing applied. ————Gwen E. Owens, NS

Mattress Interrupted Sutures

See Figure 45–32. Mattress interrupted sutures do not cross the incision line outside the skin and have two threads underlying the skin.

15. When possible, cut the visible part of the suture close to the skin at *A* and *B* in Figure 45–32, opposite the knot, and remove this small visible piece. Discard it as in step 7. In some sutures, the visible part opposite the knot may be so small that it can be cut only once.

16. Grasp the knot (*C*) with forceps. Remove the remainder of the suture beneath the skin by pulling out in the direction of the knot.

17. Follow steps 8–14.

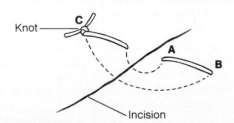

Figure 45–32

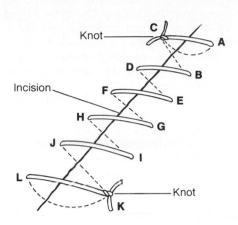

Figure 45-33

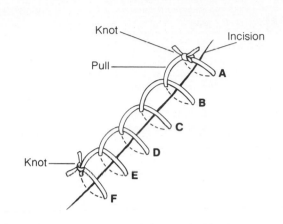

Figure 45-34

Plain Continuous Sutures

See Figure 45–32.

18. Cut the thread of the first suture opposite the knot at *A* in Figure 45–33. Then cut the thread of the second suture on that same side at *B*.

19. Grasp the knot (*C*) with the forceps, and pull. This removes the first stitch and the piece of thread beneath the skin, which is attached to the second stitch. Discard the sutures as in step 7.

20. Cut off the visible part of the second suture at *D*, and discard it.

21. Grasp the suture at *E*, and pull out the underlying loop between *D* and *E*.

22. Cut the visible part at *F*, and remove it.

23. Repeat steps 20–22 at *G–J*, until the last knot is reached. Note that, after the first stitch is removed, each thread is cut down the same side, below the original knot.

24. Cut the last suture at *L*, and pull out the last suture at *K*

25. Follow steps 10–14.

Blanket Continuous Sutures

See Figure 45–34.

26. Cut the threads that are opposite the looped blanket edge, ie, cut at *A–F* in Figure 45–34.

27. Pull each stitch out at the looped edge.

28. Follow steps 10–14.

Mattress Continuous Sutures

See Figure 45–35.

29. Cut the visible suture at both skin edges opposite the knot (at *A* and *B* in Figure 45–35) and on the suture below opposite the knot (at *C* and *D*). Remove and discard the visible portions as in step 7.

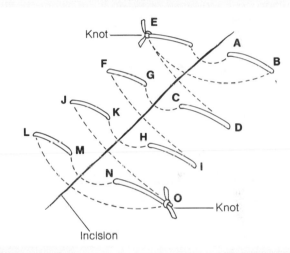

Figure 45-35

30. Pull the first suture out by the knot at *E*.

31. Lift the second suture between *F* and *G* to pull out the underlying suture between *G* and *C*. Cut off the visible part at *F* as close to the skin edge as possible.

32. Go to the opposite side between *H* and *I*. Lift out the suture between *F* and *I*, and cut off all the visible part close to the skin at *H*.

33. Lift the suture between *J* and *K* to pull out the suture between *H* and *K*, and cut the suture close to the skin at *J*.

34. Repeat steps 32–33, working from side to side of the incision, until the last suture is reached.

35. Cut the visible suture opposite the knot at *L* and *M*. Pull out all remaining pieces of suture at *O*.

36. Follow steps 10–14.

OUTCOME CRITERIA

Wound Care

The client will:

Exhibit less inflammation and drainage from the wound
Have no discomfort in the wound area
Have a normal body temperature
Exhibit no signs of wound infection

Evaluating Client Responses

Examples of outcome criteria for wound care are listed in the accompanying box.

Chapter Highlights

- There are six types of wounds: incisions, contusions, abrasions, lacerations, punctures, and penetrating wounds.
- Wounds heal by either primary intention or secondary intention, depending on the extent of tissue loss.
- Internal factors affecting wound healing include vasculature, age, immune status, nutrition, obesity, smoking, stress, and medications.
- External factors affecting wound healing include preoperative stay, preoperative preparation, and intraoperative factors.
- The main complications of wound healing are hemorrhage, infection, dehiscence, and evisceration.
- Wound assessment is an ongoing process to evaluate healing; the nurse assesses wounds by visual inspection, palpation, and the sense of smell.
- Nursing diagnoses related to wound care include potential impairment of skin integrity, potential for infection, alterations in comfort, and impaired physical mobility.
- Nurses commonly care for wounds; this care may involve changing dressings, maintaining drains, applying heat and cold, and applying bandages and binders.
- Major responsibilities of the nurse related to wound care include preventing infection, preventing further tissue damage, preventing hemorrhage, promoting healing, cleaning wounds of foreign debris, and preventing skin excoriation around draining wounds.
- The care of wounds varies considerably in accordance with the type of wound, size and location, amount of exudate, presence of complicating factors, and sometimes the personal preference of the physician.
- Open and closed methods of wound care have advantages and disadvantages that make them appropriate for different circumstances.
- Before changing dressings the nurse needs to ascertain the physician's orders, the presence of drains, the amount of wound drainage, and the cleaning solutions to be used.
- Five basic turns—spiral, circular, spiral reverse, recurrent, and figure-eight—are used in bandaging specific body parts.
- Heat and cold produce specific local physiologic responses that account for their therapeutic effects.
- Each of five common types of sutures—plain interrupted, mattress interrupted, plain continuous, mattress continuous, and blanket continuous—is removed by a specific procedure.

Selected References

Alterescue, V. May/June 1983. Toward a physiologic approach to the topical treatment of opened wounds. *Journal of Enterostomal Therapy* 10:101–7.

Brozenec, S. April 1985. Caring for the postoperative patient with an abdominal drain. *Nursing 85* 15:55–57.

Bruno, P. December 1979. The nature of wound healing: Implications for nursing practice. *Nursing Clinics of North America* 14(4):667–82.

Bruno, P., and Craven, R. F. December 1982. Age challenges to wound healing. *Journal of Gerontological Nursing* 8:686–91.

Cooper, D. M., and Schumann, D. December 1979. Postsurgical nursing intervention as an adjunct to wound healing. *Nursing Clinics of North America* 14:713–26.

Cuzzell, J. Z. February 1985. Wound care forum: Artful solutions to chronic problems. *American Journal of Nursing* 85:162–66.

———. May 1986. Wound care forum: Tell it like it is. A realistic approach to wound documentation. *American Journal of Nursing* 86:600–601.

Flynn, M. E., and Rovee, D. T. October 1982. Wound healing mechanisms. *American Journal of Nursing* 82:1544–50.

Garner, J. S. April 1986. CDC guidelines for the prevention and control of nosocomial infections: Guideline for prevention of surgical wound infections, 1985. *American Journal of Infection Control* 14:71–80.

Guyton, A. C. 1986. *Textbook of medical physiology.* 7th ed. Philadelphia: W. B. Saunders Co.

Lehmann, J. F., and DeLateur, B. J. 1982a. *Therapeutic heat and cold.* 3d ed. Baltimore: Williams and Wilkins Co.

———. 1982b. Diathermy and superficial heat and cold therapy. In Kottke, F. J.; Stillwell, G. K.; and Lehmann, J. F., editors. *Krusen's handbook of physical medicine and rehabilitation.* 3d ed. Philadelphia: W. B. Saunders Co.

Neuberger, G. B., and Reckling, J. B. February 1985. A new look at wound care. *Nursing 85* 15:34–41.

Nichols, R. L. January/February 1982. Techniques known to prevent post-operative wound infection. *Infection Control* 3:34–37.

Schumann, D. December 1979. Preoperative measures to promote wound healing. *Nursing Clinics of North America* 14:683–99.

Taylor, D. L. May 1983. Wound healing: Physiology, signs and symptoms. *Nursing 83* 13(5):44–45.

Wright, N. E. July/August 1983. Abdominal wounds: Breakdown and dehiscence. *Journal of Enterostomal Therapy* 10:143–44.

CHAPTER 46

Perioperative Care

OBJECTIVES

Describe the phases of the perioperative period.

Discuss the legal aspects of surgery.

Describe the elements of surgical risk.

Outline the various aspects of preoperative assessment.

Give examples of pertinent nursing diagnoses for surgical clients.

Identify the essential nursing responsibilities included in planning perioperative nursing care.

Describe how to teach clients to move, perform leg exercises, and perform coughing and deep breathing exercises.

Identify the essentials of preoperative skin preparation.

Explain why gastric intubation may be used for surgical clients.

Describe some of the ways to protect a client from injury.

Identify circumstances in which the nurse monitors a client.

Discuss the importance of documentation with reference to preoperative, intraoperative, and postoperative recording.

Identify potential postoperative complications and describe nursing interventions to prevent them.

Identify outcome criteria by which to evaluate the effectiveness of perioperative nursing interventions.

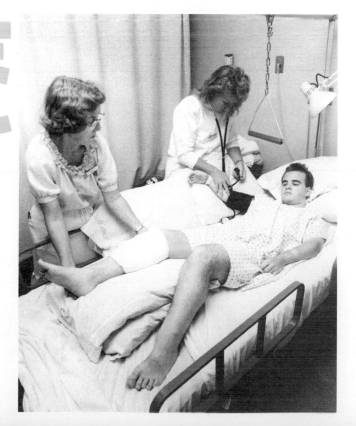

The Perioperative Period

Operations are traumatic for both clients and their support persons. Although increasing numbers of elective and minor surgical procedures are being performed in day-surgery centers, most operations still take place in hospitals, which many people associate with pain and death. Because many clients equate operations with disfigurement and pain, the nurse must be sensitive to the psychologic as well as physiologic needs of clients having operations.

The **perioperative** period is the time before, during, and after an operation; it encompasses three phases: preoperative, intraoperative, and postoperative. The **preoperative phase** begins when the decision for surgical intervention is made, and it ends when the client is transferred to the operating room bed. The preoperative client is prepared psychologically and physically for surgery. An important aspect of preoperative nursing is teaching the client what he or she needs to know. The **intraoperative phase** begins when the client is transferred to the operating room bed, and it terminates when he or she is admitted to the postanesthetic area. The main intraoperative nursing function is to maintain the client's safety.

The **postoperative phase** is the time following surgery. It begins with admission to the postanesthesia area and ends when the client has completely recovered from his or her surgery. Major postoperative nursing functions are

1. Helping the client recover from anesthesia
2. Maintaining the client's body systems
3. Preventing postoperative complications
4. Preventing undue discomfort

For a summary of nursing practice during each phase of the perioperative period see Table 46–1.

Prior to any surgical procedure clients must sign a surgical consent form. See Figure 46–1. This requirement protects clients from having any surgical procedure they do not want or do not know about. It also protects the hospital and the health personnel from a claim by client or family that permission was not granted. The consent form becomes a part of the client's record and goes to the operating room with the client.

Obtaining legal, informed consent to perform surgery is the responsibility of the surgeon. Informed consent is possible only when the client is told in advance of the character and importance of the surgery, its probable consequences, the chances for success, and alternative measures. Often a nurse is responsible for witnessing a consent. The nurse must be aware of her or his responsibilities regarding consents and be aware of the particular hospital's policies. See Chapter 6 for more information about informed consent.

Preoperative Assessment

Preoperative assessment includes clinical assessment of the client for identification of surgical risk factors and collection of a data base used during postoperative evaluation. The nurse also ensures that scheduled screening tests are completed, preparing the client beforehand and monitoring afterward when necessary. Although validating that the client has been prepared for surgery and that the client's record is correct are not really assessment activities, they are nursing responsibilities during the preoperative period.

Assessing Surgical Risk

The degree of risk involved in a surgical procedure is affected by the client's age, nutritional status, fluid and electrolyte balance, general health, use of medications, and mental health and attitude. **Elderly persons** are frequently at additional risk from surgery because of impaired circulation due to arteriosclerosis and limited cardiac function. Energy reserves are often limited, and hydration and nutritional status may be poor. In addition, the older person may be highly sensitive to medications such as morphine sulfate and barbiturates, frequently used preoperatively and postoperatively. See Table 46–2 for risk factors for the elderly surgical client.

Two **nutritional problems** that can increase surgical risk in clients of any age are obesity and malnutrition due to protein, iron, and vitamin deficiencies. Surgery for obese clients is often deferred, except in emergencies. The obese often have overtaxed hearts and elevated blood pressures. In addition, incisions in overly fatty tissue are difficult to suture and prone to infection. Nutritional deficiencies are particularly common among elderly clients and chronically ill clients. Protein and vitamins are needed for wound healing; vitamin K is essential for blood clotting.

Table 46–1 Major Areas of Nursing Practice During the Perioperative Period

Preoperative Phase	Intraoperative Phase	Postoperative Phase
Preoperative assessment	Maintain client safety	Communicate intraoperative information
Preoperative preparation	Monitor client's vital signs	Assess client's physical condition
Preoperative teaching	Provide support to client prior to anesthetic	Provide nursing interventions
Support for client and support persons		Support client and support persons

Reprinted with permission from AORN Standards and Recommended Practices for Preoperative Nursing, 1986. Copyright © AORN Inc, 10170 East Mississippi Avenue, Denver, CO 80231.

EL CAMINO HOSPITAL DISTRICT
AUTHORIZATION AND CONSENT TO SURGERY, ANESTHESIA, DIAGNOSTIC OR THERAPEUTIC PROCEDURES

Pt. Name
Hosp. No.
Rm. No.

YOUR DOCTOR IS _____

THE OPERATION(S) OR PROCEDURE(S) TO BE PERFORMED IS/ARE:

_____
(MEDICAL TERMINOLOGY)

_____
(LAY TERMINOLOGY)

1. The hospital maintains personnel and facilities to assist your doctor in his performance of various surgical operations and other special diagnostic and therapeutic procedures. These operations and procedures may all involve risks of unsuccessful results, complications, injury, or even death, from both known and unforeseen causes, and no warranty or guarantee is made as to result or cure. You have the right to be informed of such risks as well as the nature and purpose of the operation(s) or procedure(s) and the available alternative methods of treatment and this form is not a substitute for such explanations which are provided by the above named physician. Except in cases of emergency, the operation(s) or procedure(s) is/are not performed until the patient has had the opportunity to receive such explanations. You may refuse any proposed operation or procedure anytime prior to its performance.

2. Your doctor has recommended the operation(s) or procedure(s) set forth above. Upon your authorization and consent, such operation(s) or procedure(s), together with any different or further procedure(s) which in the opinion of your doctor may be indicated due to any emergency, will be performed on you. The operation(s) or procedure(s) will be performed by the doctor named above together with associates and assistants, including anesthesiologists and radiologists from the medical staff of El Camino Hospital. Your attending physician, surgeon, assistant surgeon, anesthesiologist, and other physicians are not agents, servants or employees of the hospital or your doctor but are independent contractors, and therefore your agents.

3. Your signature below authorizes the hospital pathologist to use his or her discretion in disposition of any member, organ or other tissue removed from your person during the above-named procedure(s).

4. Your signature below constitutes your acknowledgement (1) that you have read and agree to the foregoing; (2) that the operation(s) or procedure(s) set forth above has/have been adequately explained to you by your doctor and that you have received all of the information you desire concerning such operation(s) or procedure(s); (3) that you authorize and consent to the performance of the operation(s) or procedure(s); (4) and that you acknowledge receipt of a copy of this authorization.

SIGNATURE: _____
PATIENT/PARENT/LEGAL GUARDIAN

_____
DATE AND TIME

_____
RELATIONSHIP

_____
WITNESS (NOT PATIENT'S DOCTOR)

_____
REASON PATIENT UNABLE TO SIGN

Figure 46–1 A sample surgical consent form. *Source:* Courtesy of El Camino Hospital, Mountain View, California.

Fluid and electrolyte status is significant for surgical clients in that dehydration and hypovolemia predispose a client to problems during surgery. Electrolyte imbalances often accompany fluid imbalances. Imbalances in calcium, magnesium, potassium, and hydrogen ions are of particular concern during surgery. See Chapter 43.

Surgery is least risky when the client's **general**

Table 46—2 Risk Factors for the Elderly Surgical Client

Physiologic Change	Preoperative Nursing Interventions
Integumentary System	
Vulnerable skin due to venous stasis and poor venous return	Teach passive and active exercises. Measure the client for antiemboli stockings.
Cardiovascular System	
Reduced cardiac reserve due to changes in the myocardium	Determine usual pattern of ADLs and how quickly the client tires.
Tachycardia from anxiety, which is tolerated poorly in the elderly heart	Teach about and support anxiety reduction.
Decreased compliance of blood vessels due to atherosclerosis	Teach leg exercises and turning. Obtain baseline data re vital signs. Monitor blood pressure closely for hypertension.
Respiratory System	
Reduced vital capacity due to lowered expansibility of the rib cage	Teach deep breathing and coughing. Obtain baseline data re respirations.
Urinary System	
Reduced blood flow to the kidneys	Obtain baseline urine output for 24 hours.
Reduced ability to excrete toxins due to reduced glomerular filtration	Initiate fluid intake and output recordings.
Fluids and Electrolytes	
Dehydration from repeated enemas	Assess hydration status for baseline data.
Hypokalemia due to diarrhea	Monitor fluid intake and output.
Neurologic System	
Reduced sensory acuity	Orient client to surroundings.
Decreased reaction time	Allow time for client to proceed at own pace.

health is good. Any infection or pathophysiology increases the risk. Of particular concern are upper respiratory tract infections, which together with general anesthesia can adversely affect respiratory function. A recent myocardial infarction or any cardiovascular disease also can make surgery more dangerous than usual. Conditions that alter the functioning of other body organs (e.g., the kidneys, liver, or pancreas) can also increase the surgical risk.

The regular use of certain **medications** is another factor that may increase surgical risk. Examples are listed in the accompanying box.

Since some medications interact adversely with other medications and with anesthetic agents, preoperative assessment should include careful collection of a med-

ication history. Clients may be unaware of the potential adverse interactions of medications and may fail to report the use of medications used for conditions unrelated to the indication for surgery. The astute nurse interviewer may question the client and family about the use of commonly prescribed medications (and over-the-counter preparations) for specific conditions mentioned during the nursing history.

Extreme **anxiety** can increase surgical risk. The level of anxiety does not always correspond to the seriousness of the surgical procedure. The surgeon needs to know if a person **fears** that he or she will die during surgery. In some instances, professional counseling and a delay in the surgery may be indicated. Clients who have shown poor **psychologic adjustment** for some time may not be able to cope with the additional stress of surgery. People who cope only minimally in a stable, familiar environment can develop emotional problems postoperatively.

Medications Increasing Surgical Risk

Anticoagulants. Increase blood coagulation time

Tranquilizers. May cause hypotension and thus contribute to shock

Heroin and other depressants. Decrease central nervous system responses

Antibiotics. May be incompatible with anesthetic agents, resulting in untoward reactions

Diuretics. May precipitate electrolyte (especially potassium) imbalances.

Nursing Assessment

The nursing history obtained before surgery provides client data that help the nurse to plan preoperative and postoperative care. Although forms vary considerably among agencies, essential preoperative information that should be included is summarized in the accompanying box.

ASSESSMENT

Preoperative Nursing History

- *Physical condition.* General appearance (i.e., skin coloring, weight, hydration status, and energy level)
- *Mental attitude.* Mild anxiety is a normal response to surgery, severe anxiety can increase surgical risk.
- *Understanding of surgical procedure.* A well-informed client knows what to expect and in general accepts and copes more effectively with surgery and convalescence.
- *Previous experience.* May influence the physical and psychologic responses to the planned surgery.
- *Expected outcomes.* May alter a client's body image and life-style to varying degrees.
- *Medications.* List all current medications. Certain medications, such as anticonvulsants and insulin, must be continued throughout the operative period to prevent adverse effects. A physician's order to this effect is required, however.

- *Smoking.* Smokers' lung tissue may be chronically irritated, and a general anesthetic agent irritates it further.
- *Alcohol.* Heavy, consistent use can lead to problems during anesthesia, surgery, and recovery.
- *Coping resources.* Employing previously effective coping mechanisms or developing new strategies (e.g., diversional activities such as reading and relaxation exercises) may be helpful.
- *Self-concept.* A healthy, positive self-concept predisposes the client to approach a surgical experience with confidence that he or she can handle it successfully.
- *Body image.* Possible disfigurement or change in physical identity may be a concern prior to surgery. Providing accurate information often allays fears based on misconceptions.

Knowledge of the client's overall health is essential in anticipating and preventing complications. Common health problems that increase surgical risk and may lead to the decision to postpone or cancel surgery are listed in the accompanying box.

Health Problems that Increase Surgical Risk

Cardiac conditions such as angina pectoris, recent myocardial infarction, severe hypertension, and severe congestive heart failure. Well-controlled cardiac problems generally pose minimal operative risk.

Blood coagulation disorders that may lead to severe bleeding, hemorrhage, and subsequent shock.

Upper respiratory tract infections or **chronic obstructive lung diseases,** such as emphysema. These conditions, especially when exacerbated by the effects of general anesthesia, adversely affect pulmonary function. They also predispose the client to postoperative lung infections.

Renal disease that impairs the regulation of the body's fluids and electrolytes, e.g., renal insufficiency.

Diabetes mellitus, which predisposes the client to wound infection and delayed healing.

Liver disease, e.g., cirrhosis, which impairs the liver's abilities to detoxify medications used during surgery, produce the prothrombin necessary for blood clotting, and metabolize nutrients essential for healing.

Uncontrolled neurologic disease, such as epilepsy.

Screening Tests

The physician orders preoperative radiologic and laboratory tests and examinations. The nurse's responsibility is to check the orders carefully, to see that they are carried out, and to ensure that the results are obtained prior to surgery. See Table 46–3 for routine preoperative screening tests. In addition to these routine tests, diagnostic tests directly related to the client's disease are usually appropriate (e.g., stomach roentgenography to clarify the pathologic condition before gastric surgery).

In most agencies, personnel use a preoperative checklist. See Figure 46–2. The nurse checks the agency's forms and follows appropriate recording procedures. It is essential that all pertinent records (e.g., laboratory records, x-ray films, and consents) be assembled and completed so that operating and recovery room personnel can refer to them.

Nursing Diagnoses for Surgical Clients

Examples of nursing diagnoses for the surgical client are given in the accompanying box. Because surgery can both directly and indirectly involve many body systems and is a complex experience for a client, the nursing diagnoses focus on a wide variety of problems the client may encounter postoperatively. Certain diagnoses are more likely to be priorities during each of the phases of the perioperative period.

Table 46–3 Routine Preoperative Screening Tests

Test	Rationale	Test	Rationale
Urinalysis	To detect urinary tract infections and glucose in the urine	Blood grouping and cross-matching	To establish blood type for possible blood transfusion
Chest roentgenography	To identify lung pathology and heart size and location	Serum electrolytes (Na^+, K^+, MG^{++}, Ca^{++}, H^+)	To determine electrolyte imbalances
Electrocardiography (usual for clients who have cardiac pathology)	To determine cardiac pathology	Fasting blood sugar	To detect the presence of glucose in the blood, which may indicate metabolic disorders, e.g., diabetes mellitus
Complete blood count (CBC)	To determine Hgb, Hct, RBC (i.e., the blood's ability to carry oxygen), the WBC, which signals infection when elevated	Blood urea nitrogen (BUN) or creatinine	To assess urinary excretion

Form NS-68

ST. PAUL'S HOSPITAL
Vancouver, B.C.

PRE-OPERATIVE PREPARATION

EVENING PRIOR TO SURGERY—CHECK	Yes	Not Applicable
1. History—completed with signature		
2. Consultation (when necessary) on chart		
3. Treatment and operative consents—signed and witnessed		
4. Telephone no. of next of kin or friend:		
5. Identaband on wrist		
6. Allergy sign on chart and wristband		
7. Operative area prepared		
8. Pre-op bath or shower		
9. Pre-op teaching: a. Attended "Operation Tomorrow"		
b. Demonstrated deep breathing, coughing, and leg exercises		
c. Stated approximate time to OR and return to ward		
d. Stated expectations: • surgery planned		
• incision and dressing area		
• activity progression		
• pain and effect of analgesic		
• NPO, intravenous, diet progression		
• pre-op urine specimen		
e. Verbalized probable discharge plans		
10. H.S. sedation administered or refused—charted on anesthetic record		
11. Fasting sign posted		

DATE _____ SIGNATURE _____

IMMEDIATELY PRIOR TO SURGERY	Yes	Not Applicable
1. Pre-operative urine specimen sent		
2. Reports attached to chart—Lab, X-ray, ECG		
3. Old chart		
4. Addressograph plate attached		
5. Contact lens, wig, jewelry, make-up removed, prosthesis off		
6. Dentures and partial plates removed		
7. Voided _____ Catheterized—time _____ amount _____		
8. Patient in hospital gown		
9. Blood pressure, pulse and respirations taken at least an hour prior to pre-op medication—charted on clinical record		
10. Pre-medication administered and charted on the anesthetic record		
11. Notation made in nurses notes of time to surgery		

DATE _____ SIGNATURE _____

OPERATING ROOM	Yes	Not Applicable
1. Patient identified by circulating nurse		
2. Site of surgery checked by circulating nurse a. Left side _____ Right side _____		
b. Slate _____ Surgeon _____ History _____ Consent _____		

SIGNATURE _____

Figure 46–2 A sample preoperative checklist. *Source:* Courtesy of St. Paul's Hospital, Nursing Department, Vancouver, British Columbia.

NURSING DIAGNOSIS

Surgical Clients

Preoperative Period

- Anxiety related to perceived inability to deal with possible pain
- Knowledge deficit related to postoperative leg/breathing exercises
- Alterations in thought process related to fear of the unknown
- Sleep pattern disturbance related to hospitalization

Intraoperative Period

- Potential for physical injury related to inability to adapt to environmental hazards secondary to anesthetized status
- Potential fluid volume deficit related to bleeding
- Potential for infection related to accessible port of entry secondary to surgical incision

Postoperative Period

- Potential skin impairment related to immobility secondary to surgery
- Potential ineffective breathing patterns related to pain secondary to surgery
- Impaired physical mobility related to incisional pain
- Potential fluid volume deficit related to excessive wound drainage
- Potential disturbance in self-concept related to loss of right breast

Planning Perioperative Care

Planning for the perioperative period should involve the client, support persons, and the nurse. Planning includes outlining goals and selecting strategies to resolve or prevent client health problems during the preoperative, intraoperative, and postoperative periods. Planning also involves the establishment of outcome criteria to evaluate specific goals. For suggested examples, see the section on evaluation later in this chapter.

The duration of the preoperative period often affects preoperative care and planning. When the preoperative period lasts several days, nurses can draw up a nursing care plan and a teaching plan. When the preoperative period is just an hour, only the essentials can be carried out. In this case the learning needs of the client must be met prior to admission to the clinical agency during the postoperative period. The Association of Operating

Room Nurses' outcome standards for perioperative nursing are listed in the accompanying box.

Preoperative Teaching

An explanation of perioperative care informs the client and his or her support persons about the perioperative period. Usually people are anxious at this time, and many have misconceptions about surgery and surgical care. Clients often ask nurses about the operation after the surgeon has gained informed consent and left the client's room. The surgeon should be notified if the client is anxious about the procedure or has questions about the surgery that the nurse cannot answer.

Clients and their support persons need to know the time and type of surgery. The surgeon usually arranges the date and may specify it in the orders. The exact time may not be known until the surgical schedule for the hospital is distributed. If a nurse does not know the exact time of surgery, the nurse should say so and inform the client and support persons as soon as the time is decided.

It is important to listen attentively and carefully to help the client identify specific concerns or fears and talk them through. Typical questions are: What will happen during surgery? How will I feel after the operation? What will the surgeon find? How long will the hospital stay be? Some clients may worry about finances. Those whose surgery involves disfigurement may have problems with their self-image.

This is also the time to clarify any misconceptions the client may have. Providing accurate information and acting supportively will help the client deal with identified concerns. The nurse should not dismiss the client's concerns by saying, "Everything will be all right." Unknowns or misconceptions can produce unrealistic fears and anxiety.

The client also may have specific learning needs regarding postoperative care. For example, learning to attend to a colostomy or the like requires preparation

OUTCOME CRITERIA

Perioperative Clients

- The client demonstrates knowledge of the physiologic and psychologic responses to surgery.
- The client is free from infection.
- The client's skin integrity is maintained.
- The client is free from injury related to positioning, extraneous objects, or chemical, physical, and electrical hazards.
- The client's fluid and electrolyte balance is maintained.
- The client participates in the rehabilitation process.

Reprinted with permission from AORN Standards and Recommended Practices for Preoperative Nursing, 1986. Copyright © AORN Inc. 10170 East Mississippi Avenue, Denver, CO 80231.

before surgery. Pain is common postoperatively, and clients are reassured to learn *beforehand* how to minimize it (e.g., by holding a pillow against the abdomen when moving after abdominal surgery). It also is important that clients know they will receive analgesics postoperatively to minimize discomfort. Most surgical clients need to learn how to move, breathe deeply, cough, and do leg exercises after surgery. See Procedure 46–1.

PROCEDURE 46–1

Teaching Moving, Leg Exercises, and Coughing and Deep-Breathing Exercises

Intervention

Moving

After surgery, turning in bed and early ambulation are encouraged to help clients maintain blood circulation, stimulate respiratory functions, and decrease the stasis of gas in the intestines (and its resulting discomfort). Clients who practice turning before surgery usually find it easier to do postoperatively.

1. Show the client ways to turn in bed and to get out of bed. Have the client start from the supine position.
   a. Instruct a client who will have a right abdominal incision or a right-sided chest incision to turn to the left side of the bed and sit up as follows.

   ▪ Flex the knees.

   ▪ Hold the left arm and hand or a small pillow against the incision to splint the wound.

   ▪ Turn to the left while pushing with the right foot and grasping the side rail on the left side of the bed with the right hand.

   ▪ Come to a sitting position on the side of the bed by using the right arm and hand to push down against the mattress.

   b. A client with a left abdominal or left-sided chest incision can perform the same procedure but should splint with the right arm and turn to the right.
   c. For clients with orthopedic surgery (eg, hip surgery), use special aids, such as a trapeze, to assist with movement.

Leg Exercises

2. Teach the client the three exercises that follow, which contract and relax the quadriceps muscles (vastus intermedius, vastus lateralis, rectus femoris, and vastus medialis) and the gastrocnemius muscles (see Figure 46–3).
   a. Alternate dorsiflexion and plantar flexion of the feet. This exercise is sometimes referred to as calf pumping, since it alternately contracts and relaxes the calf muscles, including the gastrocnemius muscles.
   b. Flex and extend the knees, and press the backs of the knees into the bed. See Figure 46–4.
   c. Raise and lower the legs alternately from the surface of the bed. Extend the knee of the moving leg. See Figure 46–5. This exercise contracts and

relaxes the quadriceps muscles. Clients who cannot raise their legs can do isometric exercises that contract and relax the muscles.
Rationale: Leg exercises help prevent thrombophlebitis due to slowed venous circulation (venous stasis). The major danger of thrombophlebitis is that thrombi can become emboli and lodge in the arteries of the heart, brain, or lungs, causing serious injury or death.

3. Instruct the client to start exercising as soon after surgery as possible.

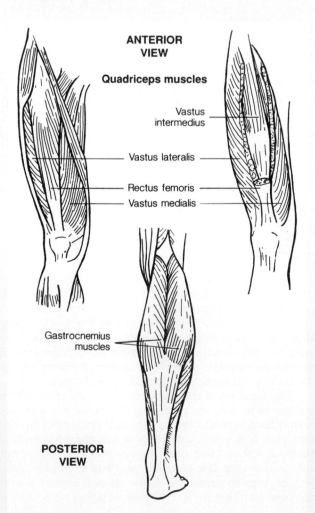

Figure 46–3

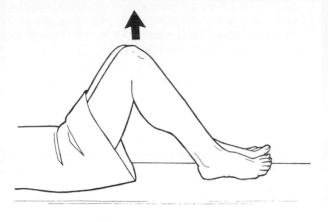

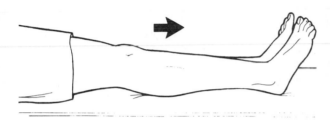

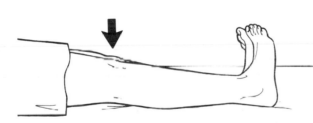

Figure 46–4

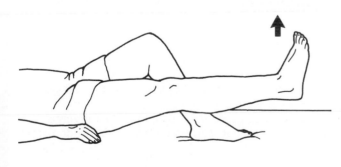

Figure 46–5

4. Encourage the client to do exercises at least once every waking hour. Note, however, that the frequency of exercising depends on the client's health status.

5. Explain that these muscle contractions will compress the veins and promote venous circulation.

Coughing and Deep-Breathing Exercises

6. Demonstrate deep-breathing (diaphragmatic) exercises as follows

   a. Place your hands palms down on the border of your rib cage, and inhale slowly and evenly through the nose until the greatest chest expansion is achieved. See Figure 46–6.

   b. Hold your breath for 2–3 seconds.

   c. Exhale slowly through the mouth.

   d. Continue exhalation until maximum chest contraction is achieved.

7. Have the client assume a sitting position and perform deep-breathing exercises while placing the palms of your hands on the border of the client's rib cage.

   Rationale: Deep-breathing exercises help remove mucus, which can form and remain in the lungs due to the effects of a general anesthetic and analgesics. These drugs depress the action of both the cilia of the mucous membranes lining the respiratory tract and the respiratory center in the brain. Deep breathing also aerates lung tissue and thereby helps prevent pneumonia, which may result from stagnation of fluid in the lungs.

8. Have the client voluntarily cough after a few deep inhalations. Have the client inhale deeply, hold the breath for a few seconds, and then cough one or two times. Ensure that the client coughs deeply and does not just clear the throat. Splinting the abdomen with clasped hands and a pillow held against the abdomen promotes effective coughing.

   Rationale: Deep breathing frequently initiates the coughing reflex. Voluntary coughing in conjunction with deep breathing facilitates the movement and expectoration of respiratory tract secretions.

9. If the client will have an incision that will be painful when coughing, demonstrate how the nurse or client can support (splint) the incision while coughing. Place the palms of your hands on either side of the incision or directly over the incision, holding the palm of one hand over the other. Also instruct the client with an abdominal incision how to splint the

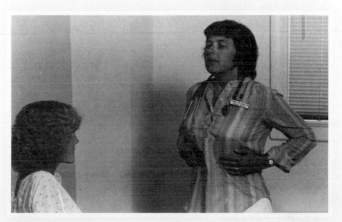

Figure 46–6

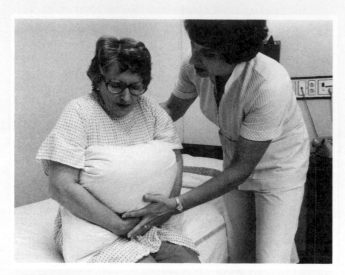

Figure 46—7

incision independently with a firmly rolled pillow. See Figure 46–9.

Rationale: Coughing uses the abdominal and other accessory respiratory muscles. Splinting the incision may reduce pain while coughing if the incision is near any of these muscles.

10. Instruct the client to start the exercises as soon after surgery as possible.

11. Encourage clients with abdominal or chest surgery to carry out deep breathing and coughing at least three or four times daily and at each session to take a minimum of five breaths. Note, however, that the number of breaths and frequency of deep breathing varies with the client's health. People who are susceptible to pulmonary problems may need deep-breathing exercises every hour. People with chronic respiratory disease may need special breathing exercises, eg, pursed-lip breathing, abdominal breathing, exercises using blow bottles and various kinds of incentive spirometers. See Chapter 42.

12. Explain to the client that deep-breathing and coughing exercises will increase lung expansion and prevent the accumulation of secretions, which may occur after anesthesia.

Nursing Roles during Surgery

Two types of nurses, the scrub nurse and the circulating nurse, assist during surgery. The scrub nurse is attired in a sterile gown, cap, mask, and gloves. The scrub nurse's responsibilities include:

1. Handing the surgeon sterile instruments and supplies from the sterile tray. Because many instruments are required during certain operations, a scrub nurse must have an extensive knowledge of all instruments and how they are used.
2. Counting sponges, needles, and instruments. Counting is done before the surgeon closes the incision so that none are left inside the client.
3. Disposing of used instruments.

The circulating nurse's responsibilities include:

1. Helping position the client on the operating room table.
2. Helping drape the client, and assisting the surgeon and scrub nurse to don sterile gowns and gloves.
3. Opening packages so that the scrub nurse can remove the sterile supplies.
4. Arranging for transfer of biopsy specimens to the laboratory.
5. Adjusting operating room lights.
6. Obtaining additional supplies and equipment.

Postoperative Planning

Most people recover from surgery without incident. Complications or problems are relatively rare, yet nurses must be aware of such possibilities and their clinical signs. See Table 46–4. Many sources of data are relevant to the planning of a client's postoperative nursing needs (e.g., the preoperative nursing history, postoperative orders, the recovery room report, and the client). See the accompanying box for significant data in the recovery room record. The nurse consults the surgeon's postoperative orders to learn:

1. Food and fluids permitted by mouth
2. Intravenous solutions and intravenous medications
3. Position in bed
4. Medications ordered, e.g., analgesics, antibiotics
5. Laboratory tests
6. Intake and output, which in some agencies are monitored for all postoperative clients
7. Activity permitted, including ambulation

The purposes of postoperative planning at this stage are to:

1. Prevent complications
2. Provide comfort and rest for the client
3. Maintain the client's safety
4. Facilitate the client's return to the highest possible level of wellness
5. Encourage exercises learned preoperatively
6. Help the client maintain a healthy attitude toward self

Recovery Room Record: Significant Data

Operation performed
Presence and location of any drains
Anesthetic used
Postoperative diagnosis
Estimated blood loss
Medications administered in the recovery room

Table 46–4 Potential Postoperative Problems

Problem	Description	Cause	Clinical Signs	Preventive Interventions
Respiratory				
Pneumonia	Inflammation of the alveoli	Commonly *Diplococcus pneumoniae,* a resident bacteria in the respiratory tract	Elevated temperature, cough, expectoration of blood-tinged or purulent sputum, dyspnea, chest pain	Deep-breathing and coughing exercises, moving in bed, early ambulation
Lobar pneumonia	Involves one or more lobes			
Bronchopneumonia	Originates in bronchi and involves patches of lung tissue	Poor lung expansion and circulation, resulting in stagnation of secretions		
Hypostatic pneumonia	Poor or stagnant circulation causing inflammation of lung tissue			
Atelectasis	Collapse of the alveoli, with retained secretions	Mucus plugs blocking bronchial passageways, inadequate lung expansion, analgesics, immobility	Marked dyspnea, cyanosis, pleural pain, prostration, tachycardia, increased respiratory rate, fever, productive cough, auscultatory crackling sounds	Deep-breathing and coughing exercises, turning, early ambulation, adequate fluid intake
Pulmonary embolism	Blood clot that has moved to the lungs and obstructs a pulmonary artery, thus inhibiting blood flow to one or more lung lobes	Stasis of venous blood from immobility, venous injury from fractures or during surgery, use of oral contraceptives high in estrogen, preexisting coagulation or circulatory disorder	Sudden chest pain, shortness of breath, cyanosis, shock (tachycardia, low blood pressure)	Deep-breathing and coughing exercises, turning, ambulation, anti-emboli stockings
Circulatory				
Hemorrhage	Bleeding internally or externally	Disruption of sutures, insecure ligation of blood vessels	Rapid weak pulse, increasing respiratory rate, restlessness, lowered blood pressure, cold clammy skin, thirst, pallor, reduced urine output	Early recognition of signs
Hypovolemic shock	Markedly reduced volume of circulating blood resulting in inadequate tissue perfusion	Hemorrhage	Same as for Hemorrhage	Early recognition of signs
Thrombophlebitis	Inflammation of the veins, usually of the legs and associated with a blood clot	Slowed venous blood flow due to immobility or prolonged sitting; trauma to vein, resulting in inflammation and increased blood coagulability	Aching, cramping pain; affected area is swollen, red, and hot to touch; vein feels hard; discomfort in calf when foot is dorsiflexed or when client walks (Homan's sign)	Early ambulation, leg exercises, anti-emboli stockings, adequate fluid intake
Thrombus	Blood clot attached to wall of vein or artery, most commonly the leg veins	Venous stasis; vein injury resulting from surgery of legs, pelvis, abdomen; factors causing increased	Same as for Pulmonary Embolism; if lodged in heart or brain, cardiac or neurologic signs	Same as for Thrombophlebitis

(continued)

Table 46—4 Potential Postoperative Problems (continued)

Problem	Description	Cause	Clinical Signs	Preventive Interventions
		blood coagulability, e.g., use of estrogen		
Embolus	Clot that has moved from its site of formation to another area of the body, e.g., the lungs, heart, or brain	Same as for Thrombus	Same as for Thrombus	Same as for Thrombophlebitis
Urinary				
Urinary retention	Accumulation of urine in the bladder and inability of the bladder to empty itself	Depressed bladder muscle tone from narcotics and anesthetics; handling of tissues during surgery on adjacent organs (rectum, vagina)	Fluid intake larger than output; inability to void or frequent voiding of small amounts, bladder distention, suprapubic discomfort, restlessness	Monitoring of fluid intake and output, interventions to facilitate voiding
Urinary infection	Inflammation of bladder	Immobilization and limited fluid intake	Burning sensation when voiding, urgency, cloudy urine, lower-abdominal pain	Adequate fluid intake, early ambulation, good perineal hygiene
Gastrointestinal				
Constipation	Infrequent or no stool passage for abnormal length of time, e.g., within 48 hours after solid diet started	Lack of dietary roughage, analgesics (decrease intestinal motility)	Absence of stool elimination, abdominal distention and discomfort	Adequate fluid intake, high-fiber diet, early ambulation
Singultus	Intermittent spasms of the diaphragm	Irritation of the phrenic nerve—for a variety of reasons, e.g., abdominal distention	Hiccups	Prevent the cause
Tympanites	Retention of gases within the intestines	Slowed motility of the intestines due to handling of the bowel during surgery and the effects of anesthesia	Obvious abdominal distention, abdominal discomfort (gas pains), absence of bowel sounds	Early ambulation, I.V. fluid progressing to clear fluids and regular diet when peristalsis returns
Nausea and vomiting		Pain, abdominal distention, ingesting food of fluids before return of peristalsis, certain medications, anxiety	Complaints of feeling sick to the stomach, retching or gagging	I.V. fluids until peristalsis returns; then clear fluids, full fluids, and regular diet; antiemetic drugs if ordered; analgesics for pain
Wound				
Wound infection	Inflammation and infection of incision or drain site	Poor aseptic technique; laboratory analysis of wound swab identifies causative microorganism	Purulent exudate, redness, tenderness, elevated body temperature, wound odor	Keeping wound clean and dry, surgical aseptic technique when changing dressings
Wound dehiscence	Separation of a suture line before the incision heals	Malnutrition (emaciation, obesity), poor circulation,	Increased incision drainage, tissues underlying skin	Adequate nutrition, appropriate incisional support and

(continued)

Table 46–4 **Potential Postoperative Problems** (*continued*)

Problem	Description	Cause	Clinical Signs	Preventive Interventions
		excessive strain on suture line	become visible along parts of the incision	avoidance of strain
Wound evisceration	Extrusion of internal organs and tissues through the incision	Same as for Wound Dehiscence	Opening of incision and visible protrusion of organs	Same as for Wound Dehiscence
Psychologic Postoperative depression	See Clinical Signs	News malignancy, severely altered body image	Anorexia, tearfulness, loss of ambition, withdrawal, rejection of others, feelings of dejection, sleep disturbances (insomnia, excessive sleeping)	Adequate rest, physical activity, opportunity to express anger and other negative feelings

For examples of outcome criteria for the postoperative client, see the section on evaluation, later in this chapter.

Implementing Planned Strategies

Just as plans are made specifically for the three phases of the perioperative period, so also are specific nursing interventions enacted in each of the phases.

Preoperative Interventions

Preoperative nursing responsibilities include monitoring nutrition and fluids, assisting with elimination, providing hygiene measures as needed, promoting rest, ensuring safety of valuables and prostheses, administering medications, preparing the skin for surgery, monitoring vital signs, and implementing special orders. Some clients may find it comforting to visit with a spiritual advisor preoperatively, and the nurse may assist the client or family to make arrangements for such a visit.

Adequate hydration and nutrition promote healing. Nurses need to record any sign of malnutrition. A perioperative record of the client's weight is one way to determine one aspect of nutritional status. If the client is receiving intravenous fluids or requires measurement of fluid intake, nurses must ensure that the fluids are carefully measured. See Chapter 43.

Because anesthetic agents depress gastrointestinal functioning and because there is a danger the client may vomit and aspirate vomitus during administration of a general anesthetic agent, the client usually fasts at least 6 to 8 hours before surgery. The surgical client and support persons need explanations to understand the necessity of fasting. Usually, the nurse removes food and fluids from the bedside and places a fasting sign at the bed the evening before surgery. The client can use a mouthwash if her or his mouth feels dry but must not swallow any. If the client ingests food or fluids during the fasting period, the nurse must notify the surgeon.

As part of the preoperative check of the client, the nurse should ascertain whether the client has emptied his or her bowels and bladder prior to surgery. If an enema is ordered, the order will specify whether it should be given the evening prior to or the day of surgery. If it is ordered for the day of surgery, it should be administered soon enough to allow the client time to expel it. A series of enemas may be needed if surgery on the bowel is planned. Sometimes a rectal suppository is ordered instead of an enema. An enema or suppository is given because anesthesia and abdominal surgery decrease bowel activity for a few days postoperatively. If a retention catheter is ordered, this is usually inserted the day of surgery. The purpose of the catheter is to ensure that the bladder remains empty, thus preventing inadvertent injury to the bladder, particularly during pelvic surgery.

Nurses may assist the client with hygiene by giving the client a complete or partial bath. In some settings clients are asked to have a bath or shower using an antimicrobial agent the evening or morning of surgery (or both). The bath includes a shampoo whenever possible. The client's nails should be trimmed and free of polish, and all cosmetics should be removed, so that the nail beds, skin, and lips are visible for assessment of circulation during and following surgery. On the day of surgery it is important to remove, or ask the client to remove, all hair pins and clips. Long hair can be braided and fastened with elastic bands to keep it in place. Hair pins and clips may cause pressure or accidental damage to the scalp when the client is unconscious.

Adequate rest helps the client manage the stress of surgery. The nurse should help the client prepare for sleep on the night before scheduled surgery. See Chapter 40 for suggested interventions. Valuables such as jewelry and money should be labeled and placed in safekeeping if support persons cannot take them home. In most hospitals, valuables can be kept in special envelopes and locked in a storage area on the unit. If a client wishes not to remove a wedding band, the nurse can tape it in place. Wedding bands must be removed, however, if there is danger of the fingers swelling after surgery. Situations warranting removal of a wedding band include surgery of or cast application to an arm and a mastectomy that involves removal of the lymph nodes. (Mastectomies may cause edema of the arm and hand.)

The nurse should check the preoperative medications the evening prior to surgery. Often a sedative is ordered to help the client get a good sleep.

Preoperative medications also may be ordered for the day of surgery. Usually a narcotic (e.g., morphine) and a medication to dry the secretions of the mouth and respiratory tract (e.g., atropine) are given by injection. Sometimes the surgeon orders oral sedatives (e.g., secobarbital) or tranquilizers to be administered before the injectable medications are given. A newer trend is to give *no* preoperative medications, or to administer preoperative medications in the preoperative holding area, when one is available, rather than premedicating the client on the nursing unit. It is essential to administer preoperative medications exactly at the time specified.

After giving the preoperative medications, the nurse informs the client that the medication will cause drowsiness and instructs him or her to remain quietly in bed. The nurse then raises the side rails, lowers the bed for safety, and places the call light within reach. Also, the nurse explains that scopolamine or atropine may cause thirst and that, although a mouthwash may be used, he or she must not have anything to drink.

All prostheses (artificial body parts, such as partial or complete dentures, contact lenses, artificial eyes, and artificial limbs) as well as eyeglasses, wigs, false eyelashes, and hearing aids must be removed before surgery. In some hospitals, dentures are placed in a locked storage area; in others, they are kept at the client's bedside. Partial dentures can become dislodged and obstruct an unconscious client's breathing. Loose teeth can become dislodged and be aspirated during anesthesia. Other prostheses may become damaged.

The purpose of preoperative skin preparation is to destroy microorganisms and thus reduce the chance of infection. It is recommended that the hair near the operative site not be removed unless absolutely necessary. In most agencies, the client's skin is "prepped" in a special room just before surgery. If hair must be removed, the Centers for Disease Control recommend that it be clipped or a depilatory be used and the area cleaned with antimicrobials just before surgery (Garner 1986, p. 77). The area prepared is generally larger than the incision area. This practice minimizes the number of microorganisms in the areas adjacent to the incision.

Preoperatively, nurses take vital signs to obtain comparative baseline data against which to assess the client's responses during and following surgery. Because any abnormality can cause postponement of surgery, the nurse promptly reports abnormalities in any of these signs (e.g., an elevated temperature) to the nurse in charge and to the surgeon. The surgeon's orders should be checked for special requirements, e.g., the administra-

tion of insulin or other medications or the insertion of a nasogastric tube prior to surgery.

Gastric intubation is the insertion of a tube into the stomach, either through the nose, the mouth, or a gastrostomy opening. A **nasogastric tube** can be passed through either the mouth or the nose; however, the nose is preferred because there is less discomfort from the gag reflex. A tube passed through the mouth is often called an **orogastric tube.**

Several types of nasogastric tubes are used for irrigation and gastric decompression. **Gastric decompression** is the reduction of the pressure within the stomach, e.g., by removal of the gastric contents. The **Levin tube** is commonly used for nasogastric intubation. It is a flexible, rubber or plastic, single-lumen tube with holes near the tip. See Figure 46–8. Inserting a Levin tube is often the nurse's responsibility. The **Salem sump tube,** also frequently used, is a nasogastric tube with a double lumen. The main reasons for inserting a gastric tube are to:

1. Prevent nausea, vomiting, and gastric distention following surgery
2. Provide a route for feeding the client
3. Remove stomach contents for laboratory analysis
4. Allow lavage of the stomach in cases of poisoning or overdose of medications

Procedure 46–2 gives detailed steps for gastric intubation.

The last preoperative nursing responsibility is validating that the client is prepared for surgery. This usually done by completing a preoperative checklist, such

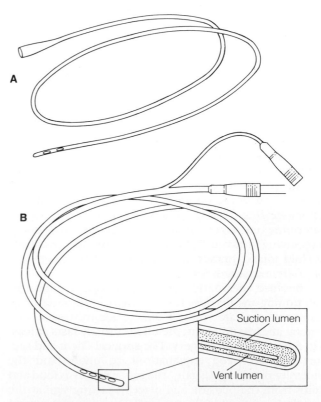

Figure 46–8 Two commonly used tubes for gastric and intestinal suction and irrigations: **A,** Levin; **B,** Salem sump

as the sample illustrated in Figure 46–2, earlier. The nurse should contact the surgeon if any screening tests results are abnormal or if there are changes in the client's current status. When the operating room transport person arrives for the client, the nurse carefully checks the client's identification bracelet against his or her chart. Generally, one staff member reads the identifying data from the bracelet while another checks it against the client's record. The nurse never relies on a drowsy client to identify himself or herself.

PROCEDURE 46–2

Inserting and Removing a Nasogastric Tube

Equipment

- A gastric tube (plastic or rubber).
- A solution basin filled with warm water or ice. Rubber tubes are placed on ice to stiffen them for easier insertion. Plastic tubes are placed in warm water to make them more flexible for insertion.
- A water-soluble lubricant.
- A 20- to 50-ml syringe with an adapter to attach to the tube. It is used to withdraw stomach contents.
- A basin in which to collect gastric contents.
- Nonallergenic adhesive tape, 2.5 cm (1 in.) wide, to secure the tube to the face.
- A clamp (optional) to close the tube after insertion.
- Suction apparatus, if ordered.
- A gauze square or a plastic specimen bag and an elastic band to cover the end of the tube.
- A safety pin and an elastic band to secure the nasogastric tube to the client's gown.
- A bib or towel to protect the client's gown.
- A glass of water and drinking straw to help the client swallow the tube.
- Facial tissues in case the client's eyes water during the procedure.
- A stethoscope to help assess placement of the tube.

Intervention

1. Before inserting a nasogastric tube, assess
   a. Any obstructions or deformities of the nostrils. Ask the client to hyperextend the head. Observe the nares, either by using a flashlight or by asking the client to breathe through one nostril while occluding the other. Select the nostril that has the greatest air flow.
   b. Intactness of the tissues of the nostrils, including any irritations or abrasions.

Inserting a Nasogastric Tube

2. Explain to the client what you plan to do. The passage of a gastric tube is not painful, but it is unpleasant because the gag reflex is activated during insertion.

3. Assist the client to a high-Fowler's position if health permits, and support the head on a pillow.
   Rationale: It is often easier to swallow in this position, and gravity helps the passage of the tube.

4. Hyperextend the head to examine the nostrils. Ask the client to breathe through each nostril while compressing the other nostril, to select the more patent one.
   Rationale: The tube is inserted through the nostril that is more patent.

5. *Determine how far to insert the tube:* Use the tube to mark off the distance from the tip of the client's nose to the tip of the earlobe and then from the tip of the earlobe to the tip of the sternum. See Figure 46–9. Mark this length with adhesive tape if the tube does not have markings.
   Rationale: This length approximates the distance from the nares to the stomach. The distance varies among individuals.

6. Lubricate the tip of the tube well with water-soluble lubricant to ease insertion.
   Rationale: A water-soluble lubricant dissolves if the tube accidentally enters the lungs. An oil-based lubricant, such as petroleum jelly, will not dissolve and could cause respiratory complications if it enters the lungs.

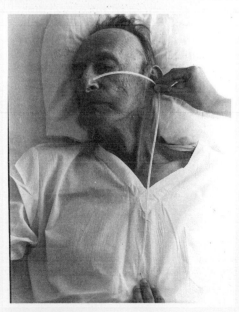

Figure 46–9

7. Insert the tube, with its natural curve toward the client, into the selected nostril.

8. Have the client hyperextend the neck, and gently advance the tube toward the nasopharynx. Direct the tube along the floor of the nostril and toward the ear on that side. Provide tissues if the client's eyes water. If the tube meets resistance, withdraw it, relubricate it, and insert it in the other nostril.
   Rationale: Hyperextension reduces the curvature of the nasopharyngeal junction. Directing the tube along the floor avoids the projections (turbinates) along the lateral wall. Slight pressure is sometimes required to pass the tube into the nasopharynx, and some clients' eyes may water at this point. Tears are a natural body response. The tube should never be forced against resistance because of the danger of injury.

9. Once the tube reaches the oropharynx (throat), have the client tilt the head forward and encourage him or her to drink and swallow. If the client gags, stop passing the tube momentarily. Have the client rest, take a few breaths, and take sips of water to calm the gag reflex.
   Rationale: The client will feel the tube in the throat and may gag and retch. Tilting the head forward facilitates passage of the tube into the posterior pharynx and esophagus rather than into the larynx; swallowing moves the epiglottis over the opening to the larynx. See Figure 46–10.

10. In cooperation with the client, pass the tube 5–10 cm (2–4 in.) with each swallow, until the indicated length is inserted. If the client continues to gag and the tube does not advance with each swallow, withdraw it slightly and inspect the throat by looking through the mouth.
    Rationale: The tube may be coiled. If so, it is withdrawn until it is straight, and the nurse tries again to insert it.

11. Aspirate the stomach contents with a syringe to determine placement of tube. See Table 46–5 for other methods.
    Rationale: If fluid is removed, the assumption is that the tube is in the stomach. (Stomach contents are usually clear or yellow with mucus.)

12. If the signs do not indicate placement in the stomach, advance the tube 5 cm (2 in.) and repeat the tests.

13. Secure the tube by taping it to the bridge of the client's nose. If the client has oily skin, wipe the nose first with alcohol.
    a. Cut 7.5 cm (3 in.) of tape and split it lengthwise at one end, leaving a 2.5-cm (1-in.) tab at the end.
    b. Place the tape over the bridge of the client's nose, and bring the split ends under the tubing and back up over the nose. See Figure 46–11.

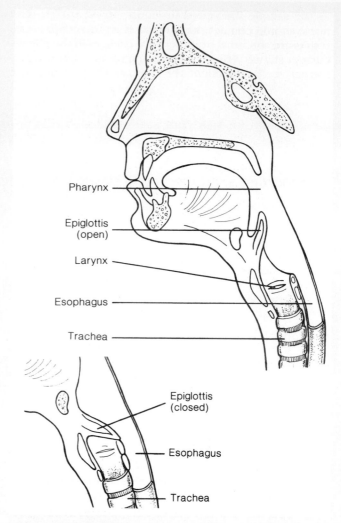

Figure 46–10

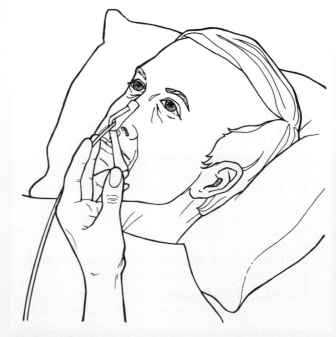

Figure 46–11

Rationale: Taping in this manner prevents the tube from pressing against and irritating the edge of the nostril.

14. Attach the end of the tubing securely to suction, if ordered.

or

15. Clamp the end of the tubing or cover it with a gauze square or plastic specimen bag and an elastic band. The tube, if inserted preoperatively, is usually clamped.

16. Attach the end of the tube to the gown by one of these two methods:

a. Loop an elastic band around the end of the tubing and attach the elastic band to the gown with a safety pin.

or

b. Attach a piece of adhesive tape to the tube, and pin the tape to the gown.

Rationale: The tube is attached to prevent it from dangling and pulling.

17. Document the insertion of the tube, means by which correct placement was determined, and assessments, eg, discomfort, abdominal distention.

18. Establish a plan for providing daily nasogastric tube care, including:

a. Inspecting the nostril for discharge and irritation.

b. Cleaning the nostril and tube with moistened, cotton-tipped applicators.

c. Applying water-soluble lubricant to the nostril if it appears dry or encrusted.

d. Changing the adhesive tape as required.

e. Giving frequent mouth care, since the client may breathe through the mouth and cannot drink.

19. If suction is applied, ensure that the patency of both the nasogastric and suction tubes is maintained. Irrigations of the tube with 30 ml of normal saline may be required at regular intervals. In some agencies, irrigations must be ordered by the physician. Managing gastrointestinal suction and irrigating a nasogastric tube are discussed in Procedure 46–5.

20. Keep accurate records of the client's fluid intake and output, and record the amount and characteristics of the drainage.

Removing a Nasogastric Tube

The removal of a nasogastric tube is ordered by a physician.

21. Turn off the suction, and disconnect the tube from suction apparatus.

22. Remove the adhesive tape securing the tube to the client's nose. Unpin the tube from the client's gown.

23. Suggest that the client keep the eyes closed while withdrawing the tube.

24. Instill 50 ml air through the tube (optional).
Rationale: The instillation of air clears the tubing of irritating gastric contents.

25. Clamp the tubing or kink it with your fingers.
Rationale: Clamping the tube prevents aspiration during removal.

26. Ask the client to take a deep breath and hold it while you steadily and quickly remove the tube.
Rationale: Holding the breath ensures closure of the glottis and prevents the possibility of aspiration.

27. Dispose of the tube in a bag or paper towel.

28. Provide tissues for the client to blow the nose, and offer mouthwash if desired.

29. Remove the suction apparatus from the bedside. Measure the amount of fluid drained. Then empty and clean the drainage bottle.

30. Document the removal of the tube, the client's response, and the amount of fluid drained.

Variation: Inserting an Orogastric Tube

Insertion of an orogastric tube through the mouth is usually done for adults prior to *gastric lavage* (aspiration of stomach contents by washing out the stomach). It is performed on adults who have no gag reflex or who may be unconscious or uncooperative. Lavage is contraindicated if corrosive substances (eg, lye and some household cleaning agents) have been swallowed. For infants who require tube feedings, orogastric tubes are preferred since infants are obligatory nose breathers. Nasogastric tube feedings can decrease oxygenation in infants. To insert an orogastric tube, the nurse lubricates the tube and passes it through the mouth toward the posterior pharynx. The client is instructed to suck on the tube as if it were a straw and to swallow at the same time. No water or ice chips are used. After the tube is inserted about 6 in., the tube is moved to the left or right cheek area between the teeth and the cheek. This maneuver helps to minimize stimulation of the gag reflex. The tube is then advanced to the premeasured mark and correct placement is assessed by aspirating stomach contents.

▪ Preparing for the Postoperative Client

While the client is in the operating room, the client's bed and room are prepared for the postoperative phase. In some agencies, the client is brought back to the unit on a stretcher and transferred to the bed in his or her room. In other agencies, the client's bed is brought to the recovery room (RR), and the client is transferred there. In the latter situation, the surgical bed needs to be made as soon as the client goes to the operating room so that it can be taken to the RR at any time. In addition, the nurse must obtain and set up special equipment as needed, such as an intravenous pole, suction, oxygen equipment, and orthopedic appliances (e.g., traction).

Table 46–5   Placement of a Nasogastric Tube

Nurse's Action	If Tube Is in the Stomach	If Tube Is in the Lungs
To Assess Placement		
Attach distal end of tube to syringe, and withdraw plunger.	Some gastric contents will fill tube.	No fluid will be in tube.
Other Indications of Placement		
Using a stethoscope, listen over the epigastric area of the abdomen while injecting 10 ml of air into tube.	Air will make a rushing sound.	There will be no sound.
Listen to distal end to tube.	There will be no sound.	There will be a crackling sound.
Ask conscious client to talk and hum.	Client will be able to talk and hum.	Client will be unable to talk or hum and will cough and/or choke.
Note unconscious client's skin color.	Color will be normal.	Client will be cyanotic.
Place end of tube in a glass of water while client exhales.	Few, if any, bubbles will appear in water.	Steady stream of bubbles will appear.

If these are not requested on the client's record, the nurse should consult with the responsible nurse. Procedure 46–3 provides instructions for making a surgical bed.

PROCEDURE 46–3

Making a Surgical Bed

Equipment

Although supplies vary from one agency to another, the following are generally needed:

- Two clean sheets
- A clean cotton drawsheet
- A clean flannelette sheet for the foundation of the bed if this is agency practice
- A clean bedspread
- A disposable incontinence or drainage pad (optional)

At some agencies these supplies are arranged in a surgical bundle.

Intervention

1. Place the supplies within easy reach in the order in which they will be used.
2. Place and leave the pillows on the bedside chair.
   Rationale: Pillows are left on a chair to facilitate transferring the client into the bed.
3. Arrange the furniture and equipment so that there is room near the bed for a stretcher or room to move the bed out of the room if the bed is to be transported to the operating room.
4. Strip the bed according to Procedure 34–13, steps 6–16.
5. Make the foundation of the bed as shown in Procedure 34–13, steps 19–31.

6. Place the flannelette sheet on the foundation of the bed, if this is agency practice.
   Rationale: A flannelette sheet provides additional warmth.
7. Place a disposable pad for the client's head (optional).
8. Spread the top covers on the bed. Do not tuck them in, miter the corners, or make a toe pleat.
9. Fold the hanging edges of the top covers up over the top of the bed so that the folds are at the mattress edge (fold the sides first, then the top and bottom). Then fanfold the covers in either of the following ways:
   a.   Fanfold them lengthwise at one side of the bed. See Figure 46–12.
   b.   Fanfold them crosswise at the bottom of the bed. See Figure 46–13.
   Rationale: The covers are fanfolded for ease in transferring the client into bed.
10. Lock the wheels of the bed if the bed is not to be moved, and leave the bed in the high position to meet the level of the stretcher.
    Rationale: Locking the wheels keeps the bed from rolling. The high position facilitates the transfer of the client.
11. Notify appropriate people that the surgical bed is ready. In some hospitals, a porter service or the like takes the bed to the recovery room.
12. Place any additional equipment, eg, suction, in readiness for use when the client returns from surgery.

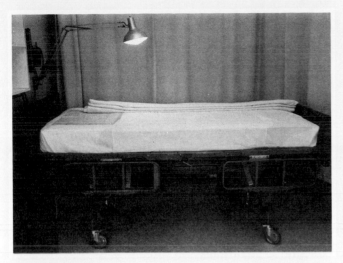

Figure 46–12

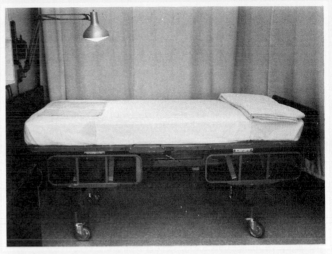

Figure 46–13

▇ Immediate Postoperative Interventions

Nursing during the postoperative phase is especially important for the client's recovery. Anesthesia impairs the ability of clients to respond to environmental stimuli and to help themselves, although the degree of consciousness of clients will vary. Moreover, surgery itself traumatizes the body by decreasing its energy and resistance. Nursing interventions include monitoring the client's cardiovascular status, fluid balance, and neurologic status; providing comfort and safety; encouraging mobility; and preventing complications. The postoperative phase can be divided into two stages: immediate postanesthetic stage and continuing postoperative stage.

Immediate postanesthetic care is usually provided in a postanesthetic room (PAR), also referred to as the recovery room (RR). Recovery room nurses have specialized skills to care for clients recovering from anesthesia and surgery. Once a client's health status has stabilized, he or she is returned to the nursing unit or, in the case of a day-surgery client, to the day-surgery area before discharge. Recovery room care is summarized in the accompanying box.

When planning immediate postoperative care, the nurse should review the client's preoperative data base and establish priorities for care based on that data as well as the surgical procedure itself.

During the immediate postanesthetic stage, an unconscious client is positioned on his or her side, with the face slightly down. A pillow is not placed under the head. In this position, gravity keeps the tongue forward, preventing occlusion of the pharynx and allowing drainage of mucus or vomitus out of the mouth rather than down the respiratory tree.

Maximum chest expansion is ensured by elevating the client's upper arm on a pillow. The upper arm is supported because the pressure of an arm against the chest reduces chest expansion potential. Once the client's reflexes return, he or she can usually assume a back-lying position. An artificial airway is maintained in place, and suction is supplied until reflexes for controlling coughing and swallowing return. Generally, the client spits out an oropharyngeal airway when coughing returns. Endotracheal tubes are not removed until the client is awake and able to maintain his or her own airway. Before any artificial airway is removed, suction is applied to the airway and the pharynx. The client is then helped to turn, cough, and take deep breaths, provided vital signs are stable. See Chapter 42 for information about artificial airways.

In the recovery room, the nurse assesses the rate, depth, and quality of respirations as well as the client's chest movements and compares the findings with the baseline data on the client's record. If respirations appear extremely shallow, the nurse should hold her or his hand in front of the client's mouth to feel for exhaled air. If exhalations are not detected, the lungs should be auscultated and any bilateral air movement noted. Oxygen should be supplied to hypoventilating clients as necessary.

After general **anesthesia**, clients usually awaken in the following sequence:

1. Responsive to stimuli (e.g., to loud noises or to their name spoken loudly)

A S S E S S M E N T

▇ Recovery Room

- Respiratory function
- Cardiovascular function (circulation)
- Fluid and electrolyte balance
- Dressings, tubes, and drains
- Neurologic status
- Pain
- Safety

2. Drowsiness
3. Awake but not oriented
4. Alert and oriented (McConnell 1977a, p. 34)

The return of the client's reflexes, such as swallowing and gagging, indicates that anesthesia is ending. Time of recovery from anesthesia varies with the kind of anesthetic agent used, its dosage, and the individual's response to it. Nurses should arouse the client by calling him or her by name, and in a normal tone of voice repeatedly tell the client that the surgery is over and that he or she is in the RR.

As the client emerges from anesthesia, it is important to assess any need for analgesics and to administer them as ordered. Analgesic dosages given in the RR are often reduced from normal levels by one-quarter to one-third, but their effects are closely evaluated. Smaller dosages of analgesics are given because respiratory and cardiovascular function are depressed by anesthesia and can be impaired further by analgesic dosages that are too high. Nurses should use judgment in withholding pain medications from hypotensive clients, for pain may be the cause of hypotension (McConnell 1977a, p. 36).

The nurse should assess the client for signs of **respiratory obstruction**, the most common recovery room emergency. It may be due to occlusion of the pharynx by the tongue, spasm or edema of the airway, accumulation of secretions in the airway, or aspiration of regurgitated vomitus. See Chapter 42 for additional information.

The client's **pulse** must be assessed for rate, rhythm, and quality every 15 minutes until signs stabilize and then every 30 minutes. Generally, the pulse is slightly faster after surgery, but a pulse above 110 beats per minute or below 60 beats per minute should be reported. A pulse rate markedly above or below the client's preoperative rate is abnormal; it may indicate internal hemorrhage or some other physiologic problem. If the radial pulse is thready, the nurse should take the apical pulse.

The client's **blood pressure** should be assessed every 15 minutes until stable and then every 30 minutes. The surgeon should be informed if the client's blood pressure falls more than 20 mm Hg after surgery or falls 5 or 10 mm Hg at each reading. This is because certain anesthetic agents and muscle relaxants may cause postoperative hypotension; it may also be a sign of hemorrhage and shock.

The client's *skin color and condition,* particularly that of the lips and nail beds, should be assessed, because the color of the lips and nail beds are indicators of **tissue perfusion** (passage of blood through the vessels). Pale, cyanotic, cool, and moist skin may be a sign of circulatory problems. In addition, the client should be assessed for signs of common circulatory problems: hemorrhage and shock, cardiac arrest, and postoperative hypotension. Disruption of sutures and insecure ligation of blood vessels can cause hemorrhage. Shock occurs as a result of massive hemorrhage or cardiac insufficiency. Signs of **hemorrhage** and **shock** are summarized in the accompanying box.

The nurse must inspect the client's dressings and the bedclothes underneath the client. Excessive bloody drainage on dressings or on bedclothes, often appearing

ASSESSMENT

Clinical Signs of Shock

- Increased pulse and respiratory rates
- Restlessness
- Lowered blood pressure
- Cold, clammy skin
- Thirst
- Pallor

underneath the client, can indicate hemorrhage. The amount of **drainage** on dressings is recorded by describing the diameter of stains. It is extremely important for the nurse to ensure that replacement of fluids lost during surgery is sufficient, to maintain blood pressure. Nurses in the RR also must determine the color, consistency, and amount of drainage from all tubes and suction apparatuses. All tubes should be patent, and tubes and suction equipment should be functioning properly.

The client's fluid **intake and output** are monitored. In addition to watching for shock, the client should also be assessed for signs of circulatory overload. See Chapter 43. During surgery, aldosterone production increases, and, as a result, the body conserves sodium and fluid. Therefore, care must be taken not to overload the body with fluid. In addition, the client is assessed for signs of fluid or electrolyte imbalance.

The surgeon may prescribe blood components to be administered in the recovery room or afterward in the surgical nursing unit. A **blood transfusion** is the introduction of whole blood or components of the blood, e.g., plasma serum, erythrocytes, or platelets, into the venous circulation. See Table 46–6 for types of blood and blood products, and indications for their use. Blood transfusions are given to:

1. Restore blood volume after severe hemorrhage
2. Restore the red blood cell level after severe and chronic anemias and to maintain blood hemoglobin levels
3. Provide plasma factors, e.g., antihemophilic factor (AHF) or coagulation factor VIII, which controls bleeding

Blood transfusions must be matched to the recipient's blood type in terms of compatible agglutinogens. See Table 46–7. Mismatched blood will cause a hemolytic reaction. Transfusion reactions can be categorized as hemolytic, febrile, and allergic. The **hemolytic reaction,** a fatal response, occurs when agglutinins and agglutinogens of the same type come in contact; e.g., A agglutinogen and anti-A agglutinin, or Type B agglutinogen and anti-B agglutinin. **Agglutination** (clumping) and **hemolysis** (rupture) of the red cells result from such contact.

To prevent hemolytic reactions, it is essential, therefore, to match the donor's blood type to the recipient's.

Table 46—6 Blood Products and Indications for Use

Type of Blood Product	Indications
Whole blood (Type A, B, AB, O, and/or Rh positive or negative)	To treat blood volume deficiencies, e.g., in acute hemorrhage; not indicated for correction of chronic anemia
Plasma	To expand blood volume; to restore circulation and renal blood flow when plasma volume is decreased but red cell mass is adequate, as in acute dehydration or burns; to replace deficient coagulation factors in bleeding disorders
Packed red cells (high hematocrit, since approximately 80% of plasma is removed)	Used when blood volume is adequate but red cell mass is inadequate, as in chronic anemia
Platelets	For clients with severe thrombocytopenia (reduced platelets); platelets plug small vascular leaks prior to clotting
Albumin	To expand blood volume when volume is reduced in clients in shock or with burns; to increase level of albumin in clients with hypoalbuminemia
Prothrombin complex (Konyne, Proplex)—contains factors VII, IX, and XI and prothrombin	For bleeding associated with deficiencies of those factors
Factor VIII fractions	For hemophiliacs
Fibrinogen preparations	For bleeding associated particularly with congenital hypofibrinogenemia (deficiency of fibrinogen, necessary for blood coagulation)

Otherwise, the agglutinins present in the recipient's plasma will agglutinate the red cells donated. Because type O blood has neither A nor B agglutinogens, it can be donated to recipients with any of the four types of blood; a person with this type is called a **universal donor.** A person with type AB blood, because it has neither anti-A nor anti-B agglutinins in plasma, is referred to as a **universal recipient,** able to receive any of the four blood types.

Febrile reactions (bacterial reactions) are rare. They occur as a result of contaminated blood or sensitivity to the donor's white blood cells. **Allergic reactions** are relatively common and are thought to be due to allergenic substances or antibodies in the donor's plasma. The signs, symptoms, and nursing actions for each type of reaction are outlined in Table 46–8.

Fifteen minutes after the transfusion has started, the nurse checks the client's vital signs. If there are no signs of a reaction, the required flow rate is established. Most adults can tolerate receiving one unit of blood in 1½ to 2 hours. The nurse continues to assess the client every 30 minutes, or more often, depending on the client's condition, including vital signs.

When the transfusion has infused, the nurse completes the requisition attached to the blood unit by fill-ing in the time the transfusion was discontinued and the amount transfused. One copy of the requisition is attached to the client's record and another to the empty blood bag. The blood bag (in a plastic transport bag) and requisiton are returned to the blood bank. The nurse records completion of the transfusion, the amount of blood absorbed, the blood unit number, and the vital signs. If the primary I.V. infusion was continued, that fact is also recorded.

Continuing Postoperative Interventions

As soon as the client returns to the nursing unit from the RR, the nurse conducts an initial assessment. See Figure 46–14 for a postoperative checklist. The sequence of these activities varies with the situation. For example, the nurse may need to check the physician's stat orders before conducting the initial assessment; in such a case, nursing interventions to implement the orders can be carried out at the same time as assessment.

The nurse records the client's condition, including the assessment, on the chart. Many hospitals have postoperative routines for regular assessment of clients. In

Table 46—7 Survey of Information on Blood Groups

Blood Type (Red Blood Cell Agglutinogens)	Agglutinins in Plasma	Possible Donors	Percentage of Human Population
A	Anti-B (beta)	Types A and O	41
B	Anti-A (alpha)	Types B and O	9
AB	None	Types AB, A, B, and O	3
O (no agglutinogen)	Anti-A and anti-B	Type O	47

Source: Adapted from A. C. Guyton. *Textbook of Medical Physiology,* 7th ed. (Philadelphia: W. B. Saunders Co., 1986) p. 70.

Table 46–8 Transfusion Reactions: Clinical Signs and Nursing Interventions

Reaction	Clinical Signs	Nursing Interventions
Hemolytic reaction	Chills, fever, headache, back pain, hemoglobinemia, hemoglobinuria, oliguria, jaundice, dyspnea, cyanosis, chest pain, vascular collapse, hypotension	1. Observe client closely for first 10 minutes of transfusion, since these reactions occur rapidly 2. Discontinue blood immediately when reaction is assessed 3. Notify physician of client's symptoms and vital signs 4. Notify laboratory to type and cross-match blood and confirm diagnosis; send donor blood back to laboratory and have specimen of recipient's blood retested 5. Maintain intravenous infusion with D5W or saline 6. Monitor vital signs every 15 minutes to assess shock and temperature 7. Record fluid intake and output to assess degree of kidney functioning 8. Save first voided specimen for laboratory analysis 9. Implement treatment as prescribed by physician
Febrile reaction	Fever, shaking, chills, warm flushed skin, headache, backache, nausea, hematemesis, diarrhea, red shock, confusion or delirium	*For mild reaction:* 1. Observe client closely for first 30 minutes of transfusion *For severe reaction:* 1. Stop transfusion 2. Maintain intravenous infusion with saline or D5W 3. Monitor client's vital signs every 30 minutes 4. Notify physician 5. Notify laboratory to take culture of client's and donor's blood 6. Implement therapy as prescribed by physician 7. Apply alcohol sponges for fever if necessary
Allergic reaction	Utricaria, occasional wheezing, arthralgia, generalized itching, nasal congestion, bronchospasm, severe dyspnea, circulatory collapse	*For mild reaciton:* 1. Slow reaction 2. Implement therapy as prescribed by physician *For severe reaction:* 1. Stop transfusion 2. Notify physician immediately 3. Maintain intravenous infusion with saline or D5W 4. Monitor vital signs frequently

some agencies, assessments are made every 15 minutes until vital signs stabilize, every hour thereafter the same day, and every 4 hours for the next 2 days. It is very important that the assessments be made as often as the client's condition requires. The nurse notifies the client's support persons that he or she has returned from surgery. It may be necessary to caution them about the client's drowsiness and about not staying too long. Special assessments should be made with older adults. See the accompanying box for postoperative risk factors.

The client's **vital signs** need to be taken at least every 4 hours, or more frequently if they are abnormal. See Table 46–4 for assistance in analyzing the meaning of altered vital signs. The client's **skin color and temperature** must be assessed. Extreme pallor and a cold, clammy skin are signs of shock.

The client should be encouraged to do **deep-breathing and coughing exercises** hourly, or at least every 2 hours, during waking hours for the first few days. The nurse should assist the client to a sitting position in bed or on the side of the bed. The client should splint the incision with a pillow when coughing, or the nurse should splint the incision for the client. These exercises help prevent respiratory complications such as hypostatic pneumonia and atelectasis. See Table 46–4. To assist clients who have difficulty with deep-breath-

ing and coughing exercises, the nurse should check about the use of blow bottles and incentive spirometers (see Chapter 42). For clients unable to cough up secretions, suctioning may be necessary (see Chapter 42).

ASSESSMENT

Postoperative Factors in Elderly Adults

- **Vulnerable** skin due to venous stasis and poor venous return
- **Reduced** cardiac reserve due to changes in the myocardium
- **Tachycardia** from anxiety, which is tolerated poorly in the elderly heart.
- **Decreased** compliance of blood vessels due to atherosclerosis
- **Reduced** vital capacity due to lowered expansibility of the rib cage
- **Reduced** blood flow to the kidneys
- **Reduced** ability to excrete toxins due to reduced glomerular filtration

1. **Time of arrival** _____
2. **Vital signs**
   Pulse _____
   Respirations _____
   Blood pressure _____
3. **Skin**
   Color _____
   Condition _____
4. **Level of consciousness**
   Conscious _____
   Semiconscious _____
   Unconscious _____
5. **Dressing**
   Dry _____
   Drainage present _____
   Blood _____
   Intact _____
6. **Intravenous**
   Type of solution _____
   Amount in bottle _____
   Drip rate _____
   Venipuncture site _____
7. **Drainage tubes**
   Type _____
   Attached to suction or drainage container _____
   Appearance and amount of drainage _____
8. **Patient position** _____
9. **Side rails** _____
10. **Pain**
    Type of analgesic _____
    Time last given _____
11. **Other discomforts** _____
    _____
    _____

Figure 46–14   A sample postoperative checklist

ASSESSMENT

Criteria for Antiemboli Stockings

Inadequate arterial blood circulation:

- Cool skin temperature in a warm environment
- Pallor
- Shiny taut skin
- Mild edema

Insufficient venous blood return:

- Thickening of the skin
- Increased pigmentation around the ankles
- Pitting edema (edema in which firm finger pressure on the skin produces an indentation, or pit, that remains for several seconds)
- Peripheral cyanosis

Posterior tibial and **dorsalis pedis pulses:** Rates, volumes, and rhythms (see Chapter 32).

Pain in the calf of the leg. The nurse dorsiflexes the client's foot abruptly and firmly while the client's knee is straight or slightly flexed to assess pain in the calf (Homan's sign). The presence of pain is a positive Homan's sign.

Distended superficial veins in the legs: Normally veins may appear distended in a dependent position but collapse when the limb is elevated.

The client should also be encouraged to do leg exercises every hour, or at least every 2 hours, during waking hours. Muscle contractions compress the veins, preventing the stasis of blood in the veins, a cause of thrombus formation and subsequent thrombophlebitis and emboli. See Table 46–4. Contractions also promote arterial blood flow.

The client should turn or be turned from side to side every 2 hours. Turning allows alternating maximum expansion of the uppermost lung. The nurse avoids placing pillows or rolls under the client's knees because pressure on the poplitcal blood vessels can slow the blood circulation to and from the lower extremities. The client should ambulate as soon as possible after surgery in accordance with the surgeon's orders. Generally, clients begin ambulation the evening of the day of surgery or the first day after surgery, unless the surgeon orders otherwise. Early ambulation prevents respiratory, circulatory, urinary, and gastrointestinal complications. It also prevents general muscle weakness. See Table 46–4. Ambulation should be scheduled for periods after the client has taken an analgesic, or when he or she is comfortable. If the client cannot ambulate, he or she should be periodically assisted to a sitting position in bed, if allowed, and turned frequently. The sitting position permits the greatest lung expansion.

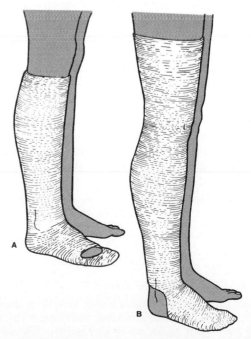

Figure 46–15   Two types of antiemboli stockings: **A,** extending to the knee, with an opening above the toes; **B,** extending to midthigh, with the heel exposed

Antiemboli (elastic) stockings are indicated for clients who have problems with circulation to their feet and legs. The elastic material compresses the veins of the legs and thereby facilitates the return of venous blood to the heart. These stockings are frequently applied preoperatively as well as postoperatively.

There are several types of stockings. One type extends from the foot to the knee and another from the foot to midthigh. These stockings usually have a partial foot that exposes either the heel or toes so that extremity circulation can be assessed. See Figure 46–15. Elastic stockings usually come in small, medium, and large sizes. The accompanying box summarizes the assessments the nurse should make before applying antiemboli stockings.

Procedure 46–4 describes how to measure and apply antiemboli stockings.

PROCEDURE 46–4

Measuring and Applying Antiemboli Stockings

Equipment

- Measuring tape
- Size chart
- Correct size of elastic stockings

Intervention

1. Assist the client to a lying position in bed. Stockings should be applied before a person arises.
   Rationale: The stockings should be donned before the veins become distended and edema occurs.

Measuring Knee-Length Stockings

2. Measure the circumference of the calf at the widest point, ie, 15 cm (6 in.) below the inferior aspect of the patella. See Figure 46–16.
3. Measure the length of the leg from the heel to the popliteal space. See Figure 46–17.

Measuring Thigh-Length Stockings

4. Measure the circumference of the calf as in step 3.
5. Measure the circumference of the thigh at the widest point, ie, 15 cm (6 in.) above the superior aspect of the patella. See Figure 46–18.
6. Measure the length of the leg from the heel to the gluteal fold. See Figure 46–19.

Measuring Waist-Length Stockings

7. Measure the circumference of the calf as in step 2.
8. Measure the circumference of the thigh as in step 5.
9. Measure the leg length from the bottom of the heel to the waist along the side of the body.

For All Types of Stockings

10. Compare the measurements to the size chart to obtain stockings of correct size.

Applying Elastic Stockings

11. Make sure the stocking is inside out; then grasp the foot and heel of the stocking, and invert the stocking over your hand, so as to turn the leg and foot portions inside out to the heel portion.

12. Remove your hand, and slip the foot portion of the stocking over the client's toes, foot, and heel. See Figure 46–20. Make sure the client's foot fits into the toe and heel portions of the stocking.

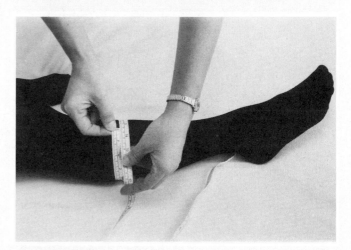

Figure 46–16

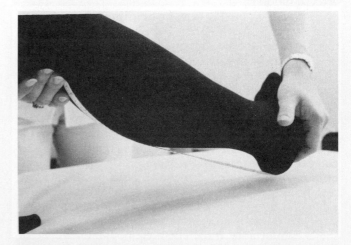

Figure 46–17

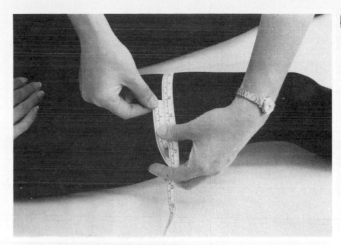

Figure 46–18

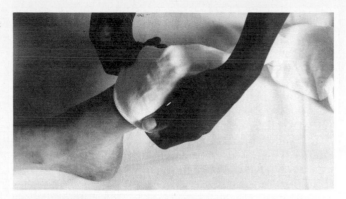

Figure 46–20

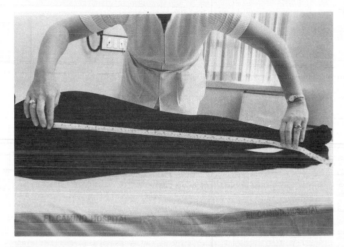

Figure 46–19

13. Pull the leg portion of the stocking over the foot and up the leg.

14. Pull the stocking up the leg evenly to its full length. Make sure there are no wrinkles or creases. Observe the lines in the material to make sure the stocking is not twisted.

    Rationale: Wrinkles and creases can irritate the skin and impede blood circulation.

15. Repeat for the other leg.

16. Inspect the stocking periodically to see that the top has not rolled and that the leg above the stocking is not swollen.

Removing a Stocking

17. Hold the top of the stocking with both hands and pull it down to the foot.

18. Supporting the foot at the ankle with one hand, pull the stocking over the foot and off.

19. Repeat for the other leg.

20. Document assessments and the time and application of the elastic stockings.

The nurse should maintain I.V. infusions as ordered. I.V. infusions are given to balance loss of body fluids during surgery (e.g., blood loss, perspiration, vomiting, and fasting). Only small sips of water should be offered to clients who can have fluids by mouth, until they establish tolerance. Large amounts of water can induce vomiting, since anesthetic agents and narcotic analgesics temporarily inhibit the motility of the stomach. Fluids are usually withheld postoperatively until peristalsis returns. Ice chips, if permitted, may be offered. The client who cannot take fluids by mouth is sometimes allowed to suck ice chips; the surgeon's orders should be checked. Mouth care should be provided, and a mouthwash should be placed at the client's bedside. Postoperative clients often complain of thirst and a dry, sticky mouth. These discomforts are a result of the preoperative fasting period, preoperative medications (such as atropine or scopolamine), and loss of body fluid.

The client's **fluid intake and output** should be measured for at least 2 days, or until fluid balance is stable without an I.V. It is important to ensure adequate fluid balance. Sufficient fluids keep the respiratory mucous membranes and secretions moist, thus facilitating the expectoration of mucus during coughing. Also, an adequate fluid balance prevents dehydration and the resulting concentration of the blood that, along with venous stasis, is conducive to thrombus formation.

The surgeon orders the client's **postoperative diet.** Depending on the extent of surgery and the organs involved, some clients may be given intravenous fluids and nothing by mouth for a few days, whereas others may progress from a diet of clear liquids to full fluids, to a light diet, and then to a regular diet within a few days, providing gastrointestinal functioning is normal. The return of peristalsis can be assessed by auscultating the abdomen. Gurgling and rumbling sounds indicate peristalsis (see Chapter 32). Anesthetic agents, narcotics, handling of the intestines during abdominal surgery, changes in fluid and food intake, and inactivity all inhibit peristalsis. Therefore, careful assessment for bowel sounds every 4–6 hours should be performed. Oral fluids and food are usually started after the return of peristalsis. The nurse may need to assist the client to eat if he or she is very weak. In addition, the nurse observes the client's tolerance of the food and fluids ingested.

The nurse may provide measures that **promote urinary elimination.** For example, the nurse helps male clients stand at the bedside, ensures that clients are free from pain, ensures that fluid intake is adequate, and helps clients walk. The nurse determines if the client has any difficulties voiding and assesses the client for bladder distention (see Chapter 41). The nurse reports to the surgeon if a client does not void within 8 hours following surgery unless another time frame is specified.

Anesthetic agents temporarily depress urinary bladder tone, which usually returns within 6 to 8 hours after surgery. Surgery in the pubic area, vagina, or rectum, during which the surgeon may manipulate the bladder, often causes urinary retention. If all measures to promote voiding fail, the physician usually orders urinary catheterization. See Chapter 41. The nurse measures the liquid intake and output of all clients with urinary cath-

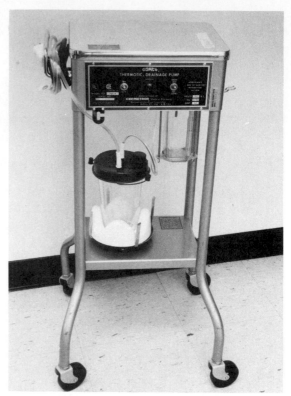

Figure 46–21 A Gomco thermotic pump.

ASSESSMENT

Ongoing Postoperative Guidelines

▪ **Acute pain.** Watch for pallor, perspiration, tension, and reluctance to perform deep-breathing and coughing exercises or to move or ambulate.

▪ Give analgesics *before* activities (e.g., ambulation or meals) or rest periods (e.g., at bedtime) and assess the effectiveness of the analgesics.

▪ **Do not assume** that the pain is caused by the incision (other causes: tight dressings, irritation from drainage tubes, or muscle strains resulting from positioning on the operating table).

▪ **Abdominal assessment.** Note and report the passage of flatus or abdominal distention.

▪ **Dressings.** Inspect regularly to ensure that they are clean, dry, and intact. Excessive drainage can indicate hemorrhage, infection, or dehiscence. See Table 46–4. Change dressings, using sterile technique as required, when they are soiled with drainage or in accordance with the surgeon's or nursing orders. (See Chapter 45.)

▪ **Wound separations.** Report promptly to the nurse in charge and the surgeon. If a large dehiscence or evisceration occurs, cover the wound with sterile, moist saline towels or dressings.

eters or other drainage devices. I & O records are kept for at least 2 days and until the client reestablishes fluid balance without a catheter in place.

Pain is usually greatest 12 to 36 hours after surgery, decreasing on the second or third day. Analgesics are usually administered every 3 or 4 hours the first day; by the third day most clients require only oral analgesics. Some may refuse to take analgesics on a regular schedule because they are not in severe pain. In this situation, the nurse assesses the need for analgesics (see Chapter 38) and, if indicated, informs the client that analgesics are most effective if given *before* pain becomes severe. The nurse also provides comfort measures to relax the client, e.g., back rubs, position changes, rest periods, and diverting activities, since tension increases pain perception and responses. Analgesics are given as ordered and as required. The accompanying box provides guidelines for ongoing postoperative assessment.

The manner in which **suction** is applied to drainage tubes depends on the type of equipment available in the agency and the amount of suction required. The following are the most commonly used:

1. *Portable electric motor suction.* Portable electric units are plugged into electric wall outlets. The units have an on-off switch, a motor that generates the negative pressure, and a drainage bottle. The bottle needs to be monitored regularly to prevent overflow of drainage into the motor, which can cause irreparable damage to the apparatus.

2. *Gomco thermotic pump.* The Gomco pump is electrically operated but consists of a pump rather than a motor. See Figure 46–21. It provides intermittent suction by alternating the air pressure, i.e., expanding and contracting the air. As the pressure alternates, red and green lights flash on and off. The amount of suction is regulated by a "high" or "low" pressure button. The pump is commonly used to suction gastrointestinal tubes.

3. *Wall suction.* In some agencies, wall suction units with piped-in negative pressure are available. These units consist of a suction pressure regulator and a drainage receptacle, which needs to be checked regularly to prevent overflow.

4. *Plastic bellows wound suction.* Plastic bellows suction equipment is commonly referred to as the *Hemovac,* or portable wound suction, since it is used to suction drainage from surgical wounds. See Procedure 45–5. Suction is created by manually compressing and releasing the sides of the apparatus.

Some clients return from surgery with a gastric or intestinal tube in place and orders to connect the tube to suction. The suction ordered can be continuous or intermittent. Intermittent suctioning is less likely to harm the mucous membrane lining near the tip of the suction tube. Procedure 46–5 details how to manage gastrointestinal suction.

PROCEDURE 46–5

Managing Gastrointestinal Suction

Equipment

Initiating and Maintaining Suction

- A gastrointestinal tube in place in the client. This may have been inserted prior to or following surgery (or prior to establishing the suction on a nonsurgical client). A Salem sump tube may be used rather than the standard single-lumen nasogastric tube. The Salem sump tube is a double-lumen tube usually made of plastic. The larger tube drains gastric contents; the smaller tube, referred to as an air vent or pigtail tube, allows for an inflow of atmospheric air. This continuous inflow of air prevents a vacuum if the gastric tube adheres to the wall of the stomach. Irritation of the gastric mucosa is thereby avoided.

- A suction device for either continuous or intermittent suction.

- A 50-ml syringe with an adapter to aspirate the stomach and the tube.

- A basin to collect the aspirated fluid.

- A connector to connect the gastrointestinal tube to the suction tubing.

- Connecting tubing.

- Cotton-tipped applicators.

- Ointment or lubricant to decrease irritation of the nostrils.

- A moisture-resistant pad.

Irrigating a Gastrointestinal Tube:

- A disposable irrigating set:
  1. A 50-ml syringe.
  2. A moisture-resistant pad.
  3. A basin to collect the irrigating solution.

  4. A graduated container.
  5. Sterile normal saline (500 ml) or the ordered solution.
  6. A stethoscope.

Intervention

1. Assess the client for
   a. Abdominal distention and discomfort by palpating.
   b. Bowel sounds by auscultating.
   c. Irritation of the nostril by the tube by inspecting the area.

Initiating Suction

2. Assist the client to the required position or to semi-Fowler's position if it is not contraindicated because of health.
   Rationale: In semi-Fowler's position the tube is not as likely to lie against the wall of the stomach and will therefore suction most efficiently. Semi-Fowler's position also prevents reflux of gastric contents, which could lead to aspiration.

3. Confirm that the tube is in the stomach by aspirating the stomach contents with the syringe and adapter. See Table 46–5.
   Rationale: The most accurate way to confirm the placement of the tube in the stomach is to withdraw stomach contents by using a syringe. Other methods listed in Table 46–5 are supplemental.

4. Set the suction at the recommended pressure and turn the suction on.
   a. Adjust the suction machine for the recommended suction pressure, in accordance with agency policy or the physician's order. Some suctions are preset and cannot be adjusted. If using a Gomco thermotic pump, the suction is usually set on intermittent "low" suction for a single-lumen nasogastric

tube or on "high" suction for a double-lumen naso-gastric tube (eg, Salem sump tube).

b. Turn on the suction machine, and check that the suction is working. The Gomco thermotic drainage pump has a red indicator light in the middle of the front panel; it blinks continuously when the machine is functioning. When using other suction machines, test for proper suctioning by holding the open end of the suction tube to the nurse's ear. Proper suctioning is confirmed by a sucking noise.

5. Connect the gastrointestinal tube to the tubing from the suction by using the connector.

6. Watch the tubing for a few minutes until the gastric contents appear to be running through the tubing into the receptacle.

7. If the suction is not working properly, check that the rubber stopper in the collection bottle and all tubing connections are tightly sealed and that the tubing is not kinked.

8. Coil and pin the tubing on the bed so that it does not loop below the suction bottle.
Rationale: If the tubing falls below the suction bottle, the suction may be obstructed because of the pressure required to push the fluid against gravity.

9. If the gastrointestinal tube has an air vent, place it beside or above the client's head. If the vent becomes blocked with gastric contents, inject 10 ml of air with a syringe to clear the vent.
Rationale: If the vent is below the client's head, ie, in a dependent position, the gastric contents can flow into the vent and block it.

10. Assess the amount, color, odor, and consistency of the drainage. Normal gastric drainage has a mucoid consistency and is either colorless or yellow-green because of the presence of bile. A coffee-grounds color and consistency may indicate bleeding. Test the gastric drainage for pH and blood (by using Hematest) when indicated. A person who has had gastrointestinal surgery can be expected to have some blood in the drainage.

11. Document initiating the suction and the time. Also record the pressure established, the color and consistency of the drainage, and nursing assessments.

Sample Recording

Date	Time	Notes
9/18/89	1400	Suction initiated 100 mm Hg. Returns watery, bright red. Abdomen firm and slightly distended. Bowel sounds are irregular and high pitched.————————————Molly Jones, RN

Maintaining Suction

12. Assess the client regularly (every 30 minutes until the system is running effectively and then every 2 hours) to ensure that the suction is functioning properly. If the client complains of fullness, nausea, or epigastric pain or if the flow of gastric secretions is absent in the tubing or the collection bottle, ineffective suctioning or blockage of the nasogastric tube is likely.

13. Inspect the suction system for patency of the system, eg, kinks or blockages in the tubing, and tightness of the connections.
Rationale: Loose connections can permit air to enter and thus decrease the effectiveness of the suction by decreasing the negative pressure.

14. To relieve blockages:
a. Milk the suction tubing.
b. Check the suction equipment. To do this, disconnect the nasogastric tube from the suction over a collecting basin (to collect gastric drainage), and then, with the suction on, place the end of the suction tubing in a basin of water. If water is drawn into the drainage bottle, the suction equipment is functioning properly, but the nasogastric tube is either blocked or positioned incorrectly.
c. Reposition the client, eg, to the other side, if permitted. This may facilitate drainage.
d. Rotate the nasogastric tube and reposition it. This step is contraindicated for clients with gastric surgery because moving the tube may interfere with gastric sutures.
e. Irrigate the nasogastric tube as agency policy advocates or on the order of the physician. See steps 21–32 later in this procedure.

15. Clean the client's nostrils every 3 hours or as needed, using the cotton-tipped applicators and water. Apply a water-soluble lubricant or ointment.

16. Provide mouth care every 3 hours or as needed. See Procedure 34–8. Some postoperative clients are permitted to suck ice chips or a moist cloth to maintain the moisture of the oral mucosa.

17. Check the drainage bottle regularly to ensure that it does not overflow.

18. Empty the drainage receptacle every 8 hours or whenever it becomes three-quarters full. To empty it:
a. Clamp the nasogastric tube and turn off the suction.
b. If the receptacle is graduated, determine the amount of drainage.
c. Disconnect the receptacle.
d. If not already measured, empty the contents into a graduated container and measure.
e. Inspect the drainage carefully for color, consistency, and presence of substances, eg, blood clots.
f. Rinse the receptacle with warm water.
g. Reattach the receptacle to the suction.
h. Turn on the suction and unclamp the nasogastric tube.
i. Observe the system for several minutes to make sure function is reestablished.

19. Encourage the client to turn from side to side and ambulate when permitted. For ambulation:
a. Turn off the suction.

b. Disconnect the gastrointestinal tube from the connector.

c. Clamp the gastrointestinal tube, and attach it to the client's gown. See Procedure 46–2, steps 15–16. Some agencies use a catheter plug, which is inserted into the lumen of the tube.

d. Ambulate the client.

e. Reestablish the suction after the client returns to bed.

20. Document assessments, supportive nursing measures, and data about the suction system.

Sample Recording

Date	Time	Notes
10/7/89	0800	250 ml light brown thick drainage. No complaints of pain. Bowel sounds hyperactive, increased pitch. Abdomen soft upon palpation. No irritation in nostrils. Nostrils cleaned with water and lubricant applied. Vital signs q.2h. BP 140/80, P 90, R 18 and stable.————R. Woo, NS

Irrigating a Gastrointestinal Tube

Nasogastric tubes are generally irrigated (a) before and after the instillation of medications, (b) before and after tube feedings, and (c) as ordered to prevent clogging. Check agency policies and practices. Nasogastric irrigation may require a physician's order. Excessive irrigation can lead to metabolic alkalosis.

21. Place the moisture-resistant pad under the end of the gastrointestinal tube.

22. Turn off the suction.

23. Disconnect the gastrointestinal tube from the connector.

24. Determine that the tube is in the stomach by using a syringe to aspirate gastric contents. If no contents can be aspirated, inject 10 ml of air while listening with a stethoscope over the epigastric region. See Table 46–5.

Rationale: This ensures that the irrigating solution enters the stomach.

25. Draw up the ordered volume of irrigating solution in the syringe; 30 ml of solution per instillation is usual, but up to 60 ml may be given per instillation if ordered.

26. Attach the syringe to the nasogastric tube and *slowly* inject the solution.

27. Gently aspirate the solution.
Rationale: Forceful withdrawal could damage the gastric mucosa.

28. If the nurse encounters difficulty in withdrawing the solution, inject 20 ml of air and aspirate again, and/or reposition the client or the nasogastric tube.
Rationale: Air and repositioning may move the end of the tube away from the stomach wall. If aspirating difficulty continues, reattach the tube to intermittent low suction and notify the nurse in charge or physician.

29. Repeat steps 25–27 until the ordered amount of solution is used.

30. Reconnect the nasogastric tube to suction. If a Salem sump tube is used, inject the air vent lumen with 10 ml of air after reconnecting the tube to suction.

31. Observe the system for several minutes to make sure it is functioning.

32. Document verification of tube placement; the time of the irrigation; the amount and type of irrigating solution used; the amount, color, and consistency of the returns; the patency of the system following the irrigation; and nursing assessments.

Sample Recording

Date	Time	Notes
9/19/89	1600	Tube placement confirmed by injecting 10 ml air. Tube irrigated with 30 ml normal saline × 2. 30 ml × 2 returns cloudy, pink with small clots. Suction running with drainage noted. Abdomen soft, no discomfort, vital signs stable.————R. Woo NS

Evaluating Client Responses

Examples of outcome criteria for a postoperative client are shown in the box on page 863.

Chapter Highlights

▪ The perioperative period includes three phases: preoperative, intraoperative, and postoperative.

▪ Nurses should assess the risk factors prior to a client's surgery whenever possible.

▪ Nursing history data are an important source for planning preoperative and postoperative care.

▪ The surgical excision of a part of the body may affect a client's self-image.

▪ Preoperative teaching should include moving, leg exercises, and coughing and deep-breathing exercises.

OUTCOME CRITERIA

Perioperative Clients

The client will:

- **Carry out** leg exercises every 4 hours as instructed
- **Turn** from side to side in bed independently
- **Cough** and deep breathe every 2 hours as instructed
- **Walk** to the end of the corridor each morning, with assistance
- **Have** normal vital signs
- **Have** no abdominal distention

Many aspects of preoperative teaching are intended to prevent postoperative complications.

Antiemboli stockings are intended to facilitate venous blood return.

A preoperative checklist provides a guide and documentation of a client's preparation before surgery.

A postoperative initial assessment checklist provides the nurse with a concise guide.

Nurses may need to set up a gastric suction postoperatively.

Selected References

Association of Operating Room Nurses. 1986. *AORN standards and recommended practices for perioperative nursing.* Denver: Association of Operating Room Nurses, Inc.

Blackwood, S. January 1986. Back to basics: The preop exam. *American Journal of Nursing* 86:39–44.

Drain, C. B. August 1984. Managing postoperative pain . . . It's a matter of sighs. *Nursing 84* 14:52–55.

Erickson, R. July 1982. Tube talk principles of fluid flow in tubes. *Nursing 82* 12:54–61.

Garner, J. S. April 1986. CDC guidelines for the prevention and control of nosocomial infections: Guideline for prevention of surgical wound infections, 1985. *American Journal of Infection Control* 14:71–80.

Kneedler, J. A., and Dodge, G. H. 1983. *Perioperative patient care.* Boston: Blackwell Scientific Publications, Inc.

LeMaitre, G. D., and Finnegan, J. A. 1980. *The patient in surgery: A guide for nurses.* 4th ed. Philadelphia: W. B. Saunders.

Luciano, K. November 1974. The who, when, where, what and how of preparing children for surgery. *Nursing 74* 4:64–65.

McConnell, E. A. March 1977a. After surgery. *Nursing 77* 7:32–39.

Mogan, J.; Wells, N.; Robertson, E. 1985. Effects of preoperative teaching on postoperative pain: A replication and expansion. *International Journal of Nursing Studies* 22(3):267–80.

Montanari, J. August 1985. Documenting your postop assessment findings. *Nursing 85* 15:31–35.

Northrop, C. 1984. Legal aspects of nursing. In McCann Flynn, J. B., and Heffron, P. B., editors. *Nursing: From concept to practice.* Bowie, Md.: Robert J. Brady Co.

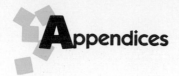

Appendices

Contents

Appendix A
Rights of Special Groups

Appendix A–1   Declaration on the Rights of Disabled Persons

1. The term "disabled person" means any person unable to ensure by himself or herself wholly or partly the necessities of a normal individual and/or social life, as a result of a deficiency, either congenital or not, in his or her physical or mental capabilities.

2. Disabled persons shall enjoy all the rights set forth in this Declaration. These rights shall be granted to all disabled persons without any exception whatsoever and without distinction or discrimination on the basis of race, colour, sex, language, religion, political or other opinions, national or social origin, state of wealth, birth or any other situation applying either to the disabled person himself or herself or to his or her family.

3. Disabled persons have the inherent right to respect for their human dignity. Disabled persons, whatever the origin, nature and seriousness of their handicaps and disabilities, have the same fundamental rights as their fellow-citizens of the same age, which implies first and foremost the right to enjoy a decent life, as normal and full as possible.

4. Disabled persons have the same civil and political rights as other human beings; article 7 of the Declaration of the Rights of Mentally Retarded Persons applies to any possible limitation or suppression of those rights for mentally disabled persons.

5. Disabled persons are entitled to the measures designed to enable them to become as self-reliant as possible.

6. Disabled persons have the right to medical, psychological and functional treatment, including prosthetic and orthetic appliances, to medical and social rehabilitation, education, vocational education, training and rehabilitation, aid, counselling, placement services and other services which will enable them to develop their capabilities and skills to the maximum and will hasten the process of their social integration or reintegration.

7. Disabled persons have the right to economic and social security and to a decent level of living. They have the right, according to their capabilities, to secure and retain employment or to engage in a useful, productive and remunerative occupation and to join trade unions.

8. Disabled persons are entitled to have their special needs taken into consideration at all stages of economic and social planning.

9. Disabled persons have the right to live with their families or with foster parents and to participate in all social, creative or recreational activities. No disabled person shall be subjected, as far as his or her residence is concerned, to differential treatment other than that required by his or her condition or by the improvement which he or she may derive therefrom. If the stay of a disabled person in a specialized establishment is indispensable, the environment and living conditions therein shall be as close as possible to those of the normal life of a person of his or her age.

10. Disabled persons shall be protected against all exploitation, all regulations and all treatment of a discriminatory, abusive and degrading nature.

11. Disabled persons shall be able to avail themselves of qualified legal aid when such aid proves indispensable for the protection of their persons or property. If judicial proceedings are instituted against them, the legal procedures applied shall take their physical and mental condition fully into account.

12. Organizations of disabled persons may be usefully consulted in all matters regarding the rights of disabled persons.

13. Disabled persons, their families and communities shall be fully informed, by all appropriate means, of the rights contained in this Declaration.

Adopted by the General Assembly of the United Nations, December 1975.

Appendix A–2 The Dying Person's Bill of Rights

- I have the right to be treated as a living human being until I die.

- I have the right to maintain a sense of hopefulness however changing its focus may be.

- I have the right to be cared for by those who can maintain a sense of hopefulness, however changing this might be.

- I have the right to express my feelings and emotions about my approaching death in my own way.

- I have the right to participate in decisions concerning my care.

- I have the right to expect continuing medical and nursing attention even though "cure" goals must be changed to "comfort" goals.

- I have the right not to die alone.

- I have the right to be free from pain.

- I have the right to have my questions answered honestly.

- I have the right not to be deceived.

- I have the right to have help from and for my family in accepting my death.

- I have the right to die in peace and dignity.

- I have the right to retain my individuality and not be judged for my decisions which may be contrary to beliefs of others.

- I have the right to discuss and enlarge my religious and/or spiritual experiences, whatever these may mean to others.

- I have the right to expect that the sanctity of the human body will be respected after death.

- I have the right to be cared for by caring, sensitive, knowledgeable people who will attempt to understand my needs and will be able to gain some satisfaction in helping me face my death.

From Amelia J. Barbus, The dying person's bill of rights, *American Journal of Nursing,* January 1975, 75:99.

Appendix A–3 Declaration on the Rights of Mentally Retarded Persons

1. The mentally retarded person has, to the maximum degree of feasibility, the same rights as other human beings.

2. The mentally retarded person has a right to proper medical care and physical therapy and to such education, training, rehabilitation and guidance as will enable him to develop his ability and maximum potential.

3. The mentally retarded person has a right to economic security and to a decent standard of living. He has a right to perform productive work or to engage in any meaningful occupation to the fullest possible extent of his capabilities.

4. Whenever possible, the mentally retarded person should live with his own family or with foster parents and participate in different forms of community life. The family with which he lives should receive assistance. If care in an institution becomes necessary, it should be provided in surroundings and other circumstances as close as possible to those of normal life.

5. The mentally retarded person has a right to a qualified guardian when this is required to protect his personal well-being and interests.

6. The mentally retarded person has a right to protection from exploitation, abuse and degrading treatment. If prosecuted for any offence, he shall have a right to due process of law with full recognition being given to his degree of mental responsibility.

7. Whenever mentally retarded persons are unable, because of the severity of their handicap, to exercise all their rights in a meaningful way or it should become necessary to restrict or deny some or all of these rights, the procedure used for that restriction or denial of rights must contain proper legal safeguards against every form of abuse. This procedure must be based on an evaluation of the social capability of the mentally retarded person by qualified experts and must be subject to periodic review and to the right of appeal to higher authorities.

Adopted by the General Assembly of the United Nations, December 1971.

▪ **A**ppendix A–4 United Nations Declaration of the Rights of the Child

Preamble

Whereas the peoples of the United Nations have, in the Charter, reaffirmed their faith in fundamental human rights, and in the dignity and worth of the human person, and have determined to promote social progress and better standards of life in larger freedom,

Whereas the United Nations has, in the Universal Declaration of Human Rights, proclaimed that everyone is entitled to all the rights and freedoms set forth therein, without distinction of any kind, such as race, colour, sex, language, religion, political or other opinion, national or social origin, property, birth or other status,

Whereas the child, by reason of his physical and mental immaturity, needs special safeguards and care, including appropriate legal protection, before as well as after birth,

Whereas the need for such special safeguards has been stated in the Geneva Declaration of the Rights of the Child of 1924, and recognized in the Universal Declaration of Human Rights and in the statues of specialized agencies and international organizations concerned with the welfare of children,

Whereas mankind owes to the child the best it has to give,

Now therefore,

The General Assembly

Proclaims this Declaration of the Rights of the Child to the end that he may have a happy childhood and enjoy for his own good and for the good of society the rights and freedoms herein set forth, and calls upon parents, upon men and women as individuals, and upon voluntary organizations, local authorities and national Governments to recognize these rights and strive for their observance by legislative and other measures progressively taken in accordance with the following principles:

Principle 1

The child shall enjoy all the rights set forth in this Declaration. Every child, without any exception whatsoever, shall be entitled to these rights, without distinction or discrimination on account of race, colour, sex, language, religion, political or other opinion, national or social origin, property, birth or other status, whether of himself or of his family.

Principle 2

The child shall enjoy special protection, and shall be given opportunities and facilities, by law and by other means, to enable him to develop physically, mentally, morally, spiritually and socially in a healthy and normal manner and in conditions of freedom and dignity. In the enactment of laws for this purpose, the best interests of the child shall be the paramount consideration.

Principle 3

The child shall be entitled from his birth to a name and a nationality.

Principle 4

The child shall enjoy the benefits of social security. He shall be entitled to grow and develop in health; to this end, special care and protection shall be provided both to him and to his mother, including adequate pre-natal and post-natal care. The child shall have the right to adequate nutrition, housing, recreation and medical services.

Principle 5

The child who is physically, mentally or socially handicapped shall be given the special treatment, education and care required by his particular condition.

Principle 6

The child, for the full and harmonious development of his personality, needs love and understanding. He shall, whenever possible, grow up in the care and under the responsibility of his parents, and, in any case, in an atmosphere of affection and of moral and material security; a child of tender years shall not, save in exceptional circumstances, be separated from his mother. Society and the public authorities shall have the duty to extend particular care to children without a family and to those without adequate means of support. Payment of State and other assistance towards the maintenance of children of large families is desirable.

Principle 7

The child is entitled to receive education, which shall be free and compulsory, at least in the elementary stages. He shall be given an education which will promote his general culture, and enable him, on a basis of equal opportunity, to develop his abilities, his individual judgement, and his sense of moral and social responsibility, and to become a useful member of society.

The best interests of the child shall be the guiding principle of those responsible for his education and guidance; that responsibility lies in the first place with his parents.

The child shall have full opportunity for play and recreation, which should be directed to the same purposes as education; society and the public authorities shall endeavour to promote the enjoyment of this right.

Principle 8

The child shall in all circumstances be among the first to receive protection and relief.

Principle 9

The child shall be protected against all forms of neglect, cruelty and exploitation. He shall not be the subject of traffic, in any form.

The child shall not be admitted to employment before an appropriate minimum age; he shall in no case be caused or permitted to engage in any occupation or employment which would prejudice his health or education, or interfere with his physical, mental or moral development.

Principle 10

The child shall be protected from practices which may foster racial, religious and any other form of discrimination. He shall be brought up in a spirit of understanding, tolerance, friendship among peoples, peace and universal brotherhood and in full consciousness that his energy and talents should be devoted to the service of his fellow men.

Adopted by the General Assembly of the United Nations, November 20, 1959.

▪ Appendix A–5 The Pregnant Patient's Bill of Rights

1. The Pregnant Patient has the right, prior to the administration of any drug or procedure, to be informed by the health professional caring for her of any potential direct or indirect effects, risks or hazards to herself or her unborn or newborn infant which may result from the use of a drug or procedure prescribed for or administered to her during pregnancy, labor, birth or lactation.

2. The Pregnant Patient has the right, prior to the proposed therapy, to be informed, not only of the benefits, risks and hazards of the proposed therapy but also of known alternative therapy, such as available childbirth education classes which could help to prepare the Pregnant Patient physically and mentally to cope with the discomfort or stress of pregnancy and the experience of childbirth, thereby reducing or eliminating her need for drugs and obstetric intervention. She should be offered such information early in her pregnancy in order that she may make a reasoned decision.

3. The Pregnant Patient has the right, prior to the administration of any drug, to be informed by the health professional who is prescribing or administering the drug to her that any drug which she receives during pregnancy, labor and birth, no matter how or when the drug is taken or administered may adversely affect her unborn baby, directly or indirectly, and that there is no drug or chemical which has been proven safe for the unborn child.

4. The Pregnant Patient has the right if cesarean section is anticipated, to be informed prior to the adminis-

tration of any drug, and preferably prior to her hospitalization, that minimizing her and in turn, her baby's intake of nonessential preoperative medicine will benefit her baby.

5. The Pregnant Patient has the right, prior to the administration of a drug or procedure, to be informed of the areas of uncertainty if there is no properly controlled follow-up research which has established the safety of the drug or procedure with regard to its direct and/or indirect effects on the physiological, mental and neurological development of the child exposed, via the mother, to the drug or procedure during pregnancy, labor, birth or lactation (this would apply to virtually all drugs and the vast majority of obstetric procedures).

6. The Pregnant Patient has the right, prior to the administration of any drug, to be informed of the brand name and generic name of the drug in order that she may advise the health professional of any past adverse reaction to the drug.

7. The Pregnant Patient has the right to determine for herself, without pressure from her attendant, whether she will accept the risks inherent in the proposed therapy or refuse a drug or procedure.

8. The Pregnant Patient has the right to know the name and qualifications of the individual administering a medication or procedure to her during labor or birth.

9. The Pregnant Patient has the right to be informed, prior to the administration of any procedure, whether that procedure is being administered to her for her

or her baby's benefit (medically indicated) or as an elective procedure (for convenience, teaching purposes or research).

10. The Pregnant Patient has the right to be accompanied during the stress of labor and birth by someone she cares for, and to whom she looks for emotional comfort and encouragement.

11. The Pregnant Patient has the right after appropriate medical consultation to choose a position for labor and for birth which is least stressful to her baby and to herself.

12. The Obstetric Patient has the right to have her baby cared for at her bedside if her baby is normal, and to feed her baby according to her baby's needs rather than according to the hospital regimen.

13. The Obstetric Patient has the right to be informed in writing of the name of the person who actually delivered her baby and the professional qualifications of that person. This information should also be on the birth certificate.

14. The Obstetric Patient has the right to be informed if there is any known or indicated aspect of her or her baby's care or condition which may cause her or her baby later difficulty or problems.

15. The Obstetric Patient has the right to have her and her baby's hospital medical records complete, accurate and legible and to have their records, including Nurses' Notes, retained by the hospital until the child reaches at least the age of majority, or alternatively, to have the records offered to her before they are destroyed.

16. The Obstetric Patient, both during and after her hospital stay, has the right to have access to her complete hospital medical records, including Nurses' Notes, and to receive a copy upon payment of a reasonable fee and without incurring the expense of retaining an attorney.

It is the obstetric patient and her baby, not the health professional, who must sustain any trauma or injury resulting from the use of a drug or obstetric procedure. The observation of the rights listed above will not only permit the obstetric patient to participate in the decisions involving her and her baby's health care, but will help to protect the health professional and the hospital against litigation arising from resentment or misunderstanding on the part of the mother.

Written by Doris B. Haire, published by the International Childbirth Education Association.

Appendix B Root Words, Prefixes, and Suffixes

Word element	Meaning	Word element	Meaning
		reni, reno, nephro	kidney
		pyelo	pelvis of kidney
		uro	urine

ROOT WORDS

Circulatory system

cardio	heart
angio, vaso	vessel
hem, hema, hemato	blood
vena, phlebo	vein
arteria	artery
lympho	lymph
thrombo	clot (of blood)
embolus	moving clot

Digestive system

bucca	cheek
os, stomato	mouth
gingiva	gum
glossa	tongue
pharyngo	pharynx
esophago	esophagus
gastro	stomach
hepato	liver
cholecyst	gallbladder
pancreas	pancreas
entero	intestines
duodeno	duodenum
jejuno	jejunum
ileo	ileum
caeco	cecum
appendeco	appendix
colo	colon
recto	rectum
ano, procto	anus

Skeletal system

skeleto	skeleton

Respiratory system

naso, rhino	nose
tonsillo	tonsil
laryngo	larynx
tracheo	trachea
bronchus, broncho	bronchus (pl. bronchi)
pulmo, pneuma, pneum	lung (sac with air)

Nervous system

neuro	nerve
cerebrum	brain
oculo, ophthalmo	eye
oto	ear
psych, psycho	mind

Urinary system

urethro	urethra
cysto	bladder
uretero	ureter

Female reproductive system

vulvo	vulva
perineo	perineum
labio	labium (pl. labia)
vagino, colpo	vagina
cervico	cervix
utero	womb; uterus
tubo, salpingo	fallopian tube
ovario, oophoro	ovary

Male reproductive system

orchido	testes

Regions of the body

crani, cephalo	head
cervico, tracheo	neck
thoraco	chest
abdomino	abdomen
dorsum	back

Tissues

cutis, dermato	skin
lipo	fat
musculo, myo	muscle
osteo	bone
myelo	marrow
chondro	cartilage

Miscellaneous

cyto	cell
genetic	formation, origin
gram	tracing or mark
graph	writing, description
kinesis	motion
meter	measure
oligo	small, few
phobia	fear
photo	light
pyo	pus
scope	instrument for visual examination
roentgen	x-ray
lapar	flank; through the abdominal wall

PREFIXES

a, an, ar	without or not
ab	away from
acro	extremities
ad	toward, to
adeno	glandular

Word element	Meaning	Word element	Meaning
aero	air	medio	middle
ambi	around, on both sides	mega, megalo	large, great
amyl	starch	meno	menses
ante	before, forward	mono	single
anti	against, counteracting	multi	many
bi	double	myelo	bone marrow, spinal cord
bili	bile	myo	muscle
bio	life	neo	new
bis	two	nephro	kidney
brachio	arm	neuro	nerve
brady	slow	nitro	nitrogen
broncho	bronchus (pl. bronchi)	noct	night
cardio	heart	non	not
cervico	neck	ob	against, in front of
chole	gall or bile	oculo	eye
cholecysto	gallbladder	odonto	tooth
circum	around	ophthalmo	eye
co	together	ortho	straight, normal
contra	against, opposite	os	mouth, bone
costo	ribs	osteo	bone
cyto	cell	oto	ear
cysto	bladder	pan	all
demi	half	para	beside, accessory to
derma	skin	path	disease
dis	from	ped	child, foot
dorso	back	per	by, through
dys	abnormal, difficult	peri	around
electro	electric	pharyngo	pharynx
en	into, in, within	phlebo	vein
encephal	brain	photo	light
entero	intestine	phren	diaphragm, mind
equi	equal	pneumo	air, lungs
eryth	red	pod	foot
ex	out, out of, away from	poly	many, much
extra	outside of, in addition to	post	after
ferro	iron	pre	before
fibro	fiber	proct	rectum
fore	before, in front of	pseudo	false
gastro	stomach	psych	mind
glosso	tongue	pyel	pelvis of the kidney
glyco	sugar	pyo	pus
hemi	half	pyro	fever, heat
hemo	blood	quadri	four
hepa, hepato	liver	radio	radiation
histo	tissue	re	back, again
homo	same	reno	kidney
hydro	water	retro	backward
hygro	moisture	rhin	nose
hyper	too much, high	sacro	sacrum
hypo	under, decreased	salpingo	fallopian tube
hyster	uterus	sarco	flesh
ileo	ileum	sclero	hard, hardening
in	in, within, into	semi	half
inter	between	sex	six
intra	within	skeleto	skeleton
intro	in, within, into	steno	narrowing, constriction
juxta	near, close to	sub	under
laryngo	larynx	super	above, excess
latero	side	supra	above
lapar	abdomen	syn	together
leuk	white	tachy	fast
macro	large, big	thyro	thyroid, gland
mal	bad, poor	trache	trachea
mast	breast	trans	across, over

Word element	Meaning	Word element	Meaning
tri	three	itis	inflammation
ultra	beyond	ize	to treat
un	not, back, reversal	lith	stone, calculus
uni	one	lithiasis	presence of stones
uretero	ureter	lysis	disintegration
urethro	urethra	megaly	enlargement
uro	urine, urinary organs	meter	instrument that measures
vaso	vessel	oid	likeness, resemblance
		oma	tumor
SUFFIXES		opathy	disease of
		orrhaphy	surgical repair
able	able to	osis	disease, condition of
algia	pain	ostomy	to form an opening or outlet
cele	tumor, swelling	otomy	to incise
centesis	surgical puncture to remove fluid	pexy	fixation
		phage	ingesting
cide	killing, destructive	phobia	fear
cule	little	plasty	plastic surgery
cyte	cell	plegia	paralysis
ectasia	dilating, stretching	rhage	to burst forth
ectomy	excision, surgical removal of	rhea	excessive discharge
emia	blood	rhexis	rupture
esis	action	scope	lighted instrument for visual examination
form	shaped like		
genesis, genetic	formation, origin	scopy	to examine visually
gram	tracing, mark	stomy	to form an opening
graph	writing	tomy	incision into
ism	condition	uria	urine

Sources: Courtesy of Margaret Ling, Director of Vocational Nursing, Santa Rosa Junior College, Santa Rosa, Calif.; B Kozier, G Erb: *Fundamentals of Nursing: Concepts and Procedures,* 3d ed., Addison-Wesley, 1987. Used by permission.

Appendix C Canada's Food Guide (1983)

Variety.   Choose different kinds of foods from within each group in appropriate numbers of servings and portion sizes.

Energy balance.   Needs vary with age, sex, and activity. Balance energy intake from foods with energy output from physical activity to control weight. Foods selected according to the Guide can supply 1000–1400 kilo-calories. For additional energy, increase the number and size of servings from the various foods groups and/or add other foods.

Moderation.   Select and prepare foods with limited amounts of fat, sugar and salt. If alcohol is consumed, use limited amounts.

Food group	Recommended number of servings (adults)	Some examples of one serving
Milk and milk products	2[a]	1 cup milk; ¾ cup yogurt; 1½ oz cheddar or process cheese
Meat, fish, poultry, and alternates	2	2–3 oz cooked lean meat, fish, poultry, or liver; 4 T peanut butter; 1 cup cooked dried peas, beans, or lentils; ½ cup nuts or seeds; 2 oz cheddar cheese; ½ cup cottage cheese; 2 eggs
Breads and cereals[b]	3–5	1 slice bread; ½ cup cooked cereal; ¾ cup ready-to-eat cereal; 1 roll or muffin; ½–¾ cup cooked rice, macaroni, spaghetti or noodles; ½ hamburger or wiener bun
Fruits and vegetables	4–5[c]	½ cup vegetables or fruits—fresh, frozen, or canned; ½ cup juice—fresh, frozen, or canned; 1 medium-sized potato, carrot, tomato, peach, apple, orange, or banana

[a]For children up to 11 years, 2–3 servings; adolescents, 3–4 servings; pregnant and nursing women, 3–4 servings.

[b]Whole grain or enriched. Whole grain products are recommended.

[c]Include at least two vegetables. Choose a variety of both vegetables and fruits—cooked, raw, or their juices. Include yellow, green, or green leafy vegetables.

Source: Minister of National Health and Welfare, Ottawa. Reproduced by permission of the Minister of Supply and Services Canada.

Appendix D   Recommended Daily Dietary Allowances (revised 1980)

Food and Nutrition Board, National Academy of Sciences—National Research Council Recommended Daily Dietary Allowances,[a] (revised 1980)*

	Age (years)	Weight (kg)	Weight (lb)	Height (cm)	Height (in)	Protein (g)	Fat-Soluble Vitamins Vitamin A (μg RE)[b]	Vitamin D (μg)[c]	Vitamin E (mg α-TE)[d]
Infants	0.0–0.5	6	13	60	24	kg × 2.2	420	10	3
	0.5—1.0	9	20	71	28	kg × 2.0	400	10	4
Children	1–3	13	29	90	35	23	400	10	5
	4–6	20	44	112	44	30	500	10	6
	7–10	28	62	132	52	34	700	10	7
Males	11–14	45	99	157	62	45	1000	10	8
	15–18	66	145	176	69	56	1000	10	10
	19–22	70	154	177	70	56	1000	7.5	10
	23–50	70	154	178	70	56	1000	5	10
	51 +	70	154	178	70	56	1000	5	10
Females	11–14	46	101	157	62	46	800	10	8
	15–18	55	120	163	64	46	800	10	8
	19–22	55	120	163	64	44	800	7.5	8
	23–50	55	120	163	64	44	800	5	8
	51 +	55	120	163	64	44	800	5	8
Pregnant						+30	+200	+5	+2
Lactating						+20	+400	+5	+3

*Designed for the maintenance of good nutrition of practically all healthy people in the U.S.A.

[a]The allowances are intended to provide for individual variations among most normal persons as they live in the United States under usual environmental stresses. Diets should be based on a variety of common foods in order to provide other nutrients for which human requirements have been less well defined.

[b]Retinol equivalents. 1 retinol equivalent = 1 μg retinol or 6 μg β carotene.

[c]As cholecalciferol. μg cholecalciferol = 400 IU of vitamin D.

[d]α-tocopherol equivalents. 1 mg d-α tocopherol = 1 α-TE.

[e]1 NE (niacin equivalent) is equal to 1 mg of niacin or 60 mg of dietary tryptophan.

Water-Soluble Vitamins							Minerals					
Vitamin C (mg)	Thiamin (mg)	Riboflavin (mg)	Niacin (mg NE)[e]	Vitamin B-6 (mg)	Folacin[f] (μg)	Vitamin B-12 (μg)	Calcium (mg)	Phosphorus (mg)	Magnesium (mg)	Iron (mg)	Zinc (mg)	Iodine (μg)
35	0.3	0.4	6	0.3	30	0.5[g]	360	240	50	10	3	40
35	0.5	0.6	8	0.6	45	1.5	540	360	70	15	5	50
45	0.7	0.8	9	0.9	100	2.0	800	800	150	15	10	70
45	0.9	1.0	11	1.3	200	2.5	800	800	200	10	10	90
45	1.2	1.4	16	1.6	300	3.0	800	800	250	10	10	120
50	1.4	1.6	18	1.8	400	3.0	1200	1200	350	18	15	150
60	1.4	1.7	18	2.0	400	3.0	1200	1200	400	18	15	150
60	1.5	1.7	19	2.2	400	3.0	800	800	350	10	15	150
60	1.4	1.6	18	2.2	400	3.0	800	800	350	10	15	150
60	1.2	1.4	16	2.2	400	3.0	800	800	350	10	15	150
50	1.1	1.3	15	1.8	400	3.0	1200	1200	300	18	15	150
60	1.1	1.3	14	2.0	400	3.0	1200	1200	300	18	15	150
60	1.1	1.3	14	2.0	400	3.0	800	800	300	18	15	150
60	1.0	1.2	13	2.0	400	3.0	800	800	300	18	15	150
60	1.0	1.2	13	2.0	400	3.0	800	800	300	10	15	150
+20	+0.4	+0.3	+2	+0.6	+400	+1.0	+400	+400	+150	h	+5	+25
+40	+0.5	+0.5	+5	+0.5	+100	+1.0	+400	+400	+150	h	+10	+50

[f]The folacin allowances refer to dietary sources as determined by *Lactobacillus casei* assay after treatment with enzymes (conjugases) to make polyglutamyl forms of the vitamin available to the test organism.

[g]The recommended dietary allowance for vitamin B-12 in infants is based on average concentration of the vitamin in human milk. The allowances after weaning are based on energy intake (as recommended by the American Academy of Pediatrics) and consideration of other factors, such as intestinal absorption.

[h]The increased requirement during pregnancy cannot be met by the iron content of habitual American diets nor by the existing iron stores of many women; therefore the use of 30–60 mg of supplemental iron is recommended. Iron needs during lactation are not substantially different from those of nonpregnant women, but continued supplementation of the mother for 2–3 months after parturition is advisable in order to replenish stores depleted by pregnancy.

Source: Committee on Dietary Allowances Food and Nutrition Board, National Research Council, National Academy of Sciences. Washington, D.C.: 1980.

Appendix E Summary Examples of Recommended Nutrient Intakes for Canadians[a,b] (1982)

Age	Sex	Average weight (kg)	Average energy needs (kcal/day)[c]	Protein (g/day)[d]	Vitamin A (RE/day)[e]	Vitamin D (μg/day)[f]	Vitamin E (mg/day)[g]	Vitamin C (mg/day)	Folacin (μg/day)[h]	Vitamin B-12 (μg/day)	Calcium (mg/day)	Magnesium (mg/day)	Iron (mg/day)	Iodine (μg/day)	Zinc (mg/day)
Months															
0–2	Both	4.5	500	11[i]	400	10	3	20	50	0.3	350	30	0.4[i]	25	2[k]
3–5	Both	7.0	700	14[i]	400	10	3	20	50	0.3	350	40	5	35	3
6–8	Both	8.5	800	16[i]	400	10	3	20	50	0.3	400	45	7	40	3
9–11	Both	9.5	950	18	400	10	3	20	55	0.3	400	50	7	45	3
Years															
1	Both	11	1100	18	400	10	3	20	65	0.3	500	55	6	55	4
2–3	Both	14	1300	20	400	5	4	20	80	0.4	500	65	6	65	4
4–6	Both	18	1800	25	500	5	5	25	90	0.5	600	90	6	85	5
7–9	M	25	2200	31	700	2.5	7	35	125	0.8	700	110	7	110	6
	F	25	1900	29	700	2.5	6	30	125	0.8	700	110	7	95	6
10–12	M	34	2500	38	800	2.5	8	40	170	1.0	900	150	10	125	7
	F	36	2200	39	800	2.5	7	40	170	1.0	1000	160	10	110	7
13–15	M	50	2800	49	900	2.5	9	50	160	1.5	1100	220	12	160	9
	F	48	2200	43	800	2.5	7	45	160	1.5	800	190	13	160	8
16–18	M	62	3200	54	1000	2.5	10	55	190	1.9	900	240	10	160	9
	F	53	2100	47	800	2.5	7	45	160	1.9	700	220	14	160	8
19–24	M	71	3000	57	1000	2.5	10	60	210	2.0	800	240	8	160	9
	F	58	2100	41	800	2.5	7	45	165	2.0	700	190	14	160	8
25–49	M	74	2700	57	1000	2.5	9	60	210	2.0	800	240	8	160	9
	F	59	1900	41	800	2.5	6	45	165	2.0	700	190	14[i]	160	8
50–74	M	73	2300	57	1000	2.5	7	60	210	2.0	800	240	8	160	9
	F	63	1800	41	800	2.5	6	45	165	2.0	800	190	7	160	8
75+	M	69	2000	57	1000	2.5	6	60	210	2.0	800	240	8	160	9
	F	64	1500	41	800	2.5	5	45	165	2.0	800	190	7	160	8
Pregnancy (additional															
1st Trimester				15	100	2.5	2	0	305	1.0	500	15	6	25	0
2nd Trimester				20	100	2.5	2	20	305	1.0	500	20	6	25	1
3rd Trimester				25	100	2.5	2	20	305	1.0	500	25	6	25	2
Lactation (additional)				20	400	2.5	3	30	120	0.5	500	80	0	50	6

[a]Recommended intakes of energy and of certain nutrients are not listed in this table because of the nature of the variables upon which they are based. The figures for energy are estimates of average requirements for expected patterns of activity. For nutrients not shown, the following amounts are recommended: thiamin, 0.4 mg/1000 kcal (0.48 mg/5000 kJ); riboflavin, 0.5 mg/1000 kcal (0.6 mg/5000 kJ); niacin, 7.2 NE/1000 kcal (8.6 NE/5000 kJ); vitamin B_6, 15μg, as pyridoxine, per gram of protein; phosphorus, same as calcium.

[b]Recommended intakes during periods of growth are taken as appropriate for individuals representative of the mid-point in each age group. All recommended intakes are designed to cover individual variations in essentially all of a healthy population subsisting upon a variety of common foods available in Canada.

[c]Requirements can be expected to vary with a range of ±30%.

[d]The primary units are grams per kilogram of body weight. The figures shown here are only examples.

[e]One retinol equivalent (RE) corresponds to the biological activity of 1 μg of retinol, 6 μg of β-carotene or 12 μg of other carotenes.

[f]Expressed as cholecalciferol or ergocalciferol.

[g]Expressed as d-α-tocopherol equivalents, relative to which β- and γ-tocopherol and α-tocotrienol have activities of 0.5, 0.1 and 0.3 respectively.

[h]Expressed as total folate.

[i]Assumption that the protein is from breast milk or is of the same biological value as that of breast milk and that between 3 and 9 months adjustment for the quality of the protein is made.

[j]It is assumed that breast milk is the source of iron up to 2 months of age.

[k]Based on the assumption that breast milk is the source of zinc for the first 2 months.

[l]After the menopause the recommended intake is 7 mg/day.

Source: Bureau of Nutritional Sciences, Food Directorate, Health Protection Branch, Ottawa. Reproduced by permission of the Minister of Supply and Services Canada.

▪ Appendix F   Equivalents

Metric Equivalents

Weights			Volume		
1 picogram	=	10^{-12} gram	1 milliliter	=	1 gram
1 nanogram	=	10^{-9} gram	1 liter	=	1 kilogram = 1000 grams
1 microgram	=	10^{-3} milligram = 10^{-6} gram			(milliliters)
1 milligram	=	1000 micrograms = 10^{-6} gram			
1 centigram	=	10 milligrams = 10^{-1} decigram = 10^{-2} gram			
1 decigram	=	100 milligrams = 10 centigrams = 10^{-1} gram			
1 gram	=	1000 milligrams = 100 centigrams = 10 decigrams			
1 kilogram	=	1000 grams			

Approximate Weight Equivalents: Metric and Apothecaries' Systems

Metric	Apothecaries'	Metric	Apothecaries'
0.1 mg	1/600 grain	30 mg	1/2 grain
1.12 mg	1/500 grain	40 mg	2/3 grain
0.15 mg	1/400 grain	50 mg	3/4 grain
0.2 mg	1/300 grain	60 mg	1 grain
0.25 mg	1/250 grain	100 mg (0.1 gm)	1-1/2 grains
0.3 mg	1/200 grain	150 mg (0.15 gm)	2-1/2 grains
0.4 mg	1/150 grain	200 mg (0.2 gm)	3 grains
0.5 mg	1/120 grain	300 mg (0.3 gm)	5 grains
0.6 mg	1/100 grain	400 mg (0.4 gm)	6 grains
0.8 mg	1/80 grain	500 mg (0.5 gm)	7-1/2 grains
1 mg	1/60 grain	600 mg (0.6 gm)	10 grains
1.2 mg	1/50 grain	1 gram	15 grains
1.5 mg	1/40 grain	1.5 gm	22 grains
2 mg	1/30 grain	2 gm	30 grains
3 mg	1/20 grain	3 gm	45 grains
4 mg	1/15 grain	4 gm	60 grains (1 dram)
5 mg	1/12 grain	5 gm	75 grains
6 mg	1/10 grain	6 gm	90 grains
8 mg	1/8 grain	7.5 gm	120 grains (2 drams)
10 mg	1/6 grain	10 gm	2-1/2 drams
12 mg	1/5 grain	30 gm	1 ounce (8 drams)
15 mg	1/4 grain	500 gm	1.1 pounds
20 mg	1/3 grain	1000 gm	2.2 pounds
25 mg	3/8 grain		1 kilogram)

Approximate Volume Equivalents: Metric, Apothecaries', and Household Systems

Metric	Apothecaries'	Household
0.06 ml	1 minim (m)	1 drop (gt)
0.3 ml	5 minims	
0.6 ml	10 minims	
1 ml	15 minims	15 drops (gtt)
2 ml	30 minims	
3 ml	45 minims	
4 ml	60 minims (1 fluid dram [f3])	60 drops (1 teaspoon [tsp])
8 ml	2 fluid drams	2 teaspoons
15 ml	4 fluid drams	4 teaspoons (1 tablespoon [Tbsp])
30 ml	8 fluid drams (1 fluid ounce [f3])	2 tablespoons
60 ml	2 fluid ounces	
90 ml	3 fluid ounces	
200 ml	6 fluid ounces	1 teacup
250 ml	8 fluid ounces	1 large glass
500 ml	16 fluid ounces (1 pint)	1 pint
750 ml	1½ pints	
1000 ml (1 liter)	2 pints (1 quart)	1 quart
4000 ml	4 quarts	1 gallon

Appendix G   Significant Events in Nursing History
Compiled by Edith P. Lewis, MN, FAAN

1–500 (circa)   Care (mostly hygienic and comfort measures) for the destitute, homeless, and sick provided mainly by early Christians, working as committed individuals or in association with an organized church.

500–1500 (circa)   Male and female religious, military, and secular orders with the primary purpose of caring for the sick came into being. Conspicuous among them were the Knights Hospitalers of St. John; the Alexian Brotherhood, organized in 1431; and the Augustinian sisters, the first purely nursing order.

1633   Sisters of Charity founded by St. Vincent de Paul in France. It was the first of many such orders with the same name (sometimes Daughters of Charity) organized under various Roman Catholic church auspices and largely devoted to caring for the sick.

1639   Augustinian sisters came to Canada, eventually establishing the Hotel Dieu in Quebec City.

1644   Jeanne Mance, known as the Florence Nightingale of Canada, founded the Hotel Dieu in Montreal.

——Mother Elizabeth Seton established the first American order of Sisters of Charity of St. Joseph, in Maryland.

1738   Mother d'Youville organized a noncloistered group of women to care for the sick in both hospitals and homes. These women became the Soeurs Grises or Grey Nuns.

1836   Theodor Fliedner reinstituted the Order of Deaconesses from earlier days, opening a small hospital and training school in Kaiserswerth, Germany. This was where Florence Nightingale received her "training" in nursing. The deaconess movement spread to four continents, the first motherhouse being established in Pittsburgh, Pennsylvania, in 1849.

1854–56   Florence Nightingale, long concerned with care of the sick, was named Superintendent of the Female Nursing Establishment of the English General Hospitals in Turkey, in charge of the nursing care of the soldiers during the Crimean War.

1859   Publication of *Notes on nursing: What it is and what it is not*, by Nightingale, in London. It was intended for the ordinary woman, not as a text for nurses.

1860   With a fund of 45,000 pounds (over $220,000 at that time) contributed by the grateful British public and soldiers, Nightingale established the first "modern" school of nursing at St. Thomas's Hospital in London. This date is considered the beginning of nursing as an organized profession. Nightingale believed not only in nursing the sick but also in promoting health.

1861–65   Dorothea Lynde Dix, better known for her earlier work in improving conditions of care for the mentally ill, was appointed superintendent of the first nurse corps of the United States Army during the Civil War.

1864   Jean Henri Dunant of Switzerland established the international conference that founded the Red Cross, for the relief of the suffering in war, in the Geneva Convention signed by 14 nations (the United States not among them).

1872   Woman's Hospital, Philadelphia, opened a training school for nurses.

——New England Hospital for Women and Children, Boston, opened a training school for nurses. Linda Richards, who graduated from the school in 1873, became known as America's first trained nurse.

——American Public Health Association established. Its primary concern at that time was with sanitary and environmental conditions. Later nurses became a significant part of its membership.

1873   First three schools of nursing patterned after (but not strictly according to) Nightingale principles were established at Bellevue Hospital, New York; Massachusetts General Hospital, Boston; and New Haven Hospital, Connecticut.

1874   First hospital training school (Mack Training School) for nurses formed in Canada at St. Catharines, Ontario.

1879   Mary Eliza Mahoney, first trained black nurse, graduated from the nursing school of New England Hospital for Women and Children.

1882   American National Red Cross organized by Clara Barton and linked with the international organization when the United States Congress ratified the Geneva Convention.

1885   Publication of *Textbook of nursing for the use of training schools, families and private students*, the first textbook written by an American nurse (Clara Weeks Shaw) for nurses.

1893   Henry Street Settlement, New York, established by Lilian D. Wald and Mary Brewster to care for the sick and poor in their homes.

——American Society of Superintendents of Training Schools for Nurses (renamed the National League of Nursing Education [NLNE] in 1912) became the first organized nursing group in the United States and Canada.

1897   Nurses' Associated Alumnae of United States and Canada organized. Renamed the American Nurses' Association (ANA) in 1911.

——Victorian Order of Nurses established in Canada by Lady Aberdeen. It conducted practically all public health nursing.

1899 International Council of Nurses (ICN) established by Mrs. Bedford Fenwick of Great Britain, United States and Canadian nurses were among its founders, and their national associations were among the first admitted to membership.

1900 *American Journal of Nursing*, first nursing journal in the United States to be owned, operated, and published by nurses, launched. Its publisher, incorporated in 1902, now also publishes *Nursing Research*, established in 1952; *Nursing Outlook*, 1953; *International Nursing Index*, 1966; *MCN: American Journal of Maternal–Child Nursing*, 1976; and *Geriatric Nursing: American Journal of Care for the Aging*, 1980.

1901 United States Army Nurse Corps formally established by act of Congress.

1903 First nurse practice acts passed in North Carolina, New Jersey, Virginia, and New York.

1905 *Canadian Nurse* journal inaugurated. By 1959 it was published in both English and French.

1908 Canadian National Association of Trained Nurses (CNATN) established. It later became the Canadian Nurses' Association (CNA).

National Association of Colored Graduate Nurses (NACGN) established.

——United States Navy Nurse Corps formed.

1912 National Organization for Public Health Nursing (NOPHN) established.

——United States Children's Bureau created by Congress as part of the Department of Commerce and Labor.

1916 Criteria for a profession, set forth by Abraham Flexner in "Is social work a profession?" (published in *School and society*, volume 1), became yardsticks for nursing and continue to serve this function.

1917 NLNE published its first *Standard curriculum for schools of nursing*; revised editions, under slightly different titles, appeared in 1927 and 1937.

1919 Ethyl Johns established the first baccalaureate degree program in nursing in the British Empire at the University of British Columbia, Vancouver.

1922 Sigma Theta Tau, national honor society of nursing in the United States, founded by six nursing students at Indiana Training School for Nurses.

1923 Publication of *Nursing and nursing education in the United States*, better known as the Goldmark (or Winslow-Goldmark) Report. Originally intended to study education for public health nursing, the study committee extended its work to include all of nursing education, criticizing the low standards, inadequate financing, and lack of separation of education from service.

——Yale University (New Haven, Connecticut) and Western Reserve University (Cleveland, Ohio), each with the aid of endowments, established independent schools of nursing. In 1934, both started requiring a baccalaureate degree for admission to the schools and granted masters of nursing degrees.

1928 Publication of *Nurses, patients, and pocketbooks*, first report of the Committee on Grading of Nursing Schools appointed two years earlier. The report indicated that there was an oversupply of nurses in general but an undersupply of adequately prepared ones.

1929 American Association of Nurse-Midwives formed, It merged in 1969 with the American College of Nurse-Midwifery to become the American College of Nurse-Midwives.

1931 Weir Report in Canada recommended integration of nursing education into the provincial education system.

1932 Association of Collegiate Schools of Nursing (ACSN) established to promote nursing education on a professional and collegiate level and to encourage research.

1933 ANA launched campaign for hospitals to employ graduate nurses instead of relying heavily on nursing students for patient care.

1934 Publication of *Nursing schools today and tomorrow*, final report of the Grading Committee (which never did grade schools publicly). It confirmed the weaknesses in nursing education pointed out in the Goldmark Report, recommended graduate instead of student nursing staffs, and called for public support of nursing education.

1939 Graduate School of Midwifery created by the Frontier Nursing Service, Hyden, Kentucky.

1940 Formation of the Nursing Council on National Defense (retitled the National Nursing Council for War Service [NNCWS] in 1941), with representation from major nursing organizations and nursing service agencies, to unify all nursing activities directly or indirectly related to war.

1942 Committee appointed to develop what became the State Board Test Pool Examination (SBTPE). By 1950 all states were using the SBTPE.

1943 United States Cadet Nurse Corps established. Through this corps, the federal government subsidized the cost of nursing education, in accelerated programs, for all students agreeing to serve after graduation in civilian or military nursing services for the duration of the war. It was discontinued in 1945.

——American Association of Industrial Nurses (now the American Association of Occupational Health Nurses) formed.

1946 ANA adopted its economic security (now economic and general welfare) program legitimizing collective bargaining for nurses through their state nurses' associations.

1947 Passage of the Taft-Hartley Act, exempting nonprofit hospitals and other charitable institutions from the obligation to bargain collectively with their employees.

1948 Publication of *Nursing for the future*, report of a far-reaching study of "who would organize, administer, and finance *professional* schools of nursing." Commissioned by the National

Nursing Council for War Services and carried out by anthropologist Esther Lucile Brown, the report recommended, among other things, that education for nursing belonged in colleges and universities, not in hospitals.

——NLNE formally established the National Nursing Accrediting Service for nursing educational programs.

——Nationwide movement toward "team nursing" started at Hartford Hospital, Connecticut.

——Metropolitan Demonstration School of Nursing in Windsor, Ontario, operated a 2-year nursing education program (from 1948 to 1952). The Lord Report in 1952 concluded that nurses could be trained at least as satisfactorily in 2 years as in 3 years.

1949 United States Air Force Nurse Corps created.

1950–53 United States nurses served in the Korean war, in Mobile Army Surgical Hospitals (M.A.S.H.).

1951 National Association of Colored Graduate Nurses dissolved itself, to be absorbed into the ANA.

1952 After years of study, the nursing profession in the United States was restructured into two national organizations: the ANA, which remained the membership organization, and the newly formed National League for Nursing (NLN), merging the former NLNE, NOPHN, and ACSN.

——Associate degree education for nursing begun in an experimental project at Teachers College, Columbia University, New York.

——*Nursing Research* launched due to the efforts of the ACSN.

1953 National Student Nurses' Association (NSNA) founded.

——United States Department of Health, Education, and Welfare (HEW) created. It became the Department of Health and Human Services (HHS) in 1980.

1954 Association of Operating Room Nurses formed.

1955 American Nurses' Foundation established by the ANA for research purposes.

1956 Federal nurse traineeship program established to aid registered nurses in advanced study.

1960 Publication of *Spotlight on nursing education* by Helen K. Mussallem, report of a pilot project for the evaluation of schools of nursing in Canada.

1963 Publication of *Toward quality in nursing*, report of the Surgeon General's Consultant Group in Nursing, another study of nursing and nursing education that projected the need for more and better prepared nurses.

1964 Ryerson Polytechnical Institute, Toronto, started the first diploma nursing program in Canada within a college institution.

——First Nurse Training Act allocated federal aid for nursing education in the United States.

1965 ANA issued its first (and famous) "Position paper on nursing education," calling for all nursing education to take place in institutions of higher education and stipulating the baccalaureate as minimum preparation for professional nursing practice, the associate degree for technical nursing practice.

1967 Pediatric nurse practitioner program initiated at University of Colorado, Boulder; a program at the University of California, San Francisco, gave nurses increased responsibility in ambulatory care. These marked the beginning of the "nurse practitioner" or "expanded role of the nurse" movement.

1969 Nurses' Association of the American College of Obstetricians and Gynecologists formed.

——American Association of Cardiovascular Nurses formed. It was broadened in 1972 to become the Association of Critical-Care Nurses.

——American Association of Colleges of Nursing (AACN) formed after two years of informal meetings.

1970 Canadian Nurses' Association established a national Testing Service (CNATS) to prepare examinations for graduate nurses seeking provincial registration.

——Publication of *An abstract for action*, report of the National Commission on Nursing and Nursing Education, and often referred to as the Lysaught report, after the study director. The report categorized nursing into episodic (illness) and distributive (preventive and health maintenance) care.

——Publication of *Extending the scope of nursing practice*, by HEW, endorsing extension of the nurse's traditional functions and responsibilities.

——Introduction of primary nursing as an alternative to team nursing.

——National Association of School Nurses formed.

1971 National Black Nurses' Association created.

——Lucille Kinlein became the first nurse to hang out her shingle as an independent practitioner. Today many nurses are in independent practice singly or in groups.

——Emergency Department Nurses' Association established.

1972 New York State amended its Nurse Practice Act to define professional nursing practice as diagnosing and treating human responses to actual or potential health problems.

——Nurses for Political Action, now Nurses' Coalition for Action in Politics (N-CAP), established to promote legislation in behalf of nursing; associated with the ANA.

1973 Federation of nursing specialty organizations and the ANA was created, after 2 years of preliminary meetings.

——ANA started certification program for nurses in specialty practice.

——American Academy of Nursing established, with appointment of 36 charter fellows. It was associated with the ANA.

——"External" associate degree program in nursing launched in New York. It permitted a degree to be awarded on the basis of independent study validated by examination. This was extended to the bachelor's degree in nursing in 1976.

——National Association of Pediatric Nurses formed.

1974 Amendments to the Taft-Hartley Act removed exemption of nonprofit institutions from the obligation to engage in collective bargaining.

——Association of Rehabilitation Nurses formed.

1975 Oncology Nursing Society started.

1976 Robert Wood Johnson Foundation launched a program of faculty fellowships in primary care.

1978 ANA House of Delegates resolved that "by 1985" minimum preparation for "entry into professional practice" would be the baccalaureate in nursing.

——Council of State Boards of Nursing separated from the ANA to form an autonomous body, the National Council of State Boards of Nursing.

1979 Committee on Credentialing in Nursing called for establishment of a free-standing national credentialing center, not endorsed by the ANA.

——Case Western Reserve University, Cleveland, initiated the first professional education program in nursing awarding the ND (Doctor of Nursing) degree.

1982 NLN endorsed the baccalaureate in nursing as minimum preparation for professional practice.

——ANA converted to a federation of constituent nurses' associations rather than an association of individual nurse members.

——National Association of Orthopedic Nurses established.

1983 Congress passed legislation changing Medicare reimbursement to hospitals to a system of prospective payment based on Diagnosis Related Groups (DRGs).

——Institute of Medicine report called for federally funded entity to place nursing research in the mainstream of scientific investigation.

1985 ANA House of Delegates voted to recommend titles for two levels of professional nursing practice: "registered nurse" for the baccalaureate-prepared nurse, and "associate nurse" for the associate degree (technical) nurse.

——National Institute of Nursing established.

1986 N-CAP (Nurses' Coalition for Action in Politics) renamed ANA-PAC.

Glossary

abdominal paracentesis removal of fluid from the peritoneal cavity

abduction movement of a bone away from the midline of the body

abductor muscle a muscle that moves a bone away from the midline of the body

ablative surgery surgery to remove a diseased organ

abrasion wearing away of a structure, such as the skin or teeth

abscess a localized collection of pus and disintegrating body tissues

abstracting forming a summary; isolating or considering separately a particular aspect of an object

acapnia a decreased level of carbon dioxide in the blood

accommodation (Piaget) the process of change in which a person's cognitive processes are sufficiently matured so that he or she can solve problems that could not be solved previously

accountability being responsible for one's actions involving clients and/or colleagues and accepting the consequences for one's behavior

accreditation a process by which an agency appraises institutions or programs to determine whether they meet established standards for service or training

acetone a flammable, colorless liquid with an ethereal odor, used to remove nail polish

acetylcholine an acetic acid ester of choline, which has an important function in the transmission of nerve impulses at the myoneural junction

aching pain a deep pain of varying degrees of intensity

acholic clay colored and free from bile

acidosis (acidemia) a condition that occurs with increases in blood carbonic acid or with decreases in blood bicarbonate; blood pH below 7.35

acne an inflammatory condition of the sebaceous glands

acromion (acromial process) the lateral projection of the scapula extending over the shoulder joint

active assistive exercise exercise carried out by the client with some assistance by the nurse

active euthanasia acts performed to shorten a person's life

active exercise exercise carried out by the client, who supplies the energy to move the body parts

active transport movement of substances across cell membranes against the concentration gradient

activity energetic action or being in a state of movement

actual health problem a health problem that currently exists

actual loss a loss identifiable by others

acupuncture a Chinese practice of piercing specific superficial nerves with needles, often to treat pain

acute sharp or severe; describing a severe condition with a sudden onset and short course (as opposed to chronic)

adaptation the process of modifying to meet new, changing, or different conditions

adaptation (Piaget) the coping behavior of a person who has the ability to handle the demands of the environment

adaptive mechanisms learned behaviors that assist an individual to adjust to the environment

addiction a term used previously to describe dependence on a drug or habit

adduction movement of a bone toward the midline of the body

adductor muscle a muscle that moves a bone toward the midline of the body

adenohypophysis the anterior part of the pituitary gland

adenosine triphosphate (ATP) a compound that stores energy from glucose oxidation

adherent sticking together, clinging

adhesion a fibrous band or structure by which parts are abnormally held together

adipose fat; of a fatty nature

adolescence a period of life beginning with the appearance of secondary sex characteristics and terminating with somatic growth, usually between ages 11 and 19

adolescent parents teenagers who assume the responsibilities of parenthood

adrenal gland an endocrine gland that is located on the superior aspect of the kidney

Adrenalin a trademark name for preparations of epinephrine

adrenocortical arising from the cortex of the adrenal gland

adrenocorticotropic hormone (ACTH) a hormone produced by the pituitary gland that stimulates the adrenal cortex to produce hormones

adsorbent an agent that attracts other materials or particles to its surface, e.g., charcoal in the stomach and intestines

adventitious breath sounds abnormal breath sounds

advocate one who pleads the cause of another or argues or pleads for a cause or proposal; *nurse advocate*—one who supports the rights of clients by making sure that they know their rights and that they have the necessary knowledge to make informed decisions about their care

aeration the process by which the blood exchanges carbon dioxide for oxygen in the lungs

aerobe an organism that requires oxygen to live

aerobic requiring oxygen

affect feelings, emotions

agglutination the process of clumping together

agglutinin a specific antibody formed in blood

agglutinogen a substance that acts as an antigen and stimulates the production of agglutinin

aggression an unprovoked attack or hostile, injurious, or destructive behavior or outlook

agnostic one who believes that the existence of God is unknown

air hunger dyspnea occurring in paroxysms

airway a passageway through which air normally circulates; a device that is inserted through the client's mouth to maintain the patency of air passages such as the trachea

alarm reaction (Selye) the initial reaction of the body to a stressor

albuminuria the presence of albumin in the urine

aldosterone a hormone produced by the adrenal cortex that regulates the level of sodium in the body

alerting as an element of anger, the act of engaging another's attention

algor mortis the gradual decrease in body temperature after death

alignment (posture) the position of body parts that facilitates body function

alkalosis (alkalemia) a condition that occurs with increases in blood bicarbonate or decreases in blood carbonic acid; blood pH above 7.45

allergy a hypersensitive state

alopecia abnormal loss of hair

altruism selfless concern for others

alveolus saclike dilation or cavity in the body (plural: alveoli)

ambulation the act of walking

amino acid one of a group of organic acids containing nitrogen that are considered the components of protein

ammonia dermatitis diaper rash

amphetamine a drug used to stimulate the central nervous system

ampule a small, sealed glass flask, usually designed to hold a single dose of a medication

anabolism a process in which simple substances are converted by the body cells into more complex substances, e.g., building tissue; positive nitrogen balance

anaerobe an organism that does not require oxygen to live

anal canal the terminal aspect of the rectum

analgesic a medication used to alter the perception and interpretation of pain

anal stage (Freud) a stage of human development usually occurring during the 2nd and 3rd years when the child is learning toilet training

analyzing (or analysis) breaking down a whole into component parts

anaphylaxis (anaphylactic shock, anaphylactic reaction) a severe allergic reaction

anasarca generalized edema throughout the body

anastomose to join or connect

anatomic position the position of normal body alignment

androgen any substance producing male characteristics

andropause (climacteric) the period of change in men when sexual activity decreases

androsperm sperm bearing a Y chromosome

anemia a condition in which the blood is deficient in red blood cells or hemoglobin

aneroid containing no liquid

anesthesia loss of sensation or feeling; induced loss of the sense of pain

anesthesiologist a physician specializing in the administration of anesthetics

anesthetist a person such as a nurse who specializes in administering anesthetics

aneurysm dilation of the wall of an artery, a vein, or the heart

anger an emotional state or a subjective feeling of animosity or strong displeasure

angiogram a diagnostic procedure enabling x-ray visualization of the vascular system after injection of a radiopaque dye

angstrom (Å) a unit of wavelength of the electromagnetic spectrum

anilingus anal stimulation provided orally

anion an ion carrying a negative charge

ankylosis permanent fixation of a joint; stiffening of a joint

anodyne a medication that relieves pain

anogenital referring to the area around the anus and the genitals

anonymity the right of a client participating in research to not be linked to the information gathered

anorexia lack of appetite

anorexia nervosa a psychologic condition in which the person eats little or nothing, leading to emaciation

anoscopy visual examination of the anal canal using a lighted instrument called an anoscope

anoxemia a condition in which the level of oxygen in the blood is below normal

anoxia systemic absence or reduction of oxygen in the body tissues below physiologic levels

antagonist muscle a muscle that acts in the opposite manner to another muscle

antecubital space the area in front of the elbow

anterior of, toward, or at the front

anthropometric measurement measurement of the size and composition of the body, e.g., height, weight, and skin folds

antibiosis an antagonistic association between organisms

antibiotic a substance produced by microorganisms that has the capacity to inhibit the growth of or kill other microorganisms

antibody a protective substance produced in the body to counteract antigens

anticipatory loss a loss experienced before it actually occurs

antidiuretic hormone (ADH) a hormone that is stored and released by the posterior pituitary gland and that controls water reabsorption from the kidney tubules; also referred to as **vasopressin**

antigen a substance capable of inducing the formation of antibodies

antipyretic a substance that is effective in relieving fever

antiseptic an agent that inhibits the growth of some microorganisms

antiserum (immune serum) a serum that contains antibodies

antrum the portion of the stomach between the fundus and the pylorus

anuria the failure of the kidneys to produce urine, resulting in total lack of urination or output of less than 100 ml per day in an adult

anus the opening of the rectum, the posterior opening of the gastrointestinal tract

anxiety a state of mental uneasiness, apprehension, or dread producing an increased level of arousal due to an impending or anticipated threat to self or significant relationships

apathy lack of interest or feeling

Apgar score a system of numerically rating the condition of a newborn infant

aphasia the inability to communicate by speech, signs, or writing, resulting from an injury or disease

apical beat the heartbeat as heard over the apex of the heart

apical-radial pulse measurement of the apical beat and the radial pulse

apnea cessation of breathing

apocrine gland a large sweat gland whose duct usually opens into a hair follicle

appetite a pleasant sensation in which one desires and anticipates food

appliance (ostomy) a device or bag that is secured to the abdomen to collect either urine or feces

approximate to bring close together (referring to wound or incision edges)

areola the circular area of different color around a central point, such as the circular pigmented area surrounding the nipple of the breast

aromatic having a spicy odor

arrector pili muscle the erector muscle attached to the hair follicle

arrhythmia an irregular pulse rhythm, also called **dysrhythmia**

arteriography x-ray filming of an arterial system after injection of a radiopaque material

arteriosclerosis a condition in which the walls of the arteries become hardened and thickened

artery forceps *see* hemostat

artificial respiration forceful movement of air into and out of the lungs by means external to the person

ascites the accumulation of fluid in the abdominal cavity

asepsis the absence of disease-producing microorganisms

asphyxia a condition resulting from a lack of oxygen in the inspired air

asphyxiation (suffocation) lack of oxygen due to interrupted breathing

aspirate to remove gases or fluids from a cavity by using suction

assault an attempt or threat to touch another person unjustifiably

assertiveness expression of oneself openly and directly without hurting others

assessing collecting, verifying, and organizing data about a client's health status

assessment an organized collection of data about a client

assimilation (of a group) the blending of attitudes and beliefs of the members

assimilation (Piaget) the process whereby humans are able to encounter and react to new situations by using the mechanisms they already possess

associative thinking a type of thinking that has little direction and often involves random thoughts (e.g., daydreaming)

asthma a disease characterized by spasmodic dyspnea, coughing, and a sense of constriction of the bronchi

astigmatism a refractive error of the eye due to an uneven curvature of the cornea

astringent an agent that causes contraction or shrinkage of tissue; usually applied topically

asymmetric lacking symmetry; showing dissimilarity of corresponding organs on opposite sides of the body

atelectasis collapse of lung tissue

atheist one who denies the existence of God

athetosis involuntary twisting and writhing movements

athlete's foot (tinea pedis) a fungal injection of the foot; ringworm

atony lack of normal muscle tone

atresia absence, closure, or degeneration of a passageway or cavity such as the primordial follicles of the ovaries

atrioventricular (AV) node the neuromuscular tissue of the heart at the base of the atrial septum that conveys impulses to the ventricles

atrioventricular valves cardiac valves between the atria and the ventricles; also referred to as the **tricuspid** and **mitral valves**

at-risk aggregate subgroup of a population who are at greater risk of illness or poor recovery

atrophy a wasting away or decrease in size of a cell, tissue, body organ, or muscle

attenuate to make thin or to weaken

attitude a feeling tone; a concomitant of behavior

audit an examination or review of records

auditory related to or experienced through hearing

auricle a chamber of the ear or the heart

auscultation the practice of examining the body by listening to body sounds

authority the right to act and command

autoantigen an antigen that originates in the person's own body

autoclave an apparatus that sterilizes, using steam under pressure

autogenous (infection) originating from the patient's own microbial flora

autoimmunity production of antibodies against the body's own tissues

autonomic self-controlling; capable of independent function

autonomy the state of being independent and self-directed without outside control

autopsy (postmortem examination) the examination of a body after death; performed by a physician

axilla the armpit (plural: axillae)

axillary line an imaginary line extending vertically from the anterior fold of the axilla

babbling prelinguistic repetitive sounds produced by infants

Babinski (plantar) reflex in infants up to 1 year, the normal fanning out of toes and dorsiflexion of the big toe elicited by stroking the sole of the foot (positive Babinski); after 1 year the normal curling of the toes at this stroking (negative Babinski)

bacteriocide an agent capable of destroying some microorganisms

bacteriostatic agent an agent that prevents the growth and reproduction of some microorganisms

balance stability; steadiness; a state of equipoise in which opposing forces counteract each other

Balkan frame a metal frame extending lengthwise over a bed and supported at either end for attaching traction or providing a means of mobility to bedridden clients

bandage a material used to wrap a body part

barbiturate a drug commonly used as a hypnotic and sedative

barium a metallic element commonly used in solution as a contrast medium for x-ray filming of the gastrointestinal tract

barium enema x-ray filming of the large intestine using a contrast medium; also called a **lower gastrointestinal series**

barium swallow x-ray filming of the esophagus, stomach, and duodenum; also referred to as an **upper gastrointestinal series**

barrel chest a chest shape in which the ratio of the anteroposterior diameter to the lateral diameter is 1 to 1

basal metabolic rate (BMR) the rate at which the body metabolizes food to produce the energy required to maintain body functions at rest

base of support the area on which an object rests

basic human need those things humans require to maintain physiologic and psychologic homeostasis

basilic vein a superficial vein that arises on the ulnar side of the dorsum of the hand, goes up the forearm, and joins the brachial vein to form the axillary vein

battery willful or negligent touching of a person or a person's clothes, which may or may not cause harm

Beau's line a deep line visible across a nail after its growth has been halted and then renewed

bedpan a receptacle used to collect urine and feces from a person confined in bed

behavioral contract a written commitment by a client to follow through with selected actions

behavior modification eliciting and rewarding externally desired behavioral responses to reduce, modify, or eliminate ineffective adaptive coping responses

belief something accepted as true by a judgment of probability rather than actuality

bereavement the state of a person who has experienced the loss of a significant other through death

beriberi a condition due to deficiency of thiamine (vitamin B_1)

bevel a slanting edge

bilateral affecting two sides

bilirubin orange pigment in the bile

bill of rights a summary of fundamental rights and privileges guaranteed to people

binder a type of bandage applied to large body areas, e.g., the abdomen or chest

biofeedback conscious control of physiologic responses under the control of the autonomic nervous system, such as heart rate and blood pressure

biologic sex sexual gender genetically determined at conception from the XX or XY chromosomal combination

biopsy the removal and examination of tissue from the living body

biorhythm an inner rhythm that appears to control a variety of biologic processes

bisexual experiencing sexual attraction to people of both genders

bleb (wheal) a small, smooth, slightly raised area on the skin, usually filled with fluid

blended family family composed of two previously existing family units; also called **reconstituted family**

blister a collection of fluid between the epidermis and the dermis

blood pressure the pressure of the blood as it pulsates through the arteries

body image an individual's perception of his or her own physical attributes, body functioning, sexuality, appearance, and state of wellness

body image disturbance negative feelings or perceptions about characteristics, functions, or limits of one's own body or body part

body mechanics the efficient and coordinated use of the body during resting activities and movement

body temperature the internal temperature of the human body

bolus a mass of food or pharmaceutical preparation ready to be swallowed; a mass passing along the gastrointestinal tract; a concentrated mass of pharmaceutical preparation given intravenously

borborygmi abnormally intense and frequent bowel sounds

boundary (of a system) a real or imaginary line that differentiates one system from another system or a system from its environment

brachial pulse a pulse located on the inner side of the biceps muscle just below the axilla; usually palpated medially in the antecubital space

bradycardia an abnormally slow heart rate, below 60 beats per minute in an adult

bradypnea abnormally slow respirations; usually fewer than 10 respirations per minute

brainstorming technique to generate ideas in which one person's idea elicits an idea from another person and so on

bronchial sounds normal loud, harsh, hollow blowing sounds heard by auscultation over the trachea and major bronchi

bronchodilator an agent that dilates the bronchi of the lungs

bronchogram an x-ray film of the bronchial tree taken after injection of an iodized oil dye, used as a contrast medium

bronchophony an increase in vocal resonance; an abnormal voice sound heard on auscultation of the chest wall

bronchopneumonia an infection that originates in the bronchi and involves patches of lung tissue

bronchoscope a lighted instrument used to visualize the bronchi of the lungs

bronchoscopy visual examination of the bronchi using a bronchoscope

bronchovesicular sounds combination of bronchial and vesicular sounds heard by auscultation over parts of the chest where a bronchus is near lung tissue

bronchus a large air passageway of the lungs (plural: bronchi)

bruit abnormal blowing, swishing, or rippling sounds heard during auscultation

bubbling gurgling sounds produced as air passes through moist secretions in the respiratory tract

buccal pertaining to the cheek

buffer an agent or system that tends to maintain constancy or that prevents changes in the chemical concentration of a substance

bulimia an uncontrollable compulsion to consume enormous amounts of food and then expel the food by self-induced vomiting

burning pain pain like the pain of burning skin

cachexia a state of weakness, emaciation, and malnutrition often seen in wasting diseases and terminal malignancies

calcitonin a hormone secreted by the thyroid gland that regulates blood calcium levels

calculus a stone composed of minerals that is formed in the body, e.g., a renal calculus formed in the kidney (plural: calculi)

calipers an instrument used to measure the thickness of folds of skin

callus hyperplasia or thickening of the horny layer of the epidermis, usually due to pressure

caloric density the number of kilocalories per unit weight of food

caloric value the amount of energy that nutrients or foods supply to the body

Calorie (large calorie, kilocalorie, C.) the amount of heat required to raise the temperature of 1 kilogram of water 1 degree Celsius

calorie (small calorie) the unit of heat required to raise the temperature of 1 gram of water 1 degree Celsius

calyx (calix) a cup-shaped organ or cavity

cancellous bone bone of spongy or latticelike structure

cannula a tube with a lumen (channel), which is inserted into a cavity or duct and is often fitted with a trocar during insertion

canthus the angle formed by the upper and lower eyelids; each eye has an inner and an outer canthus

Cantor tube a single-lumen tube inserted through the mouth into the intestines

capillary action the movement of fluid in a tube, caused by the adhesion of the fluid to the wall of the tube

capsule a soft, soluble container for a medication; an anatomic structure enclosing an organ or part of the body; (of a cell) a well-defined, gelatinous layer surrounding a bacterial cell

carbaminohemoglobin the chemical combination of carbon dioxide and hemoglobin

carbohydrate a nutrient composed of carbon, hydrogen, and oxygen, e.g., starches and sugars

carbonic acid the compound formed when carbon dioxide combines with water

cardiac arrest the cessation of heart function

cardiac board a flat board placed under a person's chest when that person requires cardiac massage and is lying on a soft surface

cardiac monitor a machine that measures and records the heart function

cardiac output the amount of blood ejected from the heart per minute by ventricular contraction

cardiopulmonary resuscitation (CPR) artificial stimulation of the heart and lungs

caries decay of a tooth or bone

carina the ridge or junction where the main bronchi meet the trachea

carminative an agent that promotes the passage of flatus from the colon

carotid arteries major arteries lying on either side of the trachea and larynx

carotid receptors nerve endings that are found in the carotid bodies and carotid sinuses and that are sensitive to blood pH, changes in blood pressure, and excessive blood CO_2

carrier a person who harbors pathogens but is not ill

cartilage a firm connective tissue found throughout the body

caster a small wheel, often made of rubber or plastic, that permits furniture such as a bed to be moved easily

catabolism a destructive process in which complex substances are broken down into simpler substances, e.g., breakdown of tissue

cataplexy partial or complete muscle paralysis that can occur during narcolepsy

cataract opacity of the lens of the eye or its capsule

cathartic a drug that induces evacuation of feces from the large intestine

catheter a tube of plastic, rubber, metal, or other material used to remove or inject fluids into a cavity such as the bladder

cation a positively charged ion

caudal anesthetic an anesthetic injected into the caudal canal, below the spinal cord

cavity a hollow space within the body or one of its organs

cecum a dilated pouch that constitutes the first part of the large intestine adjoining the small intestine

cellular fluid *see* intracellular fluid

cellulitis inflammation of cellular tissue

Celsius a thermometer scale used to measure heat; the freezing point of water is 0 C and the boiling point is 100 C

center of gravity the point at which the mass (weight) of the body is centered

central venous pressure (CVP) a measurement of the pressure of the blood, in millimeters of water, within the vena cava or the right atrium of the heart

cephalocaudal proceeding in the direction from head to toe

cerebral death death that occurs when the cerebral cortex is irreversibly destroyed

cerebrospinal fluid fluid contained within the four ventricles of the brain, the subarachnoid space, and the central canal of the spinal cord

certification the practice of determining minimum standards of competence in specialty areas

cerumen waxlike material that protects the auditory canal

cervix the lower end or neck of the uterus; projects into the vagina

chancre a papular lesion (sore) occurring at the entry of infection in some diseases; the primary sore of syphilis

change process that leads to modifications in behavior

change agent an individual, such as a nurse, or group, who operates to change the status quo in another individual or in a system

chart (medical record) a written account of a client's health history, current health status, treatment, and progress

charting (recording) the process of making written entries about a client on the medical record

cheilosis cracks or scaling at the corners of the lips

chemical thermogenesis the production of heat by chemical means, e.g., production and circulation of ephinephrine

chemoreceptor a receptor that is sensitive to chemical substances

chemosensitive pain receptors pain receptors stimulated by chemicals

chemotaxis the movement of a cell or an organism in response to a chemical gradient

Cheyne-Stokes respirations rhythmic waxing and waning of respirations from very deep breathing to very shallow breathing with periods of temporary apnea, often associated with cardiac failure, increased intracranial pressure, or brain damage

childbearing family stage of family development during which the husband and wife assume the roles of parents

childrearing family stage of family development during which the primary focus is the nurturing, education, and socialization of children

chill shivering and shaking of body with involuntary contractions of the voluntary muscles

cholangiogram an x-ray film of the biliary tract taken after the injection of a dye

cholecystogram an x-ray film of the gallbladder after the ingestion of a contrast dye; also called *oral cholecystography*

cholesterol a lipid that does not contain fatty acid but possesses many of the chemical and physical properties of other lipids

choroid plexus projections of the pia mater into the ventricles of the brain that secrete cerebrospinal fluid

chromosome a structure in the nucleus of a cell that contains DNA and transmits genetic information

chronic persisting over a long time

chyme semifluid material produced by gastric digestion of food in the stomach; it is found in the small and large intestines

cicatrix scar

cicatrization formation of a scar

cilia hairlike projections from cells, e.g., of the mucous membrane of the respiratory tract

circadian rhythm rhythmic repetition of certain phenomena each 24 hours

circa dies about a day

circulatory overload a state in which the intravascular fluid compartment contains more fluid than normal

circumcision surgical removal of part or all of the foreskin of the penis; usually performed during infancy

circumduction movement of the distal part of a bone in a circle, with the proximal end remaining fixed

circumference the outer measurement or perimeter, e.g., the distance around the chest

cisterna an enclosed space that serves as a reservoir for body fluid

cisternal puncture insertion of a needle into the subarachnoid space of the cisterna magna

citric acid cycle (Krebs cycle) a complex series of chemical reactions by which the acetyl portion of acetyl coenzyme A is broken down into carbon dioxide and hydrogen

clavicle the bone commonly known as the collarbone; it articulates with the scapula and the sternum

clean free of pathogenic organisms

clean technique a technique that maintains an area or articles free from pathogens

clergy priests, rabbis, ministers, church elders, deacons, and any other spiritual advisers

client (patient) a person seeking, waiting for, or undergoing health care

client contract a written agreement between a client and a nurse regarding a behavior change

client goal statement about the expected or desired change in a client's status after he or she receives nursing interventions

climacteric the point in development when reproduction capacity in the female terminates (menopause) and the sexual activity of the male decreases (andropause)

clinical pharmacist a person who specializes in drugs that are used for treatment, prevention, and diagnosis of disease

clitoris a small round mass of erectile tissue, blood vessels, and nerves located behind the junction of the labia minora; homologous to the penis

closed questions restrictive questions requiring only short answer

closed system a system that does not exchange energy or matter with its environment

closed wound a wound in which there is no break in the skin

clubbing (of nails) an elevation of the proximal aspect of the nail and softening of the nail bed

coagulate to clot

coccidioidomycosis a fungus disease with an acute, benign respiratory infection in the primary stage and a virulent, progressive secondary stage

cochlea a tubular structure in the inner ear that contains the organ for hearing

code of ethics formal guidelines for professional action

coercive power power derived from the perception of one's ability to threaten, harm, or punish others

cognition the process of knowing, including judgment and awareness

cognitive referring to intellectual processes such as remembering, thinking, perceiving, abstracting, and generalizing

cognitive appraisal an evaluative process that determines why and to what extent a particular transaction or series of transactions between a person and the environment are stressful

cohabiting (communal) family family unit formed by unrelated individuals or families cohabiting or living under one roof

cohesive sticking together

cohesiveness (of group) the degree of group unity or oneness

coitus sexual intercourse; from Latin, meaning "a coming together"

coitus interruptus a method of contraception during which the penis is withdrawn prior to ejaculation

colic paroxysmal intestinal cramplike pain

collaborative nursing action activity performed jointly with another member of the health care team or as a result of a joint decision by the nurse and another member of the health care team

collagen a protein found in connective tissue

colloid substances, such as large plasma protein molecules, that do not readily dissolve in true solutions

colonoscope a lighted instrument used to visualize the interior of the colon

colonoscopy visual examination of the interior of the colon with a colonoscope

colostomy an artificial abdominal opening into the colon (large bowel)

colostrum a yellow, milky fluid secreted by the mother's mammary glands a few days before or after childbirth

comatose a state of unconsciousness in which the person shows no response to maximum painful stimuli, absence of reflexes, and absence of muscle tone in the extremities

combustible able to burn; flammable

comedo a discolored mass on the skin consisting of keratin, lipids, fatty acids, and bacteria

commitment an agreement, pledge, or obligation to do something or follow a course of action

commode a portable, chairlike structure used as a toilet

common law unwritten laws that are binding and upheld by precedent in legal cases rather than statutes

communicable disease (infectious disease) a disease that can spread from one person to another

communication exchange of thoughts, ideas, or feelings between two or more people

compensation defense mechanism in which a person substitutes an activity for one that he or she would prefer doing or cannot do

compliance in learning, an individual's agreement to learn; in drug therapy, the act of carefully following the prescription

compress a moist gauze dressing that is applied frequently to an open wound; it sometimes is medicated

concave hollowed or rounded inward

concept an abstract idea or mental image of phenomena or reality generalized from particular instances

conceptual framework set of concepts and statements that integrate the concepts into a meaningful configuration

conceptual model a basic structure in which a complex of ideas is united to portray a large general idea

concurrent audit an audit to review present practices

concurrent disinfection measures taken while a client is infectious to control the spread of the microorganisms

conditioning learning in which a response previously associated with one stimulus becomes associated with another stimulus

condom a sheath or cover, usually made of rubber or plastic, worn over the penis during coitus to prevent conception or infection; it may also be used to catch urine

conduction the transfer of heat from one molecule or object to another by contact

confer to consult another person or persons for advice, information, ideas, or instructions

confidentiality the right of a client or research subject that any information revealed by that individual will not be made public or available to others

conformity actions in accordance with specified standards

confusion a mental state in which a person appears bewildered and may make inappropriate statements and answers to questions

congenital existing at, and often before, birth

congestion excessive accumulation of blood in a part of the body

congruence (communication) a state in which one's verbal and nonverbal communications convey the same message

conjunctiva the delicate membrane that covers the eyeball and lines the eyelids

conjunctivitis inflammation of the conjunctiva

consciousness a person's normal state of awareness of the environment, self, and others

consensual reaction (eyes) a reaction in which one pupil constricts quickly in response to a bright light and the other pupil constricts also, but more slowly

consent permission given voluntarily by a person in his or her right mind; **informed consent** implies that the individual is knowledgeable about the consent and understands it

constant data information that is unchanging

constipation passage of small, dry, hard stool or passage of no stool for an abnormally long time

constitutional law law stated in federal, state, or provincial constitutions

construct abstract concept derived from existing theories or observations

constructive surgery surgery to repair a congenitally malformed organ or tissue

construct validity the degree to which an instrument measures the abstract concept it was designed to measure

consultation deliberation by two or more people

consumer an individual, group, or community that uses a service or a product

contact a person who has been near an infected person and thus exposed to pathogenic microorganisms

contact lens a small, plastic corrective lens that fits on the cornea of the eye directly over the pupil

contaminated possessing pathogenic organisms

continuum a grid or graduated scale

contour position (of a bed) a position with the head and foot of the bed elevated, creating an angle of about 15 degrees

contraception the prevention of fertilization of the ovum by any method

contract a written or verbal agreement between two or more people to do or not do some lawful act

contracting family stage of family development during which the children leave the family unit, and the adult family members stabilize their roles, age, and prepare for retirement

contraction the normal active shortening or tensing of a muscle

contractual obligation a duty to render service established by a formal or informal contract

contracture permanent shortening of a muscle and subsequent shortening of tendons and ligaments

contusion a closed wound that occurs as a result of a blow from a blunt instrument; a bruise

convection transfer of heat by movement of a liquid or gas, e.g., air currents

conversion a defense mechanism in which a mental conflict is converted into a physical symptom

conversive heat heat that results from the conversion of a primary source of energy

convex curved or rounded like the external surface of a sphere

coping the process through which the individual manages the demands of the person-environment relationship that are stressful

coping behavior behavior learned in response to stress

coping mechanisms physical or emotional adaptive or defensive abilities

coping strategy an innate or acquired way of responding to a changing environment or specific problem or situation

copulation the act of coitus; from Latin, meaning "coupling or joining"

coraje a Hispanic term meaning rage in response to a particular situation

cordotomy (chordotomy) surgical severing of the spinothalamic portion of the anterolateral tract of the spinal cord, usually for the purpose of relieving pain

core-gender identity see sexual identity

corn a hardening and thickening of the skin forming a conical mass pointing downward into the corium

cornea the transparent covering of the anterior eye that connects with the sclera

corneal reflex irritation of the cornea resulting in a reflex closing of the eyelids

cornification hardening

coronal plane any line or plane dividing the body into anterior (ventral) and posterior (dorsal) portions at right angles to the sagittal plane

coroner a public official who is responsible for investigating any deaths that appear to be unnatural

cortical bone compact bone

corticoid a term applied to hormones of the adrenal cortex or substances with similar activity

cortisol the most abundant glucocorticoid; also called hydrocortisone

cortisone a hormone produced by the adrenal cortex that has antiinflammatory properties and is involved in the metabolism of glycogen to glucose

costovertebral angle the angle formed by a rib and the spine

cough a sudden expulsion of air from the lungs

counseling the process of helping a client to recognize and cope with stressful psychologic or coping problems, to develop improved interpersonal relationships, and to promote personal growth

counterirritant an agent that produces an irritation with the intent of relieving some other problem

countershock phase part of the initial stage of the general adaptation syndrome during which the body changes produced in response to a stressor are reversed

CPR *see* cardiopulmonary resuscitation

creatinine a nitrogenous waste that is excreted in the urine

creative thinking a pattern of thinking involving establishing new relationships and new concepts and solving problems innovatively

credentialing (nursing) the process of determining and maintaining competence in nursing practice

Crede's maneuver manual exertion of pressure on the bladder to force urine out

cremaster the inner layer of striated muscle and connective tissue in the scrotum

crepitus a grating sound caused by bone fragments rubbing together

creps (crepitation) a dry, crackling sound like that of crumpled cellophane, produced by air in the subcutaneous tissue or by air moving through fluid in the alveoli of the lungs

crime an act committed in violation of societal law

criminal law law that deals with actions against the safety and welfare of the public

crisis in psychosocial terms, a rapid change or event that disturbs a person's psychologic homeostasis; in fever, the sudden reduction of an elevated body temperature

criteria (of nursing care) indicators of the quality of nursing care or measures by which the nursing care is judged

criterion a standard or model that can be used in judging

critical thinking cognitive processes during which data are reviewed and explanations considered before an opinion is formed

crown (of a tooth) the exposed part of the tooth outside the gum, covered by enamel

crutch a device with hand and arm supports used to facilitate walking

crutch palsy weakness of the hand, wrist, and forearm induced by prolonged pressure of a crutch on the axillary nerves

cryptorchidism failure of the testes to descend from the abdominal cavity to the scrotal sacs

crystalline amino acids refined protein used in total parenteral nutrition (hyperalimentation) solutions

crystalloids salts that dissolve readily in true solutions

cue fact the nurse acquires by using the five senses

cultural heritage values and beliefs unique to a particular culture that influence the family's structure, methods of interaction, health care practices, and coping mechanisms

culture in microbiology, the cultivation of microorganisms or cells in a special growth medium; in sociology, the beliefs and practices that are shared by people and passed down from generation to generation

culture shock the shock that can occur when an individual changes quickly from one social setting to another where former patterns of behavior are often ineffective

cumulative effect the effect of a drug when the level builds up in the blood

cunnilingus oral stimulation of the clitoris and labia by a partner

cupula a gelatinous dome-shaped structure of the inner ear that contains sensory hair cells

curandero (female: **curandera**) a healer within the Hispanic community

curet a spoon-shaped instrument used for removing material from a body cavity

curettage removal of material from the wall of a cavity, e.g., the uterus, with a curet

cuticle the flat, thin rim of skin surrounding the nail

CVP *see* central venous pressure

cyanosis bluish discoloration of the skin, nail beds, and mucous membranes, due to reduced oxygen in the blood

cyst an enclosed cavity or sac lined by epithelium and containing liquid or semisolid material

cystic fibrosis a hereditary condition marked by the accumulation of thick and tenacious mucus in the lungs and the abnormal secretion of saliva and sweat

cystitis inflammation of the urinary bladder

cystocele protrusion of the urinary bladder through the vaginal wall

cystoscope a lighted instrument used to visualize the interior of the urinary bladder

cytoscopy visual examination of the urinary bladder with a cystoscope

cytology the study of the origin, structure, function, and pathology of cells

Dakin's solution a buffered aqueous solution of sodium hypochlorite used as a bactericide

dandruff a dry or greasy, scaly material shed from the scalp

data information

database (baseline data) all information known about a client; it includes the physician's history and physical examination, the nurse's assessment and history, and material contributed by other members of the health team

deamination the removal of the amino (NH_2) groups by hydrolysis from amino acids

debilitated having lost strength

debride to remove foreign and dying tissue from a wound so that healthy tissue is exposed

deceased dead; a person who is dead

decerebrate posturing a posture indicative of midbrain damage, consisting of extension, adduction, and internal rotation of the arms; extension of the legs with the feet in plantar flexion; and arching of the back

decibel a unit used to measure or describe sound

deciduous teeth temporary teeth that are shed

decoding the process of receiving a communication and converting the message into understandable terms

decortical posturing a posture indicative of damage to the internal capsule and corticospinal tracts above the brain stem; it consists of flexion and adduction of the fingers, wrists, and shoulders; extension and internal rotation of the legs and feet; and rigidity of all extremities

decubitus ulcer an ulcer of the skin and underlying tissues produced by prolonged pressure

decussate to cross over

deductive reasoning making specific observations from a generalization

deductive theory a theory formulated by a process in which the idea is developed first, followed by observation of relevant supportive phenomena

deep breathing inhaling the maximum amount of air possible, then exhaling

defecation expulsion of feces from the rectum and anus

defense mechanism unconscious psychologic processes that protect the person from anxiety

dehiscence a splitting open or rupture

dehydration insufficient fluid in the body

delegate to authorize another as one's representative or to entrust authority to another

delegation assigning to another aspect of client care; sharing of responsibility and authority with others and holding them accountable for performance

delirious experiencing mental confusion, restlessness, and incoherence

demineralization excessive loss of minerals or inorganic salts

demography the study of population statistics

demulcent a drug that coats the intestine, thus protecting the lining

denial a defense mechanism in which painful or anxiety-producing aspects of reality are blocked out of consciousness

dental caries tooth decay

dental floss waxed or unwaxed thread used for cleaning between the teeth and the gums

dental plaque deposits on the teeth that serve as a medium for bacterial growth

dentifrice a paste or powder used to clean or polish the teeth

dentures a natural or artificial set of teeth; usually the term designates artificial replacements for natural teeth

deoxyribonucleic acid (DNA) a nucleic acid found in all living cells; it is the carrier of genetic information

dependence reliance

dependent edema edema that collects in the lower parts of the body, where hydrostatic pressure is greatest

dependent nursing action, intervention, or **function** activity by a nurse that is a result of a physician's order

depolarize to reduce toward a nonpolarized state; to cause loss of charge

depression feelings of sadness and dejection, often accompanied by physiologic change; a decrease of functional activity, as in depression of sensorium

dermatologic preparation a medication applied to the skin

dermis (corium) true skin, containing blood vessels, nerves, hair follicles, and glands

describing as an element of anger, the process of delineating the source of the angry feelings

detrusor muscle the three layers of smooth muscle that make up the urinary bladder

detumescence the process of returning to a flaccid state, e.g., referring to the penis following ejaculation

development an individual's increasing capacity and skill in functioning, related to growth

developmental crisis a crisis that occurs as a result of stressors impeding development

developmental tasks skills and behavior patterns learned during development

dextrose a sugar; also called *glucose*

diagnosis a statement or conclusion concerning the nature of some phenomenon

diagnostic related group (DRG) a predetermined category of illnesses, injuries, surgical procedures, and/or other conditions requiring hospitalization for which the cost of care is established prior to a client's hospitalization

diagnostic surgery surgery performed to confirm a diagnosis

dialyzing membrane a membrane that permits water molecules and crystalloids in true solution to move through it but not particles in a colloid dispersion

diapedesis the movement of blood corpuscles through a blood vessel wall

diaphoresis profuse sweating

diaphragm a musculomembranous partition that separates the abdominal and thoracic (chest) cavities

diarrhea defecation of liquid feces and increased frequency of defecation

diastole the period when the ventricles of the heart are relaxed

diastolic pressure the pressure of the blood against the arterial walls when the ventricles of the heart are at rest

diathermy the production of heat in body tissues by high-frequency electric currents

diet the food and fluid regularly consumed by an individual each day

dietitian a person who is skilled in the use of diets in health and disease

diffusion movement of gases or other particles from an area of greater pressure to an area of lower pressure or concentration; the continual intermingling of molecules in liquids, gases, or solids brought about by the random movement of the molecules

diffusion coefficient the rate of solubility of gases in the respiratory membrane

digital performed with the finger

diplopia double vision

direct interview highly structured questioning that elicits specific information

direct nursing activities activities by a nurse that are carried out in the presence of the client

directed thinking a pattern of thinking that is purposeful and is used for forming judgments, problem-solving, and decision-making

disaccharide a sugar consisting of double molecules

discharge planners nurses employed by hospitals whose primary responsibility is to assess client's anticipated needs after discharge

discharge planning the process of anticipating and planning for client's needs after discharge from a hospital or other facility

disease a morbid (unhealthful) process having definite symptoms

disequilibrium a disturbed state of equilibrium, either mental or physical; an unbalanced condition

disinfectant an agent that destroys pathogens other than spores

disinfection the process by which an article is rendered free of pathogens

disorientation a state of mental confusion; loss of bearings, time, and place

displacement a defense mechanism in which an emotional reaction is transferred from one object to another less threatening object

distal farthest from the point of reference

distention (abdominal) *see* tympanites

distraction a mechanism for relieving pain in which the person's attention is drawn away from the pain

diuresis *see* polyuria

diuretic an agent that increases the production of urine

dorsal of, toward, or at the back

dorsal column stimulator an electrode attached to the dorsal column of the spinal cord for the purpose of relieving pain

dorsal flexion movement of the ankle so that the toes are pointing up

dorsalis pedis pulse a pulse located on the instep of the foot

dorsal recumbent position a back-lying position with the head and shoulders slightly elevated

drain a substance or appliance (usually made of rubber or gauze) to assist in the discharge of drainage from a wound

drainage a discharge from a wound or cavity

dressing a material used to cover and protect a wound

drug (medication) a chemical compound taken for disease prevention, diagnosis, cure, or relief or to affect the structure or function of the body

drug abuse excessive intake of a substance either continually or periodically

drug allergy a hypersensitivity to a drug; the immunologic reaction to a drug

drug dependence inability to keep the intake of a drug or substance under control

drug habituation a mild form of psychologic dependence on a drug

drug interaction the beneficial or harmful interaction of one drug with another drug

drug misuse improper use of common medications in ways that can lead to acute and chronic toxicity

drug tolerance a condition in which successive increases in the dosage of a drug are required to maintain a given therapeutic effect

drug toxicity the quality of a drug that exerts a deleterious effect on an organism or tissue

DTP diphtheria toxoid, tetanus toxoid, and pertussis vaccine

dullness (in percussion) decreased resonance or percussion sound that occurs when large amounts of fluid or pus collect in the alveoli

duodenocolic reflex a mass peristaltic movement of the colon stimulated by the presence of chyme in the duodenum

dura (dura mater) the outermost, fibrous membrane covering the brain and spinal cord

duration (of sound) the length of the sound (long or short)

dyad a two-person group

dynamic equilibrium tendency of the body to maintain a state of balance or equilibrium while continually changing

dysfunction impaired functioning

dyspareunia pain experienced by a woman during intercourse

dyspepsia indigestion

dysphagia difficulty or inability to swallow

dysphasia difficulty speaking

dyspnea difficult and labored breathing in which the client has a persistent unsatisfied need for air and feels distressed

dysrhythmia *see* arrhythmia

dysuria painful or difficult urination

ecchymosis a blotchy area or discoloration of the skin; a bruise

ecchymotic appearing like a bruise

eccrine gland a sweat gland that secretes outward via a duct

echolalia the repetition by a person of words addressed to him or her

eclampsia convulsions and coma associated with hypertension and proteinuria in pregnant women

ecology the study of the relationship of humans and the environment

ectopic pregnancy the implantation of the fertilized ovum outside the uterus

ectropion a rolling out of the eyelid

edema excess interstitial fluid

edentulous without teeth

effector organ a muscle or gland that responds to nerve impulses

efferent conveying away from the center

effluent urine or feces discharged through a stoma

ego (Freud) the part of the psyche that maintains its identity; the conscious sense of self

egocentricity concern about oneself

egocentric speech self-centered, noncommunicative speech

ego integrity feeling satisfied with one's life-style and accepting the inevitability of one's life cycle

egophony a type of bronchophony in which the voice has a nasal, bleating quality

ejaculation expulsion of semen from the penis

ejaculatory ducts short tubes that pass through the prostate gland and terminate in the urethra

elective surgery surgery performed for a person's well-being but not absolutely necessary for life

Electra complex (Freud) the female child's attraction to her father; compare with *Oedipus complex*

electrocardiogram (ECG, EKG) a graph of the electric activity of the heart

electrocardiograph a machine that measures and records impulses from the heart on an electrocardiogram

electroencephalogram (EEG) a graph of the electric activity of the brain

electroencephalograph a machine that measures and records impulses from the brain on an electroencephalogram

electrolyte a chemical substance that develops an electric charge and is able to conduct an electric current when placed in water; an ion

electromyogram (EMG) a record of the electric potential created by the contraction of a muscle

electromyograph a machine that measures and records impulses from the muscles on an electromyogram

electron a negatively charged electric particle

emaciation excessive thinness

embalming a process of preserving a body chemically

embolus a blood clot (or a substance, such as air) that has moved from its place of origin and is obstructing the circulation in a blood vessel (plural: emboli)

emesis vomit

emmetropia the normal refraction of the eye, which focuses objects on the retina

emollient an agent that soothes and softens skin or mucous membrane; often an oily substance

empacho a Hispanic term for a disease seen primarily in children that includes a swollen abdomen as a result of intestinal blockage

empathy seeing or feeling a situation the way another person sees or feels it

emphysema a chronic obstructive lung disorder in which the terminal bronchioles become distended and plugged with mucus

empirical by observation or experience

emulsification a process by which lipids are broken up and evenly dispersed in an aqueous medium

emulsion a preparation in which one liquid is distributed throughout another

encoding the selection of specific signs and symbols to transmit a message

endemic present in a community all the time

endogenous developing from within

endometrium the inner mucous membrane lining of the uterus

endorphin a polypeptide found throughout the body that is thought to relieve pain

endosteum the membrane lining a hollow bone

endothelium the layer of endothelial cells lining the blood vessels, cavities of the heart, and serous cavities

enema a solution injected into the rectum and the sigmoid colon

engorgement excessive fullness of an organ or passage

enkephalin a pentapeptide naturally occurring in the brain that has opiatelike effects

enteric referring to the intestines

enteric-coated surrounded with a special coating used for tablets and capsules that prevents release of the drug until it is in the intestines

enteric feeding a feeding administered directly into the small intestine through a tube

enteritis inflammation of the small intestine

enteroclysis the injection of a nutrient or drug into the colon

enterostomal therapist a person who specializes in ostomy care

enterostomy an opening through the abdominal wall into the intestines

entropion an inturned eyelid

enuresis bedwetting

environmental stimulus anything in the environment that arouses or incites action of a receptor (the terminus of a sensory nerve)

enzyme a biologic catalyst that speeds up chemical reactions

epidemic the occurrence of a disease in many people at the same time or in rapid succession in an area

epidemiology study of the occurrence and distribution of disease

epidermis the outermost, nonvascular layer of skin

epididymis a highly coiled duct between the seminiferous tubules of the testes and the vas deferens

epidural outside the dura mater

epidural block injection of an anesthetic between a lumbar interspace into the spinal canal (external to the dura mater)

epinephrine a hormone produced by the medulla of the adrenal glands; it is also manufactured artificially

epistaxis nosebleed

equilibrium a state of balance

equipoise a state of equilibrium

erection (penile) lengthening, widening, and hardening of the penis as it becomes congested with blood during sexual arousal

erogenous sexually sensitive

erotic stimuli sensations that cause sexual arousal

eructation ejection of gas from the stomach (belching)

erythema redness that is associated with a variety of rashes

erythematous of the nature of erythema

erythroblastosis fetalis a condition produced in second and subsequent infants borne by Rh negative mothers when the father is Rh positive

erythrocyte red blood cell

erythropoiesis the formation of red blood cells

esophagoscopy visual examination of the interior of the esophagus with a lighted instrument

esophagus the muscular tube that extends from the pharynx to the stomach

espanto a Hispanic term for a disease in which the individual is frightened by seeing supernatural spirits or events

ester a compound of alcohol and acid

estrogen a female sex hormone formed by the ovaries, the adrenal cortex, the testes, and the fetoplacental organ

ethics the rules or principles that govern right conduct

ethnic relating to races or to large groups of people with common traits and customs

ethnic group a set of individuals who share a unique cultural and social heritage passed on from one generation to another

ethnicity the condition of belonging to a specific ethnic group

ethnoscience systematic study of the way of life of a designated cultural group to obtain accurate data regarding behavior, perceptions, and interpretations of the universe

etiology cause

Eucharist *see* Holy Communion

eupnea normal respiration that is quiet, rhythmic, and effortless

eustachian (auditory) tube the tube that connects the middle ear with the nasopharynx

euthanasia the act or practice of killing for reasons of mercy

evacuator an instrument for removing fluid or small particles from a body cavity

evaluate to judge or appraise; to identify whether or to what degree a client's goals of care have been met

evaluating assessing the client's response to nursing intervention and then comparing the response to predetermined standards

evaluation the process of identifying the client's progress toward achievement of established goals, using well-defined outcome criteria; judgment or appraisal

evaporation conversion of liquid into a vapor

eversion turning outward

evisceration extrusion of the internal organs

examine to inspect or investigate

excise to cut off or out

excoriation loss of the superficial layers of the skin

excretion elimination of a waste product produced by the body cells from the body

exhalation (expiration) the act of breathing out; the outflow of air from the lungs to the atmosphere

exophthalmos protruding eyeballs

exotoxin a toxic substance formed by bacteria and found outside the bacterial cell

expanded role increased responsibility assumed by a nurse by virtue of education and experience

expanding family the stage of family development that includes the childbearing and childrearing phases

expectorate to cough and spit up mucus or other materials

expert power power derived from one's expertise, talents, and skills

expert systems computer-based models that attempts to simulate the way human experts in a particular field gather data and make decisions

expert witness one who by education or experience possesses knowledge that the ordinary layperson does not have

expiration (exhalation) the outflow of air from the lungs to the atmosphere

expiratory reserve volume the maximum amount of air exhaled after a normal exhalation

expired dead

exploratory surgery surgery performed to confirm the extent of a pathologic process and sometimes to confirm a diagnosis

extended family the nuclear family plus other relatives such as uncles, aunts, and grandparents

extension increasing the angle of a joint (between two bones); the act of straightening

extensor (muscle) a muscle that acts to straighten a joint, thus increasing the angle between two bones

external cardiac massage rhythmic massage of the heart muscle over the sternum

extracellular outside the cells

extracellular fluid (ECF) fluid found outside the body cells

extrapolating inferring facts or data from known facts or data

extrathecal outside the sheath, e.g., outside the spinal canal

extravasation the escape of blood from a vessel into the body tissues

extreme unction the sacrament of anointing the sick

exudate material, e.g., fluid and cells, that has escaped from blood vessels and is deposited in tissues or on tissue surfaces during the inflammatory process

fad a practice followed for a time with exaggerated zeal

Fahrenheit a thermometer scale used to measure heat; the freezing point of water is 32 F, and the boiling point is 212 F

family-centered nursing nursing that considers the health of the family as a unit in addition to the health of the individual family members

fantasy an adaptive mechanism in which wishes and desires are imagined as fulfilled

fasciculation abnormal contraction of a muscle involving the whole motor unit of the muscle

fastigium the highest point

fasting abstinence from eating

fat an organic substance that is greasy and insoluble in water; adipose tissue, a whitish-yellow tissue that forms soft pads between various body organs and serves as an energy reserve; an ester of glycerol with fatty acids

fatty acid the basic structural unit of fat

fear an emotional response to an actual, present danger

febrile pertaining to a fever; feverish

fecal impaction a mass of hardened feces in the folds of the rectum

fecal incontinence inability to control the passage of feces through the anus

feces body wastes and undigested food eliminated from the rectum

feedback a process that enables a system to regulate itself; the response to some of a system's output, which acts as input for the purpose of exerting influence over a process; in communication, it is the response; in learning, it is the process of relating a person's performance to the desired goal

fellatio the oral stimulation of the male genitals by licking, blowing, or sucking

felony a crime of a serious nature punishable by imprisonment

femoral anteversion the forward tipping or tilting of the femur

femoral pulse the pulse found in the groin at the midpoint of the inguinal ligament

fenestrated perforated to provide a window or opening

fetus the unborn offspring in the postembryonic stage of development

fever elevated body temperature

fiber an indigestible carbohydrate derived from plants

fibrillation involuntary contractions of a muscle; cardiac arrhythmia characterized by extremely rapid, irregular, and ineffective twitchings of the atria or ventricles

fibrin an insoluble protein formed from fibrinogen during the clotting of blood

fibrinous exudate exudate containing large amounts of fibrin

fibroplasia the formation of fibrous tissue

fibrous tissue common connective tissue composed of elastic and collagen fibers

figure-eight bandage a bandage turn usually used for flexed joints in which the bandage makes a figure-eight around and over the joint

first intention healing primary healing of a wound, which occurs when the tissue surfaces have been approximated

fissure a groove or deep fold such as that which separates the lobes of the lung

fistula an abnormal communication or passage usually between two organs or between an organ and the body surface

flaccid weak or lax

flaccid paralysis impaired muscle function with loss of muscle tone

flail chest the ballooning out of the chest wall through injured rib spaces during exhalation

flatness (in percussion) absence of resonance; extreme dullness

flatulence the presence of excessive amounts of gas in the stomach or intestines

flatus gas or air normally present in the stomach or intestines

flexion decreasing the angle of a joint (between two bones); the act of bending

flexor (muscle) a muscle that acts to bend a joint, decreasing the angle between two bones

flowsheet a record used to chart the progress of specific or specialized data, such as vital signs, fluid balance, or routine medications

flushing transient redness of the skin, often of the face and neck; it may be generalized or restricted to a particular area

follicle (hair) a pouchlike depression in the skin in which a hair is enclosed

follicle-stimulating hormone (FSH) a hormone produced by the anterior pituitary gland (adenohypophysis) that stimulates the development of the ovarian follicle

foment *see* hot pack

fomite an inanimate object other than food that can harbor pathogenic microorganisms and transmit an infection

fontanelle an unossified membranous gap in the bone structure of the skull

footboard a board placed at the foot of a bed against which a client can brace the feet

foot drop plantar flexion of the foot with permanent contracture of the gastrocnemius (calf) muscle and tendon

forceps an instrument with two blades and a handle used to grasp sterile supplies and to compress or grasp tissues

forensic medicine the application of medical knowledge to the law

foreplay physical stimulation to increase sexual arousal prior to intercourse; also called *precoital stimulation*

foreskin a covering fold of skin over the glans of the penis; also called the *prepuce*

formal operations stage (Piaget) the fourth cognitive developmental stage during ages 11 to 15 or 16 years

formulary a collection of prescriptions and formulas

Fowler's position a bed sitting position with the head of the bed raised to 45 degrees

fracture a break in the continuity of bone

fracture board a support placed under the mattress of a bed to add rigidity

framework a basic structure supporting anything

fraud false presentation of some fact or facts with the intention that the information will be acted on by another person

frenulum a fold of mucous membrane that attaches the tongue to the floor of the mouth; a fold on the lower surface of the glans penis that connects it with the prepuce

frequency (of urination) voiding at more frequent intervals than usual

friction rubbing; the force that opposes motion

friction rub *see* pleural rub

frigidity a low or nondetectable sex drive, usually applied to females

frontal plane the plane that divides the body into ventral and dorsal sections

frustration increased emotional tension due to inability to meet goals

fulcrum the fixed point of a lever

full disclosure provision of complete and truthful information to a client participating in a research study

functionalis a layer of endometrium that is shed during menstruation

functional residual capacity volume of air remaining in the lungs after a normal expiration

funnel chest (pectus excavatum) a congenital defect in which the sternum is depressed and the anteroposterior diameter of the chest is narrowed

gait the way a person walks

gastric pertaining to the stomach

gastrocolic reflex increased peristalsis of the colon after food has entered the stomach

gastroenteritis inflammation of the stomach and the intestines

gastroscope a lighted instrument used to visualize the interior of the stomach

gastroscopy visual examination of the stomach with a gastroscope

gastrostomy a surgical opening that leads through the abdomen directly into the stomach

gauge (of a needle) the diameter of the shaft of a needle

gavage administration of nourishment to the stomach through a nasogastric or orogastric tube; tube feeding

gay and lesbian families families in which the adult couple are homosexual partners

gelatinous like jelly

gender behavior behavior with masculine or feminine connotations

gender identity a person's sense of being masculine or feminine as distinct from being male or female

gender role (sexual role) all that a person says or does to indicate whether the person is male or female

gene the biologic unit of heredity, located on a chromosome

general adaptation syndrome (GAS) a general arousal response of the body to a stressor that is characterized by certain physiologic events and that is dominated by the sympathetic nervous system

generativity (Erikson) concern for establishing and guiding the next generation

genitals the reproductive organs, usually the external ones

genital stage (Freud) the final stage of maturity of an adult

genupectoral position a position in which the weight is borne by the knees and chest and the body is at a 90 degree angle to the hips

genu valgum a condition in which the medial aspects of the knees touch in the standing position while the feet remain apart; knock-knees

genu varum a condition in which, when the feet are held together, the knees remain apart; bowlegs

geographic poverty the existence of poverty in certain geographic areas of the country

geriatrics the branch of medicine pertaining to elderly people

germicidal possessing the ability to kill microorganisms

germicide an agent that kills some pathogens

gerontology the study of all aspects of aging

gingiva the gum tissue

gingivitis inflammation of the gums

glans clitoris the exposed part of the clitoris

glans penis the cap-shaped, expansive structure at the end of the penis

glaucoma an eye disease characterized by an increase in intraocular pressure that produces changes in the optic disc and the field of vision

glomerular filtrate fluid formed in the nephron of the kidney that is similar to plasma in composition; the precursor of urine

glossitis inflammation of the tongue

glottis the vocal apparatus of the larynx

glucagon a hormone produced by the alpha cells of the islands of Langerhans in the pancreas; it stimulates the breakdown of liver glycogen

glucocorticoid a hormone produced by the adrenal glands that influences the metabolism of glucose, protein, and fat

gluconeogenesis the process by which the liver converts proteins and fats into glucose

glucose a monosaccharide occurring in food

glycerol the alcohol components of fats

glycogen the chief carbohydrate stored in the body, particularly in the liver and muscles

glycogenesis formation of glycogen

glycogenolysis the breakdown of glycogen to reform glucose

glycolysis the release of energy through the breakdown of glucose

glycosuria the presence of glucose in the urine; glucosuria

goal the desired outcome of nursing interventions

gonad an ovary or testis

gonorrhea a sexually transmitted (venereal) infection due to *Neisseria gonorrhoeae*

Good Samaritan Act a law that protects physicians and

sometimes nurses when rendering aid to a person in an emergency

gout a condition characterized by excessive uric acid in the blood

governance the establishment and maintenance of social, political, and economic arrangements by which practitioners control their practice, self-discipline, working conditions, and professional affairs

granulation tissue young connective tissue with new capillaries formed in the wound healing process

gravity the force that pulls objects toward the center of the earth

grief emotional suffering often caused by bereavement

group two or more persons who have shared needs or goals

group dynamics (process) forces that determine the behavior of the group and its members

growth an increase in weight and height; an increase in physical size; the proliferation of cells

guilt the painful emotion associated with transgression of moral-ethical beliefs

gustatory referring to the sense of taste

gynecology the branch of medicine that deals with processes of the female reproductive tract

gynosperm sperm bearing an X chromosome

hair follicle a pouchlike depression in the skin enclosing the root of a hair

hair shaft the visible part of the hair

halitosis bad breath

hallucinate to perceive through the senses something unreal; such as hearing voices or seeing things that do not exist

hallucinogens drugs that cause distortion of the sensory perception

hangnail a shred of epidermal tissue at either side of the nail

haploid number the number of chromosomes (23 single) found in human sperm and egg cells

hapten a substance free of protein that can interact with other substances on antibodies but does not itself cause the formation of antibodies

Harris tube a single-lumen tube with a metal tip that is inserted through the mouth into the intestines

haustrum a saclike formation of a part of the colon, produced by contraction of both the longitudinal and the circular muscles (plural: haustra)

head mirror a mirror worn on the examiner's head that directs light onto an area being examined

health a state of being physically fit, mentally stable, and socially comfortable; it encompasses more than the state of being free of disease

health appraisal assessment of physical and psychosocial health

health behavior the action a person takes to understand his or her health state, maintain an optimal state of health, prevent illness and injury, and reach his or her maximum physical and mental potential

health beliefs concepts about health that an individual believes are true

health-illness continuum a continuum (continuous process) with high-level wellness at one end and death at the other

health maintenance organization (HMO) an organization that provides a wide range of health services on a fixed contract basis, usually geared to preventive medicine

health practice an activity that a person carries out as a result of his or her health beliefs and definition of health

health practitioner a person who provides a health care service

health problem any condition or situation in which a person requires help to maintain or regain a state of health or to achieve a peaceful death

health promotion health care aimed at enhancing the wellness of individuals through education and encouragement of behavior changes or changes in the environment

health risk appraisal (HRA) tool that indicates a client's risk of diseases or injury over time by comparing the client with a large national sample with similar demographic data

health status the health of a person at a given time

health team a group of individuals with varying skills whose cooperative efforts are designed to assist people with their health

hectic fever *see* septic fever

height a vertical measurement extending from the highest point on the head to the surface on which the individual is standing, normally measured in centimeters or inches

hemangioma a large, persistent, bright red or dark purple vascular area of the skin

hematemesis the vomiting of blood

hematocrit the percentage of red blood cell mass in proportion to whole blood

hematoma a collection of blood in a tissue, organ, or body space due to a break in the wall of a blood vessel

hematuria the presence of blood in the urine

hemiplegia the loss of movement on one side of the body

hemoglobin the red pigment in red blood cells that carries oxygen

hemoglobinuria the presence of hemoglobin in the urine

hemolysis rupture of red blood cells

hemopneumothorax a collection of blood and air or gas in the pleural cavity

hemoptysis the presence of blood in the sputum

hemorrhage bleeding; the escape of blood from the blood vessels

hemorrhoids distended veins in the rectum

hemosiderosis deposition of iron in the skin, liver, spleen, and other organs

hemostat (artery forceps) a small pair of forceps used to constrict blood vessels

hemothorax a collection of blood in the pleural cavity

heparin a substance that prevents coagulation of blood

herb a leafy plant that does not have a wood stem and is valued for its medicinal, savory, or aromatic qualities

herbalist an herb doctor; one who prescribes herbs for treating people

hereditary factors risk factors related to genetically transmitted conditions or genetic predispositions to various conditions

Hering-Breuer reflex a reflex that inhibits inspiration

hesitancy (of urination) delay and difficulty initiating voiding

hex a jinx; a spell imposed in witchcraft

high-Fowler's position a bed sitting position in which the head of the bed is elevated 90 degrees

hirsutism abnormal hairiness, particularly in women

histology the study of the structure and function of tissues

holism the view that a person is more than the sum of many parts

holistic health a model of health based on the belief that the whole is more than the sum of its parts

holophrastic speech a type of speech in which one word expresses a whole sentence

Holy Communion a memorial sacrament practiced by Christians based on the mandate of Jesus Christ at the Last Supper; it is also called the *Eucharist* or the *Lord's Supper*

home care health services provided to individuals and families in their homes

homeodynamics the continual exchange of energy between humans and the external environment

homeostasis tendency of the body to maintain a state of balance or equilibrium while continually changing

homogamy mating like with like; inbreeding; reproduction resulting from the union of two identical cells

homogeneity a high degree of likeness of attitudes and beliefs among members of a group

homosexual a person whose primary sexual orientation is to a member of the same sex

hormone a chemical substance that is produced by the body and secreted into the bloodstream and that regulates the activity of certain body organs

hospice a health care facility for the dying

hostility overt antagonism; behavior in which the individual tends to be harmful or destructive

hot pack (foment) a hot moist cloth applied to an area of the body

human chorionic gonadotropin (HCG) a hormone produced by the placenta in the first trimester of pregnancy

humanism concern for human attributes

humidity the amount of moisture in the air, expressed as a percentage

hunger an unpleasant sensation caused by deprivation of something, especially food

hyaluronidase an enzyme found in tissues; it catalyzes hydrolysis of hyaluronic acid, the cement substance of tissues

hydration the act of combining or being combined with water

hydraulics the branch of physics that deals with the physical actions of liquids

hydrocephalus a disease process resulting in excessive cerebrospinal fluid within the skull

hydrocortisone an adrenocortical steroid produced by the adrenal glands or produced synthetically; also called *cortisol*

hydrolysates hydrolyzed proteins or amino acids

hydrolysis the process of splitting a molecule in the presence of digestive enzymes with the addition of water

hydrometer an instrument used to determine the specific gravity of a fluid

hydrostatic pressure the pressure a liquid exerts on the sides of the container that holds it; also called *filtration force*

hygiene the science of health and its maintenance

hymen a thin fold of mucous membrane separating the vagina from the vestibule

hyperalgesia extreme sensitivity to pain

hyperalimentation *see* total parenteral nutrition

hypercalcemia excessive calcium in the blood plasma

hypercalciuria excessive calcium in the urine

hypercarbia (hypercapnia) accumulation of carbon dioxide in the blood

hyperemia increased blood flow to an area

hyperextension further extension between two bones or stretching out of a joint

hyperextension position a bed position with the head and foot of the bed lowered to form a 15 degree angle in the bed foundation

hyperglycemia an increased concentration of glucose in the blood

hyperkalemia excessive potassium in the blood

hypernatremia an elevated level of sodium in the blood plasma

hyperopia farsightedness

hyperphosphatemia increased phosphorous levels in the blood plasma

hyperplasia an abnormal increase in the number of cells in a tissue or an organ

hyperpnea an abnormal increase in the rate and depth of respirations

hyperpyrexia an extremely elevated body temperature

hyperreflexia an exaggeration of the reflexes

hyperresonance a lower-pitched sound than resonance

hypersensitivity an exaggerated response of the body to a foreign substance

hypersommnia excessive sleep

hypertension an abnormally high blood pressure

hyperthermia an abnormally high body temperature, sometimes induced as a therapeutic measure

hypertonicity excessive muscle tone or activity

hypertonic solution a fluid possessing a greater concentration of solutes than plasma has

hypertrophy an increase in size of a cell, tissue, or body organ such as a muscle

hyperventilation an increase in the amount of air entering the lungs, characterized by prolonged and deep breaths

hypervolemia an abnormal increase in the body's blood volume

hypnosis an abnormally induced passive state in which an individual responds to suggestions that do not conflict with the person's conscious or unconscious desires

hypnotic (drug) a drug that induces sleep

hypoalbuminemia reduction in the level of albumin in the blood

hypocalcemia decreased calcium in the blood plasma

hypocarbia (hypocapnia) depressed level of carbon dioxide in the blood

hypochloremia a reduced concentration of chlorides in the blood plasma

hypodermic *see* subcutaneous

hypodermis (subcutaneous tissue) connective tissues beneath the skin

hypodermoclysis the introduction of fluid in the subcutaneous tissues

hypofibrinogenemia an abnormally low level of fibrinogen in the blood

hypoglycemia a reduced amount of glucose in the blood

hypokalemia potassium deficit in the blood plasma

hyponatremia an abnormally low amount of sodium in the blood plasma

hypophosphatemia phosphorous deficiency in the blood

hypophysis *see* pituitary gland

hypostatic pneumonia an infection of lung tissue resulting from poor circulation or stagnation of secretions

hypotension an abnormally low blood pressure

hypothalamus the part of the brain beneath the thalamus that forms the floor and part of the wall of the third ventricle

hypothermia an abnormally low body temperature

hypothesis a statement of the relationship between two or more concepts or variables; an assumption made to test its logical or empirical consequences

hypothesizing technique of predicting which actions will solve a problem or meet a goal

hypotonicity decreased muscle tone

hypotonic solution a fluid possessing a lesser concentration of solutes than plasma has

hypoventilation a reduction in the amount of air entering the lungs, characterized by shallow respirations

hypovolemia reduction in blood volume

hypovolemic shock a state of shock due to a reduction in the volume of circulating blood

hypoxemia low partial pressure of oxygen or low saturation of oxyhemoglobin in the arterial blood

hypoxia insufficient oxygen anywhere in the body

iatrogenic caused by the physician or medical therapy

id (Freud) the unconscious part of the personality that contains primitive desires and urges and is ruled by the pleasure principle

ideational forming images or objects in the mind

identification an adaptative or defense mechanism in which one assumes the attitudes, ideas, and behavior patterns of another person or persons

identifying as an element of anger, the act of seeking a response and support from others

idiosyncratic effect a different, unexpected, or individual effect from the normal one usually expected from a medication; the occurrence of unpredictable and unexplainable symptoms

ileal conduit most commonly used urinary diversion procedure

ileocecal valve membranous folds between the distal ileum and the entrance to the large intestine (cecum)

ileostomy an artificial abdominal opening into the ileum (small bowel)

ileum the distal portion of the small intestine

illness sickness or deviation from a healthy state or the normal functioning of the total person

illness behavior the course of action a person takes to define the state of his or her health and pursue a remedy

illusion a false interpretation of some stimulus

imagination creation by the mind; forming a mental image of something not present to stimulate the senses

imitation copying the behaviors and attitudes of another person

immobility prescribed or unavoidable restriction of movement in any area of a person's life

immunity a specific resistance of the body to infection; it may be natural, endowed resistance or resistance developed after exposure to a disease agent

immunization the process of becoming immune or rendering someone immune

immunoglobulin a part of the body's plasma proteins; also called *immune bodies* or *antibodies*

immunologic reaction production of antibodies in response to an antigen; an allergic reaction

impaction a condition of being firmly wedged or lodged; in reference to feces, a collection of hardened puttylike feces in the folds of the rectum

imperforate abnormally closed; used to describe an opening, such as the anus or the hymen, that is not open

implementing putting the nursing strategies listed in the nursing care plan into action; intervening

impotence inability to achieve or to maintain an erection sufficiently to perform intercourse

impregnation fertilization of the ovum

incision a cut or wound that is intentionally made, e.g., during surgery

incoherent engaging in actions or speech that lacks cohesion, orderly continuity, relevance, or consistency

incontinence inability to control the elimination of urine (enuresis) or feces (fecal incontinence)

incorporation a process by which people or objects are internalized and become a part of one's understanding

incubation period the time between entrance of a pathogen into the body and the onset of symptoms of the infection

incurvated (ingrown) nail a nail that has grown so that it impinges into surrounding soft tissues

independence self-reliance and self-assertiveness

independent nurse practitioner a nurse who practices independently in the health care system

independent nursing action (intervention or function) an activity initiated by a nurse as a result of her or his own knowledge and skills and without the physician's direct order

indirect interview interview in which the nurse allows the client to control the purpose, subject matter, and pacing; also called *nondirect interview*

individual-client supply system (of drugs) medications supplied separately for each client in specified doses and quantities for a specified period of time

inductive reasoning making generalizations from specific data

inductive theory a theory formulated by a process in which certain phenomena are observed followed by the development of the idea relating the phenomena

induration hardening

infarct a localized area of necrosis (dead cells) usually owing to obstructed arterial blood flow to the part

infection the disease process produced by microorganisms

inference the interpretation of data from knowledge and past experience

inferential reasoning solving problems by means of inference

inferior situated below

infestation invasion of the body by insects, mites, and/or ticks

infiltration the diffusion or deposition into tissue of substances that are not normal to it

inflammation the tissue response to injury or destruction of cells

informed consent *see* consent

infradian rhythm a biorhythm that cycles monthly, such as the human menstrual cycle

infrared heat a radiant type of heat capable of penetrating body tissues to a depth of 10 mm; sources of infrared rays include heat lamps and incandescent light bulbs

infusion the introduction of fluid into a vein or part of the body

ingestion the act of taking in food or medication

ingrown toenail penetration of the edges of the toenail plate into the surrounding tissues

inhalation (inspiration) the act of breathing in; the intake of air or other substances into the lungs

inhalation therapist (respiratory therapist) a respiratory technologist skilled in therapies for individuals with respiratory problems

inhalation (aerosol) therapy deliverance of droplets of medication or moisture suspended in a gas, such as oxygen, by inhalation through the nose or mouth

inner canthus the corner of the upper and lower eyelids near the nose

inorganic having no organs; not of organic origin; in chemistry, acids or compounds that do not contain carbon

input information, material, or energy that enters a system

inquest a legal inquiry into the cause or manner of a death

insensible perspiration unnoticeable sweating that evaporates immediately once it reaches the surface of the skin

insertion (of a muscle) the more movable point of attachment of a muscle

insomnia inability to obtain a sufficient quality or quantity of sleep

inspection visual examination to detect features perceptible to the eye

inspiration (inhalation) the act of drawing air into the lungs

inspiratory capacity the maximum amount of air that can be inhaled after a normal exhalation

inspiratory reserve volume the maximum amount of air inhaled after a normal inspiration

instillation application of a medication into a body cavity or orifice

insufflator an instrument used to blow air into a part of the body, e.g., the rectum

insulator a substance or material that inhibits conduction, e.g., of heat or electricity

insulin a hormone secreted by the beta cells of the islands of Langerhans in the pancreas; also a preparation for administration

integument the skin or covering of the body

integumentary system the skin, hair, and nails

intelligence ability to learn

intensity (in percussion) the loudness or softness of a sound

intensive services level of home care services in which clients require medical and professional nursing care as an alternative to hospitalization of skilled nursing home care

intercostal between the ribs

intercostal retractions indrawing between the ribs

interdependence a balance between dependence and independence

interdigital between the digits (toes and fingers)

intermediate services level of home care services in which clients require professional nursing supervision, direct care, physical or speech therapy, regular and periodic medical supervision, or some combination of these

intermittent (quotidian) fever a fever that recurs daily

intermittent positive pressure breathing (IPPB) delivery of oxygen into the lungs at positive pressure and release of the pressure passively during expiration

intern a graduate of a basic health program who is taking planned practice experience, such as nursing or medicine, usually to obtain a license to practice

internal feedback positive or negative responses from oneself about a communication one has given either in writing or verbally

internal rotation a turning toward the midline, e.g., rotation of the hip joint

interpersonal skills verbal and nonverbal activities that people use when communicating directly with one another

interstitial between the cells of the body's tissues

interstitial cells of Leydig clusters of cells, located between the seminiferous tubules, that secrete male hormones

interstitial fluid fluid surrounding the body cells

intervention activities performed by the nurse and the client to change the effect of a problem

intervertebral between the vertebrae

interview a structured consultation used to obtain information or to evaluate the progress of a person

intestinal distention (tympanites) stretching and inflation of the intestines due to the presence of air or gas

intraarterial within or inside an artery

intracardiac within or into the heart muscle

intracellular within a cell or cells

intracellular fluid (cellular fluid, ICF) fluid found within the body cells

intractable pain pain that is resistant to cure or relief

intradermal (intracutaneous) within the skin

intrafamily communication the pattern of verbally and nonverbally transmitted messages among family members

Intralipid trademark for an intravenous fat solution that provides concentrated calories during total parenteral nutrition

intramuscular within or inside muscle tissue

intraosseous within or into the bone

intrapleural within the pleural cavity

intrapleural pressure pressure within the pleural cavity

intrapulmonic pressure pressure within the lungs

intraspinal see intravertebral

intrathecal within or into the spinal canal

intrauterine inside the uterus

intrauterine device (IUD) a device inserted into the uterus for contraception

intravascular within a blood vessel

intravascular fluid plasma

intravenous within a vein

intravenous cholangiogram an x-ray film of the bile ducts after a contrast dye has been administered intravenously

intravenous pyelogram an x-ray film of the kidneys taken after intravenous injection of a radiopaque dye

intravenous pyelography (IVP) x-ray filming of the kidney and ureters after injection of a radiopaque material intravenously; also called *intravenous urography*

intravenous urography (IVU) see intravenous pyelography

intravertebral (intraspinal) within the vertebrae

introjection unconscious acceptance and incorporation of the patterns, attitudes, and ideals of another person as one's own

introversion direction of one's energy and interest toward oneself

intubation insertion of a tube

inunction application of a topical drug to the skin or mucous membrane for absorption

inversion a turning inward

invisible poverty social and cultural deprivation

involution a rolling or turning inward of a particular organ or the entire body, e.g., the uterus after the fetus is expelled

ion an atom or group of atoms that carry a positive or negative electric charge; an electrolyte

iris the colored, circular membrane of the eye, situated behind the cornea, in the center of which is the pupil

irradiation exposure to penetrating rays, such as x-rays, gamma rays, infrared rays, or ultraviolet rays

irrational confused as to time, place, and/or person

irrigation (lavage) the washing of a body cavity or a wound

irritant a substance that stimulates unpleasant responses, that is, irritates

ischemia lack of blood supply to a body part

islands of Langerhans clusters of endocrine-secreting cells located in the pancreas

isometric having the same measure or length

isometric muscle contraction tensing of a muscle against an immovable outer resistance, which does not change muscle length or produce joint motion

isometric static exercise exercise in which a person consciously increases the tension of the muscle without moving the joint

isotonic having the same tonicity as the body fluids; the term is used to compare solutions of the same strength or concentration

isotonic exercise active exercise involving muscle contractions in which there is a marked shortening of muscle length

isotonic muscle contraction shortening of a muscle in the process of doing work that produces joint motion (e.g., range-of-motion exercises or weight lifting)

isthmus a narrow passage connecting two larger parts of an organ

jargon the technical or idiomatic terminology characteristic of a particular group

jaundice a yellowish tinge to the skin and mucous membrane

jejunum the portion of the small intestine that extends from the duodenum to the ileum

Kardex (Rand) a portable card index file that organizes data about clients in a concise way and often contains nursing care plans

Kelly forceps a type of hemostat

keratin the protein found in epidermis, hair, and nails

keratinized cells dead cells that have been converted to protein

keratotic spots horny growths, such as warts or calluses

ketogenesis the process in which deaminated amino acids are converted into fatty acids, producing ketone bodies (acetone)

ketone any compound containing the carbonyl group, CO, and having hydrocarbon groups attached to the carbonyl group

ketosis a condition in which excessive ketones are formed in the body

kilocalorie (Calorie) the amount of heat required to raise the temperature of 1 kilogram of water 1 degree Celsius

kilogram a unit of weight equal to 1000 grams or approximately 2.2 pounds

kinesiology the study of the motion of the human body

kinesthesia the sense of the position and the movement of the body parts

kinesthetic referring to awareness of body position and movement

knee-chest position see genupectoral position

Korotkoff's sounds sounds of blood produced within the artery with each ventricular contraction

kosher sanctioned by Jewish law

Kussmaul breathing (Kussmaul-Kien respiration) deep rapid breathing; a dyspnea occurring in paroxysms often preceding diabetic coma: air hunger

kwashiorkor a condition occurring in children after weaning as a result of protein and calorie malnutrition; evidenced by growth failure, potbelly, edema, and mental apathy

kyphosis an exaggerated convexity in the thoracic region of the vertebral column, resulting in a stooped posture

labia the fleshy edges of a structure, usually the female genitals

labia majora the two longitudinal folds or lips of skin extending downward and backward from the mons pubis that protect the vaginal and urethral orifices

labia minor small folds of skin lying between the labia majora and the vaginal opening

labored breathing difficult or dyspneic breathing

labyrinth a system of interconnecting canals or cavities

lacerate to tear, rather than cut, a body tissue

lacrimal fluid tears produced by the lacrimal glands that lubricate the eye

lacrimal glands organs that are situated in a depression in the frontal bone at the upper, outer angle of the eye orbit, and that secrete tears

lacrimal sac the opening connecting the tear ducts in the inner canthus of the eye to the nasolacrimal duct, which empties into the nasal cavity

lacrimation the secretion and discharge of tears

lactase an enzyme that acts as a catalyst to convert lactose into glucose and galactose

lactate salt of lactic acid that is metabolized in the liver to form bicarbonate

lactation the secretion of milk; the period of milk secretion

lactiferous conveying or producing milk

lactose a carbohydrate found in milk

lanugo fine, wooly hair or down on the shoulders, back, sacrum, and earlobes of the unborn child; it may remain for a few weeks after birth

laryngeal mirror an instrument like a dental mirror used to view the pharynx, larynx, or structures of the mouth

laryngeal stridor a harsh, crowing sound heard during expiration when there is a laryngeal obstruction

laryngoscope a lighted instrument used to visualize the larynx

laryngoscopy visual examination of the larynx with a laryngoscope

laryngospasm spasmodic closure of the larynx

larynx a structure composed of nine cartilages guarding the entrance of the trachea and containing the vocal cords

latch-key children working parents' school-age children who must care for themselves after school

latency period (Freud) the school-age years (6 to 12 years)

lateral to the side, away from the midline

lateral position a side-lying position

lavage an irrigation or washing of a body organ, such as the stomach

laxative a medication that stimulates bowel activity

leading question question that directs the client's answer

learning a permanent change in behavior

learning need a need to change behavior

learning principle an assumption thought to facilitate and maximize learning

legume the fruit or pod of a leguminous plant, such as a pea or bean

lens a transparent, convex body that is the focusing device of the eye

lesion the traumatic or pathologic interruption of a tissue or the loss of function of a body part

lethargy drowsiness; sleeping much of the time when not stimulated

leukocyte a white blood cell

leukocytosis an increase in the number of white blood cells

lever a rigid bar that moves on a fixed axis called a fulcrum

leverage force applied with the use of a lever

Levin tube a single-lumen nasogastric tube

liability the quality or state of being liable

liable legally responsible for one's obligations and actions and obliged to make financial restitution for wrongful acts

libel defamation by means of print, writing, or pictures

libido (Freud) the urge or desire for sexual activity; the energy form or life instinct; also called *sex drive* and *sexual motivation*

license a legal document authorizing an individual to offer knowledge and skills to the public

life expectancy the age to which a person is expected to live

life-style the values and behaviors adopted by a person in daily life

life-style assessment involves the appraisal of the personal life-style and habits of the client as they affect health

ligament a broad, fibrous band that holds two or more bones together

light pen penlike device that allows inputting of data into a computer by touching the computer display screen

line of gravity an imaginary vertical line running through the center of gravity

lingula (of the lung) the superior and inferior segments at the lower half of the long upper lobe of the left lung

liniment a topical liquid applied to the skin frequently to stimulate circulation or to relieve pain

lipid *see* fat

lithotomy position a back-lying position in which the feet are supported in stirrups

living will a statement of a person's wish not to be kept alive by artificial means or "heroic measures"

livor mortis discoloration of the tissues of the body after death

lobar pneumonia an infectious disease of one or more lobes of the lung

lobe a well-defined portion of an organ, e.g., of the lung or brain

local adaptation syndrome (LAS) the reaction of one organ or body part to stress

lochia the vaginal discharge that occurs during the 1st week or 2 after the birth of a baby

locus of control a measurable concept that can be used to predict which people are most likely to change their behavior

lordosis an exaggerated concavity in the lumbar region of the vertebral column

loss an actual or potential situation in which a valued ability, object, person, etc. is inaccessible or changed so that it is perceived as no longer valuable

lotion a liquid that often carries an insoluble powder

louse a parasitic insect that infests mammals (plural: lice)

lumbar puncture (LP, spinal tap) the insertion of a needle into the subarachnoid space at the lumbar region

lumen a channel within a tube, such as the channel of an artery in which blood flows

lung compliance expansibility of the lung

lung recoil the tendency of lungs to collapse away from the chest wall

lymph a transparent, slightly yellow fluid found within the lymphatic vessels

lymphadenitis inflammation of the lymph nodes

lymphangitis the inflammation of a lymphatic vessel or vessels

lymphatic referring to lymph or lymph vessels

lysis (of a fever) the gradual reduction of an elevated body temperature to normal

lysosome a minute body found in many types of cells; it is involved in intracellular digestion

lysozyme an enzyme in saliva and tears that functions as an antibacterial agent

maceration the wasting away or softening of a solid as if by the action of soaking; often used to describe degenerative changes and eventual disintegration

macrocephaly an abnormally large size of the head

macrophage a large phagocytic cell that destroys microorganisms or harmful cells

malaise a general feeling of being unwell or indisposed

mal de ojo among Hispanics, the belief that disease can result from admiring a part of another person's body, e.g., the hair

malignancy abnormal tissue with a tendency to grow and invade other tissues

malingering the willful feigning of the symptoms of illness to avoid facing something unpleasant

malleolus a rounded prominence on the distal end of the tibia or fibula

malnutrition a disorder of nutrition; insufficient nourishment of the body cells

malpractice professional misconduct or unreasonable lack of professional skill

mammary glands breast tissues that secrete nourishment for the young

mandatory licensure laws that require all persons practicing in a field, such as nursing, to be licensed

manometer an instrument used to measure the pressure of fluids or gases

manslaughter an unlawful killing without previous intent; it is a felony

margination the aggregating or lining up of substances along a surface or edge, e.g., the lining up of white blood cells against the wall of a blood vessel during the inflammatory process

marijuana an intoxicating agent from the leaves and flowers of the plant *Cannabis sativa*; commonly used in cigarettes

marital family the beginning stage of family development when the couple establishes a marital relationship and assumes the roles of husband and wife

mastectomy surgical removal of the breast

masticate to chew, e.g., food

mastication chewing

masturbation self-stimulation of the genitals or other body parts to derive erotic pleasure

material culture objects, such as eating utensils, and the ways these are used by a society

matriarchy a system of social organization in which the mother is the head of the house or family

matrilineal relating to descent through the female line

maturation the process of becoming mature or fully developed; development of inherited traits

meatus an opening, passage, or channel

mechanosensitive pain receptors pain receptors stimulated by mechanical stimuli

medial toward the middle or midline

medical asepsis practices that limit the number, growth, and spread of microorganisms; clean technique

medical examiner a physician who investigates deaths that appear unnatural and who has advanced education in pathology and forensic medicine

medical record (chart) an account of the client's health history, current health status, treatment, and progress

medication (medicine, drug) a chemical or biologic compound administered to humans or animals for disease prevention, cure, or relief, or to affect the structure or function of the body

meditation mental exercise that directs the mind to think inwardly by closing the sense organs to external stimulation

meiosis a specialized type of cell division that occurs in sperm and egg cells

melanin the dark pigment of the skin

menarche the first menstrual period, occurring sometime between the ages of 9 and 17

meniscus the crescent-shaped structure of the surface of a column of liquid; the crescent-shaped cartilage in the knee joint

menopause cessation of menstruation in the human female, usually occurring between ages 45 and 50

menses menstrual flow

mental (defense) mechanism *see* defense mechanism

mental well-being a state of contentment, peace of mind, and satisfaction with living and life

metabolism the sum of all the physical and chemical processes by which living substance is formed and maintained and by which energy is made available for use by the organism

metacarpal referring to the part of the hand between the wrist and the fingers

metaparadigm of nursing the concepts that influence nursing most significantly and determine its practice: the person, environment, health, and nursing actions

metatarsus adductus adduction of the anterior part of the foot with no deformity of the posterior part of the foot

microcephaly an abnormally small size of the head

microglia a type of nerve tissue with migratory cells that act as phagocytes to the waste products of nerve tissues

micronutrient nutrients, such as vitamins and minerals, required in small quantities by the body

microorganism minute living body visible under a microscope

micturate (urinate, void) to pass urine from the body

micturition (urination, voiding) the voluntary expulsion of urine

midclavicular line an imaginary line that runs inferiorly and vertically from the center of the clavicle

midsternal line an imaginary line that runs vertically through the middle of the sternum

milia (whiteheads) small, white nodules usually found over the nose and face of newborns

miliaria rubra a prickly heat rash of the face, neck, trunk, or perineal area of infants

Miller-Abbott tube a double-lumen tube inserted through the nose or mouth into the intestine

milliequivalent (mEq) one-thousandth of an equivalent, which is the chemical combining power of a substance

milliliter (ml) a unit of volume in the metric system approximating 1 cubic centimeter

millimol one-thousandth of a mol

mineralocorticoid a steroid hormone of the adrenal cortex that acts to retain sodium in the body and to excrete potassium

minim the least; the basic unit of volume in the apothecaries' system, equal to 0.0616 ml

misdemeanor a crime less serious than a felony and punishable by a fine or short-term imprisonment or both

mitering a method of folding the bedclothes at the bed corners to maintain them securely

mitosis the process of cell division; the process by which the body replaces cells and grows

MMR combined measles, mumps, and rubella vaccine

mobility ability to move about freely

model (paradigm) an abstract outline or a theoretical depiction of a complex phenomenon

modeling observing the behavior of people who have successfully achieved a goal that one has set for oneself and, through observing, acquiring ideas for behavior and coping strategies

mol a molar solution of a substance

mongolian spots blue or black spots of varying size found largely in the sacral area of Oriental and black infants

monologue a long speech that occurs when there is no listener or responder

monosaccharide a sugar consisting of single molecules

mons pubis a pillow of adipose tissue situated over the symphysis pubis and covered by coarse hair; also called the *mons veneris*

Montgomery's glands sebaceous glands in the areola of the nipple that become enlarged and prominent during pregnancy

Montgomery straps tie tapes used to hold dressings in place

morbidity incidence of disease

mores values of members in a group

morgue a place where dead bodies are temporarily kept before release to a mortician

morning sickness the nausea and vomiting that occur frequently in the mornings during the first trimester of pregnancy

Moro's reflex the startle reflex of infants, in which the arms and legs are extended outward and retracted in response to a sudden stimulus such as a loud noise

morphology form and structure

mortality death; the death rate

mortician a person trained in the care of the dead; also called an *undertaker*

motivation desire

mourning the process through which grief is eventually resolved or altered

mucin the chief constituent of mucus

mucolytic destroying or dissolving mucus

mucous membrane epithelial tissue that forms mucus, concentrates bile, and secretes or excretes enzymes

mucus the lubricating, free slime of the mucous membranes

murmur (cardiac) harsh, rumbling sounds resulting from turbulent blood flow

mydriatic a medication that dilates the pupils of the eyes

myelogram an x-ray film of the spinal cord, nerve roots, and vertebrae after injection of a contrast media into the subarachnoid space

myocardial infarction cardiac tissue necrosis resulting from obstruction of the blood flow to the heart

myocardium the heart muscle; the middle layer of the heart tissue

myometrium the middle, thick, smooth muscle layer of the uterus

myopia nearsightedness

narcolepsy a condition in which an individual experiences an uncontrollable desire for sleep or attacks of sleep at certain intervals

narcotic a strong analgesic

narcotic agonist-antagonist a drug with properties that simulate a narcotic and with properties that act against the effects of a narcotic

narrative charting a description (narration) of information

narrative notes records of a client's day-to-day progress that may be keyed to the SOAP format in the POMR or keyed chronologically in traditional client-records

nasogastric tube a plastic or rubber tube inserted through the nose into the stomach

nasopharynx the upper part of the pharynx adjoining the nasal passage

naturopath a nonmedical practitioner who uses such things as light, heat, and water in therapy, but not drugs

nausea the urge to vomit

nebulizer an atomizer or sprayer

necrosis nonliving cells or tissue in contact with living cells

necrotic dying

need the lack of something requisite, desirable, or useful

negative feedback (homeostasis) a mechanism in which deviations from normal are sensed and counteracted

negative nitrogen balance a nitrogen output that exceeds nitrogen intake

negligence the omission of something a reasonable person would do or the doing of something a reasonable person would not do; an unintentional tort

neonatal mortality infant death within 28 days of birth

neoplasm any growth that is new and abnormal

nephritis inflammation of a kidney

nephron the functional unit of the kidney

nephrosis a disease of the kidney in which there is malfunctioning kidney tissue without inflammation; also called *nephrotic syndrome*

nerve block chemical interruption of a nerve pathway effected by injecting a local anesthetic

neurectomy interruption of the peripheral or cranial nerves, often to relieve localized pain

neurogenous arising in the nervous system

neurohypophysis the posterior part of the pituitary gland

neurologic pertaining to the nervous system

neuron a nerve cell and its processes; the functional unit of the nervous system

neutral question question seeking information without direction or pressure from the interviewer

night terrors (pavor nocturnus) nightmares that the person is unable to recall the next morning

nitrogen balance the state of protein nutrition

nocturia (nycturia) increased frequency of urination at night not as the result of increased fluid intake

nocturnal enuresis involuntary urination at night

noncompliance (drug use) failure to follow a prescription

nondirect interview *see* direct interview

nonmaterial culture the beliefs, customs, languages, and social institutions of a society

nonpathogen a microorganism that does not produce disease under normal conditions

nonproductive cough a dry, harsh cough without secretions

non-rapid-eye-movement sleep *see* NREM sleep

nonverbal communication (body language) communication other than words, including gestures, posture, and facial expressions

norm an ideal or fixed standard; an expected standard of behavior of group members

normal saline an isotonic concentration of salt (NaCl) solution

normocephaly normal head circumference

nosocomial referring to or originating in a hospital or similar institution, e.g., a nosocomial disease

NREM sleep (non-rapid-eye-movement sleep) a deep restful sleep state; also called *slow wave sleep*

nuclear family the family unit composed of parents and children

nurse clinician a nurse with advanced skills in a particular area of nursing practice

nurse theorist a person who seeks to define the basis and principles of nursing practice systematically

nursing assessment data collected during an interview and physical examination of a client by a nurse

nursing audit the review of clients' charts to evaluate nursing competence or performance

nursing care conference a meeting of a group of nurses to discuss possible solutions to certain problems of a client

nursing care plan written guide that organizes information about a client's health, focusing on the actions nurses must take to address identified nursing diagnoses and to meet the stated goals

nursing care rounds procedure in which a group of nurses visits all or selected clients at each client's bedside

nursing diagnosis a statement describing a combination of signs or symptoms indicative of an actual or potential health problem that nurses are able, licensed, and accountable to treat

nursing goals goals stated in terms that guide the actions of the nurse

nursing order specific action that a nurse takes to help a client meet established health care goals

nursing process a five-step systematic process used in nursing

nursing research research into human responses, clinical problems, and processes of care encountered in the practice of nursing

nursing standards optimum levels of nursing care against which actual performance of a nurse is compared

nursing strategy nursing action designed to achieve established client goals

nutrient an organic or inorganic substance found in food; nutrients are digested and absorbed in the gastrointestinal tract and then used in the body's metabolic processes

nutrition what a person eats and how the body uses it

nutritionist a specialist in food and nutrition

nutritive value the nutrient content of a specified amount of food

obesity weight that is 20% greater than the ideal for height and frame

objective the aim of a maneuver or operation

objective data client information that can be determined by observation or measurement by laboratory or other means

objective symptom a sign; evidence of a disease or body dysfunction that can be observed and described by others

obligatory heat the heat produced by the body as a result of the metabolism of food

obligatory loss the essential fluid loss required to maintain body functioning

observation the act or power of observing; gathering of information by noting facts or occurrences

observe to gather data using the five senses

obstetrics the branch of medicine dealing with the birth process and related events that precede and follow it

obtunded difficult to arouse from sleep; requiring shaking or a painful stimulus to awaken

obturator a disc or instrument that closes an opening; the obturator of a tracheostomy set fits inside and closes off the end of the outer tube

occult hidden

occupation an activity in which one engages

occupational therapist an individual who helps a client develop skills necessary for the activities of daily living

Oedipus complex (Freud) the male child's attraction for his mother and accompanying hostile attitudes toward his father; compare with **Electra complex**

ointment a semisolid preparation applied externally to the body

olfactory referring to the sense of smell

oliguria production of abnormally small amounts of urine by the kidneys

opaque not admitting the passage of light

open-ended question broad question inviting a long answer

open system a system that exchanges matter, energy, and information with the environment

open wound a wound in which the continuity of the skin or mucous membrane has been interrupted

operative (intraoperative) period the time during surgery

ophthalmoscope an instrument used to examine the interior of the eye

optional surgery surgery requested by the client but not necessary for health

oral referring to the mouth

oral stage (Freud) the stage of development during the 1st year of life, when the mouth is the principal area of activity

organic referring to an organ or organs; in chemistry, referring to compounds containing carbon; arising from an organism

orgasm the climax of sexual excitement, during which physiologic and psychologic release occurs; orgasm is characterized by rhythmic spasmodic contractions of the genitals

orgasmic dysfunction the inability to achieve orgasm

orgasmic platform an increase in size of the outer one-third of the vagina and the labia minora during precoital stimulation

orientation awareness of time, place, and person

orifice an external opening of a body cavity; e.g., the anus is the orifice of the large intestine

origin (of a muscle) the fixed or least movable point of attachment to a bone

orogastric tube a tube inserted through the mouth into the stomach

oropharynx the part of the pharynx that lies between the upper aspect of the epiglottis and the soft palate

orthopnea the ability to breathe only in the upright position, i.e., sitting or standing

orthostatic hypotension low blood pressure in a standing position

orthostatism the erect standing posture of the body

osmol the number of particles in 1 gram molecular weight of a disassociated solute

osmolarity the concentration of solutes in solution; the osmolar concentration of a solution expressed in osmols per liter of solution

osmosis passage of a solvent through a semipermeable membrane from an area of lesser solute concentration to one of greater solute concentration

osmotic pressure pressure exerted by the number of non-diffusable particles in a solution; the amount of pressure needed to stop the flow of water across a membrane

osseous pertaining to bone

ossification the formation of bone or a bony substance

osteoblast a bone-building cell

osteoclast a cell associated with bone resorption and breakdown

osteomalacia the softening of the bones; decalcification of bones in adults

osteomyelitis inflammation of the bone caused by infection and resulting in bone destruction

osteoporosis decrease in bone density; demineralization of bone

-ostomy a suffix denoting the formation of an opening or outlet

otoscope an instrument used to inspect the eardrum and external ear canal

outcome (evaluative) criteria statements that describe specific, measurable, and observable responses of a client to nursing interventions; expected alterations in the health status of a client

outer canthus the corner of the upper and lower eyelids away from the nose

output the energy, matter, or information released by a system as a result of its processes

outward rotation a turning away from the midline

oval window an opening between the middle and the inner ear

ovary the female gonad (sexual gland); ova are formed in the two ovaries

overbed cradle a frame placed over a client in bed to protect the body from contact with the upper bedclothes

overhydration *see* edema

overnutrition the oversupply of calories

overweight weight that is 10% greater than the ideal for height and frame

ovulation the discharge of a mature ovum from the Graafian follicle of the ovary

ovum (egg) the female reproductive cell, which becomes the embryo after fertilization

oxyhemoglobin the compound of oxygen and hemoglobin

oxytocin a hormone secreted by the posterior pituitary gland; oxytocin helps the uterus to contract before, during, and after delivery

pace the distance covered in a step when one walks or the number of steps taken per minute

packing filling an open wound or cavity with a material such as gauze

PaCO$_2$ partial pressure of carbon dioxide (arterial blood)

pain a basically unpleasant sensation, localized or general, mild or intense, that represents the suffering induced by stimulation of specialized nerve endings; pain may be threatened or fantasied and may be induced by disease, injury, or mental derangement caused by disease or injury

pain threshold the amount of stimulation required by a person to feel pain

pain tolerance the maximum amount and duration of pain that an individual is willing to endure

palate the roof of the mouth

palliative affording relief but not cure

palliative surgery surgery to relieve the symptoms of a disease process

pallor absence of normal skin color; a whitish grayish tinge

palmar grasp reflex a reflex, normally present in newborns, that causes the fingers to curl around a small object placed in the palm of the hand

palpation the act of feeling with the hands, usually the fingers

pandemic an epidemic disease that is widespread

panic severe anxiety

PaO$_2$ partial pressure of oxygen (arterial blood)

Papanicolaou (Pap) smear a method of taking sample cervical cells for microscopic examination to detect malignancy

papule a small, superficial, round elevation of the skin

paracentesis the insertion of a needle into a cavity (usually the abdominal cavity) to remove fluid

paradigm *see* model

paradoxical breathing the ballooning out of the chest wall during expiration and depression or sucking inward of the chest wall during inspiration

paralysis the impairment or loss of motor function of a body part

paramedical having some connection with the practice of medicine

paraphrasing restating a person's message (thoughts and/or feelings) using similar words

paraplegia paralysis of the lower part of the body (including the legs) affecting both motor function and sensation

parasites plants or animals that live on or within another living organism

parasomnia a disorder that interferes with sleep, e.g., somnambulism

parasympathetic (craniosacral) nervous system a branch of the autonomic nervous system

parathyroid hormone (PTH, parathormone) the hormone produced by the parathyroid glands that regulates the calcium and phosphorous levels in the body

parenchyma the functional or essential elements of an organ

parenteral accomplished by a needle; occurring outside the alimentary tract; injected into the body through some route other than the alimentary canal, e.g., intravenously

paresthesia an abnormal sensation of burning or prickling

paronychia inflammation of the tissue surrounding the nail

parotid glands the large salivary glands located below and in front of the ears

parotitis (parotiditis) inflammation of the parotid salivary gland

paroxysm a sudden attack or sharp recurrence; a spasm

partial pressure the pressure exerted by each individual gas in a mixture according to its percentage concentration in the mixture

passive euthanasia allowing a person to die by withholding or withdrawing measures to maintain life

passive exercise exercise during which the muscles do not contract and the nurse, therapist, or client supplies the energy to move the client's body part

passivity lethargy; receptivity to outside influence; lack of energy or will

paste a semisolid dermatologic preparation that tends to penetrate the skin less than an ointment

pasteurization application of heat to milk to destroy disease-producing microorganisms

pastoral care an interpersonal relationship that focuses on the spiritual component of another person's life during distress

patent open, unobstructed, not closed

pathogen a microorganism capable of producing disease

pathogenic capable of producing disease

pathology a branch of medicine concerned with the nature of disease

patient (client) a person who is waiting for or undergoing medical treatment or care

patient (client) advocate a person who speaks on behalf of a client and can intercede on the client's behalf

patient (client) care standards *see* nursing standards

patient (client) goals goals stated as anticipated client outcomes, not as nursing activities

patriarchy a social system in which the father is the head of the household or family

patrilineal relating to descent through the male line

pavor nocturnus *see* night terrors

PCO$_2$ partial pressure of carbon dioxide (venous blood)

pectoriloquy exaggerated bronchophony

pediculosis infestation with lice

pediculosis capitis infestation with head lice

peer review an encounter between two persons equal in education, abilities, and qualifications, during which one person critically reviews the practices that the other has documented in a client's record

penetrating wound a wound created by an instrument that penetrated the skin or mucous membranes deeply into the tissues

penis the male organ of copulation and urinary excretion

Penrose drain a flexible rubber drain

perceived loss loss experienced by a person that cannot be verified by others

perception the process of understanding something new and then making it part of one's previous experience or knowledge; a person's awareness and identification of a person, thing, or situation

perception checking (consensual validation) verifying the accuracy of listening skills by giving and receiving feedback about what was communicated

percussion an assessment method in which the body surface is tapped or struck to elicit sound or vibrations from body structures below the struck area

percussion hammer an instrument shaped like a hammer with a head often made of plastic

percutaneous electric stimulation stimulation of major peripheral nerves by electricity

pericardial aspiration the removal of fluid from the pericardial sac via an inserted needle

pericardial sac (pericardium) a fibrous sac that surrounds the heart

perimetrium the thin, outer, serous layer of the uterus

perineum the area between the anus and the posterior aspect of the genitals

periodontal disease inflammation of the tissues that surround and support the teeth

perioperative period the time before, during, and after an operation

periorbital around the eye socket

periosteum the connective tissue covering all bones

periostitis inflammation of the periosteum

peripheral at the edge or outward boundary

peripheral nerve implant an electrode implanted in a major sensory nerve for the purpose of relieving pain

peristalsis wavelike movements produced by circular and longitudinal muscle fibers of the intestinal walls; it propels the intestinal contents onward

peristomal referring to the skin area that surrounds a stoma

peritoneal cavity the area between the layers of peritoneum in the abdomen; a potential space

peritoneum the membrane lining the abdominal walls

peritonitis inflammation of the peritoneum

permissive licensure the policy by which practitioners do not have to be licensed to practice but are not protected by the licensing body

personal space the physical distance people prefer to maintain in their interactions with others

perspiration the fluid secreted by the sweat glands for excreting waste products and cooling the body

petechiae pinpoint red spots on the skin

pH a measure of the relative alkalinity or acidity of a solution; a measure of the concentration of hydrogen ions

phagocyte a cell, e.g., a white blood cell, that ingests microorganisms, other cells, and foreign particles

phagocytosis the process by which cells engulf microorganisms, other cells, or foreign particles

phalanx any bone of the fingers or toes (plural: phalanges)

phallic stage (Freud) the stage of development during the 4th and 5th years when sexual and aggressive feelings come into focus associated with the genital organs

phantom pain pain that remains after the perceived location has been removed, such as pain perceived in a foot after the leg has been amputated

pharmacist an individual licensed to prepare and dispense drugs and to make up prescriptions

pharmacology the scientific study of the actions of drugs on living animals and humans

pharmacopoeia a book containing a list of drug products used in medicine, including their descriptions and formulas

pharmacy the skill of preparing, compounding, and dispensing medicines; the place where medicines are prepared and dispensed

pharmacy assistant a member of the health team who in some situations administers drugs to clients

pharynx a musculomembranous sac behind the nose and mouth that connects with the esophagus and bronchi

phenomenal field the individual's frame of reference

phimosis an extremely narrowed opening of the foreskin of the penis

phlebitis inflammation of a vein

phlebothrombosis intravascular clotting with marked inflammation of a vein

phlebotomy opening a vein to remove blood

phosphorylation the combining of glucose with phosphate inside a cell

photophobia intolerance to light

photosensitive sensitive to light

phrenic referring to the diaphragm

physiatrist a physician who specializes in rehabilitation medicine; physiatrists use physical aids such as light, heat, and apparatuses

physical pertaining to the body or to physics

physical well-being a state of having one's physical needs met appropriately for homeostasis

physiologic pertaining to body function

physiologic dependence biochemical changes occurring in the body as a result of excessive use of a drug

physiology the science concerned with the functioning of living organisms and their parts

physiotherapist (physical therapist) a member of the health team who provides assistance to clients with musculoskeletal problems

pica a craving for unnatural foods, often during pregnancy, some psychologic conditions, or extreme malnutrition

pigeon chest (pectus carinatum) a chest deformity in which there is a narrow transverse diameter, an increased anteroposterior diameter, and a protruding sternum

pilosebaceous follicle the hair follicle and sebaceous gland complex of the skin

pinna the external part of the ear

pitch (in percussion) the number of vibrations per second or the frequency of vibrations

pitting edema edema in which firm finger pressure on the skin produces an indentation (pit) that remains for several seconds

pituitary gland (hypophysis) an endocrine gland (situated in the brain) that secretes a number of hormones, including adrenocorticotropic hormone and thyrotropic hormone

placebo any form of treatment, e.g., medication, that produces an effect in the client because of its intent rather than its chemical or physical properties

placenta the tissue attached to the wall of the uterus; the fetus receives nourishment through the placenta, which is expelled as the "afterbirth" after the child is born

placing reflex a reflex of infants demonstrated when the infant is placed vertically with one foot touching the edge of a table; the infant flexes the knee and hip of the same leg and tries to place the foot on the surface of the table

planning establishing a series of steps or designing or arranging the parts of something to achieve an end or goal; process of designing nursing strategies or interventions directed toward resolving health problems

plantar flexion movement of the ankle so that the toes point downward

plantar reflex *see* Babinski reflex

plantar wart a wart on the sole of the foot that is sensitive to pressure and caused by the virus *Papovavirus hominis*

plaque a film of mucus and bacteria that forms on the teeth

plasma the fluid portion of the blood in which the blood cells are suspended

pleura the membrane around the lungs; it consists of an outer layer, the parietal pleura, and an inner layer, the visceral pleura

pleural cavity a potential space between the two layers of pleura

pleural rub (friction rub) a coarse, leathery, or grating sound produced by the rubbing together of the pleura

pleximeter the nondominant hand used in percussion

plexor the dominant hand used in percussion

plexus a network, e.g., of nerves or veins

pneumoencephalogram an x-ray film of the cerebrospinal spaces after the introduction of air

pneumonia inflammation of the lung tissue

pneumothorax accumulation of air or gas in the pleural cavity

pneumoventriculogram an x-ray film of the ventricles of the brain after the introduction of air

PO₂ partial pressure of oxygen (venous blood)

polarity the presence of two opposite poles

polarized (cardiac) electrically charged

poliomyelitis an acute viral disease that may cause paralysis

political action activities aimed toward influencing policies of the government, organizations, community, and in the workplace

politics the process of influencing the allocation of scarce resources in the spheres of government, workplace, organizations, and community

polydipsia excessive thirst

polyneuritis inflammation of many nerves

polypnea an abnormal increase in the respiratory rate

polysaccharide a carbohydrate consisting of dozens of molecules of glucose

polyunsaturated fatty acid a fatty acid that contains two or more double bonds, such as linoleic or arachidonic acid

polyuria (diuresis) the production of abnormally large amounts of urine by the kidneys

POMR (POR) *see* problem-oriented medical record

popliteal referring to the posterior aspect of the knee

population total possible membership of a specified group

population density the number of people per square mile of a given area

port an opening or entrance

portal an entrance

positive feedback (homeostasis) a control or regulating mechanism of the body that causes the production of additional hormone

positive nitrogen balance nitrogen input exceeding nitrogen output

positivism the state of being positive; a theory that positive knowledge is based on natural phenomena as verified by empirical sciences

posterior of, toward, or at the back

posterior fornix a vaultlike space at the posterior aspect of the vagina

postmortem examination *see* autopsy

postoperative bed *see* surgical bed

postoperative (postsurgical) period the time following surgery

postpartum occurring after childbirth

possible nursing diagnosis used when evidence about response is unclear or when related factors are unknown

postural drainage drainage of secretions from various lung segments by the use of specific positions and gravity

posture the bearing and position of the body; the relative arrangements of the various parts of the body

potency power; the ability of the male to engage in sexual intercourse

potential health problem the presence of risk factors that predispose persons and families to health problems

potential nursing diagnosis used when a client's responses can be predicted or when health promotion can contribute to well-being

poverty lack of sufficient economic resources to meet basic needs

power capacity to influence another person in some way or to produce change

powerlessness perceived lack of control over events

precedent a prior judicial decision used to justify or confirm a court ruling

precoital stimulation *see* foreplay

precordial thump a sharp blow of the fist to the sternum to restore heart function

precordium the area of the chest over the heart or stomach

preeclampsia an abnormal condition of late pregnancy or the early puerperium characterized by hypertension, albumin in the urine, and generalized edema

prelinguistic pertaining to sounds made by an infant that are not related to language

premature ejaculation the inability to control ejaculation prior to satisfaction of the partner or before 30 to 60 seconds after penetration

preoperational stage (Piaget) the phase of cognitive development that occurs during ages 3 to 7

preoperative period the time before an operation

preoptic center the nerve center anterior to the optic center

prepuberty the period preceding puberty

prepubic urethra the part of the male urethra that is inferior to the pubis

prepuce *see* foreskin

presbycusis loss of hearing due to aging

presbyopia inability of the lens of the eye to accommodate initially to near objects and then to far objects as a result of the aging process

prescription the written direction for the preparation and administration of a remedy

pressoreceptor (baroreceptor) a receptor that is sensitive to changes in pressure, e.g., in the carotid sinus and the arch of the aorta

pricking pain pain like the pain of a knife piercing the skin

primary care a type of practice in which the first person to meet the client, e.g., the nurse, assumes responsibility for care

primary nursing a system of nursing in which the client is assigned on admission to one nurse, who has primary responsibility for nursing care 24 hours a day

primary prevention activities directed toward the protection from or avoidance of potential health risks

primary questions questions that introduce topics or new areas in an interview

primary union (wound healing) healing that involves the production of minimal scar tissue

primigravida a woman who is pregnant for the first time

principle a fundamental law or doctrine; assumption

priority setting process of establishing a preferential order for nursing strategies

privacy a deserved degree of social retreat that provides a comfortable feeling; the right of an individual participating in a research study to behave and think without the possibility of the behavior or thoughts being used to embarrass that person later

privileged communication information given to a professional such as a physician, who is not required to disclose it in a court of law

probing asking for information chiefly out of curiosity

problem-oriented medical record (POMR, POR) a client's chart organized according to the client's problems and recording the reports of several health workers on each problem

process a series of actions directed toward a particular result; in anatomy, a prominence or projection, e.g., of a bone

processing the manipulation of data (e.g., by a computer) to achieve a specific objective

process recording a word-for-word account of a conversation, including all verbal and nonverbal interactions

proctoclysis a slow instillation of fluid into the rectum

proctoscope a lighted instrument used to visualize the interior of the rectum

proctoscopy visualization of the interior of the rectum with a proctoscope

proctosigmoidoscope a lighted instrument used to visualize the rectum and sigmoid colon

proctosigmoidoscopy visual examination of the rectum and sigmoid colon with a proctosigmoidoscope

prodromal period the stage of an illness during which there are early manifestations of the disease

productive cough a cough in which secretions are expectorated

profession work that requires special knowledge, skill, and preparation

professional a person who practices a learned profession

progesterone a hormone produced by the ovaries, placenta, and adrenal cortex

prognosis the medical opinion about the outcome of a disease

program set of instructions that direct a computer to perform certain tasks

projection a defense mechanism by which a person attributes his or her own undesired characteristics to another

proliferation rapid reproduction of parts or cells

pronation turning the palm downward; moving the bones of the forearm so that the palm of the hand turns from anterior to posterior in the anatomic position; also, flat feet

prone (prone position) lying on the abdomen with the face turned to one side

prophylaxis preventive treatment; prevention of disease

proposition statement that expresses the relationship between concepts

proprioceptor a sensory receptor that is sensitive to movement and the position of the body

prospective payment system (PPS) federal plan that establishes Medicare reimbursement rates in advance of hospitalization and according to diagnostic related groups

prostate a gland around the base of the urethra of the male

prostatectomy the removal of the prostate gland

prosthesis an artificial part, e.g., a glass eye, an artificial leg, or dentures

prostration extreme exhaustion

protein an organic substance that is composed of carbon, hydrogen, oxygen, and nitrogen and that yields amino acids upon hydrolysis

proteinuria the presence of protein in the urine

protocol written plan specifying the procedures to be followed in a particular situation

protraction moving a part of the body forward in a plane parallel to the ground

proximal closest to the point of attachment

proximal fragment the part of a fractured bone nearest the individual's head

prudent diet a diet that is likely to benefit the individual even though it may not prevent disease

pruritus intense itching

psychiatry the branch of medicine that treats behavioral, emotional, or mental disorders

psychogenic (functional) pain pain caused by psychologic factors

psychologic dependence (on a drug) a state of emotional reliance on a drug to maintain one's well-being; a feeling of need or craving for a drug

psychologic homeostasis emotional or psychologic balance or a state of mental well-being

psychology the study of mental processes and behavior

psychomotor referring to motor actions related to cerebral or psychic activity

psychosomatic concerning the mind and the body; emotional disturbances manifested by physiologic symptoms

ptyalin an enzyme in saliva

ptyalism excessive secretion of saliva

puberty the age during which the reproductive organs become active and secondary sex characteristics develop

public law rules regulating relationships between individuals and government

pudendum *see* vulva

puerperium the period from delivery to about 6 weeks after delivery

pulmonary referring to the lungs

pulmonary capacities the combinations of two or more pulmonary volumes

pulmonary embolus a blood clot that has moved to the lungs

pulmonary resuscitation *see* respiratory ventilation

pulse the wave of blood within an artery that is created by contraction of the left ventricle of the heart

pulse deficit a difference between the apical and the radial pulses

pulse pressure the difference between the systolic and the diastolic pressures

pulse rate the number of pulse beats per minute

pulse rhythm the pattern of pulse beats and of intervals between beats

pulse tension the elasticity of the arteries

pulse volume the force of the blood with each beat produced by contraction of the left ventricle

pulsus regularis equal lapses of time between beats of a normal pulse

puncture (stab) wound a wound made by a sharp instrument penetrating the skin and underlying tissues

pupil the opening at the center of the iris of the eye

Purkinje fibers a network of fibers in the ventricles of the heart that conduct stimuli from the atria to the ventricles

purulent containing pus

purulent exudate an exudate consisting of leukocytes, liquefied dead tissue debris, and dead and living bacteria

pus a thick liquid associated with inflammation and composed of cells, liquid, microorganisms, and tissue debris

pustule a small elevation of the skin or mucous membrane or a clogged pore or follicle containing pus

putrid rotten

pyelogram an x-ray film of the kidney and ureter, showing the pelvis of the kidney

pyemia a generalized, persistent blood poisoning

pyogenic pus-producing

pyorrhea purulent periodontal disease

pyrexia elevated body temperature; fever

pyrogen a substance that produces a fever

pyuria the presence of pus in the urine

quadriplegia the paralysis of all four limbs

quality (of sound) subjective description of a sound (e.g., whistling, gurgling, or snapping)

quality assessment examination of nursing services

quality assurance the evaluation of nursing services provided and the results achieved against an established standard and the efforts aimed at ensuring quality nursing care

quality assurance criteria see criteria (of nursing care)

rabbi a Jew ordained for professional religious leadership

race classification of humans into subgroups according to specific physical and structural characteristics

radial pulse the pulse point located where the radial artery passes over the radius of the arm

radiation the transfer of heat from a warm object to a cooler object by means of electromagnetic waves, without contact between the two objects; electromagnetic waves used in diagnostic tests and some kinds of therapy

radiation therapy therapy involving x-rays, radium, or other radioactive substances

radiology technologist a member of the health team who takes roentgenograms and assists with other related tests

radiopaque able to block the passage of radiant energy, such as x-rays

rales bubbling or rattling sounds audible on inhalation as air moves through accumulated moist secretions in the lungs

random sample a study sample in which all members of a population have an equal chance of being included

range of motion the degree of movement possible for each joint

rationale the scientific reason for selecting a specific nursing action

rationalization a defense mechanism in which good reasons, acceptable to the conscious mind, are given for behavior or circumstances instead of the real reason

reaction formation a defense mechanism in which one behaves exactly opposite to the way one is feeling

readiness the state of being ready; it is used to describe the developmental maturation and growth necessary before one can perform some activities, e.g., walking

receptor (sensor) the terminal of a sensory nerve that is sensitive to specific stimuli

reconstituted family see blended family

reconstitution the technique of adding a solvent to a powdered drug to prepare it for injection

reconstructive surgery surgery to repair tissues whose function or appearance is damaged

record a collection of related data items about one file member

recording (charting) the process of making entries on clients' records

recovery bed see surgical bed

recovery index the sum of three 30-second pulse rates taken after increasing intervals of activity

recreational therapist a member of the health team who assists clients with activities for recreation

rectocele (proctocele) a protrusion of part of the rectum into the vagina

rectum the distal portion of the large intestine

recumbent length the distance from the soles of the feet to the vertex of the head of a person lying on the back

reduced hemoglobin hemoglobin that has released its oxygen

reduction realignment of fractured bone fragments to their normal position

reexamining (reevaluating) the process of reassessing and replanning

referred pain pain perceived to be in one area but whose source is another area

referent power power derived from an individual's own vision and sense of self, and his or her ability to communicate these so that others are motivated to follow

referring the transfer of a client's care to another person

reflex an involuntary activity in response to a stimulus

reflexive vocalization nondescriptive sounds infants make in response to various stimuli and environmental conditions

reflexogenic erection an erection of the penis that occurs without apparent sexual stimuli

refractory period the period immediately following orgasm when males cannot respond to sexual stimuli

regeneration the replacement of destroyed tissue cells by cells that are identical or similar in structure and function

regimen a regulated pattern of activity

registration the recording or entering of certain information about individuals

regression a defense mechanism in which one adapts behavior that was comforting earlier in life to overcome the discomfort and insecurity of the present situation

rehabilitation the restoration of a person who is ill or injured to the highest possible capacity

rehabilitative services see intermediate services

relapsing fever a fever characterized by periods of normal temperature, lasting 1 or more days, between periods of fever

religion an organized system of worship

remittent fever a fever characterized by a wide range of temperatures, all above normal, over a 24-hour period

REM sleep sleep during which the person experiences rapid eye movement; also called *paradoxical sleep*

renal relating to the kidney

renal dialysis a process in which blood flows from an artery through an artificial membrane that removes impurities; the blood then returns to the client through a vein

renal pelvis the funnel-shaped upper end of each ureter

renin a substance secreted by the kidneys when blood sodium levels are low; it controls aldosterone secretion

repolarized (cardiac) requiring an electric charge

repression a defense mechanism in which painful events are excluded from consciousness

research in nursing study of the nursing profession, including historic, ethical, and political areas

research-practice gap the separation between research and the clinical practice arena

research process a series or steps of phases, which are dynamic, flexible, and expandable, aimed toward generating useful knowledge

reservoir a source of pathogens

residual urine the amount of urine remaining in the bladder after a person voids

residual volume (air) the amount of air remaining in the lungs after a person exhales both tidal and expiratory reserve volumes

resistive behaviors behaviors that inhibit involvement, cooperation, or change

resistive exercise exercise in which the client contracts a muscle against an opposing force, e.g., a weight

resonance a low-pitched, rich sound produced over normal lung tissue when the chest is percussed

respiration the act of breathing; transport of oxygen from the atmosphere to the body cells and transport of carbon dioxide from the cells to the atmosphere

respiratory acidosis (hypercapnia) a state of excess carbon dioxide in the body

respiratory alkalosis a state of excessive loss of carbon dioxide from the body

respiratory arrest the sudden cessation of breathing

respiratory membrane the alveolar walls and the surrounding blood capillaries

respiratory technologist a person who provides diagnostic and therapeutic measures for clients with respiratory problems

respiratory therapist *see* inhalation therapist

respiratory ventilation (pulmonary resuscitation) the inhalation of air into the lungs by artificial means

responsibility reliability and trustworthiness

rest calmness or relaxation without emotional stress

restitution an adaptive mechanism in which one performs restorative acts to relieve guilt

resuscitate to restore life; to revive

resuscitation the application of measures to reestablish breathing

retching the involuntary attempt to vomit without producing emesis

retention (urinary) the accumulation of urine in the bladder and the inability of the bladder to empty itself

retention (stay) suture a large plain suture that attaches to underlying tissues of fat and muscle in addition to the skin; retention sutures are used to support incisions

retina the membrane that lines the back of the eye, receives the image, and is connected to the brain by the optic nerve

retraction moving a part of the body backward in a plane parallel to the ground; the act of drawing back

retrograde pyelogram an x-ray film taken after a contrast medium is injected through ureteral catheters into the kidneys

retroperitoneal behind the peritoneum

retrospective audit an audit of past events

reverse Trendelenburg's position a position with the head of the bed raised and the foot lowered, while the bed foundation remains unbroken

Rh factor antigens present on the surface of some people's erythrocytes; persons who possess this factor are referred to as *Rh positive,* while those who do not are referred to as *Rh negative*

rhinitis inflammation of the mucous membrane of the nose

rhizotomy interruption of the anterior or posterior nerve root between the ganglion and the spinal cord, often for the purpose of relieving pain

rhonchi coarse, dry, wheezy, or whistling sounds, more audible during exhalation, as the air moves through tenacious mucus or a constricted bronchus

rickets a bone disorder resulting from a deficiency of vitamin D and calcium; decalcification of bone

right a just claim

rights of human subjects the just claims of individuals who participate in research studies for full disclosure, self-determination, privacy, and confidentiality and to not be harmed

rigidity stiffness or inflexibility of a muscle

rigor mortis the stiffening of the muscles after death

risk assessment *see* health risk appraisal

risk factor a phenomenon that increases a person's chance of acquiring a specific disease

risk of harm exposure to the possibility of injury going beyond everyday situations

risk reduction planning and implementing nursing interventions to reduce health risks when possible or to optimize an individual's current health status when risks cannot be reduced

ritualistic behavior (ritualism) a series of repetitive acts performed compulsively, often to relieve anxiety

roentgen the unit of measurement of gamma rays (γ) or x-radiation

roentgenogram a film produced by photography with x-rays

role the pattern of behavior expected of an individual in a situation or particular group

role conflict a clash between the beliefs, behaviors, etc. imposed by two or more roles fulfilled by one person

rooting reflex a reflex that causes newborns to turn their heads toward the side of a stimulated cheek or lip

rotation turning a bone around its central axis either toward the midline of the body (*internal rotation*) or away from midline of the body (*external rotation*)

round window an opening from the middle ear to the inner ear

rubefacient reddening the skin; a substance that reddens the skin

ruga a ridge or fold in the lining of an organ such as the vagina or the stomach (plural: rugae)

sacrum a triangular bone at the base of the vertebral column

sagittal plane a vertical line or plane dividing the body or its parts into right and left portions

Salem sump tube a double-lumen nasogastric tube

sample a subset of the population selected for study

sanction punishment or a measure used to enforce normative behavior of group members

sanguineous bloody

sanguineous exudate an exudate containing large amounts of red blood cells

saphenous vein either of two superficial veins of the leg; the greater one extends from the foot to the inguinal region, while the lesser one extends from the foot up the back of the leg to the knee joint

sarcoidosis a disease in which affected tissues develop epithelioid cell tubercles; commonly affected organs are the lymph nodes, liver, spleen, lungs, skin, eyes, and small bones in the feet and hands

satiety a feeling of fullness as a result of satisfying the desire for food

saturated fat a fat whose molecular structure is saturated with hydrogen, such as fats in meat, butter, and eggs

scab the crust over a superficial wound

scan a specialized type of x-ray procedure involving the use of a scanning device (probe), a computer, a printout machine, and a viewing apparatus

scapula the shoulder blade, a flat, triangular bone at the back of the shoulder

scar (cicatrical) tissue dense fibrous tissue derived from granulation tissue

scientific inquiry process in which observable, verifiable data are systematically collected to describe, explain, and/or predict events and phenomena

scientific method a logical, systematic approach to solving problems

sclera the white covering of the eye that joins with the cornea

sclerosis a process of hardening that occurs from inflammation and disease of the interstitial substance; the term is used to describe hardening of nervous tissues and arterioles

scoliosis a lateral curvature of a part of the vertebral column

scored marked with a line or groove

scrotum the sac suspended down and behind the penis that contains and protects the testes

scultetus binder an abdominal binder applied in strips that overlap each other

scurvy a condition resulting from vitamin C deficiency

sebaceous gland a gland of the dermis that secretes sebum

seborrheic dermatitis a chronic disease of the skin, characterized by scaling and crusted patches on various body areas, e.g., the scalp

sebum the oily, lubricating secretion of sebaceous glands in the skin

secondary questions probing-type questions

secondary union (second intention) healing that requires the formation of considerable granulation tissue

secretion the product of a gland, e.g., saliva is the secretion of the salivary glands

secretory (luteal) stage see postovulatory stage

sedative an agent that tends to calm or tranquilize

segmentation contractions contractions of segments of the intestine in contrast to contractions of large areas of the intestine

self-actualization (Maslow) the highest level of personality development

self-care activities performed by individuals in their own behalf to maintain health and well-being

self-concept the combination of beliefs and feelings one holds about oneself at a given time

self-consistency the aspect of self that strives to maintain a stable self-image

self-determination the right of clients to feel free from undue influence

self-esteem self-acceptance; self-worth

self-expectancy what a person wants to become; the power a person perceives he or she has to meet self-expectations

self-image a person's perception of self at a specific time or over a period of time

self-terminating order on a client's record, an order whose termination time is implicit

semantics the study of the meaning of words

semen seminal plasma combined with sperm

semicircular canals passages shaped like half circles in the inner ear that control the sense of balance by the effect of fluid moving against hairlike nerves

semicomatose pertaining to a state of unconsciousness characterized by reflex movement only when painful stimuli are applied and, in some instances, by decortical or decerebrate posturing

semi-Fowler's position a bed sitting position in which the head of the bed is elevated at least 30 degrees, with or without knee flexion

semilunar valves crescent-shaped valves that guard the entrances from the cardiac ventricles into the aorta and pulmonary trunk

seminal plasma substances that are produced by the seminal vesicles, prostate, and Cowper's glands and that energize the sperm and enhance their transport

seminiferous tubules highly coiled tubes that manufacture sperm within each testis

senescence the process of growing old

senility feebleness or loss of mental, emotional, or physical control that occurs in old age

sensitivity quick response, often referring to the response of microorganisms to an antibiotic

sensorimotor stage (Piaget) the initial phase of cognitive development between birth and 2 years

sensorium a sensory nerve center

sensory deficit partial or complete impairment of any sensory organ

sensory deprivation (input deficit) insufficient sensory stimulation for a person to function

sensory overload an overabundance of sensory stimulation

serosanguineous composed of serum and blood

serous of or like serum

serous exudate a watery exudate composed mainly of serum

serum (blood) blood plasma from which the fibrinogen has been separated during clotting

sex maleness or femaleness; sexual intercourse

sex behavior the behavior associated with sexual intercourse, including physiologic responses and sexual dysfunctions

sex chromosome pair the pair of chromosomes, one from the sperm and one from the ovum, that determine whether gonads develop into testes or ovaries; the sex chromosome pair is designated XX (female) or XY (male)

sex drive see libido

sex-typed behavior the action that typically elicits different rewards for one sex or the other

sexual differentiation biologic sex determination of the fetus, during which male genitals or female genitals develop

sexual dimorphism the average differences between males and females in any given species

sexual dysfunction a perceived problem in achieving desired satisfaction of sexuality

sexual identity (core-gender identity) a person's inner feeling or sense of being male or female

sexuality what constitutes male and female; the constitution of an individual in relation to sexual attitudes or activities

sexually transmitted (venereal) disease a disease that can be passed on through intercourse with an infected person

sexual motivation *see* libido

sexual role behavior sexual behavior and gender behavior

shiatsu form of massage in which firm, gentle pressure is applied to the acupuncture points of the body; also referred to as *acupressure*

shock acute circulatory failure

shock phase initial stage of the general adaptation syndrome during which the stressor may be perceived consciously or unconsciously and large amounts of epinephrine and cortisone are released in the body

shroud a large rectangular or square piece of plastic or cloth used to enclose a body after death

sick role behavior actions directed at getting well taken by the person who considers himself or herself ill

sickle cell anemia a genetic defect of hemoglobin synthesis that accounts for abnormally crescent-shaped erythrocytes; common to Afro-Americans

side effect (of a drug) an outcome that is not intended, such as an unintended action or complication of a drug

sigmoid colon the lower portion of the descending colon of the large intestine; it is shaped like the letter S

sigmoidoscope a lighted instrument used to examine the sigmoid colon

sigmoidoscopy examination of the interior of the sigmoid colon with a sigmoidoscope

Sims' position semiprone position

single-parent family a family unit in which only one parent is present

sings healing ceremonies or rituals carried out by some Native Americans

singultus hiccups

sinoatrial (SA) node the pacemaker of the heart; the collection of Purkinje's fibers in the right atrium of the heart where the rhythm of contraction is initiated

Skene's glands paraurethral glands that open into the urethra just within the external urinary meatus

slander defamation by spoken words

sleep a state of unconsciousness from which a person can be aroused by appropriate sensory or other stimuli

sleep apnea periodic cessation of breathing during sleep

slipper pan a bedpan with a flattened end to ease placement under the client; also called a *fracture pan*

smear material spread across a glass slide in preparation for microscopic study

smegma a thick, white, cheeselike secretion that collects between the labia and under the foreskin

SOAP the format used in the POR to record the client's progress; it has four components: Subjective data, Objective data, Assessment, and Planning

socialization the process by which individuals learn the knowledge, skills, and dispositions of their social group or society

socialized speech the exchange of thoughts between individuals, including questions, answers, commands, and criticisms of others

social support network others outside the immediate family unit who provide strength, encouragement, and assistance to the family, especially during a crisis

social worker an individual who assists persons and families with social problems

sociogram a diagram of the flow of verbal communication within a group during a specified period

sociology the study of social relationships and social institutions, such as marriage or education

sociopath a person who is unable to follow society's moral and ethical standards; one who has an antisocial personality

sodium cotransport theory a hypothesis about the mechanism for glucose transport in the presence of sodium

soixante-neuf (69) simultaneous oral-genital stimulation between two persons

solute a substance dissolved in a solution

solvent the component of a solution that can dissolve a solute

somatic referring to the physical body

somatogenic (organic) pain pain of physical origin

somnambulism sleepwalking

sordes the accumulation of foul matter (food, microorganisms, and epithelial elements) on the teeth and gums

souffle a blowing sound heard by auscultation

source-oriented medical record a traditional client's chart, organized according to the source of records (i.e., the person or department reporting); it includes separate records for the doctor, the nurse, the social worker, etc.

spasm involuntary contraction of a muscle or muscle group

spastic describing the sudden, prolonged involuntary muscle contractions of clients with damage to the central nervous system

special (therapeutic) diet a diet in which the amount of food, kind of food, or frequency of eating is prescribed

specific gravity the weight or degree of concentration of a substance compared with the weight of an equal amount of another substance used as a standard (e.g., water used as a standard has a specific gravity of 1, while urine in comparison has a specific gravity of 1.010 to 1.025)

speculum a funnel-shaped instrument used to widen and examine canals of the body, e.g., the vagina or nasal canal

sperm the male germ cell (reproductive cell)

spermatogenesis production of sperm

spermicide foam, jelly, or cream inserted in the vagina before intercourse to destroy the sperm chemically

sphincter a ringlike muscle that opens or closes a natural orifice, such as the urethra, when it relaxes or contracts

sphygmomanometer an instrument used to measure the pressure of the blood in the arteries

spinothalamic tract the nerve pathway of the spinal cord in which impulses ascend to the brain

spiral bandage a bandage applied to parts of the body extremities that are of uniform circumference

spiral reverse bandage a bandage applied to extremities of the body that are not of uniform circumference

spiritual belief a belief in a higher power, creative force, divine being, or infinite source of energy; the belief may or may not be associated with an organized religion

spiritual need what a client needs to maintain, increase, or restore his or her beliefs and faith and to fulfill religious obligations

spirometry the measurement of pulmonary volumes and capacities using a spirometer

splint a rigid bar or appliance used to stabilize a body part

spore a round or oval structure highly resistant to destruction that is formed in some bacterial cells

sprain injury of the ligaments and associated structure of a joint by wrenching or twisting; associated structures include tendons, muscles, nerves, and blood vessels

spreader block (bar) a block of wood or metal that spreads traction tape away from the medial and lateral aspects of the foot in a traction such as a Buck's extension

sputum the mucous secretion from the lungs, bronchi, and trachea that is ejected through the mouth

stab wound *see* puncture wound

stamina staying power or endurance

stammer involuntary repetitions and stops in vocal utterances

standard (norm) a measure of quantity, quality, weight, extent, or value that is set up as a rule

standards in nursing, optimum levels of care against which actual performance is compared

standing order written document about policies, rules, regulations, or orders regarding client care that gives the nurse authority to carry out specific actions under certain circumstances, often when a physician is not available

stasis stagnation or stoppage of flow of body fluids, such as intestinal fluids, urine, or blood

static electricity stationary electric charges

station stance; the way a person stands

stature the height of a standing person

statutory law a law passed by a legislature (state, provincial, or federal)

stenosis constriction or narrowing of a body canal or opening

stereotype something that conforms to a fixed pattern; an oversimplified judgment or attitude about a person or group

sterile free from microorganisms, including pathogens

sterile field a specified area that is considered free from microorganisms

sterile technique *see* surgical asepsis

sterilization a process that destroys all microorganisms, including spores

sternum the breastbone, a flat elongated bone lying between the ribs and over the heart

stertor snoring or sonorous respiration, usually due to a partial obstruction of the upper airway

stethoscope an instrument used to listen to various sounds inside the body, such as the heartbeats

stimulus anything that arouses or incites action from a receptor

stock supply (of drugs) medications stocked in relatively large quantities in a nursing unit; individual doses are taken from the large supply

stoma an artificial opening in the abdominal wall; it may be permanent or temporary

stomatitis inflammation of the entire mouth

stool (feces) waste products excreted from the large intestine

stopcock a valve that controls the flow of fluid or air through a tube

storage device equipment used to retain data after processing by a computer

strabismus squinting or crossing of the eyes; uncoordinated eye movements

strain (of a muscle) overexertion or overstretching of a muscle or part of a muscle

stress an event or set of circumstances causing a disrupted response; the disruption caused by a noxious stimulus or stressor

stressor any factor that produces stress or alters the body's equilibrium

stress syndrome *see* general adaptation syndrome (GAS)

stretch receptors nerve receptors sensitive to changes in pressure, i.e., in the aorta and carotid sinus; also called *presoreceptors* or *baroreceptors*

striae gravidarum colorless streaks or lines on the abdomen, breasts, or thighs caused by pregnancy; stretch marks

stricture a narrowing of a passageway or canal

stridor a shrill, harsh, crowing sound made on inhalation due to constriction of the upper airway or laryngeal obstruction

stroke volume the amount of blood ejected from the heart with each ventricular contraction

stroma tissue that forms the framework or structure of an organ

structural-functional theory a framework for studying the family unit that focuses on family membership and relationships among family members as well as the functions of the family

stupor a condition of partial or nearly complete unconsciousness; stuporous clients are never fully awakened even when painfully stimulated

stuttering a speech problem evidenced by the repetition of letters or words and prolonged pauses

stylet a metal or plastic probe inserted into a needle or cannula to render it stiff and to prevent occlusion of the lumen by particles of tissue

subarachnoid space the area between the arachnoid membrane and the pia mater

subcostal below the ribs

subcutaneous (hypodermic) beneath the layers of the skin

subcutaneous tissue *see* hypodermis

subjective data client information that only the patient personally can give, such as thoughts or feelings

sublimation the channeling of sexual and aggressive desires into socially acceptable forms of behavior

sublingual under the tongue

suborbital beneath the cavity or orbit

subscapular below the scapula

substantia gelatinosa gray matter in the dorsal horns of the spinal cord where pain fibers terminate

substernal retractions indrawing beneath the breastbone

substitution replacing one thing with another; an adaptive mechanism in which unattainable or unacceptable goals are replaced with ones that are attainable or acceptable

subsystem the low-level components of a system

suctioning aspiration of secretions by a catheter connected to a suction machine or outlet

sudden infant death syndrome (SIDS) a condition of some children during the first year, resulting in death during sleep

sudoriferous gland a gland of the dermis that secretes sweat

suicide the taking of one's own life

sulcular technique a dental hygiene technique for removing plaque and cleaning under the gingival margins

superego (Freud) an unconscious part of the psyche that monitors the id and the ego; concerned primarily with ethics, conscience, and social standards

supination turning the palm upward; moving the bones of the forearm so that the palm of the hand turns from posterior to anterior in the anatomic position

supine (supine position) lying on the back with the face upward without support for the head and shoulders; also called *dorsal position*

support system the people and activities that can assist a person at a time of stress

suppository a solid, cone-shaped, medicated substance inserted into the rectum, vagina, or urethra

suppression the willful exclusion of a thought or feeling from consciousness; the sudden stoppage of a secretion or an excretion, e.g., urine

suppuration the formation of pus

supraclavicular retractions indrawing above the clavicles

supraoptic above the eye

supraorbital above the orbit of the eye

suprapubic above the pubic arch

suprasternal retractions indrawing above the breastbone

surfactant a lipoprotein mixture secreted in the alveoli that reduces surface tension of the fluid lining the alveoli

surgical asepsis measures that render and maintain objects free from microorganisms (sterile)

surgical bed (anesthetic, recovery, or postoperative bed) a bed with the top covers fanfolded to one side or to the end of the bed

susto among Hispanics, a disease of emotional origin; fright caused by natural phenomena such as lightning or loud noises

suture in surgery, a surgical stitch used to close accidental or surgical wounds; in anatomy, a junction line of the skull bones

symbolization an adaptive mechanism by which objects are used to represent ideas or emotions too painful for a person to express; the creation of a mental image to stand for something

sympathectomy the severing of pathways of the sympathetic nervous system, often to relieve pain of a vascular origin

symphysis pubis the fibrocartilagenous line of union of the bodies of the pubic bones in the median plane

symptom (covert data) *see* subjective data

synapse the junction between two neurons, where nerve impulses are transmitted from one neuron to another

syncope fainting or temporary loss of consciousness

syndrome a group of signs and symptoms resulting from a single cause and constituting a typical clinical picture, such as the shock syndrome

synergist an agent that enhances the action of another so that their combined effect is greater than the effect of either

synovial joint a freely movable joint surrounded by a capsule enclosing a cavity that contains a transparent, viscid fluid

synthesis the process of putting together; assembling the parts of a whole

syphilis a sexually transmitted (venereal) disease caused by the microorganism *Treponema pallidum*

syringe an instrument used to inject or withdraw liquids

system a set of identifiable parts or components

systemic pertaining to the body (or other system) as a whole

systole the period when the ventricles of the heart are contracted

systolic pressure the pressure of the blood against the arterial walls when the ventricles of the heart contract

tablet a medication in solid form that is often compressed and molded

tachycardia an excessively rapid pulse or heart rate, over 100 beats per minute in the adult

tachypnea abnormally fast respirations, usually more than 24 per minute, marked by quick, shallow breaths

tactile pertaining to the sense of touch

tactile (vocal) fremitus vibrations, palpable with the palms of the hands, originating in the larynx and transmitted to the chest wall during speech

talipes equinovarus clubfoot; a foot is malpositioned in plantar flexion at the ankle, with inversion and adduction of the heel and forefoot

Talmud the authoritative written body of Jewish tradition

Taoism Chinese mystical philosophy

tartar the film on teeth, often formed from plaque; dental calculus

taxonomy a classification system or set of categories, such as nursing diagnoses

T-binder a cloth in the shape of a T often used to retain dressings in the genital region

teaching an interactive process between a teacher and one or more learners in which specific learning objectives or desired behavior changes are achieved

team nursing the delivery of individualized nursing care to clients by a nursing team led by a professional nurse

technical assault and battery assault and battery without the intent to injure, e.g., when giving a hypodermic injection

temporal pulse a pulse point where the temporal artery passes over the temporal bone of the skull

tenacious sticky, adhesive

tendon a fibrous cord that attaches a muscle to a bone

tenesmus straining; painful, ineffective straining during defecation or urination

terminal hair long, coarse, pigmented body hair

territoriality the pattern of behavior arising from an individual's feeling that certain spaces and objects belong to him or her

testes the male gonads

testosterone a testicular hormone that stimulates the growth of the genitals and the development of male secondary sexual characteristics

tetany a syndrome manifested by muscle twitching, cramps, convulsions, and sharp flexion of the wrist and ankle joints

thalamus the larger and middle portion of the diencephalon of the brain

theory a scientifically acceptable general principle that governs practice or is proposed to explain observed facts

therapeutic healing; supportive of health

therapeutic effect (of a drug) the primary effect desired, or the reason the drug is prescribed

therapy remedial treatment

thermal trauma injury caused by excessive heat or cold

thermosensitive pain receptors pain receptors sensitive to heat and cold

thoracocentesis insertion of a needle into the pleural cavity for diagnostic or therapeutic purposes

thorax the chest cavity

thought disorganization a mental condition evidenced by difficulty remembering what one is saying, confusion about time, inappropriate verbal responses, and sensory distortions

thrombocytopenia an abnormal reduction in the number of platelets in the blood

thrombophlebitis inflammation of a vein followed by formation of a blood clot

thrombosis the development of a blood clot

thrombus a solid mass of blood constituents in the circulatory system; a clot (plural: thrombi)

thyroid hormone a hormone produced by the thyroid gland consisting of thyroxine and triiodothyronine

thyroid-stimulating hormone (TSH, thyrotropic hormone) a hormone produced by the anterior pituitary gland that stimulates the thyroid gland to produce thyroxine

thyroxine a hormone produced by the thyroid gland

tic a repetitive twitching of the muscles, often of the face or upper trunk

tick a small parasite that bites into tissue and sucks blood

tidal volume the volume of air that is normally inhaled and exhaled

tinea pedis *see* athlete's foot

tinnitus a ringing or buzzing sensation in the ears that is purely subjective

tissue perfusion passage of fluid, e.g., blood, through a specific organ or body part

tolerance the ability to endure without ill effects; the term is often used with reference to taking medications

tomography a scanning procedure during which several x-ray beams pass through the body part from different angles

tonicity the normal condition of tension or tone, e.g., of a muscle

tonometer an instrument used to assess the pressure inside the eye

tonsillectomy the surgical removal of a tonsil or tonsils

tonus the slight, continual contraction of muscles

topical applied externally, e.g., to the skin or mucous membranes

torsion twisting

tort a wrong committed by a person against another person or the other person's property

torticollis limited range of motion of the neck, with lateral inclination and rotation of the head away from the midline of the body

tortuous twisted

total lung capacity the maximum volume to which the lungs can be expanded

total parenteral nutrition (TPN) intravenous hyperalimentation (IVH); administration of a hypertonic solution of carbohydrates, amino acids, and lipids by an indwelling intravenous catheter placed into the superior vena cava via the jugular or subclavian vein

tourniquet a device, e.g., a rubber strip, that is wrapped around a body area to compress the blood vessels

toxemia a generalized intoxication due to the absorption of toxins in the body

toxemia of pregnancy a metabolic disturbance during pregnancy; *see* eclampsia, preeclampsia

toxin a poison produced by some microorganisms, animals, and plants

toxoid a modified exotoxin that is no longer toxic but still has the ability to stimulate the production of antibodies

trachea a membranous tube, composed of cartilage, descending from the larynx and branching into the right and left bronchi

tracheal tug an indrawing and downward pulling of the trachea during inhalation

tracheostomy a procedure by which an opening is made in the anterior portion of the trachea and a cannula is introduced into the opening

traction the exertion of a pulling force

traditional family family unit in which both parents reside in the home with their children—the mother playing the nurturing role and the father providing necessary economic support

traditional health care mode of health care in which activities are aimed toward identifying and correcting a health problem that already exists

transcutaneous electrical stimulation the placement of electrodes on the surface of the skin over a peripheral nerve pathway for the purpose of relieving pain

transfusion (blood) the introduction of whole blood or its components, e.g., serum, erythrocytes, or platelets, into the venous circulation

transudation the passage of serum or other body fluids through a membrane or tissue

transverse plane a horizontal line or plane dividing the body or its parts into superior and inferior portions

trapeze bar a triangular handgrip suspended from an overbed frame

trauma injury

tremor an involuntary muscle contraction, e.g., quivering, twitching, or convulsions

trend prevailing tendency or approach

Trendelenburg's position a bed position with the head of the bed lowered and the foot raised, while the bed foundation remains unbroken; in some agencies, the position involves elevation of the knees, with the feet lowered and the head lowered

triage picking, choosing, sorting, and selecting

trial legal proceedings during which all relevant facts are presented to a jury or judge

triglyceride a simple lipid or neutral fat consisting of three fatty acids for each glycerol base

trigone the triangular area at the base of the urinary bladder

trimester a period of 3 months

trocar a sharp, pointed instrument that fits inside a cannula and is used to pierce body cavities

trochanter either of two processes below the neck of the femur

trochanter roll a rolled towel support placed against the hips to prevent external rotation of the legs

troche a lozenge

tubal ligation a surgical tying of the fallopian tubes, rendering the female sterile

tubercle a rounded eminence of bone

tumor an uncontrolled and progressive growth of cells

tunica albuginea a dense, white, fibrous capsule encasing each testis

tunica dartos the middle layer of smooth muscle and tough connective tissue in the scrotum

tuning fork an instrument shaped like a two-pronged fork and made of metal; the prongs vibrate when struck

turgor normal fullness and elasticity

two-career family family in which both the husband and wife are employed

tympanic membrane a membrane separating the external and the middle ear

tympanites (distention) swelling of the abdomen due to the presence of excessive flatus in the intestines or peritoneal cavity

tympany a musical drumming sound produced on percussion over organs that contain gas or air

ulcer a localized sloughing of skin tissue or mucous membrane commonly associated with varicosities or hyperactivity of the gastrointestinal tract

ultradian rhythm a biologic cycle completed in minutes or hours

ultrasound high-frequency, mechanical, radiant energy

ultraviolet referring to radiation having wavelengths shorter than violet rays and longer than x-rays; ultraviolet radiation has powerful chemical properties

umbilicus the navel; the site where the umbilical cord was attached to the fetus

unconscious incapable of responding to sensory stimuli; insensible

unconscious mind (Freud) the mental life of which a person is unaware

uncontrolled variable variable other than the independent variable that might affect the outcome of a study

undernutrition inadequate caloric intake or nourishment

unilateral affecting one side

unit dose system (of drugs) prepackaged and labeled individual doses of medication for each client; the amount of medication the client is to receive at a prescribed hour

universal donor a person with type O blood

universal recipient a person with type AB blood

unpalatable distasteful, unpleasant to the taste

unsterile containing microorganisms; unsterile material may be clean or contaminated

untoward adverse

urban relating to or constituting a city

urea a substance found in urine, blood, and lymph; the main nitrogenous substance in blood

urea frost (uremic frost) the appearance of the skin when the salt crystals remain after the evaporation of the sweat in urhidrosis

uremia the retention in the blood of excessive amounts of the by-products of protein metabolism

ureter the fibrous, muscular tube extending from the kidneys to the urinary bladder

ureteroileosigmoidostomy an artificial opening into the ureters in which a segment of the ileum is resected and connected to the sigmoid colon and the ureters are implanted into this ileal pouch

ureterosigmoidostomy an artificial opening into the ureters in which the ureters are implanted into the sigmoid colon

ureterostomy an artificial opening into the ureter

urethra the canal extending from the urinary bladder to the outside of the body

urethritis inflammation of the urethra

urgency a feeling that one must urinate

urgent surgery surgery necessary for the client's health

urhidrosis a condition in which urinous materials, e.g., uric acid and urea, are present in the sweat

urinal a receptacle used to collect urine

urinalysis laboratory analysis of the urine

urinary diversion *see* urostomy

urine the fluid of water and waste products excreted by the kidneys

urobilin the oxidized form of urobilinogen, a compound formed from bilirubin, that is found in feces and occasionally in urine

urostomy (ureterostomy, urinary diversion) an opening through the abdominal wall into the urinary tract that permits the drainage of urine

urticaria an allergic reaction marked by smooth, reddened, slightly elevated patches of skin and intense itching

uterus the womb; the hollow, muscular organ in the female in which the fertilized ovum develops

uvula a small fleshy mass projecting from the soft palate above the base of the tongue

vaccine a suspension of killed, attenuated, or living microorganisms administered to prevent or treat an infectious disease

vagina the canal of the female reproductive tract

vaginal diaphragm a round rubber cup inserted over the cervix of the uterus for contraception

vaginal orifice the external opening of the vagina

vaginal smear vaginal cells placed on a glass slide for laboratory analysis

vaginismus painful, irregular, and involuntary contraction of the muscles around the outer third of the vagina during coitus

Valsalva maneuver forceful exhalation against a closed glottis, which increases intrathoracic pressure and thus interferes with venous return to the heart

value something of worth; a belief held dearly by a person

values clarification a process by which individuals define their own values

vaporization evaporation; conversion of a solid or liquid into a gas (vapor)

variable data information that is changeable or apt to be changeable

varicosity the state of having swollen, distended, and knotted veins, especially in the legs

vas deferens a long tube that extends from the scrotum, curves around the urinary bladder, and empties into the ejaculatory ducts

vasectomy ligation and cutting of the vas deferens, rendering the male sterile

vasoconstriction a decrease in the caliber (lumen) of blood vessels

vasodilation an increase in the caliber (lumen) of blood vessels

vasopressor an agent that causes the blood pressure to rise

vasospasm spasm or constriction of the blood vessels

vector an insect or other animal that transfers pathogens from one host to another

vehicle a transporting agent or medium

vellus fine, nonpigmented body hair

venereal disease *see* sexually transmitted disease

ventilation the movement of air; the act of breathing

ventral of, toward, or at the front; anterior

ventricle a small cavity, such as those located in the brain or the heart

ventriculogram an x-ray film of the ventricles of the brain taken after the introduction of an opaque medium

ventriculography radiologic examination of the ventricles of the brain following the insertion of air or a radiopaque medium

verbal communication communication by the spoken or written word

verdict (legal) the outcome of a trial rendered by a jury

vermin external animal parasites, e.g., ticks, lice, and fleas

vernix caseosa the white, cheesy, greasy, protective material found on the skin of newborns

vertex the top of the head

vertigo dizziness

vesicostomy an artificial opening into the bladder in which the anterior wall of the bladder is sutured to the abdominal wall and a stoma is formed from the bladder wall

vesicular sounds normal, quiet, rustling, or swishing respiratory sounds heard over the terminal bronchioles and alveoli during auscultation

vestibule a space or cavity at the entrance to a canal; the cleft between the labia containing the vaginal and urethral orifices, hymen, and openings of several ducts

viable fetus a fetus capable of extrauterine life

vial a glass medication container with a sealed rubber cap, for single or multiple doses

vibration a technique of rapid agitation of the hands while pressing on a body area

violence exertion of physical force to injure or abuse

virulence ability to produce disease

virus minute infectious agents smaller than bacteria

viscera large interior organs in body cavities, e.g., the liver and stomach (singular: viscus)

visceral referring to viscera

visceral pain pain originating in the viscera

viscosity the quality of being viscous

viscous thick, sticky

visible poverty lack of money or material resources

visual relating to the sense of sight

vital capacity maximum amount of air that can be exhaled following a maximum inhalation

vital (cardinal) signs measurements of physiologic functioning, specifically temperature, pulse, respirations, and blood pressure

vitamins organic chemical substances found in food and essential for normal metabolism and life

vocal resonance vibrations of the larynx transmitted during speech through the respiratory system to the chest wall

vocation the work that a person regularly performs and that especially suits a person

void urinate, micturate

volatile evaporating readily

vomitus material vomited; emesis

voodoo the practice of witchcraft or magic

vulnerable subjects individuals who because of diminished physical or mental capacity may be unable to give free and informed consent

vulva the external female genitals that surround the vaginal orifice and the urethra; also called the *pudendum*

walker a metal, rectangular frame used as an aid to ambulation

weight the heaviness of a body or object, normally measured in kilograms or pounds

well-being active state of an individual in which he or she becomes aware of and makes choices that lead to a more successful existence

wellness the ongoing process of behaving in ways that lead to improved health; subjective perception of balance, harmony, and vitality

wheal *see* bleb

wheeze a whistling sound on exhalation that usually indicates narrowing of the bronchial air passages

will a declaration of how a person wishes to distribute his or her property after death

xiphoid process the lower portion of the sternum

xeromammography x-ray of the breasts using lower doses of radiation

x-rays electromagnetic radiations with extremely short wavelengths

yang in Chinese folk medicine, a positive force that regulates health; it represents the male, warmth, light, and fullness

yin in Chinese folk medicine, a negative force that regulates health; it represents the female, coldness, darkness, and emptiness

yoga an Indian science that involves various physical postures and stationary exercises as well as psychologic measures to improve one's mental, social, and spiritual states

zygote the fertilized ovum

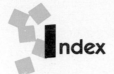

Index

Note: Italicized page numbers refer to figures and/or illustrations.

Some SI Units Applicable to Health

Quantity	SI Unit	Symbol	Customary Unit	Typical Application
Length	kilometer meter millimeter micrometer	km m cm mm (10^{-3} m) μm (10^{-6} m)	mile yard, foot inch	Distance, distance in visual acuity, body linear measurement, size of bacteria
Surface area	square centimeter square meter	cm^2 m^2	square inch square foot	Surface area, body surface area
Mass	kilogram gram milligram microgram	kg g mg μg	lb, oz	Body mass, pharmaceutical and chemical products
Temperature	degree Celsius*	°C	°F or degree Fahrenheit	Body temperature, clinical thermometer
Time	day hour minute second	d h min s		Expression of point in time in a health record, 24 h clock, time of medication
Volume and capacity	liter milliliter	L mL	qt cc, fluid oz, teaspoon	Fluid or gas, measuring vessel, baby formula, oral dosage
Power	watt	W	horsepower	Mechanical power, bicycle ergometer tests
Energy	joule kilojoule	J kJ	calorie, kilocalorie, Calorie	Food energy, metabolic energy, kinetic energy
Catalytic activity	katal†	kat	International Units	Measurement of enzyme
Pressure	pascal kilopascal	Pa kPa	millimeter of mercury, inches of water	Ocular, cerebrospinal, and blood pressure
Frequency	hertz	Hz	cycle per second	Audio, radio, and x-ray frequencies
Substance concentration	mole/liter	mol/L	milligram percent, milli-equivalent per liter	Composition of body fluid
Dose equivalent	sievert	Sv	rem	Radiation protection
Absorbed dose	gray	Gy	rad	Absorbed dose of ionizing radiation
Activity	becquerel	Bq	curie	Activity of radionuclides
Exposure (in air)	no special SI name	C/kg of air (coulomb per kilogram)	roentgen	Specialized applications

*The degree Celsius: Note that the unit of temperature is the degree Celsius (not degree centigrade). This has been accepted because the kelvin has limited application in medicine. The symbol for degree Celsius is °C. Although the scale origins of kelvin and Celsius differ, the degree Celsius equals the kelvin in magnitude, thus, a rise in body temperature of 1.0 K is equivalent to a rise of 1.0 °C. 0 °C is defined as 273.15 K, 98.6 °F—37 °C—310.15 K.

†Not yet an approved SI unit